TISSUE OPTICS

Light Scattering Methods and Instruments for Medical Diagnosis

SECOND EDITION

TISSUE OPTICS

Light Scattering Methods and Instruments for Medical Diagnosis

SECOND EDITION

Valery Tuchin

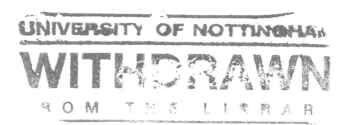
SPIE
PRESS

Bellingham, Washington USA

Library of Congress Cataloging-in-Publication Data

Tuchin, V. V. (Valerii Viktorovich)
  Tissue optics : light scattering methods and instruments for medical diagnosis / Valery V. Tuchin.
-- 2nd ed.
     p. ; cm.
  Includes bibliographical references and index.
  ISBN-13: 978-0-8194-6433-0
  ISBN-10: 0-8194-6433-3
  1. Tissues--Optical properties. 2. Light--Scattering. 3. Diagnostic imaging. 4. Imaging systems
in medicine. I. Society of Photo-optical Instrumentation Engineers. II. Title.
  [DNLM: 1. Diagnostic Imaging. 2. Light. 3. Optics. 4. Spectrum Analysis. 5. Tissues--
radiography. WN 180 T888t 2007]

QH642.T83 2007
616.07'54--dc22
                                                                                              2006034872

Published by   **1005601702**

SPIE
P.O. Box 10
Bellingham, Washington 98227-0010 USA
Phone: +1 360 676 3290
Fax: +1 360 647 1445
Email: spie@spie.org
Web: http://spie.org

The content of this book reflects the work and thought of the author(s).
Every effort has been made to publish reliable and accurate information herein,
but the publisher is not responsible for the validity of the information or for any
outcomes resulting from reliance thereon.

Printed in the United States of America.

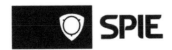

To My Grandkids

Dasha, Zhenya, and Stepa

Contents

Nomenclature

$2l$	separation between two point light sources formed in the nodal plane
$2R_a$	diameter of circular aperture
$A = \log 1/R_d$	apparent absorbance
$\bar{a}$	numerical coefficient depending on the form of the diffusion equation
a	radius of a scatterer (particle), nm or µm
A	signal amplitude in the frequency-domain measuring technique
A	acoustic amplitude
$A = \langle i \rangle^2$	square of the mean value of the photocurrent (the base line of the autocorrelation function)
a'	the largest dimension of a nonspherical particle, nm or µm
A_0	initial amplitude due to the instrumental response
A_{ac}	ac component of the amplitude of the photon-density wave
A_{dc}	dc component of the amplitude of the photon-density wave
a_m	more probable scatterer radius, µm
a_n and b_n	Mie coefficients
$A(\mathbf{r})$	describes the optical absorption properties of the tissue at $\mathbf{r}$
a_T	thermal diffusivity of the medium, m^2/s
B_d	detection bandwidth
b_s	accounts for additional irradiation of upper layers of a tissue due to backscattering (photon recycling effect)
c	velocity of light in the medium, cm/c
c_0	velocity of light in vacuum, cm/c
C_1 and C_2	concentrations of molecules in two spaces separated by a membrane
$C_a(x,t)$	concentration of the agent
C_{a0}	initial concentration of the agent
c_{ab}	concentration of absorber in µmol, mmol, or mol
c_b	blood specific heat, J/kg K
C_{Hb}	hemoglobin concentration
$C_f(x,t)$	fluid concentration
c_P	specific heat capacity for a constant pressure, J/kg K
c_s	relative concentration of the scattering centers
$\overline{C}_S$	average concentration of dissolved matter in two interacting solutions

c_V	specific heat capacity for a constant volume, J/kg K
C_n^α	Gegenbauer polynomials
$\langle C \rangle$	average blood concentration
$\langle C \rangle V_{rms}$	blood flux or perfusion
$D = z\lambda/\pi L_\phi^2$	wave parameter
D	photon diffusion coefficient, cm^2/c
D_A	diattenuation (linear dichroism)
D_a	agent diffusion coefficient, cm^2/c
D_B	coefficient of Brownian diffusion, cm^2/c
D_f	fluid coefficient of diffusion, cm^2/c
d	sample (tissue layer or slab) thickness, cm
$\mathbf{D}^{-1}$	inverse of the measurement matrix
$D_\perp$	dimension of incident light beam across the area where the total radiant energy fluence rate is maximal (determined from the $1/e^2$ level), cm
$D_\parallel$	dimension of incident light beam along the area where the total radiant energy fluence rate is maximal (determined from the $1/e^2$ level), cm
$d\Omega$	unit solid angle about a chosen direction, sr
d_{av}	average size of a speckle in the far-field zone
D_f	fractal (volumetric) dimension
D_I	structure function of the fluctuation intensity component
d_p	length of the space where the exciting and the probe laser beams are overlapped, cm
d_s	mean distance between the centers of gravity of the particles
D_T	coefficient of translation diffusion
D_{Tf}	coefficient of translation diffusion for fast process
D_{Ts}	coefficient of translation diffusion for slow process
D_V	diameter of a microvessel
$d\bar{n}/d\lambda$	material dispersion, 1/nm
dn/dT	medium (tissue) refractive index temperature gradient, 1/°C
DPF	differential path length factor accounting for the increase in photon migration paths due to scattering
dS	thermoelastic deformation, cm
E	incident pulse energy, J
e	electron charge
E_0	incident laser pulse energy at the sample surface (J/cm^2)
E_{0j}	scattering amplitude of an isolated particle, V/m
$\vec{E}_{\perp i}$	electric field component of the incident light perpendicular to the scattering plane, V/m
$\vec{E}_{\parallel i}$	electric field component of the incident light parallel to the scattering plane, V/m
$E_{\parallel s}$	electric field component of the scattered light parallel to the scattering plane, V/m

$E_{\perp s}$	electric field component of the scattered light perpendicular to the scattering plane, V/m
$\vec{E}_s$	scattered electric field vector, V/m
E_s	amplitude of a scattered wave, V/m
E_T	absorbed pulse energy, J
$E(0)$	subsurface irradiance (J/cm^2)
$F(Hct)$	packing function of RBC
$F(\vec{r})$	radiant flux density or irradiance, W/cm^2
$f(t, t')$	describes the temporal deformation of a δ-shaped pulse following its single scattering
$f_{1,2}$	volume fractions of tissue components
f_a	frequency of acoustic oscillations, Hz
f_c	volume fraction of the collagen in tissue
f_{cp}	volume fraction of the fluid in the tissue contained inside the cells
f_{cyl}	surface fraction of the cylinders' faces
f_D	Doppler frequency
f_{Ds}	Doppler frequency shift
f_f	volume fraction of the fibers in the tissue
f_{ge}	oscillator strength of transition between the ground and excited states
$F_{int}(\theta)$	interference term taking into account the spatial correlation of particles
$f_n = g^n$	n'th order moment of the phase function
f_{nc}	volume fraction of the nuclei in the tissue contained inside the cells
f_{or}	volume fraction of the organelles in the tissue contained inside the cells
f_p	pulse repetition rate
f_r	fixed reference (lock-in) frequency
f_{RBCi}	volume fraction of RBCs
f_s	volume fraction of scatterers
f_T	focal length of the "thermal lens," cm
F_v	total volume fraction of the particles
f_σ	material fringe value
$g_1(\tau)$	first-order autocorrelation function (normalized autocorrelation function of the optical field)
$g_2(\Delta\xi)$	autocorrelation function of intensity fluctuations
G	domain where radiative transport is examined
g	scattering anisotropy parameter (the mean cosine of the scattering angle θ, $\langle\cos(\theta)\rangle$)
$G_1(\tau)$	autocorrelation function of the scalar electric field, $E(t)$, of the scattered light
$G(f)$	power spectrum with a Gaussian envelope

$g(r)$	radial distribution function of scattering centers (local-to-average density ratio for scattering centers)
$G(\mathrm{r})$	binary density-density correlation function
$\tilde{g}_2$	autocorrelation function of the fluctuation intensity component
g_d	scattering anisotropy factor of dermis
g_e	scattering anisotropy factor of epidermis
G_s	attenuation factor accounting for scattering and geometry of the tissue
G_V	gradient of the flow rate
H or Hct	blood hematocrit
H	tissue hydration
h	Planck's constant
h	apparent energy transfer coefficient
$H(\mathbf{r}, \bar{t})$	heating function defined as the thermal energy per time and volume deposited by the light source in the close proportion to the optical absorption coefficient of interest
$h\nu$	photon energy
$h(x, y)$	spatial variations in the thickness of the RPS
$I(\theta)/I(0)$ $\equiv p(\theta)$	normalized scattering indicatrix, 1/sr
$I(\theta)$	scattering indicatrix (angular dependence of the scattered light intensity), W/cm^2 sr $i = (-1)^{1/2}$
I_{AS}, I_S	intensity of the anti-Stokes and Stokes Raman lines for a given vibration state
I_F	fluorescence intensity
I_i	irradiance or intensity of the incident light beam, W/cm^2
$\langle I \rangle$	mean value of the intensity fluctuations
I	refers to the irradiance or intensity of the light, W/cm^2
$I_\perp(t)$	intensity of the scattered light polarized orthogonal to the incident light
$I(\bar{r}, \bar{s})$	radiance (or the specific intensity)—average power flux density at a point $\bar{r}$ in the given direction $\bar{s}$, W/cm^2 sr
$I(\bar{r}, \bar{s}, t)$	time-dependent radiance (or the specific intensity), W/cm^2 sr
$I(0)$	intensity at the center of the beam
$I(d)$	intensity of light transmitted by a sample of thickness d measured using a distant photodetector with a small aperture (on line or collimated transmittance), W/cm^2
$I, Q, U,$ and V	Stokes parameters
$I_H, I_V, I_{+45°},$ $I_{-45°}, I_R,$ and I_L	are the light intensities measured with a horizontal linear polarizer, a vertical linear polarizer, a +45° linear polarizer, a −45° linear polarizer, a right circular analyzer, and a left circular analyzer in front of the detector, respectively
$I_{\mathrm{in}}(\eta_c)$	incident radiance angular distribution

$I_\Sigma(\theta)$	angular distribution of the scattered intensity of a system of N particles
$I_\Sigma(x, y)$	intensity of light transmitted by an RPS
$I_\parallel$ and $I_\perp$	intensities of the transmitted (scattered) light polarized in parallel or perpendicular to linear polarization of the incident light, respectively
$I(\theta)$	angular distribution of the scattered light by a particle, W/cm^2 sr
$I(2\omega)$	SHG signal intensity
$I_0(\lambda)$	spectrum of the incident light
I_0	incident light intensity, W/cm^2
I_b	intensity of the uniform background light
$I_c(x, y)$	intensity of light transmitted in the forward direction (the specular component)
$I_{F\parallel}$ and $I_{F\perp}$	fluorescence intensities of light polarized in parallel or perpendicular to the exciting electric field vector
I_{par} and I_{per}	intensity images for light polarized in parallel or perpendicular to linear polarization of the incident light, respectively
$I_r(r)$ and $I_s(r)$	intensity distributions of the reference and signal fields
I_{rest} and I_{test}	light intensity detected when an object is at rest (brain tissue, skeletal muscle, etc.) and test (induced brain activity, cold or visual test, training, etc.)
$I_s(x, y)$	intensity of the scattered component
I_{sp}	mean intensity of speckles
J	flux of matter, mol/s/cm^2
J_0	zero-order Bessel function
J_1	first-order Bessel function
J_S	dissolved matter flux
J_W	water flux
$k = 2\pi/\lambda$	wavenumber
k_a	acoustic wave vector
k_F	rate constant of the fluorescence transition to the ground state S_0 (including its vibrational states)
k_{ET}	rate constant of non-radiative energy transfer to adjacent molecules
K, S	Kubelka–Munk parameters
$K_\phi(\Delta x)$	correlation coefficient of phase fluctuations of the boundary field
k_B	Boltzmann constant
k_{bvo}	modification factor for reducing the crosstalk between changes of blood volume and oxygenation
k_G	gas heat conductivity, W/K
$k_i(\omega)$	imaginary part of the photon-density wave vector, 1/cm
$k_r(\omega)$	real part of the photon-density wave vector, 1/cm
k_{IC}	rate constant of internal conversion to the ground state S_0

k_{ISC}	rate constant of intersystem crossing from the singlet to the triplet state T_1
k_T	heat conductivity, W/K
L	total mean path length of a photon
L	tissue slab thickness
$L = D\lambda/2l$	period of interferential fringes (D is the mean distance between eye nodal plane and retina)
L_D	phenomenological coefficient characterizing the interchange flux induced by osmotic pressure
L_ϕ	correlation length of the phase fluctuations of the scattered field
l_0	amplitude of longitudinal harmonic vibrations
L_c	correlation length of the inhomogeneities (random relief)
l_c	coherence length of a light source
$l_d = \mu_{eff}^{-1}$	diffusion length, cm
l_e	depth of light penetration into a tissue
L_p	phenomenological coefficient indicating that the volumetric flux can be induced by rising hydrostatic pressure
L_{pd}	phenomenological coefficient indicating on the one hand the volumetric flux that can be induced for the membrane by the osmotic pressure, and on the other, the efficiency of the separation of water molecules and dissolved matter
$l_{ph} = \mu_t^{-1}$	photon mean free path, cm
$l_s = l/\mu_s$	scattering length, cm
$l_t = (\mu_s' + \mu_a)^{-1}$	photon transport mean free path (MFP), cm
l_T	length of thermal diffusivity (thermal length), cm
M	molecule weight
$m \equiv n_s/n_0$	relative refractive index of the scatterers
$M = I_1/I_0$	intensity modulation depth defined as the ratio between the intensity at the fundamental frequency I_1 and the unmodulated intensity I_0
$\mathbf{M}$	normalized 4×4 scattering matrix (intensity or Mueller's matrix) (LSM)
M_0	zero-moment of the power density spectrum $S(\nu)$ of the intensity fluctuations
M_1	first-moment of the power density spectrum $S(\nu)$ of the intensity fluctuations
m_I	intensity modulation depth of the incident light
M_{ij}	LSM elements, $i, j = 1$–4, 16 elements
$\overline{M}_{ij}$	LSM element normalized to the first one
M_{ij}^0	LSM elements of an isolated particle
m_{RBC}	relative index of refraction of RBC
m_t	amount of dissolved matter at the moment t
m_∞	amount of dissolved matter at the equilibrium state

$m_U \equiv AC_{detector}/$ $DC_{detector}$	modulation depth of scattered light intensity
n	relative mean refractive index of tissue and surrounding media
n''	imaginary part of index of refraction
$\bar{n}$	mean refractive index of the scattering medium
N	number of scatterers (particles)
$N = \theta/2\pi$	fringe order (θ is the optical phase)
N_0	number of scatterers in a unit volume
$N_1(z) = z \times \mu_s^{ex}$	average number of scattering events experienced by the excitation light before it reached the fluorophore (z is the distance of fluorophore location)
$N_2(z) = z \times \mu_s^{em}$	average number of scattering events experienced by the emitted light before it exited the medium (z is the distance of fluorophore location)
$\overline{N}$	outside vector normal to ∂G
n_{2f}	rate of two-photon excitation
n_0	refractive index of the ground matter
$\bar{n}_0$	average background index of refraction
n_c	refractive index of collagen fibers
n_{cp}	refractive index of the cytoplasm
n_e	extraordinary refractive index
n_f	refractive index of tissue fibers (collagen and elastin)
n_{g0}	refractive index of the ground material of a tissue
$\bar{n}_{g1}$	effective (mean) group refractive index of a tissue
n_{g2}	group refractive index of the homogeneous reference medium (air)
n_g	group refractive index
n_{gs}	group refractive index of the scatterers
n_{H_2O}	refractive index of water
$N_i = f_{RBCi}/$ V_{RBCi}	number of RBC in a unit volume of blood
$N_{int} =$ $[arcsin(\lambda/$ $2l)]^{-1}$	density of interferential fringes per a degree of the view angle (an angular resolving power of the eye or retinal visual acuity)
n_{is}	refractive index of the interstitial fluid
n_{nc}	refractive index of cell nucleus
n_o	ordinary refractive index
n_{or}	refractive index of cell organelles
N_p	number of particle diameters
n_s	refractive index of the scattering centers
$\bar{n}_s$	refractive index of a scattering particle received by averaging of refractive indices of tissue components
$\bar{n}_{sc}$	average refractive index of eye sclera
N_{sp}	number of speckles within the receiving aperture

NA	numerical aperture of the objective or fiber
$n(x, y)$	spatial variations in the refractive index of the RPS
$\bar{n}_t$	average refractive index of the tissue
OD	optical density
osm	osmolarity
p	packing dimension
p	porosity coefficient
P	laser beam power, W
P	induced polarization
P_a	coefficient of permeability
P_0	average incident power, W
$P_C = V/I = [Q^2 + U^2]^{1/2} /I$	degree of circular polarization
$P_{FL} = (I_{F\parallel} - I_{F\perp})/ (I_{F\parallel} + I_{F\perp})$	degree of linear polarization of fluorescence
$P_L = (I_{\parallel} - I_{\perp})/ (I_{\parallel} + I_{\perp})$	degree of linear polarization
$P_L^r(\lambda)$	residual polarization degree spectra
P_{min}	minimal detectable signal power
$p(I)$	intensity probability density distribution function
$p(s)$	distribution function of photon migration paths in the medium
$p(\bar{s}, \bar{s}') = p(\theta)$	scattering phase function (the probability density function for scattering in the direction $\bar{s}'$ of a photon travelling in the direction $\bar{s}$), 1/sr
$p_{gk}(\theta)$	Gegenbauer kernel phase function (GKPF)
$p_{hg}(\theta)$	Henyey-Greenstein phase function (HGPF)
PI	polarization degree image
$P_n^1(\cos\theta)$	Legendre polynomials
$p(\Delta L)$	probability density distribution function of relief variations
$p(r, \bar{t})$	the acoustic wave
$\vec{q}$	scattering vector
$|\vec{q}|$	value of scattering vector
$q(\bar{r})$	source function (i.e., the number of photons injected into the unit volume)
Q, U, and V	represent the extent of horizontal liner, 45° linear, and circular polarization, respectively
Q_a	asymmetry parameter of the intensity fluctuations
q_b	blood perfusion rate (1/s), defined as the volume of blood flowing through unit volume of tissue in one second
Q_s	factor of scattering efficiency
$\mathbf{r}$	transverse spatial coordinate
$r = \frac{I_{\parallel} - I_{\perp}}{I_{\parallel} + 2I_{\perp}}$	polarization anisotropy

$r_F = (I_{F\parallel} - I_{F\perp})$ fluorescence polarization anisotropy
$/(I_{F\parallel} + 2I_{F\perp})$

$\mathbf{R}(\phi)$	Stokes rotation matrix for angle ϕ
$\bar{r}$	radius vector of a scatterer or of a given point where the radiance is evaluated, cm
$r_{\perp\parallel}(\tau)$	cross-correlation function (correlation coefficient) for two polarization states
$R_{\parallel}(\lambda)$ and $R_{\perp}(\lambda)$	reflectance spectra at in parallel and perpendicular orientations of polarization filters
$\hat{R}$	reflection operator
$\bar{R}$	4×1 response vector corresponding to the four retarder/ analyzer settings
R_a	reflectance from the backward surface of the sample impregnated by an agent
$R_\theta(\lambda)$	spectrum of light scattered under the angle $(\theta + d\theta)$
r_0	radius of the incident light beam, cm
R_{bd}	distance between the axis of exciting laser beam and the acoustic detector, cm
R_d	diffuse reflectance
$R_F = [(n-l)/ (n+l)]^2$	coefficient of Fresnel reflection
R_G	gas cell radius, cm
r_h	hydrodynamic radius of a particle
R_o	dimension (radius for a cylinder form) of a bioobject, cm
r_p	radius of the pinhole
r_{RBC}	radius of RBC
r_s	radius of the scattered beam in the observation plane
R_s	reflectance from the backward surface of the control sample
r_{sd}	distance between light source and detector at the tissue surface (source-detector separation), cm
$R(\eta_c', \eta_c)$	reflection redistribution function
$RT\Delta C_S$	osmotic pressure
$R(z)$	optical backscattering or reflectance
s	total photon path length (or mean path length of a photon)
S	hemoglobin oxygen saturation
S	heat source term, W/m^3
S	sample area
S_D	surface of detection
$\mathbf{S}$	Stokes vector
$\bar{S}$	Stokes vector calculated on the basis of experimental data
$\mathbf{S}_s$	Stokes vector of the scattered light
$\mathbf{S}_i$	Stokes vector of the incident light
$\bar{s}$ and $\bar{s}'$	directions of photon travel or unit vectors for incident and scattered waves

$\|\bar{s}\| = 2k\sin(\theta/2)$	magnitude of the scattering wave vector $k = 2\pi\bar{n}/\lambda_0$
$\vec{S}_0$	unit vector of the direction of the incident wave
$\vec{S}_1$	unit vector of the direction of the scattered wave
$S(\bar{r},\bar{s})$	incident light distribution at ∂G
$S(f)$	power spectrum of intensity fluctuations of the speckle field
$S(q)$	structure factor
$S_3(\theta)$	3-D structure factor
$S_2(\theta)$	2-D structure factor
$S(\omega)$	spectrum of intensity fluctuations
$S_{1\text{-}4}$	elements of the amplitude scattering matrix (S-matrix) or Jones matrix
$S_r(t)$	surface radiometric signal
$S(\bar{t})$	describes the shape of the irradiating pulse
T_a	acoustic period
$T_\theta(\lambda)$	transmission spectrum when a measuring system with a finite angle of view is used (the collimated light beam with some addition of a forward-scattered light in the angle range 0 to θ is detected)
t_0	spatially independent amplitude transmission of the RPS
t_1	the first moment of the distribution function $f(t,t')$; time interval of an individual scattering act, s
$t_2 = 1/(\mu_t c)$	average interval between interactions, s
T	absolute temperature
T	exposure time, s
$T(\mathbf{r})$	change in tissue temperature at point $\mathbf{r}$
$T(\eta'_c,\eta_c)$	transmission redistribution function
T_a	arterial blood temperature, K
t_b	blood temperature
$T_c(\lambda)$	collimated transmission spectrum
T_c	collimated transmittance
T_d	diffuse transmittance
T_s and T_e	temperature of the tissue surface and environment, respectively
$t_s(x,y)$	amplitude transmission coefficient of an RPS
$T_t = T_c + T_d$	total transmittance
$T_t(\lambda)$	total transmission spectrum
t	time, s
$U(\bar{r})$	total radiant energy fluence rate, W/cm^2
$\langle U \rangle$	averaged amplitude of the output signal of the homodyne interferometer
U_m	maximum of the total radiant energy fluence rate, W/cm^2
V	illuminated volume
V	volume of the tissue sample
v	velocity of motion of the object with respect to the light beam
V_C	volume of collagen fibers

V_e	volume of an erythrocyte
V_M	molecular volume
$\overline{V}(z)$	contrast of average-intensity fringes
V_Φ	phase velocity of a photon-density wave, cm/s
V_0	contrast of the interference pattern in the initial laser beam
v_a	velocity of acoustic waves in a medium, m/s
V_I	contrast of the intensity fluctuations
v_p	radius (in optical units) of conjugate pinholes of a confocal microscopic system
V_P	contrast of the polarization image
V_{RBC}	RBC volume, μm^3
V_{rms}	root-mean-square speed of moving particles
V_s	velocity of a moving particle
$\overline{V}_S$	partial mole volumes of dissolved matter
v_{sh}	shear rate
V_V	parameter directly proportional to the flow velocity
$\overline{V}_W$	partial mole volumes of water
w	laser (Gaussian) beam radius (or radius of a cylinder illuminated by a laser beam), cm
w_p	probing laser beam radius, cm
w_0	radius of the Gaussian beam waist
x^0	fixed point at the plane where speckles are observed
$x = 2\pi a/\lambda$	size (diffraction) parameter
z	linear coordinate (depth inside the medium), cm
$\mathbf{Z}$	normalized phase matrix $z_0 = (\mu_s')^{-1}$, cm

Greek

$\alpha(z)$	reflectivity of the sample at the depth of z
α_{Hb}	spectrally-dependent coefficient of proportionality of hemoglodin imaginary refractive index on its concentration
α_i	incidence angle of the beam, angular degrees
β	coefficient of volumetric expansion, 1/K
β	modulation depth of photoelectric signal of the interferometer
$\langle\beta\rangle$	orientation averaged first molecular hyperpolarizability
β_{sb}	parameter of self-beating efficiency
Γ	Grüneisen parameter (dimensionless, temperature-dependent factor proportional to the fraction of thermal energy converted into mechanical stress)
Γ_{eff}	effective shear rate
Γ_T	relaxation parameter
$\gamma = c_P/c_V$	ratio of specific heat capacities
$\gamma_{11}(\Delta t)$	degree of temporal coherence of light
$\Delta\psi$	phase shift in a measuring interferometer, degrees

Δa	halfwidth of the radii distribution
$\Delta E_{vib} = h\nu_{vib}$	energy of the molecular vibration state
ΔF	width of the averaged spectrum
$\Delta \tilde{k}$	wavenumber shift
$\Delta L = \Delta(nh)$	optical length (relief) variations
Δn	refractive indices difference
Δn_{oe}	refractive indices difference due to birefringence of form
Δp	change of pressure, Pa
Δp	hydrostatic pressure, Pa
$\Delta R^r(\lambda)$	differential residual polarization spectra
ΔV	change of illuminated volume caused by local temperature increase, m^3
Δw	change of radius of a cylinder illuminated by a laser beam caused by local temperature increase, cm
Δx	linear shift of the center of maximal diffuse reflection, cm
Δz	longitudinal displacement of the object
ΔT	local temperature increase, °C
ΔT	optical clearing (enhancement of transmittance)
Δx_T	amplitude of mechanical oscillations, cm
$\langle \Delta n \rangle$	mean refractive index variation
$\Delta \Phi_0$	initial phase due to the instrumental response
$\Delta \theta$	angular width of the coherent peak in backscatter, angular degrees
$\Delta \lambda$	bandwidth of a light source
$\Delta \xi$	change in variable
$\Delta \Psi_I(r)$	deterministic phase difference of the interfering waves
$\Delta \Phi$	phase shift relative to the incident light modulation phase (phase lag), degrees
$\langle \Delta r^2(\tau) \rangle$	mean-square displacement of a particle within time interval τ
$\Delta \Phi_I(r)$	random phase difference
ΔT_S	temperature change of a sample, °C
ΔT_G	temperature change of a surrounding gas, °C
Δt	time shift of the transmitted pulse peak
$\Delta \Phi_I(r)$	time-dependent phase difference related to the motion of an object
$\delta = 2\pi d \Delta n/\lambda_0$	phase delay (retardance) of optical field
δ_n and δ_d	parameters related to the average contributions per photon free path and per scattering event, respectively, to the ultrasonic modulation of light intensity
$\delta_{oe} = 2\pi d \Delta n_{oe}/\lambda_0$	phase delay of optical field due to birefringence
$\delta p(\omega)$	amplitude of harmonically modulated pressure, Pa
$\delta p(t)$	time-dependent change of pressure, Pa
∂G	boundary surface of the domain G

$\partial n/\partial p$	adiabatic piezo-optical coefficient of the tissue
Δz_{opt}	optical path length
ε_{ab}	absorption coefficient measured in $\text{mol}^{-1}\,\text{cm}^{-1}$
ε_λ^d	extinction coefficient of deoxyhemoglobin measured in $\text{mol}^{-1}\,\text{cm}^{-1}$
ε_λ^o	extinction coefficient of oxyhemoglobin measured in $\text{mol}^{-1}\,\text{cm}^{-1}$
ε_λ	extinction coefficient at the wavelength λ in $\text{mol}^{-1}\,\text{cm}^{-1}$
η	absolute viscosity of the medium
$\eta(a)$ or $\eta(2a)$	radii (a) or diameter $(2a)$ distribution function of scatterers
η_c	cosine of the polar angle
η_F	fluorescence quantum yield
η_q	quantum efficiency of the detector
$\eta'(2a)$	correlation-corrected distribution $\eta(2a)$
θ	scattering angle, angular degrees
θ_I	angle between the wave vectors of the interfering fields
θ_{rnd}^{GK}	GKPFrandom scattering angle
θ_{rnd}^{HG}	HGPF random scattering angle
$\Lambda = \frac{\sigma_{\text{sca}}}{\sigma_{\text{ext}}} = \frac{\mu_s}{\mu_t}$	albedo for single scattering (characterizes the relation of scattering and absorption properties of a tissue)
$\Lambda' = \frac{\mu_s'}{\mu_a + \mu_s'}$	transport albedo
Λ_Φ	photon-density wavelength, cm
Λ_I	spacing of interference fringes
$\lambda = \lambda_0/\bar{n}$	wavelength in the scattering medium, nm
λ_0	wavelength of the light in vacuum, nm
λ_p	wavelength of the probe beam, nm
μ_a'	absorption coefficient at the thermal radiation emission wavelength, 1/cm
μ_a	absorption coefficient, 1/cm
μ_b	volume-averaged backscattering coefficient, 1/cm sr
$\mu_{\text{eff}} = [3\mu_a(\mu_s' + \mu_a)]^{1/2}$	effective attenuation coefficient or inverse diffusion length, 1/cm
μ_{ge}	change in dipole moment between the ground and excited states
μ_n	$n$order statistical moment $(n = 1, 2, 3 \ldots)$
$\mu_s' = (1 - g)\mu_s$	reduced (transport) scattering coefficient, 1/cm
μ_s	scattering coefficient, 1/cm
μ_s^{ex}	scattering coefficient of the excitation light, 1/cm
μ_s^{em}	scattering coefficient of the emitting light, 1/cm
$\mu_t = \mu_a + \mu_s$	extinction coefficient (interaction or total attenuation coefficient), 1/cm
$\mu_t' = \mu_a + \mu_s'$	transport coefficient
$|\mu(z)|$	modulus of the transverse correlation coefficient of the complex amplitude of the scattered field

ν_I	exponential factor of the spatial intensity fluctuations
$\xi \equiv x$ or t	spatial or temporal variable
ξ_I	characteristic depolarization length for linearly ($i = L$) and circularly ($i = C$) polarized light
ρ	medium density, kg/m^3
ρ	polarization azimuth
ρ_a	volume density of absorbers, 1/cm^3
ρ_b	blood density (kg/m^3)
ρ_G	gas density, kg/m^3
ρ_s	volume density of the scatterers, 1/cm^3
$\rho(s)$	probability density function of the optical paths
σ	halfwidth of the particle size distribution
$\sigma = -(L_{pd}/L_p)$	molecular reflection coefficient
$(\sigma_1 - \sigma_2)$	difference in the in-plane principle stress
σ_{abs}	absorption cross-section of a particle, cm^2
$\bar{\sigma}_{abs}$	specific absorption coefficient, cm^{-1}
σ_{ext}	extinction cross section of a particle, cm^2
σ_f	photon absorption cross-section
σ_h	standard deviation of the altitudes (depths) of inhomogeneities
σ_I	standard deviation of the intensity fluctuations
σ_L	standard deviation of relief variations (in optical lengths)
σ_m	width of the skewed logarithmic distribution function for the volume fraction of particles of diameter $2a$
$\sigma_s(2a_i)$	optical cross-section of an individual particle with diameter $2a_i$ and volume v_i, cm^2
σ_{sca}	scattering cross-section of a particle, cm^2
$\overline{\sigma}_{sca}$	specific scattering coefficient, cm^{-1}
Σ_{sca}	scattering cross-section for the system of particles, cm
σ_ϕ	standard deviation of the phase fluctuations of the scattered field
σ_I^2	variance of the intensity fluctuations
σ_s^2	*spatial* variance of the intensity in the speckle pattern
σ_U^2	variance of the output signal of the homodyne interferometer
τ	delay time
τ	lifetime of the excited state
$\tau = \int_0^s \mu_t ds$	optical thickness
$\tau_a = 1/\mu_a c$	average travel time of a photon before being absorbed, s
τ_c	correlation time of intensity fluctuations in the scattered field
τ_d	time delay between optical and acoustical pulses, s
τ_L	duration of a laser pulse, s
τ_p	pulse duration
τ_r	time constant of rotational diffusion
τ_{th}	time delay for the "thermal lens" technique, s
τ_T	thermal relaxation time of the photoacoustic cell, s

$\tau_B^{-1} \equiv \Gamma_T$	characterizes the random (Brownian) flow
$\tau_S^{-1} \cong$ $0.18 G_V |\bar{q}| l_t$	characterizes the directed flow
$\Phi(x, y)$	random phase shift introduced by the RPS at the (x, y) point
$\Phi_p(\omega)$	phase-lag of harmonically modulated pressure, degrees
$\phi(t)$	phase shift defined by a scatterer position
φ	angle of observation and azimuthal angle, angular degrees
φ_d	deflection angle of a probe laser beam, angular degrees
Ω	solid angle, sr
Ω_v	frequency of harmonic vibrations
$\omega = 2\pi f$	modulation frequency, 1/s
ω_a	fundamental acoustic frequency
ω_{ge}	energy difference between the ground and excited states
ω_p	packing factor of a medium filled with a volume fraction f_s of scatterers
$(\omega t - \theta)$	phase of the photon-density wave
$\chi^{(n)}$	the nth order nonlinear susceptibility

Acronyms

ac	alternating current
ADC	amplitude-digital convertor
AF	autocorrelation function
AF	autofluorescence
AHA	α-hydroxy acid
AO	acoustooptical
AOM	acoustooptic modulator
AOT	AO tomography
APD	avalanch photodetector
ALA	δ-aminolevulenic acid
ATR-FTIR	attenuated total reflectance Fourier transform infrared
AW	acoustic waves
BEM	boundary-element method
BSA	bovine serum albumin
BW	birefringent wedges
CBF	cerebral blood flow
CCD	charge-coupled device
CDI	coherent detection imaging
CFD	constant-fraction discriminator
CIE	Commission Internationale de l'Eclairage which is the French title of the International Commission on Illumination
CIN	cervical intraepithelial neoplasia
CIS	carcinoma *in situ*
CM	confocal microscopy
CMOS	complementary metal-oxide-semiconductor
CP OCT	cross-polarization OCT
CPU	central processing unit
CSF	cerebrospinal fluid
CT	computed tomography
CW	continuous wave
DBM	double-balanced mixer
dc	direct current
DG	delay generator
DIS	double integrating sphere
DMSO	dimethyl sulfoxide
DNA	deoxyribonucleic acid

DOCP	degree of circular polarization
DOLP	degree of linear polarization
DOP	degree of polarization
DOPA	3,4-dihydroxyphenylalanine
DOPE	dioleylphosphatidylethanolamine
DPF	differential path length factor
DPS OCT	differential phase-sensitive OCT
DT	diffusion theory
DWS	diffusion wave spectroscopy
EDL	extensor digitorum longus
EDTA	ethylenediaminetetraacetic acid
EEM	excitation-emission map
ESR	erythrocyte sedimentation rate
FAD	flavin dinucleotide
FD	frequency domain
FDA	Food Drug Administration
FD-LUM	frequency-domain luminescence
FD-OTR	frequency-domain OTR
FDPM	frequency-domain photon migration
FDTD	finite-difference time-domain
FFT	fast Fourier transform
FG	function generator
FMN	flavin mononucleotide
FRAP	fluorescence recovery after photobleaching
FWHM	full width half maximum
GHb	glycated hemoglobin
GK	Gergenbauer kernel
GKPF	Gegenbauer kernel phase function
GPM	goniophotometric measurements
GRIN	gradient index
Hb	hemoglobin
HEM	human epidermal membrane
HCM	human cervical mucus
Hct	hematocrit
HPD	hematoporphirin derivative
HG	Henyey-Greenstein
HGPF	Henyey-Greenstein phase function
HWHM	half width half maximum
IAD	inverse adding–doubling
ICG	indocyanine green
IF	intermediate frequency
IFS	interfibrillar spacing
IMC	inverse Monte Carlo
IMS	intermolecular spacing

IC25	Infracyanine 25
IQ	in-phase quadrature
IR	infrared
IS	integrating sphere
KDP	kalium dihydrophosphate
KMM	Kubelka-Munk model
LASCA	laser speckle contrast analysis
LD	laser diode
LDA	laser Doppler anemometer
LDI	laser Doppler imaging
LDM	laser Doppler microscope
LED	light-emitting diode
LID	lattice of islet damage
LIPT	laser-induced pressure transient
LITT	laser-induced interstitial thermal therapy
LO	local oscillator
LPF	low-pass filter
LSI	laser speckle imaging
LSM	light-scattering matrix
LSMM	laser scattering matrix meter
LSS	light scattering spectroscopy
LVDS	low-voltage differential signaling
MAR	modified amino resin
MB	methylene blue
MBG	mean blood glucose
MC	Monte Carlo
MCA	multichannel analyzer
MCP-PMT	multichannel plate-photomultiplier tube
MED	minimal erythema dose
MFP	mean free path length
MIM	multispectral imaging micropolarimeter
MIR	middle infrared
MO	microobjective
MONSTIR	multichannel optoelectronic near-infrared system for time-resolved image reconstruction
MPS	maximum permissible exposure
MR	magnetic resonance
MRI	MR imaging
MTT	meal tolerance test
NA	numerical aperture
NAD	nicotinamide adenine dinucleotide
NAD$^+$	oxidized form of NAD
NADH	reduced form of NAD
NIR	near infrared

OA	optoacoustic
OAT	OA tomography
OCA	optical clearing agent
OCI	optical coherence interferometry
OCM	optical coherence microscopy
OCP	optical clearing potential
OCT	optical coherence tomography
OD	optical density
OGTT	oral glucose tolerance test
OMA	optical multichannel analyzer
OT	optothermal
OTR	optothermal radiometry
PA	photoacoustic
PAM	photoacoustic microscopy
PBS	phosphate buffered saline
PC	personal computer
PD	photodetector
PDF	probability distribution function
PDMD	phase-delay measurement device
PDT	photodynamic therapy
PDWFCS	photon-density wave-fluctuation correlation spectroscopy
PEG	polyethylene glycol
PG	propylene glycol
PHA	pulse-height analysis
PM	polarization-maintaining
PMT	photomultiplier tube
POS	polyorganosiloxane
PPG	polypropylene glycol
PRS	polarized reflectance spectroscopy
PS OCT	polarization-sensitive OCT
PS-OLCR	phase-sensitive optical low-coherence reflectometer
PT	photothermal
PTFC	PT flow cytometry
PTM	PT microscopy
PTR	PT radiometry
PVDF	polyvinyldenefluoride
PY	Percus-Yevick
QELS	quasi-elastic light scattering
RBC	red blood cell
RC	relative contrast
RCM	reflection confocal microscopy
RF	radio frequency
RGA	Rayleigh-Gans approximation
rms	root mean square

RNA	ribonucleic acid
RNFL	retinal nerve fiber layer
ROI	region of interest
RPS	random phase screen
RSODL	rapid scanning optical delay line
RTE	radiative transfer equation
RTT	radiation transfer theory
SC	stratum corneum
SEM	standard error of the mean
SERS	surface-enhanced Raman scattering
SHG	second harmonic generation
SMF	skeletal muscle fibers
SL	sonoluminescence
SLD	superluminescent diode
SLT	SL tomography
SMLB	spatially-modulated laser beam
SNR	signal-to-noise ratio
SPR	spatially resolved reflectance
SSB	single sideband
SRR	spatially resolved reflectance
ST	*Staphylococcus* toxin
TAC	time-to-amplitude convertor
TD	time-domain
TDM	time division multiplex
TDM	transillumination digital microscopy
TEWL	transepidermal water loss
TGS	thermal gradient spectroscopy
THb	total hemoglobin
TMP	trimethylolpropanol
TOAST	time-resolved optical absorption and scattering tomography
TRS	time-resolved spectroscopy
US	ultrasound
UV	ultraviolet
VOA	variable optical attenuator
WP	Wollaston prism
VRTE	vector radiative transfer equation
VTW	virtual transparent window
WDM	wavelength division multiplex
WHO	World Health Organization

Preface to First Edition

Many up-to-date medical technologies are based on recent progress in physics, including optics.[1–102] An interesting example relevant to the topic of this tutorial is provided by computer tomography.[1,4] X-ray, magnetic resonance, and positron-emission imaging techniques are extensively used in high-resolution studies of both anatomical structures and local metabolic processes. Another safe and technically simple tool currently in use is diffuse optical tomography.[1,3,4,6,15,28,71]

From the viewpoint of optics, biological tissues and fluids (blood, lymph, saliva, mucus, gastric juice, urine, aqueous humor, semen, etc.) can be separated into two large classes.[1–69,92–97,101] The first class includes strongly scattering (opaque) tissues and fluids, such as skin, brain, vessel walls, eye sclera, blood, and lymph. The optical properties of these tissues and fluids can be described within the framework of the model of multiple scattering of scalar or vector waves in a randomly nonuniform absorbing medium. The second class consists of weakly scattering (transparent) tissues and fluids, such as cornea, crystalline lens, vitreous humor, and aqueous humor of the front chamber of the eye. The optical properties of these tissues and fluids can be described within the framework of the model of single scattering (or low-step scattering) in an ordered isotropic or anisotropic medium with closely packed scatterers with absorbing centers.

The vector nature of light waves is especially important for transparent tissues, although much attention has been recently focused also on the investigation of polarization properties of light propagating in strongly scattering media.[3,5,6,8–10,23,28,43,59–64,69,70] In scattering media, the vector nature of light waves is manifested as polarization of an initially nonpolarized light beam or as depolarization (generally, the change in the character of polarization) of an initially polarized beam propagating in a medium. Similar to coherence properties of a light beam reflected from or transmitted through a biological object, polarization parameters of light can be employed as a selector of photons coming from different depths in an object.

The problems of optical diagnosis and spectroscopy of tissues are concerned with two radiation regimes: continuous wave and time-resolved.[1,3,4,6,12,14,15,28,31,71,92] The latter is realized by means of the exposure of a scattering object to short laser pulses ($\sim 10^{-10}$ to 10^{-12} s) and the subsequent recording of scattered broadened pulses (the time-domain method), or by irradiation with modulated light, usually in the frequency range 50 MHz to 1000 MHz and recording the depth of modulation of scattered light intensity and the corresponding phase shift at modulation frequencies (the frequency-domain or phase method). The time-resolved regime is based on the excitation of the photon-density wave spectrum in a strongly scattering medium, which can be described in the framework of the nonstationary radiation transfer theory (RTT). The continuous radiation regime is described by the stationary RTT.

Many modern medical technologies employ laser radiation and fiber-optic devices.[1–7] Since the application of lasers in medicine has both fundamental and technical purposes, the problem of coherence is very important for the analysis of the interaction of light with tissues and cell ensembles. On the one hand, this problem can be considered in terms of the loss of coherence due to the scattering of light in a randomly nonuniform medium with multiple scattering, or the change in the statistics of speckle structures of the scattered field. On the other hand, this problem can be interpreted in terms of the appearance of an amplified, coherent, sharply directed component in backscattered radiation under conditions when a tissue is probed with an ultrashort laser pulse.[1,3,73,74] The coherence of light is of fundamental importance for the selection of photons that have experienced a small number of scattering events or none, as well as for the generation of speckle-modulated fields from scattering phase objects with single and multiple scattering.[1,3,75–77] Such approaches are important for coherent tomography, diffractometry, holography, photon-correlation spectroscopy, laser Doppler anemometry, and speckle interferometry of tissues and fluxes of biological fluids.[1,3,5,15,22,28,76–83] The use of optical sources with a short coherence length opens up new opportunities in coherent interferometry and tomography of tissues, organs, and blood flows.[1,3,8,17,18,77,84]

The transparency of tissues reaches its maximum in the near infrared (NIR), which is associated with the fact that living tissues do not contain strong intrinsic chromophores that would absorb radiation within this spectral range. Light penetrates into a tissue for several centimeters, which is important for the transillumination of thick human organs (brain, breast, etc.). However, tissues are characterized by strong scattering of NIR radiation, which prevents one from obtaining clear images of localized inhomogeneities arising in tissues due to various pathologies, e.g., tumor formation, a local increase in blood volume caused by a hemorrhage or the growth of microvessels. Strong scattering of NIR radiation also imposes certain requirements on the power of laser radiation, which should be sufficient to ensure the detection of attenuated fluxes. Special attention in optical tomography and spectroscopy is focused on the development of methods for the selection of image-carrying photons or detection of photons providing the information concerning the optical parameters of the scattering medium. These methods employ the results of fundamental studies devoted to the propagation of laser beams in scattering media.[1,3,4,6,15,28,31,71,92]

Another important area in which deep tissue probing is practiced is reflecting spectroscopy, e.g., optical oxymetry for the evaluation of the degree of hemoglobin oxygenation in working muscular tissue, the diseased neonatal brain, or the active brain of adults.[1,3,4]

This tutorial is primarily concerned with light-scattering techniques recently developed for quantitative studies of tissues and optical cell ensembles. It discusses the results of theoretical and experimental investigations into photon transport in tissues and describes methods for solving direct and inverse scattering problems for random media with multiple scattering and quasi-ordered media with single scattering, in order to model different types of tissue behavior. The theoretical consideration is based on stationary and nonstationary radiation transfer theories for strongly scattering tissues, the Mie theory for transparent tissues, and the numerical Monte Carlo method, which is employed for the solution of direct and inverse problems of photon transport in multilayered tissues with complicated boundary conditions.

These are general approaches extensible to the examination of a large number of abiological scattering media. It is worthwhile to note that many known methods of scattering media optics (e.g., the integrating sphere technique) were brought to perfection when used in biomedical research. Concurrently, new measuring systems and algorithms for the solution of inverse problems have been developed that are useful for scattering media optics in general. Moreover, the improvement of certain methods was undertaken only because they were needed for tissue studies; this is especially true of the diffuse photon-density waves method, which is promising for the examination of many physical systems: aqueous media, gels, foams, air, aerosols, etc.

Based on such fundamental optical phenomena as elastic and quasi-elastic (static and dynamic) scattering, diffraction, and interference of optical fields and photon density waves (intensity waves), we will discuss optical methods and instruments offering much promise for biomedical applications. Among these are spectrophotometry and polarimetry; time-domain and frequency-domain spectroscopy and imaging systems; photon-correlation spectroscopy; speckle interferometry; coherent topography and tomography; phase, confocal, and heterodyne microscopy; and partial coherence interferometry and tomography.

I am grateful to Terry Montonye, Donald O'Shea, Alexander Priezzhev, Barry Masters, and Rick Hermann for their valuable suggestions and comments on preparation of this tutorial.

I am very thankful to Andre Roggan, Lihong Wang, and Alexander Oraevsky for their valuable comments and constructive criticism of the manuscript.

I greatly appreciate the cooperation and contribution of all my colleagues, especially D. A. Zimnyakov, V. P. Ryabukho, S. S. Ul'yanov, I. L. Maksimova, V. I. Kochubey, S. R. Uts, I. V. Yaroslavsky, A. B. Pravdin, G. G. Akchurin, I. L. Kon, E. I. Zakharova, A. A. Bednov, A. A. Chaussky, S. Yu. Kuz'min, K. V. Larin, I. V. Meglinsky, A. A. Mishin, I. S. Peretochkin, and A. N. Yaroslavskaya.

I am very thankful to attendees of my short courses on biomedical optics, which I have giving during SPIE Photonics West International Symposia since 1992, for their good questions, fruitful discussions, and critical evaluations of presented materials. Their responses were very valuable for preparation of this volume. I am especially grateful to Michael DellaVecchia, Hatim Carim, Sandor Vari, M. Pais Clemente, Haishan Zeng, Leon Sapiro, and Zachary Sacks, who became my good friends and colleagues for many years.

Prolonged collaboration with the University of Pennsylvania, my fruitful discussions with Britton Chance, Shoka Nioka, Arjun Yodh, David Boas, and many others were very helpful in writing this book.

My joint chairing with Halina Podbielska, Ben Ovryn, and Joe Izatt of the SPIE Conference on Coherence Domain Optical Methods in Biomedical Science and Clinical Applications also was very helpful.

The original part of this work was supported within the program "Leading Scientific Schools" of the Russian Foundation for Basic Research (Project No. 96-15-96389), USA–Russia CRDF grant RB1-230, and ISSEP grants p97-372, p98-768, and p99-703 within the program "Soros Professors."

I would like to thank all my numerous colleagues and friends all over the world who kindly sent me reprints of their papers, which were used in this tutorial and made my work much easier, especially Y. Aizu, J. D. Briers, Z. Chen, B. Devaraj, A. F. Fercher, M. Ferrari, J. G. Fujimoto, M. J. C. van Gemert, E. Gratton, J. Greve, A. H. Hielscher, S. L. Jacques, R. G. Johnston, G. W. Kattawar, M. Keijzer, S. M. Khanna, A. Ya. Khairulllina, A. Knuettel, J. R. Lakowicz, M. W. Lindner, Q. Luo, R. L. McCally, W. P. van de Merwe, G. Mueller, F. F. M. de Mul, M. S. Patterson, B. Pierscionek, H. Rinneberg, P. Rol, W. Rudolph, B. Ruth, J. M. Schmitt, W. M. Star, R. Steiner, H. J. C. M. Sterenborg, L. O. Svaasand, J. E. Thomas, B. J. Tromberg, A. J. Welch, and J. R. Zip.

I would like to say a few words in memory of Pascal Rol, my good friend and colleague with whom I have organized many SPIE meetings. Pascal died suddenly on January 10, 2000. The reader will find many of his excellent results on scleral tissue optics in this tutorial. He has made many outstanding contributions to biomedical optics, and I will always remember him as a good scientist and friendly person.

I am very thankful to Ruth Haas, Erika Wittmann, and Sue Price for their assistance in editing and production of the book, and to S. P. Chernova and E. P. Savchenko for their help in the preparation of the figures.

Last, but not least, I express my gratitude to my wife, Natalia, and all my family for their support, understanding, and patience.

Valery Tuchin
April 2000

Preface to the Second Edition

This is the second edition of the tutorial *Tissue Optics: Light Scattering Methods and Instruments for Medical Diagnosis* first published in 2000. The last seven years, since the printing of the first edition, have seen intensive growth of research and development in tissue optics, particularly in the field of tissue diagnostics and imaging.[103–147] Further developments of light-scattering techniques for the quantitative evaluation of optical properties of normal and pathological tissues and cell ensembles have occurred. New results on theoretical and experimental investigations into light transport in tissues and methods for solving direct and inverse scattering problems for random media with multiple scattering and quasi-ordered media have been found. A few specific fields, such as optical coherence tomography (OCT)[108–111,115,116,126,127,129,130,136,142] and polarization-sensitive technologies,[129,130,135,136,138,139] which are very promising for optical medical diagnostics and imaging, have developed rapidly over the last few years. The optical clearing method, based on reversible reduction of tissue scattering due to refractive index matching of scatterers and ground matter, has also been of great interest for research and application since the last edition.[129,132,136,139,140] Further developments of Raman and vibrational spectroscopies[104,105,123,130,132,136,143] and multiphoton microscopy[114,119,122,130,132,136,137] applied to morphology and the functioning of living cells and tissues have been provided by many research groups.

This new edition of this book is conceptually the same as the first one. It is also divided into two parts: Part I describes tissue optics fundamentals and basic research, and Part II presents optical and laser instrumentation and medical applications. The author has corrected misprints, updated the references, and added some new results mostly on tissue optical properties measurements (Chapter 2) and polarized light interaction with turbid tissues (Section 1.4). Recent results on polarization imaging and spectroscopy techniques (Chapter 7), as well as on OCT developments and applications (Chapter 9) are also overviewed. Materials on controlling tissue optical properties (Chapter 5) and optothermal and optoacoustic interactions of light with tissues (Section 1.5) are updated. Brief descriptions of fluorescent, nonlinear, and inelastic light scattering spectroscopies are provided in Chapter 1.

I am grateful to Sharon Streams for her suggestion to prepare the second edition of the tutorial and for her assistance in editing of the book. I also would like to thank Merry Schnell for her assistance on the final stage of book editing and production.

I am very thankful to attendees of my short courses "Coherence, Light Scattering, and Polarization Methods and Instruments for Medical Diagnosis," "Tissue Optics and Spectroscopy," "Tissue Optics and Controlling of Tissue Optical Properties," and "Optical Clearing of Tissues and Blood," which I have given during

SPIE Photonics West Symposia, SPIE/OSA European Conferences on Biomedical Optics, and OSA CLEO/QELS Conferences over last seven years, for their stimulating questions, fruitful discussions, and critical evaluations of presented materials. Their responses were very valuable for preparation of this edition. My joint chairing with Joseph A. Izatt and James G. Fujimoto of the SPIE Conference on Coherence Domain Optical Methods and Optical Coherence Tomography in Biomedicine also was very helpful.

The original part of this work was supported within the Russian and international research programs by grant N25.2003.2 of President of Russian Federation "Supporting of Scientific Schools," grant N2.11.03 "Leading Research-Educational Teams," contract No. 40.018.1.1.1314 "Biophotonics" of the Ministry of Industry, Science and Technologies of RF, grant REC-006 of CRDF (U.S. Civilian Research and Development Foundation for the Independent States of the Former Soviet Union) and the Russian Ministry of Education, the Royal Society grants for a joint projects between Cranfield University (UK) and Saratov State University, grants of National Natural Science Foundation of China (NSFC), grant of Federal Agency of Education of RF No. 1.4.06, RNP.2.1.1.4473, CRDF grants BRHE RUXO-006-SR-06 and RUB1-570-SA-04, and by Palomar Medical Technologies Inc., MA, USA.

I greatly appreciate the cooperation, contributions, and support of all my colleagues from Optics and Biomedical Physics Division of Physics Department and Research-Educational Institute of Optics and Biophotonics of Saratov State University, especially A. N. Bashkatov, I. V. Fedosov, E. I. Galanzha, E. A. Genina, I. L. Maksimova, I. V. Meglinski, V. I. Kochubey, V. P. Ryabukho, A. B. Pravdin, G. V. Simonenko, Yu. P. Sinichkin, S. S. Ul'yanov, D. A. Yakovlev, and D. A. Zimnyakov.

I would like to thank all my numerous colleagues and friends all over the world for collaboration and sending materials which were used in this tutorial and made my work much easier, especially P. E. Andersen, J. F. de Boer, Z. Chen, P. M. W. French, J. G. Fujimoto, V. M. Gelikonov, P. Gupta, C. K. Hitzenberger, J. A. Izatt, S. L. Jacques, A. Kishen, S. J. Kirkpatrick, A. Knüttel, J. R. Lakowicz, K. V. Larin, G. W. Lucassen, Q. Luo, B. R. Masters, K. Meek, G. Mueller, F. F. M. de Mul, L. T. Perelman, A. Podoleanu, A. V. Priezzhev, F. Reil, J. Rodriguez, H. Schneckenburger, A. M. Sergeev, A. N. Serov, N. M. Shakhova, B. J. Tromberg, L. V. Wang, R. K. Wang, A. J. Welch, A. N. Yaroslavskaya, I. V. Yaroslavsky, P. Zhakharov, and V. P. Zharov, R. Myllylä, S. A. Boppart, M. Meinke, A. Mahadevan-Jansen, T. Troy, L. Oliveira, M. Pais Clemente, and X. H. Hu.

I express my gratitude to my wife, Natalia, and all my family, especially to my daughter, Nastya, and grandchildren, Dasha, Zhenya, and Stepa, for their indispensable support, understanding, and patience during my writing this book.

Valery Tuchin
June 2007

Part I
An Introduction to Tissue Optics

1

Optical Properties of Tissues with Strong (Multiple) Scattering

This first chapter introduces the problem of light (laser beams) transport within strongly (multiple) scattering tissues such as skin, breast, brain, and vessel walls. Basic principles and theoretical descriptions using radiation transfer theory or Monte Carlo (MC) simulation are considered. The propagation of short pulses and photon-density diffusion waves in scattering and absorbing media is analyzed, and the prospects of these methods for tissue spectroscopy and tomography are discussed. Tissue structure and anisotropy, polarization phenomena, optothermal, optoacoustic, and acoustooptical interactions in strongly scattering tissues are described. A discrete-particle model of soft tissue is presented. Fluorescence and inelastic light scattering, including multiphoton fluorescence and vibrational and Raman spectroscopies, are discussed. The design and characterization of tissuelike phantoms for optical diagnostics and light dosimetry are described.

1.1 Propagation of continuous-wave light in tissues

1.1.1 Basic principles, and major scatterers and absorbers

Biological tissues are optically inhomogeneous and absorbing media whose average refractive index is higher than that of air. This is responsible for partial reflection of the radiation at the tissue/air interface (Fresnel reflection), while the remaining part penetrates the tissue. Multiple scattering and absorption are responsible for laser beam broadening and eventual decay as it travels through a tissue, whereas bulk scattering is a major cause of the dispersion of a large fraction of radiation in the backward direction. Therefore, light propagation within a tissue depends on the scattering and absorption properties of its components: cells, cell organelles, and various fiber structures.[1–3,15,129,130,134,138] The size, shape, and density of these structures; their refractive index relative to the tissue ground substance; and the polarization states of the incident light all play important roles in the propagation of light in tissues.[1–3,15,129,130,134,138,145–153]

In view of the great diversity and structural complexity of tissues, the development of adequate optical models that account for the scatter and absorption of light is often the most complex step of a study. Two approaches are currently used for tissue modeling. In the framework of the first one, tissue is modeled as a medium with a continuous random spatial distribution of optical parameters;[3,129,154,155] the second one considers tissue as a discrete ensemble of scatterers.[1–3,15,129,130,134,138,156]

The choice of the approach is dictated by both the structural specificity of the tissue under study and the kind of light scattering characteristics that are to be obtained.

Most tissues are composed of structures with a wide range of sizes, and most can be described as a random continuum of inhomogeneities of the refractive index with a varying spatial scale.[154,155] Phase contrast microscopy has been used in particular to show that the structure of the refraction index inhomogeneities in mammalian tissues is similar to the structure of frozen turbulence in a number of cases.[154] This fact is of fundamental importance for understanding the peculiarities of light propagation in tissue, and it may be a key to the solution of the inverse problem of tissue structure reconstruction. This approach is applicable for tissues with no pronounced boundaries between elements that feature significant heterogeneity. The process of scattering in these structures may be described under certain conditions using the model of a phase screen.[75,136,155,157]

The second approach to tissue modeling is its representation as a system of discrete scattering particles. In particular, this model has been advantageously used to describe the angular dependence of the polarization characteristics of scattered radiation.[145,146,148,150,158] Blood is the most important biological example of a disperse system that entirely corresponds to the model of discrete particles.[48,101,159]

Biological media are often modeled as ensembles of homogeneous spherical particles, since many cells and microorganisms, particularly blood cells, are close in shape to spheres or ellipsoids. A system of noninteracting spherical particles is the simplest tissue model. Mie theory rigorously describes the diffraction of light in a spherical particle.[148,160] The development of this model involves taking into account the structures of the spherical particles, namely, the multilayered spheres and the spheres with radial nonhomogeneity, anisotropy, and optical activity.[145,146]

Because connective tissue consists of fiber structures, a system of long cylinders is the most appropriate model for it. Muscular tissue, skin dermis, *dura mater*, eye cornea, and sclera belong to this type of tissue formed essentially by collagen fibrils. The solution of the problem of light diffraction in a single homogeneous or multilayered cylinder is also well understood.[148]

The sizes of cells and tissue structure elements vary in size from a few tenths of nanometers to hundreds of micrometers.[47,58,94–96,129,130,135,138,149–153,161–180] Blood cells (erythrocytes, leukocytes, and platelets) exhibit the following parameters. A normal erythrocyte in plasma has the shape of a concave-concave disk with a diameter varying from 7.1 to 9.2 μm, a thickness of 0.9–1.2 μm in the center and 1.7–2.4 μm on the periphery, and a volume of 90 μm^3. Leukocytes are formed like spheres with a diameter of 8–22 μm. Platelets in the bloodstream are biconvex disklike particles with diameters ranging from 2 to 4 μm. Normally, blood has about 10 times as many erythrocytes as platelets and about 30 times as many platelets as leukocytes.

Most other mammalian cells have diameters in the range of 5–75 μm. In the epidermal layer, the cells are large (with an average cross-sectional area of about 80 μm^2) and quite uniform in size. Fat cells, each containing a single lipid droplet that nearly fills the entire cell and therefore results in eccentric placement of the cytoplasm and nucleus, have a wide range of diameters, from a few microns to 50–75 μm. Fat cells may reach diameters of 100–200 μm in pathological cases.

There are a wide variety of structures within cells that determine tissue light scattering (see Fig. 1.1). Cell nuclei are on the order of 5–10 μm in diameter; mitochondria, lysosomes, and peroxisomes have dimensions of 1–2 μm; ribosomes are on the order of 20 nm in diameter; and structures within various organelles can have dimensions of up to a few hundred nanometers. Usually, the scatterers in cells are not spherical. The models of prolate ellipsoids with a ratio of the ellipsoid axes between 2 and 10 are more typical.

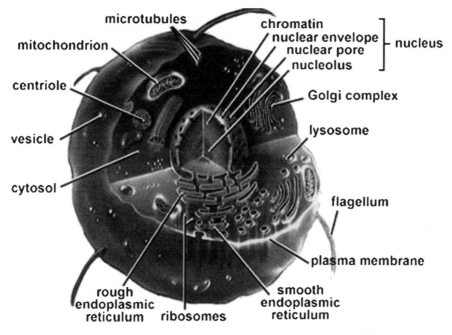

Figure 1.1 Major organelles and inclusions of the cell.[129]

The hollow organs of the body are lined with a thin, highly cellular surface layer of epithelial tissue, which is supported by underlying, relatively acellular connective tissue. In healthy tissues, the epithelium often consists of a single well-organized layer of cells with en face diameter of 10–20 μm and height of 25 μm (see Fig. 1.2). In dysplastic epithelium, cells proliferate and their nuclei enlarge and appear darker (hyperchromatic) when stained.[150] Enlarged nuclei are primary indicators of cancer, dysplasia, and cell regeneration in most human tissues.

In fibrous tissues or tissues containing fiber layers (cornea, sclera, *dura mater*, muscle, myocardium, tendon, cartilage, vessel wall, retinal nerve fiber layer, etc.) and composed mostly of microfibrils and/or microtubules, typical diameters of the cylindrical structural elements are 10–400 nm. Their length is in a range from 10–25 μm to a few millimeters.

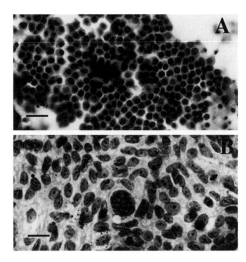

Figure 1.2 Microphotograph of the isolated normal intestinal epithelial cells (a) and intestinal malignant cell line T84 (b). Note the uniform nuclear size distribution of the normal epithelial cell (a) in contrast to the T84 malignant cell line, which at the same magnification shows larger nuclei and more variation in nuclear size (b). Solid bars equal 20 μm in each panel (from Ref. 150 © 1999 IEEE).

The dominant scatterers in an artery may be the fibers, cells, or subcellular organelles. Muscular arteries have three main layers. The inner intimal layer consists of endothelial cells with a mean diameter of less than 10 μm. The medial layer consists mostly of closely packed smooth muscle cells with a mean diameter of 15–20 μm; small amounts of connective tissue, including elastin, collagenous, and reticular fibers, as well as a few fibroblasts, are also located in the medial. The outer adventitial layer consists of dense fibrous connective tissue that is largely made up of 1- to 12-μm-diameter collagen fibers and thinner, 2- to 3-μm-diameter elastin fibers.

Another two examples of complex scattering structures are the myocardium and the retinal nerve fiber layer. The myocardium consists mostly of cardiac muscle, which is comprised of myofibrils (about 1 μm in diameter) that in turn consist of cylindrical myofilaments (6–15 nm in diameter) and aspherical mitochondria (1–2 μm in diameter). The retinal nerve fiber layer comprises bundles of unmyelinated axons that run across the surface of the retina. The cylindrical organelles of the retinal nerve fiber layer are axonal membranes, microtubules, neurofilaments, and mitochondria. Axonal membranes, like all cell membranes, are thin (6–10 nm) phospholipid bilayers that form cylindrical shells enclosing the axonal cytoplasm. Axonal microtubules are long tubular polymers of the protein tubulin with an outer diameter of ≈25 nm, an inner diameter ≈15 nm, and a length of 10–25 μm. Neurofilaments are stable protein polymers with a diameter ≈10 nm. Mitochondria are ellipsoidal organelles that contain densely involved membranes of lipid and protein. They are 0.1–0.2 μm thick and 1–2 μm long.

For some tissues, the size distribution of the scattering particles may be essentially monodispersive, and for others it may be quite broad. Two opposing examples are a transparent eye cornea stroma, which has a sharply monodispersive distribution, and a turbid eye sclera, which has a rather broad distribution of collagen fiber diameters.[129,130] There is no universal distribution size function that would describe all tissues with equal adequacy. In optics of dispersed systems, Gaussian, gamma, or power size distributions are typical.[171] Polydispersion for randomly distributed scatterers can be accounted for by using the gamma-distribution or the skewed logarithmic distribution of scatterers' diameters, cross sections, or volumes.[61,129,154,156,165,172] In particular, for turbid tissues such as eye sclera, the gamma radii distribution function is applicable.[61,172]

Absorbed light is converted to heat or radiated in the form of fluorescence; it is also consumed in photobiochemical reactions. The absorption spectrum depends on the type of predominant absorption centers and water content of tissues (see Figs. 1.3–1.7). Absolute values of absorption coefficients for typical tissues lie in the range 10^{-2} to 10^4 cm^{-1}.[1–4,6,9–15,28,29,31,37–42,56,57,72,86–91] In the ultraviolet (UV) and infrared (IR) ($\lambda \geq 2000$ nm) spectral regions, light is readily absorbed, which accounts for the small contribution of scattering and the inability of radiation to penetrate deep into tissues (only through one or two cell layers). Short-wave visible light penetrates typical tissues as deep as 0.5–2.5 mm, whereupon it undergoes an e-fold decrease of intensity. In this case, both scattering and absorption occur, with 15–40% of the incident radiation being reflected. In the 600–1600-nm wavelength range, scattering prevails over absorption, and light penetrates to a depth of 8–10 mm. Simultaneously, the intensity of the reflected radiation increases to 35–70% of the total incident light (due to backscattering).

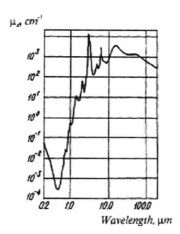

Figure 1.3 The absorption spectrum of water.[56]

Light interaction with a multilayer and multicomponent skin is a very complicated process.[57] The horny-skin layer (stratum corneum) reflects about 5–7% of the incident light. A collimated light beam is transformed to a diffuse one by microscopic inhomogeneities at the air/horny-layer interface. A major part of reflected light results from backscattering in different skin layers (stratum corneum,

Molar extinction coefficient, x10^5, *L mol*$^{-1}$ *cm*$^{-1}$

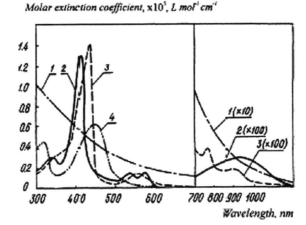

Wavelength, nm

Figure 1.4 Molar attenuation spectra for solutions of major visible light-absorbing human skin pigments: 1, DOPA-melanin (H_2O); 2, oxyhemoglobin (H_2O); 3, hemoglobin (H_2O); 4, bilirubin ($CHCl_3$).[57]

Transmission, %

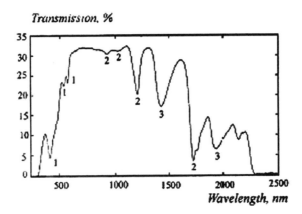

Wavelength, nm

Figure 1.5 The transmittance spectrum of a 3-mm-thick slab of female breast tissue. A spectrometer with an integrating sphere was used. The contributions of absorption bands of the tissue components are marked: 1, hemoglobin; 2, fat; and 3, water.[50]

epidermis, dermis, blood, and fat). The absorption of diffuse light by skin pigments is a measure of bilirubin content, hemoglobin concentration, and its saturation with oxygen, and the concentration of pharmaceutical products in blood and tissues; these characteristics are widely used in the diagnosis of various diseases (see Fig. 1.4). Certain phototherapeutic and diagnostic modalities take advantage of ready transdermal penetration of visible and near-infrared (NIR) light inside the body in the wavelength region, corresponding to the therapeutic or diagnostic window (600–1600 nm) (Fig. 1.7).

Another example of heterogeneous multicomponent tissue is a female breast (which is principally composed of adipose and fibrous tissues). The absorption bands of hemoglobin, fat, and water are clearly seen *in vitro* in the measured spec-

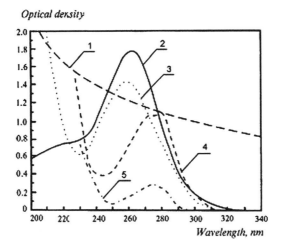

Figure 1.6 UV absorption spectra of major chromophores of human skin: 1, DOPA-melanin, 1.5 mg % in H_2O; 2, urocanic acid, 10^4 M in H_2O; 3, DNA, calf thymus, 10 mg % in H_2O (pH = 4.5); 4, tryptophane, 2×10^4 M (pH = 7); 5, tyrosine, 2×10^4 M (pH = 7).[57]

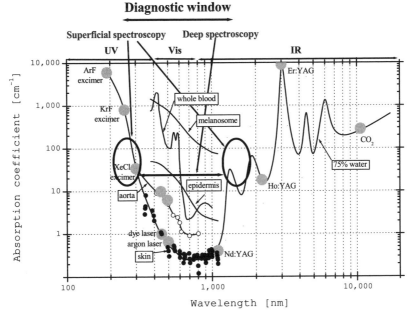

Figure 1.7 Absorption spectra of skin and aorta; spectra of tissue components—water (75%), epidermis, melanosome, and whole blood are also presented; diagnostic lasers and their wavelengths as well as diagnostic/therapeutic window and wavelength ranges suitable for superficial and deep spectroscopy are shown (adapted from Ref. 36).

trum of a 3-mm slab of breast tissue presented in Fig. 1.5.[50] Measurement was done using the integrating sphere spectrometer. There is a wide window between

700 and 1100 nm, and narrow ones at about 1300 and 1600 nm, where the lowest percentage of light is attenuated.

Solid tissues such as ribs and the skull, as well as whole blood, are also easily penetrable by visible and NIR light.[1–4,6,9–16,36,91,129,130] The relatively good transparency of skin for long-wave UV light (UVA) depends on DNA, tryptophane, tyrosine, urocanic acid, and melanin absorption spectra and underlies selected methods of photochemotherapy of skin tissues using UVA irradiation (see Fig. 1.4).[3,6,10,57,86,129,130]

A collimated (laser) beam is attenuated in a thin tissue layer of thickness d in accordance with the Bouguer-Beer-Lambert exponential law as[37]

$$I(d) = (1 - R_F)I_0 \exp(-\mu_t d), \tag{1.1}$$

where $I(d)$ is the intensity of transmitted light measured using a distant photodetector with a small aperture (on-line or collimated transmittance), W/cm^2; R_F is the coefficient of Fresnel reflection; at the normal beam incidence, $R_F = [(n-1)/(n+1)]^2$; n is the relative mean refractive index of tissue and surrounding media; I_0 is the incident light intensity, W/cm^2;

$$\mu_t = \mu_a + \mu_s \tag{1.2}$$

is the extinction coefficient (interaction or total attenuation coefficient), 1/cm, where μ_a is the absorption coefficient, 1/cm, and μ_s is the scattering coefficient, 1/cm. Strictly speaking, Eq. (1.1) is valid only for a highly absorbing media, when $\mu_a \gg \mu_s$.

The extinction coefficient is connected with the extinction cross section σ_{ext} as

$$\mu_t = \rho_s \sigma_{ext}, \tag{1.3}$$

where ρ_s is the density of particles (tissue and cell compounds). For a system of particles with absorption,

$$\sigma_{ext} = \sigma_{sca} + \sigma_{abs}, \tag{1.4}$$

and

$$\mu_s = \rho_s \sigma_{sca}, \quad \mu_a = \rho_s \sigma_{abs}. \tag{1.5}$$

The average scattering cross section per particle can be presented in a form suitable for experimental evaluations:[148]

$$\sigma_{sca} = \left(\frac{\lambda^2}{2\pi}\right)\left(\frac{1}{I_0}\right)\int_0^\pi I(\theta)\sin\theta d\theta, \tag{1.6}$$

where I_0 is the intensity of the incident light, $I(\theta)$ is the angular distribution of the scattered light by a particle, and θ is the scattering angle. For macroscopically isotropic and symmetric media, the average scattering cross section is independent of the direction and polarization of the incident light. The average extinction, σ_{ext}, and absorption, σ_{abs}, cross sections are also independent of the direction and polarization state of the incident light.

The probability that a photon incident on a small volume element will survive is equal to the ratio of the scattering and extinction cross sections, and is called the "albedo" for single scattering, Λ:

$$\Lambda = \frac{\sigma_{sca}}{\sigma_{ext}} = \frac{\mu_s}{\mu_t}. \tag{1.7}$$

The albedo ranges from zero for a completely absorbing medium to unity for a completely scattering medium.

The mean free path length (MFP) between two interactions is denoted by

$$l_{ph} = \mu_t^{-1}. \tag{1.8}$$

1.1.2 Theoretical description

To analyze light propagation under multiple scattering conditions, it is assumed that absorbing and scattering centers are uniformly distributed across the tissue. UV-A, visible, or NIR radiation is normally subject to anisotropic scattering characterized by a clearly apparent direction of photons undergoing single scattering, which may be due to the presence of large cellular organelles [mitochondria, lysosomes, and inner membranes (Golgi apparatus)].[3,58,85,95,96,129,130,135,150–153]

When the scattering medium is illuminated by unpolarized light and/or only the intensity of multiply scattered light needs to be computed, a sufficiently strict mathematical description of continuous wave (CW) light propagation in a medium is possible in the framework of the scalar stationary radiation transfer theory (RTT).[1,3,6,12–16,129,130,135,136,145,146,181–197]

This theory is valid for an ensemble of scatterers located far from one another and has been successfully used to work out some practical aspects of tissue optics. The main stationary equation of RTT for monochromatic light has the form[1]

$$\frac{\partial I(\bar{r}, \bar{s})}{\partial s} = -\mu_t I(\bar{r}, \bar{s}) + \frac{\mu_s}{4\pi} \int_{4\pi} I(\bar{r}, \bar{s}')p(\bar{s}, \bar{s}')d\Omega', \tag{1.9}$$

where $I(\bar{r}, \bar{s})$ is the radiance (or specific intensity)—average power flux density at point $\bar{r}$ in the given direction $\bar{s}$, W/cm^2 sr; $p(\bar{s}, \bar{s}')$ is the scattering phase function, 1/sr; and $d\Omega'$ is the unit solid angle about the direction $\bar{s}'$, sr. It is assumed that there are no radiation sources inside the medium.

The scalar approximation of the radiative transfer equation (RTE) gives poor accuracy when the size of the scattering particles is much smaller than the wavelength, but provides acceptable results for particles comparable to and larger than the wavelength.[146,184] There is ample literature on the analytical and numerical solutions of the scalar radiative transfer equation.[1,3,15,129,130,184–197]

If radiative transport is examined in a domain $G \subset R^3$, and ∂G is the domain boundary surface, then the boundary conditions for ∂G can be written in the following general form:

$$I(\bar{r}, \bar{s})\big|_{(\bar{s}\bar{N})<0} = S(\bar{r}, \bar{s}) + \hat{R} I(\bar{r}, \bar{s})\big|_{(\bar{s}\bar{N})>0},\qquad(1.10)$$

where $\bar{r} \in \partial G$, $\bar{N}$ is the outside normal vector to ∂G, $S(\bar{r}, \bar{s})$ is the incident light distribution at ∂G, and $\hat{R}$ is the reflection operator. When both absorption and reflection surfaces are present in the domain G, conditions analogous to Eq. (1.10) must be given at each surface.

For practical purposes, integrals of the function $I(\bar{r}, \bar{s})$ over certain phase space regions $(\bar{r}, \bar{s})$ are of greater value than the function itself. Specifically, optical probes of tissues frequently measure the outgoing light distribution function at the medium surface, which is characterized by the radiant flux density or irradiance (W/cm^2):

$$F(\bar{r}) = \int_{(\bar{s}\bar{N})>0} I(\bar{r}, \bar{s})(\bar{s}\bar{N})d\Omega,\qquad(1.11)$$

where $\bar{r} \in \partial G$.

In problems of optical radiation dosimetry in tissues, the measured quantity is actually the total radiant-energy-fluence rate $U(\bar{r})$. It is the sum of the radiance over all angles at a point $\bar{r}$ and is measured by watts per square centimeter:

$$U(\bar{r}) = \int_{4\pi} I(\bar{r}, \bar{s})d\Omega.\qquad(1.12)$$

The phase function $p(\bar{s}, \bar{s}')$ describes the scattering properties of the medium and is in fact the probability density function for scattering in the direction $\bar{s}'$ of a photon traveling in the direction $\bar{s}$; in other words, it characterizes an elementary scattering act. If scattering is symmetric relative to the direction of the incident wave, then the phase function depends only on the scattering angle θ (angle between directions $\bar{s}$ and $\bar{s}'$), i.e.,

$$p(\bar{s}, \bar{s}') = p(\theta).\qquad(1.13)$$

The assumption of random distribution of scatterers in a medium (i.e., the absence of spatial correlation in the tissue structure) leads to normalization:

$$\int_0^\pi p(\theta)2\pi \sin\theta d\theta = 1.\qquad(1.14)$$

In practice, the phase function is usually well approximated with the aid of the postulated Henyey-Greenstein function:[1,3,12–16,70,129,130,164]

$$p(\theta) = \frac{1}{4\pi}\frac{1-g^2}{(1+g^2-2g\cos\theta)^{3/2}},\qquad(1.15)$$

where g is the scattering anisotropy parameter (mean cosine of the scattering angle θ):

$$g \equiv \langle \cos \theta \rangle = \int_0^\pi p(\theta) \cos \theta \cdot 2\pi \sin \theta d\theta. \tag{1.16}$$

The value of g varies in the range from -1 to 1:[145,146] $g = 0$ corresponds to isotropic (Rayleigh) scattering, $g = 1$ to total forward scattering (Mie scattering at large particles), and $g = -1$ to total backward scattering.

The integrodifferential Eq. (1.9) is too complicated to be employed for the analysis of light propagation in scattering media. Therefore, it is frequently simplified by representing the solution in the form of spherical harmonics. Such simplification leads to a system of $(N + 1)^2$ connected differential partial derivative equations known as the P_N approximation. This system is reducible to a single differential equation of order $(N + 1)$. For example, four connected differential equations reducible to a single diffusion-type equation are necessary for $N = 1$.[191-197] It has the following form for an isotropic medium:

$$(\nabla^2 - \mu_{\text{eff}}^2)U(\bar{r}) = -Q(\bar{r}), \tag{1.17}$$

where

$$\mu_{\text{eff}} = [3\mu_a(\mu_s' + \mu_a)]^{1/2} \tag{1.18}$$

is the effective attenuation coefficient or inverse diffusion length, $\mu_{\text{eff}} = 1/l_d$, $1/\text{cm}$;

$$Q(\bar{r}) = (cD)^{-1}q(\bar{r}), \tag{1.19}$$

where $q(\bar{r})$ is the source function (i.e., the number of photons injected into the unit volume), and

$$D = \frac{1}{3(\mu_s' + \mu_a)} \tag{1.20}$$

is the photon diffusion coefficient, cm^2/c;

$$\mu_s' = (1 - g)\mu_s \tag{1.21}$$

is the reduced (transport) scattering coefficient, $1/\text{cm}$, and c is the velocity of light in the medium. The transport mean free path of a photon (cm) is defined as

$$l_t = (1/\mu_t') = (\mu_a + \mu_s')^{-1}, \tag{1.22}$$

where $\mu_t' = \mu_a + \mu_s'$ is the transport coefficient.

It is worthwhile to note that the transport mean free path (MFP) in a medium with anisotropic single scattering significantly exceeds the MFP in a medium with isotropic single scattering, $l_t \gg l_{ph}$ [see Eq. (1.8)]. The transport MFP l_t is the distance over which the photon loses its initial direction.

Diffusion theory provides a good approximation in the case of a small scattering anisotropy factor $g \leq 0.1$ and large albedo $\Lambda \to 1$. For many tissues, $g \approx 0.6\text{--}0.9$, and can be as large as $0.990\text{--}0.999$, for example, for blood.[48,49,87,129] This significantly restricts the applicability of the diffusion approximation. It is argued that this approximation can be used at $g < 0.9$, when the optical thickness τ of an object is of the order 10–20:

$$\tau = \int_0^d \mu_t ds, \tag{1.23}$$

where d is the tissue depth (thickness) in the direction s.

However, the diffusion approximation is inapplicable for beam input near the object's surface where single or low-step scattering prevails. When a narrow light beam is normally incident upon a semi-infinite turbid medium with anisotropic scattering, it can be considered as converted into an isotropic point source at the depth of one transport MFP l_t [Eq. (1.22)] below the surface. The strength of this point source is the original source strength multiplied by the transport albedo[193]

$$\Lambda' = \frac{\mu_s'}{\mu_a + \mu_s'}. \tag{1.24}$$

It was confirmed that diffusion theory is accurate for describing photon migration in infinite, homogeneous, turbid media.[34,46,51,93,191,198–206] However, another procedure of diffusion equation derivation, described in Refs. 34, 51, and 191, in spite of leading to the basic Eq. (1.20) gives a more general expression for the photon diffusion coefficient:

$$D = \frac{1}{3(\mu_s' + \bar{a}\mu_a)}, \tag{1.25}$$

where $\bar{a}$ is the numerical coefficient depending on the form of the diffusion equation (on the scattering anisotropy factor).

Systematic approximation schemes lead to recommendations[34,51,191] of $\bar{a} = 0, 1/5, 1/3, 1$. Any of these $\bar{a}$ values gives significantly better agreement with random-walk simulations than the diffusion equation at $\bar{a} = 0$, with $\bar{a} = 1/3$ being slightly better than the two others.[191] Because values $\bar{a} = 1/5$ and $\bar{a} = 1$ lead to the wrong pulse-front propagation speeds, and only the intermediate value $\bar{a} = 1/3$ gives the correct speed, the photon-diffusion coefficient should be taken in the form[191]

$$D \cong \frac{1}{3\mu_s' + \mu_a}. \tag{1.26}$$

This expression in general gives a better agreement between the diffusion equation and RTE, but in practice it is useful only for highly absorbing tissues or tissue components, when $\mu_a/\mu'_s > 0.01$.[199]

For accurate use of diffusion theory, one must accurately convert the narrow light beam into isotropic photon sources that must be sufficiently deep in the medium comparable with photon-transport length l_t; and the absorption coefficient μ_a should be much less than the reduced scattering coefficient μ'_s.[198]

Measurement of diffusely reflected light is often used to infer bulk tissue optical properties for the aims of tissue spectroscopy and imaging. To provide such measurements, an adequate calculating algorithm should be derived. The diffusion equation solved subject to boundary conditions at the interfaces is one of the bases for the calculation algorithm.[46,93,204–206] These boundary conditions are derived by considering Fresnel's laws of reflection and balancing the fluence rate and photon current crossing the interface. For the source term modeled as a point scattering source at a depth of one transport MFP, l_t, and extrapolated boundary approach satisfying the boundary condition, the spatially resolved steady-state reflectance per incident photon $R(r_{sd})$ is expressed as[205,206]

$$
R(r_{sd}) = \frac{F_U}{4\pi}\left[l_t\left(\mu_{eff} + \frac{1}{r_1}\right)\frac{\exp(-\mu_{eff}r_1)}{r_1^2}\right.
$$
$$
\left. + (l_t + 2z_b)\left(\mu_{eff} + \frac{1}{r_2}\right)\frac{\exp(-\mu_{eff}r_2)}{r_2^2}\right]
$$
$$
+ \frac{F_F}{4\pi D}\left[\frac{\exp(-\mu_{eff}r_1)}{r_1} - \frac{\exp(-\mu_{eff}r_2)}{r_2}\right], \qquad (1.27)
$$

where r_{sd} is the distance between light source and detector at the tissue surface (source-detector separation), cm; $r_1 = \sqrt{l_t^2 + r_{sd}^2}$; $r_2 = \sqrt{(l_t + 2z_b)^2 + r_{sd}^2}$; $z_b = 2AD$ is the distance to the extrapolated boundary; $A = (1 + R_{eff})/(1 - R_{eff})$; R_{eff} is the effective reflection coefficient, which can be found by integrating the Fresnel reflection coefficient over all incident angles;[204] and D is the diffusion coefficient [see Eq. (1.26)]. The parameters F_U and F_F represent the fractions of the fluence rate and the flux that exit the tissue across the interface. These values are obtained by integration of the radiance over the backward hemisphere[205] and depend on a refractive index mismatch on the boundary.[206]

Some limitations of the diffusion theory, in particular connected with bad description of the fluence rate if one gets to the source, can be gotten over when it is modified on the basis of accurate but simple Grosjean's equation, which describes the light distribution in infinite isotropically scattering turbid media.[201] A new diffusion approximation to the RTE for a scattering medium with a spatially varying refractive index is derived in Ref. 203.

Now, let us briefly review other solutions of the transport equation. The first-order solution is realized for optically thin and weakly scattering media

$(\tau < 1, \Lambda < 0.5)$, when the intensity of a transmitting (coherent) wave is described by Eq. (1.1) or a similar expression:[192]

$$I(s) = (1 - R_F)I_0 \exp(-\tau), \qquad (1.28)$$

where the incident intensity I_0 (W/cm^2) is defined by the incident radiant-flux density or irradiance [see Eq. (1.11)] F_0 and a solid angle delta function pointed in the direction $\overline{\Omega}_0$: $I_0 = F_0 \delta(\overline{\Omega} - \overline{\Omega}_0)$.

Given a narrow beam (e.g., a laser), this approximation may be applied to denser tissues $(\tau > 1, \Lambda < 0.9)$. However, certain tissues have $\Lambda \approx 1$ in the therapeutic/diagnostic window wavelength range, which makes the first-order approximation inapplicable even at $\tau \ll 1$.

A more strict solution of the transport equation is possible by the discrete ordinates method (multiflux theory) in which Eq. (1.9) is converted into a matrix differential equation for illumination along many discrete directions (angles).[183] The solution approximates an exact one as the number of angles increases. It was shown above that the fluence rate can be expanded in powers of spherical harmonics, separating the transport equation into components for spherical harmonics. This approach also leads to an exact solution, provided the number of spherical harmonics is sufficiently large. For example, a study of tissues made use of up to 150 spherical harmonics,[207] and the resulting equations were solved by the finite-difference method.[208] However, this approach requires tiresome calculations if a sufficiently exact solution is to be obtained. Moreover, it is hardly suitable for δ-shaped phase scattering functions.[212]

The P3-approximation is an approximate solution to the RTE [see Eq. (1.9)], which expresses the radiance algebraically in a truncated series of Legendre polynomials. Star was the first to use the advances in computer power to compare the P3-approximation to Monte Carlo calculations in a slab geometry.[209,210] The further development of the P3-approximation for a spherical geometry that is more practical for application in tissue study is described in Ref. 211.

Tissue optics extensively employs simpler methods for the solution of transport equations, e.g., the two-flux Kubelka-Munk theory[212] or three-, four-, and seven-flux models.[56,183,192] Such representations are natural and very fruitful for laser tissue probing. Specifically, the four-flux model[213] is actually two diffuse fluxes traveling to meet each other (Kubelka-Munk model) and two collimated laser beams, the incident one and the one reflected from the rear boundary of the sample. The seven-flux model is the simplest three-dimensional representation of scattered radiation and an incident laser beam in a semi-infinite medium.[56] Of course, the simplicity and the possibility of expeditious calculation of the radiation dose or rapid determination of tissue optical parameters (solution of the inverse scattering problem) is achieved at the expense of accuracy.

1.1.3 Monte Carlo simulation techniques

The development of new methods for the solving forward and inverse radiation transfer problems in media with arbitrary configurations and boundary conditions is crucial for the reliable layer-by-layer measurements of laser radiation inside tissues and is necessary for practical purposes such as diffuse optical tomography and the spectroscopy of biological objects. The Monte Carlo (MC) method appears to be especially promising in this context, being widely used for the numerical solution of the RTT equation in different fields of knowledge (astrophysics, atmosphere and ocean optics, etc.).[214] It has recently been applied to tissue optics.[1–3,12–16,29,33,41,198,213,215–247] The method is based on the numerical simulation of photon transport in scattering media. Random migrations of photons inside a sample can be traced from their input until absorption or output. Known algorithms allow a few tissue layers with different optical properties to be characterized along with the final incident beam size and the reflection of light at interfaces. Typical examples of multilayer tissues are skin, vascular tissue, urinary bladder, and uterine walls.

For all its high accuracy and universal applicability, the MC method has one major drawback, which is that it consumes too much computation time needed to trace a large number of photons to get an acceptable variance due to the statistical nature of modeling. The MC simulations are especially computationally expensive when the absorption coefficient is much less than the scattering coefficient of the media, in which photons may propagate over a long distance before being absorbed.

Depending on the problem to be solved, the MC technique is used to either simulate the diffuse reflectance or transmittance for one wavelength or for a whole spectrum; other optical characteristics at various experimental geometries also can be modeled.[1–3,12–16,29,33,41,198,213,215–247] Because the implicit photon capturing technique is used during the MC simulation, a photon packet with an initial weight of unity is launched perpendicularly to the tissue surface along the direction of the light beam for the problem of pencil beam propagation, and isotropically for the problem of light distribution of an isotropic light source inserted into a tissue. Other geometries are also possible. Then, a step size is chosen statistically using the expression[198]

$$l = \frac{-\ln(\xi)}{\mu_a + \mu_s}, \qquad (1.29)$$

where ξ is a random number equidistributed between 0 and 1 ($0 < \xi \leq 1$). Because of absorption in the system, the photon packet loses some of its weight at the end of each step. The amount of weight lost is the photon weight at the beginning of the step multiplied by $(1 - \Lambda)$, where Λ is the albedo [see Eq. (1.7)]. The photon with the remaining weight is scattered. A new photon direction is statistically determined by a phase function [see Eq. (1.13)], which according to the scattering anisotropy factor g can be taken in the form of the Henyey-Greenstein postulated function [see Eq. (1.15)]. A new step size is then generated by Eq. (1.29), and the process is repeated. When the photon does try to leave the medium, the probability of an internal reflection is calculated using Fresnel's equation.[204,230] When the photon weight is less than a preset threshold (usually 10^{-4}), a form of "Russian roulette" is used to determine whether the photon should be terminated or propagated further with an increased weight. If the photon packet crosses the surface boundary into the ambient medium, the photon weight contributes to the diffuse reflectance or transmittance. If a reflection occurs, then the photon packet is reflected back into the medium the appropriate distance and migration continues. Otherwise, the migration of that particular photon packet halts and a new photon is launched into the medium at the predefined source location. Multiple photon packets are used to obtain statistically meaningful results; at present 1–10 million photon packets are usually used. For example, three-dimensional MC code, designed for photon migration through complex heterogeneous media, allows one to obtain a SNR greater than 100 up to distances of 30 mm with a 1 mm^2 detector with 10^8 photons propagated within 5–10 hr of computer time on a Pentium III 1000 MHz CPU.[245]

Although advanced computer facilities and software systems have reduced the time needed, further developments in laser diagnostic and therapeutic tools require more effective, relatively simple, and reliable algorithms of the MC method. For instance, the condensed MC method allows one to obtain the solution for any albedo based on the results of modeling for a single albedo, which substantially facilitates computation.[226] Also, the development of very economical hybrid models currently underway is intended to combine the accuracy of the MC method and the high performance of diffusion theories or approximating analytic expressions.[198,225,229,230]

The original MC code that allows one to obtain information required to reconstruct an internal structure of highly scattering objects with size of 1000 scattering lengths and more was recently designed based on the path-integration technique and Metropolis algorithm.[248] The path-integral apparatus first suggested by Feynman for the alternative description of quantum mechanics can be also used to describe the movement of photons in a turbid medium as if they are particles undergoing collisions at a given collision frequency with a mean deflection in trajectory per collision.[249–254] The integral over all possible paths using a set of nested integrals is called a "path integral." This approach offers analytical solutions to the RTE in the framework of Perelman's approximation that is valid for a relatively weak scattering.[250] The path-integral model described in Ref. 249 is derived from first principles and does not include Perelman's approximation. The path-integral technique was applied to numerical calculations in the model of photon "random walk" within a three-dimensional discrete grid.[254] In the context of the MC approach, the path-integral technique may be seen as an extreme form of variance reduction, when instead of finding the most likely paths by random sampling, the path-integral formalism sets out to identify them directly.[248,249] Therefore, the elimination of "uninformative" photon paths from the calculations may provide a few-orders-higher calculation rate.[248]

Let us consider human-skin optics as an example.[37,38,57,213,221,222,224,227,228,236,237,243,246,255–262] In order to calculate distributions of the radiant-flux density $F(\bar{r})$ and the total radiant-energy-fluence rate $U(\bar{r})$ by the MC method [see Eqs. (1.11) and (1.12)], let us represent the skin as a plane multilayer scattering and absorbing medium (Fig. 1.8), with a laser beam falling normally onto its surface. Let us further assume that each ith layer is characterized by the following parameters: μ_{ai}, μ_{si}, $p_i(\theta)$, the thickness d_i, and the refractive index of the filler medium n_i. It should be noted that a more general approach to MC simulation that accounts for the interfaces between the dermal layers as quasi-random periodic surfaces and spectral skin response is also available.[243,246]

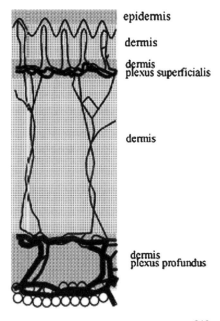

epidermis

dermis

dermis plexus superficialis

dermis

dermis plexus profundus

Figure 1.8 A model of human skin.[213]

Using the MC algorithm described in Refs. 213, 224, 261, and 262 to simulate the distribution of Gaussian light beams in the skin (see Fig. 1.8 and Table 1.1), the total fluence rate at wavelengths 337, 577, and 633 nm was obtained as shown in Fig. 1.9, along with the dependencies of the maximum total radiant-energy-fluence rate U_m and the maximum fluence rate area $D_\parallel \times D_\perp$ on the incident beam radius r_0 at 633 nm (Fig. 1.10). $D_\parallel$ and $D_\perp$ are defined at the $1/e^2$ level of U along and across the incident light beam, respectively. It is readily seen that the illumination maximum is formed at a certain depth inside the tissue, and the total fluence rate at the point of maximum U_m may be significantly higher than that in the middle of the beam incident to the surface of the medium (U_0). This was noticed by many authors (see, for instance, Refs. 1, 3, 37, and 210), who emphasized the strong correlation between the U_m/U_0 ratio and the optical properties of the medium, the incident beam radius, and boundary properties. It appears from Fig. 1.10(b) that an

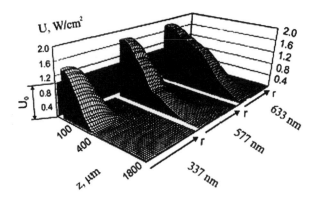

Figure 1.9 Results of Monte Carlo simulation of the total radiant-energy-fluence rate distribution U (W/cm^2) in skin irradiated by Gaussian laser beams with different wavelengths ($\lambda = 633$, 577, and 337 nm), equal radius on the skin surface ($r_0 = 1.0$ mm), and equal intensity at the beam center ($U_0 = 1$ W/cm^2).[6] z is the linear coordinate (depth inside the skin) and r is the coordinate across the light beam.

Table 1.1 Optical parameters of skin.[6,213]

N	Skin layer	λ, nm	μ_a, cm^{-1}	μ_s, cm^{-1}	g	n	d, μm
1.	Epidermis	337	32	165	0.72	1.5	100
		577	10.7	120	0.78	1.5	
		633	4.3	107	0.79	1.5	
2.	Dermis	337	23	227	0.72	1.4	200
		577	3.0	205	0.78	1.4	
		633	2.7	187	0.82	1.4	
3.	Dermis with *plexus superficialis*	337	40	246	0.72	1.4	200
		577	5.2	219	0.78	1.4	
		633	3.3	192	0.82	1.4	
4.	Dermis	337	23	227	0.72	1.4	900
		577	3.0	205	0.78	1.4	
		633	2.7	187	0.82	1.4	
5.	Dermis with *plexus profundus*	337	46	253	0.72	1.4	600
		577	6	225	0.78	1.4	
		633	3.4	194	0.82	1.4	

increase in the incident beam radius leads to a broadening of the illuminated area inside the tissue, with the enhancement rate in the transversal direction exceeding that along the beam.

For practical purposes, such calculations for human skin and other multilayered soft tissues are necessary to correctly choose the irradiation doses for photochemical, photodynamic, and photothermal therapy of cancer and many other

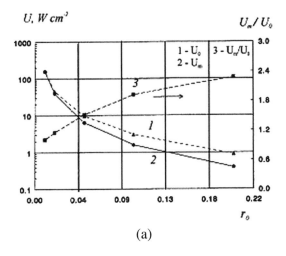

(a)

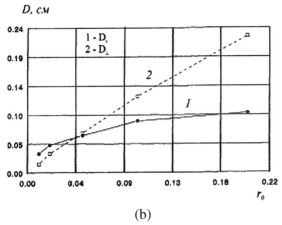

(b)

Figure 1.10 Parameters of the maximum illumination area as functions of the incident beam radius. A beam with a Gaussian profile, wavelength 633 nm, power 25 mW. (a) 1, Total illumination in the center of the incident beam U_0; 2, maximal total illumination U_m; 3, U_m/U_0. (b) 1, The size of the maximally illuminated area (at the $1/e^2$ level) along the beam axis, $D_{\parallel}$; 2, size of the maximally illuminated area (at the $1/e^2$ level) across the beam axis $D_{\perp}$.[213]

diseases, and the laser coagulation of the superficial blood vessels or transscleral cyclophotocoagulation.[2,3,10–16,22,29,32,33,37,57,72,90,91,210,258–268]

In particular, based on the results of MC simulation presented in Figs. 1.9 and 1.10, attenuation of a wide laser beam of intensity I_0 at depths $z > l_d = 1/\mu_{eff}$ [see Eq. (1.18)] in a thick tissue may be described as

$$I(z) \approx I_0 b_s \exp(-\mu_{eff} z),\qquad(1.30)$$

where b_s accounts for additional irradiation of upper layers of a tissue due to backscattering (photon recycling effect). Respectively, the depth of light penetration into a tissue is

$$l_e = l_d[\ln b_s + 1]. \qquad (1.31)$$

Typically, for tissues $b_s = 1$–5 for beam diameter of 1–20 mm.[210,265] Thus, when wide laser beams are used for irradiation of highly scattering tissues with low-absorption, CW light energy is accumulated in tissue due to the high multiplicity of chaotic long-path photon migrations. A highly scattering medium works as a random cavity, providing the capacity of light energy. The light power density within the superficial tissue layers may substantially (up to fivefold) exceed the incident power density and cause the overdosage during photodynamic therapy or overheating during interstitial laser thermotherapy. On the other hand, the photon recycling effect can be used for more effective irradiation of undersurface lesions at relatively small incident power densities.

1.2 Short pulse propagation in tissues

1.2.1 Basic principles and theoretical background

Based on the time-dependent radiation-transfer theory (RTT), it is possible to analyze the time response of scattering tissue. Such an analysis is important to provide a rationale for noninvasive optical diagnostic methods using time-resolved measurement of reflectance and transmittance in tissues.[1,3,31,42,44,71,92,129,130,199,200,203,205,248–254,269–302] In its general form, the time-dependent RTT equation for time-dependent radiance (or the specific intensity) $I(\bar{r}, \bar{s}, t)$ can be written as:[269,301]

$$\frac{\partial}{\partial S} I(\bar{r}, \bar{s}, t) + \mu_t t_2 \frac{\partial}{\partial t} I(\bar{r}, \bar{s}, t) = -\mu_t I(\bar{r}, \bar{s}, t)$$

$$+ \frac{\mu_s}{4\pi} \int_{4\pi} \left[\int_{-\infty}^{t} I(\bar{r}, \bar{s}', t') f(t, t') dt' \right] p(\bar{s}, \bar{s}') d\Omega'. \qquad (1.32)$$

Compared with the CW equation (1.9), the following notation is introduced into Eq. (1.32): t is time, $t_2 = l/(\mu_t c)$ is the average interval between interactions, where c is the velocity of light in the medium; $f(t, t')$ describes the temporal deformation of a δ-shaped pulse following its single scattering and can be represented in the form of an exponentially decaying function as

$$f(t, t') = \frac{1}{t_1} \exp\left(-\frac{t - t'}{t_1}\right), \qquad (1.33)$$

where t_1 may be a function of $\bar{r}$, and t_1 is the first moment of the distribution function $f(t, t')$ that describes the time interval of an individual scattering act at $t_1 \to 0$, $f(t, t') \to \delta(t - t')$. The radiance $I(\bar{r}, \bar{s}, t)$ in Eq. (1.32) contains two components: the attenuated incident radiation and the diffuse. This equation meets the boundary conditions [see Eq. (1.10)] at $(\bar{r}, \bar{s}) \rightarrow (\bar{r}, \bar{s}, t)$.

When probing the plane-parallel layer of a scattering medium with an ultra-short laser pulse, the transmitted pulse consists of a ballistic (coherent) component, a group of photons having zigzag trajectories, and a highly intensive diffuse component (see Fig. 1.11).[1,3,31] Both unscattered photons and photons undergoing forward-directed single-step scattering contribute to the intensity of the ballistic component (composed of photons traveling straight along the laser beam). This component is subject to exponential attenuation with increasing sample thickness [see Eq. (1.1)]. This accounts for the limited utility of ballistic photons for practical diagnostic purposes in medicine.

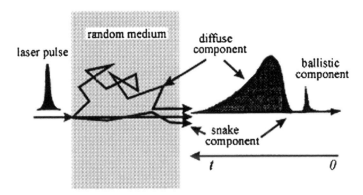

Figure 1.11 An ultrashort laser pulse propagating through a random medium spreads into a diffuse component, a snake with zigzag paths, and a ballistic component.[1]

The group of snake photons with zigzag trajectories includes photons that have experienced only a few collisions each. They propagate along trajectories that deviate only slightly from the direction of the incident beam and form the first-arriving part of the diffuse component. These photons carry information about the optical properties of the random medium and parameters of any foreign object that they may happen to come across during their progress.

The diffuse component is very broad and intense since it contains the bulk of incident photons after they have participated in many scattering acts and therefore migrate in different directions and have different path lengths. Moreover, the diffuse component carries information about the optical properties of the scattering medium, and its deformation may reflect the presence of local inhomogeneities in the medium. The resolution obtained by this method at a high light-gathering power is much lower than in the method measuring straight-passing photons. Two probing schemes are conceivable, one recording transmitted photons and the other taking advantage of their backscattering (see Fig. 1.12).

If in the diffusion approximation (valid at $\mu_a \ll \mu_s'$) the tissue is homogeneous and semi-infinite, the size of both the source and the detector is small compared with the distance r_{sd} between them at the tissue surface, and the pulse may be

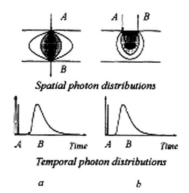

Figure 1.12 Typical schemes for time-resolved tissue studies:[1] (a) Recording transmitted photons; (b) backscattering regime. A, Probing beam; B, detected radiation. The dark area in the center of the scattering layer is a local inhomogeneity (tumor). Spatial and temporal photon distributions in the medium are shown.

regarded as single; then the light distribution is described by the time-dependent diffusion equation:[272,273]

$$\left(\nabla^2 - c\mu_a D^{-1} - D^{-1}\frac{\partial}{\partial t}\right) \cdot U(\vec{r}, t) = -Q(\vec{r}, t),\tag{1.34}$$

which is in fact the generalization of the CW Eq. (1.17). It is worth noting that the diffusion equation is equivalent to the equation for thermal conductivity.[286] The solution of Eq. (1.34) yields the following relation for the number of backscattered photons at the surface for unit time and from unit area $R(r_{sd}, t)$:[272,273]

$$R(r_{sd}, t) = \frac{z_0}{(4\pi D)^{3/2}} t^{-5/2} \exp\left(-\frac{r_{sd}^2 + z_0^2}{2Dt}\right) \exp(-\mu_a ct),\tag{1.35}$$

and correspondingly for transmittance

$$T(r_{sd}, d, t) = (4\pi D)^{-3/2} t^{-5/2} \exp\left(\frac{-r_{sd}^2}{4Dt}\right) \left\{ (d - z_0) \exp\left[-\frac{(d - z_0)^2}{4Dt}\right]\right.$$

$$- (d + z_0) \exp\left[-\frac{(d + z_0)^2}{4Dt}\right] + (3d - z_0) \exp\left[-\frac{(3d - z_0)^2}{4Dt}\right]$$

$$\left. - (3d + z_0) \exp\left[-\frac{(3d + z_0)^2}{4Dt}\right] \right\} \exp(-\mu_a ct),\tag{1.36}$$

where $z_0 = (\mu_s')^{-1}$, and d is the tissue thickness.

In practice, μ_a and μ_s' are estimated by fitting Eq. (1.35) or Eq. (1.36) with the shape of a pulse measured by the time-resolved photon counting technique. Experimentally measured optical parameters of many tissues and model media obtained by the pulse method can be found in Refs. 1, 3, 6, 12–15, 31, 88, 89, 129,

130, 245, 272–289, and 300. An important advantage of the pulse method is its applicability to *in vivo* studies owing to the possibility of the separate evaluation of μ_a and μ'_s using a single measurement in the backscattering or transillumination regimes. It seems appropriate to mention that a search for more adequate approaches to describing tissue responses to laser pulses is underway (see, for instance, Refs. 199, 200, 203, 204, 248–254, and 291–302). Many publications are devoted to image transfer in tissues and the evaluation of the resolving power of optical tomographic schemes that make use of the first-transmitted photons of ultrashort pulses.[1,3,71,129,130,245,270,271,279–284,294,297–302]

1.2.2 Principles and instruments for time-resolved spectroscopy and imaging

The main principle of enhanced viewing through a turbid medium (tissue) using a time-resolved approach is well illustrated in Fig. 1.13.[1,31] A contrast image of an object in a scattering medium can be provided by electronic or optical time-gating of the earliest-arriving, minimally scattered light (ballistic and snake photons), which contains geometric information.[1,3,31,71] The typical optical schemes using the selection of the earliest-arriving photons are presented in Figs. 1.14 and 1.15. The first group of schemes (see Fig. 1.14) uses the electronic time-gating procedure. The time-correlated single-photon-counting technique explores a high-repetition-rate picosecond laser (for example, a cavity-dumped mode-locked dye laser). At the detection of the earliest-arriving photons, the time delay is measured with a time-to-amplitude converter [see Fig. 1.14(a)] and a histogram of the arrival

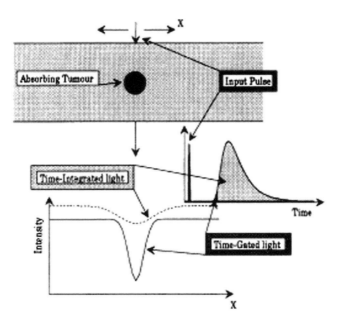

Figure 1.13 Gated viewing through tissue. An enhanced spatial resolution is obtained by selecting "early" light only.[1]

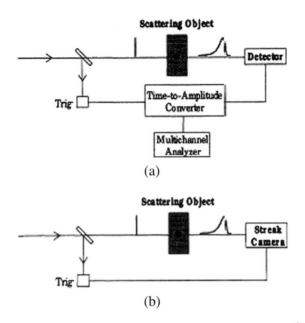

Figure 1.14 Techniques for electronically gated viewing.[1]

times is built up using a large number of low-energy pulses. The time resolution of such a technique is limited to about 50 ps. For more energetic pulses from lasers with a lower repetition rate, the use of streak cameras allows for a time resolution down to 1 ps [see Fig. 1.14(b)]. If a synchroscan streak camera is employed, even a high-repetition rate source with low-energy pulses can be used.

The second group of techniques uses optical nonlinear effects to select photons (see Fig. 1.15).[1] For a scheme with an optical Kerr gate, an energetic laser is used. Part of the pulse is transmitted into the tissue and part opens the shutter by use of the optical Kerr effect (the cell with CS_2) [see Fig. 1.15(a)]. Since the gate width is determined only by the length of the laser pulse, subpicosecond gate times can be achieved. The Raman-amplifier-gating technique also uses energetic laser pulses. A Stokes wave generated by stimulated Raman scattering in a gas cell is used to probe the tissue [see Fig. 1.15(b)]. The low-intensity transmitted light is amplified in a Raman amplifier, which in turn is pumped by an ultrashort laser pulse. This pulse has the proper time delay to strobe on the desired early temporal part of the light under investigation. The third scheme uses a time-correlated frequency-doubling technique and is often used in optical autocorrelators for monitoring laser pulse characteristics [see Fig. 1.15(c)]. It can be used directly for optical gating of signal photons.

1.2.3 Coherent backscattering

The use of ultrafast laser pulses gives rise to a local peak of intensity backscattered within a narrow solid angle owing to scattered light interference.[31,73,74] In the exact backward direction, the intensity of the scattered light is normally twice

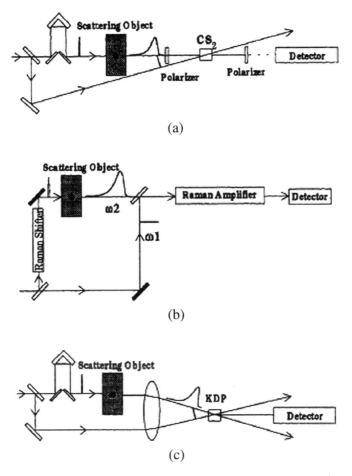

Figure 1.15 Gated-viewing technique using nonlinear optical phenomena:[1] CS_2 is the optical Kerr cell filled by CS_2; KDP is the nonlinear crystal for frequency doubling.

the diffuse intensity. Such interference in coherence arises from the time reversal symmetry among various scattered light paths in the backscattering direction. This phenomenon is known as weak localization. The profile of the angular distribution of the coherent peak depends on the transport mean path l_t and the absorption coefficient μ_a. The angular width of the peak is directly related to l_t as[74]

$$\Delta\theta \approx \frac{\lambda}{2\pi l_t}. \tag{1.37}$$

In many hard and soft tissues such as human fat tissue, lung cancer tissue, normal and cataractous eye lens, and myocardial, mammary, and dental tissues, the backscattered coherent peak occurs when the probing laser pulse is shorter than 20 ps.[74]

1.3 Diffuse photon-density waves

1.3.1 Basic principles and theoretical background

The frequency-domain (FD) method has been proposed for photon migration studies in scattering media. The method is designed to evaluate the dynamic response of scattered light intensity to modulation of the incident laser beam intensity in a wide frequency range, usually in tissue research using 50 to 1000 MHz.[1,3,4,6,10,52,53,71,129,130,285,286,301–337] The FD method measures the modulation depth of scattered light intensity $m_U \equiv ac_{detector}/dc_{detector}$ (see Fig. 1.16) and the corresponding phase shift relative to the incident light modulation

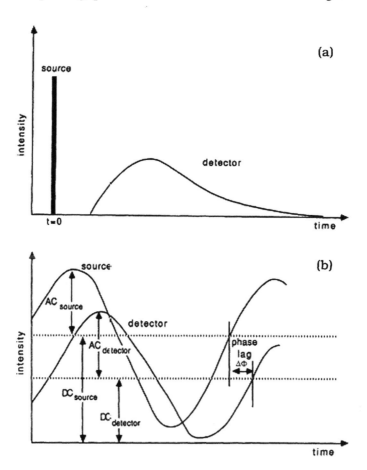

Figure 1.16 Schematic representation of the time evolution of the light intensity measured in response to (a) a very narrow light pulse and (b) a sinusoidally intensity-modulated light transversing an arbitrary distance in a scattering and absorbing medium. (a) If the medium is strongly scattering, there are no unscattered components in the transmitted pulse. (b) The transmitted photon density wave retains the same frequency as the incoming wave in the medium. The reduced amplitude of the transmitted wave arises from attenuation related to the scattering and absorption processes. The demodulation is the ratio ac/dc normalized to the modulation of the source.[314]

phase $\Delta\Phi$ (phase lag). Compared with the time-domain (TD) measurements described earlier, this method is more simple and reliable in terms of data interpretation and immunity from noise. These happen because FD equipment involves amplitude modulation at low peak power, slow rise time [compare Figs. 1.16(a) and 1.16(b)], and hence smaller bandwidths than TD instruments; higher SNRs are attainable as well. Medical FD equipment is more economic and portable, and can be built on the basis of measuring devices used in optical telecommunication systems and studies of optical fiber dispersion.[4,328] However, the FD technique suffers from the simultaneous transmission and reception of signals and requires special attempts to avoid unwanted cross talk between the transmitted and detected signals. The current measuring schemes are based on heterodyning of optical and transformed signals.[1,3,4,6,10,52,53,71,129,130,285–290,301–323,334,335]

The development of the theory underlying this method resulted in the discovery of a new type of wave: photon-density waves or waves of progressively decaying intensity. Microscopically, individual photons make random migrations in a scattering medium, but collectively they form a photon-density wave at a modulation frequency ω that moves away from a radiation source (see Figs. 1.16 and 1.17). Diffuse waves of this type are well known in other fields of physics (for example, thermal waves are excited upon absorption of modulated laser radiation in various media, including biological ones[5,6,25]). Photon-density waves possess typical wave properties; e.g., they undergo refraction, diffraction, interference, dispersion, and attenuation.[1,3,4,6,71,52,53,129,130,285,301,303,307–310,313–315,334]

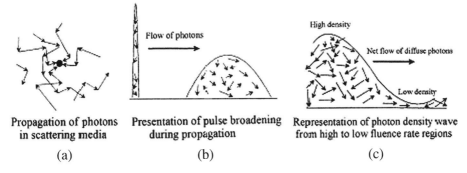

Propagation of photons in scattering media	Presentation of pulse broadening during propagation	Representation of photon density wave from high to low fluence rate regions
(a)	(b)	(c)

Figure 1.17 Schematic representation of photons propagation in scattering media induced by (a) a CW, (b) a pulse, and (c) a sinusoidally intensity-modulated light source.[315]

In strongly scattering media with weak absorption far from the walls and a source or a receiver of radiation, the light distribution may be regarded as a decaying diffusion process described by the time-dependent diffusion equation for photon density [see Eq. (1.34)]. When a point light source with harmonic intensity modulation is used, placed at the point $\bar{r} = 0$,

$$I(0, t) = I_0[1 + m_I \exp(j\omega t)], \qquad (1.38)$$

where m_I is the intensity modulation depth of the incident light.

The solution of Eq. (1.34) for a homogeneous infinite medium can be presented in the form[71]

$$U(\bar{r}, t) = U_{dc}(\bar{r}) + U_{ac}(\bar{r}, w) \exp(j w t), \qquad (1.39)$$

where

$$U_{dc} = \left(\frac{I_0}{4\pi D\bar{r}}\right) \exp\left(\frac{-\bar{r}}{l_d}\right), \qquad (1.40)$$

$$U_{ac}(\bar{r}, w) = \tilde{U}_{ac}(\bar{r}, w) \exp[-i k_r(w)\bar{r}], \qquad (1.41)$$

$$\tilde{U}_{ac}(\bar{r}, w) = m_I \left[\frac{I_0}{4\pi D\bar{r}}\right] \exp[-k_i(w)\bar{r}], \qquad (1.42)$$

and $w = 2\pi v$ is the modulation frequency, $l_d = \mu_{eff}^{-1}$ is the diffusion length [see Eq. (1.18)], and $k_r(w)$ and $k_i(w)$ are the real and imaginary parts of the photon-density wave vector, respectively:

$$k = k_r - i k_i = -i[(\mu_a c + i w)/D]^{0.5}, \qquad (1.43)$$

$$k_{r,i} = l_d^{-1} \left\{ \frac{[1 + (w\tau_a)^2]^{0.5} \mp 1}{2} \right\}^{0.5}, \qquad (1.44)$$

$$\tau_a^{-1} = \mu_a c, \qquad (1.45)$$

where $\tau_a = 1/(\mu_a c)$ is the average travel time of a photon before being absorbed.

An alternating component of this solution is a retreating spherical wave with its center at the point $\bar{r} = 0$ that oscillates at a modulation frequency v and undergoes a phase shift relative to the phase value at point $\bar{r} = 0$ equal to

$$\Delta\Phi = k_r(w)\bar{r}. \qquad (1.46)$$

Constant and time-dependent components of the photon-density wave fall with distance as $\exp(-\bar{r}/l_d)$ and $\exp[-k_i(w)\bar{r}]$, respectively. The length of a photon-density wave is defined by

$$\Lambda_\Phi = \frac{2\pi}{k_r} = \left(\frac{2\pi}{w}\right)(2c D \mu_a \{1 + [1 + (w\tau_a)^2]^{1/2}\})^{1/2}, \qquad (1.47)$$

and its phase velocity is

$$V_\Phi = \Lambda_\Phi \nu. \tag{1.48}$$

It follows that photon-density waves are capable of dispersion.

For biomedical applications, in particular, optical mammography, we can easily estimate that for $\omega/2\pi = 500$ MHz, $\mu'_s = 15$ cm^{-1}, $\mu_a = 0.035$ cm^{-1}, and $c = (3 \times 10^{10}/1.33)$ cm/s; the wavelength is $\Lambda_s \cong 5.0$ cm and the phase velocity is $V_s \cong 1.77 \times 10^9$ cm/s.

For weakly absorbing media, when $\omega\tau_a \gg 1$,

$$\Lambda_\Phi^2 = \frac{8\pi^2 D}{\omega}; \quad V_\Phi^2 = 2D\omega, \tag{1.49}$$

$$m_U(\bar{r}, \omega) \equiv \frac{\tilde{U}_{ac}(\bar{r}, \omega)}{U_{dc}(\bar{r})} = m_I \exp\left(\bar{r}\sqrt{\frac{D}{c\mu_a}}\right)\exp\left(-\bar{r}\sqrt{\frac{\omega}{2D}}\right), \tag{1.50}$$

$$\Delta\Phi(\bar{r}, \omega) = \bar{r}\left(\frac{\omega}{2D}\right)^{0.5}. \tag{1.51}$$

It clearly follows from Eq. (1.50) that in order to support the transport of a photon-density wave in a medium, light scattering is needed (see first exponential term); but in contrast, high scattering turns a photon density wave to decay (see second exponential term).

Measuring $m_U(\bar{r}, \omega)$, $\Delta\Phi(\bar{r}, \omega)$ allows one to separately determine the transport scattering coefficient μ'_s and the absorption coefficient μ_a, and evaluate the spatial distribution of these parameters.

1.3.2 Principles of frequency-domain spectroscopy and imaging of tissues

Evidently, there is a close relationship between the two time-resolved methods for the assessment of optical properties of tissues. In the case of pulse probing of a scattering medium, Fourier instrumental or computer-aided analysis of scattered pulses allows us to simultaneously obtain the amplitude-phase response of the medium for a continuous set of harmonics.[1,3,4,71,286,301–303,311] Figure 1.18 illustrates the typical behavior of the amplitude-phase response in a tissuelike phantom (whole or diluted milk).[71] Such characteristics are useful for the spectroscopic examination of tissues, e.g., for *in vivo* evaluation of hemoglobin oxygenation[321,338] or blood glucose level.[339–341]

The spatial resolution available using photon-density waves is crucial for the visualization of macroinhomogeneities. Theoretical considerations illustrated by

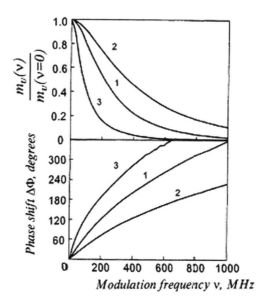

Figure 1.18 (a) Amplitude and (b) phase responses of a model medium [unskimmed (1, 3) and 40% diluted (2) milk] obtained by the Fourier transformation of experimental pulse responses; 1, 2, recording transmitted pulses, 2-cm-thick cuvette; 3, backscattering regime (large volume of unskimmed milk). The distance between irradiating and detecting optic fibers is $r_{sd} = 2$ cm.[71]

Fig. 1.19 for two absorbing macroinhomogeneities in a scattering medium provide evidence that their separate identification is feasible if the accuracy of the phase and wave amplitude measurements is not less than 1.0 and 2.0%, respectively.[310,330] The predicted resolving power of diffuse tomography using photon-density waves is close to 1 mm; i.e., it is comparable to that of positron-emission and magneto-resonance tomography.[4,285] Important advantages of optical tomography are technical simplicity, the enhancement of an object's contrast by molecular dyes, and the visualization of local metabolic processes.

Figure 1.20 presents images of tumor-containing female breast tissue outlined by contour lines for μ_a and μ'_s that were obtained by exposure to modulated visible and near-IR radiation.[71] The tumor is readily discernible because of its high absorption and scattering coefficients.

In principle, a record-breaking resolving power of less than 1 mm can be achieved by taking advantage of the interference of photon-density waves excited by spaced sources.[4,53,302,330,342] Not only a good spatial resolution, but also a high contrast and low sensitivity to the movements and geometry of the object under study should be provided to get a high-quality image. A tissue immersion technique can be used to improve image quality.[129,324,328] When the imaged tissue is surrounded with a medium of matched scattering and absorption properties, a uniform transillumination image is obtained and the maximum dynamic range is available to examine variations within the tissue. In addition, it allows one to eliminate the influence of the boundary conditions and geometry for objects with a

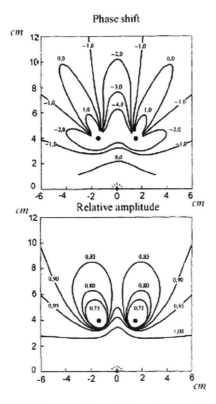

Figure 1.19 Theoretical distributions of the relative phase shift and intensity modulation at 200 MHz in an irradiated system of two absolute absorbers (balls 0.5 cm in diameter) placed in a homogeneous scattering medium ($\mu_s' = 10$ cm^{-1}, $\mu_a = 0.02$ cm^{-1}). The source is located at the origin and the absorbers are located at points $(-2, 4)$ and $(2, 4)$.[310]

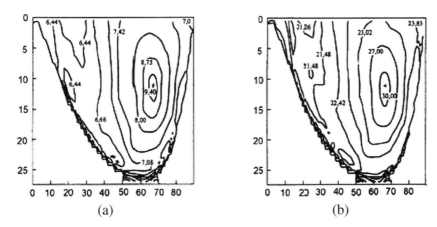

(a)   (b)

Figure 1.20 Reconstructed optical images of human cancerous breast tissue obtained by exposure to modulated radiation in the visible and NIR wavelength regions. (a) The image outlined by contour lines for the absorption coefficient μ_a (10^{-2} cm^{-1}). (b) The same for the transport scattering coefficient μ_s' (cm^{-1}). The tumor is located near the point (70, 10); the coefficients have relative values.[71]

complex shape and structure. It also allows one to achieve optical matching of the probe laser beam and tissue, to considerably reduce the influence of external and internal movements (breathing, heartbeats, muscle tremor, etc.) of the object during the imaging process, and to calibrate measurements using well-known optical properties of the immersion medium. Sometimes, such a simple technique is a good alternative for more sophisticated imaging techniques based on multifrequency analysis.

Apart from the visualization of macroinhomogeneities in breast tissues, the FD method is useful in examining other tissue, e.g., brain and lungs. It also provides an insight into many physiological processes dependent on oxygen consumption by tissues and organs and related hemodynamic changes. One of the most important areas of application may be the evaluation of the oxygen distribution in a functioning brain.[4,285,302,303] Another example is the monitoring of neoplastic growth patterns, including enhanced blood volume and blood deoxygenation, increased intracellular organelle content, and tissue calcification, which may be important for the differentiation between benign and malignant tumors.[285,302,303]

To conclude, it should be emphasized that high tissue density sometimes necessitates taking into consideration the time interval of an individual scattering act t_1 [see Eqs. (1.32) and (1.33)], which may prove comparable to the mean time interval between interactions t_2.[301,327] Moreover, the widely used diffusion approximation imposes important constraints on the analysis of the optical properties of tissues. Therefore, the development of more universal models of photon-density wave dispersion is well under way using new MC algorithms.[301–303,327]

1.4 Propagation of polarized light in tissues

1.4.1 Introduction

Up to this point, we have ignored the vector nature of light transport in scattering media such as tissues because we assumed it to be rapidly depolarized during propagation in a randomly inhomogeneous medium. It is a common belief that the randomness of tissue structure results in fast depolarization of light propagating in tissues. Therefore, polarization effects are usually ignored. However, in certain tissues (transparent tissues such as eye tissues, cellular monolayers, mucous membrane, and superficial skin layers), the degree of polarization of transmitted or reflected light remains measurable, even when the tissue has a considerable thickness. In such a situation, the information about the structure of tissues and cell ensembles can be extracted from the registered depolarization degree of initially polarized light, the polarization state transformation, or the appearance of a polarized component in the scattered light.[3,5,6,59,67–70,105,129,135,138,145,146,148,149,155,159,166,186,343]

In regard to practical implications, polarization techniques are believed to give rise to simplified schemes of optical-medical tomography compared with time-resolved methods, and also provide additional information about the structure of tissues.[343–396]

1.4.2 Tissue structure and anisotropy

Many biological tissues are optically anisotropic.[3,9,10,24,29,43,59–70,97,127–130,135,138,150,151,166,168,176,177,397–440] Tissue birefringence results primarily from the linear anisotropy of fibrous structures, which forms the extracellular media. The refractive index of a medium is higher along the length of a fiber than along the cross section. A specific tissue structure is a system composed of parallel cylinders that create a uniaxial birefringent medium with the optic axis parallel to the cylinder axes. This is called birefringence of form. A large variety of tissues such as eye cornea, tendon, cartilage, eye sclera, *dura mater*, testis, muscle, nerve, retina, bone, teeth, myelin, etc. exhibit form birefringence. All of these tissues contain uniaxial and/or biaxial birefringent structures. For instance, in bone and teeth, these are mineralized structures originating from hydroxyapatite crystals, which play an important role in hard tissue birefringence. In particular, dental enamel is an ordered array of such crystals surrounded by a protein/lipid/water matrix.[65,66,97,423,425,426] Fairly well oriented hexagonal crystals of hydroxyapatite of approximately 30–40 nm in diameter and up to 10 μm in length are packed into an organic matrix to form enamel prisms (or rods) with an overall cross section of 4–6 μm. Enamel prisms are roughly perpendicular to the tooth surface. Tooth dentin is a complex structure, honeycombed with dentinal tubules, which are shelled organic cylinders with a highly mineralized shell. Tubules diameters are 1–5 μm, and their number density is in the range $(3–7) \times 10^6$ cm^{-2}.[65,66,97,423]

Tendon consists mostly of parallel, densely packed collagen fibers arranged in parallel bundles interspersed with long, elliptical fibroblasts. In general, tendon fibers are cylindrical in shape with diameters ranging from 20 to 400 nm.[176,177] The ordered structure of collagen fibers running parallel to a single axis makes tendon a highly birefringent tissue.

Arteries have a more complex structure than tendons. The medial layer consists mostly of closely packed smooth muscle cells with a mean diameter of 15–20 μm. Small amounts of connective tissue, including elastin, collagenous, and reticular fibers, as well as a few fibroblasts, are also located in the media. The outer adventitial layer consists of dense fibrous connective tissue. The adventitia is largely made up of collagen fibers, 1–12 μm in diameter, and thinner elastin fibers, 2–3 μm in diameter. As with tendon, the cylindrical collagen and elastin fibers are ordered mainly along one axis, thus causing the tissue to be birefringent.

Myocardium, on the other hand, contains fibers oriented along two different axes. Myocardium consists mostly of cardiac muscle fibers arranged in sheets that wind around the ventricles and atria. In pigs, the myocardium cardiac muscle is comprised of myofibrils (about 1 μm in diameter) that in turn consist of cylindrical myofilaments (6–15 nm in diameter) and aspherical mitochondria (1–2 μm in diameter). Myocardium is typically birefringent since the refractive index along the axis of the muscle fiber is different from that in the transverse direction.[176,177]

Form birefringence arises when the relative optical phase between the orthogonal polarization components is nonzero for forward-scattered light. After multiple forward scattering events, a relative phase difference accumulates and a delay (δ_{oe}) similar to that observed in birefringent crystalline materials is introduced between orthogonal polarization components. For organized linear structures, an increase in phase delay may be characterized by a difference (Δn_{oe}) in the effective refractive index for light polarized along, and perpendicular to, the long axis of the linear structures. The effect of tissue birefringence on the propagation of linearly polarized light is dependent on the angle between the incident polarization orientation and the tissue axis. Phase retardation δ_{oe} between orthogonal polarization components is proportional to the distance d traveled through the birefringent medium:[416]

$$\delta_{oe} = \frac{2\pi d \, \Delta n_{oe}}{\lambda_0}.$$ (1.52)

A medium of parallel cylinders is a positive uniaxial birefringent medium [$\Delta n_{oe} = (n_e - n_o) > 0$] with its optic axis parallel to the cylinder axes [see Fig. 1.21(a)]. Therefore, a case defined by an incident electrical field directed parallel to the cylinder axes will be called "extraordinary," and a case with the incident electrical field perpendicular to the cylinder axes will be called "ordinary." The difference $(n_e - n_o)$ between the extraordinary index and the ordinary index is a measure of the birefringence of a medium comprised of cylinders. For the Rayleigh limit ($\lambda \gg$ cylinder diameter), the form birefringence becomes[399,402]

$$\Delta n_{oe} = (n_e - n_o) = \frac{f_1 f_2 (n_1 - n_2)^2}{f_1 n_1 + f_2 n_2},$$ (1.53)

where f_1 is the volume fraction of the cylinders; f_2 is the volume fraction of the ground substance; and n_1, n_2 are the corresponding indices. For a given index difference, maximal birefringence is expected for approximately equal volume fractions of thin cylinders and ground material. For systems with large diameter cylinders ($\lambda \ll$ cylinder diameter), the birefringence goes to zero.[402]

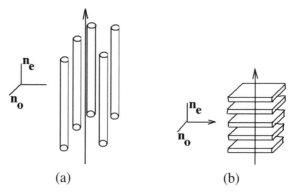

(a)   (b)

Figure 1.21 Models of tissue birefringence: (a) system of long dielectric cylinders, (b) system of thin dielectric plates.[442]

For a system of thin plates [see Fig. 1.21(b)], the following equation is obtained:[160]

$$n_e^2 - n_o^2 = -\frac{f_1 f_2 (n_1 - n_2)}{f_1 n_1^2 + f_2 n_2^2},$$

(1.54)

where f_1 is the volume fraction occupied by the plates; f_2 is the volume fraction of the ground substance; and n_1, n_2 are the corresponding indices. This implies that the system behaves like a negative uniaxial crystal with its optical axis aligned normally with the plate surface.

Form birefringence is used in biological microscopy as an instrument for studying cell structure. The sign of the observed refractive index difference points to the particle shape closest to that of the rod or the plate, and if n_1 and n_2 are known, one can then assess the volume fraction occupied by the particles. To separate the birefringence of the form and the particle material, the refractive indices of the particles and the ground substance should be matched, because form birefringence vanishes with $n_1 = n_2$.

Linear dichroism (diattenuation), i.e., different wave attenuation for two orthogonal polarizations, in systems formed by long cylinders or plates is defined by the difference between the imaginary parts of the effective indices of refraction. Depending on the relationship between the sizes and the optical constants of the cylinders or plates, this difference can take both positive and negative values.[160]

Reported birefringence values for tendon, muscle, coronary artery, myocardium, sclera, cartilage, and skin are on the order of 10^{-3} (see, for instance, Refs. 400, 409, 410, and 412–416). The measured refractive index variations for the fast and slow axes of rabbit cornea show that its birefringence varies within the range of 0 at the apex, or top of the cornea, to 5.5×10^{-4} at the base of the cornea, where it attaches to the sclera.[398,404] The predominant orientation of collagenous fibers in different regions of the cornea results in birefringence and dichroism.[403] Based on experimental results, it has been assumed that the birefringent portions of the corneal surface all have a relatively universal fast axis located approximately 160 deg from the vertical axis, defined as a line that runs from the apex of the cornea through the pupil.[404]

A new technique—polarization-sensitive optical-coherence tomography (PS OCT)—allows for the measurement of linear birefringence in turbid tissue with high precision.[412–416,418] The following data have been reported using this technique: for rodent muscle, 1.4×10^{-3} (Refs. 415 and 416); for normal porcine tendon, $(4.2 \pm 0.3) \times 10^{-3}$ and for thermally treated (90°C, 20 s), $(2.24 \pm 0.07) \times 10^{-3}$; for porcine skin, 1.5×10^{-3}–3.5×10^{-3}; for bovine cartilage, 3.0×10^{-3} (Ref. 418); and for bovine tendon, $(3.7 \pm 0.4) \times 10^{-3}$ (Ref. 413). Such birefringence provides 90% phase retardation at a depth on the order of several hundred micrometers.

The magnitude of birefringence and diattenuation are related to the density and other properties of the collagen fibers, whereas the orientation of the fast axis indicates the orientation of the collagen fibers. The amplitude and orientation of birefringence of the skin and cartilage are not as uniformly distributed as in tendon. In other words, the densities of collagen fibers in skin and cartilage are not as uniform as in tendon, and the orientation of the collagen fibers is not distributed in as orderly a fashion.[418]

In addition to linear birefringence and dichroism (diattenuation), many tissue components show optical activity. In polarized light research, the molecule's chirality, which stems from its asymmetric molecular structure, results in a number of characteristic effects generically called optical activity.[430,434] A well-known manifestation of optical activity is the ability to rotate the plane of linearly polarized light about the axis of propagation. The amount of rotation depends on the chiral molecular concentration, the path length through the medium, and the light wavelength. For instance, chiral asymmetrically encoded in the polarization properties of light transmitted through a transparent media enables very sensitive and accurate determination of glucose concentration. Tissues containing chiral components display optical activity.[404,428,429] Interest in chiral turbid media is driven by the attractive possibility of noninvasive *in situ* optical monitoring of the glucose in diabetic patients.[105,138] Within turbid tissues, however, where the scattering effects dominate, the loss of polarization information is significant and the chiral effects due to the small amount of dissolved glucose are difficult to detect.

In complex tissue structures, chiral aggregates of particles, in particular spherical particles, may be responsible for optical activity of tissue (see Fig. 1.22). More sophisticated anisotropic tissue models can also be constructed. For example, the cornea can be represented as a system of plane anisotropic layers (plates, i.e., lamellas), each of which is composed of densely packed long cylinders (fibrils) [see Fig. 1.21(a)] with their optical axes oriented along a spiral (see Fig. 2.2). This fibrilar-lamellar structure of the cornea is responsible for the linear and circular dichroism and its dependence on the angle between the lamellas.[403]

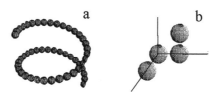

Figure 1.22 Examples of chiral aggregates of spherical particles.

1.4.3 Light scattering by a particle

Let us now consider the transformation of any polarization type (linear, circular, or elliptical) in a scattering medium with typical tissue parameters, and compare the penetration depth of circular and linear polarization in different media. To this end, let us examine a monochromatic plane wave incident on an isolated scatterer.[43,148,149] The geometry needed to describe the scattering of light by a particle is shown in Fig. 1.23. The incident monochromatic plane wave comes from below and travels along the positive z-axis. Some of the light is scattered by the particle along the direction indicated by the vector $\vec{S}_1$ toward a detector located a distance r from the particle. The scattering direction is defined by the scattering angle θ and azimuthal angle φ. The scattering plane is originated by the vector $\vec{S}_1$ and the z-axis. The electrical field of the incident light is in the x-y plane and can be resolved into components parallel, $\vec{E}_{\|i}$, and perpendicular, $\vec{E}_{\perp i}$, to the scattering plane. The electrical-field vector and the intensity of the incident light beam are given by

$$\vec{E}_i = \vec{E}_{\|i} + \vec{E}_{\perp i}, \tag{1.55}$$

$$I_i = \langle E_{\|i} E^*_{\|i} + E_{\perp i} E^*_{\perp i} \rangle, \tag{1.56}$$

where the asterisk denotes complex conjugation and the angular brackets denote a time average.

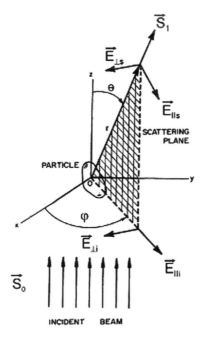

Figure 1.23 Geometry of the scattering of light by a particle located at the origin.[148] The incident light beam is parallel to the z-axis. A detector is located a distance r from the origin along the vector $\vec{S}_1$.

The electrical field of the scattered light wave is perpendicular to $\vec{S}_1$ and can be resolved into components $E_{\|s}$ and $E_{\perp s}$, which are parallel and perpendicular, respectively, to the scattering plane. The scattered electrical-field vector is given by

$$\vec{E}_s = \vec{E}_{\|s} + \vec{E}_{\perp s}.$$ (1.57)

There is a linear relationship between the incident and scattered field components, defined by Eqs. (1.55) and (1.57):[43,148,149]

$$\begin{bmatrix} E_{\|s} \\ E_{\perp s} \end{bmatrix} = \frac{e^{ik(r-z)}}{-ikr} \begin{bmatrix} S_2 & S_3 \\ S_4 & S_1 \end{bmatrix} \begin{bmatrix} E_{\|i} \\ E_{\perp i} \end{bmatrix},$$ (1.58)

where $k = 2\pi/\lambda$ is the wave number, $\lambda = \lambda_0/\bar{n}$ is the wavelength in the scattering medium; $\bar{n}$ is the mean refractive index of the scattering medium; λ_0 is the wavelength of the light in vacuum; $i = \sqrt{-1}$; r is the distance from the scatterer to the detector; and z is the position coordinate of the scatterer. The complex numbers S_{1-4} are the elements of the amplitude scattering matrix (S-matrix) or Jones matrix.[43,148,149,160,443–449] They each depend on scattering and azimuthal angles θ and φ, and contain information about the scatterer. Both amplitude and phase must be measured to quantify the amplitude scattering matrix. The direct measurements of matrix elements can be done using a two-frequency Zeeman laser, which produces two laser lines with a small frequency separation (about 250 kHz) and orthogonal linear polarizations,[149] or by the coherence optical tomography (OCT) technique.[418]

1.4.4 Polarized light description and detection

Definitions of polarized light and its properties, as well as production and detection techniques, are well described in literature.[135,160,443–448] Polarization refers to the pattern described by the electric-field vector as a function of time at a fixed point in space. When the electrical-field vector oscillates in a single, fixed plane all along the beam, the light is said to be linearly polarized. This linearly polarized wave can be resolved into components parallel and perpendicular to the scattering plane [see Eqs (1.55) and (1.57) and Fig. 1.23]. If the plane of the electrical field rotates, the light is said to be elliptically polarized because the electrical-field vector traces out an ellipse at a fixed point in space as a function of time. If the ellipse happens to be a circle, the light is said to be circularly polarized. The connection between phase and polarization can be understood as follows: circularly polarized light consists of equal amounts of linear mutually orthogonal polarized components that oscillate exactly 90 deg out of phase. In general, light of arbitrary elliptical polarization consists of unequal amplitudes of linearly polarized components, and the electrical fields of the two polarizations oscillate at the same frequency but have some constant phase difference.

Light of arbitrary polarization can be represented by four numbers known as the Stokes parameters, I, Q, U, and V. I refers to the irradiance or intensity of the light; the parameters Q, U, and V represent the extent of horizontal linear, 45 deg linear, and circular polarization, respectively.[135,160,443–448]

In polarimetry, the Stokes vector $\mathbf{S}$ of a light beam is constructed based on six flux measurements obtained with different polarization analyzers in front of the detector:

$$\mathbf{S} = \begin{pmatrix} I \\ Q \\ U \\ V \end{pmatrix} = \begin{pmatrix} I_H + I_V \\ I_H - I_V \\ I_{+45°} - I_{-45°} \\ I_R - I_L \end{pmatrix}, \tag{1.59}$$

where I_H, I_V, $I_{+45°}$, $I_{-45°}$, I_R, and I_L are the light intensities measured with a horizontal linear polarizer, a vertical linear polarizer, a $+45°$ linear polarizer, a $-45°$ linear polarizer, a right circular analyzer, and a left circular analyzer in front of the detector, respectively. Because of the relationship $I_H + I_V = I_{+45°} + I_{-45°} = I_R + I_L = I$, where I is the intensity of the light beam measured without any analyzer in front of the detector, a Stokes vector can be determined by four independent measurements, for example, I_H, I_V, $I_{+45°}$, and I_R:

$$\mathbf{S} = \begin{pmatrix} I_H + I_V \\ I_H - I_V \\ 2I_{+45°} - (I_H + I_V) \\ 2I_R - (I_H + I_V) \end{pmatrix}. \tag{1.60}$$

From the Stokes vector, the degree of polarization (DOP), the degree of linear polarization (DOLP), and the degree of circular polarization (DOCP) are derived as

$$\mathrm{DOP} = \frac{\sqrt{Q^2 + U^2 + V^2}}{I},$$

$$\mathrm{DOLP} = \frac{\sqrt{Q^2 + U^2}}{I}, \tag{1.61}$$

$$\mathrm{DOCP} = \frac{\sqrt{V^2}}{I}.$$

If the DOP of a light field remains at unity after transformation by an optical system, this system is nondepolarizing; otherwise, the system is depolarizing.

The values of the normalized Stokes parameters, which correspond to a certain type of polarization, are presented in Table 1.2.

The Mueller matrix $\mathbf{M}$ of a sample transforms an incident Stokes vector $\mathbf{S}_{\mathrm{in}}$ into the corresponding output Stokes vector $\mathbf{S}_{\mathrm{out}}$ as

$$\mathbf{S}_{\mathrm{out}} = \mathbf{M}\mathbf{S}_{\mathrm{in}}. \tag{1.62}$$

Table 1.2 Polarization types.[149]

Stokes parameter	Horizontal (linear)	Vertical (linear)	+45° (linear)	−45° (linear)	Right (circular)	Left (circular)
I	1	1	1	1	1	1
Q	1	−1	0	0	0	0
U	0	0	1	−1	0	0
V	0	0	0	0	1	−1

Obviously, the output Stokes vector varies with the state of the incident beam, but the Mueller matrix is determined only by the sample and the optical path. Conversely, the Mueller matrix can fully characterize the optical polarization properties of the sample. The Mueller matrix can be experimentally obtained from measurements with different combinations of source polarizers and detection analyzers. In the most general cases, a 4×4 Mueller matrix has 16 independent elements; therefore, at least 16 independent measurements must be acquired to determine a full Mueller matrix.

The normalized Stokes vectors for the four incident polarization states, H, V, +45 deg, and R, are, respectively,

$$\mathbf{S}_{Hi} = \begin{pmatrix} 1 \\ 1 \\ 0 \\ 0 \end{pmatrix}, \quad \mathbf{S}_{Vi} = \begin{pmatrix} 1 \\ -1 \\ 0 \\ 0 \end{pmatrix}, \quad \mathbf{S}_{+45°i} = \begin{pmatrix} 1 \\ 0 \\ 1 \\ 0 \end{pmatrix}, \quad \mathbf{S}_{Ri} = \begin{pmatrix} 1 \\ 0 \\ 0 \\ 1 \end{pmatrix}, \quad (1.63)$$

where H, V, +45°, and R, represent horizontal linear polarization, vertical linear polarization, +45 deg linear polarization, and right circular polarization, respectively. We may express the 4×4 Mueller matrix as $\mathbf{M} = [\mathbf{M}_1 \ \mathbf{M}_2 \ \mathbf{M}_3 \ \mathbf{M}_4]$, where $\mathbf{M}_1$, $\mathbf{M}_2$, $\mathbf{M}_3$, and $\mathbf{M}_4$ are four column vectors of four elements each. The four output Stokes vectors that correspond to the four incident polarization states, H, V, +45 deg, and R, are denoted, respectively, by $\mathbf{S}_{Ho}$, $\mathbf{S}_{Vo}$, $\mathbf{S}_{+45°o}$, and $\mathbf{S}_{Ro}$. These four output Stokes vectors are experimentally measured based on Eq. (1.60) and can be expressed as

$$\begin{cases} \mathbf{S}_{Ho} = \mathbf{M}\mathbf{S}_{Hi} = \mathbf{M}_1 + \mathbf{M}_2 \\ \mathbf{S}_{Vo} = \mathbf{M}\mathbf{S}_{Vi} = \mathbf{M}_1 - \mathbf{M}_2 \\ \mathbf{S}_{+45°o} = \mathbf{M}\mathbf{S}_{+45°i} = \mathbf{M}_1 + \mathbf{M}_3 \\ \mathbf{S}_{Ro} = \mathbf{M}\mathbf{S}_{Ri} = \mathbf{M}_1 + \mathbf{M}_4 \end{cases}. \quad (1.64)$$

The Mueller matrix can be calculated from the four output Stokes vectors as[449]

$$\mathbf{M} = \frac{1}{2}[\mathbf{S}_{Ho} + \mathbf{S}_{Vo} \quad \mathbf{S}_{Ho} - \mathbf{S}_{Vo} \quad -2\mathbf{S}_{+45°o}(\mathbf{S}_{Ho} + \mathbf{S}_{Vo}) \quad 2\mathbf{S}_{Ro} - (\mathbf{S}_{Ho} + \mathbf{S}_{Vo})]. \quad (1.65)$$

In other words, at least four independent Stokes vectors must be measured to determine a full Mueller matrix, and each Stokes vector requires four independent intensity measurements with different analyzers.

1.4.5 Light interaction with a random single scattering media

In terms of the electrical-field components, the Stokes parameters from Eqs. (1.59) and (1.60) are given by

$$
\begin{aligned}
I &= \langle E_\| E_\|^* + E_\perp E_\perp^* \rangle \\
Q &= \langle E_\| E_\|^* - E_\perp E_\perp^* \rangle \\
U &= \langle E_\| E_\perp^* + E_\perp E_\|^* \rangle \\
V &= \langle i (E_\| E_\perp^* - E_\perp E_\|^*) \rangle
\end{aligned}
\tag{1.66}
$$

All Stokes parameters have the same dimension—energy per unit area per unit time per unit wavelength. For an elementary monochromatic plane or spherical electromagnetic wave,[145]

$$
I^2 \equiv Q^2 + U^2 + V^2.
\tag{1.67a}
$$

For an arbitrary light beam, as in the case of a partially polarized quasi-monochromatic light that is due to the fundamental property of additivity, the Stokes parameters for the mixture of the elementary waves are sums of the respective Stokes parameters of these waves. Equation (1.67a) is replaced by the inequality[145,148]

$$
I^2 \geq Q^2 + U^2 + V^2.
\tag{1.67b}
$$

The degree of polarization (DOP), the degree of linear polarization (DOLP), and the degree of circular polarization (DOCP) for the incident and scattered light are defined by Eq. (1.61). In particular, for the DOLP (P_L) and the DOCP (P_C) of the scattered light, we have

$$
P_L = \frac{I_\| - I_\perp}{I_\| + I_\perp} = \frac{\sqrt{Q_s^2 + U_s^2}}{I_s},
\tag{1.68a}
$$

$$
P_C = \frac{\sqrt{V_s^2}}{I_s}.
\tag{1.68b}
$$

In the far field, the polarization of the scattered light is described by the Stokes vector $\mathbf{S}_s$ connected with the Stokes vector of the incident light $\mathbf{S}_i$ [see Eq. (1.62)][148]

$$
\mathbf{S}_s = \mathbf{M} \cdot \mathbf{S}_i,
\tag{1.69}
$$

where $\mathbf{M}$ is the normalized 4×4 scattering matrix (intensity or Mueller's matrix)

$$\mathbf{M} = \begin{bmatrix} M_{11} & M_{12} & M_{13} & M_{14} \\ M_{21} & M_{22} & M_{23} & M_{24} \\ M_{31} & M_{32} & M_{33} & M_{34} \\ M_{41} & M_{42} & M_{43} & M_{44} \end{bmatrix}. \tag{1.70}$$

Elements of the light-scattering matrix (LSM) depend on the scattering angle θ, the wavelength, and geometrical and optical parameters of the scatterers. M_{11} is what is measured when the incident light is unpolarized, the scattering angle dependence of which is the phase function of the scattered light. It provides only a fraction of the information theoretically available from scattering experiments. M_{11} is much less sensitive to chirality and long-range structure than some of the other matrix elements.[148,149] M_{12} refers to the degree of linear polarization of the scattered light; M_{22} displays the ratio of depolarized light to the total scattered light (a good measure of the scatterers' nonsphericity); M_{34} displays the transformation of 45-deg obliquely polarized incident light to circularly polarized scattered light (which is uniquely characteristic for different biological systems); the difference between M_{33} and M_{44} is a good measure of the scatterers' nonsphericity.

In addition to the degree of light polarization, defined by Eqs. (1.61), (1.68a), and (1.68b), diattenuation (linear dichroism) is introduced as

$$D_A = \frac{P_1^2 - P_2^2}{P_1^2 + P_2^2} = \frac{\sqrt{M_{12}^2 + M_{13}^2 + M_{14}^2}}{M_{11}}, \tag{1.71}$$

where P_1 and P_2 are the principal coefficients of the amplitude transmission for the two orthogonal polarization eigenstates.

In general, all 16 elements of the LSM are nonzero. However, there are only seven independent elements (out of 16) in the scattering matrix of a single particle with fixed orientation, and nine relations, which connect the others together.[145,146] For scattering by a collection of randomly oriented scatterers, there are 10 independent elements.

The LSM for macroscopically isotropic and symmetric media has the well-known block-diagonal structure[182]

$$\mathbf{M}(\theta) = \begin{bmatrix} M_{11}(\theta) & M_{12}(\theta) & 0 & 0 \\ M_{12}(\theta) & M_{22}(\theta) & 0 & 0 \\ 0 & 0 & M_{33}(\theta) & M_{34}(\theta) \\ 0 & 0 & -M_{34}(\theta) & M_{44}(\theta) \end{bmatrix}. \tag{1.72}$$

It follows that only eight LSM elements are nonzero and only six of these are independent. Moreover, there are special relationships for two specific scattering angles 0 and π:[145]

$$M_{22}(0) = M_{33}(0), \quad M_{22}(\pi) = -M_{33}(\pi),$$

$$M_{12}(0) = M_{34}(0) = M_{12}(\pi) = M_{34}(\pi) = 0, \qquad (1.73)$$

$$M_{44}(\pi) = M_{11}(\pi) - 2M_{22}(\pi).$$

Rotationally symmetric particles have an additional property:[145]

$$M_{44}(0) = 2M_{22}(0) - M_{11}(0). \qquad (1.74)$$

The structure of the LSM further simplifies for spherically symmetric particles, which are homogeneous or radially inhomogeneous (composed of isotropic materials with a refractive index that depends only on the distance from the particle center), because in this case[145]

$$M_{11}(\theta) \equiv M_{22}(\theta), \ M_{33}(\theta) \equiv M_{44}(\theta). \qquad (1.75)$$

The phase function, i.e., the M_{11} element, for scattering symmetric relative to the direction of the incident wave depends only on the scattering angle θ and satisfies the normalization condition [see Eq. (1.14)][145,148]

$$2\pi \int_0^\pi M_{11}(\theta) \sin\theta d\theta = 1, \qquad (1.76)$$

which corresponds to assumption of random distribution of scatterers in a medium.

The scattering anisotropy parameter (mean cosine of the scattering angle θ) or the asymmetry parameter of the phase function [see Eq. (1.16)] is expressed now as

$$g \equiv \langle \cos\theta \rangle = 2\pi \int_0^\pi M_{11}(\theta) \cos\theta \sin\theta d\theta. \qquad (1.77)$$

If a particle is small with respect to the wavelength of the incident light, its scattering can be described as the reemission of a single dipole. This Rayleigh theory is applicable under the condition that $m(2\pi a/\lambda) \ll 1$, where m is the relative refractive index of the scatterers, $(2\pi a/\lambda)$ is the size parameter, a is the radius of the particle, and λ is the wavelength of the incident light in a medium.[148] For the visible and NIR light and scatterers with a typical (for biological tissue) refractive index relative to the ground matter $m = 1.05$–1.11, the maximum particle radius must be about 12–14 nm for Rayleigh theory to remain valid. For this theory, the scattered irradiance is inversely proportional to λ^4 and increases as a^6; the angular distribution of the scattered light is isotropic.

The Rayleigh-Gans or Rayleigh-Debye theory addresses the problem of calculating the scattering by a special class of arbitrary shaped particles. It requires $|m - 1| \ll 1$ and $(2\pi a'/\lambda)|m - 1| \ll 1$, where a' is the largest dimension of the particle.[129,145,146,149] These conditions mean that the electrical field inside the particle must be close to that of the incident field and that the particle can be viewed as a collection of independent dipoles that are all exposed to the same incident field. A biological cell might be modeled as a sphere of cytoplasm with a higher refractive index ($n_{cp} = 1.37$) relative to that of the surrounding water medium ($n_{is} = 1.35$); then $m = 1.015$, and for the NIR light, this theory is valid for particle dimensions up to $a' = 0.8$–1.0 μm. This approximation has been applied extensively to calculations of light scattering from suspensions of bacteria.[149] It can be applicable for describing light scattering from cell components (mitochondria, lysosomes, peroxisomes, etc.) in tissues due to their small dimensions and refraction.[58,96,150–153,163,166]

For describing the forward scattering caused by large particles (on the order of 10 μm), the Fraunhofer diffraction approximation is useful.[149] According to this theory, the scattered light has the same polarization as that of the incident light and the scatterer pattern is independent of the refractive index of the object. For small scattering angles, the Fraunhofer diffraction approximation can accurately represent the change in irradiance as a function of particle size. That is why this approach is applicable in laser flow cytometry. The structures in a biological cell, such as cell membrane, nuclear texture, and granules in the cytoplasm, can be detected by variations in optical density. An optical Fourier transform of the diffraction pattern can be performed by a lens. Spatial variations in optical density in the object plane are converted by a Fourier transform into spatial frequency variations in the Fourier transform plane in the rear focal plane of the lens.[149] If the optical density changes slowly across the object, the Fourier transform places most of the scattered light near zero angles (low spatial frequency) in the Fourier transform plane. This is a good model of a cell with clear cytoplasm (constant optical density). If the optical density changes rapidly across the object, the Fourier transform moves more of the energy to larger scattering angles (higher spatial frequency) in the Fourier transform plane. This is a good model of a cell with highly granular cytoplasm (rapid changes in optical density across the cytoplasm). It was shown that the transforms of abnormal cells have significantly high spatial frequency compared with the transforms of normal cells, in particular single cells in cervical smears. Fourier optical microscopes were developed for such studies. The technique is applicable for a positive photographic transparency of the cell, single cells on slides, and cells in flows.[149]

Mie or Lorenz-Mie scattering theory is an exact solution of Maxwell's electromagnetic field equations for a homogeneous sphere.[148,160] In the general case, light scattered at a particle becomes elliptically polarized. For spherically symmetric particles of an optically inactive material, the Mueller scattering matrix is given by Eqs. (1.72) and (1.75). Mie theory has been extended to arbitrary coated spheres and to arbitrary cylinders.[145,146,149] In the Mie theory, the electromagnetic fields of the incident, internal, and scattered waves are each expanded in a series.[160] A linear transformation can be made between the fields in each of the regions. This approach can also be used for nonspherical objects such as spheroids.[145,146] The linear transformation is called the transition matrix (T-matrix). The T-matrix for spherical particles is diagonal.

Thus far, Stokes vectors have been defined for the case of a monochromatic plane wave, and the Mueller matrix for single scattering. These concepts have been generalized to more complicated situations. The Stokes vector was defined for a quasi-monochromatic wave.[181] Then in the case of partially polarized light, the inequality, described by Eq. (1.67b), is valid.[148]

When Mueller matrices from an ensemble of particles differing in size, orientation, morphology, or optical properties are added incoherently, six of the above-mentioned equalities became inequalities.[381] For an ensemble of interacting particles in the single scattering approximation,[5,6,10,442] LSM elements have the form

$$M_{ij}(\theta) = M_{ij}^0(\theta)NF_{\text{int}}(\theta), \qquad (1.78)$$

where M_{ij}^0 are the LSM elements of an isolated particle, N is the number of scatterers, and $F_{\text{int}}(\theta)$ is the interference term, taking into account the spatial correlation of particles. Note that the normalized elements (M_{ij}/M_{11}) in a monodisperse system weakly depend on whether account is taken of the spatial correlation of scatterers, and this ratio is close to that for isolated particles.[442]

1.4.6 Vector radiative transfer equation

As it was already shown, the majority of tissues are turbid media showing a strong scattering and much less absorption (up to two orders less than scattering in the visible and NIR ranges). Moreover, in their natural state (nonsliced), tissues are rather thick. Therefore, multiple scattering is a specific feature of a wide class of tissues.[1–3,6,24,31,129,130]

Polarization effects at light propagation through various multiply scattering media, including tissues, are fully described by the vector radiative transfer equation (RTE).[59,145,146,188,344–366] The radiative transfer theory (RTT) originated as a phenomenological approach based on considering the transport of energy through a medium filled with a large number of particles and ensuring energy conservation.[182–185] This medium, composed of discrete, sparsely, and randomly distributed particles, is treated as continuous and locally homogeneous. Discussed above, the concept of single scattering and absorption by an individual particle is thus replaced in this subsection by the concept of single scattering and absorption by a small homogeneous volume element. In the framework of the RTT, the scattering and absorption of the small volume element follow from the Maxwell equations and are given by the incoherent sums of the respective characteristics of the constituent particles; the result of scattering is not the transformation of a plane incident wave into a spherical scattered wave but the transformation of the specific intensity vector (Stokes) of the incident light into the specific intensity vector of the scattered light.[146,188]

For macroscopically isotropic and symmetric plane-parallel scattering media, the vector radiative transfer equation (VRTE) can be substantially simplified as follows:[146,188]

$$\frac{dS(\bar{r}, \vartheta, \varphi)}{d\tau(\bar{r})} = -S(\bar{r}, \vartheta, \varphi)$$

$$+ \frac{\Lambda(\bar{r})}{4\pi} \int_{-1}^{+1} d(\cos\vartheta') \int_{0}^{2\pi} d\varphi' \overline{Z}(\bar{r}, \vartheta, \vartheta', \varphi - \varphi')S(\bar{r}, \vartheta', \varphi'),$$

$$(1.79)$$

where S is the Stokes vector defined by Eq. (1.59); $\bar{r}$ is the position vector; ϑ, φ are the angles characterizing incident direction, respectively, the polar (zenith) and the azimuth angles;

$$d\tau(\bar{r}) = \rho(\bar{r})\langle\sigma_{ext}(\bar{r})\rangle ds \qquad (1.80)$$

is the optical-path-length element, ρ is the local particle-number density, $\langle\sigma_{ext}\rangle$ is the local ensemble-averaged extinction coefficient, ds is the path-length element measured along the unit vector of the direction of light propagation; Λ is the single scattering albedo; ϑ', φ' are the angles characterizing scattering direction, respectively, the polar (zenith) and the azimuth angles; $\overline{Z}$ is the normalized phase matrix

$$\overline{Z}(\bar{r}, \vartheta, \vartheta', \varphi - \varphi') = R(\Phi)M(\theta)R(\Psi), \qquad (1.81)$$

where $M(\theta)$ is the single scattering Mueller matrix, defined by Eq. (1.62); θ is the scattering angle, and $R(\phi)$ is the Stokes rotation matrix for angle ϕ:

$$R(\phi) = \begin{bmatrix} 1 & 0 & 0 & 0 \\ 0 & \cos 2\phi & -\sin 2\phi & 0 \\ 0 & \sin 2\phi & \cos 2\phi & 0 \\ 0 & 0 & 0 & 1 \end{bmatrix}. \qquad (1.82)$$

Every Stokes vector and Mueller matrix are associated with a specific reference plane and coordinates. In the Mie theory, the Mueller matrix of a single scattering event is defined in the scattering plane that is formed by the incident light vector and the scattered light vector (see Fig. 1.23). For a general coordinate system associated with this scattering plane, the z-axis is along the direction of photon propagation. The x-axis is within the reference plane and is perpendicular to the z-axis. The y-axis is perpendicular to both the z-axis and the reference plane.

There is a local coordinate system associated with each incident photon packet, and its Stokes vector S_{in} is associated with this local coordinate system. The local coordinate system of the photon before scattering is (x, y, z). After the scattering event, the photon propagates along the z'-axis with θ as the polar scattering angle and φ as the azimuth angle. The scattering plane is formed by the z-axis and the z'-axis, which is the new reference plane.

To calculate the Stokes vector of the scattered light, Eq. (1.59) is used. Because the Mueller matrix of the scattering event defined in the reference plane [see

Eq. (1.62)], we need first to transform the Stokes vector of the incident light to the coordinate system associated with the reference plane. This transformation can be done by rotating the local coordinate system (x, y, z) by ϕ about the z-axis, where the rotation matrix is defined by Eq. (1.82). The new Stokes vector is obtained by

$$\mathbf{S}'_{in} = \mathbf{R}(\phi)\mathbf{S}_{in}. \tag{1.83}$$

The local coordinate system of the photon packet is tracked in the process. The transformation can be divided into two steps. The first step is rotating the (x, y, z) system by ϕ about the z-axis, and the second step is to rotate the coordinate by θ about the rotated y-axis to get (x', y', z'). After the transformation, the z'-axis is aligned with the new light vector. The transformation matrix is

$$\begin{bmatrix} x' \\ y' \\ z' \end{bmatrix} = \begin{bmatrix} \cos\theta & 0 & -\sin\theta \\ 0 & 1 & 0 \\ \sin\theta & 0 & \cos\theta \end{bmatrix} \begin{bmatrix} \cos\phi & \sin\phi & 0 \\ -\sin\phi & \cos\phi & 0 \\ 0 & 0 & 1 \end{bmatrix} \begin{bmatrix} x \\ y \\ y \end{bmatrix}. \tag{1.84}$$

After a photon packet passes through the turbid medium, its Stokes vector is recorded and accumulated. The local coordinate system is tracked in the simulation. In order to record the Stokes vector, the local coordinate system of each photon packet needs to be transformed into the laboratory coordinate system. In the laboratory coordinate system (e_1, e_2, e_3), the local photon coordinate can be written as

$$\begin{bmatrix} x \\ y \\ z \end{bmatrix} = \begin{bmatrix} e_{1x} & e_{2x} & e_{3x} \\ e_{1y} & e_{2y} & e_{3y} \\ e_{1z} & e_{2z} & e_{3z} \end{bmatrix} \begin{bmatrix} e_1 \\ e_2 \\ e_3 \end{bmatrix}. \tag{1.85}$$

To transform the photon Stokes vector from the local coordinate system into the laboratory coordinate system, the local coordinate system is rotated about its z-axis so that the new x-axis lies within the (e_2, e_3) plane in the laboratory coordinate. The rotation angle is

$$\phi = \tan^{-1}\left(\frac{e_{1x}}{e_{1y}}\right). \tag{1.86}$$

The rotation matrix and the new Stokes vector can be obtained from Eqs. (1.82) and (1.83).

The phase matrix, Eq. (1.81), links the Stokes vectors of the incident and scattered beams, specified relative to their respective meridional planes. To compute the Stokes vector of the scattered beam with respect to its meridional plane, one must calculate the Stokes vector of the incident beam with respect to the scattering plane, multiply it by the scattering matrix (to obtain the Stokes vector of the scattered beam with respect to the scattering plane), and then compute the Stokes vector of the scattered beam with respect to its meridional plane. Such a procedure involves two rotations of the reference plane: $\Phi = -\phi$; $\Psi = \pi - \phi$ and $\Phi = \pi + \phi$;

and $\Psi = \phi$. The scattering angle θ and the angles Φ and Ψ are expressed via the polar and the azimuth incident and scattering angles:

$$\cos\theta = \cos\vartheta' \cos\vartheta + \sin\vartheta' \sin\vartheta \cos(\varphi' - \varphi),$$

$$\cos\Phi = \frac{\cos\vartheta - \cos\vartheta' \cos\theta}{\sin\vartheta' \sin\theta}, \qquad (1.87)$$

$$\cos\Psi = \frac{\cos\vartheta' - \cos\vartheta \cos\theta}{\sin\vartheta \sin\theta}.$$

The first term on the right-hand side of the VRTE [Eq. (1.79)] describes the change in the specific intensity vector over the distance ds caused by extinction and dichroism, the second term describes the contribution of light illuminating a small volume element centered at $\bar{r}$ from all incident directions and scattered into the chosen direction. For real systems, the form of the VRTE tends to be rather complex and often intractable. Therefore, a wide range of analytical and numerical techniques have been developed to solve the VRTE. Because of the important property of the normalized phase matrix, Eq. (1.81), being dependent on the difference of the azimuthal angles of the scattering and incident directions rather than on their specific values,[146,188] an efficient analytical treatment of the azimuthal dependence of the multiply scattered light, using a Fourier decomposition of the VRTE, is possible. The following techniques and their combinations can be used to solve the VRTE: transfer matrix method, the singular eigenfunction method, the perturbation method, the small-angle approximation, the adding-doubling method, the matrix operator method, the invariant embedding method, and the Monte Carlo method.[129,138,145,146,187,188,344–368]

When the medium is illuminated by unpolarized light and/or only the intensity of multiply scattered light needs to be computed, the VRTE can be replaced by its approximate scalar counterpart. In that case, in Eq. (1.79), the Stokes vector is replaced by its first element (i.e., radiance) [see Eq. (1.9)] and the normalized phase matrix by its (1, 1) element (i.e., the phase function) [see Eq. (1.13)]. The scalar approximation gives poor accuracy when the size of the scattering particles is much smaller than the wavelength, but provides acceptable results for particles comparable to and larger than the wavelength.[146,184] There is ample literature[1,3,15,129,130,185,188–190] on the analytical and numerical solutions of the scalar RTE, Eq. (1.9).

1.4.7 Monte Carlo simulation

The Monte Carlo (MC) method, being widely used for the numerical solution of the RTT equation[368–370] in different fields (astrophysics, atmosphere and ocean optics, etc.), appears to be especially promising for the solution of direct and inverse radiation transfer problems for media with arbitrary configurations and boundary conditions, in particular for the purposes of the medical polarization optical tomography and spectroscopy.[1,3,15,41,129,213,215,349,357,361–367] The method is based on the numerical simulation of photon transport in scattering media. Random migrations of photons inside a sample can be traced from their input until absorption or output occur.

The straightforward simulation using the MC method has the following advantages: (1) one can employ any scattering matrix; (2) there are no obstacles for the use of strongly forward directed phase functions or experimental single scattering matrices; (3) the polarization calculation takes only a twofold increase in computation time over that needed for the evaluation of intensity; (4) any reasonable number of detectors can be accounted for without noticeable increase of the computation time; (5) there are no difficulties in determining the radiation parameters inside the medium; (6) it is possible to model media with complex geometry where radiance depends not only on the optical depth, but also on the transverse coordinates.

The liability of the obtained results to statistical variations on the order of a few percent at an acceptable computation time is the main disadvantage of the MC technique. For a twofold increase of the accuracy, one needs a fourfold increase in the computation time. The MC method is also impractical for great optical depths $(\tau > 100)$.

A few MC codes for modeling of polarized light propagation through a scattering layer are available in the literature (see, for example, Refs. 349, 357, and 361–367). To illustrate the MC simulation technique, the algorithm described in Ref. 366 and applied to model the angular dependencies of the scattering matrix elements is discussed. Let a flux of photons within an infinitely narrow beam be incident exactly upon the center of the spherical volume filled up by the scattering particles.[366] The path of a single photon migration in the medium is accounted for in a process of computer simulation. The photons are considered in this case as ballistic particles. Different events possible in the course of the photon migration are estimated by the appropriate probability distributions. In the model under study, the photons would either be elastically scattered or absorbed under their collisions with the medium particles. A certain outcome of every event is found by a set of uniformly distributed random numbers. The probability of scattering in the given direction is determined in accordance with scattering by a single particle. One is able to specify the cross section of scattering and values of the scattering matrix elements for every photon interaction with a scatterer.

When an incident photon enters a scattering layer, it is allowed to travel a free path length, l. The l value depends on the particle concentration ρ and extinction cross section σ_{ext}. The free path length l is a random quantity that takes any positive values with the probability density $p(l)$:

$$p(l) = \rho \sigma_{ext} e^{-\rho \sigma_{ext} l}. \tag{1.88}$$

The particular realization of the free path length l is dictated by the value of a random number ξ that is uniformly distributed over the interval $[0, 1]$:

$$\int_0^l p(l)dl = \xi.$$ (1.89)

Substituting Eq. (1.88) into Eq. (1.89) yields the value l of the certain realization in the form

$$l = -\frac{1}{\rho\sigma_{\text{ext}}} \ln \xi.$$ (1.90)

If the distance l is larger than the thickness of the scattering system, then this photon is detected as transmitted without any scattering. If, having passed the distance l, the photon remains within the scattering volume, then the possible events of photon-particle interaction (scattering or absorption) are randomly selected.

Within the spherical system of coordinates, the probability density of photon scattering along the direction specified by the angle of scattering θ between the directions of the incident and scattered photons and by the angle ϕ between the previous and new scattering planes is given as

$$p(\theta, \phi) = \frac{I_s(\theta, \phi) \sin \theta}{\int_0^{2\pi} \int_0^\pi I_s(\theta, \phi) \sin \theta d\theta d\phi},$$ (1.91)

where $I_s(\theta, \phi)$ is the intensity of the light scattered in the direction (θ, ϕ) with respect to the previous direction of the photon, defined by angels ϑ and φ [see Eqs. (1.79) and (1.80)]. For spherical particles, this intensity is given by the Mie formulas with allowance for the state of polarization of each photon. An integral $I_s(\theta, \phi)$ over all scattering directions, similar to Eq. (1.6), determines the scattering cross section

$$\sigma_{\text{sca}} = \int_0^{2\pi} \int_0^\pi I_s(\theta, \phi) \sin \theta d\theta d\phi.$$ (1.92)

The probability density of photon scattering along the specified direction, $p(\theta, \phi)$, depends on the Mueller matrix of the scattering particle $\mathbf{M}(\theta, \phi)$ (a single scattering matrix) and the Stokes vector $\mathbf{S}$ associated with the photon [Eqs. (1.59) and (1.69)]. The single scattering Mueller matrix $\mathbf{M}(\theta, \phi)$ links the Stokes vectors of the incident $[\mathbf{S}_i(0, 0)]$ and scattered $[\mathbf{S}_s(\theta, \phi)]$ light. For spherical scatterers, the elements of this matrix may be factorized:

$$\mathbf{M}(\theta, \phi) = \mathbf{M}(\theta)\mathbf{R}(\phi).$$ (1.93)

The single scattering matrix $\mathbf{M}(\theta)$ of spherical particles has the form described by Eqs. (1.72) and (1.75). The elements of this matrix are given by the Mie formulas,[148,160] which are functions of the scattering angle θ and diffraction parameter $x = 2\pi a/\lambda$, where a is the radius of the spherical particle, and λ is the wavelength in the medium.

The matrix $\mathbf{R}(\phi)$ describes the transformation of the Stokes vector under rotation of the plane of scattering through the angle ϕ, which is defined by Eq. (1.82). Thus, the intensity of the light scattered by spherical particles is determined by the expression

$$I_s(\theta, \phi) = [M_{11}(\theta)I_i + (Q_i \cos 2\phi + U_i \sin 2\phi)M_{12}(\theta)], \qquad (1.94)$$

where Q_i and U_i are components of the Stokes vector of the incident light [see Eqs. (1.59) and (1.66)]. As it follows from this equation, the probability $p(\theta, \phi)$ [Eq. (1.91)], unlike the scattering matrix (Eq. 1.93), cannot be factorized, it appears to be parametrized by the Stokes vector associated with the scattered photon. In this case, one should use a rejection method to evaluate $p(\theta, \phi)$.

The following method of generating pairs of random numbers with the probability density $p(\theta, \phi)$ may be used.[366] In a three-dimensional space, the function $p(\theta, \phi)$ specifies some surface. The values (θ, ϕ) corresponding to the distribution $p(\theta, \phi)$ are chosen using the following steps: (1) a random direction (θ_ξ, ϕ_ξ) with a uniform spatial distribution is selected, the values of the random quantities θ_ξ, and ϕ_ξ distributed over the intervals $(0, \pi)$ and $(0, 2\pi)$, respectively, are found from the equations

$$\phi_\xi = 2\pi\xi, \cos \theta_\xi = 2\xi - 1, \qquad (1.95)$$

where ξ is a random number uniformly distributed over the interval $(0, 1)$; (2) the surface specified by the function $p(\theta, \phi)$ is surrounded by a sphere of radius $\hat{R}$, equal to the maximum value of the function $p(\theta, \phi)$, and a random quantity $r_\xi = \xi \hat{R}$ is generated; (3) the direction (θ_ξ, ϕ_ξ) is accepted as the random direction of the photon scattering at this stage, provided the condition $r_\xi \leq p(\theta_\xi, \phi_\xi)$ is satisfied. In the opposite case, steps 1 and 2 are repeated again.

The migration of the photon in the scattering medium can be described by a sequence of transformations for the related coordinate system. Each scattering event is accompanied by a variation of the Stokes vector associated with the photon. The new Stokes vector $\mathbf{S}_{n+1}$ is a product of the preceding Stokes vector, transformed to the new scattering plane, and the Mueller matrix $\mathbf{M}_k(\theta)$ of the scattering particle:

$$\mathbf{S}_{n+1} = \mathbf{M}_k(\theta)\mathbf{R}_n(\phi)\mathbf{S}_n, \qquad (1.96)$$

where the matrix $\mathbf{R}_n(\phi)$ [see Eq. (1.82)] describes rotation of the Stokes vector around the axis specifying the direction of propagation of the photon before the interaction.

For the chosen scattering direction, the Stokes vector is recalculated using Eqs. (1.69), (1.72), (1.75), and (1.96), and expressions for elements of the single-scattering Mueller matrix for a homogeneous sphere made of an optically inactive material.[135,148,160] The value thus obtained is renormalized so that the intensity remains equal to unity. Thus, the Stokes vector associated with the photon contains information only about the variation of the state of polarization of the scattered photon. Real intensity is determined by the number of detected photons in the chosen direction within the detector aperture.

The above procedure is repeated as long as the photon appears to be outside the scattering volume. In this case, if the photon propagation direction intersects the surface of the detector, the photon is detected. Upon detection, the Stokes vector is rotated from the current plane of the last scattering to the scattering plane of laboratory coordinate system. The values obtained are accumulated in the appropriate cells of the detector whose number is defined by the photon migration direction. Furthermore, with registering, the photon is classified in accordance with the scattering multiplicity and the length of a total path. For every nonabsorbed photon, the direction and the coordinates of a point at which it escapes the scattering volume, as well as the number of scattering acts it has experienced, were also recorded. The spatial distribution of radiation scattered by the scattering volume can be obtained with regard to polarization by analyzing the above data for a sufficiently great number of photons.

To find the full LSM of an object, one has to detect the light scattering for four linearly independent states of polarization of the incident light, $\mathbf{S}_{1i}$, $\mathbf{S}_{2i}$, $\mathbf{S}_{3i}$, and $\mathbf{S}_{4i}$. This allows one to construct the following system of linear equations:

$$\mathbf{CM'} = \mathbf{S'}, \tag{1.97}$$

where $\mathbf{M'}$ is the column matrix composed of matrix elements of the LSM of the object, and $\mathbf{S'}$ is the 16-element vector containing the Stokes vector elements recorded upon light scattering for the four independent states of the incident light polarization. The transformation matrix $\mathbf{C}$ is determined by the choice of the initial set of the Stokes vectors of the incident light. Having solved this system of equations for the set of Stokes vectors, $\mathbf{S}_{1i} = (1, 1, 0, 0)$, $\mathbf{S}_{2i} = (1, -1, 0, 0)$, $\mathbf{S}_{3i} = (1, 0, 1, 0)$, and $\mathbf{S}_{4i} = (1, 0, 0, 1)$, one finds the desired LSM of the object, $\mathbf{M'} = \mathbf{M}$:

$$\mathbf{M} = \frac{1}{2} \begin{bmatrix} I_1 + I_2 & I_1 - I_2 & 2I_3 - (I_1 + I_2) & 2I_4 - (I_1 + I_2) \\ Q_1 + Q_2 & Q_1 - Q_2 & 2Q_3 - (Q_1 + Q_2) & 2Q_4 - (Q_1 + Q_2) \\ U_1 + U_2 & U_1 - U_2 & 2U_3 - (U_1 + U_2) & 2U_4 - (U_1 + U_2) \\ V_1 + V_2 & V_1 - V_2 & 2V_3 - (V_1 + V_2) & 2V_4 - (V_1 + V_2) \end{bmatrix}, \tag{1.98}$$

where the elements of the Stokes vectors of the scattered light obtained in each of these four cases are denoted as $\mathbf{S}_n = (I_n, Q_n, U_n, V_n)$, $(n = 1, 2, 3, 4)$. As a result, one may calculate the angular dependencies for all elements of the LSM with allowance for the contributions of multiple scattering.

The simulation was performed for the systems of spherical particles with relative index of refraction $m = 1.2$, which are uniformly distributed within a spherical volume at volume fraction $f = 0.01$.[366] In the calculations, the illuminating beam was assumed to be infinitely narrow and incident exactly upon the center of the scattering volume in the zero angle direction and the scattered radiation is detected at different scattering angles in the far zone by a detector with the full angular aperture of 1 deg in the scattering plane and 5 deg in a plane that is perpendicular to the scattering one.

The calculated angular distributions of the total scattering intensity for different scattering systems of spherical particles with small radius, $a = 50$ nm, or large radius, $a = 300$ nm, are presented in Fig. 1.24. The average multiplicity of scattering of the detected radiation increases with increasing dimensions of the scattering system. For systems of small particles at illumination in the visible range (633 nm), approximation of the Rayleigh scattering is applicable. For rather small dimensions of the scattering volume of 1 mm of diameter, the contribution of single scattering is predominant. This follows from the intensity angular dependence, which is rather isotropic [Fig. 1.24(a)]. As the dimensions of the scattering system increase, the fraction of contributions of the higher multiplicity scattering grows as well. For a 20-mm diameter system, the detected light contains noticeable contributions of scattering of the 10th–20th multiplicity. With a further increase of the system dimensions, most of the incident light is scattered in the backward direction and the scattering intensity in the forward half plane vanishes. For this reason, beginning from a certain value, the dimensions of the scattering system hardly affect the shape of the diagram of the scattering multiplicity distribution.

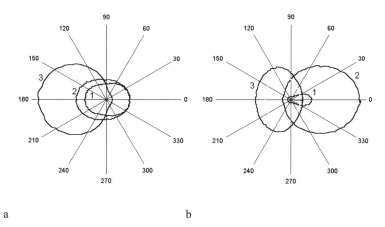

a   b

Figure 1.24 Angular distributions of the total scattering intensity for the multiply scattering systems of spherical particles that have a relative refractive index $m = 1.2$ and uniformly distributed within a spherical volume at volume fraction $f = 0.01$: (a) particles with small radius, $a = 50$ nm, diameter of the system is equal to (1) 1, (2) 2, and (3) 20 mm; and (b) particles with large radius, $a = 300$ nm, diameter of the system is equal to (1) 0.002, (2) 0.2, and (3) 2 mm; the infinitely narrow unpolarized light beam incidents exactly upon the center of the scattering volume in the zero-angle direction (not shown); the wavelength is 633 nm.[366]

Systems composed of particles with a size on the order of the wavelength [Fig. 1.24(b)] also show an increase in the contributions of higher-order scattering with increasing dimensions of the scattering system. The system transforms

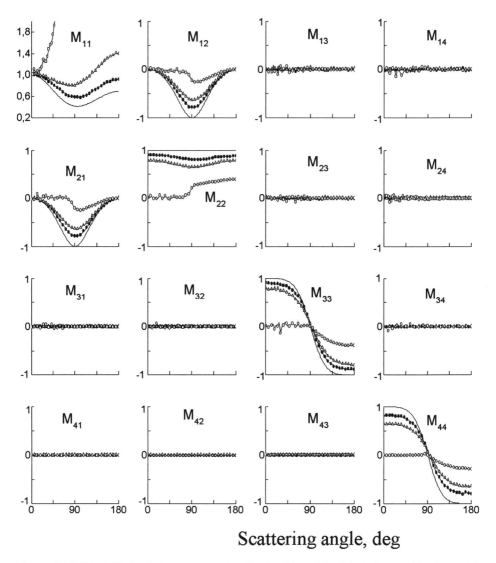

Figure 1.25 The MC simulation: the angular distributions of the LSM elements for the multiple scattering systems of small spherical particles ($a = 50$ nm, $m = 1.2$) uniformly distributed within a spherical volume ($f = 0.01$); diameter of the system is equal to 1 mm (–●–), 2 mm (–△–), and 20 mm (–○–); the solid line shows the results of calculations in the approximation of single scattering; the infinitely narrow unpolarized light beam incidents exactly upon the center of the scattering volume in the zero-angle direction (not shown); the wavelength is 633 nm.[366]

from the forward to backward directed scattering mode at rather small thickness, 2-mm diameter.

As it is seen, the intensity of unpolarized light at the higher scattering multiplicity weakly depends on the scattering angle and carries almost no information about the size of the scattering particles. Note that systems of small particles at triple scattering may already be considered as nearly isotropic, while angular dis-

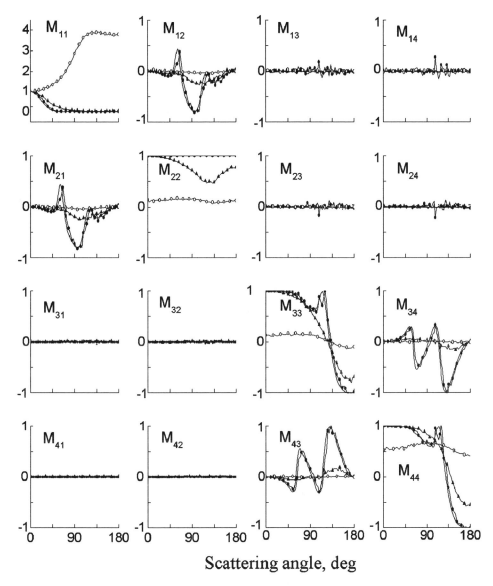

Figure 1.26 The MC simulation: the angular distributions of the LSM elements for the multiple scattering systems of large spherical particles ($a = 300$ nm, $m = 1.2$) uniformly distributed within a spherical volume ($f = 0.01$); diameter of the system is equal to 0.002 mm (–●–), 0.2 mm (–△–), and 2 mm (–○–); the solid line shows the results of calculations in the approximation of single scattering; the infinitely narrow unpolarized light beam incidents exactly upon the center of the scattering volume in the zero angle direction (not shown); the wavelength is 633 nm.[366]

tributions for the large particles, strongly elongated in the forward direction at single scattering, remain anisotropic for sufficiently high scattering multiplicity [four to six scattering events for the system of 0.2 mm diameter, Fig. 1.24(b)].

The view of the LSM elements' angular dependences under the conditions of multiple scattering differs substantially from that for the LSM of a single-scattering system. It is seen from Figs. 1.25 and 1.26 that the multiple scattering flattens the angular dependences of the LSM elements. The solid line shows the result of calculation of a normalized LSM for an isolated spherical particle with a similar radius and relative index of refraction. All elements of the LSM are normalized to the M_{11} element (total scattering intensity) along the given direction, and the element M_{11} is presented in the plot as normalized to unity in the forward direction; its actual intensity distributions are presented in Fig. 1.24.

Since the single scattering angular distribution for particles with sizes substantially exceeding the Rayleigh limit is strongly asymmetric, the scattering intensity at large angles is very low. For this reason, one must trace the trajectories of a great number of photons to obtain good accuracy in this angular range. Therefore, to demonstrate the fine structure of the angular dependence of the matrix elements, one needs to use in the simulation 10^7–10^8 photons.[363,366]

For the scattering by particle suspensions in a spherical volume of small diameter, almost all the detected photons are singly scattered. An increase in the optical thickness considerably enhances the contribution of multiple scattering. The angular dependences of the LSM elements have a form close to the single scattering LSM, provided that the optical thickness of the scattering system τ does not exceed unity for the systems of large particles considered ten or above for systems of small particles.

The multiple-scattering intensity (the element M_{11}) for a volume of large diameter decreases with increasing scattering angle slower that the single-scattering intensity. As the cell diameter further increases, the backward scattering becomes predominant (see Figs. 1.24–1.26). In the systems of small particles (see Fig. 1.25), the growth of the multiple scattering contributions is accompanied by a gradual decrease in magnitude of all the elements except for M_{11}; i.e., the form of the LSM approaches that of the ideal depolarizer. In particular, the magnitudes of the elements M_{12} and M_{21} decrease in nearly the same way; the elements M_{33} and M_{44} also decrease in magnitude, but M_{44} decreases faster. As a result, multiple scattering gives rise to a difference in the detected values of the elements M_{33} and M_{44}, even for the systems of spherical particles. The value of the element M_{22} becomes smaller than unity, this decrease being more substantial in the range of scattering angles close to 90 deg. Thus, the manifestation of the effect of multiple scattering in monodisperse systems of spherical particles, which is revealed in the appearance of nonzero values of the differences $|M_{33} - M_{44}|$ and $|1 - M_{22}|$, is similar to the manifestation of the effect of nonsphericity of the scatterers observed under conditions of single scattering.[158]

For large particle systems, the multiple scattering also decreases the magnitudes and smoothes out the angular dependences of the normalized elements of the LSM (see Fig. 1.26). The corresponding angular dependences, as compared to the LSM of small particles, show the following specific features: the minimum value of the element M_{22} is reached not at 90 deg, but rather at large scattering angles; the fine structures of the angular dependences for all elements are smeared even in the presence of a small fraction of the multiply scattered light; and, finally, a very important result that the element M_{44}, unlike the other elements, in the limit of high scattering multiplicity, tends to 0.5 rather than to zero for all scattering angles. Such a form of the LSM means that the radiation scattered by the large particles holds the preferential circular polarization at higher scattering multiplicities. This result may serve as a confirmation of preferential survival of different types of polarization under conditions of multiple scattering for different sizes of scattering particles or tissue structures.[59,345,348,438]

The process of multiple scattering of the photons during their migration is considered as a series of successive rotations of their coordinate systems, determined by the scattering planes and directions. Since these rotations are random, the detected photons are randomly polarized and, hence, the detected light is partially depolarized. The depolarization will increase with the increasing multiplicity of scattering. For the moderate optical thicknesses (0.2 mm, $f = 0.01$), the depolarizing ability is strongly different for different directions. The scattered light may be almost completely polarized in the region of small scattering angles, completely depolarized at large angles ($\theta = 120$ deg), and be partly polarized in the backward direction. The angular range of the strongest depolarization corresponds to the angle at which the element M_{22} acquires minimum values (see Fig. 1.26).

The simulated dependences allow one to estimate the limits of applicability of the single scattering approximation when interpreting the results of experimental studies of disperse scattering systems. It follows from these simulations that modifications of the LSM of monodisperse systems of spherical particles due to the effects of multiple scattering have much in common with modification of the LSM of singly scattering systems upon deviation of the shape of the particles from spherical. This fact imposes serious limitations on the application of the measured LSM of biological objects for the inverse problem solving to determine particle nonsphericity. The appropriate criteria to distinguish the effects of multiple scattering and particle nonsphericity have to be developed.

It is important to note that the comparison of MC simulation accounting for all orders of multiple scattering with the analytical double-scattering model indicated no essential change in the backscattering polarization patterns.[350,351] This is due to the fact that the main contribution comes from near-double-scattering trajectories in which light suffers two wide-angle scatterings and many near-forward scatterings among multiple-scattering trajectories. The contributions of such multiple but near-double scattering trajectories are obviously well approximated by the contributions of the corresponding double-scattering trajectories.

The above MC technique of photon trajectory modeling is well suited to the simulation of multiple scattering effects in a system of randomly arranged particles. Furthermore, this scheme allows for an approximate approach to describe the interference effects caused by space particle ordering. To this end, one should include the interference of scattered fields into calculations of the single scattering Mueller matrix and integral cross sections for a particle. In other words, at the first stage one accounts for the interference effects for simulation of the *single scattering* properties, and then uses these properties in the MC simulation of *multiple scattering*. Such an approach is admissible if the size of a region of the local particle ordering is substantially smaller than the mean free-photon path length.

In general, for polarized light propagated in a strongly scattering medium, the multiple scattering decreases the magnitudes and smooths out the angular dependences of the normalized LSM elements, characterizing polarized light interaction with the medium. For media composed of large particles, specified by a high degree of single scattering anisotropy or considerable photon transport length, the scattered radiation holds the preferential circular polarization at higher scattering multiplicities. This theoretical result serves as a confirmation of preferential survival of different types of polarization under conditions of multiple scattering for different sizes of scattering particles or tissue structures.

1.4.8 Strongly scattering tissues and phantoms

Given the known character of the Stokes vector transformation for each scattering act, the state of polarization following multiple light scattering in a highly scattering medium can be found using various approximations of the multiple scattering theory or the MC method. For small particles, the effects of multiple scattering are apparent as the broken symmetry relationship between LSM elements [see Eqs. (1.72)–(1.75)], $M_{12}(\theta) \neq M_{21}(\theta)$, $M_{33}(\theta) \neq M_{44}(\theta)$, and a significant reduction of linear polarization of the light scattered at angles close to $\pi/2$.[450]

For a system of small spatially uncorrelated particles, the degree of linear $(i = L)$ and circular $(i = C)$ polarization in the far region of the initially polarized (linearly or circularly) light transmitted through a layer of thickness d is defined by the relation[345]

$$P_i \cong \frac{2d}{l_s} \sinh\left(\frac{l_s}{\xi_i}\right) \exp\left(-\frac{d}{\xi_i}\right), \tag{1.99}$$

where $l_s = 1/\mu_s$ is the scattering length,

$$\xi_i = \left(\frac{\zeta_i l_s}{3}\right)^{0.5} \tag{1.100}$$

is the characteristic depolarization length for a layer of scatterers, $d \gg \xi_i$, $\zeta_L = l_s/[\ln(10/7)]$, and $\zeta_C = l_s/(\ln 2)$.

As can be seen from Eq. (1.99), the characteristic depolarization length for linearly polarized light in tissues that can be represented as ensembles of Rayleigh particles is approximately 1.4 times greater than the corresponding depolarization length for circularly polarized light. One can employ Eq. (1.99) to assess the depolarization of light propagating through an ensemble of large-scale spherical particles whose sizes are comparable with the wavelength of incident light (Mie scattering). For this purpose, one should replace l_s by the transport length $l_t \cong 1/\mu_s'$ [see

Eq. (1.22)] and take into account the dependence on the size of scatterers in ζ_L and ζ_C. With the growth in the size of scatterers, the ratio ζ_L/ζ_C changes. It decreases from ~1.4 down to 0.5 as $2\pi a/\lambda$ increases from 0 up to ~4, where a is the radius of scatterers and λ is the wavelength of the light in the medium; it remains virtually constant at the level of 0.5 when $2\pi a/\lambda$ grows from ~4 to 15.

Monte Carlo numerical simulations and model experiments in aqueous latex suspensions with particles of various diameters demonstrate that there are three regimes of the dependence of the ratio of the degree of linear polarization to the circular polarization for transmitted light, P_L/P_C, on d/l_t (Fig. 1.27).[345] In the Rayleigh range, P_L/P_C grows linearly with the increase of d/l_t. In the intermediate range, this ratio remains constant. In the range of Mie scattering, this quantity decreases linearly. Such behavior of this quantity is associated with the transition of the system under study from isotropic scattering to anisotropic scattering. Qualitatively, the physical mechanism behind the change in the depolarization is associated with the fact that a considerable probability of backward scattering in each event of light-medium interaction (isotropic scattering) does not distort linear polarization, whereas backward scattering for circular polarization is equivalent to the reversal of polarization direction (similar to reflection from a mirror), i.e., it is equivalent to depolarization. For the same reason, in the case of a strongly elongated scattering phase function, the degree of circular polarization in an individual scattering event (anisotropic scattering) for light propagating in a layer should remain nonzero for lengths greater than the degree of linear polarization.

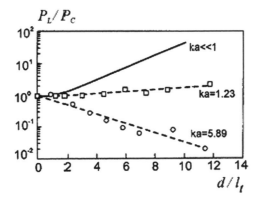

Figure 1.27 Semilogarithmic dependencies of the degree of polarization ratio P_L/P_C on d/l_t for three ka values, $k = 2\pi/\lambda$. The solid line corresponds to Rayleigh scattering ($ka \ll 1$) and the dashed lines indicate a correspondence between experimental findings and Eq. (1.99) at $l_s = l_t$. The experimental points are measurements for aqueous suspensions of polystyrol latex spherical particles having diameter 0.22 (□) and 1.05 (○) μm, where $\lambda_0 = 670$ nm.[345]

These arguments also follow from the above MC simulation of polarized light interaction with multiply scattering systems[366] and experimental works.[429,438] For example, at high scattering multiplicities the radiation scattered by the large particles holds the preferential circular polarization (LSM element M_{44} is far from zero for all scattering angles, see Fig. 1.26). At multiple scattering, the LSM for a monodisperse system of randomly distributed spherical particles is modified to be approximately identical to the single-scattering LSM of the system containing nonspherical particles, or optically active spheres.[366]

Thus, different tissues or the same tissues in various pathological or functional states should display different responses to a probe with linearly and circularly polarized light. This effect can be employed in both optical-medical tomography and for determining optical and spectroscopic parameters of tissues. As follows from Eq. (1.99), the depolarization length in tissues should be close to the mean transport path length l_t of a photon because this length characterizes the distance within which the direction of light propagation and, consequently, the polarization plane of linearly polarized light becomes totally random after many sequential scattering events.

Since the length l_t is determined by the parameter g, characterizing the anisotropy of scattering, the depolarization length should also substantially depend on this parameter. Indeed, the experimental data of Ref. 371 demonstrate that the depolarization length l_p of linearly polarized light, which is defined as the length within which the ratio $I_\parallel/I_\perp$ decreases down to 2, displays such a dependence. The ratio mentioned above varied from 300 to 1, depending on the thickness of the sample and the type of tissue (Fig. 1.28). These measurements were performed within a narrow solid angle ($\sim 10^{-4}$ sr) in the direction of the incident laser beam. The values of l_p differed considerably for the white matter of brain and tissue from the cerebral cortex: 0.19 and 1.0 mm for $\lambda = 476$–514 nm and 0.23 and 1.3 mm for $\lambda = 633$ nm, respectively. Human skin dermis (bloodless) has a depolarization length of 0.43 mm ($\lambda = 476$–514 nm) and 0.46 mm ($\lambda = 633$ nm). The depolarization length at $\lambda = 476$–514 nm decreases in response to a pathological change

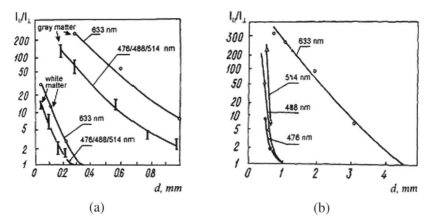

(a)   (b)

Figure 1.28 Dependence of the depolarization degree ($I_\parallel/I_\perp$) of laser radiation (He:Ne laser, $\lambda = 633$ nm; Ar laser, $\lambda = 476/488/514$ nm) on the penetration depth for (a) brain tissue (gray and white matter) and (b) whole blood (low hematocrit).[371] Measurements were performed within a small solid angle (10^{-4} sr) along the axis of a laser beam 1 mm in diameter. A strong influence of fluorescence was seen in blood irradiated by the Ar laser.

in aorta wall tissue: 0.54 mm for normal tissue, 0.39 mm for the stage of tissue calcification, and 0.33 mm for the stage of necrotic ulcer. Whole blood with a low hematocrit is characterized by a considerable depolarization length (about 4 mm) at $\lambda = 633$ nm, which is indicative of the dependence on the parameter g, whose value for blood exceeds the values of this parameter for tissues of many other types, estimated as 0.966–0.997.[2,40,48,164]

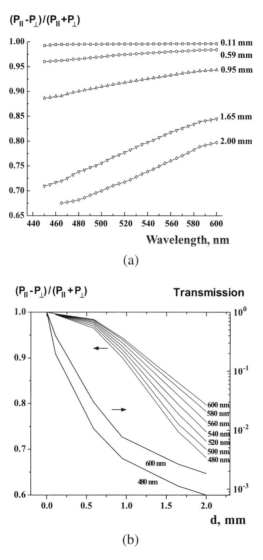

Figure 1.29 (a) Polarization spectra of light transmitted in the forward direction and (b) the relevant dependencies on the layer thickness d for a gelatin-milk (20%) phantom.[374]

In contrast to depolarization, the attenuation of collimated light is determined by the total attenuation coefficient μ_t [see Eq. (1.1)]. For many tissues, μ_t is much greater than μ'_s. Therefore, in certain situations, it is impossible to detect pure ballistic photons (photons that do not experience scattering), but the forward-scattered photons retain their initial polarization and can be used for imaging.[372,373] This is illustrated by Figs. 1.29 and 1.30, which present the experimental data for decay of the degree of linear polarization P_L [see Eq. (1.68a)] obtained for a gelatin-milk phantom (a model of bloodless dermis) within a broad wavelength range,[77,374] and for various tissues and blood as a function of light transmission.[438] The kink in the characteristics of polarization decay [Fig. 1.29(b)], which can be observed for a small thickness of 0.6 mm, can be attributed to the transition of a medium to the regime of multiple scattering.

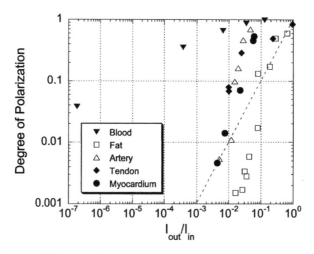

Figure 1.30 Degree of linear polarization in different tissues as a function of the sample optical transmittance, $I_{out}/I_{in} \equiv T$, on 633 nm. Each point is an average of three measurements.[438] The error bars representing standard deviation of measurements are smaller than the used symbols.

The authors of Ref. 375 experimentally demonstrated that laser radiation retains linear polarization on the level of $P_L \le 0.1$ within $2.5 l_t$. Specifically, for skin irradiated in the red and NIR ranges, we have $\mu_a \cong 0.4$ cm^{-1}, $\mu'_s \cong 20$ cm^{-1}, and $l_t \cong 0.48$ mm. Consequently, light propagating in skin can retain linear polarization within a length of about 1.2 mm. Such an optical path in a tissue corresponds to a time delay on the order of 5.3 ps, which provides an opportunity to produce polarization images of macroinhomogeneities in a tissue with a spatial resolution equivalent to the spatial resolution that can be achieved by the selecting of photons using more sophisticated time-resolved techniques. In addition to the selection of diffuse-scattered photons, polarization imaging makes it possible to eliminate specular reflection from the surface of a tissue, which allows one to use this technique to image microvessels in facile skin and detect birefringence and optical activity in superficial tissue layers.[138,376–378,382,383]

Polarization imaging is a new direction in tissue optics.[36,129,135,138,344–368,] [371–424,428,429,435–442,450,451] The most prospective approaches for polarization tissue imaging, in particular linear-polarization-degree mapping, two-dimensional backscattering Mueller matrix measurements, polarization-sensitive optical coherence tomography (OCT), and a full-field polarization-speckle technique, will be discussed in this and the following chapters.

The registration of two-dimensional polarization patterns for the backscattering of a polarized incident narrow laser beam is the basis for the polarization imaging technique.[375,382,383] The major informative images can be received using the backscattering Mueller matrix approach.[351,361–367,380,381,385–387] To determine each of the 16 experimental matrix elements, a total of 16 images should be taken at various combinations of input and output polarization states.

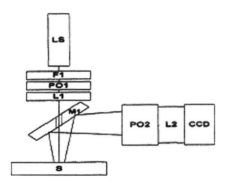

Figure 1.31 Schematic diagram of the experimental setup for polarization imaging:[351,381] LS, 10 mW He:Ne laser (633 nm); F1, 10% neutral density filter; PO1, polarization optics (set 1); L1, focusing lens ($f = 10$ cm); M1, mirror; S, sample; PO2, polarization analyzer optics (set 2); L2, imaging lens system; CCD, imaging camera.

A schematic view of the experimental setup used for collection of the diffuse backscattered images is shown in Fig. 1.31.[351,381] A collimated laser light beam is polarized via various polarization optics (PO1, linear and circular polarizers) to obtain the desired input polarization. This polarized light is then focused through a hole (about 2 mm in diameter) in a mirror (M1) mounted onto the sample at 45 deg. The diffusely backscattered light from the sample is then imaged through a polarization analyzer (PO2) using a cooled 12-bit CCD camera. The polarization analyzer consists of a variety of optics that were interchanged in order to analyze a specific state of polarization (vertical; horizontal; ±45 deg linear; and left, right circular) for a respective image used to reconstruct the Mueller matrix.

To determine each of the 16 experimental matrix elements, a total of 49 images ($49 - 16 = 33$ are dependent) were taken at various combinations of input and output analyzer polarization states.[351,381] Each of the 16 experimental elements was calculated by adding or subtracting a series of images. Each image was collected using an exposure time of 1.7 s, having the speckle effect averaged out (the estimated correlation time of the laser-induced speckles was generally of the order of 10 ms).

A comparison of the measurements of the Mueller matrix elements with the Monte Carlo calculations is presented in Fig. 1.32.[351,381] For the MC simulations, the average number of collisions per photon trajectory was 10. A good agreement between the experimental and calculated patterns, especially azimuthal dependence, can clearly be seen. For the suspensions studied, the transport mean free path l_t is about 1 cm. It appears that for distances exceeding two transport mean free paths, the azimuthal dependence of the images becomes less pronounced because multiple scattering tends to randomize the polarization state of the light. It was shown both theoretically and experimentally that only seven matrix elements are independent and the rest can be obtained by simple rotations. The nature of such symmetry is quite general: the scattering medium should be invariant under rotations around the initial laser beam direction and should contain an ensemble (or a finite number of different ensembles) of identical (possibly asymmetric) scatterers in random orientations.[351,381] The polarization images of tissuelike phantoms, cancerous and noncancerous cell suspensions, and living tissues (human skin, bone) are presented in Refs. 351, 353–357, 362, and 375–390.

It should be noted that in media containing large-scale scatterers (a common tissue model), depolarization is a higher-order effect ($\sim\theta^4$, $\theta < 1$) than polariza-

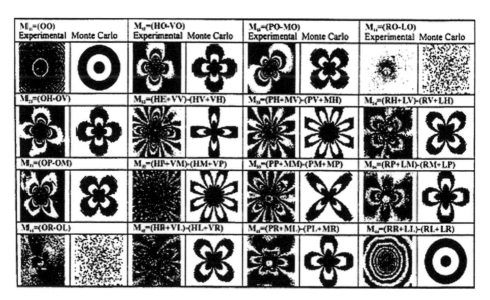

Figure 1.32 Experimental and Monte Carlo backscattered Mueller matrix:[351,381] The individual images are represented by a two-letter combination that denotes the input polarizer and output analyzer orientation (see Fig. 1.31). HV denotes horizontal input polarized light and a vertical polarization analyzer; V, vertical; H, horizontal; P, +45 deg; M, −45 deg; R, right; L, left; and O, open polarization optics or none. The approximate size of each image is 1.6 × 1.6 cm. The tissuelike phantom was composed of a suspension of 2.02 μm polysterene spheres in water: $\mu_s' \cong 12$ cm^{-1}, $g = 0.912$, $\mu_a \approx 0$.

tion ($\sim \theta^2$).[70] In the literature, the polarization state of multiply scattered light is analyzed either under conditions of spatial diffusion of photons, when the angular spectrum of radiation is virtually isotropic (see, for example, Refs. 184, 393, and 450) or in the case of small-angle scattering in media with large-scale inhomogeneities.[70,186,345,450] It should be emphasized, following Ref. 70, that the analysis of polarization state in the case of small-angular multiple scattering is important for many problems pertaining to optical diagnosis of biological media that can be represented as random systems with long-range correlation of fluctuations of dielectric permittivity. Such systems display coherent scattering effects[73,74,391] or may be expected to show fluctuations of polarization similar to those in disordered media with large-scale inhomogeneities.[392–396]

In weakly absorbing media that shows a small-angular multiple scattering, the degree of linear polarization for a Henyey-Greenstein phase function [see Eq. (1.15)] is described by the following formula:[70]

$$P_L = -\left[\frac{(\mu_s' z)^4}{2\theta^2}\right]\left[\sqrt{1 + \left(\frac{\theta}{\mu_s' z}\right)^2} - 1\right]^2\left[1 + \left(\frac{\theta}{\mu_s' z}\right)^2\right]. \qquad (1.101)$$

This means that in a very small angle range ($\theta \ll \mu_s' z$), the degree of polarization does not depend on the depth (z)

$$P_L = -\frac{\theta^2}{8}. \qquad (1.102)$$

At the wings of the scattering angle dependence ($\theta \gg \mu_s' z$), it tends toward

$$P_L = -\frac{\theta^2}{2}, \qquad (1.103)$$

which equals the degree of polarization of singly scattered light.

1.5 Optothermal and optoacoustic interactions of light with tissues

1.5.1 Basic principles and classification

The optothermal (OT) method detects the time-dependent heat generated in a tissue via interaction with pulsed or intensity modulated optical radiation.[5,6,25,452–518]

Such interaction induces a number of thermoelastic effects in a tissue; in particular, it causes the generation of acoustic waves. The detection of acoustic waves is the basis of optoacoustic (or photoacoustic) methods.[5,6,25,455–489,511,512,514–518] The informative features of this method allow one to estimate tissue thermal, optical, and acoustical properties that depend on peculiarities of tissue structure.

Three modes can be used for excitation of tissue thermal response as follows:[5,6,25,455]

(1) A pulse of light (usually pulsed laser) excites the sample and the signal is detected in the time domain with a fast detector attached to a wideband amplifier. In this case, signal averaging and gating techniques are used to increase the SNR.

(2) An intensity-modulated (usually harmonic modulation) light source (high-intensity lamp or CW laser) and a low-frequency transducer is used. The measurement is in the frequency domain; phase-sensitive detection (lock-in-amplification of the signal at the modulation frequency) is used for noise suppression.

(3) CW excitation generates a photochemical reaction and the heat evolved through a particular reaction can be detected as a temperature rise.

In every case, the thermal waves generated by the heat release result in several effects that have given rise to various techniques as follows:[5,6,25,455]

- Optoacoustics (OA) or photoacoustics (PA) (direct or indirect sound wave generation)
- Optothermal radiometry (OTR) or photothermal radiometry (PTR) (detection of infrared thermal emission)
- Photorefractive techniques such as thermal blooming, thermal lensing, probe beam refraction, interferometry, and deflectometry (detection of refractive index gradients above and inside the sample)
- The optogeometric technique (surface deformation in solids, volume changes in fluids)
- Optical calorimetry or laser calorimetry (temperature rise)

The term "optoacoustics" refers primarily to the time-resolved technique utilizing pulsed lasers and measuring the profiles of pressure in tissue; the term "photoacoustics" describes primarily spectroscopic experiments with CW-modulated light and a photoacoustic cell.

A schematic representation of some OT and OA techniques applied to tissue study is given in Fig. 1.33. An excitation laser beam falls onto the sample surface, the light wavelength is tuned to an absorption line of the tissue component of interest, and the optical energy is absorbed by the medium. In a condensed medium, the collisional quenching rate in the component is significantly higher than the radiative rate; therefore, most of the energy transforms to heat. The time-dependent heating leads to all of the above-mentioned thermal and thermoelastic effects. In OA or PA techniques (see 1 in Fig. 1.33), a microphone or a piezoelectric transducer that is in acoustic contact with the sample is used as a detector to measure the amplitude or phase of the resultant acoustic wave.[5,6,455] In the OTR technique (see 2 in Fig. 1.33), distant IR detectors and array cameras are employed for estimating the temperature of the sample surface and its image.[5,6,25,455,490–501] Heating the medium changes its refractive index. The change in the refractive index of the sample or surrounding gas can be detected either directly by means of an interferometer, or by a probe laser beam that changes its shape, either converging or

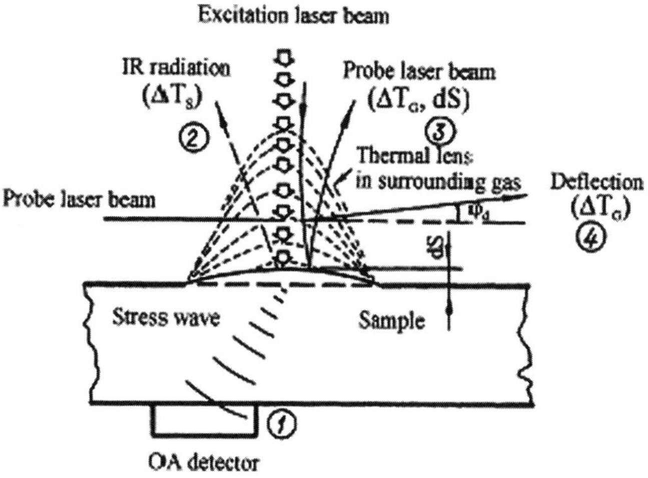

Figure 1.33 Schematic representation of some optothermal techniques used in a tissue study:[6] ΔT_S is the temperature change of a sample; ΔT_G is the temperature change of a surrounding gas; dS is the thermoelastic deformation; φ_d is the deflection angle of a probe laser beam. 1, OA technique; 2, OTR technique; 3, thermal lens technique; 4, deflection technique.

diverging (thermal lens, see 3 in Fig. 1.33), or is deflected (see 4 in Fig. 1.33) when it passes the region excited by the pump beam.[502–508]

The intensity of the signals obtained with any of the OT or OA techniques depends on the amount of energy absorbed and transformed into heat, and on the thermoelastic properties of the sample and its surroundings. Assuming that non-radiative relaxation is the main process in light beam decay and extinction is not very high, $\mu_a d \ll 1$ (d is the length of a cylinder within the sample occupied by a pulse laser beam), the absorbed energy can be estimated on the basis of Beer's law as[5,6,25]

$$E_T \cong E\mu_a d, \tag{1.104}$$

where E is the incident pulse energy, and μ_a is the absorption coefficient.

Energy absorption causes an increase in the local temperature ΔT, which is defined by the relation[5,6,25]

$$\Delta T = \frac{E_T}{c_P V \rho} \cong \frac{E\mu_a d}{c_P V \rho}, \tag{1.105}$$

where c_P is the specific heat capacity for a constant pressure, $V = \pi w^2 d$ is the illuminated volume, w is the laser beam radius, and ρ is the medium density. Assuming an adiabatic expansion of an illuminated volume at a constant pressure, one can calculate the change in this volume as

$$\Delta V = \pi(w + \Delta w)^2 d - \pi w^2 d = \beta V \Delta T \cong \frac{\beta E\mu_a d}{c_P \rho}, \tag{1.106}$$

where Δw is the change in radius of a cylinder illuminated by a laser beam caused by a local temperature increase and β is the coefficient of volumetric expansion.

This expansion induces a wave propagating in a radial direction with the speed of sound. The corresponding change of pressure Δp is proportional to the amplitude of mechanical oscillations $\Delta x_T \sim \Delta w$:

$$\Delta p = 2\pi f_a v_a \rho \Delta x_T \sim f_a v_a \rho \Delta w, \tag{1.107}$$

where f_a is the frequency of acoustic oscillations and v_a is the velocity of acoustic waves in a medium.

Using Eq. (1.107) and taking into account that $\Delta w \ll w$, we can finally find:

$$\Delta p \sim \left(\frac{f_a}{w}\right)\left(\frac{\beta v_a d}{c_P}\right) E \mu_a. \tag{1.108}$$

Equations (1.105)–(1.108) present the principles of various OT and OA techniques. Information on the absorption coefficient μ_a at a specific wavelength can be obtained from direct measurements of the temperature change ΔT (optical calorimetry), volume change ΔV (optogeometric technique), or pressure change Δp (OA and PA techniques). Using the connections between the focal length of the "thermal lens" f_T, the deflection angle of a probe laser beam φ_d, and the phase shift in a measuring interferometer $\Delta \psi$ with the change in a sample temperature ΔT, the approximate expressions describing the photorefractive methods can be written in the form[5,6,25] for a "thermal lens" technique as

$$\frac{1}{f_T} \approx d_p \left(\frac{dn}{dT}\right)\left(\frac{\Delta T}{w^2}\right), \tag{1.109}$$

a probe beam deflection technique

$$\varphi_d \approx \left(\frac{1}{n}\right)\left(\frac{dn}{dT}\right)\Delta T, \tag{1.110}$$

and a phase shifting (interferometry) technique

$$\Delta \psi \approx \left(\frac{2\pi d_p}{\lambda_p}\right)\left(\frac{dn}{dT}\right)\Delta T, \tag{1.111}$$

where dn/dT is the medium (tissue) refractive index temperature gradient, d_p is the length of the space where the exciting and the probe laser beams are overlapped, and λ_p is the wavelength of the probe beam.

The effects considered are possible in gases, liquids, and solids. Usually, a tissue under study is surrounded by a gas (composition of gases, like air) or by a liquid (blood, cerebrospinal fluid, aqueous humor, etc.); therefore, a variety of OT and OA effects can be monitored concurrently due to transport of optical intensity, thermal, and acoustic waves in this tissue and its surroundings.[5,6,25]

The time delay between optical and thermal (acoustic) pulses is an important parameter of the OT (or OA) techniques, defining the SNR. For example, the pulse OA method can be characterized by the time delay between optical and acoustical pulses as[455]

$$\tau_d \cong R_{bd}/v_a, \tag{1.112}$$

where R_{bd} is the distance between the axis of the exciting laser beam and the acoustic detector.

The time delay for the "thermal lens" technique is defined by the time of the thermal wave propagation transverse to the probing laser beam with a radius w_p,[455]

$$\tau_{th} \approx \frac{(w_p/2.4)^2}{a_T}, \tag{1.113}$$

where

$$a_T \approx \frac{k_T}{\rho c_P} \tag{1.114}$$

is the thermal diffusivity of the medium, k_T is the heat conductivity, and ρ is the density of the medium. When the duration of a laser pulse τ_L is much less than τ_{th}, focusing the probe laser beam allows one to improve the transit time of this method.

It should be noted that the values of thermal parameters (the heat conductivity k_T and the specific heat capacity for a constant pressure c_P) and the density ρ for many tissues are given in Refs. 2 and 87.

1.5.2 Photoacoustic method

For molecular gas systems when the rate of nonradiative relaxation of the excited states prevails, the time dependent PA signal for excitation by a pulse with the energy E has a form[5,6]

$$\delta p(t) \approx (\gamma - 1)\left(\frac{E\mu_a}{\pi R_G^2}\right)\exp\left(\frac{-t}{\tau_T}\right), \tag{1.115}$$

where $\delta p(t)$ is the time-dependent change in pressure and t is the time; $\gamma = c_P/c_V$ and c_V is the specific heat capacity for a constant volume; R_G is the gas PA cell radius;

$$\tau_T \approx \left[\frac{(R_G/2.4)^2}{a_T}\right] \tag{1.116}$$

is the thermal relaxation time of the PA cell, and

$$a_T \approx \frac{k_G}{\rho_G c_V},$$ (1.117)

where a_T is defined in Eq. (1.114) for a condensed matter, ρ_G is the gas density, and k_G is the gas heat conductivity.

The length of thermal diffusivity (thermal length) is an important parameter, which for the pulse excitation is estimated as[5,6]

$$l_T \approx (4a_T \tau_L)^{1/2},$$ (1.118)

where τ_L is the duration of a laser pulse.

Quantitative PA images and spectroscopic studies of tissues can be provided in a frequency-domain mode, when a laser beam of power P intensity modulated at frequency ω irradiates the sample and the acoustic detector registers the modulation amplitude $\delta p(\omega)$ and the phase lag $\Phi_p(\omega)$ of the acoustic signal.[5,6,25,455,460] In that case, the following expressions for $\delta p(\omega)$ and $\Phi_p(\omega)$ can be derived:[5,6,25]

$$\delta p(\omega) \approx \frac{(\sqrt{2}/2)(\gamma - 1)(P\mu_a/\pi R_G^2)\tau_T}{[1 + (\omega \tau_T)^2]^{1/2}},$$ (1.119)

$$\Phi_p(\omega) \approx -\tan^{-1}(\omega \tau_T),$$ (1.120)

where τ_T is defined by Eq. (1.116). These expressions are applicable within the same limits as Eq. (1.115); the notations also coincide with those of Eq. (1.115).

A gas cell PA method is widely seen and used to study optical and thermal properties of condensed materials (liquids and solids).[5,6,25,455,457] Light intensity modulated at frequency ω is absorbed by condensed matter and partially converted into heat, which induces perturbations of the surrounding gas pressure, which in its turn can be registered by a microphone. For a description of the PA signal, three characteristic lengths are usually used: the geometric d, the mean free path of photon $l_{ph} \cong 1/\mu_a$ (when $\mu_a \gg \mu_s$), and the "thermal" (thermal diffusion) l_T,

$$l_T = (2a_T/\omega)^{1/2},$$ (1.121)

where a_T is defined by Eq. (1.114) or (1.117), depending on the measuring method used. Six various modes of a gas-microphone method can be used, based on different relations between these three lengths. Evidently for optically and thermally thick samples $(d > l_T \approx l_{ph})$, the PA signal generated can be saturated, and such situations should be avoided.[25] For a given sample, l_T is defined by modulation frequency ω or pulse duration [see Eq. (1.118)]. For optically and thermally transparent samples $(d \approx l_{ph} + l_T)$, the PA response also includes a back surface of the sample; therefore, besides the six modes mentioned, some others can be used.

When light is assumed to be absorbed at the sample surface and heat flow is approximated by the one-dimensional model, the phase lag can be written in the form[460]

$$\tan \Phi_p = \tan\left(\frac{d}{l_T}\right)\frac{1 + R_b \exp(-2d/l_T)}{1 - R_b \exp(-2d/l_T)},\tag{1.122}$$

where $R_b = (1 - b)/(1 + b)$, $b = (k_{Tb}\rho_b c_{pb}/k_T \rho c_p)^{1/2}$, l_T is the thermal diffusion length of tissue [see Eq. (1.121)], and d is the geometric length of the sample (parameters of the backing material are denoted by the subscript b).

Equation (1.122) shows that Φ_p is linear with $\omega^{1/2}$, provided $R_b \exp(-2d/l_T) \ll 1$. This condition is generally fulfilled for thermally thick objects ($d \gg l_T$). However, it is even valid for a thermally thin case if the effusivity of the sample and the backing material are close to each other ($b \approx 1$):

$$\Phi_p \approx d/l_T \sim \omega^{1/2}.\tag{1.123}$$

In that case, the images reflect only the thermal diffusivity of the samples. The PA cell was employed in the laser imaging system described in Ref. 460. It has two plane glass windows separated by 1 mm with a silicone sheet spacer. To ensure surface absorption, a sample was covered with copper foil 5-µm thick and placed on the rear window. An intensity-modulated (970 Hz) light beam from an argon laser (200 mW) irradiated the sample from the foil side and was absorbed at its surface. Then, generated heat traveled through the sample and showed the phase lag at the air/sample boundary, which was detected as the PA signal with a microphone. Transparent liquid paraffin was injected between the sample and window to prevent generation of the PA signal on the foil surface. It also worked as a backing material. The sample was embedded in paraffin and sectioned to approximately a 5-µm thick film and placed on copper foil. The observed area of the sample was scanned in increments of 25 µm over 100×100 points transverse to a laser beam focused up to 40 µm.

A few types of tissues were studied: a slice of a canine eye and a mouse kidney. From PA phase images, the thermal diffusivity for each point can be obtained. For example, the thermal diffusivity of the optical nerve was estimated as 1.9×10^{-7} m^2/s. The accuracy of the thermal diffusivity measured was about a few tens of percent, primarily due to the difficulty of determining the exact thickness. The calculated thermal diffusion length was about 8 µm. Thus, lateral resolution was limited only by the laser beam diameter and the minimal scanning step. This method may be interesting for examining the relationship between the thermal properties and physiological functions of natural biological microtextures because, in principle, it requires no fixation. The method belongs to PA microscopy (PAM).

The basic principles of PAM are very simple.[25,461] Spatially coherent laser radiation serves as a probe beam that can be focused at least to about 1 µm. The scanning of a focused laser beam across the object's surface and the registration of the PA signal induced using a microphone or piezotransducer give the distributions of the optical, thermal, and acoustic properties of the object.

The PAM allows profiling of the object in depth. When the wavelength of the light source is changed, the penetration depth of the light is also changed and the PA signal is generated at different depths. It should also take into account the spectral properties of absorbers and their distribution within the tissue. Another way of depth profiling is to change the modulation frequency. This property is a specific one and characteristic only for PAM. The depth of profiling is defined by the thermal diffusion length of the medium [see Eq. (1.121)] for a given modulation frequency. For example, for a highly absorptive sample ($\mu_a \approx 10^6$ cm^{-1}), a PA signal can be generated at different depths from 10^{-1} to 10^3 µm when the modulation frequency is changed in the range from 100 MHz to 1 Hz.

1.5.3 Time-resolved optoacoustics

Measurement of the stress-wave profile and amplitude using an OA spectrometer (see Fig. 1.34), combined with measurement of the total diffuse reflectance, allows one to separately extract both absorption and scattering coefficients of the sample. The absorption coefficient in a turbid medium can be estimated from the acoustic transient profile only if the subsurface irradiance is known. For turbid media irradiated with wide laser beams (> 0.1 mm), the effect of backscattering causes a higher subsurface fluence rate compared with the incident laser fluence (see, for example, Figs. 1.9 and 1.10 for skin). Therefore the z-axial light distribution in tissue and the corresponding stress distribution have a complex profile, with a maximum at a subsurface layer. However, the stress amplitude adjacent to the irradiated surface $\delta p(0)$ and the stress exponential tail into the depth of the tissue sample can be expressed as[467] [see also Eq. (1.30)]

$$\delta p(0) = \Gamma \mu_a E(0), \text{ at surface } (z=0), \tag{1.124}$$

$$\delta p(z) = \Gamma \mu_a b_s E_0 \exp(-\mu_{\text{eff}} z), \quad \text{for } z > \frac{1}{\mu_{\text{eff}}}, \tag{1.125}$$

where $\Gamma = \beta v_a^2 / c_T$, c_T is the specific heat of the tissue, b_s is the factor that accounts for the effect of backscattered irradiance that increases the effective energy absorbed in the subsurface layer, μ_{eff} is defined in Eq. (1.18), $E(0)$ is the subsurface irradiance, and E_0 is the incident laser pulse energy at the sample surface (J/cm^2); the rest of the parameters are given in Eqs. (1.105)–(1.108). For optically thick samples,[458,467]

$$E(0) \approx (1 + 7.1 R_d) E_0, \tag{1.126}$$

where R_d is the total diffuse reflection.

The Grüneisen parameter Γ is a dimensionless temperature-dependent factor proportional to the fraction of thermal energy converted into mechanical stress. For water, it can be expressed with an empirical formula (see Ref. 467) as

$$\Gamma = 0.0043 + 0.0053T, \tag{1.127}$$

where temperature T is measured in degrees Celsius; for $T = 37°C$ $\Gamma \approx 0.2$.

Equations (1.124) and (1.125) are strictly valid only when the heating process is much faster than expansion of the medium. The stress is temporarily confined during laser heat deposition when the duration of the laser pulse is much shorter than the time of stress propagation across the depth of light penetration in the tissue sample. Such conditions of temporal pressure confinement in a volume of irradiated tissue allow for the most efficient pressure generation.[458,459,467]

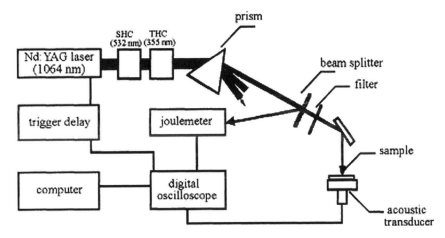

Figure 1.34 Optoacoustic spectrometer for *in vitro* measurement of optical parameters of tissues:[467] SHC, second harmonic converter (532 nm); THC, third harmonic converter (355 nm).

The OA method described and instruments presented in Figs. 1.34 and 1.35 were successfully used for measurement of the optical parameters of some tissues.[467,468] The main advantage of this three-wavelengths laser OA spectrometer for measuring tissue optical properties is the $LiNbO_3$ acoustic detector (Fig. 1.35), which provides high sensitivity (~ 100 nV/Pa) combined with a broad ultrasonic frequency range (to 300 MHz) and long-term stability, and thus accurate absolute calibration.[467] From OA measurements for human aorta samples (advanced fibrous atheroma), tissue optical properties were evaluated as $\mu_a = 16.5, 3.53$, and 0.15 cm^{-1}, and $\mu_s' = 72.1, 36.5$, and 4.85 cm^{-1}, respectively, at wavelengths 355, 532, and 1064 nm for sample thicknesses of $\sim 3, 7$, and 12 mm, and estimated root-mean-square (rms) values of the measurements, respectively, $\sim 10, 15$, and 50%. One can measure the absorption and scattering coefficients by using a combination of diffuse reflectance and OA techniques.[468] Those measurements at wavelength 1064 nm gave $\mu_a = 0.53 \pm 0.03$ cm^{-1} and $\mu_s' = 7.56 \pm 0.92$ cm^{-1} for

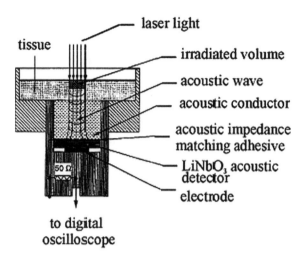

laser light

tissue

irradiated volume

acoustic wave

acoustic conductor

acoustic impedance
matching adhesive

LiNbO$_3$ acoustic
detector

electrode

to digital
oscilloscope

Figure 1.35 Scheme of an acoustic transducer.[467]

native canine liver. For coagulated tissue, a 1.3-fold increase in absorption coefficient ($\mu_a = 0.71 \pm 0.30$ cm^{-1}) and a 2.6-fold increase in scattering coefficient ($\mu_s' = 19.9 \pm 6.2$ cm^{-1}) were observed. The determination of optical properties of soft tissue in the NIR using OA spectroscopy is also described in Ref. 472. Some data for the optical parameters received using the OA method are given in Table 2.1.

The systematic outline of OA techniques, starting with production and extending to the propagation and detection of OA waves, are presented in Ref. 514. The focal point was the production of acoustic waves with maximal amplitude and minimal distortion. Receiving of the maximal amplitude is important for AO spectroscopy and minimal signal distortion is the key to the determination of optical distribution and imaging in tissues.

1.5.4 Grounds of OA tomography and microscopy

The concept of OA tomography (OAT)[458,459,465,466,470,473,475–484] is illustrated in Figs. 1.36 and 1.37. Short laser pulses ensure the temporal confinement of the transient pressure generated in the irradiated volume of tissue as a consequence of laser heating. This means that laser-induced acoustic waves do not move noticeably during laser heating of a tissue volume under study. As a result, the substantial fraction of energy deposited in the target volume (tumor) will generate an ultrasonic wave before it can escape at the speed of sound, and the profile of the laser-induced pressure precisely resembles the distribution of the laser energy absorbed.

If the optical pumping pulse duration is much shorter than the thermal diffusion time, thermal diffusion can be neglected; this is known as the assumption of thermal confinement. In this case, the acoustic wave $p(\mathbf{r}, \bar{t})$, which reaches a detector at position $\mathbf{r}$ and time $\bar{t}$, is related to the optical energy absorption $H(\mathbf{r}, \bar{t})$ by the

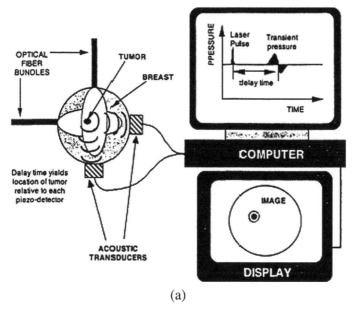

(a)

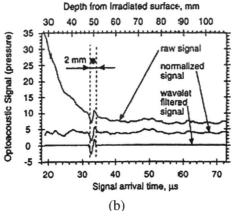

(b)

Figure 1.36 Principal schematic diagram of laser OA imaging system for breast cancer diagnostics in (a) transmission mode and (b) temporal pressure profiles recorded upon laser irradiation of the breast phantom with a small "tumor" (the upper profile) and the same profile filtered using a MatLab wavelet transform method.[459,465] The x-axis displays the time of transient acoustic wave arrival at the transducer. The "time" axis can be converted into the "depth" axis because depth = time × speed of sound (1.5 mm/μs).

following wave equation:[456,517]

$$\frac{\partial^2 p(\mathbf{r}, \bar{t})}{\partial \bar{t}^2} - \nabla^2 p(\mathbf{r}, \bar{t}) = \frac{\beta v_a}{c_T} \frac{\partial H(\mathbf{r}, \bar{t})}{\partial \bar{t}}, \qquad (1.128)$$

where $\bar{t} = t v_a$, acoustic speed v_a is assumed to be constant, $H(\mathbf{r}, \bar{t})$ is the heating function defined as the thermal energy per time and volume deposited by the light

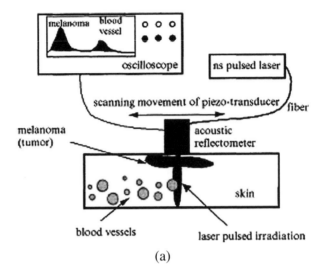

(a)

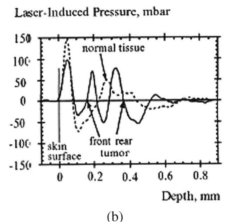

(b)

Figure 1.37 Principal schematic diagram of laser OA imaging system for skin cancer diagnostics in (a) reflection mode and (b) OA signals (pressure transients) measured *in vivo* in tumor tissue (solid line) and normal tissue (dashed line) in a mouse model of breast carcinoma.[459,465] During the experiment, tissues were compressed by an attached acoustic transducer; therefore, all depths appear slightly smaller than they actually were.

source in the close proportion to the optical absorption coefficient of interest, and the other parameters are defined earlier. Equation (1.128) can be rewritten in terms of $H(\mathbf{r}, \bar{t})$ as

$$p(\mathbf{r}, \bar{t}) = \frac{\beta v_a}{4\pi c_T} \iiint \frac{\partial H(\mathbf{r}', t')}{\partial t'} \frac{d\mathbf{r}'}{|\mathbf{r} - \mathbf{r}'|}, \qquad (1.129)$$

where $t' = \bar{t} - |\mathbf{r} - \mathbf{r}'|$. The source term $H(\mathbf{r}, \bar{t})$ can be further rewritten as the product of a purely spatial (optical absorption function) and a purely temporal (function of laser energy) component, i.e.,

$$H(\mathbf{r}, \bar{t}) = I_0 A(\mathbf{r}) S(\bar{t}), \tag{1.130}$$

where I_0 is a scaling factor, proportional to the incident radiation intensity; $A(\mathbf{r})$ describes the optical absorption properties of the tissue at $\mathbf{r}$; and $S(\bar{t})$ describes the shape of the irradiating pulse. Substituting Eq. (1.130) into (1.131) results in

$$p(\mathbf{r}, \bar{t}) = \frac{I_0 \beta v_a}{4\pi c_T} \iiint A(\mathbf{r}') \frac{dS(t')}{dt'} \frac{d\mathbf{r}'}{|\mathbf{r} - \mathbf{r}'|}. \tag{1.131}$$

This equation shows the solution to the forward problem-prediction of the pressure outside the tissue if the absorption properties of the medium and the profile of the laser pulse are known.

For imaging, the inverse problem needs to be solved. Exact inverse solutions in planar, spherical, and cylindrical geometries are available (see references in Ref. 517). These exact solutions are computationally intensive and can be approximated to more efficient solutions in most cases.[517] In practice, the distance between the OA sources and the detector is much longer than the wavelength of the high-frequency OA waves that are useful for imaging. Under this condition, the following back-projection algorithm is a good approximate of the inverse solution[517]

$$A(\mathbf{r}) = C \int_{S_D} \int dS_D \cos(\varphi_D) \frac{1}{t} \frac{\partial p(\mathbf{r}_0, t)}{\partial t} |_{t=|\mathbf{r}_0 - \mathbf{r}|/v_a}, \tag{1.132}$$

where C is a constant, S_D is the surface of detection, and φ_D is the angle between the normal of dS_D and $\mathbf{r} - \mathbf{r}_0$ (the vector pointing from a point of detection to a point of reconstruction).

It should be noted that this is a modified back-projection of the quantity $(1/t)[\partial p(\mathbf{r}_0 t)/\partial t]$. This back-projection is analogous to that in x-ray computed tomography (CT). In x-ray CT, the back-projection is along the paths of x-ray propagation; as in OAT, the back-projection is along spherical shells that are centered at the detector and have a radius determined by the acoustic time of flight.

In contrast to photon density waves, acoustic waves (AWs) can provide minimally distorted diagnostic information from sufficient depths in tissue to the surface of a human organ due to their much lower (two to three orders) scatter in tissues than optical waves.[517] This is a key point of laser OA imaging and is explained by the independence of its resolution to light scattering. In addition, its low sensitivity to light scattering helps to create more homogeneous light distribution in the volume of diagnostic interest. Light as a carrier of tissue structure information is replaced with a transient AW, which resembles the initial profile of light distribution and can bring this profile to the acoustic detector unaltered. The imaging contrast is based primarily on the optical properties of tissue (absorption), and the imaging resolution is based primarily on the acoustic waves. Wideband ultrasonic detection permits the accurate reproduction of the initial pressure distribution in the irradiated volume. Profiles of the pressure transients detected and the time of their arrival carry information on dimensions, optical properties, and location of tumors. Owing to the sensitive detection of AW (5 V/bar), a temperature rise of only 0.1 mK in a 2-mm tumor located at a depth of 5 cm will be sufficient for the generation of pressure signals with amplitudes of 10 times the noise level.[458,459,465]

Figures 1.36 and 1.37 present two types of OAT, in a transmission mode and in a reflection mode. The first one can be applied in breast cancer diagnosis and the second one in the detection of skin cancer. A matrix of fiber-optic bundles delivers NIR laser energy from a pulse Nd:YAG laser to the breast surface [see Fig. 1.36(a)]. A matrix of piezoelectric transducers reads temporal profiles of laser-induced acoustic waves. An electronic system digitizes the detected signal profiles and amplifies, filters, and transmits them to a computer for further data processing and image reconstruction. As an example, Fig. 1.36(b) shows a pressure profile recorded for the breast phantom (turbid collagen gel with "tumor" inserted into a 2-mm gel sphere colored with hemoglobin). The bipolar signal that came from a depth of about 5 cm represents a 2-mm spherical "tumor." The slope of the general pressure profile is due to the exponential decrease in laser energy absorbed in the phantom medium. The normalized and filtered final signal is free of high-frequency noise and other distortions and can be used for image reconstruction. Reconstructed 3D images can be obtained after a minimum of two OA signal matrixes are measured at 90 deg relative to each other.

The reflection-type OAT system contains a fiber-optic light delivery system with a single piezoelectric transducer, so that AWs can be detected at the site of laser irradiation [see Fig. 1.37(a)].[458,459,465] The emphasis in this imaging system is on high spatial resolution (up to several microns) and therefore the acoustic detector bandwidth must be the widest possible (about 300 MHz). Correspondingly, the laser wavelength and pulse duration should be chosen to generate pressure profiles with a maximum contrast in tissue layers. Figure 1.37(b) shows z-axial profiles of transient pressure signals measured *in vivo* in a mouse. One mammary gland of the mouse had a tumor (duct carcinoma) located underneath the skin with a diameter of about 5–6 mm and a thickness of about 0.5 mm (histology was performed after the experiments). The tumor had an advanced microcirculation developed as a sphere around it. Two surfaces of the tumor are depicted as two maxima in the OA signal on the axial profile. To obtain 3D images, one needs to scan the OA reflectometer along the area of diagnostic interest. An endoscopic version of the system is possible.

1.5.5 Optothermal radiometry

Pulse laser heating of a tissue causes temperature perturbations and the corresponding modulation of its thermal (infrared) radiation. This is the basis for pulse optothermal radiometry (OTR).[491–501] The maximum intensity of the thermal radiation of living objects falls at the wavelength range close to 10 µm. A detailed analysis of OTR signal formation requires knowledge of the internal temperature distribution within the tissue sample, the tissue thermal diffusivity, and its absorption coefficients at the excitation μ_a and emission μ'_a (10 µm) wavelengths. At the same time, knowledge of some of the parameters mentioned allows one to use the measured OTR signal to reconstruct, for example, the depth distribution of μ_a.[491,497]

The characteristic thermal time response of a bio object is defined by its dimension R_0 (the radius for a cylinder form) and the thermal diffusivity of its material a_T [see Eqs. (1.113) and (1.116)] as

$$\tau_T \sim \frac{(R_0)^2}{a_T}. \tag{1.133}$$

Experimental values for the thermal diffusivity a_T of some human tissues are presented in Table 1.3. For many soft tissues, these values lie within the rather narrow range defined by the thermal diffusivity of tissue components: type I hydrated collagen (50% water), 1.03×10^{-7} m^2/s; and pure water, 1.46×10^{-7} m^2/s.[494,495] Therefore, the characteristic thermal time response for various organs is mainly

Table 1.3 Experimental values for thermal diffusivity a_T of human tissues.[2]

Tissue	a_T, 10^{-7} m^2/s	Remarks
Muscle, underarm	0.60	*In vivo*, 0.45 mm
	1.00	*In vivo*, 0.90 mm
	1.30	*In vivo*, 0.90 mm
Muscle, thigh	0.545	*In vivo*, 0...1 mm
	0.963	*In vivo*, 1...2 mm
Skin	0.4...1.6	*In vivo*
	0.82...1.2	*In vitro*, room to body temperature
Kidney	1.32	*In vitro*, 5°C, 84% water
Heart	1.48	*In vitro*, 5°C, 81% water
Spleen	1.38	*In vitro*, 5°C, 80% water
Liver	1.50	*In vitro*, 5°C, 77% water
Brain	0.44...1.4	*In vitro*, room to body temperature
Brain, white matter	1.35	*In vitro*, 5°C, 71% water
Brain, gray matter	1.43	*In vitro*, 5°C, 83% water
Brain, whole	1.37	*In vitro*, 5°C, 78% water
Blood, hemolyzed	1.19	Power measurement, use of thermal model
Blood, plasma	1.21	
Teeth	4.09	–

defined by their dimensions and can be estimated as 10^{-3} s for a cell, 3×10^{-2} s for a small blood vessel, 10^2 s for a finger, and more than 10^4 s for a whole arm.

For a laser pulse duration much shorter than the thermal relaxation time of the sample τ_T, the normalized to incident radiant exposure and initial temperature OTR signal (the normalized surface temperature) induced in homogeneous absorbing-only and turbid samples is defined by the following expressions derived, respectively, on the basis of Beer's law and diffusion approximation:[497]

$$S_r(t) = \frac{\delta}{1-\delta^2}[\exp(\delta^2\alpha t)\mathrm{erfc}(\delta\sqrt{\alpha t}) - \delta\exp(\alpha t)\mathrm{erfc}(\sqrt{\alpha t})], \qquad (1.134)$$

$$S_r(t) = \delta \left\{ \begin{array}{l} \dfrac{A}{1-\delta_d^2}[\exp(\delta_d^2\alpha t)\mathrm{erfc}(\delta_d\sqrt{\alpha t}) - \delta_d\exp(\alpha t)\mathrm{erfc}(\sqrt{\alpha t})] \\[2mm] + \dfrac{B}{1-\delta_t^2}[\exp(\delta_t^2\alpha t)\mathrm{erfc}(\delta_t\sqrt{\alpha t}) - \delta_t\exp(\alpha t)\mathrm{erfc}(\sqrt{\alpha t})] \end{array} \right\}.$$

$$(1.135)$$

Here, $\delta = \mu_a/\mu_a'$, $\alpha = (\mu_a')^2 a_T$, $\delta_d = \mu_d/\mu_a'$, $\delta_t = (\mu_a + \mu_s')/\mu_a'$, $\mathrm{erfc}(x) = (2/\sqrt{\pi})\int_0^x e^{-\xi^2}d\xi$, is the complementary error function, and A and B are defined in diffusion theory. The corresponding temperature distributions inside the homogeneous and layered samples are presented in Ref. 497.

The surface radiometric signal $S_r(t)$ at any time t is the sum of the contributions from all depths in the tissue at time t. The radiation from deeper depths is attenuated by the infrared absorption of the sample before reaching the detector. Since the initial surface temperature is known, the temperature distribution into the sample depth can be extracted from the $S_r(t)$ measurement. An inverse OT method to convert surface temperatures as a function of time into internal temperatures as a function of depths is described in Ref. 497.

Figure 1.38 shows the results of pulse OTR experiments conducted on skin using a 577-nm, 1-μs pulsed dye laser.[497] Radiometric signals were collected from visibly healthy areas of the wrist and also from a port wine stain on the wrist of a Caucasian volunteer. The laser energy was maintained at 100 mJ over an area of about 20 mm^2. The infrared thermal signal from the irradiated area was monitored using a 1-mm^2 HgCdTe photoconductive detector with a wavelength detection range of 8 to 12 μm. The detector signal was conditioned using a dc to 1.5 MHz amplifier impedance matched to the detector. The signal was then recorded on a digital oscilloscope. The sampling rate was 10 to 50 μs per point, and 10,000 data points were collected after the laser pulse. The detector response was about 50 mV/°C. Twenty pulses were averaged to reduce the noise.

The calculated internal temperature distributions for a healthy area on the wrist and for a port wine stain are presented in Figs. 1.38(a) and 1.38(b). There is a noticeable peak in the temperature profile at around 80 μm, indicating a subsurface absorber. The limitations of this technique are that absorption profiles can only be made to a depth of 500 μm before the signal decays too much. Fortunately, most interesting structures in the skin are found between 0 and 600 μm from the skin

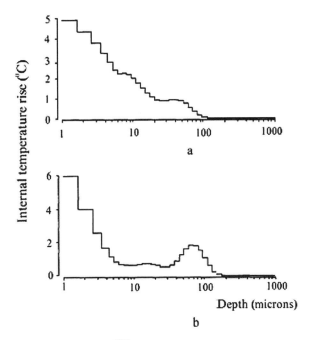

Figure 1.38 Depth profiling for skin.[497] The graph shows the temperature distribution for (a) a healthy area of the skin and (b) for a port wine stain. A temperature peak is evident at around 80 μm, indicating the presence of a subsurface absorber.

surface. The uncertainty in the location of the internal temperature layers increases with the depth of the layer.[497]

However, the single-wavelength pulsed OTR technique is applicable for the accurate determination of port wine stain depth if blood vessels are deeper than 100 μm.[498] When blood vessels are close or partially overlap the epidermal melanin layer, a two-wavelength (585 and 600 nm) technique is a superior method to determine lesion depth. It was demonstrated both theoretically and experimentally in *in vivo* measurements that the two-wavelength method should be appropriate for a wider range of port wine stain patients with various blood volume fractions, blood vessel size, and depth distribution.[498,499] This is due to the direct-difference approach used in which vessel depth is determined from a weighted difference of temperature profiles reconstructed independently from two-wavelength measurements.

It was also demonstrated both theoretically and experimentally how morphological information can be extracted from a simplified 2D model of a blood vessel if pulsed OTR imaging is performed and multidimensional analysis of the data is carried out.[513]

The pulse OTR method has good potentialities in the study of the optical and thermal properties of tissues *in vitro* and *in vivo*.[490–497] Some data received for the optical parameters are given in Table 2.1. Sequences (pairs) of infrared emission images recorded following pulsed laser irradiation were used to determine the thermal diffusivity of the biomaterial with a high precision.[495] The mean thermal diffusivity of an *in vitro* Type I hydrated (50% water) collagen film structure (a model skin phantom) at room temperature (22°C) deduced from 60 recorded infrared emission image pairs is equal to $a_T = (1.03 \pm 0.07) \times 10^{-7}$ m^2/s. Application of the method to *in vivo* tissues study was discussed.

The time-resolved OTR was used to determine the absorption coefficients of dental enamel and dentin at 2.79, 2.94, 9.6, and 10.6 μm.[454] These data are presented in Table 2.1 and are potentially important in the application of erbium [Er:YSGG (2.79 μm) and Er:YAG (2.94 μm)], or CO$_2$ (9.6 and 10.6 μm) lasers for the ablation of hard dental tissue. On the other hand, the OTR technique may serve for the online monitoring of tooth ablation or hard tissue depth profilometry for the inspection of dental defects.

The frequency-domain OTR technique uses an intensity-modulated laser radiation for inducing modulation frequency-dependent infrared optothermal radiometric (FD-OTR) signals from tissue lesions or defects.[500,501] The significance to dentistry of this technique is caused by its potentiality to monitor dental lesions at the early stages of carious decay where lateral and subsurface spatial resolution on the order of the crack sizes and subsurface depths investigated in Refs. 500 and 501 (100–300 μm) may be required. FD-OTR exhibits a much higher SNR than its pulsed counterpart and a fixed probe depth with the use of a single modulation frequency. For an image to be formed, either the source or the detector must be localized. Photothermal imaging generally falls into the category of scanned microscopy with a localized source. The temperature modulation allows for thermal energy to reach the surface diffusively from a depth approximately equal to a thermal length, described by Eq. (1.118). Scatterers located within a fraction of a thermal length from the source dominate the contrast of radiometric images. In this way, when the thermal length is varied, e.g., by changing the laser beam modulation frequency, the region of the specimen that contributes to the image is also varied.

In dental practice, it is often desirable to obtain detailed local information on potential lesions, and inside pits and fissures with high spatial resolution, such as that achieved with a focused laser source. To meet these objectives, recently a combination of FD-OTR and FD-LUM (luminescence) was used as a fast dental diagnostic tool to quantify sound enamel or dentin as well as subsurface cracks in human teeth.[500,501] Under laser excitation and modulation frequencies in the range from 10 Hz to 10 kHz, it was found that OTR images are complementary to LUM images as a direct result of the complementary nature of nonradiative (thermal) and radiative (fluorescence) de-excitation processes, which are responsible for the OTR and LUM signal generation, respectively. Measurements were performed at the 488, 659, and 830 nm wavelengths.

A probe beam deflection technique detecting the thermally induced refractive index gradient inside the sample was described [see Eq. (1.110)].[502] From the He:Ne laser probe beam deflection measurements and refractive index gradient estimates, it was found that a diode laser (1480 nm) beam produces superheated water of ~200°C. The temperature profile in the diode laser beam and vicinity is predicted as a function of laser pulse duration and power. An optimal (safe) regime to dissect the zona pellucida (shell) of preembryos by a focused laser beam (1480 nm) was defined as the pulse duration of ≤ 5 ms and laser power of ~ 100 mW.

1.5.6 Acoustooptical interactions

Acoustooptical tomography (AOT) or ultrasound-modulated optical tomography is based on the acoustic [ultrasound (US)] modulation of coherent laser light traveling in tissue.[517,519–524] An acoustic wave (AW) is focused into tissue and laser light is irradiating the same volume within the tissue, for instance, such as it is shown in Fig. 1.39. Any light that is encoded by the ultrasound, including both singly and multiply scattered photons, contributes to the imaging signal. Axial resolution along the acoustic axis can be achieved with US-frequency sweeping and subsequent application of the Fourier transformation,[517,521] whereas lateral resolution can be obtained by focusing the AW. Three possible mechanisms have been identified for the acoustic modulation of light in scattering tissues[517,520,524] (see Fig. 1.40). The first mechanism is based on US-induced variations of the optical properties of a tissue caused by spatially and temporally dependent tissue compression or rarifying at propagation of the AW. These variations in tissue density cause the corresponding oscillations of tissue optical properties, including absorption and scattering coefficients, and refractive index. Accordingly, the detected intensity of light varies with the AW. However, US modulation of incoherent light has been too weak to be observed experimentally.

The second mechanism is based on variations of the optical properties in response to US-induced displacement of scatterers. The displacements of scatterers,

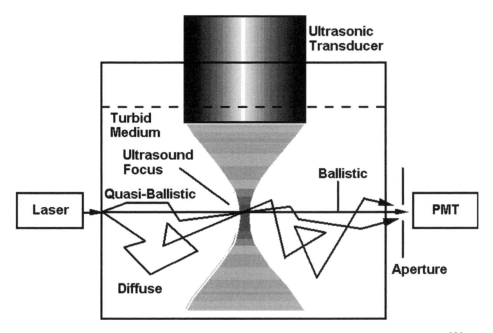

Figure 1.39 Illustration of the principle of acoustic-modulated optical tomography.[520]

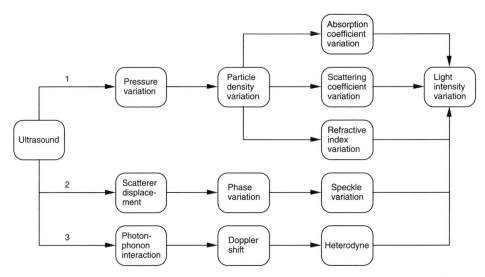

Figure 1.40 List of possible mechanisms of acoustic modulation of light in tissues.[520]

assumed to follow AW amplitudes, modulate the physical path lengths of light traveling through the acoustic field. Multiply scattered light accumulates modulated physical path lengths along its path. Consequently, the intensity of the speckles formed by the multiply scattered light fluctuates with the AW. The modulated component of the speckle pattern carries spatial information determined by the US and can be utilized for tomographic imaging.

The third mechanism is caused by photon-phonon interactions, where light is considered as an ensemble of photons and AW—as an ensemble of phonons. The photon-phonon interactions cause a Doppler shift in the classical sense to the frequency of the photons by the acoustic frequency and its harmonics. An optical detector functions as a heterodyning device between the Doppler-shifted light and unshifted light and produces an intensity signal at the acoustic frequency and its harmonics.

Both the second and the third mechanisms require the use of coherent light and both may be associated with the speckle effect. The modulation of the speckles in the second mechanism is caused by the acoustic modulation of scatterer displacements, while the modulation of the speckles in the third mechanism is caused by the acoustic modulation of the refractive index of the tissue. The acoustic modulation of the refractive index also appears in both the first and third mechanisms. However, in the first mechanism, the variation of refractive index causes light that may or may not be coherent to fluctuate in intensity, whereas in the second, the variation of refractive index causes fluctuation in phase of the coherent light, which is converted to fluctuation in intensity by a square-law detector. Thus, as a result of acoustic modulation of the refractive index, the optical phase between two consecutive scattering events is modulated, multiply scattered light accumulates modulated phases along its path, and the modulated phase causes the intensity of the speckles formed by the multiply scattered light to vary with the AW.

The intensity modulation depth M is defined as the ratio between the intensity at the fundamental frequency I_1 and the unmodulated intensity I_0

$$M = I_1/I_0. \tag{1.136}$$

The spectral intensity I_1 at fundamental acoustic frequency w_a is calculated from[517]

$$I_n = \left(\frac{1}{T_a}\right) \int_0^{T_a} \cos(nw_a\tau) G_1(\tau) d\tau \tag{1.137}$$

at $n = 1$; here, T_a is the acoustic period. In Eq. (1.137), the autocorrelation function of the scalar electric field, $E(t)$, of the scattered light calculated in the approximation of weak scattering (the optical MFP is much longer than the optical wavelength) and weak modulation (the acoustic amplitude is much less than the optical wavelength) has a view[517]

$$G_1(\tau) = 1 - \left(\frac{1}{6}\right)\left(\frac{L}{l_t}\right)\varepsilon[1 - \cos(w_a\tau)], \tag{1.138}$$

where

$$\varepsilon = 6(\delta_n + \delta_d)(n_0 k_0 A)^2,$$

$$\delta_n = (\alpha_{n1} + \alpha_{n2})\eta^2,$$

$$\alpha_{n1} = \frac{k_a l_t \tan^{-1}(k_a l_t)}{2},$$

$$\alpha_{n2} = \frac{\alpha_{n1}}{(k_a l_t)/\tan^{-1}(k_a l_t) - 1},$$

$$\delta_d = \frac{1}{6}.$$

L is the tissue slab thickness, n_0 is the background refractive index, k_0 is the optical wave vector in a vacuum, A is the acoustic amplitude, k_a is the acoustic wave vector, and l_t is the photon transport mean free path. Parameter η is related to the adiabatic piezo-optical coefficient of the tissue $\partial n/\partial p$, the density ρ, and the acoustic velocity v_a: $\eta = (\partial n/\partial p)\rho(v_a)^2$. The parameters δ_n and $\delta_d (= 1/6)$ are related to the average contributions per photon free path and per scattering event, respectively, to the ultrasonic modulation of light intensity. The contribution from the index of refraction δ_n increases with $k_a l_t$ because a longer photon free path, relative to the acoustic wavelength, accumulates a greater phase modulation. By contrast, the contribution from displacement δ_d stays constant at $1/6$, independent of k_a and l_t. The contribution from the index of refraction above a critical point at $k_a l_t = 0.559$, where contributions from refractive index and displacement are equal, increases with $k_a l_t$ and can significantly outmatch the contribution from displacement.

Accounting for Eq. (1.138), the modulation depth of intensity fluctuations can be presented as

$$M = \left(\frac{1}{6}\right)\left(\frac{L}{l_t}\right)^2 \varepsilon \propto A^2. \tag{1.139}$$

This equation shows a quadratic relationship between the intensity modulation depth M and the acoustic amplitude A. Only the nonlinear terms of phase accumulation contribute to the acoustic modulation of coherent light at multiple scattering. The linear term vanishes as a result of optical random walk in scattering media. In the ballistic (nonscattering) regime, M is proportional to A due to nonaveraged contributions from the linear term of phase accumulation. In the quasi-ballistic (minimal scattering) regime, M may show a mixed behavior with A.

It is important to note that the quadratic relationship described by Eq. (1.139) can be experimentally observed if a spectrometer, such as a Fabry-Perot interferometer, is used as a detector. In many cases, the measured modulation depth M' is defined as the ratio between the observed ac and dc signals, where the ac signal is originated from the beats between the electric field at the fundamental frequency of the modulated light ($w_0 \pm w_a$) and the electric field at the intrinsic unmodulated optical frequency (w_0). As a result, the measured modulation depth is approximately described by

$$M' \propto \left(\frac{I_1}{I_0}\right)^{1/2} = M^{1/2} \propto A, \tag{1.140}$$

indicating that the measured modulation depth is proportional to the acoustic amplitude.

A frequency-swept (chirped) AW is used to encode a laser beam that crosses the acoustic axis of the US transducer with various frequencies.[517] Decoding the transmitted light in the frequency domain allows one to image objects buried inside the scattering media. Such images are resolved along the acoustic axis. This encoding scheme is analogous to that of MRI.

A parallel AOT uses a CCD camera for detection of a US-modulated signal pixel by pixel.[517] A schematic of the experimental arrangement is shown in Fig. 1.41(a). The z-axis is on the acoustic axis pointing from the US transducer to the sample, the y-axis is along the optical axis pointing to the diode laser, and the x-axis is perpendicular to both the acoustic and optical axes. The AOT system, described in Ref. 517, had the following parameters: a focused US transducer

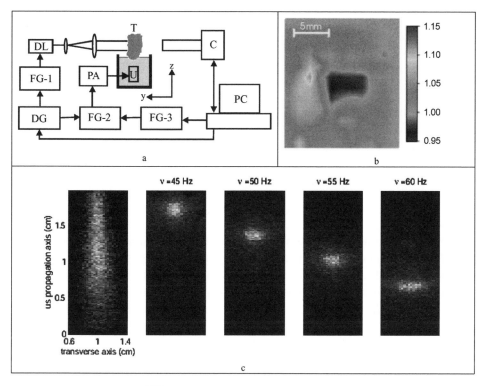

Figure 1.41 Parallel AOT.[517] (a) Schematic of the experimental setup: DL, diode laser; C, CCD camera; U, ultrasonic transducer; FG-1, FG-2, and FG-3, function generators; DG, delay generator; PA, power amplifier; T, tissue sample. (b) Experimental two-dimensional image of 1.2-cm-thick chicken breast tissue containing a buried object; the horizontal and vertical axes are along the x- and z-axes, respectively. (c) Demonstration of the virtual source of ultrasound-modulated light; left frame, the entire virtual source; following frames, virtual sources corresponding to various values of y obtained by adjusting the frequency f_h.

with a 2.54-cm focal length in water, a 1-MHz central response frequency, and the peak focal pressure of $\sim 2 \times 10^5$ Pa (less below the damage threshold for tissue); a diode laser with 690-nm wavelength, average power 12 mW and coherence length ~ 7 cm; the laser beam was expanded to 1.6×0.3 cm and projected onto the tissue sample; and a high-speed 12-bit digital CCD camera. The tissue sample was partially immersed in water to provide good acoustic coupling. The light transmitted through the sample produced a speckle pattern, which was detected by the CCD camera. Three function generators, FG-1, FG-2, and FG-3, shared the same time base to ensure synchronization. FG-1 and FG-2 generated chirp functions to modulate the laser and to excite the US transducer, respectively. A delay generator (DG) controlled the time delay between the trigger signals to FG-1 and FG-2.

If no amplitude modulation is provided by FG-3, the frequency of the heterodyne signal received from location z along the US axis is defined by

$$f_h(z, \tau) = b\left(\tau - \frac{z}{v_a}\right), \tag{1.141}$$

where b is the rate of the frequency sweep and τ is the time delay between the two chirps from FG-2 and FG-1. By producing a reference sinusoidal wave with a frequency equal to $f_h(z, \tau)$, which modulates the amplitude of the chirp, FG-3 implements the source-synchronized lock-in measurement. The signal in a single CCD pixel can be represented as

$$I_i(\phi_i) \propto I_b + I_m \cos(\phi_s + \phi_r), \tag{1.142}$$

where I_b is the background intensity, I_m is the signal intensity related to the ultrasound-modulated component, ϕ_i is the randomly distributed initial phase of the speckle that does not provide useful information in this imaging system, and ϕ_r is the initial phase of the reference sinusoidal wave from FG-3. The modulation depth, $M' = I_m/I_b$, which reflects the local optical and acoustic properties, can be calculated from four consequent frames of CCD taken at ϕ_r equal to 0, 90, 180, and 270 deg, using the following expression:[517]

$$M' = \frac{1}{2I_b}\sqrt{[I_i(90°) - I_i(270°)]^2 + [I_i(0°) - I_i(180°)]^2}. \tag{1.143}$$

To recover M', calculations should be performed for each pixel and a total $N \times N$ pixel data points should be averaged to produce a single data point for the image.

For fixed reference (lock-in) frequency f_r from FG-3, the US-modulated light from a specific spatial location z_0 that corresponds to the heterodyne frequency f_r and the time delay τ can be detected, where z_0 is derived from Eq. (1.141) as

$$z_0 = v_a\left(\tau - \frac{f_r}{b}\right). \tag{1.144}$$

The US-modulated light from the other locations have different frequencies and hence are rejected by the CCD camera. One-dimensional images along the US axis are obtained by electronically scanning the time delay τ, as well as 2D tomographic images by additional mechanically scanned the US transducer along the x-axis.

Figure 1.141(b) illustrates 2D image of the object buried inside a chicken breast tissue sample. The buried object, which has little acoustic absorption, is clearly visible in the background. The image resolution along the x-axis is $\sim$2 mm, which is determined by the 2-mm focal diameter of the US transducer. The spatial resolution along the US axis (z-axis) Δz is determined by the frequency span Δf of the chirp function and the US velocity v_a as follows:

$$\Delta z \approx v_a/\Delta f, \tag{1.145}$$

where $v_a \approx 1{,}500$ m/s, and for $\Delta f = 800$ kHz is $\sim$2 mm.

The special measurements with the laser beam illuminating the sample obliquely at 10 deg to the z-axis has shown that images were also the same as those measured in the case of normal incidence.[517] Hence, AOT depends primarily on scattered photons, and ballistic photons are not the major contributors to the signal.

Figure 1.41(c) shows a series of images of the virtual light sources defined by the US. As follows from Eq. (1.141), the frequency of the heterodyned signal is related to the source location y; thus, these images correspond to various values of y obtained by adjusting the frequency f_h. When the virtual source propagates through a scattering medium, a direct view of the virtual source is blurred. However, if the virtual source is detected immediately without further propagation, a clear view of the virtual source can be acquired. This demonstration clearly illustrates the importance of US tagging of light that enhances the spatial resolution of the imaging.

1.5.7 Thermal effects

Thermal imaging is based on sensing the IR radiation that is emitted by all objects at any temperature above absolute zero temperature.[525] Such emission is due to molecular transitions from a high-energy to a low-energy state and for condensed media its energy distribution between different wavelengths is described by the Planck curve. At the normal temperature of the human body, the peak of the Planck curve occurs in the mid-IR between 9- and 10-μm wavelengths.

The Planck function is exponentially nonlinear in temperature; it follows from this function that the lower-temperature objects emit orders of magnitude less energy than do higher-temperature objects. The human body belongs to the lower-temperature objects; therefore, accurate detection of IR radiation from the body is not simple. Moreover, usually a human body and its surroundings emit comparable amounts of IR energy, which leads to additional difficulties in measurements. Often the SNR is low and to detect a signal specialized background correction instrumentation, lock-in signal processing techniques, and careful analysis of the resulting data are required.[525] The technologies of IR array detectors, associated electronics, image processing, and noise reduction have been significantly improved over the last 10 years. Infrared cameras suitable for medical thermal imaging are reviewed in Ref. 525. At present, the accuracy with which temperature and temperature changes can be measured has reached 10^{-3} K.

The steady-state form of the bioheat equation originated from the energy balance and describes the change in tissue temperature $T(\mathbf{r})$ at point $\mathbf{r}$ in the tissue[2,3,42,525–530]

$$\nabla(k_T \nabla T) + S + \rho_b c_b q_b (T_a - T) = 0, \qquad (1.146)$$

where k_T is the thermal conductivity of the tissue (W/K); S is the heat source term (W/m^3), defined by the metabolic heat generation rate at point $\mathbf{r}$; ρ_b is the blood density (kg/m^3); c_b is the blood specific heat (J/kgK); q_b is the blood per-fusion rate (1/s), defined as the volume of blood flowing through unit volume of tissue in one second; T_a is the arterial blood temperature (K), and T is the local temperature of the tissue, all at point $\mathbf{r}$ in the tissue. The first term describes any heat conduction (typically away from point $\mathbf{r}$), the source term accounts for heat generation due to metabolic processes, and the last term describes the heat transfer caused by blood perfusion. The temperature of the arterial blood is approximated to be the core temperature of the body.

In many practical cases, it may often be assumed that only the heat transfer process normal to the surface need to be taken into account as a one-dimensional problem[530]

$$\frac{1}{r^n}\frac{\partial}{\partial r}\left(k_T r^n \frac{\partial T}{\partial r}\right) + S + \rho_b c_b q_b (T_a - T) = 0, \qquad (1.147)$$

where $n = 0, 1, 2$ are for slab, cylinder, and sphere, respectively.

To solve this equation the boundary conditions must be accounted for. The boundary conditions depend on tissue and environment states. The tissue exchanges energy (and mass) with the environment through a combination of convection, radiation, evaporation, and conduction. The driving forces for these exchanges are the differences in temperature and water vapor partial pressure between the tissue and the surroundings. The boundary conditions for heat transfer at the tissue surface can be taken in the general form[530]

$$-k_T \frac{\partial T}{\partial r}\Big|_s = h(T_s - T_e), \qquad (1.148)$$

where h is the apparent energy transfer coefficient, which may be dependent on temperature, pressure, relative humidity, tissue insulation, etc.; T_s and T_e are the temperature of the tissue surface and environment, respectively. A deep boundary condition, supposing that the temperature remains constant at the depth R_0 and equal to the core body temperature (or arterial blood temperature T_a), is

$$T|_{R_0} = T_a. \qquad (1.149)$$

The bioheat equation of the general form, Eqs. (1.146) and (1.147), can be applied to each tissue and surrounding material layer to set up a partial differential equation group coupled by the conditions, which ensures the continuity of temperature and heat fluxes at any interface between adjacent layers. Methods of solving the bioheat equation can be found in Refs. 2, 3, 42, 261, 262, and 525–530.

The metabolic heat generation rate may be significantly different for normal tissue and for tumor. For example, for normal breast tissue $S(\mathbf{r})$ was estimated as 450 W/m^3 and for tumor 29,000 W/m^3, and the corresponding blood perfusion rate q_b as 0.00018 s^{-1} for normal tissue and 0.00900 s^{-1} for a pathological one.[525] Theoretical modeling using these data and Eq. (1.146) for the normal breast and breast with a tumor as a spherical inclusion of radius 1.1 cm with its center located at 2.1 cm beneath the skin surface showed a temperature rise of the skin surface caused by the tumor of about 2°C, from ∼32°C for the normal breast to ∼34°C for the breast with tumor. This is a most significant result because tumor introduces a local temperature rise on the breast surface that is accurately detectable by modern IR cameras. Furthermore, inverse bioheat transfer calculations may provide a method of locating the tumor using the surface thermograms.[525]

For different normal tissues, the blood perfusion rate q_b is evaluated as the highest for kidney choroids, 0.05–0.10 s^{-1}; as the midlevel for brain cortex, 0.007–0.02 s^{-1}, skin, 0.002–0.007 s^{-1}, and muscle, 0.0003–0.002 s^{-1}; and as the lowest for fat, 0.0001–0.0003 s^{-1}.[526]

A simplified 3D bioheat equation describing the effect of blood flow on blood-tissue heat transfer was proposed in Ref. 529. This equation contains a remarkably simple expression for the tensor conductivity of the tissue as a function of the local vascular geometry and flow velocity in the thermally significant countercurrent vessels, which was derived using the concept of anisotropic heat transfer. The concept is based on the statement that the primary mechanism for blood-tissue energy exchange is incomplete countercurrent exchange in the thermally significant microvessels.

Many applications of IR thermal imaging have been reported, some of which are overviewed in Ref. 525. The basic measurements involve tissue temperature distributions resulting from a variety of internal and external conditions affecting blood microcirculation and metabolic processes. Thermal imaging was used for detection of breast cancer, monitoring of the inflammatory state of human gingiva, for identifying the health status of the thyroid gland, for indication of ectodermal dysplasia, to measure the depth of burns, in the management of pain, in monitoring surgical tendon repair, to measure brain activity, to image atherosclerotic plaque, for detecting anxiety, etc. The temperature increase of thermally insulated skin measured by IR radiometry provides useful information about its blood flow and the blood temperature.[530,531]

The main disadvantages of thermal imaging for monitoring of any disease state, including breast cancer, is its nonspecific nature connected with tissue blood perfusion response and tissue metabolic activity, and providing only surface temperature measurements. Therefore, this technique must be used as an adjunct to other diagnostic techniques and in conjunction with newly designed instrumentation and analytical and numerical computational tools.[525]

1.5.8 Sonoluminescence

A sonoluminescence (SL) signal generated internally in media with a 1-MHz continuous-wave ultrasound (US) can be used to produce two-dimensional images of objects imbedded in turbid media.[532,533] This technique is based on a light emission phenomenon connected with the driving of small bubbles by US collapse. The bubbles start out with a radius of several microns and expand to ∼50 µm, owing to a decrease in acoustic pressure in the negative half of a sinusoidal period; after the AW reaches the positive half of the period, the resulting pressure difference leads to a rapid collapse of the bubbles, accompanied by a broadband emission of light—SL. Such emission is of a short duration (in tens of picoseconds), repeatable with each cycle of sound, and has the spectrum containing molecular emission bands (with peaks near 300–500 nm) associated with the liquid, mostly water, in which the SL occurs.

SL tomography (SLT) as a new approach for optical imaging of dense turbid media (biological tissues) is described in Refs. 532 and 533. The major advantages of SLT include: (1) high SNR due to the internally generated probe optical signal; (2) high contrast of imaging; (3) good spatial resolution, which is limited by the US focal size; and (4) low cost of equipment. It was shown experimentally that there is a threshold of SL generation at applied US pressure, when the peak pressure at the US focus was ~2 bars (~100 V, see Fig. 1.42). The rapid increase of the SL intensity with the acoustic pressure above the threshold indicates that the SL signal would be a sensitive measure of the local acoustic pressure. It is also seen in Fig. 1.42 that generation of SL is not affected by the addition of Intralipid and trypan blue, but is significantly affected by the addition of polystyrene spheres. Because SL is a broadband emission, the scattering and the absorption spectra of tissues and immersion liquids should be accounted for in imaging algorithms.[533] On the basis of the calculated diffuse transmittance of the polystyrene phantom near 400 nm, the SL power at the source was estimated to be greater than 1 pW. The turbid media (tissue) functions as a filter that modifies the spectrum of the SL signal. For a cubic object made from rubber buried in the Intralipid phantom, the spatial resolution of the edges was estimated to be 2–3 mm, and an excellent imaging contrast was observed.[533]

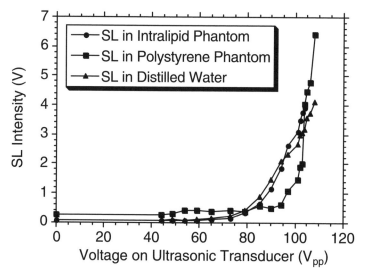

Figure 1.42 SL intensity versus the driving voltage on the US transducer.[533]

SLT is based on several contrast mechanisms:[533] (1) for the objects with US contrast relative to the background, the SL signal originating from the object differs from that originating from the background medium, the SL generation is affected by the local US intensity (see Fig. 1.42); (2) for the objects with contrast in optical properties, the SL signal from the object is attenuated differently because the SL light must propagate through the object; (3) for objects with the ability to generate SL, the SL from the object is different, even if the local US pressure is the same.

It should be noted that the peak pressure at the US focus is typically less than $\sim$2 bars (1.3 W/cm^2 in spatial-peak-temporal-peak power), which is one order in magnitude less than the safety limit set by the US FDA (23 bars) and two orders less than the tissue damage threshold (400 and 900 W/cm^2 at 1 MHz for brain and muscle, respectively).[533]

1.5.9 Prospective applications and measuring techniques

It was recently shown that OA imaging allows one to perform highly resolved 3D images of artificial blood vessels in a tissue phantom with $\sim$20-μm depth resolution and $\sim$200-μm resolution in a lateral direction.[477] The designed measuring technique and reconstruction algorithm were applied to image a vascular tree from a Wistar rat *in vitro*[480] and human wrist skin blood vessels *in vivo*.[481] In Ref. 481, a double-ring OA sensor together with measurements of a cross-correlation between the signals detected by the two rings were used to provide a narrow angular aperture of the system. The depth position of the observed vessels of the human wrist was about 1.5 to 2 mm below the skin surface. It was also demonstrated that besides skin and superficial blood vessels, the underlying bone was also identified, at a depth of about 3 mm below the skin surface.[481] The total data acquisition time for getting a 2D image with 101 measurement positions (A-scans) was about 5 min for laser with a pulse repetition rate of 10 Hz. The maximum depth at which vessels can be detected is dependent on parameters such as the illuminating light intensity, the wavelength used, and the sensitivity of the OA sensor.

The feasibility of using the OA method for the monitoring of glaucoma treatment by application of a laser cyclophotocoagulation technique was proved recently.[488] From described results it follows that the laser OA method seems to be a promising tool for localization of the ciliary body and monitoring of the coagulating process. In order to optimize fundus laser treatments of the eye, an online noninvasive OA technique for monitoring of fundus temperature was designed.[489] It was found that the OA method can be used to noninvasively determine retinal temperatures during pulsed laser treatment of the eye. This technique can also be adapted to CW photocoagulation, photodynamic therapy and transpupillary thermotherapy, or other fields of laser-heated tissue.

Optoacoustics is used for the characterization of layered tissue structures in the near and far fields[471] that is important to provide in-depth measurements of port wine stain of the human skin.[474] The OA method can be also used to perform *in vivo* tomographic images of small animals. The 2D OA images[475] as well as slices of a 3D image[476] of sacrificed mice were reported. A system capable of performing OA structural and functional imaging in rat brain was developed.[483,484] One more important application of the time-resolved OA technique is monitoring tissue mechanical response and ablation.[511]

Measurement of the pressure transient or displacement at the tissue surface is the most commonly provided by the use of piezoelectric sensors.[458,459,481] Although piezoelectric sensors have the advantage that broadband sensors are easy to construct and their sensitivity is rather high, optical methods may sometimes be preferable in *in vivo* studies due to their ability to provide noncontact measurements (see Fig. 1.33).[473,485–487] A minimally invasive noncontact interferometric technique to accurately measure the effective optical attenuation depth of a sample is described.[486,487] This technique measures the time-resolved tissue surface displacement that results from absorption of a short laser pulse. The surface motion is caused by thermoelastic stress relaxation, whose time constant is proportional to the optical attenuation depth of the sample. The magnitude of expansion is a function of the incident radiant exposure and thermophysical properties of the sample. This technique is complementary to interferometric photothermal spectroscopy, a method that determines the effective optical attenuation depth through time-resolved measurements of surface displacement resulting from the thermal diffusion that follows the thermoelastic stress relaxation process.[509,510] The interferometric system utilizes a time-resolved high-resolution interferometer capable of angstrom-level displacement resolution and nanosecond temporal resolution to detect subsurface blood vessels within a human forearm *in vivo*.[486,487]

High resolution and minimal artifacts of the images are characteristic for the circular-scanning OA computed tomography with a full 360-deg scan about an object with elevated geometry, such as brain and breast.[483,484,517,518] Planar reflection-mode techniques[458,459,465,477] are not limited by the shape of the sample, but they may suffer from the strong OA waves emitted from optical absorbers near the surface, such as hair follicles and melanin granules in the skin, whose acoustic reverberations can potentially overshadow the much weaker OA signals from structures deep in the tissue. A reflection-mode microscopic OA imaging technique that uses dark-field illumination prevents the occurrence of such artifacts.[518] High image resolution and high sensitivity were achieved by utilizing a high-frequency, large-numerical-aperture (NA) spherically focused ultrasonic transducer that is coaxial and confocal with the optical illumination. Both a wide bandwidth and a large NA provide the high resolution of the acoustic detector; however, the increasing of frequency is limited because of a corresponding decrease of the acoustic wave penetration depth (attenuation in a tissue is of 0.7–3 dB/cm/MHz). Therefore, the OA sensor with a large NA ($= 0.44$) and frequency range from 32.5 to 67.5 MHz was used by the authors of Ref. 518 in *in vitro* and *in vivo* studies of rat skin. These parameters of the OA sensor provide lateral resolution of 45–120 μm (defined by the NA) and axial resolution of $\sim$15 μm (defined by the frequency range). The system is capable of imaging optical-absorption contrast as deep as 3 mm in tissue.

In monitoring and determining chemical traces, the time-resolved OA technique and other optothermal techniques may be prospective procedures to be used in noninvasive monitoring of glucose[534–546] and blood hemoglobin volume and oxygenation.[516,547,548]

In the low-scattering mode when aqueous glucose solutions were irradiated by NIR laser pulses at wavelengths that corresponded to NIR absorption of glucose (1.0–1.8 μm), OA signal generation was assumed to be due to initial light absorption by the glucose molecules.[536] A linear relationship between the OA signal and glucose concentration was found. It was also shown that the OA signal tracks change in glucose concentration in human measurements. No specific advantages of OA spectroscopy over an NIR measurement of glucose are expected in this case.[534]

Another approach of OA glucose detection is based on the glucose property to change scattering parameters of tissues.[172,339–341,534,549–551] As follows from Eq. (1.125), the OA signal from the tissue depth is defined by optical attenuation μ_{eff}, which is related to changes in the refractive index of the medium induced by changes in glucose concentration. Decreasing scattering increases the energy density in the OA sound source and induces higher OA signals.[541] OA temporal profiles induced by 355-nm laser pulses in *in vivo* rabbit sclera at intravenous glucose administering demonstrated that a 1 mM increase in glucose concentration resulted in up to a 5% decrease of μ_{eff}.[537] The UV light used in this experiment allowed one to increase the absolute value of the OA signal and its sensitivity to scattering change due to much higher absorption and scattering of tissues in UV than in the visible and NIR [see Eq. (1.125)].

However, in the NIR range, the effect of glucose on the scattering properties of tissue phantoms is also detectable by using the OA technique.[540,541] At 905 nm, a 1% (1 g dl^{-1}) change in glucose concentration increased the OA signal by 2.0% in distilled water, 5.4% in 3% milk, and 2.5% in bloodless tissue, and at 1064 nm the similar change in glucose concentration increased the OA signal by 2.7% in 1% Intralipid. It was also found that the glucose-induced change in the OA signal was larger in blood than in Intralipid, amounting to 6.0%/0.5 g dl^{-1} of added glucose at 532 nm and 11.4%/0.5 g dl^{-1} of added glucose at 1064.[540] Glucose-induced changes in the 1% Intralipid can be explained by a matching of refractive indices of phospholipid micelles and water with added glucose, whereas the observed changes in blood may be additionally influenced by the changes in the size and shape of red blood cells due to changes of blood plasma osmolarity.[48,538,540,552]

Besides the increase in the peak-to-peak value of the OA signal as a function of glucose concentration, a corresponding shift in the position of the OA signal maximum toward earlier times at higher glucose concentrations, produced by changes in the sound velocity of the sample at glucose addition, was found.[540,543] The other two parameters in Eq. (1.125), the thermal expansion coefficient β and tissue or blood specific heat c_T, also may be changed with a glucose concentration change. Estimations done in Ref. 541 showed that variations of these two parameters are not so high and do not seriously influence the OA signal in the limits of physiological glucose concentrations. As for the sound velocity dependence on glucose concentration, it may be excluded from the measurements of the OA temporal profile and give additional information on glucose concentration.

One of the drawbacks of the OA technique is that measurement of sound propagation in tissue is dependent on mechanical coupling between the tissue and the measuring probe and on the pressure of the probe on the tissue surface. This effect is quite similar to ultrasound propagation in tissue where coupling gels are used to decrease sound reflections.

Still further work is needed to understand OA signal origination and propagation in tissue and its use for glucose sensing. At present, the OA technique based on scattering measurements also does not offer any noticeable advantage over other scattering methods.[534] However, a few groups and companies, such as Glucon, Inc.,[542] are developing different new approaches for OA glucose sensing, including techniques based on combining ultrasound and OA spectroscopy.[534]

Thermal gradient spectroscopy (TGS) is based on measuring the fundamental absorption bands of glucose at 9.1–10.5 μm using the body's naturally emitted IR radiation as an internal source of radiation.[534,544–546] The cooling-induced skin transparency allows for monitoring of IR emission from the interstitial fluid and cutaneous layers.[544,545] A linear response between *in vivo* TGS detected glucose and reference blood glucose values has been reported in clinical studies for several individuals with Type 1 diabetes.[544] Different modifications of this method and corresponding instrumentation for more precise quantifying of glucose in a human body are described in the literature.[534,545,546] The simplicity of this method makes it quite appealing; however, the overlap between the effect of glucose on the signal and temperature variations due to circadian periodicity, as well as temperature and blood flow response to glucose change, should be eliminated or accounted for.[534]

An OA laser system for noninvasive monitoring of cerebral venous oxygenation in the superior sagittal sinus based on a *Q*-switched nanosecond Nd:YAG laser (wavelength 1064 nm, pulse repetition rate 1 Hz) was designed.[516] The authors demonstrated that the amplitude and temporal profile of OA waves are linearly dependent on blood oxygenation in the wide range of blood oxygenation from 24% to 92%. The designed system was capable of real-time and continuous measurements of blood oxygenation despite optical and acoustic attenuation by thick bone.

The use of an OA technique for noninvasive and real-time continuous monitoring of total hemoglobin concentration (THb) was recently proposed.[547,548] It was shown that the OA technique may provide accurate measurements of THb by detection and analysis of OA signal temporal profiles induced by short optical pulses in blood circulating in arteries or veins. A portable OA system based on a 10-ns Nd:YAG laser (1064 nm) was designed for the monitoring of THb in the radial artery. Results of *in vitro* and *in vivo* studies demonstrated that (1) the slope of OA waves induced in blood in the transmission mode is linearly dependent on THb in the range from 6.2 to 12.4 g/dl; (2) OA signals can be detected despite optical attenuation in turbid tissue phantoms with a thickness of 1 cm; and (3) the OA system detects signals induced in blood circulating in the radial artery. Clinical studies for healthy volunteers, described in Ref. 548, showed that the amplitude of

OA signal generated in the radial artery closely followed the THb (rapidly changed at infusion of intravenous saline) measured directly in concurrently collected blood samples.

The photothermal microscopy (PTM) technique shows the capability to visualize absorbing cellular structures of living cells *in vitro* without labeling,[503–506] as well as to image moving unlabeled cells in real time *in vivo* in studies of circulating red and white blood cells in capillaries and lymph microvessels of rat mesentery.[507,508] We will briefly discuss some potential applications of this optical tool called PT flow cytometry (PTFC).[508] The imaging of single cells *in vivo* is potentially important for the early diagnosis of diseases (e.g., cancer and diabetes) or for the study of the influence of various factors (e.g., drugs, smoking, ionizing radiation) on individual cells.

To realize PTFC, a nonscanning fast PTM system was used because of cells crossing the area of detection in 0.1–0.01 s for even relatively slow flow in capillaries.[508] Such a system was built on the basis of a pulsed pumping tunable optical parametric oscillator (420–570 nm, pulse width of 8 ns, pulse energy of 0.1–400 μJ; Lotis Ltd.). Laser-induced temperature-dependent variations of the refractive index in the cell were detected using a phase-contrast imaging technique (Olympus BX51 microscope with a CCD camera; AE-260E, Apogee Inc.) with illumination by a low-energy collinear probe pulse (Raman shifter, wavelength 639 nm, pulse width of 13 ns, and pulse energy of 2 nJ). The diameters of the pump- and probe-beam spots, with stable, smooth intensity profiles, ranged from 20 to 50 μm and 15 to 50 μm, respectively, and thus covered entire single cells and even whole microvessels. A spatial resolution of $\sim$0.7 μm was provided. The acquisition procedure included illumination of the cell with three pulses: an initial probe pulse followed by a 0.08-s delay to the pump pulse, and then a second probe pulse with a tunable time delay (0–5000 ns) to the pump pulse. The PT image, calculated as the difference between the two probe-pulse images, depends only on absorption contrast transformed by the pump laser pulse into refractive contrast.[508]

To experimentally prove the concept of *in vivo* PTFC, a rat mesentery model was chosen among various animal models (e.g., ears, lips, etc.) because of its unique anatomic structure consisting of thin, transparent, duplex connective tissue with a single layer of blood and lymph microvessels. Using transillumination digital microscopy (TDM) RBCs and lymphocytes traveling through blood and/or lymph vessels, lymphatic valves, and other mesenteric structures were imaged (Fig. 1.43). It was found that in most intact lymph vessels (diameter of 50–150 μm), lymphocytes in flow had an average velocity of $\sim$211 $\pm$ 11 μm/s. In comparison, the velocity of RBCs was significantly higher, up to 2 mm/s in blood vessels with a diameter of 20–30 μm and from 100 to 500 μm/s for capillaries with diameter less than 10 μm. The high spatial resolution of TDM (300 nm at 100$\times$, NA = 1.25 with immersion) allowed roughly estimating the cell size and even shape (Fig. 1.44, left). Because of its low absorption sensitivity, however, TDM was not suitable for visualizing absorbing cellular structures. In contrast, the PTFC mode (navigated by TDM) allowed the obtaining of images of moving lymphocytes and RBCs (Fig. 1.44, right) that showed structures specific to PT images and

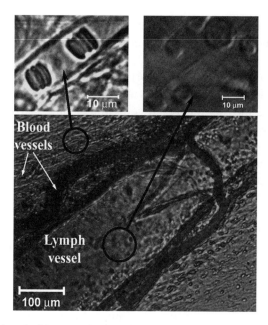

Figure 1.43 Typical optical image of a lymph microvessel of rat mesentery with blood microvessels along the lymphatic walls (bottom), RBCs in a capillary (top left), and single cells in lymph flow (top right).[508]

associated with the spatial distribution of absorbing cellular chromophores (e.g., hemoglobin in RBCs, or cytochromes in lymphocytes). Currently, PTFC's rate of ~10 cells/s is limited by the repetition rate of the pump laser (10 Hz).

Potential applications of *in vivo* PTFC may include: (1) identification of cells with differences in natural absorptive properties (e.g., the counting of white cells in blood flow or of rare RBCs among lymphocytes in microlymphatic vessels); (2) monitoring of the circulation and distribution of absorbing nanoparticles used for PT probing or photosensitizing; (3) study of laser-cell interactions; and (4) study of the influence of different environmental factors on cells.

The main technical difficulty of the time-resolved measurements of OA profiles is associated with correct detection of acoustic signals, which requires simultaneously high temporal resolution equal to or higher than the laser pulse duration and wideband frequency detection extending into low-frequency ultrasound.[458] Wideband piezoelectric transducers with short-circuit or open-circuit operating modes, being low-noise detectors, have proved to be most suitable for this purpose. The transducer operating in the short-circuit mode has substantial thickness that is larger than the spatial width of the detected ultrasonic transient. The transducer thickness limits the lower limit of detected ultrasonic frequencies and duration of the detection window. An excessively thick piezoelement would: (1) lead to a more prominent acoustic diffraction at lower ultrasonic frequencies in the detected signal, and (2) reduce the electric capacity to a value below the electric capacity of the electronic circuitry. It is difficult to design acoustic transducers operating in short-circuit mode for detection of OA profiles longer than 1–2 μs. However, these

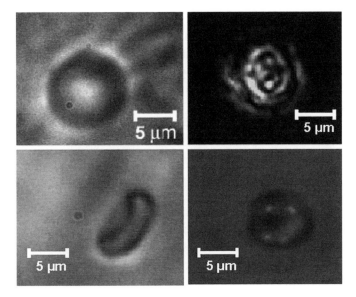

Figure 1.44 Optical transmission (left column) and PT (right column) images *in vivo* of a single, moving lymphocyte (top row) and RBCs (bottom row) in lymph flow in rat mesentery (vessel diameter 105 μm, velocity ∼120 μm/s). Pump pulse parameters: wavelength, 525 nm; pulse width, 8 ns; and pulse energy, 30 μJ and 0.5 μJ (right column, top and bottom, respectively); time delay between pump and probe pulses, 10 ns.[508]

transducers would be most optimal for detection of submicrosecond and nanosecond OA signals. The upper limit of ultrasonic frequency is defined by the discharge time of the transducer capacity. The ultrasonic detection band could reach several hundred megahertz. This type of transducer does not require backing material to reduce resonant vibrations.

In the case of an acoustic transducer operating in the open-circuit mode, it is necessary that the thickness of piezoelectric element be smaller than the acoustic wavelength detected in its upper ultrasonic frequency limit.[458] The lower limit of detectable ultrasonic frequencies is defined by the discharge time of the transducer electric capacity through the input resistor of the electronic preamplifier. In order to design acoustic transducers operating in the open-circuit mode with very wide ultrasonic detection band (≥100 MHz), one has to employ piezoelectric elements that are a few microns thick. The choice of appropriate backing material is crucial for widening the frequency band. Design of the backing layer acoustically matched with the piezoelectric material for effective damping of transducer resonances is one of the most important technical problems. The sensitivity of open-circuit transducers is greater than that of short-circuit transducers due to longer holding of the electric charge at the piezoelement.

Another technical difficulty in providing high temporal resolution in the detection of OA profiles is the need for precise adjustment of the detector face with respect to the wavefront of the arriving optoacoustic signal.[458] Obviously, the time difference between the instances of the laser-induced pressure transient (LIPT) arrival to the opposite edges of the piezoelectric element should be shorter than the temporal resolution of this transducer. Therefore, the angle between the direction of the LIPT wavefront propagation and the normal to the piezoelectric detector must be as small as possible. For example, to achieve temporal resolution of $\Delta\tau$ ~10 ns, the LIPT has to be incident with angle by less than ~3 min relative to the sensitive area aperture of ~3 mm.

The highest possible piezoelectric efficiency for wideband piezoelectric detection can be achieved with piezoceramics, such as PZT-5H.[458] A lower sensitivity could be obtained with polyvinyldenefluoride (PVDF) or PVDF copolymers. Quartz and lithium niobate have significantly lower sensitivity for wideband ultrasonic detection.

Low acoustic impedance, which is similar to that in biological tissues, makes PVDF suitable for applications in medical and biological sensing.[458] Design of effective backing for PVDF transducers does not represent a great problem and makes detected OA signals clear from reverberations within the piezoelement.

There are a number of designs of wideband acoustic and OA transducers that may be employed for a variety of applications in biomedicine (see Fig. 1.35).[458,467,518] Two-dimensional OA images can be provided either by using a stationary array of acoustic transducers or by scanning a single transducer along the tissue surface.[459] The arc-shaped array containing 32 ultrawideband piezoelectric transducers with 1×12.5-mm size and a distance of 3.85 mm between the elements is described.[459] The 110-μm-thick piezoelectric polymer PVDF was used to provide an ability to operate in a wide ultrasonic frequency band. The transducers were mounted on the arc surface with a radius of 60 mm; thus, such geometry provided optimal resolution in the entire 60×60-mm field of view within the image plane. The shape and length of individual piezoelements determine spatial resolution of this array in the plane perpendicular to the image plane. The flat elements used provided a resolution equal to the linear size of the element. This 32-element array was used for the acquiring of two-dimensional OA images of breast tumors.[459] Two images at two different laser wavelengths of 1064 and 757 nm were acquired in succession at irradiation with sixteen 100-ns pulses at each wavelength over the course of 0.8 s. Image reconstruction took about 1 s. Resolution of the image visualization was ~1 mm along the depth axis and 1.5 mm in the lateral direction, which is comparable to that of x-ray mammography and ultrasound.

Three-dimensional OA imaging can be provided using the system designed by LaserSonix Technologies, Inc. which is based on a bifocal array of 64 piezoelectric transducers and corresponding 64 data acquisition channels.[459] This system has close-to-real-time image acquisition and data processing with a resolution of about 3 mm in the plane perpendicular to the image plane, so that thin frontal slices of the breast can be visualized. Full-field-of-view 3D images can be reconstructed by fusing sixty 2D slices. A fast OA imaging system based on a 320-transducer linear array was also recently developed and tested.[553]

A high-resolution confocal OA transducer that provides subsurface imaging in the scanning mode is applicable when a superhigh resolution on the cellular or subcellular level is needed.[459] An ultrawide band of ultrasonic detection realized in front-surface transducers yields an in-depth resolution close to 15 μm. In incident optical beam focusing, a comparable lateral resolution is also achievable. The confocal OA transducer provides sharp focusing of the optical beam and a long narrow waist of acoustic focus in the ultrasonic detection system. The distributions of focused light and the caustic of the ultrasonic detection define the measuring volume of the confocal transducer.

Another modification of an OA sensor used in the dark-field reflection-mode imaging system, containing an optical fiber that is coaxially positioned with a focused ultrasonic transducer and attached to a concave lens, is described in Ref. 518. A variety of OA probes suitable or already tested for OA spectroscopy and imaging of biological tissues and blood are described in Refs. 512, 515, 516, 540, 541, 547, 548, and 553–557.

1.5.10 Conclusion

OTR, OA, and PA transient techniques provide a convenient means for *in vitro*, or even *in vivo* and *in situ*, monitoring of optical and thermal properties of a variety of human tissues, including skin. In particular, water content and surface concentration and diffusion of topically applied substances (drugs and sunscreens) can be measured.[460,490–492] The main difficulty of the PA method in the case of *in vivo* measurements is the requirement for a closed sample cell that can efficiently guide the acoustic signal from sample to microphone.

The use of pulsed OA and OTR techniques is more appropriate for *in vivo* and *in situ* experiments. The optothermal and optothermoelastic responses of a living tissue on pulse laser excitation discussed are the basis for a novel approach in medical tomography that combines achievements of optical, thermal, and acoustical probing of a tissue.[458,459,517]

A variety of tissue imaging techniques are suggested on the basis of US and light beams interacting within an inhomogeneous medium that occurs through the change in optical properties of the medium resulting from its compression by the US.[517,519–542] These are so-called acousto optical (AO) interactions and imaging technologies.

To OA and AO signals contribute any scattered photons (singly and multiply); therefore, the imaging depth is extended compared with other ballistic or quasi-ballistic imaging modalities, such as OCT or confocal microscopy.

The OA and AO tomographies (OAT and AOT) provide:[517] (1) a combination of high optical contrast and high acoustic resolution; (2) a potential for simultaneous functional imaging of blood oxygenation and blood volume; (3) a high ratio between imaging depth and resolution; (4) no speckle artifacts; (5) scalable resolution and imaging depth by varying the US frequency; (6) an ability to simultaneously acquire OAT/AOT images and pure US images from the same cross sections of the sample for added diagnostic value; and (7) nonionizing laser and US radiation within the safety limits for biological tissues.

However, OAT and AOT have some limitations mostly associated with the usage of US technology. They are: contact measurements, which are required for acoustic coupling, and strong US wavefront aberrations induced by some heterogeneous tissues and organs. In the case when acoustic heterogeneity is strong, concurrent US imaging may be useful for providing the acoustic properties that are needed for image reconstruction in OAT or AOT.

1.6 Discrete particle model of tissue

1.6.1 Introduction

Although it follows from the preceding discussion that the optical properties of tissue are related to its microstructure and refractive index distribution, the nature of the relationship should be discussed in more detail. It has been shown that the contribution of mitochondria and spatial variations in the refractive index of cells and other tissue components, such as collagen and elastin fibers, to the scattering properties of tissue can be estimated theoretically and experimentally.[58,85,96,154,156,558] However, the quantitative model that relates the microscopic properties of cells and other tissue components to the scattering coefficients of bulk tissue is still not completed. Ideally, such a model should be able to predict the absolute magnitudes of the optical scattering coefficients as well as their wavelengths and angle dependencies.[156] The model should provide insight into how the scattering properties are influenced by the numbers, sizes, and arrangement of the tissue components in order to be useful for inverse problem solving. This section presents a framework for a particulate model of soft tissue that satisfies at least a few of these requirements. The model was developed by the authors of Ref. 156; their paper is discussed.

1.6.2 Refractive-index variations of tissue

Soft tissue is composed of closely packed groups of cells entrapped in a network of fibers through which water percolates. At a microscopic scale, the tissue components have no pronounced boundaries. They appear to merge into a continuous structure with spatial variations in the refractive index. To model such a complicated structure as a collection of particles, it is necessary to resort to a statistical approach.

It has been shown that the tissue components that contribute most to the local refractive-index variations are the connective tissue fibers (bundles of elastin and collagen), cytoplasmic organelles (mitochondria, lysosoms, and peroxisomes), cell nuclei, and melanin granules.[58,154,156] Figure 1.45 shows a hypothetical index profile formed by measuring the refractive index along a line in an arbitrary direction through a volume of tissue. The widths of the peaks in the index profile are proportional to the diameters of the elements, and their heights depend on the refractive index of each element relative to that of its surroundings. In accordance with this model, the origin of the index variations will be presented by a statistically equivalent volume of discrete particles having the same index but different sizes.

The refractive indices of tissue structure elements, such as the fibrils, the interstitial medium, nuclei, cytoplasm, organelles, and the tissue itself, can be derived using the law of Gladstone and Dale, which states that the resulting value represents an average of the refractive indices of the components related to their volume fractions as[442]

$$\bar{n} = \sum_{i=1}^{N} n_i f_i, \quad \sum_i f_i = 1, \tag{1.150}$$

where n_i and f_i are the refractive index and volume fraction of the individual components, respectively, and N is the number of components.

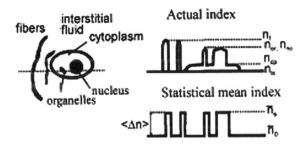

Figure 1.45 Spatial variations of the refractive index of a soft tissue. A hypothetical index profile through several tissue components is shown, along with the profile through a statistically equivalent volume of homogeneous particles. The indices of refraction labeling of the profile are defined in the text.[156]

The statistical mean index profile in Fig. 1.45 illustrates the nature of the approximation implied by this model. The average background index is defined as the weighted average of the refractive indices of the cytoplasm and the interstitial fluid, n_{cp} and n_{is}, as

$$\bar{n}_0 = f_{cp} n_{cp} + (1 - f_{cp}) n_{is}, \tag{1.151}$$

where f_{cp} is the volume fraction of the fluid in the tissue contained inside the cells. Literature data presented in Ref. 58 allow one to estimate $n_{cp} = 1.367$ and $n_{is} = 1.355$. Since approximately 60% of the total fluid in soft tissue is contained in the intracellular compartment, it follows from Eq. (1.151) that $\bar{n}_0 = 0.6(1.367) + 0.4(1.355) = 1.362$. The refractive index of a particle can be defined as the sum of the background index and the mean index variation,

$$\bar{n}_s = \bar{n}_0 + \langle \Delta n \rangle, \tag{1.152}$$

which can be approximated by another volume-weighted average,

$$\langle \Delta n \rangle = f_f(n_f - n_{is}) + f_{nc}(n_{nc} - n_{cp}) + f_{or}(n_{or} - n_{cp}). \tag{1.153}$$

Here, the subscripts f, is, nc, cp, and or refer to the fibers, interstitial fluid, nuclei, cytoplasm, and organelles, respectively, which were identified above as the major contributors to index variations. The terms in parentheses in this expression are the differences between the refractive indices of the three types of tissue component and their respective backgrounds; the multiplying factors are the volume fractions of the elements in the solid portion of the tissue. The refractive index of the connective-tissue fibers is about 1.47 (see Table 2.2), which corresponds to about 55% hydration of collagen, its main component. The nucleus and the cytoplasmic organelles in mammalian cells that contain similar concentrations of proteins and nucleic acids, such as mitochondria and the ribosomes, have refractive indices that lie within a relative narrow range (1.38–1.41).[58] Taking this into account and assuming that $n_{nc} = n_{or} = 1.40$, the mean index variation can be expressed in terms of only the fibrous-tissue fraction c_f as

$$\langle \Delta n \rangle = f_f(n_f - n_{is}) + (1 - f_f)(n_{nc} - n_{cp}). \tag{1.154}$$

Collagen and elastin fibers compose approximately 70% of the fat-free dry weight of dermis, 45% of the heart, and 2–3% of nonmuscular internal organs (see Refs. 14–16 in Ref. 156). Therefore, depending on tissue type, f_f may be as small as about 0.02 or as large as 0.7. For $n_f - n_{is} = 1.470 - 1.355 = 0.115$ and $n_{nc} - n_{cp} = n_{or} - n_{cp} = 1.400 - 1.367 = 0.033$, the mean index variations that correspond to these two extremes are $\langle \Delta n \rangle = 0.02(0.115) + (1 - 0.02)(0.033) = 0.035$ and $\langle \Delta n \rangle = 0.7(0.115) + (1 - 0.7)(0.033) = 0.09$.

1.6.3 Particle size distributions

For some tissues, the size distribution of the scattering particles may be essentially monodispersive and for others it may be quite broad. Two opposite examples are transparent eye cornea stroma, which has a sharply monodispersive distribution, and turbid eye sclera, which has a rather broad distribution of collagen fiber diameters.[129] There is no universal distribution size function that describes all tissues with equal adequacy. In the optics of dispersed systems, Gaussian, gamma, or power size distributions are typical.[171] Polydispersion for randomly distributed scatterers can be accounted for by using the gamma distribution or the skewed logarithmic distribution of scatterers' diameters, cross sections, or volumes.[61,129,154,156,165,172] In particular, for turbid tissues such as eye sclera, the following gamma radii distribution function is applicable:[61,172]

$$\eta(a) = a^\mu \exp(-\mu\beta), \tag{1.155}$$

where $\sigma/a_m = 2.35\mu^{-0.5}$, $\beta = a/a_m$, σ is the half-width of the distribution, and a_m is the more probable scatterer radius.

A two-phase system made up of an ensemble of equally sized small particles, and a minor fraction of larger ones, provides a good model of pathological tissue, e.g., a cataractous lens.[173]

For epithelial cells and their nuclei scattering structures, log-normal size distributions of spherical or slightly prolated ellipsoidal particles are characteristic as[166]

$$\eta(a) = \left(\frac{1}{a\sigma\sqrt{2\pi}}\right)\exp\left\{-\frac{[\ln(a) - \ln(a_m)]^2}{2\sigma^2}\right\}. \tag{1.156}$$

In particular, for epithelial cells and their nucleus components, two log-normal size distributions for small and big spherical scatterers with the following parameters were found in a certain line of rat prostate carcinoma cells:[166] $a_{m1} = 0.012$ µm, $\sigma_1 = 1.15$ µm, and $a_{m2} = 0.59$ µm, $\sigma_2 = 0.43$ µm.

For the description of scattering characteristics of a particle with a complex shape, different from a sphere or long cylinder, some special procedures, for example, the method of T-matrices, can be applied.[145,146,166] Complexly shaped scatterers, like cells themselves, may be modeled as aggregates of spherical particles.

The scattering centers in turbid tissue have a wide range of dimensions and tend to aggregate into complex forms suggestive of fractal objects. The skewed logarithmic distribution function is used extensively in particle-size analysis as being the most plausible on physical grounds. The skewed logarithmic distribution function for the volume fraction of particles of diameter $2a$ is[156]

$$\eta(2a) = \frac{F_v}{C_m}(2a)^{3-D_f}\exp\left\{-\frac{[\ln(2a) - \ln(2a_m)]^2}{2\sigma^2}\right\}, \tag{1.157}$$

where

$$C_m = \sigma\sqrt{2\pi}(2a_m)^{4-D_f}\exp\left[\frac{(4 - D_f)^2\sigma^2}{2}\right]$$

is the normalizing factor;

$$F_v = \int_0^\infty \eta(2a)d(2a)$$

is the total volume fraction of the particles, and the quantities $2a_m$ and σ set the center and width of the distribution, respectively; D_f is the (volumetric) fractal dimension.

In the limit of an infinitely broad distribution of particle sizes,

$$\eta(2a) \approx (2a)^{3-D_f}. \tag{1.158}$$

For $3 < D_f < 4$, this power-law relationship describes the dependence of the volume fractions of the subunits of an ideal mass fractal on their diameter, $2a$. These size distributions expand the size distributions described by Eqs. (1.155) and (1.156) to account for the fractal properties of tissues.

Scatterers in the epidermal layer of the skin also exhibit a log-normal size distribution, whereas the spatial fluctuations in the index of refraction of dense fibrous tissues, such as the dermis, and many other tissues follow a power law.[107,165]

1.6.4 Spatial ordering of particles

A discrete particle ensemble is characterized by the packing density or, in other words, by the volume fraction occupied by particles. Evidently, in addition to particle size, the volume fraction of particles is also essential for the optical properties of an ensemble due to its influence on the refractive index distribution [see Eqs. (1.150)–(1.154)], optical anisotropy [see Eqs. (1.53) and (1.54)], and other structure characteristics. The volume fraction of particles for a certain tissue may be experimentally found using electron micrographs of tissue slices. Estimations of a volume fraction occupied by scattering particles may also be accomplished by the weighting of a native tissue and dry rest.

The volume fraction occupied by the scattering particles in tissues, such as muscle, cornea, sclera, and eye lens, covers from 20 to 40%. Conventionally, whole blood contains $(4–5) \times 10^6$ erythrocytes, $(4–9) \times 10^3$ leukocytes, and $(2–3) \times 10^5$ platelets in 1 mm^3. Cells make up 35–45% of the blood volume. The volume fraction f of erythrocytes in the blood is called the hematocrit H. For normal blood, $H = 0.4$. The remaining 60% of the blood volume is mostly the plasma—an essentially transparent water solution of salts.

Most tissues are comprised of cellular and subcellular structures located in close proximity to each other. In general, densely packed structures are likely to exhibit correlation scattering, an effect that has been observed, for instance, in corneal stroma.[63,129,432,433,435,436] Cornea is comprised of individual collagen fibrils that are closely packed and parallel to one another in a lamella. If each fibril in the lamella scattered light independently, then the scattering cross section of the lamella should be the product of the cross section of a single fibril and the number of fibrils in the lamella. If all of the cornea fibers scattered light independently, the cornea would scatter 90% of the light incident on it, and we would see essentially nothing. However, the fibrils do not scatter independently and the coherent scattering (interference) effects cannot be neglected. Accordingly, correlated polarization effects can be observed.[63,435–438] For example, in spherical particle suspensions, as the particle concentration increases beyond a concentration at which independent scattering can be assumed, the degree of polarization increases (rather than decreases) as the scatterer concentration increases.[437,438]

Thus, the spatial organization of the particles forming a tissue plays a substantial role in the propagation of light. As mentioned above, with very small packing densities, incoherent scattering by independent particles occurs. If the volume fraction occupied by the particles is equal to or more than 0.01–0.1, coherent concentration effects appear. The concentration of scattering particles is adequate in most tissues to allow spaces between individual scatterers that are comparable to their sizes. If, however, the particle-size distribution is rather narrow, then dense packing entails a certain degree of order in the arrangement of the particles.

Spatial ordering is of utmost importance in optical eye tissue.[63,64,129,403,432,433,435,436] In a large variety of other tissues, spatial ordering is also more or less inherent, particularly in tendon, cartilage, *dura mater*, skin, or muscle. The high degree of order in densely packed scatterers ensures high transmission in the cornea and eye lens. Tissue structures with statistically ordered periodical variations in the index at characteristic scales of light wavelength, like photonic crystals,[440] exhibit high-transmission spectral regions and bands for which the propagation of electromagnetic waves is forbidden. The position and depth of these bands depend on the size, refractive index, and spatial arrangement of the scattering particles.

To account for the interparticle correlation effects, which are important for systems with volume fractions of scatterers higher than 1–10% (dependent on particle dimensions), the following expression for the packing factor of a medium filled with a volume fraction f_s of scatterers with different shapes is valid:[148]

$$w_p = \frac{(1 - f_s)^{p+1}}{[1 + f_s(p - 1)]^{p-1}}, \tag{1.159}$$

where p is a packing dimension that describes the rate at which the empty space between scatterers diminishes as the total density number increases. The packing of spherical particles is described well by packing dimension $p = 3$. The packing of sheetlike and rod-shaped particles is characterized by dimensions that approach 1 and 2, respectively. The elements of tissue have all of these different shapes and may exhibit cylindrical and spherical symmetry simultaneously, and the packing dimension may lie anywhere between 1 and 5. When one calculates the optical coefficients at high concentrations of particles, the size distribution $\eta(2a)$ [Eqs. (1.155)–(1.158)] should be replaced by the correlation-corrected distribution[156]

$$\eta'(2a) = \frac{[1 - \eta(2a)]^{p+1}}{[1 + \eta(2a)(p - 1)]^{p-1}}\eta(2a). \tag{1.160}$$

Most of the observed scattering properties of soft tissue that are explained in the model treat tissue as a collection of scattering particles whose volume fractions are distributed according to a skewed log-normal distribution modified by a packing factor, to account for correlated scattering among densely packed particles.[156]

1.6.5 Scattering by densely packed particle systems

The spatial correlation of individual scatterers results in a necessity to consider the interference of multiply scattered waves. The particle reradiation in the densely packed disperse system induces the distinction of an effective optical field in a medium from the incident one. Under these conditions, the statistical theory of multiple wave scattering seems to be most promising for describing the collective interaction between an ensemble of particles and electromagnetic radiation.[75,442,559]

The rigorous theory of wave multiple scattering is constructed on the basis of fundamental differential equations for the fields followed by using statistical considerations.[75] The total field $\vec{E}(\vec{r})$ at the point $\vec{r}$ is the sum of the incident field $\vec{E}_i(\vec{r})$ and the scattered fields from all particles with regard to their phases,

$$\vec{E}(\vec{r}) = \vec{E}_i(\vec{r}) + \sum_{j=1}^{N} \vec{E}_j^s(\vec{r}), \qquad (1.161)$$

where $\vec{E}_j^s(\vec{r})$ is the scattered field of the jth particle. The field scattered by the jth particle is defined by the parameters of this particle and by the effective field incident on the particle.

Twersky has derived a closed system of integral equations describing the processes of multiple scattering.[560] A rigorous solution in a general form has not yet been found for this problem. In actual calculations, various approximations are exploited in order to perform the averaging of Eq. (1.161) over statistical particle configurations. For example, the quasi-crystalline approximation proposed for densely packed media by Lax[561] is used most efficiently in tissue optics.[442]

Averaging of Eq. (1.161) over statistical particle configurations results in an infinite set of equations that is truncated at the second step by applying the quasi-crystalline approximation. The closed system of equations obtained for the effective field is reduced to a system of linear equations by expansion in terms of vector spherical or cylindrical harmonics. The explicit expressions[562,563] for the expansion coefficients involve the radial distribution function as well as the Mie coefficients for a single particle. The equality to zero for the determinant of this system of linear equations yields the dispersion relation for the effective propagation constant k_{eff} of this medium.[564] For the systems of particles whose sizes are small compared with the wavelength, the expression for k_{eff} obtained in this way has the form[442,562]

$$k_{eff}^2 = k^2 + \frac{3fy}{D}k^2\left[1 + i\frac{2}{3}\frac{k^2a^2y}{D}S_3(\theta = 0)\right], \qquad (1.162)$$

where

$$y = \frac{n_1^2 - n_0^2}{n_1^2 + 2n_0^2}, \, D = 1 - fy, \, S_3(\theta = 0) = \frac{1}{1 - H_3}, \, H_3 = -24f\left(\frac{\alpha}{3} + \frac{\beta}{4} + \frac{\delta}{6}\right),$$

(1.163)

in which f is the volume fraction occupied by particles with the radius a and the refractive index n_1, and the α, β, and δ values are found according the approximation of hard spheres

$$\alpha = \frac{(1 + 2f)^2}{(1 - f)^4}, \quad \beta = -6f\frac{(1 + 0.5f)^2}{(1 - f)^4}, \quad \delta = \frac{1}{2}f\frac{(1 + 2f)^2}{(1 - f)^4}.$$

(1.164)

The calculated effective index of refraction[442]

$$n_{eff} = n'_{eff} + in''_{eff}$$

(1.165)

is complex, even if the particles and a base substance surrounding them exhibit no intrinsic absorption. The imaginary part of the effective index of refraction n''_{eff} describes the energy diminishing for an incident plane wave due to scattering in all directions. The transmittance of this layer with thickness z is

$$T = \exp\left(-\frac{4\pi}{\lambda}n''_{eff}z\right).$$

(1.166)

The quantity $\mu_t = 4\pi n''_{eff}/\lambda$ is the extinction coefficient. The value of the imaginary part of the effective index of refraction grows for these systems with a higher radiation frequency and it nonmonotonously depends on the particle concentration in the layer. As a result, the transmittance of the disperse layer decreases for small particle concentrations with a greater concentration of particles and, starting at $f \approx 0.1$, the transmittance grows and the so-called clearing effect takes place. The real portion of the effective index of refraction in this approximation is essentially independent of the wavelength and alters monotonously with growing particle concentration to approach the refractive index of the particles. The near ordering in the scatterers' arrangement with their greater concentration not only provides for conditions for the manifestation of the secondary scattered wave interference, but it also changes the regime of propagation of noncoherent multiply scattered light.[565] This may be accompanied by the so-called concentration effects of clearing and darkening.

The optical softness of tissues enables one to employ under calculation an expansion by scattering multiplicities with restriction by low orders. In Ref. 566, an expression was obtained for the effective index of refraction of the eye cornea modeled by the system of cylinder scatterers in the form of expansion by the scattering multiplicities, and the effects of polarization anisotropy were analyzed with respect to the double scattering contributions.

Using the theory of multiple scattering, Twersky[567] succeeded in deriving the approximate expressions for the absorption μ_a and scattering μ_s coefficients that describe the light propagation in the blood. The blood hematocrit Hct is related to the erythrocyte concentration ρ and to the volume of an erythrocyte V_e by the following ratio:[183,567]

$$\rho = Hct/V_e. \tag{1.167}$$

Thus, the absorption factor μ_a is

$$\mu_a = \left(\frac{Hct}{V_e}\right)\sigma_a. \tag{1.168}$$

For sufficiently small values of Hct ($Hct < 0.2$), the scattering coefficient is given by the equation

$$\mu_s = \left(\frac{Hct}{V_e}\right)\sigma_s. \tag{1.169}$$

For $Hct > 0.5$, the particles become densely packed and the medium is almost homogeneous. In this case, the blood may be considered as a homogeneous medium containing hemoglobin in which scattering particles formed by plasma surrounding red blood cells are embedded. Within the limits of $Hct \rightarrow 1$, "plasma particles" disappear and the scattering coefficient should tend to zero. This results in the following approximate equation for μ_s:[183,568]

$$\mu_s \approx \frac{Hct(1 - Hct)}{V_e}\sigma_s, \tag{1.170}$$

where the coefficient $(1 - Hct)$ regards the scattering termination with $Hct \rightarrow 1$. However, the absolute dense packing ($Hct = 1$) is not attainable in reality; for example, for the hard sphere approximation, Hct may not exceed 0.64. Considering this fact and keeping in mind the physiological conditions, the affect of cell packing on light scattering might be described by a more complex function as

$$\mu_s = \left(\frac{Hct}{V_e}\right)\sigma_s F(Hct), \tag{1.171}$$

where the packing function $F(Hct)$ accounts for physiological conditions of red blood cells, in particular, cell deformability at high concentration.

Although the equations from Twersky's wave-scattering theory[560,567] agree reasonably well with measured optical density data for a whole blood layer,[568] researchers have had to resort to curve-fitting techniques to evaluate the parameters in Twersky's equations. This theory also does not describe the spatial distribution of the reflected and transmitted light, and therefore does not accommodate light detectors and sources that do not share a common optical axis. By contrast, the radiative transfer theory discussed above—in particular, its more simple diffusion approximation—overcome listed limitations of the wave-scattering theory; but to be applied to densely packed tissues, this theory should account for particle inter-action and size distribution effects. The combination with other theories describing particle interactions and the usage of empirical data can be considered as a fruitful and practical approach for modeling of the optical properties of tissues.

For example, using the diffusion theory, Steinke and Shepherd[568] have cor-rected the dependence [Eq. (1.170)] of the scattering coefficient μ_s for a thin blood layer on the hematocrit Hct, as the following:

$$\mu_s \approx \left(\frac{Hct}{V_e}\right)\sigma_s(1 - Hct)(1.4 - Hct). \qquad (1.172)$$

Using the concept of combination of photon-diffusion theory and particle rep-resentation of a tissue, a microoptical model that explains most of the observed scattering properties of soft tissue has been developed.[156] The model treats the tis-sue as a collection of scattering particles whose volume fractions are distributed according to a skewed log-normal distribution modified by a packing factor p to account for correlated scattering among densely packed particles [see Eqs. (1.157), (1.158), and (1.160)]. Assuming that the waves scattered by the individual particles in a thin slice of the modeled tissue volume add randomly, then the scattering coef-ficient of the volume can be approximated as the sum of the scattering coefficients of the particles of a given diameter as

$$\mu_s = \sum_{i=1}^{N_p} \mu_s(2a_i), \qquad (1.173)$$

where

$$\mu_s(2a_i) = \frac{\eta(2a_i)}{v_i}\sigma_s(2a_i), \qquad (1.174)$$

N_p is the number of particle diameters; $\eta(2a_i)$ is the volume fraction of particles of diameter $2a_i$ [see Eqs. (1.157), (1.158), and (1.160)]; and $\sigma_s(2a_i)$ is the opti-cal cross section of an individual particle with diameter $2a_i$ and volume v_i. The volume-averaged phase function $p(\theta)$ (and scattering anisotropy parameter g) of the tissue slice is the sum of the angular-scattering functions $p_i(\theta)$ (and anisotropy parameters, g_i) of the individual particles weighted by the product of their respec-tive scattering coefficients,

$$p(\theta) = \frac{\sum_{i=1}^{N_p} \mu_s(2a_i)p_i(\theta)}{\sum_{i=1}^{N_p} \mu_s(2a_i)}, \qquad (1.175)$$

$$g = \frac{\sum_{i=1}^{N_p} \mu_s(2a_i) g_i(2a_i)}{\sum_{i=1}^{N_p} \mu_s(2a_i)}. \qquad (1.176)$$

The reduced scattering coefficient is usually defined as $\mu_s' = \mu_s(1-g)$. The volume-averaged backscattering coefficient can be defined as the sum of the particle cross sections weighted by their angular-scattering functions evaluated at 180 deg:

$$\mu_b = \sum_{i=1}^{N_p} \frac{\eta(2a_i)}{v_i} \sigma_s(2a_i) p_i(180°). \qquad (1.177)$$

The product of μ_b $(\text{cm}^{-1}/\text{sr})$ and the thickness of the tissue slice yield the fraction of the incident irradiance backscattered per unit solid angle in the direction opposite to the incident light.

The evaluation of the model by applying Mie theory to a collection of spheres with a wide range of sizes gave a set of parameters for the distribution and packing of the particles: volumetric fractal dimension $D_f = 3.7$, mean refractive index of tissue grounds $\bar{n}_0 = 1.352$, mean refractive index of scatterers (particles) $\bar{n}_s = 1.420$, total volume fraction of the particles $F_v = 0.2$, center of particle size distribution $2a_m = 1.13$ μm, width of this distribution $\sigma = 2$ μm, and packing factor $p = 3$ [see Eqs. (1.152), (1.157)–(1.160)], which yields credible estimates of the scattering coefficients and scattering anisotropy parameters of representative soft tissues. Table 1.4 summarizes the optical properties predicted by the model at three wavelengths (633, 800, and 1300 nm) for a soft tissue containing different dry-weight fractions of connective tissue fibers ($f_f = 0.03$, 0.3, and 0.7). The coefficients μ_s, μ_s', μ_b, and g were computed for specific parameters of the particle system. In general, these calculations fit the experimental data well for *in vitro* and even *in vivo* measurements of optical parameters of soft tissues.

Table 1.4 Optical coefficients of model tissues with three different dry-weight fiber fraction (f_f), for $D_f = 3.7$.[156]

Wavelength, nm	633			800			1300		
f_f	0.03	0.3	0.7	0.03	0.3	0.7	0.03	0.3	0.7
μ_s (cm^{-1})	105	224	402	69	146	274	29	63	119
μ_s' (cm^{-1})	8.0	20	45	5.7	14	32	3.0	7.5	16.5
μ_b $(\text{cm}^{-1}/\text{sr})$	0.8	2.2	5.0	0.5	1.3	3.1	0.3	0.9	2.0
g	0.92	0.91	0.89	0.92	0.90	0.88	0.90	0.88	0.86

By using the model to describe a soft tissue, the authors of Ref. 156 have shown the following: (1) as an optical medium, tissue is represented best by a volume of scatterers with a wide distribution of sizes; (2) fixing the total volume fraction of particles and their refractive indices places upper and lower bounds on the magnitude of the scattering coefficient; (3) the scattering coefficient decreases with wavelength approximately as $\mu_s \sim \lambda^{2-D_f}$ for $600 \leq \lambda \leq 1400$ nm, where D_f is the limiting fractal dimension; and (4) scatterers in tissue with diameters between $\lambda/4$ and $\lambda/2$ are the dominant backscatterers and the scatterers that cause the greatest extinction of forward-scattered light have diameters between 3λ and 4λ.

As it follows from Ref. 107, the fractal dimension D_f is highly dependent on how the continuous size distribution is discretized. In the ten-sphere discrete model by Schmitt and Kumar,[156] the fractal dimension between $3 < D_f < 4$ was found, in contrast to the model of spheres ranging from 5 nm to 30,000 nm, at an interval of 5 nm, described by Wang,[107] where the range of fractal dimension such as $4 < D_f < 5$ was determined. In Wang's model, the scattering coefficient decreases with wavelength as $\mu_s \sim \lambda^{3-D_f}$ for $600 \leq \lambda \leq 1500$ nm; therefore, both models give the similar power law for dependence of the scattering coefficient on the wavelength, which is in the range from $\mu_s \sim \lambda^{-1}$ to $\mu_s \sim \lambda^{-2}$. The magnitude of the scattering coefficient increases as the fractal dimension decreases because the larger particles, which have the largest optical cross sections, contribute relatively more to the total optical cross section of the tissue. Wang's model also confirms that particles with diameters between $\lambda/4$ and $\lambda/2$ are the dominant backscatterers; but in comparison with the model by Schmitt and Kumar, it predicts a wider range for scatterers' diameters for which the greatest extinction of forward scattering is characteristic, i.e., between λ and 10λ.

The reduced scattering coefficient decreases with an increase in wavelength in accordance with a power law that was experimentally demonstrated for normal, dehydrated, and coagulated human aorta in an *in vitro* study as[569,570]

$$\mu_s' \propto \lambda^{-h}. \tag{1.178}$$

Experimental data for normal human (control) and processed samples of human aorta are presented in Table 1.5. At direct heating (100°C), h was reduced from 1.38 for the normal tissue sample to 1.06 for the heated one. An *in vitro* study of rat skin impregnated by glycerol also showed a power wavelength dependence of the reduced scattering coefficient in the range 500–1200 nm with $h = 1.12$ for normal skin, and with subsequent decrease in h with increased time in glycerol (mostly dehydration effect).[571] These values were 1.09 for 5 min, 0.85 for 10 min, 0.52 for 20 min, and 0.9 for the rehydrated sample.[571]

In vivo backscattering measurements for human skin and underlying tissues have also demonstrated the power law for the wavelength dependence of the reduced scattering coefficient:[572]

$$\mu_s' = q\lambda^{-h} \; (\text{cm}^{-1}, \; \lambda \text{ in } \mu m). \tag{1.179}$$

In particular, for reflectance spectra from the human forearm in the wavelength range 700–900 nm, constants q and h were determined as 5.50 ± 0.11 and 1.11 ± 0.08, respectively. From Mie theory, it follows that the power constant h

Table 1.5 Power relationship between wavelength and the reduced scattering coefficient and the significance of h [see Eq. (1.178)] values for control and experimental reduced scattering spectra (400–1300 nm) for human aorta as obtained from a t-test (rms values in parentheses).[569,570]

Description	$h_{control}$	h_{exper}	Significance, %
Dehydration	1.15 (0.10)	1.22 (0.13)	~15
Heating at 60°C	1.21 (0.12)	1.28 (0.04)	~25
Heating at 70°C	1.30 (0.01)	1.10 (0.10)	<5
Heating at 100°C (direct heating)	1.38 (0.11)	1.06 (0.07)	<5
Heating at 100°C (wrapped heating)	1.26 (0.08)	1.03 (0.05)	<5

is related to an averaged size of the scatterers: the Mie-equivalent radius a_M. Once h is determined, this radius can be derived from[572]

$$h = -1109.5a_M^3 + 341.67a_M^2 - 9.36961a_M - 3.9359 (a_M < 0.23 \ \mu m), \quad (1.180)$$

$$h = 23.909a_M^3 - 37.218a_M^2 + 19.534a_M - 3.965 (0.23 < a_M < 0.60 \ \mu m). \quad (1.181)$$

These relations were determined for a relative refractive index between spheres and the surrounding medium, $m = 1.037$. The *in vivo* measured constant $h = 1.11$ leads to an a_M value of 0.30 μm, which is about two times smaller than the mean radius (0.57 μm) used in the above-discussed model of a collection of packed spheres with a wide range of sizes.[156]

1.7 Fluorescence and inelastic light scattering

1.7.1 Fluorescence

One of the fundamental mechanisms of interaction between light and biological objects is luminescence, which is subdivided into fluorescence, corresponding to an allowed optical transition with a rather high quantum yield and a short (nanosecond) lifetime, as well as phosphorescence, corresponding to a "forbidden" transition with low quantum yield and long decay times in the microsecond–millisecond range.[573–575]

Absorption of light is connected with an electronic transition from a ground state to an excited state of a molecule. Light passing through a layer of thickness d is thereby attenuated according to the equation[574]

$$I(\lambda) = I_0 \exp(-\mu_a d) = I_0 10^{-\varepsilon_\lambda c_{ab} d}, \quad (1.182)$$

with $I(\lambda)$ being the transmitted light intensity, I_0 the incident intensity, ε_λ the molar extinction coefficient, and c_{ab} the concentration of absorbing molecules. In scattering samples, the absorption coefficient μ_a and the scattering coefficient μ_s [omitted in Eq. (1.182)] sum up, thus causing further reduction of transmitted light, as described in detail above.

Fluorescence arises upon light absorption and is related to an electronic transition from the excited state to the ground state of a molecule. Its intensity (quantum flux) corresponds to[574]

$$I_F(\lambda) = I_0[1 - 10^{-\varepsilon_\lambda c_{ab} d}]\eta_F \frac{\Omega}{4\pi}, \tag{1.183}$$

with η_F being the fluorescence quantum yield, and Ω the angle of detection of isotropic fluorescence radiation. In the case of thin samples, e.g., cell monolayers or biopsies with a few micrometers in thickness, Eq. (1.183) can be approximated by

$$I_F(\lambda) = I_0 \ln 10 \varepsilon_\lambda c_{ab} d \eta_F \frac{\Omega}{4\pi}. \tag{1.184}$$

This implies that fluorescence intensity is proportional to the concentration and the fluorescence quantum yield of the absorbing molecules. In scattering media, the path lengths of scattered and unscattered photons within the sample are different, and Eqs. (1.183) and (1.184) have to be modified. However, in virtually homogenous thin samples, the linearity between I_F, c_{ab}, and η_F is still fulfilled.

Energies of the electronic states of a molecule are complex functions of the nuclear distances of relevant atoms, usually forming "potential wells," as shown in Fig. 1.46 for the ground state (S_0) and the first excited state (S_1). Each well contains a larger number of vibrational levels ν_i that further split into numerous rotational levels (omitted in Fig. 1.46) of the molecule. Electronic transitions occur in the "vertical direction" because during their short duration nuclear coordinates do not change (Franck-Condon principle). Electronic transitions usually originate from vibronic ground states (excitation, S_0 and ν_0; fluorescence, S_1 and ν_0). The probability of each transition corresponds to the square of the transition dipole moment, and is determined by an overlap of the corresponding electronic wave functions in the ground state and the excited state of the molecule. Therefore, absorption and fluorescence spectra originate from a superposition of several transitions, often resulting in broad spectral bands. From Fig. 1.46, one can deduce that the so-called 0-0 transition between the lowest vibrational levels is only slightly pronounced, since the overlap between corresponding wave functions is very low. Therefore, fluorescence spectra are usually shifted to lower energies ΔW corresponding to higher wavelengths $\lambda = \Delta W / hc$ as compared with absorption or excitation spectra (h is Planck's constant, c is the velocity of light). This phenomenon is called the "Stokes shift."

If the potential curves are plotted without regard to the variable nuclear distances, the different molecular states can be illustrated in a Jablonski diagram, as

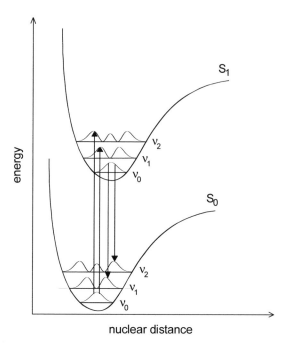

Figure 1.46 Potential diagram of electronic states (S_0, S_1) and vibrational levels (ν_i). Electronic wave functions and optical transitions are indicated (excitation: $S_0\nu_0 \rightarrow S_1\nu_n$; fluorescence: $S_1\nu_0 \rightarrow S_0\nu_n$).[574]

shown in Fig. 1.47. Excitation usually occurs from the singlet ground state S_0 to various vibronic levels of the excited singlet states S_n, from where fast nonradiative transitions ("internal conversion") occur within the femtosecond time range to the lowest excited state S_1. From S_1, various transitions can be distinguished: fluorescence to the ground state S_0 (including its vibrational states) with a rate k_F, internal conversion to the ground state S_0 (rate k_{IC}), intersystem crossing from the singlet to the triplet state T_1 (rate k_{ISC}), and nonradiative energy transfer to adjacent molecules (rate k_{ET}). All these rates sum up according to

$$k = k_F + k_{IC} + k_{ISC} + k_{ET} = \frac{1}{\tau}, \qquad (1.185)$$

where τ is the lifetime of the excited state S_1. The ratio k_F/k corresponds to the fluorescence quantum yield η_F. Although by optical spectroscopy only radiative transitions can be monitored, changes of k_{IC} or k_{ET} are often deduced from fluorescence lifetime measurements. It should be noted that the radiative transition $T_1 \rightarrow S_0$ is spin forbidden, and only within a few specific molecules is this transition becoming prominent.

Transition dipole moments have defined orientations within a molecule. Upon excitation with linear polarized light, one preferentially excites those molecules, whose transition dipoles are parallel to the electric field vector of incident light. This selective excitation of an oriented population of molecules results in par-

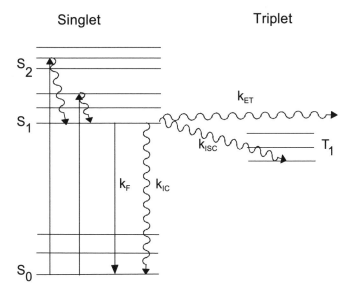

Figure 1.47 Jablonski diagram of molecular energy levels and transition rates. Straight lines, radiative transitions; wavy lines, nonradiative transitions.[574]

tially polarized fluorescence, which is described by the degree of polarization [see Eq. (1.68a)] as

$$P_{FL} = (I_{F\parallel} - I_{F\perp})/(I_{F\parallel} + I_{F\perp}) \qquad (1.186)$$

or by fluorescence anisotropy[573]

$$r_F = \frac{I_{F\parallel} - I_{F\perp}}{I_{F\parallel} + 2I_{F\perp}}, \qquad (1.187)$$

with $I_{F\parallel}$ and $I_{F\perp}$ being the fluorescence intensities of light polarized parallel or perpendicular to the exciting electric-field vector, respectively. Usually, P_{FL} and r_F depend on the time interval between excitation and fluorescence detection, since during the lifetime of their excited states, many molecules change their orientation by rotation ("rotational diffusion"). From time-resolved measurements of fluorescence anisotropy, a time constant τ_r of rotational diffusion can be determined that is correlated with the volume V_M of the molecule and the viscosity η of its environment according to

$$\tau_r = \frac{\eta V_M}{k_B T}, \qquad (1.188)$$

where k_B is the Boltzmann constant and T is the absolute temperature. Time constants of rotational diffusion of about 13 ns were correlated with a molecular weight of proteins around 50,000 daltons,[573] whereas a time constant around

300 ps was attributed to an aggregated species of a photosensitizing porphyrin (protoporphyrin) with a 1.6 nm diameter.[574]

At excitation of biological objects by ultraviolet light ($\lambda \leq 370$ nm), fluorescence of proteins as well as of nucleic acids can be observed. Fluorescence quantum yields of all nucleic acid constituents, however, are around 10^{-4}–10^{-5}, corresponding to lifetimes of the excited states in the picosecond time range. Autofluorescence (AF) of proteins is related to the amino acids tryptophan, tyrosin, and phenylalanine with absorption maxima at 280 nm, 275 nm, and 257 nm, respectively, and emission maxima between 280 nm (phenylalanine) and 350 nm (tryptophan).[573–575] The protein spectrum is usually dominated by tryptophan. Fluorescence from collagen or elastin is excited between 300 and 400 nm and shows broad emission bands between 400 and 600 nm with maxima around 400 nm, 430 nm, and 460 nm. In particular, fluorescence of collagen and elastin can be used to distinguish various types of tissues, e.g., epithelial and connective tissue.[31,92,98,574–581]

The reduced form of coenzyme nicotinamide adenine dinucleotide (NADH) is excited selectively in a wavelength range between 330 and 370 nm. NADH is most concentrated within mitochondria, where it is oxidized within the respiratory chain located within the inner mitochondrial membrane, and its fluorescence is an appropriate parameter for detection of ischemic or neoplastic tissues.[574,581] Fluorescence of free and protein-bound NADH has been shown to be sensitive on oxygen concentration. Flavin mononucleotide (FMN) and dinucleotide (FAD) with excitation maxima around 380 nm and 450 nm have also been reported to contribute to intrinsic cellular fluorescence.[574]

Porphyrin molecules, e.g., protoporphyrin, coproporphyrin, uroporphyrin, or hematoporphyrin, occur within the pathway of biosynthesis of hemoglobin, myoglobin, and cytochromes. Abnormalities in heme synthesis, occurring in the cases of porphyrias and some hemolytic diseases, may enhance the porphyrin level within tissues considerably. Several bacteria, e.g., *Propionibacterium acnes*, or bacteria within dental plaque (biofilm), such as *Porphyromonas gingivalis*, *Prevotella intermedia*, and *Prevotella nigrescens*, accumulate considerable amounts of protoporphyrin.[582,583] Therefore, acne or oral and tooth lesion detection based on measurements of intrinsic fluorescence appears to be a promising method.

Recently, a number of theoretical computer modeling and experimental studies of fluorescence intensity distributions accounting for light scattering effects were performed.[584–592] In particular, a diffusion theory model of spatially resolved fluorescence from depth-dependent fluorophore concentration was described in Ref. 585. In Ref. 586, three-dimensional epithelial tissue phantoms suitable for fluorescence spectroscopy, collagen cross-linking studies, and cancer diagnosis were presented. Some principle features of near-infrared fluorescence tomography such as three-dimensional image reconstruction from sparse and noisy data sets[587] and localization of fluorescent masses deeply embedded in tissue[588] were discussed. A few experimental approaches for recovery of scattering free fluorescence from measured fluorescence[589] and validation of Monte Carlo modeling of fluorescence in tissues in the UV-visible spectrum[590] were developed. Monte Carlo simulations of some practical cases such as the effect of fiber-optic probe geometry on depth-resolved fluorescence measurements from epithelial tissues[591] and spatial fluorescence distribution in the skin[592] were also performed.

At present, various exogenous fluorescing dyes can be applied for probing of cell anatomy and cell physiology.[574,593–597] For instance, subcellular localization of sulfonated tetraphenyl porphines in colon carcinoma cells was studied by spectrally resolved fluorescence imaging.[593]

In humans, such dyes as fluorescein and indocyanine green are in use for fluorescence angiography or blood volume determination. Novel fluorescent contrast agents for optical imaging of *in vivo* tumors based on a receptor-targeted dye-peptide conjugate[595] and green fluorescent protein[596] platforms were recently described. Fluorescence properties of such dyes as albumin blue 633 and 670 in plasma and whole blood were studied.[594] Exogenous specific fluorescence markers for *in vivo* quantitative three-dimensional localization of tumors were studied in Ref. 597.

Fluorescence spectra often give detailed information on fluorescent molecules, their conformation, binding sites, and interaction within cells and tissues. Fluorescence intensity can be measured either as a function of the emission wavelength or of the excitation wavelength. The fluorescence emission spectrum $I_F(\lambda)$ is specific for any fluorophore and is commonly used in fluorescence diagnostics.

For many biomedical applications, an optical multichannel analyzer (OMA) (a diode array or a CCD camera) as a detector of emission radiation is preferable because spectra can be recorded very rapidly and frequently with sequences in the millisecond range. Fluorescence spectrometers for *in vivo* diagnostics are commonly based on fiber-optic systems.[133,574–577,591] The excitation light of a lamp or a laser is guided to the tissue (e.g., some specific organ) via fiber using appropriate optical filters. Fluorescence spectra are usually measured either via the same fiber or via a second fiber or fiber bundle in close proximity to the excitation fiber.

Various comprehensive and powerful fluorescence spectroscopies, such as microspectrofluorimetry, polarization anisotropy, time-resolved with pulse excitation and frequency domain, time-grated, total-internal-reflection fluorescence spectroscopy and microscopy, the fluorescence resonant energy transfer method, confocal laser scanning microscopy, and their combinations are available now.[573–601] These methods allows one to provide the following:

- 3D topography of specimens measured in the reflection mode for morphological studies of biological samples
- High resolution microscopy measured in the transmission mode
- 3D fluorescence detection of cellular structures and fluorescence bleaching kinetics
- Time-resolved fluorescence kinetics
- Studies of motions of cellular structures
- Time-grated imaging in order to select specific fluorescent molecules or molecular interactions

- Fluorescence lifetime imaging
- Spectrally resolved imaging

The potential of time-gated fluorescence spectroscopy is shown in Fig. 1.48.[574,593] Shown fluorescence spectra of *Saccharomyces cerevisiae* are very similar to the fluorescence spectra of various cell cultures. An emission maximum at 460–465 nm, corresponding to free NADH, is clearly identified within a time gate of 0–5 ns, whereas emission maxima around 435 nm (bound NADH) and 515 nm (flavins) are resolved at later time gates. In contrast, CW spectra of autofluorescence are broad and exhibit only little substructure.

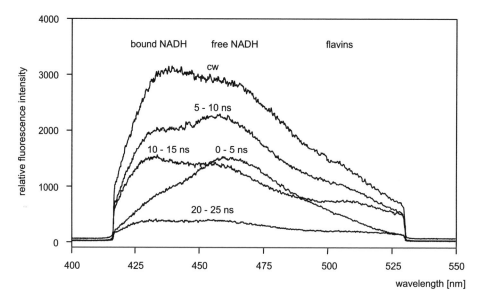

Figure 1.48 CW and time-gated fluorescence spectra of *Saccharomyces cerevisiae* after excitation at 365 nm (upper curve) and 355 nm (other curves).[593]

Using time-resolved fluorescence detection, free and bound NADH could be studied separately; time-gated fluorescence spectroscopy includes studies of the tumor-localizing porphyrins within tissues of strong autofluorescence; and the fluorescence energy transfer method can be used to selectively measure mitochondrial depolarization, which may precede mitochondrial autophagy, apoptosis, and necrotic cell death.[574] Analytical models and solutions for time-resolved fluorescence lifetime quantitative spectroscopy and imaging in turbid media and tissue were recently developed.[598–601]

Principles of optical clinical chemistry based on the measuring of changes of fluorescence intensity, wavelength, polarization anisotropy, and lifetime are described in Ref. 573. Various fluorescence techniques of selective oxygen sensing and blood glucose and blood gases detection are available.[573]

A few examples of fluorescence (autofluorescence) imaging and spectroscopy of normal and pathological tissues such as normal and malignant mucosa in patients with head and neck cancer,[602] carotid atherosclerotic plaque,[603] cervical precancerous tissue,[604] normal and neoplastic human breast tissue,[605] and basal cell carcinomas in the skin[606] should be mentioned. A real-time calibrated autofluorescence technique for *in vivo* imaging of neoplastic growths was realized.[607] Autofluorescence-based methods and instruments designed for ophthalmic diagnostics are overviewed in Ref. 608.

Currently, reflectance and fluorescence spectroscopies are probably the most developed among the available optical methods for investigating skin *in vivo*. Reflectance and fluorescence from skin carry information on the structure of epidermis and dermis, on the quantity and density of blood vessels, on the concentration and spatial distribution of chromophores and fluorophores in skin, and on the nature of skin metabolic processes. Typical applications include the *in vivo* quantitative analysis of skin erythema and pigmentation, determination of cutaneous color variation, monitoring of dermatological treatment effects, determination of skin photoaging, diagnosis of skin tumors, and study of skin biophysics.[57,575,578–580,606]

The absorption and scattering properties of the skin affect both the AF and the reflectance spectra. Therefore, the combined use of fluorescence and reflectance may provide additional information for the analysis of skin tissue. The potential advantages and possible uses of the combined use of reflectance and fluorescence spectroscopy of skin for the evaluation of the erythema and pigmentation indices, the determination of the hemoglobin oxygenation and concentration, and the investigation of the efficacy of topical sunscreens are discussed in Ref. 575.

One of the goals of fluorescence spectroscopy is the identification of excitation wavelengths suitable for the differentiation of various pathological conditions. This is closely related to the identification of the chromophores responsible for this differentiation. Most of the biological components, which are either related to the skin tissue structure or are involved in metabolic and functional processes, generate fluorescence emission in the UV-visible spectral region. As a result, different morphofunctional conditions of the skin related to histological, biochemical, and physiochemical alterations can be characterized, in principle, on the basis of information available in the fluorescence excitation-emission maps (EEMs) (see Fig. 1.49).[575,577,579] The fluorescence maximum in the range 320–370 nm with the peak at 340 nm arises with excitation in the 250–290 nm range (peak at 280 nm). AF in the UVA range is dominated by the fluorescence bands of aromatic amino acids, namely, tyrosine and tryptophan. There is only a slight variation in the UVA fluorescence of the skin between different skin sites. This may be attributed to the absence of AF attenuation by melanin, which is deposited mainly within the epidermis. Tyrosine and tryptophan content in epidermis is more than twice that of the whole skin, and this is why epidermis has a high AF in the UVA range.

Among the endogenous skin fluorophores are also different forms of NAD and keratin located in the epidermis and dermal collagen. The reduced (NADH) and oxidized (NAD$^+$) forms of NAD take part in cellular metabolism, and the intensity of their specific fluorescence (fluorescence maxima near 460 nm and 435 nm,

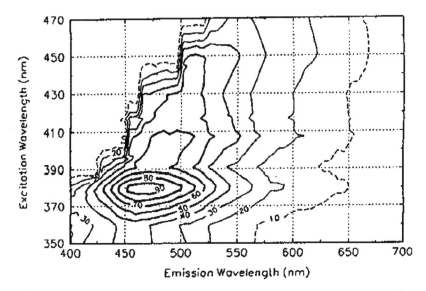

Figure 1.49 Excitation-emission maps of the *in vivo* skin AF emission.[579]

respectively) is used not only for the differential diagnostics of the metabolism dysfunction, but also in quantitative NADH detection.[575]

For collagen and elastin, which are located predominantly within the papillary and reticular layers of dermis, both excitation and emission light is attenuated because of absorption by melanin and fluorescence intensity in the 400–480 nm range is subject to attenuation by other skin chromophores: hemoglobin, porphyrins, carotenoids, etc. Both the total intensity and the spectral features may be affected. The AF spectrum of human skin and the fluorescence spectrum of collagen are essentially identical following optical filtering through the dermal blood plexus.[575,580] Figure 1.50 represents the temporal dynamics of the AF skin spectra involved in the process of the UV-erythema formation. The main part of the change observed is a significant decrease of the AF intensity during the erythema formation caused by the optical filtering effect of blood (early stage) and induced melanin (latter stage).

1.7.2 Multiphoton fluorescence

A new direction in laser spectroscopy and imaging of biological objects is associated with multiphoton (two- and three-photon) fluorescence scanning microscopy, which makes it possible to image functional states of an object or, in combination with autocorrelation analysis of the fluorescence signal, determine the intercellular motility in small volumes.[114,122,131,137,609–618] The two-photon technique employs both ballistic and scattered photons at the wavelength of the second harmonic of incident radiation coming to a wide-aperture photodetector exactly from the focal area of the excitation beam (see Fig. 1.51).[609] A unique advantage of two-photon microscopy is the possibility of investigating three-dimensional distributions of

Fluorescence intensity, arb. units

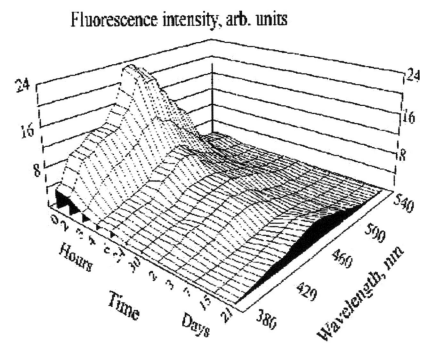

Figure 1.50 3D plot of human skin AF after UV irradiation with four minimal erythema doses (MEDs).[575,580]

chromophores excited with ultraviolet radiation in thick samples. Such an investigation becomes possible because chromophores can be excited (e.g., at the wavelength of 350 nm) with laser radiation whose wavelength falls within the range (700 nm) where a tissue has a high transparency. Such radiation can reach deeply lying layers and produces less damage in tissues. Fluorescent emission in this case lies in the visible range (>400 nm) and comparatively easily emerges from a tissue and reaches a photodetector, which registers only the legitimate signal from the focal volume without any extraneous background.

In a two-photon excitation process, the rate of excitation is proportional to the average squared photon density. This quadratic dependence follows from the requirement that the fluorophore must simultaneously absorb two photons per excitation process. Multiphoton absorption processes are shown in Fig. 1.52. To demonstrate that a multiphoton excitation process has occurred, it is necessary to measure the intensity of fluorescence as a function of the intensity of the excitation light. A two-photon excitation process is characterized by a slope of two on a log-log plot of measured intensities; a three-photon excitation process is characterized by a slope of three.

The rate of two-photon excitation can be described analytically as[614]

$$n_{2f} \approx \frac{P_0^2 \sigma_f}{\tau_p f_p^2} \left[\frac{\pi (NA)^2}{hc\lambda} \right]^2, \tag{1.189}$$

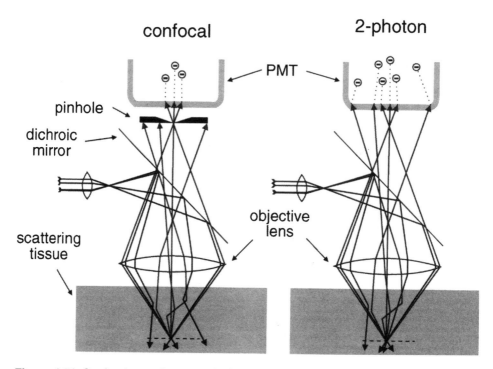

Figure 1.51 Confocal one-photon excitation imaging compared with two-photon imaging in scattering tissue.[609] Because of the longer wavelength, less excitation light is lost to scattering when using two-photon excitation. Ballistic and diffusing fluorescence photons can be used in the two-photon case, but only ballistic photons can be used in the confocal case.

where τ_p is the pulse duration, f_p is the repetition rate, P_0 is the average incident power, σ_f is the photon absorption cross section, h is Planck's constant, c is the speed of light, NA is the numerical aperture of the focusing lens, and λ is the wavelength. This rate is expressed as the number of photons absorbed per fluorophore per pulse and is a function of the pulse duration, the pulse repetition rate, the photon absorption cross section, and the numerical aperture of the microscope objective that focuses the light.[137,614] The derivation of this equation assumes negligible saturation of the fluorophore and that the paraxial approximation is valid.

The laser light in a two-photon excitation microscope is focused by the microscope objective to a focal volume. Only in this focused volume is there sufficient intensity to generate appreciable excitation. The low photon flux outside the focal volume results in a negligible amount of fluorescence signal. The origin of the optical sectioning capability of a two-photon excitation microscope is due to the nonlinear quadratic dependence of the excitation process and the strong focusing capability of the microscope objective. Most specimens are relatively transparent to near-infrared light. The focusing of the microscope objective results in two-photon excitation of ultraviolet absorbing fluorophores in a small focal volume. It is possible to move the focused volume through the thickness of the sample and

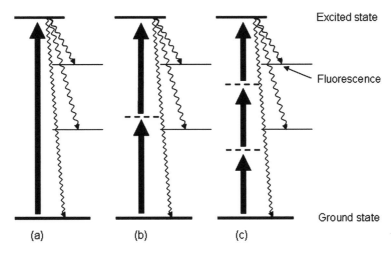

Figure 1.52 Multiphoton fluorescence. Diagram showing the absorption and fluorescence processes for a molecule with (a) one-photon absorption, (b) two-photon absorption, and (c) three-photon absorption. The solid and dashed horizontal lines represent, respectively, real and virtual molecular energy states; the solid vertical arrows, photon absorption pathways; and wavy arrows, fluorescence.

thus achieve optical sectioning in three dimensions. Thus, the optical sectioning in a two-photon excitation microscope occurs during the excitation process.

Investigations of tissues and cells by means of two-photon microscopy are characterized by the following typical parameters of laser systems: the wavelength ranges from 700 to 960 nm, the pulse duration is on the order of 150 fs, the pulse repetition rate is 76–80 MHz, and the mean power is less than 10 mW. Such parameters can be achieved with mode-locked dye lasers pumped by a Nd:YAG laser or with titanium sapphire lasers pumped by an argon laser. Diode-pumped solid-state lasers also hold much promise for the purpose of two-photon microscopy.[609] Virtually the same parameters of lasers are required for three-photon fluorescence microscopy of tissue, which possesses the same advantages as two-photon microscopy but ensures a somewhat higher spatial resolution and provides an opportunity to excite chromophores with shorter wavelengths.[612]

1.7.3 Vibrational and Raman spectroscopies

Middle and far infrared (IR) and Raman spectroscopies use light-excited vibrational energy states in molecules to get information about the molecular composition, molecular structures, and molecular interactions in a sample.[30,99,104,105,115,123,143,619–629] In Fig. 1.53, the IR and Raman processes are depicted in a molecular energy level diagram. In IR-spectroscopy infrared light from a broadband source [usually in the wavelength range of 2.5–25 μm or in wavenumbers $(1/\lambda)$ of 4000–400 cm^{-1}] is directly absorbed to excite the molecules to higher vibrational states.[624] When the absorbed energy $h\nu$ matches the energy needed

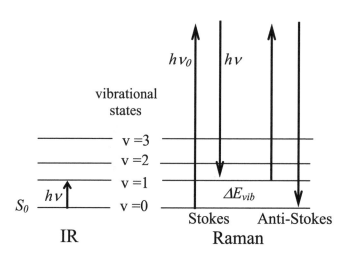

Figure 1.53 Illustration of an IR absorption process and a Raman scattering process in a molecular energy level diagram.[624]

for an allowed infrared excitation of a molecular vibration, an absorption peak is observed in the IR spectrum.

In a Raman scattering event, light is inelastically scattered by a molecule when a small amount of energy is transferred from the photon to the molecule (or from the molecular to the photon). This leads to an excitation of the molecule from usually its lowest vibrational energy level in the electronic ground state S_0 to a higher vibrational state of the same electronic state. The Raman spectrum displays the intensity of scattered light as a function of the difference in frequency between the scattered and the incident light. Since each molecular species has its own unique set of molecular vibrations, the Raman spectrum of a particular species consists of a series of peaks or bands of scattered light, each shifted from the incident light frequency by one of the characteristic vibrational frequencies of that molecule. The energy (frequency) difference between incident ($h\nu_0$) and scattered photon ($h\nu$) is expressed as a wave-number shift:[624]

$$\Delta \tilde{k} = \frac{1}{\lambda_0} - \frac{1}{\lambda}. \tag{1.190}$$

When the energy of the Raman scattered photons is lower than the energy of the incident photons, the process is called Stokes-Raman scattering. When a photon interacts with a molecule in a higher vibrational level, anti-Stokes Raman scattering can occur, in which the energy of the Raman scattered photons is higher than the energy of the incident photons (see Fig. 1.53). The intensity ratio of the anti-Stokes (I_{AS}) and Stokes (I_S) Raman lines for a given vibrational state is given by[624]

$$\frac{I_{AS}}{I_S} = \frac{(\nu_0 + \nu_{vib})^4}{(\nu_0 - \nu_{vib})^4} \exp\left(-\frac{h\nu_{vib}}{k_B T}\right), \tag{1.191}$$

where $\Delta E_{vib} = h\nu_{vib}$ is the energy of the molecular vibrational state. It follows that at room temperature the intensity of Stokes-Raman lines in the most informative spectral region (>400 cm^{-1}) is much higher than that of the anti-Stokes-Raman lines. In its turn, the intensity of Stokes-Raman scattered light is very low, typically 10^{-7} to 10^{-15} times the intensity of the excitation light. The real-time detection of Raman scattering spectra became practical because of the commercial development of lasers and subsequent advances in detector technology.

Different selection rules apply for excitation of molecular vibrational states through absorption of an IR photon or through Raman scattering of an incident photon.[115,123,621,624] Some vibrations can be excited by both Raman and IR processes; others can only be excited by either a Raman scattering process or by IR absorption. For symmetric molecules, the selection rules are mutually exclusive for all vibrations. Molecules exhibit IR activity when, during the vibration, a change in the molecular dipole moment occurs. Raman activity occurs when there is a change in polarizability. Therefore, the band intensity in IR and Raman spectra of the same molecular vibrational frequency can be quite different; symmetric vibrational modes are often strong in Raman, whereas antisymmetric vibrational modes are strong in IR. Depending on the polarization state of the incident and observed light, information on the symmetry of the molecules can be obtained.

In most tissues, the fluorescence cross section, when excited by visible or near UV wavelengths (within 300–700 nm), is about six orders of magnitude stronger than the Stokes Raman cross section; moreover, the fluorescence is a broadband signal within the same spectral range as the Stokes-Raman spectrum.[143,624] Fortunately, at different excitation wavelengths, UV, visible, and NIR, Raman scattering produces the same change in vibrational energy, while NIR light has a frequency too low to excite fluorescence and UV-excited fluorescence has much lower frequency than the Raman scattered light frequency. Hence, the usage of NIR or UV excitation can reduce fluorescence background in the Raman spectrum. Especially for tissue studies, NIR excitation is preferable due to the high penetration depth.

The IR and Raman spectroscopy techniques are successfully applied in various areas of clinical studies such as cancerous tissues examination, the mineralization process of bone and teeth tissue monitoring, glucose sensing in blood, noninvasive diagnosis of skin lesions on benign or malignant cells, and monitoring of treatments and topically applied substances (e.g., drugs, cosmetics, moisturizers, etc.) in skin.[30,99,104,105,143,619,620,622–626]

Raman spectroscopy is widely used in biological studies, ranging from studies of purified biological compounds to investigations at the level of single cells.[621,623,625,627,629] At present, combinations of spectroscopic techniques such as IR and Raman with microscopic imaging techniques are explored to map molecular distributions at specific vibrational frequencies to locally characterize tissues or cells.[620,623,624,629] Spectral biochemical imaging will become more and more important in the clinical diagnosis; in particular, for differentiation of cancerous and noncancerous cells. The measured IR spectra depend on various aspects of sample preparation, i.e., the degree of hydration and homogeneity, and on the physiological state of cells (exponential phase of growth or plateau); therefore, measurements accounting for named artifacts and cell status should be provided.[629] As it was shown recently, the accurate measurement of vibrational spectra of mammalian cells is possible for the homogeneous aqueous cell suspensions; these IR spectra can be closely reproduced with a linear combination of DNA, RNA, phospholipid, glycogen, and protein spectra.[629]

Because of a penetration depth of middle IR (MIR) light in tissue to only a few micrometers, the attenuated total reflectance Fourier transform infrared spectroscopy (ATR-FTIR) method is suited to study changes of the outermost cell layers of the tissue.[624] As an example, sequential hydrated-human-skin stratum-corneum ATR-FTIR spectra measured during occlusion each minute for half an hour are shown in Fig. 1.54. Hydration of the skin is obtained by keeping the forearm pressed against the ATR-FTIR crystal. During occlusion, water in the skin cannot evaporate and accumulates in the skin stratum corneum.

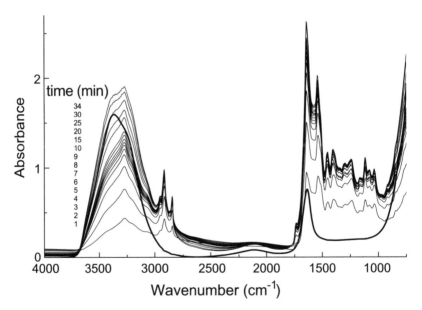

Figure 1.54 Sequential hydrated-human-skin stratum-corneum MIR ATR-FTIR spectra measured during occlusion each minute for half an hour.[624] The thick line represents the water spectrum (scaled twice). Spectral changes can be clearly identified: increased contribution of the water-bending mode at 1640 cm^{-1} and pronounced increase of the OH stretches in the high wave number band around 3300 cm^{-1}. Also, the water combination band around 2125 cm^{-1} is clearly visible in the hydrated spectra. A Nicolet-800 Fourier Transform spectrometer with a "high-top" model ATR with a ZnSe ($n = 2.42$) crystal of rectangular shape (10 × 80 mm) with 45-deg entrance and exit facets is used to record spectra. The ATR-FTIR spectrum is obtained by the Fourier transform of 64 and 128 interferograms. The acquisition time for 64 scans at a resolution of 8 cm^{-1} is about 20 s. Spectra were recorded on the volar part of the forearm by slight pressure on the ZnSe crystal.

The Raman technique possesses certain characteristics that make it particularly suitable for studying the skin, both *in vitro* and *in vivo*.[622,624] *In vivo* confocal Raman spectra of the skin show a considerable decrease in the absolute signal intensity if the distance from the laser focus to the skin surface is increased. This is mainly due to diffuse light scattering, which is a much stronger effect in the skin than light absorption. Confocal detection is therefore particularly useful in the study of outer skin layers, i.e., the stratum corneum and the viable epidermis. The *in vivo* Raman signal of the dermis is strongly reduced due to scattering in the epidermis; therefore, the dermis requires considerably longer signal collection times than for the epidermis. However, since the dermis is much thicker than the epidermis (1–4-mm thick), it can easily be studied using a nonconfocal detection scheme with a detection volume that is large compared to the thickness of the epidermis. In this case, the dermis will be the dominant source of the Raman signal, which is illustrated by Fig. 1.55.[624] The figure shows the confocal spectrum measured using a confocal spectrometer and a nonconfocal spectrum measured with a fiber-optic probe. Both spectra were scaled to equal intensity. It is clear that the spectrum obtained with the fiber-optic probe is almost entirely determined by the Raman signal of the dermis. For equal signal collection time, the SNR of the dermis spectrum obtained with the fiber-optic probe is considerably higher than that of the spectrum that was measured confocally.[624]

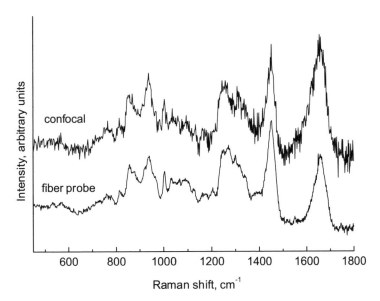

Figure 1.55 *In vivo* Raman spectra of the dermis, as obtained by confocal detection and by nonconfocal detection (fiber-optic probe). Experimental conditions for the confocal spectrum and the nonconfocal spectrum: signal collection time 2 min, laser power 100 mW. The spectra are scaled to equal intensities.[624]

Near-infrared Raman spectroscopy also has a number of advantages in *in vivo* detection of cervical tissue pathologies, in particular precancer predictions.[30,626]

Surface-enhanced Raman scattering (SERS) is based on a strong increase in Raman signals from molecules if those molecules are attached to submicron metallic structures. Two effects are believed to contribute to the SERS enhancement mechanisms: electromagnetic effects and chemical effects.[620,627] For a smooth metal surface, there is only a small (on the order of 10 times or less) enhancement of Raman intensity compared with that in the absence of the surface, but for a rough surface due to excitation of electromagnetic resonances by the incident radiation, such enhancement may be of a few orders. These resonances appear due to collective excitation of conduction electrons in the small metallic structures and are also called surface plasmon resonances. Both the excitation and Raman scattered fields contribute to this enhancement; thus, the SERS signal is proportional to the fourth power of the field enhancement factor.[620]

The surface roughening effect can be achieved by isolated metal particles, by gratings, by assemblies of particles on surfaces, and randomly roughened surfaces. All these structures provide enhancement if the metal involved has narrow plasmon resonances at convenient frequencies for Raman measurements.[627] The "chemical mechanisms" include enhancements that arise from interactions between molecule and metal. The most commonly considered interaction that requires overlap between molecular and metal wave numbers occurs when charge transfer between the surface and molecule leads to the formation of excited states that serve as resonant intermediates in Raman scattering.[620,627] Interactions that do not require overlap between molecular and metal wave numbers arise from electromagnetic coupling between the vibrating molecule and the metal. These interactions can occur either at the vibrational frequency or at optical frequencies. The combined enhancement factors can be as high as 10^{14}, which is enough to observe SERS spectra from single molecules.

1.8 Tissue phantoms

1.8.1 Introduction

Phantoms that model the transport of visible and infrared light in tissue are needed to evaluate techniques, to calibrate equipment, to optimize procedures, and for quality assurance.[31,46,47,93–95,219,220,233,236,237,263,277,284,467,494,495,511,572,630–646] They have been used in all fields of optical diagnostics, particularly for testing instruments for time- and frequency-domain transillumination tomography[284,639] and spatially resolved reflectance measurements,[46,93,637,638] to evaluate the fluorescence spectroscopic technique,[632,633,636,641–643] and to test theoretical predictions experimentally.[47,94,95,219,220,634,636] Tissue models have been developed for tissue noninvasive glucose monitoring,[339–341,535,536,540,541,630,631,635] oxygenation monitoring and oxymetry,[516,644] optoacoustics,[467,511,516,535,536,540,541] pulsed photothermal measurements,[491,495,497] and measuring of polarization degree decay.[374,645] Tissuelike phantoms have also been taken up in areas of research connected with therapeutic implementation of optical radiation, among them being light dosimetry,[646] laser ablation,[511] and PDT.[640,646]

1.8.2 Concepts of phantom construction

To describe the concepts of constructing phantoms, we will draw upon Refs. 632–634 and 636. Phantoms consist of a scattering medium, an absorbing medium, a diluent, and in some cases fluorophores.[632,633,636] Some common scattering media are Intralipid, Nutralipid, and Liposyn. These intravenously administered nutrients are fat emulsions that contain soybean oil, egg phospholipids, and glycerol. Other common scatterers are milk or micron-sized latex (polystyrene) spheres. Polystyrene microspheres exhibit low fluorescence, and some of their optical properties can be calculated from Mie theory. Absorbing media include some biological stains such as trypan blue, Evans blue, indocyanine green, methylene blue, and Photofrin II, as well as black India ink. The diluent is usually deionized water, although isotonic phosphate-buffered saline has been used.

An optical phantom is developed by mixing the correct proportions of the scattering and absorbing media in the diluent, so that the resulting suspension has the desired intrinsic optical properties of the simulated tissue. These optical properties include the absorption coefficient μ_a, the scattering coefficient μ_s, and the anisotropy factor g. For soft tissues, typical optical properties are $\mu_a \approx 0.5$ to 5.0 cm^{-1}, $\mu_s \approx 0.2$ to 400 cm^{-1}, and $g = 0.9$ for visible and NIR wavelengths (see Table 2.1).

A liquid phantom system is very easy to prepare; however, it cannot be used to make samples of realistic complexity. Solid phantom samples have been made using either transparent hosts, such as polymers, silicone, or gelatin; or using inherently light-scattering materials, such as wax. Polymer-based phantoms have been reported to crack if they are too large or to shrink during polymerization, which limits their applicability. Gels contain a solvent that evaporates, changing the dimensions and optical properties of the sample within a short period of time.

Steps toward realistic complex geometries have been the application of layered samples, inserted inhomogeneities, and phantoms mimicking whole organs.[46,47,93–95,233,236,237,277,284,632–636] Some phantom systems have realistic optical properties over a wide wavelength range.[47,94,95,236,237] When the task is to model tissue with complex architecture, or even a whole organ, or to prepare the test object for evaluation of imaging techniques, the "macroscopic" geometry of the natural object should be reproduced in phantom. One of the most commonly encountered features is a layered tissue structure. Multilayered phantoms have been developed in the past to mimic, for example, the skin,[497] the human head,[647,648] and the cervix.[641–643]

A realistic tissue phantom should satisfy the following requirements:[632,633]

- It should model the geometry and optical parameters of the physiological structures that are relevant for the transport of light.
- All components must be compatible with each other regarding chemical stability and spectroscopic properties.
- The relevant parameters of radiation transport must be both reproducible and predictable from the sample composition.

- The physical parameters of the phantom sample should be temporally stable (evaporation, diffusion, aging) and independent of environmental influence.
- The phantom should allow the construction of inhomogeneous samples by stacking phantom slabs or by elaborate molding techniques.
- Sample preparation should be simple, quick, and safe.

The strategy for systematic design of tissue phantom systems showing realistic optical properties over a broad wavelength range is based on the discrete particle model of tissue.[632,633] Light scattering and absorption of particles composing tissue (phantom) are calculated by Mie theory. The relevant parameters are the size (radius a) and shape of the particles; their complex refractive index

$$n_s(\lambda_0) = n'_s(\lambda_0) + in''_s(\lambda_0), \tag{1.192}$$

the refractive index of the dielectric host (ground material) $n_0(\lambda_0)$, and the relative refractive index of the scatterers and the ground materials, $m = n_s/n_0$; λ_0 is the wavelength in a vacuum. The imaginary part of the complex refractive index of scatterer material is responsible for light losses due to absorption. Mie theory yields the absorption and scattering efficiencies and the phase function from which the absorption and scattering coefficients, $\mu_s = \rho\sigma_{sca}$ and $\mu_a = \rho\sigma_{abs}$, and the scattering anisotropy factor g are calculated; ρ is the scatterers (particles) density. In the framework of Mie theory, the expressions for the scattering and the absorption cross sections can be written in the form[148]

$$\sigma_{sca} = \left(\frac{\lambda_0^2}{2\pi n_0^2}\right)\sum_{n=1}^{\infty}(2n+1)\left(|a_n|^2 + |b_n|^2\right), \tag{1.193}$$

$$\sigma_{abs} = \left(\frac{\lambda_0^2}{2\pi n_0^2}\right)\sum_{n=1}^{\infty}(2n+1)\left[\text{Re}(a_n + b_n) - \left(|a_n|^2 + |b_n|^2\right)\right], \tag{1.194}$$

$$g = \frac{\lambda_0^2}{\pi n_0^2 \sigma_{sca}}\left[\sum_{n=1}^{\infty}\frac{2n+1}{n(n+1)}\text{Re}(a_n b_n^*) + \sum_{n=1}^{\infty}\frac{n(n+2)}{n+1}\text{Re}\left(a_n a_{n+1}^* + b_n b_{n+1}^*\right)\right], \tag{1.195}$$

where an asterisk indicates the complex conjugate; and a_n and b_n are Mie coefficients, which are functions of the relative complex refractive index of particles (m) and parameter $2\pi a n_0/\lambda_0$ to be taken as

$$a_n = \frac{\psi_n(\alpha)\psi'_n(m\alpha) - m\psi_n(m\alpha)\psi'_n(\alpha)}{\xi(\alpha)\psi'_n(m\alpha) - m\psi_n(m\alpha)\xi'_n(\alpha)}, \tag{1.196}$$

$$b_n = \frac{m\psi'(m\alpha)\psi_n(\alpha) - \psi_n(m\alpha)\psi'_n(\alpha)}{m\psi'_n(m\alpha)\xi_n(\alpha) - \psi_n(m\alpha)\xi'_n(\alpha)}, \tag{1.197}$$

$$m = \frac{n_p}{n_0}; \quad \alpha = \frac{2\pi a n_0}{\lambda_0}, \tag{1.198}$$

where a is the radius of spherical scattering particles, λ_0 is the light wavelength in vacuum, ψ_n, ξ_n, ψ'_n, ξ'_n are the Riccati-Bessel functions of the first or second kind, n_0 is the refractive index of the ground (host) material, and n_p is the refractive index of scattering particle material.

The introduction of the specific scattering and absorption coefficients extrapolated to a volume fraction of 100% is useful for describing scattering and absorption properties of the medium under construction.[632,633] In that case and when the particles are sufficiently diluted to prevent dependent scattering, the scattering, transport scattering, and absorption coefficients are proportional to the dimensionless volume fraction of scatterers c_s,

$$\mu_s = c_s \overline{\sigma}_{sca}, \quad \mu'_s = c_s \overline{\sigma}_{sca}[1 - g(\lambda_0, a)], \quad \mu_a = c_s \overline{\sigma}_{abs}, \tag{1.199}$$

where the specific scattering and absorption coefficients $\overline{\sigma}_{sca}$ and $\overline{\sigma}_{abs}$ are expressed in cm^{-1}. The optical parameters of broadband particle size distributions are values averaged over the distribution weighted by the volume fractions of particles with different diameters. The relative frequencies of the corresponding particle size are determined from images made with an electron microscope. The resulting specific optical coefficients are the averaged values and can be defined analogously to Eqs. (1.173)–(1.176). The mean distance d_s between the centers of gravity of the particles is determined by their radius a and volume fraction c_s as

$$d_s = \frac{2a}{\sqrt[3]{c_s}}. \tag{1.200}$$

Mie theory predicts that scattering introduced by spherical micrometer-sized particles is strongest if the particle radius and wavelength are of the same order of magnitude. Mie theory is strictly only applicable to particles of particular regular shapes, but results are still useful if the shape is irregular. The oscillatory structure of the scattering coefficient and anisotropy factor as a function of particle size, which is observed with spherical particles (Fig. 1.56), is averaged out.[148] The transport scattering coefficient increases strongly with the ratio n'_s/n_0. In turn, the scattering anisotropy factor is maximal when this ratio approaches 1 (Fig. 1.56). A trade-off has to be made between maximizing scattering (to prevent dependent scattering) and optimizing the scattering anisotropy factor when constructing certain phantoms.

For the matched refractive indices of scatterers and background material, the scattering coefficient goes to zero, which means that only absorption is responsible now for the light beam extinction [see Eq. (1.1)]. However, as it follows from Mie theory, absorbing particles suspended in an index-matched medium cause strongly forward-directed resonance scattering. Light absorption by such particles is smaller than expected from their bulk absorption coefficient.[632,633] For 1-μm diameter particles with $n_s = 1.6$ and a bulk absorption coefficient of their material equal to 10^4 cm^{-1} in an index-matched medium, the particle system absorption coefficient $\mu_a = c_s \times 4120$ cm^{-1}.

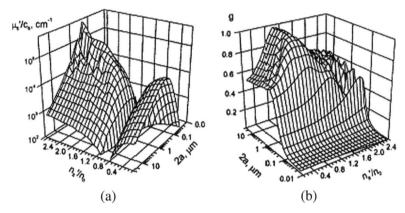

(a)   (b)

Figure 1.56 Designing of a tissue phantom. The scattering properties of nonabsorbing particles at a wavelength of 633 nm are calculated by Mie theory.[632,633] The transport scattering coefficient (a) strongly depends on both the particle size and relative refractive index. This graph is approximately symmetric. The axis of symmetry is at $n'_s/n_0 = 1$. While the transparent scattering coefficient equals zero there, in (b) the scattering anisotropy factor is maximal. In some parts of the range shown, the functions are not monotonous, but rapidly oscillating.

The wavelength dependencies of scattering parameters are shown in Fig. 1.57. The spectral variation of the relative index has been neglected in calculations, but may be relevant in practice. If particle size and ratio of refractive indices are fixed, the wavelength dependencies are caused by the spectral variation of the ratio of particle size and wavelength. For particles with a refractive index close to that of the host (see Fig. 1.57), the scattering coefficient of the particle system with a diameter of particles smaller than the wavelength decreases with wavelength, while that of the system with a diameter of particles larger than the wavelength is almost constant. The scattering anisotropy factor depends less on the wavelength. There are plateaus if the particles are much smaller (isotropic scattering) or larger (highly anisotropic scattering) than the wavelength, with a steep increase between.

Biological tissue shows increasing scattering toward shorter wavelengths and high scattering anisotropy. These cannot be realized using monodisperse particles. Therefore, a mixture of large particles contributing high scattering anisotropy and small particles with increasing scattering toward shorter wavelengths should be a good approximation for the elaborating of a tissuelike phantom.[179,632,633]

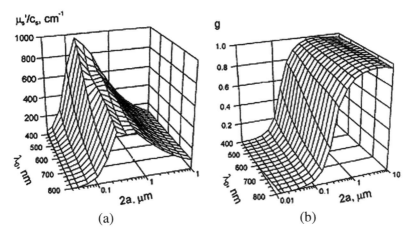

(a)   (b)

Figure 1.57 Designing of a tissue phantom. The wavelength dependencies of scattering by nonabsorbing particles at $n'_s/n_0 = 1.07$ are calculated by Mie theory.[632,633] The specific transport scattering coefficient (a) of particles smaller than the wavelength increases strongly toward shorter wavelengths. Particles with a diameter larger than the wavelength have an almost constant specific transport scattering coefficient over the whole visible spectral range. The scattering anisotropy factor (b) scarcely depends on the wavelength, but very much on the particle size.

1.8.3 Examples of designed tissue phantoms

Optical phantoms at 1064 nm on the basis of Intralipid and India ink mixtures have been developed using the preliminary experimentally determined absorption coefficient, scattering coefficient, and anisotropy factor of the components.[634] For evaluation of the optical parameters of phantom components and phantoms themselves, the integrating sphere technique together with the collimated light transmission measurements and the inverse adding-doubling (IAD) algorithm were used. The average optical properties from all the data for the phantom components are shown in Table 1.6. A comparison of the predicted, measured, and calculated optical properties of the two phantoms are shown in Table 1.7. In Table 1.8, the predicted (Mie theory) and measured (IAD algorithm) data for two phantoms (804-nm diameter polystyrene sphere and water suspensions) are presented.

Table 1.6 Average optical properties in dependence on concentration of India ink, 10% Intralipid, and water at 1064 nm.[634]

Scattering media	$\mu_s/\%$, cm^{-1}/%	$\mu_a/\%$, cm^{-1}/%	g
India ink	4.64 ± 2.07	35.99 ± 4.28	0.30 ± 0.18
Intralipid	1.30 ± 0.047	0.054 ± 0.02	0.50 ± 0.02
Water	–	0.0018	–

Note: The absorption results of Intralipid are corrected for water absorption.

Table 1.7 Predicted and measured optical properties of phantoms.[634]

Phantoms	μ_s, cm^{-1}	μ_a, cm^{-1}	g
Phantom 1 (Intralipid and India ink)			
Predicted	8.82	0.32	0.48
Measured	9.69 ± 0.22	0.76 ± 0.01	0.56 ± 0.00
Calculated	8.75	0.89	0.50
Phantom 2 (Intralipid only)			
Predicted	8.82	0.00	0.48
Measured	8.84 ± 0.03	0.33 ± 0.01	0.51 ± 0.00
Calculated	8.70	0.53	0.50

Note: The predicted values for phantoms 1 and 2 assume that Intralipid and water do not absorb and that ink does not scatter 1064-nm light. The calculated values were determined from the concentration values found in Table 1.6.

Table 1.8 Predicted and measured optical properties of phantoms (804-nm diameter polystyrene sphere and water suspensions) at 1064 nm.[634]

Phantoms	μ_s, cm^{-1}	μ_a, cm^{-1}	g
Phantom 1			
Predicted	2.23	–	0.807
Measured	1.99 ± 0.12	0.28 ± 0.02	0.775 ± 0.04
Phantom 2			
Predicted	2.96	–	0.807
Measured	3.15 ± 0.01	0.25 ± 0.01	0.811 ± 0.004

Note: The predicted values for phantoms 1 and 2 were calculated using the Mie theory. The absorption coefficients were not corrected for water absorption.

All these data clearly show that liquid phantom systems allow the design of controlled tissuelike phantoms and their optical properties on at least one wavelength are well predicted theoretically. In particular, by knowing the dependence of scattering and absorption of the India ink and Intralipid, a phantom with predicted optical properties can be constructed. However, the constructed phantom's final optical properties should be measured for an accurate determination of phantom optical parameters. Unfortunately, the scattering properties of diluted Intralipid correspond to those of tissues that have a relatively low scattering anisotropy factor of about $g = 0.56$. A more realistic value of an anisotropy factor can be obtained by water suspensions of polystyrene spheres with a diameter close to the wavelength. A comparison of the constructed phantom's optical properties at 1064 nm with the corresponding optical parameters of human tissues, presented in Table 2.1, shows that the absorption properties of these phantoms are well matched to many tissues, but the scattering properties are much lower than for tissues.

To check the validity of analyzing the optical properties of human skin by using *in vivo* reflectance measurements, liquid phantoms consisting of Intralipid-10% as a scatterer and Evans blue as an absorber in phosphate-buffered saline were applied.[572] Concentrations of Intralipid-10% in the range 10–50% and Evans blue up to 0.01 g/l were used. In an *ex vivo* study of human skin in the NIR range, phantoms composed of aqueous solutions of 1.27-µm polystyrene microspheres and infrared dye (S109564 Zeneca) were used.[236,237] The accuracy and the limitations of the experimental system for spatially resolved absolute diffuse reflectance measurements were tested using tissue-simulating phantoms that consisted of Liposyn-20% stock solution and trypan blue dye as the absorber.[46,93] For a 1% volume concentration of Liposyn (without trypan blue) at 633 nm, $\mu'_s = 14.0 \pm 0.5$ cm^{-1}, $g = 0.8$, and $\mu_a = 0.005$ cm^{-1} were found.

Comparing the experimental results for absorption length, transport length, and anisotropy factor against wavelength obtained for a 2% Intralipid-10% stock solution with Mie theory, it was found that one can use the following approximations:[31,92]

$$\mu'_s(\lambda) \approx 1.6 \times 10^3 \lambda^{-1} \ (\text{cm}^{-1}) \ \text{and} \ g(\lambda) \approx 1.1 - 0.58 \times 10^{-3}\lambda, \qquad (1.201)$$

for wavelengths from 400 to 1100 nm. To obtain a solution with $\mu'_s = 76.9$ cm^{-1} and $\mu'_s = 10$ cm^{-1} at 550 nm, the stock solution of Intralipid-10% was diluted as 1:2 and 1:15, respectively.[31,92]

Sometimes, in the constructing of phantoms with precise optical properties in a wide range of wavelengths, the dependencies of refractive indices of phantoms' components should be included. For example, for water-polystyrene suspension phantoms, to include the wavelength dependence of the refractive indices of water and polystyrene particles, the dispersion functions for water (w) and polystyrene (p) valid in the visible and NIR should be used as[630]

$$n_w(\lambda) = 1.31848 + \frac{6.662}{\lambda[\text{nm}] - 129.2}$$

$$\cong 1.3199 + \frac{6878}{\lambda^2} - \frac{1.132 \times 10^9}{\lambda^4} + \frac{1.11 \times 10^{14}}{\lambda^6}. \qquad (1.202)$$

$$n_p = 1.5626 + \frac{11690}{\lambda^2} - \frac{1.25 \times 10^9}{\lambda^4} + \frac{1.72 \times 10^{14}}{\lambda^6}, \qquad (1.203)$$

where λ is in nanometers.

To study laser-induced stress transients in a nonscattering homogeneously absorbing liquid where a theoretical description of optoacoustic phenomena is straightforward, an aqueous solution of potassium chromate (K_2CrO_4) was used.[467,511] This solution does not fluoresce, and the total absorbed laser energy is therefore converted into heat; it is photochemicaly stable, and its optical properties are not altered, even at high laser fluences. A solution of 35 mg of K_2CrO_4 per cubic centimeter yields an absorption coefficient of $\sim$1000 cm^{-1} at 355 nm. Dilution of the initial solution allows one to control the light penetration depth and, therefore, the acoustic frequency of laser-induced stress waves.[467]

Laser-induced stress generation, propagation, and detection in tissues can be well modeled with the help of turbid absorbing gels.[467] A warm water solution (90 cm^3) was mixed with 10 g of gelatin powder to prepare gel phantoms. These gels were colored with potassium chromate and made turbid with polystyrene microspheres (0.9 μm in diameter). A 10% polystyrene sphere solution has a scattering coefficient of $\mu_s = 6090$ cm^{-1} and an anisotropy factor $g = 0.918$ at 355 nm, yielding a reduced scattering coefficient of $\mu_s' = 499$ cm^{-1}; the absorption coefficient at 355 nm is defined by the concentration of K_2CrO_4 and can be very high, up to 1000 cm^{-1}. However, the spectral range of importance for biomedical optics is from visible to NIR, in which diagnostics, imaging, and photodynamic therapy treatments are performed. Therefore, the polystyrene sphere concentration can be chosen to be approximately 2% in the experimental gels, which yields $\mu_s' = 99$ cm^{-1}. A typical μ_s'/μ_a ratio for biological tissues at 600–1000-nm wavelength is from 70 to 100, which can be easily realized for such phantoms. Soft elastic collagen gel phantoms can be prepared using milk as a scatterer and can be colored with hemoglobin or even whole blood. They allow for easy embedding of inclusions modeling various pathology states (for instance, an absorbing sphere simulating tumor) or modeling the specificity of tissue structure (for instance, a vessel network).

Adding a small percentage of agarose to solidify the well-characterized and easily available water solutions of Intralipid and ink is a good alternative for more complicated solid phantoms.[284] Solutions of such phantom consist of 1% agarose in distilled water, with Intralipid and black ink added. The agarose produces a gelatin that can be easily manufactured in order to create and embed an inclusion. In addition, gelatin (collagen) gel phantoms with different optical properties can be stacked on top of each other to yield a layered-tissue structure model.[277,641–643] TiO_2 particles can be used as scatterers and India ink can be used as an absorber in the constructing of gelatin (collagen) gel phantoms.

TiO_2 particles 0.3 μm in diameter and Projet 900NP dye (Zeneca) were used as scatterers and absorber in solid phantoms composed of Araldite epoxy resin (Ciba Polymers).[236,237] These phantoms also allow one to combine optical properties by stacking slabs with different optical parameters. As a homogeneous solid scattering phantom for calibration of a microspectrophotometric optical system, a composite consisting of highly dispersed SiO_2 particles (diameter < 10 μm, volume-filling fraction, 43%) in an organic methacrylate matrix was used.[263]

Temporally stable samples were made from a phantom system based on polyorganosiloxane (POS, silicone) as a host, which has been described in detail elsewhere.[632,633] Highly hydrophobic POS is supplied in monomeric form as a two-component system. It is especially suited to the modeling of fine structures. When a cross-linking component is added, POS starts to polymerize in an additional reaction; it takes typically less than 30 min at 80°C in a drying oven. There is no shrinking or cracking. Particles as small as 40 nm in diameter are immobilized in the rubber meshwork. The resulting rubber is mechanically stable and transparent in the visible range. Its refractive index equals 1.40 at 589 nm. This method of phantom preparation allows one to construct multilayer phantoms with stepwise varying optical properties without any gap between homogeneous layers, and to include fine tissue details such as structured surfaces and tiny holes, modeling tissue surface and blood vessels, respectively. Various types of particles can be used to induce scattering. Some of them with negligible absorption in the visible spectral region are presented in Table 1.9. This table illustrates the range of values for the relative refractive indices that can be provided in two phantom systems considered.

To achieve homogeneous dispersion, particles should be dispersed in a host media by an ultracentrifuge. The authors of Refs. 632 and 633 used spherical porous

Table 1.9 Relative refractive indices of substances with negligible absorption in the visible spectral range.[632,633]

Substance	In aqueous gel	In POS
SiO_2	1.10	1.04
γ-Al_2O_3	1.20	1.14
$BaSO_4$	1.23	1.17
MgO	1.31	1.24
α-Al_2O_3	1.33	1.26
TiO_2	1.95	1.86

Note: The relative refractive index is given for an aqueous gel ($n_0 = 1.33$) and POS ($n_0 = 1.40$ at 589 nm) for a host. The particles are assumed to be massive.

Table 1.10 Comparison of the results of integrating sphere measurements and Mie calculation based on isolated characterization.[632,633]

Wavelength, nm	Method	Porous aluminium oxide particles		Iron particles	
		$\overline{\sigma}_{sca}$, cm^{-1}	$\overline{\sigma}_{abs}$, cm^{-1}	$\overline{\sigma}_{sca}$, cm^{-1}	$\overline{\sigma}_{abs}$, cm^{-1}
546	Mie theory	$210(50)^a$	–	$3000(600)^c$	$4500(900)^c$
546	Measured	$200(10)^b$	<0.7	$3500(900)^a$	$3800(200)^a$
633	Mie theory	$210(50)^a$	–	$3000(600)^c$	$4500(900)^c$
633	Measured	$190(10)^b$	<0.7	$2800(800)^a$	$3900(200)^a$

Note: The assumption was that the pores of the particles are completely filled with POS and the average refractive index of particles was estimated. Spherical porous aluminium oxide particles have a symmetrical size distribution, with the mean value 5.3 ± 1.0 μm, and spherical iron particles have an asymmetrical size distribution: 16% of the volume fraction is contributed by particles of diameter up to 2.0 μm, 50% by particles up to 3.0 μm, and 84% by particles up to 3.6 μm.

Errors are given in parentheses in units of the last digit(s) and are: [a] the upper limit error caused by uncertain refractive index (particle composition); [b] sum of error of measurement, limited reproducibility of sample production, error of sample thickness, and systematic error of diffusion theory; [c] variations of reported values.

aluminium oxide, iron, and modified amino resin (MAR) particles to obtain an appropriate scattering. Some data that allow one to compare the optical properties predicted by Mie theory, taking into account the optical properties of isolated particles and their size distributions, and the optical properties of POS phantoms measured using the integrating sphere technique are presented in Table 1.10. These phantoms were designed for modeling the fluorescence of tissue components, in particular, protoporphyrin IX fluorescence.

Various phantoms have been designed to determine the accuracy of *in vivo* optical monitoring of glucose concentration in blood and tissues.[339–341,535,536,540, 541,630,631,635]

1.8.4 Examples of whole organ models

Models of whole organs are described in the literature.[636,647,648] For example, human skin was modeled by a film (50 to 150 μm) of hydrated Type I collagen.[494,495] This film contained variable amounts of subsurface absorbers positioned at a given depth and simulated discrete chromophores buried in multilayered composite human skin. The chromophores were constructed by staining a film with triphenylmethane dye, which absorbs optimally at 585 nm. Discrete chromophores were prepared by cutting a stained collagen film (125-μm thick) with known optical absorption ($\mu_a = 400$ cm^{-1}) into a number of thin strips (100- to 300-μm width). A model skin phantom was constructed by positioning variably spaced (50 to 700 μm) absorbing thin strips underneath a known thickness (110 μm) of a nonabsorbing collagen film. The absorbing thin strips and nonabsorbing films were positioned on a 10-mm thick collagen sponge to simulate an infinite half-space as in living skin.

Another example of whole organ modeling consists of models of the adult head.[233,647,648] The models[233] consist of three- or four-layered slabs, the latter incorporating a clear cerebrospinal fluid (CSF) layer. The most sophisticated model also incorporates slots that imitate sulci on the brain surface. Using these models, it was shown that light propagation in the adult head is highly affected by the presence of the clear CSF layer, and both the optical path length and the spatial sensitivity profile of the models with a CSF layer are quite different from those without the CSF layer. However, the geometry of the sulci and the boundary between the gray and the white matter have little effect on the light distribution detected.

2

Methods and Algorithms for the Measurement of the Optical Parameters of Tissues

Methods and algorithms for solving the inverse problem of finding tissue and blood optical parameters such as absorption and scattering coefficients, anisotropy factor, and refractive index are presented. Advantages and drawbacks of these methods are analyzed. Widespread measuring techniques such as integrating sphere, spatially, time-, and angular-resolved, and OCT, as well as inverse methods, such as Kubelka-Munk, multiflux, adding-doubling and inverse Monte Carlo, are overviewed. Exhaustive data on optical properties of human tissue and blood measured *in vitro*, *ex vivo*, and *in vivo* are presented.

2.1 Basic principles

Methods for determining the optical parameters of tissues can be divided into two large groups, direct and indirect methods.[1–4,9–16,29,32,33,37,38,40,46,48,49,56,72,87–90, 98,129,130,164,179,182,213,221,222,226–228,231–233,236–238,255,263,369,572,649–726] Direct methods include those based on some fundamental concepts and rules such as the Bouguer-Beer-Lambert law [see Eq. (1.1)], the single-scattering phase function [see Eqs. (1.13) and (1.15)] for thin samples, or the effective light penetration depth for slabs. The parameters measured are the collimated light transmission T_c and the scattering indicatrix $I(\theta)$ (angular dependence of the scattered light intensity, W/cm^2 sr) for thin samples or the fluence rate inside a slab. The normalized scattering indicatrix is equal to the scattering phase function $I(\theta)/I(0) \equiv p(\theta)$, 1/sr. These methods are advantageous in that they use very simple analytic expressions for data processing. Their disadvantages are related to the necessity to strictly fulfill experimental conditions dictated by the selected model (single scattering in thin samples, exclusion of the effects of light polarization and refraction at cuvette edges, etc.); in the case of slabs with multiple scattering, the recording detector (usually a fiber light guide with an isotropically scattering ball at the tip end) must be placed far from both the light source and the medium boundaries.

Indirect methods obtain the solution of the inverse scattering problem using a theoretical model of light propagation in a medium. They are in turn divided into iterative and noniterative models. The former use equations in which the optical properties are defined through parameters directly related to the quantities being evaluated. The latter are based on the two-flux Kubelka-Munk model and multiflux models.[40,46,56,93,183,192,213,255,661,674] In indirect iterative methods, the optical properties are implicitly defined through measured pa-

143

rameters. Quantities determining the optical properties of a scattering medium are enumerated until the estimated and measured values for reflectance and transmittance coincide with the desired accuracy. These methods are cumbersome, but the optical models currently in use may be even more complicated than those underlying noniterative methods [examples include the diffusion theory,[40,183,198–203] inverse adding-doubling (IAD),[266,267,646,652,667,675–677] and inverse MC (IMC)[213,226,236–238,242,244,255,263,264,369,650,655,656,662,665,678,719,720] methods].

The optical parameters of tissue samples (μ_a, μ_s, and g) are measured by different methods. *In vitro* evaluation is most often achieved by the double integrating sphere method combined with collimated transmittance measurements (see Fig. 2.1 and Table 2.1). This approach implies either sequential or simultaneous determination of three parameters: collimated transmittance $T_c = I(d)/I(0)$ [see Eq. (1.1)], total transmittance $T_t = T_c + T_d$ (T_d being diffuse transmittance), and diffuse reflectance R_d. The optical parameters of the tissue are deduced from these measurements using different theoretical expressions or numerical methods (two-flux and multiflux models, the IMC or IAD methods) relating μ_a, μ_s, and g to the parameters being investigated.

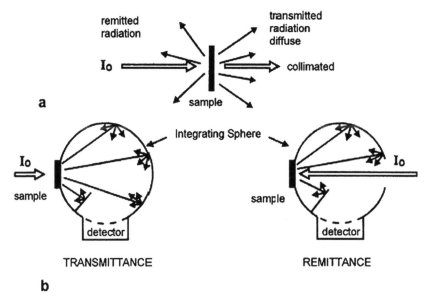

Figure 2.1 Measurement of (a) collimated and (b) total transmittance, and diffuse reflectance using an integrating sphere. The integrating surface of the sphere is coated with $BaSO_4$ or MgO, which have nearly 100% diffuse remittance over the entire optical spectrum.[6,57]

Any three measurements from the following five are sufficient for the evaluation of all three optical parameters:[40]

• Total (or diffuse) transmittance for collimated or diffuse radiation.

Table 2.1 Optical properties of human tissues measured *in vitro*, *ex vivo*, and *in vivo* (rms. values are given in parentheses).

Tissue	λ, nm	μ_a, cm^{-1}	μ_s, cm^{-1}	μ_s', cm^{-1}	g	Remarks
In vitro measurements						
Aorta:						
Normal	308	33	—	77	—	*Post mortem* (6 hr), excised, in
Normal coagulated	308	44	—	270	—	4°C saline, slab, water bath
Fibrous plaque	308	24	—	81	—	(85°C), integrating sphere (IS)
Fibrous plaque coagulated	308	34	—	272	—	technique, inverse adding doubling (IAD) method, data from Ref. 40
Normal	1064	0.53 (0.09)	239 (45)	23.9	0.9	*Post mortem*, slab, 70°C water
Coagulated	1064	0.46 (0.18)	293 (73)	29.3	0.9	bath, 10 min, IS, inverse Monte Carlo (IMC) method, goniophotometric measurements (GPM), data from Ref. 40
Fibro-fatty	355	17.7	—	64.9	—	*Post mortem*, resected, slab
	532	3.6	—	24.8	—	(24 hr), photoacoustic (PA),
	1064	0.09	—	7.7	—	data from Ref. 40
Normal	633*	0.52	316	41	0.87	*Post mortem*, slab, IS, GPM,
	1064**	0.5	239	23.9	0.9	*diffusion theory (DT), **IMC,
	1064*	0.7	—	22.4	—	data from Ref. 40
	1320**	2.2	233	23.3	0.9	
	1320*	4.3	—	17.8	—	
Normal	470	5.3 (0.9)	—	42.6 (6.0)	—	Thin sections (250 µm, intima
	476	5.1 (0.9)	—	41.9 (5.9)	—	and media), kept in saline.[569]
	488	4.5 (0.9)	—	39.9 (5.6)	—	IS, DT.
	514.5	3.7 (0.9)	—	36.9 (5.4)	—	Corrected data (see Ref. 3,
	580	2.8 (0.9)	—	31.1 (4.9)	—	p. 379)
	600	2.6 (0.9)	—	29.6 (4.7)	—	

Table 2.1 (Continued).

Tissue	λ, nm	μ_a, cm^{-1}	μ_s, cm^{-1}	μ_s', cm^{-1}	g	Remarks
Adventitia	633	2.6 (0.9)	—	27.4 (4.4)	—	Frozen sections, IS, DT,
	1064	2.7 (0.5)	—	15.5 (2.8)	—	Ref. 218
	476	18.1	267	69.4	0.74	
	580	11.3	217	49.9	0.77	
	600	6.1	211	46.4	0.78	
	633	5.8	195	37.1	0.81	
	1064	2.0	484	—	0.97	Double IS (DIS), DT, data
						from Ref. 691
Intima	476	14.8	237	45.0	0.81	Frozen sections, IS, DT,
	580	8.9	183	34.8	0.81	Ref. 218
	600	4.0	178	33.8	0.81	
	633	3.6	171	25.7	0.85	
	1064	2.3	165	—	0.97	DIS, DT, data from Ref. 691
Media	476	7.3	410	45.1	0.89	Frozen sections, IS, DT,
	580	4.8	331	33.1	0.90	Ref. 218
	600	2.5	323	35.5	0.89	
	633	2.3	310	31.0	0.90	
	1064	1.0	634	—	0.96	DIS, DT, data from Ref. 691
Bladder:						
Integral	633	1.40	88.0	3.52	0.96	Excised, kept in saline, Ref. 40
Integral	633	1.40	29.3	2.64	0.91	DIS, DT, data from Refs. 2
Mucous	1064	0.7	7.5	—	0.85	and 691
Wall	1064	0.9	54.3	—	0.85	
Integral	1064	0.4	116	—	0.90	
Blood:						
HbO$_2$ (Hct = 0.41)	665	1.30	1246	6.11	0.995	Whole blood; absorbance,
HbO$_2$ (Hct = 0.41)	685	2.65	1413	14.13	0.990	radial reflectance, and/or GPM;
HbO$_2$ (Hct = 0.41)	960	2.84	505	3.84	0.992	Mie theory, transport theory, or

Table 2.1 (Continued).

Tissue	λ, nm	μ_a, cm^{-1}	μ_s, cm^{-1}	μ_s', cm^{-1}	g	Remarks
HbO$_2$ (Hct = 0.4)	810	4.5	—	6.6	—	IMC; data from Refs. 691 and 40
HbO$_2$ (Hct = 0.4)	1064	3.0	—	3.4	—	
Hb (Hct = 0.41)	960	16.8	668	5.08	0.992	
Hb (Hct = 0.4)	810	4.5	—	3.9	—	
Hb (Hct = 0.4)	1064	0.3	—	6.6	—	
Hct = 0.47	450	381	2940	8.3	0.9972	Whole blood; IAD and Beer's
(partially oxygenated)	488	133	3190	4.0	0.9987	law; data by Jacques (1993)
	514	116	3320	4.1	0.9988	from Ref. 40
	577	301	3140	7.3	0.9977	
	630	14.3	3660	8.9	0.9976	
	760	15.5	2820	7.9	0.9972	
(Hct = 0.45–0.46,	633	15.5	644.7	—	0.982	DIS, Henyey-Greenstein phase
oxygenation > 98%)	710	4 (0.8)	737 (75)	—	0.986 (0.006)	function (HGPF), IMC,[665,666]
	765	5.3 (0.6)	725 (75)	—	0.991 (0.002)	data from graphs of
	810	6.5 (0.5)	690 (80)	—	0.989 (0.002)	Refs. 164, 724; whole blood
	865	7.2 (0.3)	649 (25)	—	0.990 (0.001)	
	910	8.9 (0.4)	649 (25)	—	0.992 (0.002)	
	965	9.3 (0.6)	650 (25)	—	0.991 (0.001)	
	1010	8.3 (0.4)	645 (25)	—	0.992 (0.001)	
	1065	5.6 (0.3)	645 (25)	—	0.992 (0.001)	
	1110	4.2 (0.3)	630 (20)	—	0.993 (0.001)	
	1165	4.1 (0.7)	655 (15)	—	0.993 (0.001)	
	1210	5.5 (0.5)	654 (20)	—	0.995 (0.001)	
(Hct = 0.421,	260	375.5 (9.0)	631.5 (57.6)	136.4 (28.0)	0.784 (0.030)	IS, fresh erythrocytes from a
oxygenation > 99%)	350	368.1	559.5	82.5	0.852	healthy blood donor diluted in
	375	338.6 (4.2)	542.8 (66.5)	69.5 (12.7)	0.872 (0.007)	PBS, pH 7.4, hemoglobin
	415	782.5 (62.9)	390.3 (61.2)	129.5 (17.0)	0.668 (0.008)	concentration 129 g/l, the
	450	263.0	682.6	52.5	0.923	temperature was kept constant

Table 2.1 (Continued).

Tissue	λ, nm	μ_a, cm^{-1}	μ_s, cm^{-1}	μ_s', cm^{-1}	g	Remarks
	490	106.8	793.8	30.4	0.962	at 20°C, turbulence-free cuvette
	520	120.4 (6.9)	766.2 (42.4)	24.9 (7.6)	0.967 (0.009)	with a laminar flow and a
	540	232.3	655.6	35.8	0.945	sample thickness of 116 μm,
	555	178.9	709.3	33.0	0.953	constant wall share rate of
	575	231.6	658.0	31.7	0.952	600 s^{-1}; in the wavelength
	585	160.2 (10.3)	751.7 (46.1)	33.5 (9.7)	0.955 (0.007)	region around 415 nm a cuvette
	620	4.14	905.3	23.3	0.974	of 40 μm in thickness was used;
	630	2.51 (0.09)	894.6 (28.6)	22.3 (3.3)	0.975 (0.004)	Reynolds-McCormick phase
	670	1.22	892.3	21.5	0.976	function ($\alpha = 1.7$), IMC, data
	700	1.25	879.3	21.1	0.976	were presented by the authors of
	750	1.99	840.8	20.6	0.975	Ref. 1271.
	780	2.85	821.5	20.5	0.975	
	800	3.27 (0.12)	809.9 (66.4)	20.2 (5.4)	0.975 (0.003)	
	830	4.90	798.7	20.1	0.975	
	850	4.65	799.5	20.1	0.975	
	870	5.10	784.4	20.1	0.974	
	900	5.43	751.4	19.9	0.973	
	950	6.15 (0.35)	712.0 (69.8)	20.8 (2.7)	0.971 (0.002)	
	980	6.79	685.9	20.8	0.970	
	1000	6.51	680.8	20.5	0.970	
	1050	4.91 (0.12)	661.3 (12.8)	19.91 (0.67)	0.9699 (0.0006)	
	1100	3.74	639.5	18.85	0.970	
Brain:						
Astrocytoma (grade III WHO, $n = 7$, different spots on the sample)	400	10*	84*	—	0.9*	Microspectrophotometry, IMC, slab 600 μm,[263] *data from graphs
	633	6.3 (1.6)	67 (8)	—	0.883 (0.011)	
	700	4*	50*	—	0.88*	
	800	3*	50*	—	0.88*	
Glioma	415	16.6	—	6		Ref. 39, data from graphs

Table 2.1 (Continued).

Tissue	λ, nm	μ_a, cm^{-1}	μ_s, cm^{-1}	μ_s', cm^{-1}	g	Remarks
(male, 65 yr, 4 hr *post mortem*)	488	12.5	—	3	—	
	630	3.0	—	3	—	
	800–1100	≈1.0	—	>1–2	—	
Gray matter (male, 71 yr, 24 hr *post mortem*)	514	19.5	—	85	—	
	585	14.5	—	63	—	
	630	4.3	—	52	—	
	800–1100	≈1.0	—	45–20	—	
Melanoma (male 71 yr, 24 hr *post mortem*)	585	2	—	158	—	
	630	20.0	—	75	—	
	800	8.0	—	40	—	
	900	4.0	—	30	—	
	1100	2.0	—	25	—	
White matter (female, 32 yr, 24 hr *post mortem*)	415	2.1	—	24	—	
	488	1.0	—	60	—	
	630	0.2	—	32	—	
	800–1100	0.2–0.3	—	40–20	—	
White matter (female, 63 yr, 30 hr *post mortem*)	488	2.7	—	25	—	
	630	0.9	—	22	—	
	800–1100	1.0–1.5	—	20–10	—	
Gray matter	633	2.7 (2)	354 (37)	20.6 (2)	0.94 (0.004)	Freshly resected, slabs; data
	1064	5.0 (5)	134 (14)	11.8 (9)	0.90 (0.007)	from Ref. 40
White matter	633	2.2 (2)	532 (41)	91 (5)	0.82 (0.01)	
	1064	3.2 (4)	469 (34)	60.3 (2.5)	0.87 (0.007)	
Gray matter	800	0.25	—	25	—	Ref. 233
White matter	800	0.05	—	60	—	
Gray matter ($n=7$)	360	3.33 (2.19)	141.3 (42.6)	—	0.818 (0.093)	DIS, IMC[665,666]
	640	0.17 (0.26)	90.1 (32.5)	—	0.89 (0.04)	
	1060	0.56 (0.7)	56.8 (18.0)	—	0.90 (0.05)	

Table 2.1 (Continued).

Tissue	λ, nm	μ_a, cm^{-1}	μ_s, cm^{-1}	μ_s', cm^{-1}	g	Remarks
Gray matter coagulated ($n = 7$)	360	9.39 (1.70)	426 (122)	–	0.868 (0.031)	DIS, IMC; 2 hr, 80°C[665,666]
	740	0.45 (0.27)	–	–	–	
	1100	1.0 (0.45)	179.8 (32.6)	–	0.954 (0.001)	
Gray matter	456	9	686	34.3	0.95	IS, δ-Eddington
	514	11.7	578	17.34	0.97	approximation;[698]
	630	1.4	473	33.11	0.93	data from Ref. 264
	675	0.6	364	32.76	0.91	
	1064	1.9	267	10.7	0.96	
White matter	456	8.1	923	73.84	0.92	
	514	5.0	1045	73.15	0.93	
	630	1.5	386	54.04	0.86	
	675	0.7	436	56.68	0.87	
	1064	1.6	513	25.65	0.95	
White matter ($n = 7$)	360	2.53 (0.55)	402.0 (91.8)	–	0.702 (0.093)	DIS, IMC[665,666]
	640	0.8 (0.2)	408.2 (88.5)	–	0.84 (0.05)	
	860	0.97 (0.4)	353.1 (68.1)	–	0.871 (0.028)	
	1060	1.08 (0.51)	299.5 (70.1)	–	0.889 (0.010)	
White matter coagulated ($n = 7$)	360	8.3 (3.65)	604.2 (131.5)	–	0.800 (0.089)	DIS, IMC; 2 hr, 80°C[665,666]
	860	1.7 (1.3)	417.0 (272.5)	–	0.922 (0.025)	
	1060	2.15 (1.34)	363.3 (226.8)	–	0.930 (0.015)	
White matter	800	0.8 (0.16)	140 (14)	–	0.95 (0.02)	DIS, IMC; samples 0.5–3 hr
	1064	0.4 (0.08)	110 (11)	–	0.95 (0.02)	*post mortem*, fast frozen and
White matter coagulated	800	0.9 (0.18)	170 (17)	10.2	0.94 (0.02)	homogenized; coagulation in
	1064	0.5 (0.1)	130 (13)	9.1	0.93 (0.02)	a bath at 75°C[662]
Gray matter ($n = 7$)	450	0.7	117	14.04	0.88	IS, IMC, quasi-Newton inverse
	510	0.4	106	12.72	0.88	algorithm,
	630	0.2	90	9.9	0.89	HGPF;

Table 2.1 (Continued).

Tissue	λ, nm	μ_a, cm^{-1}	μ_s, cm^{-1}	μ'_s, cm^{-1}	g	Remarks
White matter (n = 7)	670	0.2	84	8.4	0.90	hemoglobin free cryosections (<48 hr *post mortem*): gray matter—100–200 μm; white matter—80–150 μm; coagulation: saline bath 80°C, 2 hr;[264] data from tables of Ref. 264
	1064	0.5	57	5.7	0.90	
	450	1.4	420	92.4	0.78	
	510	1.0	426	80.94	0.81	
	630	0.8	409	65.44	0.84	
	670	0.7	401	60.15	0.85	
	850	1.0	342	41	0.88	
	1064	1.0	296	32.56	0.89	
White matter coagulated (n = 7)	850	0.9	300	36.0	0.88	
	1064	0.1	270	29.7	0.89	
Astrocytoma (grade II WHO, n = 4)	400	18.8 (11.3)	198.4 (55.6)	–	0.93 (0.03)	IS, IMC, quasi-Newton inverse algorithm, HGPF; hemoglobin free cryosections of normal tissues (<48 hr *post mortem*): cerebellum, gray matter, pons, and thalamus—100–200 μm; white matter—80–150 μm; and
	490	2.5 (0.9)	158.5 (53.7)	–	0.96 (0.02)	
	600	1.2 (0.7)	132.4 (49.0)	–	0.96 (0.02)	
	700	0.5 (0.3)	113.2 (41.8)	–	0.96 (0.02)	
	800	0.7 (0.2)	96.7 (41.8)	–	0.96 (0.01)	
	900	0.3 (0.2)	86.4 (34.6)	–	0.96 (0.01)	
	1000	0.5 (0.3)	79.0 (34.2)	–	0.96 (0.01)	
	1100	0.6 (0.2)	73.8 (29.6)	–	0.96 (0.01)	
Cerebellum (n = 7)	400	4.7 (0.8)	276.7 (19.1)	–	0.80 (0.03)	tumors excised from patients of ≈300 μm in thickness; coagulation: saline bath 80°C, 2 hr;[264] data from graphs of Ref. 264, taken from Ref. 696 with corrections
	500	1.4 (0.2)	277.5 (32.6)	–	0.85 (0.02)	
	600	0.8 (0.2)	272.1 (12.3)	–	0.87 (0.02)	
	700	0.6 (0.1)	266.8 (12.1)	–	0.89 (0.01)	
	800	0.6 (0.1)	250.3 (17.2)	–	0.90 (0.01)	
	900	0.7 (0.1)	229.6 (15.8)	–	0.90 (0.01)	
	1000	0.8 (0.1)	215.4 (14.7)	–	0.90 (0.01)	
	1100	0.7 (0.1)	202.1 (13.9)	–	0.90 (0.01)	
Cerebellum coagulated (n = 7)	400	19.3 (7.7)	560.0 (25.5)	–	0.61 (0.01)	
	500	5.1 (1.7)	512.2 (47.8)	–	0.77 (0.02)	

Table 2.1 (Continued).

Tissue	λ, nm	μ_a, cm^{-1}	μ_s, cm^{-1}	μ_s', cm^{-1}	g	Remarks
	600	2.9 (1.4)	458.2 (65.6)	—	0.78 (0.01)	
	700	1.7 (0.4)	489.9 (70.1)	—	0.85 (0.01)	
	800	1.1 (0.2)	458.2 (54.0)	—	0.87 (0.02)	
	900	1.1 (0.3)	458.2 (65.6)	—	0.89 (0.02)	
	1000	1.0 (0.4)	419.1 (49.4)	—	0.90 (0.03)	
	1100	1.1 (0.5)	428.5 (40.0)	—	0.91 (0.03)	
Gray matter ($n = 7$)	400	2.6 (0.6)	128.5 (18.4)	—	0.87 (0.02)	
	500	0.5 (0.2)	109.9 (13.0)	—	0.88 (0.01)	
	600	0.3 (0.1)	94.1 (13.5)	—	0.89 (0.02)	
	700	0.2 (0.1)	84.1 (12.0)	—	0.90 (0.02)	
	800	0.2 (0.1)	77.0 (11.0)	—	0.90 (0.02)	
	900	0.3 (0.2)	67.3 (9.6)	—	0.90 (0.02)	
	1000	0.6 (0.3)	61.6 (5.7)	—	0.90 (0.02)	
	1100	0.5 (0.3)	55.1 (6.5)	—	0.90 (0.02)	
Gray matter coagulated ($n = 7$)	400	7.5 (0.4)	258.6 (18.8)	—	0.78 (0.04)	
	500	1.8 (0.2)	326.5 (7.7)	—	0.85 (0.03)	
	600	0.7 (0.1)	319.0 (15.2)	—	0.87 (0.03)	
	700	0.7 (0.1)	319.0 (7.5)	—	0.88 (0.03)	
	800	0.8 (0.1)	252.7 (18.3)	—	0.87 (0.02)	
	900	0.9 (0.1)	214.6 (10.3)	—	0.87 (0.02)	
	1000	1.4 (0.2)	191.0 (18.7)	—	0.88 (0.03)	
	1100	1.5 (0.2)	186.6 (13.5)	—	0.88 (0.03)	
Meningioma ($n = 6$)	410	4.1 (0.5)	197.4 (19.8)	—	0.88 (0.02)	
	490	1.3 (0.2)	188.2 (18.8)	—	0.93 (0.01)	
	590	0.7 (0.2)	171.1 (12.7)	—	0.95 (0.01)	
	690	0.3 (0.1)	155.5 (15.6)	—	0.95 (0.01)	
	790	0.2 (0.1)	141.3 (14.2)	—	0.96 (0.01)	

Table 2.1 (Continued).

Tissue	λ, nm	μ_a, cm^{-1}	μ_s, cm^{-1}	μ_s', cm^{-1}	g	Remarks
Pons ($n = 7$)	910	0.2 (0.1)	116.8 (8.6)	—	0.95 (0.01)	
	990	0.4 (0.2)	163.5 (15.3)	—	0.96 (0.01)	
	1100	0.6 (0.2)	133.7 (19.2)	—	0.97 (0.01)	
	400	3.1 (0.7)	163.5 (15.3)	—	0.89 (0.02)	
	500	0.9 (0.3)	133.7 (19.2)	—	0.91 (0.01)	
	600	0.6 (0.2)	109.4 (18.5)	—	0.91 (0.01)	
	700	0.5 (0.2)	93.5 (20.9)	—	0.91 (0.01)	
	800	0.6 (0.3)	83.6 (21.0)	—	0.91 (0.01)	
	900	0.7 (0.3)	74.8 (18.7)	—	0.92 (0.01)	
	1000	1.0 (0.4)	69.9 (17.5)	—	0.91 (0.01)	
	1100	0.9 (0.4)	64.0 (17.8)	—	0.92 (0.01)	
Pons coagulated ($n = 7$)	410	17.2 (1.6)	685.7 (63.7)	—	0.85 (0.02)	
	510	8.5 (0.8)	627.5 (73.6)	—	0.89 (0.01)	
	610	7.7 (0.5)	510.5 (70.5)	—	0.89 (0.01)	
	710	6.9 (0.6)	402.5 (67.7)	—	0.89 (0.01)	
	810	6.5 (0.6)	329.7 (55.4)	—	0.89 (0.01)	
	910	5.9 (1.0)	276.0 (46.4)	—	0.88 (0.01)	
	1010	5.7 (1.0)	241.6 (34.4)	—	0.88 (0.01)	
	1100	6.5 (0.9)	221.1 (31.5)	—	0.88 (0.01)	
Thalamus ($n = 7$)	410	3.2 (1.0)	146.7 (49.4)	—	0.86 (0.03)	
	510	0.9 (0.3)	188.7 (31.9)	—	0.87 (0.03)	
	610	0.6 (0.2)	176.3 (34.5)	—	0.88 (0.02)	
	710	0.5 (0.3)	169.0 (28.7)	—	0.89 (0.03)	
	810	0.7 (0.3)	158.5 (35.3)	—	0.89 (0.02)	
	910	0.7 (0.3)	155.4 (22.3)	—	0.90 (0.02)	
	1010	0.8 (0.3)	139.3 (34.9)	—	0.90 (0.02)	
	1100	0.8 (0.3)	146.0 (36.6)	—	0.91 (0.02)	

Table 2.1 (Continued).

Tissue	λ, nm	μ_a, cm^{-1}	μ_s, cm^{-1}	μ_s', cm^{-1}	g	Remarks
Thalamus coagulated ($n = 7$)	400	15.0 (3.3)	391.1 (56.1)	—	0.83 (0.04)	
	500	4.2 (0.9)	399.9 (67.7)	—	0.90 (0.01)	
	600	1.6 (0.6)	365.7 (43.2)	—	0.92 (0.01)	
	700	1.4 (0.3)	327.0 (30.6)	—	0.92 (0.01)	
	800	1.1 (0.3)	286.0 (33.8)	—	0.93 (0.01)	
	900	1.1 (0.3)	267.4 (31.6)	—	0.93 (0.01)	
	1000	1.4 (0.4)	233.8 (39.7)	—	0.93 (0.01)	
	1100	1.5 (0.4)	223.6 (32.1)	—	0.94 (0.01)	
White matter ($n = 7$)	400	3.1 (0.2)	413.5 (21.4)	—	0.75 (0.03)	
	500	0.9 (0.1)	413.5 (43.9)	—	0.80 (0.02)	
	600	0.8 (0.1)	413.5 (21.4)	—	0.83 (0.02)	
	700	0.8 (0.1)	393.1 (30.9)	—	0.85 (0.02)	
	800	0.9 (0.1)	364.5 (28.6)	—	0.87 (0.01)	
	900	1.0 (0.1)	329.5 (35.0)	—	0.88 (0.01)	
	1000	1.2 (0.2)	305.4 (15.9)	—	0.88 (0.01)	
	1100	1.0 (0.2)	283.2 (22.2)	—	0.88 (0.01)	
White matter coagulated ($n = 7$)	410	8.7 (1.7)	568.7 (111.9)	—	0.83 (0.03)	
	510	2.9 (0.6)	513.2 (116.9)	—	0.87 (0.02)	
	610	1.7 (0.4)	500.2 (129.9)	—	0.90 (0.02)	
	710	1.4 (0.5)	475.2 (108.3)	—	0.91 (0.01)	
	810	1.5 (0.5)	440.0 (114.3)	—	0.92 (0.01)	
	910	1.7 (0.6)	407.4 (92.8)	—	0.93 (0.01)	
	1010	1.9 (0.6)	367.7 (95.5)	—	0.93 (0.01)	
	1100	2.4 (0.5)	358.4 (81.6)	—	0.93 (0.01)	
Gray matter ($n = 25$)	400	9.778	—	25.878	—	IS, IAD, fixed the anisotropy factor
	418	14.873	—	26.593	—	$g = 0.85$ and the refractive index
	428	16.722	—	26.709	—	$n = 1.40$ were assumed for every

Table 2.1 (Continued).

Tissue	λ, nm	μ_a, cm⁻¹	μ_s, cm⁻¹	μ_s', cm⁻¹	g	Remarks
	450	5.161	—	19.389	—	wavelength and for every sample; brain
	488	2.272	—	15.957	—	tissue samples were acquired during open
	500	2.206	—	15.283	—	craniotomy for tumor resection or temporal
	550	2.955	—	13.315	—	lobectomy, hemoglobin free cryosections
	600	1.460	—	11.367	—	with thickness from 0.22 to 1.25 mm were
	632	0.925	—	10.370	—	studied, measurements were done at 25°C,
	670	0.809	—	9.480	—	pH 7.4; data were presented by the authors
	700	0.733	—	8.907	—	of Ref. 1272
	750	0.599	—	8.481	—	
	800	0.507	—	7.886	—	
	830	0.485	—	7.707	—	
	850	0.472	—	7.555	—	
	870	0.479	—	7.351	—	
	900	0.503	—	7.055	—	
	950	0.521	—	6.868	—	
	1000	0.585	—	6.059	—	
	1064	0.502	—	5.333	—	
	1100	0.502	—	5.197	—	
	1150	0.815	—	5.070	—	
	1200	1.010	—	4.882	—	
	1250	0.865	—	4.669	—	
	1300	0.894	—	4.560	—	
White matter ($n = 19$)	400	9.134	—	88.611	—	
	418	13.603	—	83.304	—	
	428	15.417	—	80.905	—	
	450	3.958	—	77.053	—	
	488	1.869	—	70.112	—	
	500	1.834	—	68.318	—	

Table 2.1 (Continued).

Tissue	λ, nm	μ_a, cm^{-1}	μ_s, cm^{-1}	μ_s', cm^{-1}	g	Remarks
	550	2.584	–	62.383	–	
	600	1.175	–	56.759	–	
	632	0.801	–	53.179	–	
	670	0.711	–	50.067	–	
	700	0.674	–	47.626	–	
	750	0.649	–	45.061	–	
	800	0.622	–	41.878	–	
	830	0.626	–	40.634	–	
	850	0.643	–	39.658	–	
	870	0.666	–	38.785	–	
	900	0.684	–	37.607	–	
	950	0.785	–	35.851	–	
	1000	0.883	–	32.603	–	
	1064	0.752	–	30.161	–	
	1100	0.762	–	29.219	–	
	1150	1.135	–	27.951	–	
	1200	1.420	–	26.646	–	
	1250	1.268	–	25.310	–	
	1300	1.274	–	24.250	–	
Glioma ($n = 39$)	400	12.393	–	39.009	–	
	418	17.496	–	37.867	–	
	428	16.124	–	37.076	–	
	450	4.891	–	32.340	–	
	488	2.592	–	28.933	–	
	500	2.352	–	28.057	–	
	550	2.768	–	25.300	–	
	600	1.149	–	22.514	–	
	632	0.846	–	21.068	–	

Table 2.1 (Continued).

Tissue	λ, nm	μ_a, cm^{-1}	μ_s, cm^{-1}	μ_s', cm^{-1}	g	Remarks
	670	0.741	—	19.608	—	
	700	0.709	—	18.543	—	
	750	0.679	—	17.343	—	
	800	0.656	—	15.969	—	
	830	0.662	—	15.481	—	
	850	0.670	—	15.133	—	
	870	0.685	—	14.749	—	
	900	0.707	—	14.138	—	
	950	0.768	—	13.646	—	
	1000	0.938	—	11.588	—	
	1064	0.822	—	10.344	—	
	1100	0.831	—	10.005	—	
	1150	1.231	—	9.654	—	
	1200	1.518	—	9.282	—	
	1250	1.379	—	8.813	—	
	1300	1.412	—	8.523	—	
Breast (female):						
Fatty normal	749	0.18 (0.16)	8.48 (3.43)	—	—	Excised, kept in saline, 37°C,
($n = 23$)	789	0.08 (0.10)	7.67 (2.57)	—	—	Ref. 232
	836	0.11 (0.10)	7.27 (2.40)	—	—	
Fibrous normal ($n = 35$)	749	0.13 (0.19)	9.75 (2.27)	—	—	
	789	0.06 (0.12)	8.94 (2.45)	—	—	
	836	0.05 (0.08)	8.10 (2.21)	—	—	
Infiltrating carcinoma ($n = 48$)	749	0.15 (0.14)	10.91 (5.59)	—	—	
	789	0.04 (0.08)	10.12 (5.05)	—	—	
	836	0.10 (0.19)	9.10 (4.54)	—	—	
Mucinous carcinoma ($n = 3$)	749	0.26 (0.20)	—	6.15 (2.44)	—	
	789	0.016 (0.072)	—	5.09 (2.42)	—	

Table 2.1 (Continued).

Tissue	λ, nm	μ_a, cm^{-1}	μ_s, cm^{-1}	μ_s', cm^{-1}	g	Remarks
Ductal carcinoma	836	0.023 (0.108)	—	4.78 (3.67)	—	
in situ (n = 5)	749	0.076 (0.068)	—	13.10 (2.85)	—	
	789	0.023 (0.034)	—	12.21 (2.45)	—	
	836	0.039 (0.068)	—	10.46 (2.65)	—	Homogenized tissue, Ref. 660
Glandular tissue (n = 3)	540	3.58 (1.56)	—	24.4 (5.8)	—	
	700	0.47 (0.11)	—	14.2 (3.0)	—	
	900	0.62 (0.05)	—	9.9 (2.0)	—	
Fatty tissue (n = 7)	540	2.27 (0.57)	—	10.3 (1.9)	—	
	700	0.70 (0.08)	—	8.6 (1.3)	—	
	900	0.75 (0.08)	—	7.9 (1.1)	—	
Fibrocystic (n = 8)	540	1.64 (0.66)	—	21.7 (3.3)	—	
	700	0.22 (0.09)	—	13.4 (1.9)	—	
	900	0.27 (0.11)	—	9.5 (1.7)	—	
Fibroadenoma (n = 6)	540	4.38 (3.14)	—	11.1 (3.0)	—	
	700	0.52 (0.47)	—	7.2 (1.7)	—	
	900	0.72 (0.53)	—	5.3 (1.4)	—	
Carcinoma (n = 9)	540	3.07 (0.99)	—	19.0 (5.1)	—	
	700	0.45 (0.12)	—	11.8 (3.1)	—	
	900	0.50 (0.15)	—	8.9 (2.6)	—	
Carcinoma	580	4.5 (0.8)	—	—	—	Tissue slices of thickness
	850	0.4 (0.5)	—	—	—	5–5.3 mm, Ref. 223
	1300	0.5 (0.8)	—	—	—	
Adjacent healthy tissue	580	2.6 (1.1)	—	—	—	
	850	0.3 (0.2)	—	—	—	
	1300	0.8 (0.6)	—	—	—	
Fatty tissue	700	—	—	13 (5)	0.95 (0.02)	
Fibroglandular tissue	700	—	—	12 (5)	0.92 (0.03)	
Carcinoma (central part)	700	—	—	18 (5)	0.88 (0.03)	

Table 2.1 (Continued).

Tissue	λ, nm	μ_a, cm^{-1}	μ_s, cm^{-1}	μ_s', cm^{-1}	g	Remarks
Fatty tissue	625	0.06 (0.02)	—	14.3 (2.1)	—	Ref. 31
Benign tumor	625	0.33 (0.06)	—	3.8 (0.3)	—	Spatially resolved reflectance
Invasive ductal	450	2.55 (0.30)	—	31.5 (2.5)	—	(SRR); diffusion approximation;
carcinoma ($n = 10$, 9 in	460	2.62 (0.34)	—	31.0 (2.4)	—	source-detector separation,
the age group 55–65 yr	470	2.44 (0.25)	—	30.7 (2.2)	—	$r_{sd} > 1.2$ mm; fibers with core
and 1–35 yr)	480	2.32 (0.26)	—	30.3 (2.4)	—	diameter 400 μm; tissue slices
	490	2.23 (0.25)	—	29.9 (2.4)	—	of thickness ~10 mm[699]
	500	2.22 (0.22)	—	29.5 (2.2)	—	
	510	2.16 (0.24)	—	29.1 (2.3)	—	
	520	2.12 (0.22)	—	29.0 (2.3)	—	
	530	2.07 (0.22)	—	28.7 (2.0)	—	
	540	1.99 (0.21)	—	28.0 (2.1)	—	
	550	2.13 (0.23)	—	28.4 (2.0)	—	
	560	2.09 (0.21)	—	27.7 (2.0)	—	
	570	2.09 (0.25)	—	27.5 (1.9)	—	
	580	2.07 (0.21)	—	27.3 (2.0)	—	
	590	2.01 (0.22)	—	27.1 (1.7)	—	
	600	1.90 (0.19)	—	26.8 (1.8)	—	
	610	1.82 (0.18)	—	26.8 (1.6)	—	
	620	1.71 (0.18)	—	2.64 (1.8)	—	
	630	1.64 (0.17)	—	26.2 (1.5)	—	
	640	1.55 (0.17)	—	25.9 (1.4)	—	
	650	1.48 (0.15)	—	25.7 (1.3)	—	
	633	—	—	—	0.96 (0.01)	GPM, tissue slices of 20 μm; HGPF; $\theta = 10°–165°$; radius of Mie scatterer— $a_M = 0.64 (0.06)$ μm[699]

Table 2.1 (Continued).

Tissue	λ, nm	μ_a, cm^{-1}	μ_s, cm^{-1}	μ_s', cm^{-1}	g	Remarks
	633	—	—	—	0.86 (0.02)	GPM, tissue slices of 20 μm; double HGPF $[g = f(1 - g_1) + (1 - f)g_2]$; $\theta = 52°-165°$; $a_M = 0.28$ (0.02) μm[699]
Adjacent healthy tissue	450	1.45 (0.22)	—	21.7 (2.1)	—	SRR; diffusion approximation; $r_{sd} > 1.2$ mm; fibers with core diameter 400 μm; tissue slices of thickness ~ 10 mm[699]
($n = 10$; 9 in the age	460	1.48 (0.21)	—	21.3 (2.2)	—	
group 55–65 yr and	470	1.42 (0.21)	—	20.8 (1.9)	—	
1–35 yr)	480	1.35 (0.19)	—	20.3 (1.8)	—	
	490	1.26 (0.21)	—	19.9 (2.0)	—	
	500	1.24 (0.21)	—	20.1 (1.8)	—	
	510	1.23 (0.19)	—	19.1 (1.9)	—	
	520	1.19 (0.18)	—	18.7 (1.8)	—	
	530	1.14 (0.17)	—	18.4 (1.8)	—	
	540	1.19 (0.22)	—	18.0 (1.8)	—	
	550	1.16 (0.26)	—	18.2 (1.6)	—	
	560	1.14 (0.17)	—	17.4 (1.5)	—	
	570	1.13 (0.16)	—	17.2 (1.5)	—	
	580	1.17 (0.17)	—	16.9 (1.3)	—	
	590	1.07 (0.17)	—	16.6 (1.4)	—	
	600	1.00 (0.12)	—	16.4 (1.5)	—	
	610	0.95 (0.12)	—	16.2 (1.5)	—	
	620	0.89 (0.11)	—	15.9 (1.3)	—	
	630	0.82 (0.07)	—	15.7 (1.3)	—	
	640	0.79 (0.08)	—	15.5 (1.2)	—	
	650	0.74 (0.08)	—	15.3 (1.2)	—	

Table 2.1 (Continued).

Tissue	λ, nm	μ_a, cm^{-1}	μ_s, cm^{-1}	μ_s', cm^{-1}	g	Remarks
	633	–	–	–	0.88 (0.01)	GPM, tissue slices of 20 μm; HGPF; $\theta = 10°–165°$; $a_M = 0.32\ (0.02)$ μm[699]
	633	–	–	–	0.76 (0.01)	GPM, tissue slices of 20 μm; double HGPF $[g = f(1 - g_1) + (1 - f)g_2]$; $\theta = 52°–165°$; $a_M = 0.19\ (0.02)$ μm[699]
Colon:						
Muscle	1064	3.3	238	–	0.93	Data from Ref. 691
Submucous	1064	2.3	117	–	0.91	
Mucous	1064	2.7	39	–	0.91	
Integral	1064	0.4	261	–	0.94	
Esophagus	633	0.4	–	12	–	2.5-mm slab, Ref. 40
Esophagus (mucous)	1064	1.1	83	–	0.86	Data from Ref. 691
Fat:						
Abdominal	1064	3.0	37	–	0.91	Data from Ref. 691
Subcutaneous	1064	2.6	29	–	0.91	
Gallstones:						
Porcinement	351	102 (16)	–	–	–	Dehydrated, embedded in plastic, and sliced in 1-mm slab, pulsed photothermal radiometry technique, data from Ref. 40
	488	179 (28)	–	–	–	
	580	125 (29)	–	–	–	
	630	85 (11)	–	–	–	
	1060	121 (12)	–	–	–	
Cholesterol	351	88 (7)	–	–	–	
	488	62 (15)	–	–	–	
	580	36 (7)	–	–	–	

Table 2.1 (Continued).

Tissue	λ, nm	μ_a, cm^{-1}	μ_s, cm^{-1}	μ_s', cm^{-1}	g	Remarks
Head (adult):						
Dura mater ($n = 8$), post mortem, <24 hr	630	44 (10)	—	—	—	IS, IAD; excised tissue slabs, stored at $-12°$C; measurements at room temperature; in the spectral ranges 480–550 and 600–700 nm: $\mu_s' = 4.54 \times 10^4 \lambda^{-1.23}$, $[\lambda] =$ nm; Refs. 703 and 704
	1060	60 (9)	—	—	—	
	400	3.08 (0.15)	—	22.35 (0.89)	—	
	450	1.51 (0.08)	—	22.89 (0.92)	—	
	500	1.09 (0.05)	—	21.60 (0.86)	—	
	550	1.10 (0.05)	—	18.48 (0.74)	—	
	600	0.80 (0.04)	—	17.11 (0.68)	—	
	650	0.70 (0.04)	—	15.51 (0.62)	—	
	700	0.74 (0.04)	—	13.99 (0.56)	—	
Scalp and skull	800	0.4	—	20	—	Ref. 233
Cerebral spinal fluid	800	0.01	—	0.1	—	
Scalp ($n = 3$)	805	0.52 (0.04)	—	14.09 (1.74)	—	Adult scalp post mortem (<12 hr), excised, slab, IS, IAD; data averaged for three tissue samples with thicknesses of 6 ± 0.5 mm, 3.5 ± 0.15 mm and 3.5 ± 0.12 mm[738,739]
	900	0.40 (0.02)	—	15.66 (2.06)	—	
	950	0.39 (0.03)	—	16.44 (2.63)	—	
	1000	0.33 (0.03)	—	16.83 (2.77)	—	
	1100	0.19 (0.04)	—	17.10 (2.69)	—	
	1200	0.65 (0.04)	—	16.70 (2.89)	—	
	1300	0.50 (0.07)	—	14.70 (2.59)	—	
	1400	1.98 (0.31)	—	14.28 (3.69)	—	
	1430	2.19 (0.29)	—	13.15 (3.07)	—	
	1500	2.04 (0.35)	—	14.40 (3.75)	—	
	1600	1.43 (0.22)	—	14.16 (3.41)	—	
	1700	1.87 (0.28)	—	14.71 (3.51)	—	
	1800	1.73 (0.22)	—	13.36 (2.91)	—	
	1900	2.57 (0.28)	—	12.15 (3.05)	—	
	1930	2.52 (0.25)	—	11.52 (2.57)	—	
	2000	2.09 (0.29)	—	12.00 (2.91)	—	

Table 2.1 (Continued).

Tissue	λ, nm	μ_a, cm^{-1}	μ_s, cm^{-1}	μ_s', cm^{-1}	g	Remarks
Scull bone ($n = 8$)	801	0.11 (0.02)	—	19.48 (1.52)	—	Adult head *post mortem* (24 hr), excised, slab from the occipital part, IS, IAD; data averaged for 8 tissue samples $\mu_s' = 1.53 \times 10^3 \lambda^{-0.65}$, $[\lambda] = $ nm (spectral range from 1130 to 1910 nm is excluded)[738,739]
	900	0.15 (0.02)	—	18.03 (1.19)	—	
	980	0.23 (0.03)	—	17.38 (1.01)	—	
	1000	0.22 (0.03)	—	17.10 (0.91)	—	
	1100	0.16 (0.03)	—	15.92 (0.76)	—	
	1180	0.67 (0.07)	—	16.53 (0.83)	—	
	1200	0.67 (0.07)	—	16.77 (0.85)	—	
	1300	0.54 (0.05)	—	14.78 (0.80)	—	
	1400	2.43 (0.24)	—	17.22 (1.73)	—	
	1465	3.33 (0.31)	—	16.84 (1.88)	—	
	1500	3.13 (0.26)	—	15.96 (1.37)	—	
	1600	2.47 (0.40)	—	15.84 (3.05)	—	
	1700	2.77 (0.46)	—	16.12 (3.72)	—	
	1740	2.98 (0.54)	—	15.82 (3.79)	—	
	1800	2.97 (0.62)	—	15.42 (3.98)	—	
	1900	4.39 (1.33)	—	11.37 (2.76)	—	
	1930	4.97 (1.52)	—	10.92 (2.17)	—	
	2000	4.47 (1.18)	—	11.48 (2.01)	—	
Heart:						
Endocard	1060	0.07	136	—	0.97	Excised, kept in saline, Ref. 40
Epicard	1060	0.35	167	—	0.98	Data from Ref. 691
Myocard	1060	0.3	177.5	—	0.96	
Epicard	1060	0.21	127.1	—	0.93	
Aneurysm	1060	0.4	137	—	0.98	
Trabecula	1064	1.4	424	—	0.97	
Myocard	1064	1.4	324	—	0.96	Ref. 369
Myocard	1060	0.52	—	4.48	—	

Table 2.1 (Continued).

Tissue	λ, nm	μ_a, cm^{-1}	μ_s, cm^{-1}	μ_s', cm^{-1}	g	Remarks
Kidney:						
Pars conv.	1064	2.4	72	–	0.86	Data from Ref. 691
Medulla ren.	1064	2.1	77	–	0.87	
Liver	515	18.9 (1.7)	285 (20)	–	–	Frozen sections[657]
	635	2.3 (1.0)	313 (136)	100	0.68	
	1064	0.7	356	–	0.95	
	630	3.2	414	–	0.95	Ref. 369
Lung	515	25.5 (3.0)	356 (39)	–	–	Frozen sections,[657]
	635	8.1 (2.8)	324 (46)	81	0.75	data from Ref. 691
	1064	2.8	39	–	0.91	
Muscle	515	11.2 (1.8)	530 (44)	–	–	Frozen sections,[657]
	1064	2.0	215	–	0.96	data from Ref. 691
Meniscus	360	13	–	108	–	Frozen, thawed, slab,
	400	4.6	–	67	–	data from Ref. 40
	488	1	–	30	–	
	514	0.73	–	26	–	
	630	0.36	–	11	–	
	800	0.52	–	5.1	–	
	1064	0.34	–	2.6	–	
Prostate:						
Normal	850	0.6 (0.2)	100 (20)	–	0.94 (0.02)	Shock frozen sections of
	980	0.4 (0.2)	90 (20)	–	0.95 (0.02)	60–500 μm, 0.5–3 hr post
	1064	0.3 (0.2)	80 (20)	–	0.95 (0.02)	mortem, Ref. 691
Coagulated	850	7.0 (0.2)	230 (30)	–	0.94 (0.02)	Sections of 60–500 μm,
	980	5.0 (0.2)	190 (30)	–	0.95 (0.02)	0.5–3 hr post mortem, water
	1064	4.0 (0.2)	180 (30)	–	0.95 (0.02)	bath (75°C, 10 min), Ref. 691
Normal	1064	1.5 (0.2)	47 (13)	0.64	0.862	Freshly excised, slab, water bath

Table 2.1 (Continued).

Tissue	λ, nm	μ_a, cm^{-1}	μ_s, cm^{-1}	μ_s', cm^{-1}	g	Remarks
Coagulated	1064	0.8 (0.2)	80 (12)	1.12	0.861	(70°C, 10 min), Ref. 40
Normal ($n = 3$)	695	0.8	330 (30)			0.95	P3 approximation; thick slabs; <36 hr *post mortem*; fiber probe[211]
Sclera	650	0.08		25	—	Ref. 315
Sclera ($n = 5$)	404	5.00 (0.50)		81.40 (8.14)	—	IS, IAD; excised tissue slabs, <24 hr *post mortem*, stored in saline at 4°C; measurements at room temperature; $\mu_s' = 8.95 \times 10^4 \lambda^{-1.16}$, $[\lambda] = $ nm; Ref. 703
	449	3.99 (0.40)		73.34 (7.33)	—	
	499	2.96 (0.30)		65.17 (6.52)	—	
	549	2.26 (0.23)		58.00 (5.80)	—	
	599	1.95 (0.19)		53.16 (5.32)	—	
	649	1.74 (0.17)		48.21 (4.82)	—	
	699	1.67 (0.17)		44.15 (4.42)	—	
	749	1.65 (0.17)		40.10 (4.01)	—	
	799	1.58 (0.16)		37.64 (3.76)	—	
Skin:						
Stratum corneum	193	6000		—	—	Frozen sections[40]
	250	1150	2600	260	0.9	Data from graphs of Ref. 37; μ_s' is calculated
	308	600	2400	240	0.9	
	337	330	2300	230	0.9	
	351	300	2200	220	0.9	
	400	230	2000	200	0.9	
Epidermis	250	1000	2000	616	0.69	Data from graphs of Ref. 37; μ_s' and g are calculated using Eqs. (1.21) and (2.23)
	308	300	1400	407	0.71	
	337	120	1200	338	0.72	
	351	100	1100	306	0.72	
	415	66	800	206	0.74	
	488	50	600	143	0.76	

Table 2.1 (Continued).

Tissue	λ, nm	μ_a, cm^{-1}	μ_s, cm^{-1}	μ_s', cm^{-1}	g	Remarks
	514	44	600	139	0.77	
	585	36	470	99	0.79	
	633	35	450	88	0.80	
	800	40	420	62	0.85	
Dermis	250	35	833	257	0.69	Data from graphs of Ref. 37;
	308	12	583	170	0.71	values are transformed in
	337	8.2	500	141	0.72	accordance with data for
	351	7	458	127	0.72	$\lambda = 633$ nm[658] (bloodless
	415	4.7	320	82	0.74	tissue, hydration—85%), μ_s' and
	488	3.5	250	60	0.76	g are calculated
	514	3	250	58	0.77	
	585	3	196	41	0.79	
	633	2.7	187.5	37	0.80	
	800	2.3	175	30	0.85	
Epidermis	517	19	480	—	0.787	Averaged using data of
	585	19	470	—	0.790	Verkruysse et al. (1993) and
	590	19	460	—	0.800	van Gemert et al. (1992);
	595	19	460	—	0.800	oxygenated blood[259,260]
	600	19	460	—	0.800	
Dermis	517	2.2	210	—	0.787	
	585	2.2	205	—	0.790	
	590	2.2	200	—	0.800	
	595	2.2	200	—	0.800	
	600	2.2	200	—	0.800	
Blood	517	354	468	—	0.995	
	585	191	467	—	0.995	
	590	69	466	—	0.995	

Table 2.1 (Continued).

Tissue	λ, nm	μ_a, cm^{-1}	μ_s, cm^{-1}	μ_s', cm^{-1}	g	Remarks
Dermis (leg)	595	43	465	–	0.995	Frozen sections[657]
	600	25	464	–	0.995	
Dermis	635	1.8 (0.2)	244 (21)	78	0.68	Frozen sections, DIS[232]
	749	0.24 (0.19)	–	23.1 (0.75)	–	
	789	0.75 (0.06)	–	22.8 (1.29)	–	
	836	0.98 (0.15)	–	15.9 (2.16)	–	
Dermis	633	<10	–	11.64	0.97	Treweek and Barbenel (1996)[236]
Dermis	700	2.7 (1.0)	–	21.3 (3.7)	–	Analysis of data from Hardy et al. (1956)[228]
Dermis	633	1.9 (0.6)	–	23.8 (3.3)	–	Analysis of data from Ref. 658.[228]
Dermis	633	1.5	–	50.2	–	Prahl (1988)[236]
Skin and underlying tissues including vein wall (leg)	633	3.1	70.7	11.4	0.8	Tissue sections[335]
Caucasian male skin ($n = 3$)	500	5.1	–	50	–	IS, IAD; sample thickness: 0.40, 0.23, 0.25 mm[667]
	810	0.26	–	15.8	–	
Caucasian male skin ($n = 3$), external pressure 0.1 kg/cm^2	500	15.3	–	167.4	–	IS, IAD, sample thickness: 0.15, 0.05, 0.13 mm[667]
	810	0.63	–	52.7	–	
Caucasian male skin ($n = 3$), external pressure 1 kg/cm^2	500	13.6	–	156.7	–	IS, IAD; sample thickness: 0.12, 0.05, 0.13 mm[667]
	810	0.57	–	53.4	–	
Caucasian female skin ($n = 3$)	500	5.2	–	23.9	–	IS, IAD; sample thickness: 0.42, 0.50, 0.50 mm[667]
	810	0.97	–	8.2	–	

Table 2.1 (Continued).

Tissue	λ, nm	μ_a, cm^{-1}	μ_s, cm^{-1}	μ_s', cm^{-1}	g	Remarks
Caucasian female skin (n = 3), external pressure 0.1 kg/cm²	500	7.4	—	31.5	—	IS, IAD; sample thickness: 0.30, 0.30, 0.34 mm[667]
	810	1.4	—	11.3	—	
Caucasian female skin (n = 3), external pressure 1 kg/cm²	500	10.0	—	40.2	—	IS, IAD; sample thickness: 0.27, 0.20, 0.23 mm[667]
	810	1.7	—	13.1	—	
Hispanic male skin (n = 3)	500	3.8	—	24.2	—	IS, IAD; sample thickness: 0.70, 0.78, 0.63 mm[667]
	810	0.87	—	7.5	—	
Hispanic male skin (n = 3), external pressure 0.1 kg/cm²	500	5.1	—	37.6	—	IS, IAD; sample thickness: 0.35, 0.62, 0.48 mm[667]
	810	0.93	—	11.4	—	
Hispanic male skin (n = 3), external pressure 1 kg/cm²	500	6.2	—	40.4	—	IS, IAD; sample thickness: 0.28, 0.48, 0.33 mm[667]
	810	0.87	—	10.2	—	
Caucasian skin (n = 21)	400	3.76 (0.35)	—	71.79 (9.42)	—	IS, IAD; tissue slabs, 1–6 mm; post-mortem; <24 hr after death; stored at 20°C in saline; measurements at room temperature; in the spectral range 400–2000 nm: $\mu_s' = 1.1 \cdot 10^{12}\lambda^{-4} + 73.7\lambda^{-0.22}$, $[\lambda] = $ nm; Ref. 726
	500	1.19 (0.16)	—	32.46 (4.21)	—	
	600	0.69 (0.13)	—	21.78 (2.98)	—	
	700	0.48 (0.11)	—	16.69 (2.27)	—	
	800	0.43 (0.11)	—	14.02 (1.89)	—	
	900	0.33 (0.02)	—	15.66 (2.06)	—	
	1000	0.27 (0.03)	—	16.83 (2.77)	—	
	1100	0.16 (0.04)	—	17.11 (2.69)	—	
	1200	0.54 (0.04)	—	16.71 (2.89)	—	
	1300	0.41 (0.07)	—	14.69 (2.59)	—	
	1400	1.64 (0.31)	—	14.28 (3.69)	—	
	1500	1.69 (0.35)	—	14.41 (3.75)	—	
	1600	1.19 (0.22)	—	14.16 (3.41)	—	

Table 2.1 (Continued).

Tissue	λ, nm	μ_a, cm^{-1}	μ_s, cm^{-1}	μ_s', cm^{-1}	g	Remarks
	1700	1.55 (0.28)	—	14.71 (3.51)	—	
	1800	1.44 (0.22)	—	13.36 (2.91)	—	
	1900	2.14 (0.28)	—	12.15 (3.05)	—	
	2000	1.74 (0.29)	—	12.01 (2.91)	—	
Epidermis	370	1.35 (0.16)	—	11.56 (1.25)	0.8	IS, IMC, slabs, Ref. 1273
	420	1.20 (0.12)	—	9.82 (0.99)	0.8	
	470	0.84 (0.06)	—	7.96 (0.82)	0.8	
	488	0.76 (0.07)	—	7.41 (0.74)	0.8	
	514	0.63 (0.07)	—	6.67 (0.66)	0.8	
	520	0.60 (0.07)	—	6.51 (0.64)	0.8	
	570	0.39 (0.08)	—	5.52 (0.55)	0.8	
	620	0.28 (0.07)	—	4.90 (0.47)	0.8	
	633	0.26 (0.07)	—	4.76 (0.45)	0.8	
	670	0.26 (0.08)	—	4.48 (0.43)	0.8	
	720	0.24 (0.07)	—	4.11 (0.39)	0.8	
	770	0.19 (0.06)	—	3.79 (0.37)	0.8	
	820	0.15 (0.06)	—	3.60 (0.35)	0.8	
	830	0.14 (0.06)	—	3.56 (0.35)	0.8	
	870	0.10 (0.05)	—	3.41 (0.34)	0.8	
	920	0.07 (0.04)	—	3.32 (0.34)	0.8	
	970	0.06 (0.03)	—	3.15 (0.34)	0.8	
	1020	0.04 (0.03)	—	3.02 (0.33)	0.8	
	1064	0.02 (0.02)	—	2.97 (0.32)	0.8	
	1070	0.02 (0.02)	—	2.97 (0.32)	0.8	
	1120	0.02 (0.02)	—	2.86 (0.32)	0.8	
	1170	0.06 (0.04)	—	2.71 (0.31)	0.8	
	1220	0.07 (0.04)	—	2.63 (0.31)	0.8	

Table 2.1 (Continued).

Tissue	λ, nm	μ_a, cm^{-1}	μ_s, cm^{-1}	μ_s', cm^{-1}	g	Remarks
	1270	0.06 (0.04)	—	2.62 (0.31)	0.8	
	1320	0.11 (0.05)	—	2.53 (0.30)	0.8	
	1370	0.56 (0.14)	—	2.50 (0.31)	0.8	
	1420	2.36 (0.35)	—	3.01 (0.41)	0.8	
	1470	2.96 (0.42)	—	3.08 (0.45)	0.8	
	1520	1.89 (0.29)	—	2.66 (0.39)	0.8	
	1570	1.01 (0.20)	—	2.39 (0.34)	0.8	
Dermis	370	0.98 (0.14)	—	8.76 (1.36)	0.8	IS, IMC, slabs, Ref. 1273
	420	0.85 (0.11)	—	6.85 (0.89)	0.8	
	470	0.43 (0.06)	—	5.36 (0.60)	0.8	
	488	0.36 (0.05)	—	4.90 (0.51)	0.8	
	514	0.31 (0.04)	—	4.32 (0.41)	0.8	
	520	0.30 (0.04)	—	4.20 (0.39)	0.8	
	570	0.22 (0.03)	—	3.50 (0.31)	0.8	
	620	0.15 (0.02)	—	3.07 (0.28)	0.8	
	633	0.15 (0.02)	—	2.99 (0.27)	0.8	
	670	0.15 (0.02)	—	2.78 (0.26)	0.8	
	720	0.15 (0.02)	—	2.54 (0.24)	0.8	
	770	0.13 (0.02)	—	2.33 (0.24)	0.8	
	820	0.11 (0.02)	—	2.18 (0.23)	0.8	
	830	0.11 (0.02)	—	2.15 (0.23)	0.8	
	870	0.09 (0.02)	—	2.05 (0.22)	0.8	
	920	0.08 (0.02)	—	1.99 (0.23)	0.8	
	970	0.08 (0.02)	—	1.90 (0.22)	0.8	
	1020	0.07 (0.02)	—	1.84 (0.22)	0.8	
	1064	0.05 (0.02)	—	1.80 (0.21)	0.8	
	1070	0.05 (0.02)	—	1.79 (0.21)	0.8	

Table 2.1 (Continued).

Tissue	λ, nm	μ_a, cm^{-1}	μ_s, cm^{-1}	μ_s', cm^{-1}	g	Remarks
	1120	0.06 (0.02)	—	1.74 (0.21)	0.8	
	1170	0.12 (0.02)	—	1.69 (0.20)	0.8	
	1220	0.13 (0.02)	—	1.65 (0.20)	0.8	
	1270	0.10 (0.02)	—	1.63 (0.20)	0.8	
	1320	0.15 (0.03)	—	1.61 (0.19)	0.8	
	1370	0.48 (0.04)	—	1.66 (0.19)	0.8	
	1420	1.76 (0.18)	—	2.03 (0.21)	0.8	
	1470	2.19 (0.20)	—	2.13 (0.21)	0.8	
	1520	1.41 (0.11)	—	1.87 (0.20)	0.8	
	1570	0.85 (0.07)	—	1.65 (0.19)	0.8	
Subcutaneous fat	370	1.18 (0.21)	—	5.27 (0.69)	0.8	IS, IMC, slabs, Ref. 1273
	420	1.65 (0.33)	—	4.59 (0.59)	0.8	
	470	0.75 (0.09)	—	3.92 (0.50)	0.8	
	488	0.63 (0.08)	—	3.69 (0.47)	0.8	
	514	0.47 (0.07)	—	3.37 (0.43)	0.8	
	520	0.44 (0.07)	—	3.31 (0.42)	0.8	
	570	0.31 (0.09)	—	2.89 (0.36)	0.8	
	620	0.15 (0.03)	—	2.59 (0.31)	0.8	
	633	0.14 (0.03)	—	2.54 (0.30)	0.8	
	670	0.13 (0.03)	—	2.40 (0.27)	0.8	
	720	0.12 (0.02)	—	2.22 (0.24)	0.8	
	770	0.11 (0.02)	—	2.07 (0.21)	0.8	
	820	0.10 (0.02)	—	1.98 (0.20)	0.8	
	830	0.10 (0.02)	—	1.96 (0.20)	0.8	
	870	0.09 (0.02)	—	1.89 (0.19)	0.8	
	920	0.09 (0.02)	—	1.81 (0.18)	0.8	
	970	0.09 (0.03)	—	1.76 (0.18)	0.8	

Table 2.1 (Continued).

Tissue	λ, nm	μ_a, cm^{-1}	μ_s, cm^{-1}	μ_s', cm^{-1}	g	Remarks
	1020	0.08 (0.02)	—	1.72 (0.16)	0.8	
	1064	0.07 (0.02)	—	1.69 (0.15)	0.8	
	1070	0.07 (0.02)	—	1.68 (0.15)	0.8	
	1120	0.08 (0.02)	—	1.65 (0.15)	0.8	
	1170	0.14 (0.03)	—	1.63 (0.15)	0.8	
	1220	0.15 (0.03)	—	1.61 (0.15)	0.8	
	1270	0.10 (0.03)	—	1.59 (0.14)	0.8	
	1320	0.12 (0.03)	—	1.58 (0.14)	0.8	
	1370	0.27 (0.04)	—	1.60 (0.15)	0.8	
	1420	0.93 (0.14)	—	1.77 (0.18)	0.8	
	1470	1.08 (0.18)	—	1.81 (0.19)	0.8	
	1520	0.70 (0.12)	—	1.70 (0.17)	0.8	
	1570	0.43 (0.07)	—	1.60 (0.16)	0.8	
Infiltrative basal cell carcinoma	370	0.68 (0.08)	—	6.52 (0.92)	0.8	IS, IMC, slabs, Ref. 1273
	420	0.67 (0.11)	—	5.89 (0.52)	0.8	
	470	0.33 (0.04)	—	4.88 (0.36)	0.8	
	488	0.29 (0.05)	—	4.50 (0.33)	0.8	
	514	0.26 (0.06)	—	4.04 (0.30)	0.8	
	520	0.25 (0.06)	—	3.95 (0.30)	0.8	
	570	0.20 (0.07)	—	3.33 (0.28)	0.8	
	620	0.15 (0.06)	—	2.90 (0.28)	0.8	
	633	0.15 (0.05)	—	2.81 (0.28)	0.8	
	670	0.14 (0.05)	—	2.59 (0.28)	0.8	
	720	0.13 (0.05)	—	2.35 (0.28)	0.8	
	770	0.11 (0.04)	—	2.12 (0.26)	0.8	
	820	0.09 (0.04)	—	1.96 (0.25)	0.8	
	830	0.09 (0.04)	—	1.92 (0.25)	0.8	

Table 2.1 (Continued).

Tissue	λ, nm	μ_a, cm^{-1}	μ_s, cm^{-1}	μ_s', cm^{-1}	g	Remarks
	870	0.07 (0.03)	—	1.80 (0.24)	0.8	
	920	0.06 (0.03)	—	1.66 (0.20)	0.8	
	970	0.08 (0.03)	—	1.50 (0.15)	0.8	
	1020	0.07 (0.03)	—	1.36 (0.11)	0.8	
	1064	0.08 (0.04)	—	1.26 (0.09)	0.8	
	1070	0.08 (0.04)	—	1.25 (0.09)	0.8	
	1120	0.10 (0.06)	—	1.19 (0.09)	0.8	
	1170	0.16 (0.07)	—	1.15 (0.09)	0.8	
	1220	0.17 (0.09)	—	1.09 (0.10)	0.8	
	1270	0.18 (0.12)	—	1.05 (0.11)	0.8	
	1320	0.27 (0.15)	—	1.04 (0.10)	0.8	
	1370	0.69 (0.27)	—	1.09 (0.10)	0.8	
	1420	2.21 (0.46)	—	1.54 (0.25)	0.8	
	1470	2.75 (0.54)	—	1.66 (0.32)	0.8	
	1520	1.90 (0.47)	—	1.33 (0.27)	0.8	
	1570	1.12 (0.31)	—	1.11 (0.16)	0.8	
Nodular basal cell carcinoma	370	0.87 (0.29)	—	4.62 (0.61)	0.8	IS, IMC, slabs, Ref. 1273
	420	0.73 (0.20)	—	4.36 (0.38)	0.8	
	470	0.40 (0.12)	—	3.85 (0.22)	0.8	
	488	0.34 (0.12)	—	3.60 (0.20)	0.8	
	514	0.28 (0.11)	—	3.27 (0.18)	0.8	
	520	0.27 (0.11)	—	3.20 (0.18)	0.8	
	570	0.18 (0.09)	—	2.71 (0.16)	0.8	
	620	0.13 (0.06)	—	2.34 (0.13)	0.8	
	633	0.12 (0.06)	—	2.27 (0.12)	0.8	
	670	0.09 (0.05)	—	2.07 (0.11)	0.8	
	720	0.07 (0.04)	—	1.84 (0.10)	0.8	

Table 2.1 (Continued).

Tissue	λ, nm	μ_a, cm^{-1}	μ_s, cm^{-1}	μ_s', cm^{-1}	g	Remarks
	770	0.04 (0.03)	—	1.66 (0.09)	0.8	
	820	0.02 (0.02)	—	1.52 (0.07)	0.8	
	830	0.02 (0.01)	—	1.49 (0.07)	0.8	
	870	0.01 (0.01)	—	1.40 (0.07)	0.8	
	920	0.01 (0.00)	—	1.31 (0.06)	0.8	
	970	0.01 (0.01)	—	1.25 (0.06)	0.8	
	1020	0.00 (0.00)	—	1.20 (0.06)	0.8	
	1064	0.00 (0.00)	—	1.16 (0.06)	0.8	
	1070	0.00 (0.00)	—	1.15 (0.06)	0.8	
	1120	0.00 (0.00)	—	1.09 (0.05)	0.8	
	1170	0.01 (0.01)	—	1.04 (0.04)	0.8	
	1220	0.02 (0.01)	—	1.01 (0.04)	0.8	
	1270	0.01 (0.01)	—	1.00 (0.04)	0.8	
	1320	0.05 (0.01)	—	0.97 (0.04)	0.8	
	1370	0.32 (0.03)	—	1.03 (0.06)	0.8	
	1420	1.46 (0.20)	—	1.44 (0.13)	0.8	
	1470	1.86 (0.16)	—	1.59 (0.15)	0.8	
	1520	1.19 (0.07)	—	1.31 (0.10)	0.8	
	1570	0.67 (0.04)	—	1.06 (0.08)	0.8	
Squamous cell carcinoma	370	0.94 (0.20)	—	4.36 (0.61)	0.8	IS, IMC, slabs, Ref. 1273
	420	1.21 (0.23)	—	4.21 (0.50)	0.8	
	470	0.41 (0.06)	—	3.38 (0.47)	0.8	
	488	0.34 (0.05)	—	3.13 (0.43)	0.8	
	514	0.32 (0.04)	—	2.80 (0.39)	0.8	
	520	0.32 (0.04)	—	2.74 (0.38)	0.8	
	570	0.29 (0.04)	—	2.35 (0.32)	0.8	
	620	0.14 (0.02)	—	1.95 (0.26)	0.8	

Table 2.1 (Continued).

Tissue	λ, nm	μ_a, cm^{-1}	μ_s, cm^{-1}	μ_s', cm^{-1}	g	Remarks
	633	0.13 (0.02)	—	1.88 (0.25)	0.8	
	670	0.11 (0.02)	—	1.71 (0.23)	0.8	
	720	0.09 (0.02)	—	1.52 (0.20)	0.8	
	770	0.07 (0.02)	—	1.35 (0.18)	0.8	
	820	0.05 (0.02)	—	1.24 (0.16)	0.8	
	830	0.05 (0.02)	—	1.22 (0.15)	0.8	
	870	0.04 (0.01)	—	1.16 (0.14)	0.8	
	920	0.03 (0.01)	—	1.09 (0.13)	0.8	
	970	0.04 (0.02)	—	1.02 (0.12)	0.8	
	1020	0.04 (0.02)	—	0.94 (0.12)	0.8	
	1064	0.04 (0.02)	—	0.88 (0.12)	0.8	
	1070	0.04 (0.02)	—	0.88 (0.12)	0.8	
	1120	0.04 (0.02)	—	0.85 (0.12)	0.8	
	1170	0.10 (0.03)	—	0.84 (0.11)	0.8	
	1220	0.11 (0.03)	—	0.81 (0.11)	0.8	
	1270	0.11 (0.03)	—	0.78 (0.11)	0.8	
	1320	0.17 (0.04)	—	0.77 (0.11)	0.8	
	1370	0.43 (0.05)	—	0.85 (0.11)	0.8	
	1420	1.70 (0.12)	—	1.29 (0.18)	0.8	
	1470	2.35 (0.21)	—	1.44 (0.23)	0.8	
	1520	1.50 (0.15)	—	1.16 (0.16)	0.8	
	1570	0.92 (0.12)	—	0.92 (0.13)	0.8	
Spleen	1064	6.0	137	—	0.90	Data from Ref. 691
Stomach:						
Muscle	1064	3.3	29.5	—	0.87	Data from Ref. 691
Mucous	1064	2.8	732	—	0.91	
Integral	1064	0.8	128	—	0.91	

Table 2.1 (Continued).

Tissue	λ, nm	μ_a, cm^{-1}	μ_s, cm^{-1}	μ_s', cm^{-1}	g	Remarks
Tooth:						
Dentin	543	4	180	—	—	IS, GPM*, Refs. 66 and 97, see also Ref. 426
	633	4	130	—	—	
Enamel	633	6.0*	1200*	672*	0.44*	
	543	<1	45	—	—	
	633	<1	25	—	—	
Dentin	543	3–4	280 (84)	—	0.93 (0.02)	GPM, double HGPF, fractions of isotropic scatterers are 0–2% for dentin and 60–35% for enamel; polished plane-parallel sections of 30–2000 μm[426]
	633	3–4	280 (84)	—	0.93 (0.02)	
	1053	3–4	260 (78)	—	0.93 (0.02)	
Enamel	543	<1	105 (30)	—	0.96 (0.02)	
	633	<1	60 (18)	—	0.96 (0.02)	
	1053	<1	15 (5)	—	0.96 (0.02)	
Enamel	200	≈10	≈450	—	—	Compiled data of a few papers, from graphs of Ref. 454
	300	≈5	≈270	—	—	
	400	≈1	≈150	—	—	
	500	<1	≈73	—	—	
	600	<1	≈64	—	—	
	700	<1	≈50	—	—	
	800	<1	≈33	—	—	
	1000	<1	≈16	—	—	
Dentin	2940	2200	—	—	—	Time-resolved radiometry, data from graphs of Ref. 454
	2790	1500	—	—	—	
	9600	6500	—	—	—	
	10600	800	—	—	—	
Enamel	2940	800	—	—	—	
	2790	400	—	—	—	
	9600	8000	—	—	—	
	10600	800	—	—	—	

Table 2.1 (Continued).

Tissue	λ, nm	μ_a, cm^{-1}	μ_s, cm^{-1}	μ_s', cm^{-1}	g	Remarks
Dentin	2790	988 (111)	—	—	—	Transmission measurements, Ref. 454
	10300	1198 (104)	—	—	—	
	10600	813 (63)	—	—	—	
Enamel	2940	768 (27)	—	—	—	
	2790	451 (29)	—	—	—	
	10300	1168 (49)	—	—	—	
	10600	819 (62)	—	—	—	
Uterus	635	0.35 (0.1)	394 (91)	122	0.69	Frozen sections[657]
Vein (femoral)	1064	3.2	487	—	0.97	Data from Ref. 691
Ex vivo measurements						
Aorta:						
Normal ($n=4$)	1300	—	150–360	—	0.9–1	Optical coherence tomography (OCT)[711]; 4 hr of autopsy; $g_{\text{eff}} = \cos\theta_{\text{rms}}$, θ_{rms}—rms scattering angle, $g_{\text{eff}} \geq g$
Lipid rich ($n=4$)	1300	—	0–200	—	0.6–1	
Fibrous ($n=3$)	1300	—	50–400	—	0.6–1	
Fibrocalcific ($n=3$)	1300	—	0–200	—	0.8–1	
Fat:						
Abdominal ($n=2$)	360	3.12 (0.78)	—	32.59 (3.26)	—	IS, IAD; tissue slabs, <12 h after surgery, stored at 4°C in saline; measurements at room temperature; in the spectral range 600–1600 nm: $\mu_s' = 1.23 \times 10^3 \lambda^{-0.59}$, $[\lambda]$ = nm; Ref. 705
	400	3.97 (0.99)	—	25.62 (2.56)	—	
	500	2.37 (0.59)	—	28.23 (2.82)	—	
	600	1.90 (0.47)	—	28.58 (2.86)	—	
	700	1.84 (0.46)	—	26.27 (2.63)	—	
	800	1.87 (0.47)	—	25.74 (2.57)	—	
	900	1.80 (0.45)	—	21.21 (2.12)	—	
	1000	1.77 (0.44)	—	20.14 (2.01)	—	
	1100	1.68 (0.42)	—	19.05 (1.90)	—	
	1200	1.79 (0.45)	—	17.55 (1.76)	—	

Table 2.1 (Continued).

Tissue	λ, nm	μ_a, cm^{-1}	μ_s, cm^{-1}	μ_s', cm^{-1}	g	Remarks
	1300	1.52 (0.38)	—	17.42 (1.74)	—	
	1400	1.75 (0.44)	—	17.15 (1.71)	—	
	1500	1.63 (0.41)	—	17.08 (1.71)	—	
	1600	1.47 (0.37)	—	16.41 (1.64)	—	
	1700	2.11 (0.53)	—	17.21 (1.72)	—	
	1800	1.92 (0.48)	—	17.40 (1.74)	—	
	1900	2.48 (0.62)	—	20.38 (2.04)	—	
	2000	2.12 (0.53)	—	19.44 (1.94)	—	
	2100	1.74 (0.43)	—	18.72 (1.87)	—	
	2200	1.65 (0.41)	—	18.95 (1.89)	—	
Subcutaneous ($n = 6$)	400	2.26 (0.24)	—	13.39 (2.78)	—	IS, IAD; tissue slabs, 1–3 mm;
	500	1.49 (0.06)	—	13.82 (4.00)	—	<6 hr after surgery; stored at
	600	1.18 (0.02)	—	13.39 (4.65)	—	20°C in saline; measurements at
	700	1.11 (0.05)	—	12.17 (4.41)	—	room temperature; in the
	800	1.07 (0.11)	—	11.62 (4.63)	—	spectral range 600–1500 nm:
	900	1.07 (0.07)	—	9.97 (3.42)	—	$\mu_s' = 1.05 \times 10^3 \lambda^{-0.68}$,
	1000	1.06 (0.06)	—	9.39 (3.32)	—	$[\lambda] =$ nm; Ref. 726
	1100	1.01 (0.05)	—	8.74 (3.28)	—	
	1200	1.06 (0.07)	—	7.91 (3.17)	—	
	1300	0.89 (0.07)	—	7.81 (3.19)	—	
	1400	1.08 (0.03)	—	7.51 (3.31)	—	
	1500	1.05 (0.02)	—	7.36 (3.42)	—	
	1600	0.89 (0.04)	—	7.16 (3.21)	—	
	1700	1.26 (0.07)	—	7.53 (3.33)	—	
	1800	1.21 (0.01)	—	7.50 (3.48)	—	
	1900	1.62 (0.06)	—	8.72 (4.15)	—	
	2000	1.43 (0.09)	—	8.24 (4.03)	—	

Table 2.1 (Continued).

Tissue	λ, nm	μ_a, cm^{-1}	μ_s, cm^{-1}	μ_s', cm^{-1}	g	Remarks
Forearm:						
Fat	633	0.026	—	12.0	0.9$^\Delta$	SRR; ($^\Delta$) from literature[260]
Muscle	633	0.96	—	5.3	0.9$^\Delta$	
Mucous of maxillary sinus	400	4.89 (0.92)	—	36.01 (6.41)	—	IS, IAD; tissue slabs, 1–2 mm;
at antritis ($n=10$)	500	1.13 (0.18)	—	17.69 (2.84)	—	<6 hr after surgery; stored at
	600	0.45 (0.23)	—	13.81 (2.43)	—	20°C in saline; measurements at
	700	0.16 (0.24)	—	11.53 (2.02)	—	room temperature; in the
	800	0.13 (0.16)	—	9.79 (1.68)	—	spectral range 600–1300 nm:
	900	0.12 (0.09)	—	7.62 (0.92)	—	$\mu_s' = 4.4 \times 10^5\lambda^{-1.62}$, [$\lambda$] = nm;
	1000	0.27 (0.21)	—	6.14 (0.74)	—	Ref. 726
	1100	0.16 (0.14)	—	5.19 (0.58)	—	
	1200	0.57 (0.31)	—	4.43 (0.43)	—	
	1300	0.67 (0.35)	—	3.89 (0.38)	—	
	1400	4.84 (1.79)	—	5.07 (0.71)	—	
	1500	6.06 (2.38)	—	4.95 (1.21)	—	
	1600	2.83 (1.01)	—	3.13 (0.55)	—	
	1700	2.26 (0.79)	—	2.83 (0.51)	—	
	1800	3.04 (1.15)	—	3.04 (0.57)	—	
	1900	9.23 (2.69)	—	7.01 (3.57)	—	
	2000	9.31 (2.28)	—	6.26 (3.56)	—	
Oral mucosa	855	—	27 (11)	—	—	Optical coherence microscopy:
	855	—	39 (6)	—	—	normal tissue;
	855	—	60 (9)	—	—	dysplastic tissue;
						squamous cell carcinoma;
						Ref. 1274
Skin:						
Caucasian dermis ($n=12$)	633	0.33 (0.09)	—	27.3 (5.4)	0.9	A single integrating sphere
	700	0.19 (0.06)	—	23.2 (4.1)	0.9	"comparison" method, IMC;

Table 2.1 (Continued).

Tissue	λ, nm	μ_a, cm^{-1}	μ_s, cm^{-1}	μ_s', cm^{-1}	g	Remarks
Negroid dermis ($n = 5$)	900	0.13 (0.07)	—	16.3 (2.5)	0.9	samples from abdominal and breast tissue obtained from plastic surgery or *post mortem* examinations, $g = 0.9$ is supposed value in calculations[236,237]
	633	2.41 (1.53)	—	32.1 (20.4)	0.9	
	700	1.49 (0.88)	—	26.8 (14.1)	0.9	
	900	0.45 (0.18)	—	18.1 (0.4)	0.9	
Subdermis (primarily globular fat cells) ($n = 12$)	633	0.13 (0.05)	—	12.6 (3.4)	0.9	
	700	0.09 (0.03)	—	12.1 (3.2)	0.9	
	900	0.12 (0.04)	—	10.8 (2.7)	0.9	
Muscle ($n = 1$)	633	1.21	—	8.9	0.9	
	700	0.46	—	8.3	0.9	
	900	0.32	—	5.9	0.9	
Sample/subject—01/01; female (F), age = 51 yr; back of knee, left leg; moderate inflammation in dermis; SC = 40–70 μm; E = 40–150 μm; D = 300 μm	1460	17.88 (1.12)	—	10.74 (0.49)	—	DIS, IAD; slabs containing stratum corneum (SC), epidermis (E), and dermis (D), taken from 14 subjects; measured within 24 hr of excision; heated to 37°C; three measurements on each side of the sample; 2.5-cm-diameter sample ports on the setup, for small sample size reduced to 1.3 cm*; totally data for 52 wavelengths in the range 1000–2200 nm are available[677]
	1600	5.35 (0.24)	—	8.06 (0.29)	—	
	2200	7.46 (0.56)	—	7.17 (0.26)	—	
02/01; F, age = 51 yr; back of knee, left leg; moderate inflammation in dermis; SC = 40–70 μm; E = 40–140 μm; D = 300 μm	1460	18.70 (1.13)	—	11.39 (0.65)	—	
	1600	5.46 (0.27)	—	8.62 (0.34)	—	
	2200	8.86 (0.46)	—	8.15 (0.26)	—	
03/02; F, age = 66 yr; lower back, right side; mild solar damage; SC = 20–50 μm; E = 30 μm; D = 200 μm	1460	16.01 (0.56)	—	9.83 (0.59)	—	
	1600	4.91 (0.10)	—	6.78 (0.45)	—	
	2200	10.94 (0.23)	—	9.00 (0.54)	—	

Table 2.1 (Continued).

Tissue	λ, nm	μ_a, cm^{-1}	μ_s, cm^{-1}	μ_s', cm^{-1}	g	Remarks
04/02; F, age = 66 yr; lower back, right side; mild solar damage; SC = 20–50 μm; E = 30 μm; D = 200 μm	1460	12.65 (0.96)	—	8.61 (0.63)	—	
	1600	3.86 (0.28)	—	6.04 (0.29)	—	
	2200	8.58 (0.55)	—	7.74 (0.23)	—	
05/03; F, age = 67 yr; shin, right leg; mild solar damage, chronic inflammation; SC = 20–50 μm; E = 30–50 μm; D = 200 μm	1460	16.58 (3.26)	—	11.68 (1.41)	—	
	1600	5.15 (0.60)	—	8.89 (1.11)	—	
	2200	9.65 (1.17)	—	10.31 (0.81)	—	
06/03; F, age = 67 yr; shin, right leg; mild solar damage, chronic inflammation; SC = 20–50 μm; E = 30–50 μm; D = 200 μm	1460	18.07 (0.42)	—	13.13 (0.63)	—	
	1600	5.60 (0.17)	—	10.34 (0.52)	—	
	2200	11.26 (0.16)	—	12.20 (0.88)	—	
07/04; M, age = 64 yr; thigh, right leg; mild chronic dermatitis; SC = 20–30 μm; E = 50–90 μm; D = 300 μm	1000	0.69 (0.01)	—	10.45 (0.61)	—	
	1460	16.64 (0.95)	—	10.75 (0.81)	—	
	1600	4.96 (0.27)	—	7.72 (0.40)	—	
	2200	13.04 (2.36)	—	9.42 (1.57)	—	
08/05; M, age = 75 yr; lower thigh, left leg; normal skin; SC = 8–12 μm; E = 20–60 μm; D = 200 μm	1000	0.83 (0.03)	—	12.25 (1.20)	—	
	1460	19.06 (1.22)	—	11.46 (1.09)	—	
	1600	5.75 (0.27)	—	8.31 (0.76)	—	
	2200	11.92 (0.41)	—	10.34 (0.76)	—	
09/05; M, age = 75 yr; lower thigh, left leg; normal skin; SC = 8–12 μm; E = 20–60 μm; D = 200 μm	1000	0.85 (0.02)	—	11.66 (0.96)	—	
	1460	18.03 (2.01)	—	11.19 (1.51)	—	
	1600	5.61 (0.56)	—	7.87 (0.81)	—	
	2200	11.85 (0.83)	—	10.03 (0.90)	—	

Table 2.1 (Continued).

Tissue	λ, nm	μ_a, cm^{-1}	μ_s, cm^{-1}	μ_s', cm^{-1}	g	Remarks
10/06; F, age = 42 yr; groin, left side; mild chronic inflammation; SC = 5 μm; E = 25–30 μm; D = 200 μm	1000	0.80 (0.01)	—	14.17 (0.71)	—	
	1460	20.49 (0.89)	—	13.64 (1.44)	—	
	1600	5.85 (0.14)	—	10.05 (0.55)	—	
	2200	12.46 (0.42)	—	11.79 (0.69)	—	
11/06; F, age = 42 yr; groin, left side; mild chronic inflammation; SC = 5 μm; E = 25–30 μm; D = 200 μm	1000	0.77 (0.03)	—	13.95 (1.12)	—	
	1460	20.24 (1.04)	—	13.18 (1.72)	—	
	1600	5.76 (0.28)	—	9.48 (0.91)	—	
	2200	12.71 (0.58)	—	10.89 (1.20)	—	
12/07; M, age = 33 yr; posterior thigh, right side; mild chronic dermatitis; SC = 2–5 μm; E = 5–10 μm; D = 300 μm	1000	0.82 (0.02)	—	14.35 (0.81)	—	
	1460	19.01 (1.28)	—	13.30 (0.91)	—	
	1600	5.81 (0.33)	—	10.14 (0.49)	—	
	2200	11.13 (1.21)	—	9.00 (0.33)	—	
13/08; F, age = 52 yr; axillary, right side; mild perivascular chronic inflammation; SC = 5–7 μm; E = 25 μm; D = 100 μm	1000	0.97 (0.08)	—	13.70 (0.35)	—	
	1460	21.39 (1.25)	—	12.54 (0.72)	—	
	1600	6.17 (0.30)	—	9.94 (0.78)	—	
	2200	12.53 (0.84)	—	9.45 (0.84)	—	
14/09; M, age = 37 yr; back of thigh, upper left; mild chronic dermatitis; SC = 3 μm; E = 13 μm; D = 300 μm	1000	0.82 (0.02)	—	15.00 (0.49)	—	
	1460	23.31 (0.71)	—	12.32 (0.51)	—	
	1600	6.68 (0.11)	—	10.01 (0.37)	—	
	2200	15.19 (1.37)	—	8.54 (0.52)	—	
15/10; M, age = 70 yr; scalp; mild chronic dermatitis w/solar elastosis; SC = 4–15 μm; E = 8–10 μm; D = 200 μm	1000	1.04 (0.02)	—	12.26 (0.44)	—	
	1460	15.95 (0.99)	—	10.75 (1.20)	—	
	1600	5.09 (0.23)	—	8.83 (0.92)	—	
	2200	12.65 (0.52)	—	8.83 (1.94)	—	

Table 2.1 (Continued).

Tissue	λ, nm	μ_a, cm^{-1}	μ_s, cm^{-1}	μ_s', cm^{-1}	g	Remarks
16/11*; M, age = 61 yr; scalp; mild chronic dermatitis w/solar elastosis; SC = 2–4 μm; E = 6 μm; D = 300 μm	1000	0.79 (0.02)	—	13.11 (0.61)	—	—
	1460	16.47 (1.05)	—	12.45 (0.56)	—	—
	1600	5.11 (0.24)	—	10.43 (0.57)	—	—
	2200	13.30 (1.48)	—	9.89 (0.79)	—	—
17/12*; F, age = 68 yr; scalp/facial tissue; mild solar damage, chronic inflammation; SC = 2 μm; E = 8–10 μm; D = 200 μm	1000	1.06 (0.03)	—	8.79 (1.18)	—	—
	1460	12.81 (1.84)	—	9.60 (0.57)	—	—
	1600	4.26 (0.50)	—	6.93 (0.75)	—	—
	2200	11.32 (1.52)	—	8.14 (0.81)	—	—
18/12*; F, age = 68 yr; scalp/facial tissue; sever solar damage, mild chronic inflammation; SC = 2 μm; E = 8–10 μm; D = 150 μm	1000	1.32 (0.05)	—	8.63 (1.91)	—	—
	1460	12.68 (5.07)	—	8.74 (1.26)	—	—
	1600	4.31 (1.34)	—	6.60 (0.92)	—	—
	2200	11.33 (3.05)	—	7.30 (0.24)	—	—
19/13*; F, age = 53 yr; scalp/facial tissue; mild chronic inflammation; SC = 4 μm; E = 10 μm; D = 200 μm	1000	1.55 (0.02)	—	11.96 (0.65)	—	—
	1460	16.13 (1.38)	—	11.52 (0.64)	—	—
	1600	5.38 (0.31)	—	8.65 (0.54)	—	—
	2200	13.84 (1.02)	—	9.67 (0.65)	—	—
20/13; F, age = 53 yr; scalp/facial tissue; mild solar damage; SC = 4 μm; E = 10 μm; D = 200 μm	1000	1.53 (0.02)	—	12.89 (0.77)	—	—
	1460	16.82 (1.13)	—	12.01 (0.81)	—	—
	1600	5.57 (0.19)	—	9.47 (0.60)	—	—
	2200	13.46 (0.58)	—	10.41 (0.71)	—	—
21/14; F, age = 52 yr; abdomen; mild chronic inflammation; SC = 4–5 μm; E = 10 μm; D = 200 μm	1000	0.88 (0.03)	—	14.96 (1.28)	—	—
	1460	18.21 (2.51)	—	14.20 (0.71)	—	—
	1600	5.74 (0.68)	—	10.58 (0.44)	—	—
	2200	11.33 (0.76)	—	10.40 (0.47)	—	—

Table 2.1 (Continued).

Tissue	λ, nm	μ_a, cm^{-1}	μ_s, cm^{-1}	μ_s', cm^{-1}	g	Remarks
22/14; F, age = 52 yr; abdomen; mild chronic inflammation; SC = 4–5 μm; E = 10 μm; D = 200 μm	1000	0.94 (0.02)	—	15.26 (0.63)	—	
	1460	18.46 (1.64)	—	15.10 (1.01)	—	
	1600	5.76 (0.31)	—	11.05 (0.39)	—	
	2200	13.72 (0.52)	—	13.72 (0.42)	—	
Uterus:						
Postmenopausal	630	0.515 (0.054)	—	9.1 (1.7)	—	Frequency-domain (FD); intact
Premenopausal	630	0.193 (0.013)	—	7.3 (0.9)	—	uteri were obtained by
	630	0.314 (0.030)	—	8.9 (1.5)	—	hysterectomy; during
	630	0.213 (0.024)	—	6.0 (0.8)	—	measurement period (3–4 hr)
	630	0.197 (0.030)	—	7.3 (1.5)	—	wet gauze was applied, Ref. 318
Fibroid	630	0.0824 (0.0075)	—	7.2 (0.9)	—	
In vivo measurements						
Adenocarcinoma (multiple subcutaneous large-cell, male 62 yr):						FD, r_{sd} = 2.2 cm[306,308]
Abdominal, normal tissue	674	0.0589 (0.0036)	—	8.94 (0.19)	—	
	811	0.0645 (0.0032)	—	8.82 (0.18)	—	
	849	0.0690 (0.0025)	—	8.77 (0.14)	—	
	956	0.1110 (0.015)	—	7.00 (0.62)	—	
Abdominal, tumor	674	0.169 (0.02)	—	8.48 (0.73)	—	
	811	0.190 (0.015)	—	8.30 (0.49)	—	
	849	0.276 (0.03)	—	9.93 (0.87)	—	
	956	—	—	—	—	
Back, normal tissue	674	0.0883 (0.006)	—	10.7 (0.4)	—	
	811	0.0892 (0.005)	—	9.99 (0.27)	—	
	849	0.0915 (0.0030)	—	9.65 (0.15)	—	
	956	0.127 (0.03)	—	6.3 (0.9)	—	

Table 2.1 (Continued).

Tissue	λ, nm	μ_a, cm^{-1}	μ_s, cm^{-1}	μ_s', cm^{-1}	g	Remarks
Back, tumor	674	0.174 (0.02)	—	10.4 (0.9)	—	
	811	0.177 (0.013)	—	9.23 (0.5)	—	
	849	0.190 (0.01)	—	9.20 (0.33)	—	
	956	0.186 (0.16)	—	4.7 (2.7)	—	
Brain:						
Normal cortex, temporal	674	>0.2	—	10 (1)	0.92	SRR; measurements during brain
and frontal lobe	849	>0.2	—	9.2 (1)	0.92	surgery, Ref. 655
	956	>0.2	—	8.5 (1)	0.92	
Normal optic nerve	674	0.60 (0.25)	—	18 (1)	0.92	
	849	0.75 (0.25)	—	17 (1)	0.92	
	956	0.65 (0.25)	—	16 (1)	0.92	
Astrocytoma of optic nerve	674	1.6 (1)	—	14 (1)	0.92	
	849	1.1 (1)	—	8.5 (1)	0.92	
	950	1.8 (1)	—	8.5 (1)	0.92	
Normal cortex, frontal lobe	674	<0.2	—	10 (0.5)	—	SRR; measurements during brain
	811	<0.1	—	9.1 (0.5)	—	surgery,[695] data from Ref. 696
	849	<0.1	—	9.2 (0.5)	—	
	956	0.15 (0.1)	—	8.9 (0.5)	—	
Normal cortex, frontal lobe	674	0.2 (0.1)	—	10 (0.5)	—	
	811	0.2 (0.1)	—	8.2 (0.5)	—	
	849	<0.1	—	8.2 (0.5)	—	
	956	0.25 (0.1)	—	8.2 (0.5)	—	
Normal optic nerve	674	0.6 (0.3)	—	17.5 (2)	—	
	849	0.8 (0.3)	—	16 (2)	—	
	956	0.7 (0.3)	—	15.2 (2)	—	
Astrocytoma of optic	674	1.4 (0.3)	—	12.5 (1)	—	
nerve	811	1.2 (0.3)	—	9.5 (1)	—	

Table 2.1 (Continued).

Tissue	λ, nm	μ_a, cm^{-1}	μ_s, cm^{-1}	μ_s', cm^{-1}	g	Remarks
Normal white matter	849	0.9 (0.3)	—	7.6 (1)	—	
	956	1.5 (0.3)	—	7.3 (1)	—	
	674	2.5 (0.5)	—	13.5 (1)	—	
	849	0.95 (0.2)	—	8.5 (1)	—	
	956	0.9 (0.2)	—	7.8 (1)	—	
White matter with scar	674	<0.2	—	6.5 (0.5)	—	
	849	<0.2	—	8 (0.5)	—	
Medulloblastoma	674	2.6 (0.5)	—	14 (1)	—	
	849	1 (0.2)	—	10.7 (1)	—	
	956	0.75 (0.2)	—	4 (1)	—	
Breast (female): Normal (30 Japanese women, averaged for all ages)	753	0.046 (0.014)	—	8.9 (1.3)	—	Time domain (TD), μ_a (cm^{-1}) $\approx 0.087 - 8.31 \times 10^{-4}x$, μ_s' (cm^{-1}) $\approx 13 - 0.08x$, where x = age (20–80 yr)[289]
Normal (6 women, 26–43 yr)	800	0.017–0.045	—	7.2–13.5	—	TD, μ_s' (cm^{-1}) ≈ 16.7–$7.9 \times 10^{-3}\lambda$, $\lambda = 500$–1060 nm, Ref. 288
Normal (6 women, tissue thickness, 33–49 mm at light compression)	580	0.70 (0.12)	—	—	—	Measurements of transmission, $g \approx 0.92$–0.95, $\mu_s' = 12$–13 cm^{-1}, Ref. 223
	780	0.23 (0.02)	—	—	—	
	850	0.27 (0.03)	—	—	—	
Breast cancer (5 patients)	630	0.305 (0.16)	—	9.41 (7.35)	—	SRR; relapsed cancer, HPD (72 hr)[659]
Normal (56 yr)	674	0.04	—	8.5	—	FD, $r_{sd} = 2.2$ cm[306,308]
	811	0.035	—	7.4	—	
	849	0.035	—	7.0	—	
	956	0.085	—	6.5	—	

Table 2.1 (Continued).

Tissue	λ, nm	μ_a, cm^{-1}	μ_s, cm^{-1}	μ_s', cm^{-1}	g	Remarks
Fibroadenoma with ductal hyperplasia (56 yr)	674	0.055	—	9	—	
	811	0.06	—	8	—	
	849	0.055	—	7.6	—	
	956	0.12	—	7.5	—	
Normal (27 yr)	674	0.035	—	11.1	—	
	811	0.03	—	9.6	—	
	849	0.038	—	9.6	—	
	956	0.09	—	9.7	—	
Fluid-filled cyst (27 yr)	674	0.07	—	7.9	—	
	811	0.07	—	7.0	—	
	849	0.08	—	7.0	—	
	956	0.16	—	7.0	—	
Papillary cancer (55 yr)	690	0.084 (0.014)	—	15.0 (0.3)	—	FD, diffusion approximation[707]
	825	0.085 (0.017)	—	12.7 (0.3)	—	
Normal (67 yr)	674	0.057	—	9.5	—	FD, diffusion approximation; tumor 1.8 × 0.9 cm; segmented reconstruction[714]
	782	0.050	—	9.4	—	
	803	0.047	—	9.0	—	
	849	0.054	—	8.9	—	
Ductal carcinoma *in situ* (67 yr)	674	0.17	—	4.1	—	
	782	0.18	—	3.6	—	
	803	0.15	—	4.2	—	
	849	0.21	—	3.3	—	
Calf (11 subjects, 14 measurements)	800	0.17 (0.05)	—	9.4 (0.7)	—	μ_s' (cm^{-1}) $\approx$ 16–8.9 × 10$^{-3}\lambda$, λ = 760–900 nm, Ref. 274

Table 2.1 (Continued).

Tissue	λ, nm	μ_a, cm^{-1}	μ_s, cm^{-1}	μ_s', cm^{-1}	$g/\mu_{bs}/\gamma$	Remarks
Cervical stromal tissue	849	0.34	61.1	–	0.9	Ref. 700; data from Ref. 242
Cervical tissue:		μ_{bs}			μ_{bs}	$\mu_{bs} = \mu_s p_b$. p_b—probability of backscattering[716-718]
Epithelium ($n = 36$)	1300	–	10–140	–	0.1–11	OCT, two-layered model,[716]
Stroma ($n = 36$)	1300	–	30–290	–	1.5–12	genetic inverse algorithm [716]
Dysplasia II-III	1300	–	40–65	–	1.4–3.6	OCT, single-layered model,
Leukoplakia	1300	–	16–32	–	1.3–2.0	genetic inverse algorithm[718]
Epithelium	1300	–	80 (25)	–	0.28 (0.08)	OCT, genetic inverse algorithm
Stroma	1300	–	210 (30)	–	3.0 (2)	two-layered model
Cancer	1300	–	300 (20)	–	1.2 (0.6)	single-layered model[717,718]
Gastrointestinal tract:					$\gamma = (1 - g_2)/(1 - g_1)$	
Mucosa in the antrum	500	2.5 (0.8)	–	16.8 (3.4)	1.98 (0.20)	Endoscopic SRR, r_{sd} from 0.3
	550	3.6 (1.3)	–	13.8 (3.4)	1.93 (0.15)	to 1.35 mm; IMC, two-moments
	600	1.0 (0.6)	–	12.8 (2.1)	1.90 (0.12)	HGPF [see Eq. (2.18)];
	650	0.5 (0.5)	–	11.7 (1.8)	1.87 (0.12)	35 patients (21 females and
	700	0.4 (0.4)	–	10.7 (1.6)	1.86 (0.12)	14 males, aged from 23 to 87),
	750	0.45 (0.45)	–	9.7 (1.6)	1.85 (0.12)	for each patient, four sites were
	800	0.5 (0.4)	–	9.0 (1.6)	1.85 (0.12)	usually selected—two in the
	850	0.7 (0.5)	–	8.8 (1.6)	1.85 (0.12)	antrum and two in the fundus,
	900	0.8 (0.5)	–	8.3 (1.5)	1.86 (0.12)	average data for normal tissue
Mucosa in the fundus	500	3.3 (0.8)	–	21.7 (3.1)	2.12 (0.26)	from graphs of Ref. 683
	550	4.4 (1.5)	–	18.6 (3.1)	2.04 (0.24)	
	600	1.8 (0.5)	–	16.5 (2.1)	2.00 (0.19)	
	650	0.8 (0.4)	–	15.0 (2.1)	1.97 (0.17)	
	700	0.7 (0.4)	–	13.8 (1.7)	1.98 (0.15)	
	750	0.7 (0.5)	–	12.4 (1.6)	1.98 (0.15)	
	800	0.7 (0.3)	–	11.7 (1.6)	1.95 (0.12)	

Table 2.1 (Continued).

Tissue	λ, nm	μ_a, cm^{-1}	μ_s, cm^{-1}	μ_s', cm^{-1}	$g/\mu_{bs}/\gamma$	Remarks
Head (7 subjects, 10 measurements)	850	0.7 (0.3)	—	11.0 (1.4)	1.92 (0.12)	μ_s' (cm^{-1}) $\approx$ 14.5 − 6.5 × 10$^{-3}\lambda$, λ = 760–900 nm, Ref. 274
	900	0.8 (0.4)	—	10.3 (1.4)	1.94 (0.12)	
	800	0.16 (0.01)	—	9.4 (0.7)	—	TD, μ_s' (cm^{-1}) $\approx$ 11 − 5.1 × 10$^{-3}\lambda$, λ = 760–900 nm[232]
Forearm (5 subjects, 14 measurements)	800	0.23 (0.04)	—	6.8 (0.8)	—	FD; r_{sd}—a few cm; data from Ref. 701
Forearm	715	0.18	—	3.7	—	
	825	0.24	—	3.0	—	
Forehead	715	0.16	—	7.3	—	
	825	0.16	—	6.9	—	
Skin:						
Dermis	660	0.07–0.2	—	9–14.5	—	SRR, IMC[228]
Skin	633	0.62	—	32	—	Dognitz and Wagnieres (1998) (see Ref. 572)
	700	0.38	—	28.7	—	
Skin (0–1 mm)	633	0.67	—	16.2	—	Ref. 260
Skin (1–2 mm)	633	0.026	—	12.0	—	
Skin (>2 mm)	633	0.96	—	5.3	—	
Forearm:						
Epidermis	633	8$^{\Delta}$	—	17.5	0.9$^{\Delta}$	SRR; (Δ) from literature[260]
Dermis	633	0.15	—	17.5	0.9$^{\Delta}$	
Epidermis and dermis	750	0.375	—	15	—	SRR; diffusion approximation[702] (from Ref. 692)
Subcutaneous fat	750	0.03	—	10	—	
Arm	633	0.17 (0.01)	—	9.08 (0.05)	—	SRR, 9 detecting 600-μm fibers; mean separation 1.7 mm; Mie phase function[572]
	660	0.128 (0.005)	—	8.68 (0.05)	—	
	700	0.090 (0.002)	—	8.14 (0.05)	—	

Table 2.1 (Continued).

Tissue	λ, nm	μ_a, cm^{-1}	μ_s, cm^{-1}	μ_s', cm^{-1}	$g/\mu_{bs}/\gamma$	Remarks
Foot sole	633	0.072 (0.002)	—	11.17 (0.09)	—	
	660	0.053 (0.003)	—	10.45 (0.09)	—	
	700	0.037 (0.001)	—	9.52 (0.08)	—	
Forehead	633	0.090 (0.009)	—	16.72 (0.09)	—	
	660	0.052 (0.003)	—	16.16 (0.08)	—	
	700	0.0240 (0.002)	—	15.38 (0.06)	—	
Abdominal skin:						
chosen direction	810	0.014	—	20	—	SRR; CCD detector, $r_{sd} \leq 10$ mm; diffusion approximation[692]
perpendicular direction (along collagen fibers)	810	0.07	—	10	—	
Forearm (light skin, $n = 7$): skin temperature—22°C	590	2.372 (0.282)	—	9.191 (0.931)	—	SRR; MC-generated grid[681]
	750	0.966 (0.110)	—	7.340 (0.901)	—	
	950	0.981 (0.073)	—	6.067 (0.847)	—	
skin temperature—38°C	590	2.869 (0.289)	—	9.613 (0.894)	—	
	750	1.157 (0.106)	—	7.649 (0.971)	—	
	950	1.135 (0.123)	—	6.234 (0.928)	—	
Dermis of a lower arm	1300	—	47	—	—	OCT[13]
Stratum corneum of finger	1300	—	12	—	—	
Volar side of lower arm:						
epidermis	1300	—	15–20	—	—	OCT[712]
upper dermis	1300	—	80–100	—	—	
Palm of hand:						
stratum corneum	1300	—	10–15	—	—	
epidermis:						
grandular layer	1300	—	60–70	—	—	
basal layer	1300	—	40–50	—	—	

Table 2.1 (Continued).

Tissue	λ, nm	μ_a, cm^{-1}	μ_s, cm^{-1}	μ_s', cm^{-1}	$g/\mu_{bs}/\gamma$	Remarks
upper dermis	1300	–	50–80	–	–	OCT[713]; depth up to 350 μm; skin treated with a detergent
Volar side of lower arm (epidermis and dermis)						solution (2% of anionic tensides in water)
Normal	1300	–	140	–	–	
Treated	1300	–	80	–	–	
Skull	674	<0.2	–	9 (1)	–	SRR; measurements during
	849	<0.1	–	9 (1)	–	brain surgery;[695] data from
	956	0.15 (0.1)	–	8.5 (1)	–	Ref. 696

- Total (or diffuse) reflectance for collimated or diffuse radiation.
- Absorption by a sample placed inside an integrating sphere.
- Collimated transmittance (of unscattered light).
- Angular distribution of radiation scattered by the sample.

Iterative methods normally take into account discrepancies between refractive indices at sample boundaries as well as the multilayer nature of the sample. The following factors are responsible for the errors in the estimated values of optical coefficients and need to be borne in mind as a comparative analysis of optical parameters obtained in different experiments:[40]

- The physiological conditions of tissues (the degree of hydration, homogeneity, species-specific variability, frozen/thawed or fixed/unfixed state, *in vitro/in vivo* measurements, smooth/rough surface)
- The geometry of irradiation
- The matching/mismatching interface refractive indices
- The orientation of detecting optical fibers inside the sample relative to the source fibers
- The numerical aperture of the recording fibers
- The angular resolution of photodetectors
- The separation of radiation experiencing forward scattering from unscattered radiation
- The theory used to solve the inverse problem

2.2 Integrating sphere technique

One of the indirect methods to determine optical properties of tissues *in vitro* is the integrating sphere technique.[6,48,49,57,649,650,652,656,661–668,672,674,675,677,678,691,719,720,724–726] Diffuse reflectance R_d, total transmittance T_t, and collimated transmittance T_c are measured. In general, absorption coefficient μ_a, scattering coefficient μ_s, and anisotropy factor g can be obtained from these data using an inverse method based on radiative transfer theory. When the scattering phase function $p(\theta)$ is available from goniophotometry, g can be readily calculated. In this case, for the determination of μ_a and μ_s, it is sufficient to measure R_d and T_t only. Sometimes, in experiments with tissue and blood samples, a double-integrating sphere configuration is preferable. In this case both reflectance and transmittance can be measured simultaneously and less degradation of the sample is expected during measurements (see Fig. 2.2). Nevertheless, in the case of a double-integrating sphere arrangement of the experiment in addition to the single-integrating sphere corrections of measured signals, multiple exchanges of light between the spheres should be accounted for.[264,663,664] The collimated transmittance measurement is usually carried out as shown in Fig. 2.1(a).

The integrating sphere technique was used by a number of investigators to determine the absorption coefficient, the scattering coefficient, the anisotropy

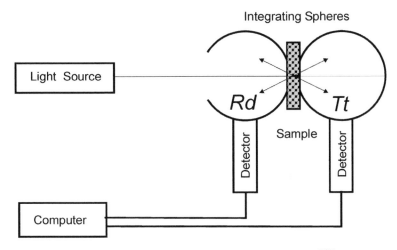

Figure 2.2 The double-integrating sphere setup.[725]

factor, and/or the reduced scattering coefficient of tissues and blood.[6,48,49,57,649–651,656,661–668,672,674,675,677,678,691,719,720,724–726] Barium-sulfate or Spectralon integrating spheres are used in the experiments. As monochromatic light sources, a laser, a Xe-lamp, and/or a Hg-lamp combined with a monochromator are used, while a photomultiplier or a Si-photodiode is employed as a detector. Sometimes, a white light source is used as the irradiator and a CCD fiber-optic spectrometer as a detector.[719]

Some tissues (for instance, melanin-containing) and blood have high total attenuation coefficients in the visible and near-infrared spectral ranges. Therefore, the collimated transmittance measurement for such samples (for example, the undiluted blood layer with a moderate thickness, ≈0.1 mm[48]) is a technically difficult task. To solve this problem, a powerful light source combined with a sensitive detector must be used.[49] Alternatively, it is possible to collect the collimated light together with some forward-scattered light using the third integrating sphere.[672] In this case, the collimated transmittance is separated from the scattered flux on the stage of the data processing using, for example, a Monte Carlo technique[665] or a small angle approximation.[673]

2.3 Kubelka-Munk and multiflux approach

To separate the light beam attenuation due to absorption from the loss due to scattering, the one-dimensional, two-flux Kubelka-Munk model (KMM) can be used as the simplest approach to solve the problem. This approach has been widely used to determine the absorption and scattering coefficients of biological tissues, provided the scattering is significantly dominant over the absorption.[1,2,36,37,40,212,649,661,674,691] The KMM assumes that light incident on a slab of tissue because of interaction with the scattering media can be modeled by two fluxes, counterpropagating in the tissue slab. The optical flux, which propagates in the same direction as the incident flux, is decreased by absorption and scattering processes and is also increased by back-scattering of the counterpropagating flux in the same direction. Changes in counterpropagating flux are determined in an analogous manner. The fraction of each flux lost by absorption per unit path length is denoted as K, while the fraction lost due to scattering is called S. The main assumptions of the KMM: K and S parameters are assumed to be uniform throughout the tissue slab; all light fluxes are diffuse; and the amount of light lost from the edges of the sample during reflectance measurements is negligible. Basic KMM does not account for reflections at boundaries, at which index of refraction mismatches exist.

Following the KMM and diffusion approximation of the RTE, the KMM parameters were expressed in terms of light transport theory: the absorption and scattering coefficients and scattering anisotropy factor.[37,40] Thus, when scattering significantly prevails on absorption, a simple experimental method using modified KMM expressions can be successfully employed as

$$S = \frac{1}{bd} = \ln\left[\frac{1 - R_d(a - b)}{T_d}\right],$$

$$K = S(a - 1), \quad a = \frac{1 - T_d^2 + R_d^2}{2R_d}, \quad b = \sqrt{a^2 - 1}, \qquad (2.1)$$

$$K = 2\mu_a, \quad S = \frac{3}{4}\mu_s(1 - g) - \frac{1}{4}\mu_a,$$

$$\mu_t = \mu_a + \mu_s; \quad \mu_s' = \mu_s(1 - g) > \mu_a,$$

where μ_t is determined based on Eq. (1.1) from measured values of collimated transmittance T_c. Thus, all three parameters (μ_a, μ_s, g) can be found from the experimental data for total transmittance T_t, diffuse reflectance R_d, and collimated transmittance T_c of the sample.

The further modifications of the KMM were undertaken to account for reflections at the sample boundaries.[213,227,674] The use of one of the measuring modalities in question can be illustrated by determining the optical parameters of human-skin epidermis. Transmittance and reflectance spectra of thin epidermal slices (stripping samples, 20–50-μm thickness) measured in the wavelength range of 240–400 nm on a spectrophotometer with an integrating sphere were used to calculate the absorption $\mu_a(\lambda)$ and scattering $\mu_s(\lambda)$ coefficients based on a four-flux model, taking into consideration collimated reflection at the sample boundaries[213,227] (see Fig. 2.3). The differences between the absorption coefficients in the considered wavelength range for normal human epidermis and samples containing psoriatic plaques are due to variations in skin metabolism (see UV absorption spectra of major skin epidermal chromophores, Fig. 1.6). The epidermis of psoriatic skin is characterized by a marked optical inhomogeneity caused by structural changes of the tissue in the psoriatic plaques and the appearance of air-filled microspaces between parakeratotic scales, accounting for a 10–15% rise in the diffuse reflection coefficient (for stripping samples of normal epidermis, this coefficient at 240–400 nm increases by 6–10% at most).

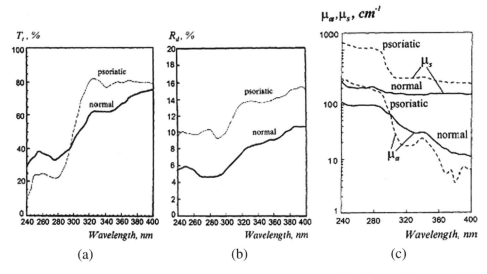

Figure 2.3 Experimental spectra for (a) total transmittance and (b) diffuse reflectance. Calculated spectra for (c) the absorption (μ_a) and scattering (μ_s) coefficients derived from experimental transmittance and diffuse reflectance spectra of stripped human epidermis using the four-flux model. Solid lines, normal skin; dotted lines, psoriatic skin.[213,227]

Often, such simple methods as the KMM[48] or δ-Eddington approximation[665,724] are used as the first step of the inverse algorithm for estimation of the optical properties of tissues and blood. The estimated values of the optical properties are then used to calculate the reflected and transmitted signals, employing one of the more sophisticated models of light propagation in tissue or blood. At the next step, the calculated values are compared with the measured ones. If the required accuracy is not achieved, the current optical properties are altered using one of the optimization algorithms. The procedures of altering the optical properties and calculating the reflected and transmitted signals are repeated until the calculated values match the measured values with the required accuracy.

2.4 The inverse adding-doubling (IAD) method

The IAD method provides a tool for the rapid and accurate solution of the inverse scattering problem.[266,267,725,652,666,667,675–677,691] It is based on the general method for the solution of the transport equation for plane-parallel layers suggested by van de Hulst[182] and introduced to tissue optics by Prahl.[679,680] An important advantage of the IAD method when applied to tissue optics is the possibility of rapidly obtaining iterative solutions with the aid of up-to-date microcomputers; moreover, it is flexible enough to take into account anisotropy of scattering and the internal reflection from the sample boundaries. The method includes the following steps:

(1) The choice of optical parameters to be measured,
(2) counting reflections and transmissions,
(3) comparing calculated and measured reflectance and transmittance, and
(4) repeating the procedure until the estimated and measured values coincide with the desired accuracy.

In principle, the method allows any intended accuracy to be achieved for all the parameters being measured, provided the necessary computer time is available. An error of 3% or less is considered acceptable.[652] Also, the method may be used to directly correct experimental findings obtained with the aid of integrating spheres. The term "doubling" in the name of the method means that the reflection and transmission estimates for a layer at certain in-going and out-going light angles may be used to calculate both the transmittance and reflectance for a layer twice as thick by means of superimposing one upon the other and summing the contributions of each layer to the total reflectance and transmittance. Reflection and transmission in a layer that has an arbitrary thickness are calculated in consecutive order, first for the thin layer with the same optical characteristics (single scattering), then by consecutive doubling of the thickness, for any selected layer. The term "adding" indicates that the doubling procedure may be extended to heterogeneous layers for modeling multilayer tissues or taking into account internal reflections related to abrupt changes in refractive index.[652]

The adding-doubling technique is a numerical method for solving the one-dimensional transport equation in slab geometry.[652,679,680,725,726] It can be used for media with an arbitrary phase function and arbitrary angular distribution of the spatially uniform incident radiation. Thus, finite beam size and side losses of light cannot be taken into account. The method is based on the observation that for an arbitrary incident radiance angular distribution $I_{in}(\eta_c)$, where η_c is the cosine of the polar angle, the angular distribution of the reflected radiance (normalized to an incident diffuse flux) is given by[652,679,680,725]

$$I_{ref}(\eta_c) = \int_0^1 I_{in}(\eta_c')R(\eta_c', \eta_c)2\eta_c'd\eta_c', \tag{2.2}$$

where $R(\eta_c', \eta_c)$ is the reflection redistribution function determined by the optical properties of the slab.

The distribution of the transmitted radiance can be expressed in a similar manner, with obvious substitution of the transmission redistribution function $T(\eta_c', \eta_c)$.

If M quadrature points are selected to span over the interval $(0, 1)$, the respective matrices can approximate the reflection and transmission redistribution functions as

$$R(\eta'_{ci}, \eta_{cj}) \rightarrow R_{ij}, \quad T(\eta'_{ci}, \eta_{cj}) \rightarrow T_{ij}. \tag{2.3}$$

These matrices are referred to as the reflection and transmission operators, respectively. If a slab with boundaries indexed as 0 and 2 is comprised of two layers, (01) and (12), with an internal interface 1 between the layers, the reflection and transmission operators for the whole slab (02) can be expressed as

$$
\begin{aligned}
\mathbf{T}^{02} &= \mathbf{T}^{12}(\mathbf{E} - \mathbf{R}^{10}\mathbf{R}^{12})^{-1}\mathbf{T}^{01}, \\
\mathbf{R}^{20} &= \mathbf{T}^{12}(\mathbf{E} - \mathbf{R}^{10}\mathbf{R}^{12})^{-1}\mathbf{R}^{10}\mathbf{T}^{21} + \mathbf{R}^{21}, \\
\mathbf{T}^{20} &= \mathbf{T}^{10}(\mathbf{E} - \mathbf{R}^{12}\mathbf{R}^{10})^{-1}\mathbf{T}^{21}, \\
\mathbf{R}^{02} &= \mathbf{T}^{10}(\mathbf{E} - \mathbf{R}^{12}\mathbf{R}^{10})^{-1}\mathbf{R}^{12}\mathbf{T}^{01} + \mathbf{R}^{01},
\end{aligned}
\tag{2.4}
$$

where $\mathbf{E}$ is the identity matrix defined in this case as

$$E_{ij} = \frac{1}{2\eta_{ci}w_i}\delta_{ij}, \tag{2.5}$$

where w_i is the weight assigned to the ith quadrature point and δ_{ij} is a Kroneker delta symbol, $\delta_{ij} = 1$ if $i = j$, and $\delta_{ij} = 0$ if $i \neq j$.

The definition of the matrix multiplication also slightly differs from the standard. Specifically,

$$(\mathbf{AB})_{ik} \equiv \sum_{j=1}^{M} A_{ij}2\eta_{cj}w_j B_{jk}. \tag{2.6}$$

Equations (2.4) allow one to calculate the reflection and transmission operators of a slab when those of the comprising layers are known. The idea of the method is to start with a thin layer for which the RTE can be simplified and solved with relative ease, producing the reflection and transmission operators for the thin layer, then to proceed by doubling the thickness of the layer until the thickness of the whole slab is reached. Several techniques exist for layer initialization. The single-scattering equations for reflection and transmission for the Henyey-Greenstein function are given in Refs. 182 and 679. The refractive index mismatch can be taken into account by adding effective boundary layers of zero thickness and having the reflection and transmission operators determined by Fresnel's formulas. The total transmittance and reflectance of the slab are obtained by straightforward integration of Eq. (2.2). Different methods of performing the integration are discussed in Ref. 679. The IAD program provided by Prahl[680] allows one to obtain the absorption and the scattering coefficients from the measured diffuse reflectance

R_d and diffuse transmittance T_d of the tissue slab. This program is the numerical solution to the steady-state RTE [see Eq. (1.9)] realizing an iterative process, which estimates the reflectance and transmittance from a set of optical parameters until the calculated reflectance and transmittance match the measured values. Values for the anisotropy factor g and the refractive index n must be provided to the program as input parameters.

It was shown that using only four quadrature points, the IAD method provides optical parameters that are accurate to within 2–3%,[652] as was mentioned early; higher accuracy, however, can be obtained by using more quadrature points, but it would require increased computation time. Another valuable feature of the IAD method is its validity for the study of samples with comparable absorption and scattering coefficients,[652,675,676] since other methods based only on diffusion approximation are inadequate. Furthermore, since both the anisotropic phase function and Fresnel reflection at boundaries are accurately approximated, the IAD technique is well suited to optical measurements for biological tissues and blood held between two glass slides.[49,652,675]

The IAD method has been successfully applied to determining optical parameters of blood; human and animal dermis; ocular tissues such as retina, choroids, sclera, conjunctiva, and ciliary body; aorta; and other soft tissues in a wide range of wavelengths.[49,266,381,267,667,676–678]

The adding-doubling method provides accurate results in cases when the side losses are not significant, but it is less flexible than the Monte Carlo (MC) technique.

2.5 Inverse Monte Carlo method

Both the real geometry of the experiment and the tissue structure can be complicated. Therefore, the MC method should be used if reliable estimates are to be obtained. A number of algorithms for using the inverse MC (IMC) method are available now in the literature.[2,213,217,226,228,236–238,244,369,638,654,655,662,678,681–684,691,719,720,725] Many researchers use the MC simulation program provided by Jacques.[684] Among the first designed IMC algorithms, two similar algorithms for determining all three optical parameters of the tissue (μ_a, μ_s, and g) based on the *in vitro* evaluation of the total transmittance, diffuse reflectance, and collimated transmittance using a spectrophotometer with integrating spheres, can be mentioned.[213,650,656,662,691,719] The initial approximation (to speed up the procedure) was achieved with the help of the Kubelka-Munk theory, specifically its four-flux variant.[213,656] Both algorithms take into consideration the sideways loss of photons, which becomes essential in sufficiently thick samples. Similar results were obtained using the condensed IMC method.[226,228]

The MC technique is employed as a method to solve the forward problem in the inverse algorithm for the determination of the optical properties of tissues and blood. The MC method is based on the formalism of the RTT (see Chapter 1), where the absorption coefficient is defined as a probability of a photon to be absorbed per unit length, and the scattering coefficient is defined as the probability of a photon to be scattered per unit length. Using these probabilities, a random sampling of photon trajectories is generated.

The basic algorithm for the generation of photon trajectories can be shortly described as follows.[725] A photon described by three spatial coordinates and two angles (x, y, z, θ, ϕ) is assigned its weight $W = W_0$ and placed in its initial position, depending on the source characteristics. The step size l of the photon is determined using Eqs. (1.88)–(1.90). The direction of the photon's next movement is determined by the scattering phase function substituted as the probability density distribution. Several approximations for the scattering phase function of tissue and blood have been used in MC simulations. These include the two empirical phase functions widely used to approximate the scattering phase function of tissue and blood, the Henyey-Greenstein phase function (HGPF) [see Eq. (1.15)] and the Gegenbauer kernel phase function (GKPF),[727] and theoretical Mie phase function.[148] The HGPF has one parameter g that may be represented as the infinite series of Legendre polynomials $P_n^1 (\cos \theta)$,

$$p_{hg}(\theta) = \frac{1}{4\pi} \sum_{n=0}^{\infty} (2n + 1) f_n P_n^1 (\cos \theta),$$

(2.7)

where $f_n = g^n$ is the nth order moment of the phase function.

The GKPF has two variable parameters, α and g:

$$p_{gk}(\theta) = K \left[1 + g^2 - 2g \cos(\theta) \right]^{-(\alpha+1)},$$

(2.8)

where $K = \alpha g \pi^{-1} (1 - g^2)^{2\alpha} [(1 + g)^{2\alpha} - (1 - g)^{2\alpha}]^{-1}$, $\alpha > -1/2$, $|g| \leq 1$.

The GKPF is a generalization of the HGPF and can be reduced to HGPF by setting $\alpha = 0.5$. The GKPF may be represented as the infinite series of Gegenbauer polynomials, C_n^α:[727,728]

$$p_{gk}(\theta) = \frac{2K}{(1 - g^2)} \sum_{n=0}^{\infty} \left(1 + \frac{n}{\alpha} \right) C_n^\alpha [\cos(\theta)] g^n.$$

(2.9)

The HGPF and GKPF are widely employed in radiative transport calculations for the description of the single-scattering process in whole blood because of their mathematical simplicity.[48,729,730] However, it is clear that the HGPF and GKPF cannot be used for accurate calculations of the angular light distribution scattered by a single erythrocyte. For some calculations, the theoretical Mie phase function may be useful,[148]

$$p(\theta) = \frac{1}{k^2 r^2} \left(|S_1|^2 + |S_2|^2 \right),$$

(2.10)

where S_1 and S_2 are functions of the polar scattering angle and can be obtained from Mie theory as

$$S_1(\theta) = \sum_{n=1}^{\infty} \frac{2n+1}{n(n+1)} [a_n \pi_n (\cos \theta) + b_n \tau_n (\cos \theta)],$$

$$S_2(\theta) = \sum_{n=1}^{\infty} \frac{2n+1}{n(n+1)} [b_n \pi_n (\cos \theta) + a_n \tau_n (\cos \theta)].$$

(2.11)

The parameters π_n and τ_n represent

$$\pi_n (\cos \theta) = \frac{1}{\sin \theta} P_n^1 (\cos \theta),$$

$$\tau_n (\cos \theta) = \frac{d}{d\theta} P_n^1 (\cos \theta),$$

(2.12)

where $P_n^1 (\cos \theta)$ is the associated Legendre polynomial. The following recursive relationships are used to calculate π_n and τ_n:

$$\pi_n = \frac{2n-1}{n-1} \pi_{n-1} \cos \theta - \frac{n}{n-1} \pi_{n-2},$$

$$\tau_n = n \pi_n \cos \theta - (n+1) \pi_{n-1},$$

(2.13)

and the initial values are

$$\begin{cases} \pi_1 = 1, & \pi_2 = \cos \theta, \\ \tau_1 = \cos \theta, & \tau_2 = 3 \cos 2\theta. \end{cases}$$

(2.14)

The coefficients a_n and b_n are defined in Eqs. (1.196)–(1.198).

For the HGPF, the random scattering angle θ_{rnd}^{HG} is given by[217]

$$\theta_{rnd}^{HG} = \arccos \left\{ \frac{1}{2g} \left[1 + g^2 - \left(\frac{1 - g^2}{1 - g + 2g\xi} \right)^2 \right] \right\},$$

(2.15)

where ξ is a random number uniformly distributed over the interval $(0, 1)$ [see Eq. (1.89)].

For the GKPF, the random scattering angle θ_{rnd}^{GK} is determined as[164]

$$\theta_{rnd}^{GK} = \arccos \left[\frac{(1 + g^2 - 1/\sqrt[\alpha]{\zeta_{rnd}})}{2g} \right],$$

(2.16)

where $\zeta_{rnd} = 2\alpha g \xi / K + (1+g)^{-2\alpha}$, and α and K are defined in Eq. (2.8).

If the experimental scattering phase function is known for the discrete set of scattering angles θ_i, $f(\theta) = f(\theta_i)$, it can be determined in the total angular range using the spline-interpolation technique.[726] Then, the value of the function $F_n = \int_0^{\theta_n} f(\theta)d\theta$ can be calculated numerically for any value of θ_n. It is easy to see that F_n is a nondecreasing function that is mapping the interval $(0, 1)$. Therefore, when random value γ is sampled, θ_{rnd}^{exp} is determined by setting $F_n = \xi$.

The Mie phase function can be tabulated and treated in the same way as the experimental phase function.[164] In most cases azimuthal symmetry is assumed. This leads to $p(\phi) = 1/2\pi$ and, consequently, $\phi_{rnd} = 2\pi\xi$. At each step, the photon loses part of its weight due to absorption: $W = W(1 - \Lambda)$, where Λ is the albedo of the medium.

When the photon reaches the boundary, part of its weight is transmitted according to the Fresnel equations. The amount transmitted through the boundary is added to the reflectance or transmittance. Since the refraction angle is determined by Snell's law, the angular distribution of the out-going light can be calculated. The photon with the remaining part of the weight is specularly reflected and continues its random walk.

When the photon's weight becomes lower than a predetermined minimal value, the photon can be terminated using a "Russian roulette" procedure.[217,224] This procedure saves time, since it does not make sense to continue the random walk of the photon, which will not essentially contribute to the measured signal. On the other hand, it ensures that the energy balance is maintained throughout the simulation process.

The MC method has several advantages over the other methods because it may take into account mismatched medium-glass and glass-air interfaces, losses of light at the edges of the sample, any phase function of the medium, and the finite size and arbitrary angular distribution of the incident beam. If the collimated transmittance is measured, then the contribution of scattered light into the measured collimated signal can be accounted for.[665] The only disadvantage of this method is the long time needed to ensure good statistical convergence, since it is a statistical approach. The standard deviation of a quantity (diffuse reflectance, transmittance, etc.) approximated by the MC technique decreases proportionally to $1/\sqrt{N}$, where N is the total number of launched photons.

Values of coefficients μ_a, μ_s, and g for the human brain, canine prostate, and porcine liver at 800 and 1064 nm as well as μ_a and μ_s spectra at 350–1050 nm for some strongly scattering eye tissues (sclera, retina) obtained by the IMC method from *in vitro* reflection and transmission measurements have been reported in Refs. 650 and 662 (some of these data for human tissues are presented in Table 2.1). It is worthy of note that stable operation of the algorithm was maintained by generation of from 10^5 to 5×10^5 photons per iteration. Two to five iterations were usually necessary to estimate the optical parameters with approximately 2% accuracy. The computer time required can be reduced not only by the condensed IMC method but also by means of graphical solutions of the inverse problem following a preliminary MC simulation.[369,681–683]

In general, *in vivo* μ_a and μ_s' values for human skin proved to be significantly smaller than those obtained *in vitro* (about 10 and 2 times, respectively).[228,236–238,572] For μ_a, the discrepancy may be attributed to the low sensitivity of the double-integrating sphere, and goniometric techniques have been applied for *in vitro* measurements at weak absorption combined with strong scattering ($\mu_a \ll \mu_s$) and sample preparation methods. For μ_s', the discrepancy may be related to the strong dependence of the method on variations in the relative refractive index of scatterers and the ground medium of the tissue m, $\mu_s' \sim (m - 1)^2$, which can be quite different for living and sampled tissue.[179,681] *Ex vivo* measurements using the single-integrating sphere "comparison" technique, the corresponding IMC model, and very carefully prepared human skin samples allow for accurate evaluation of μ_a and μ_s' that are very close to *in vivo* measurements[236–238] (see Table 2.1). This technique has the advantage over the conventional double-sphere method in that no corrections are required for the sphere properties, and measurements are therefore sufficiently accurate to recover the absorption coefficient reliably.

2.6 Spatially resolved and OCT techniques

For many tissues, *in vivo* measurements are possible only in the geometry of the backscattering. The spatially resolved reflectance $R(r_{sd})$ is defined as the power of the backscattered light per unit of area detected by a receiver at the surface of the tissue at a distance r_{sd} from the source. $R(r_{sd})$ depends on the optical properties of the sample, i.e., the absorption coefficient μ_a, the scattering coefficient μ_s, and the phase function $p(\theta)$, the refractive index, and the NA of the receiving system.[683,685] The corresponding relation for the backscattering intensity as a function of source and detector positions and optical parameters can be written on the basis of a diffusion approximation. For a semi-infinite medium and source and detector probes (for instance, optical fibers) separated by a distance r_{sd} and normally oriented to the sample surface, the reflecting flux is given by[685]

$$R = \frac{z_0 A}{2\pi} \left[\frac{\mu_{eff}}{r_{sd}^2 + z_0^2} + \frac{1}{(r_{sd}^2 + z_0^2)^{3/2}} \right] \exp\left[-\mu_{eff} (r_{sd}^2 + z_0^2)^{1/2} \right], \qquad (2.17)$$

where $z_0 = K/\mu_s'$ is the extrapolation length, K is a dimensionless constant with a magnitude that depends on the anisotropy parameter of the scatterers and the reflection coefficient at the surface, A is the area of detector, and μ_{eff} is defined by Eq. (1.18).

The measurement of the intensity of a back-reflected light from a tissue for different source-detector separations r_{sd} is the basis of the spatially resolved technique, which allows one to evaluate the absorption and the scattering coefficients using, for example, the analytical expression (2.17), valid for highly scattering thick tissues.

When optical parameters of skin or mucosa are under investigation, the small source-detector separations should be used, where the diffusion approximation is not valid due to the proximity to the tissue boundary.[46,47,93,94,170,180,228,572,620,654, 681–683,686,692,695,731–735] In that case, more sophisticated approximations of the RTE solution should be employed; in particular, a numerical solution of the inverse problem by the MC method is prospective. For example, the authors of Ref. 655 studied the parameters of the spatial distribution of radiation transmitted through a tissue (halfwidth, etc.) while the condensed IMC method was employed in Ref. 228 to process *in vivo* estimates of radiation reflected from a tissue that were obtained with the aid of a special sensor consisting of two light diodes (660 and 940 nm) and three spaced photodetectors. Such a spatially resolved reflectance technique can also be implemented using multifiber probes with a number of fixed source-detector separations[572] or using a CCD with a special optical system,[46,93] allowing for the depth profiling of the optical properties of tissue if enough fibers or pixels are employed. For example, in Ref. 572, a fiber-optical probe with one signal and nine detecting 600-μm core diameter fibers with an averaged interfiber distance of 1.7 mm was used for the *in vivo* study of the optical properties of human skin in the wide spectral range of 400–1050 nm. The CCD system described in Refs. 46 and 93 provides absolute diffuse reflectance measurements when the reflectance images are referenced to images of the incident beam using a mirror. Such internal calibration leads to about three times less uncertainty in the determined absorption and reduced scattering coefficients in comparison with the usually used relative measurements. This system also provides copolarized and cross-polarized measurements of the back reflectance relative to the linear polarization of the incident light. The light-guiding effect for muscle tissue was determined on the basis of polarization measurements.

The effective endoscopic fiber-optic system and the optimized algorithm for the automatic spectral determination of tissue optical properties locally and superficially were recently described.[683] The optical probe was made of 11 optical fibers, one for illumination and ten for detection [see Fig. 2.4(e)]. The fibers used had an NA of 0.22 and a core diameter of 0.2 mm. The ten detecting fibers were placed at various distances (noted as ρ_i, $i = 1$–10, $\rho \equiv r_{sd}$) from the illumination fiber, ranging approximately from 0.3 to 1.35 mm with a step of approximately 0.1 mm.

To provide the absolute reflectance spectra recording, a two-step calibration procedure was performed. First, the effect of the spectral responses of the light source, fibers, grating, and detector was corrected by performing a measurement on a spectrally flat reflectance standard using an integrating sphere made of Spectralon. Second, the effective source intensity was obtained by performing a series of measurements on a solid turbid siloxane phantom with known scattering and absorption properties.

The model developed for extraction of tissue optical parameters from the spatially resolved measurements takes into account the specific influence of the phase function, does not require any assumption about the optical properties of the tissue, and could accommodate more complex models that account for multilayer geometries.[683,687] The accuracy of the evaluated optical properties depends significantly on the phase function used, when the reflectance measurements close to the light source are provided.[683,686] The phase function $p(\theta)$ can be expanded into a series of Legendre polynomials $P_n^1(\cos \theta)$ [see Eq. (2.7)]. The received expression contains as the coefficients the different order moments of the phase function

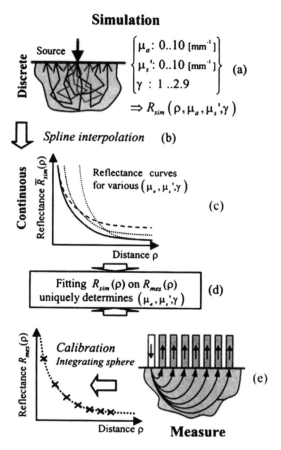

Figure 2.4 Diagram of the algorithm for the automatic spectral determination of tissue optical properties. (a) First, a set of reflectance curves simulated by the MC method is produced for a wide range of discrete values for each optical coefficient [i.e., μ_a, μ'_s, and $\gamma = (1 - g_2)/(1 - g_1)$]. (b) Second, the simulated curves are interpolated by cubic B-splines to provide a reflectance curve (c) for any value of μ_a, μ'_s, and γ. Finally, for each wavelength of the spectrum, a fit (d) of the measured reflectance curve (e) is performed onto the interpolated set of simulated curves, allowing for the determination of μ_a, μ'_s, and γ. The fitting method used is the Levenberg–Marquardt algorithm.[683]

ranged from unity to infinity, g_n, where g_1 is the conventional anisotropy factor, generally noted as g.

The diffusion approximation generally holds for $\mu'_s \rho > 5$ and $\mu'_s > 100\mu_a$. For shorter source-detector separations, typically when $0.5 < \mu'_s \rho < 5$, the second moment of the phase function g_2 must also be accounted for.[688] It can be shown that besides the refractive index, only three parameters are needed to accurately describe the light propagation at such small source-detector distances: μ_a, μ'_s, and γ, where

$$\gamma = \frac{1 - g_2}{1 - g_1} \tag{2.18}$$

and γ depends on the scatterers' relative refractive index and on the ratio between the scattering size and the wavelength; γ varies between 0.9 (Rayleigh-type scattering) and values larger than 2 (large scatterers compared to wavelength). For a Henyey-Greenstein phase function, $g_2 = (g_1)^2$ and, therefore, $g = g_1 = \gamma - 1$.[683] The authors of Ref. 683 showed that for fractal distribution, γ is related to the fractal power of the size distribution of the scatterers.

Approximately 40 discrete values were chosen by the authors of Ref. 683 for μ_a and μ_s', ranging, respectively, from 0.003 to 10 mm^{-1} and from 0.5 to 10 mm^{-1}; 20 values were chosen for γ, ranging from 1.0 to 2.9. This resulted in a four-dimensional matrix of simulated reflectance curves, noted as $R_{\text{sim}}(\rho_i, \mu_a, \mu_s', \gamma)$, each coefficient taking only discrete values [see Fig. 2.4(a)]. Using these parameters, 32,000 reflectance curves have been computed, each for a specific triplet of optical coefficients (μ_a, μ_s', γ). Since the path lengths and exit positions of each simulated photon were stored, a full MC simulation was required only for each different value of γ (thus, only 20 simulations). Assuming the tissue is homogeneous, scaling relationships allow one to derive any reflectance curve $R_{\text{sim}}(\rho_i, \mu_a, \mu_s', \gamma)$ from a single simulation $R_{\text{sim}}(\rho_i, \mu_a = 0, \mu_s' = 1, \gamma)$, γ being kept constant.[683]

Clinical measurements performed endoscopically *in vivo* in the stomach of human subjects were provided using the described technique and algorithm.[683] The absorption and scattering properties were found to be significantly different in the antrum and in the fundus (see Table 2.1) and were correlated with histopathologic observations.

In the six-detector fiber system made of 0.4-mm core diameter optical fiber that is described in Ref. 681, typical source-detector distances were: $r_{\text{sd}} = 0.44, 0.78, 0.92, 1.22, 1.40$, and 1.84 mm. The authors performed MC simulations using a program provided by Jacques.[684] In the course of their *in vivo* studies, temperature dependences of the absorption and the reduced scattering coefficients of human forearm skin were determined (see Table 2.1).

Another six-detector fiber system made of 0.2-mm core diameter optical fiber with the following range of the source-detector separations: 0.23, 0.67, 1.12, 1.57, 2.01, and 2.46 mm, and a corresponding algorithm based on the MC simulation of light propagation and multivariate calibration models using a feed-forward artificial neural network or partial least-squares procedures were applied to the determination of optical properties in highly attenuating tissue.[682] An absolute accuracy of the scattering and absorption coefficients' determination, respectively, on the level of ± 2 and ± 3 cm^{-1} (rms) was achieved. The method was applied to estimation of the optical properties of *ex vivo* bovine liver samples. The absorption and scattering coefficients, determined as $\mu_a = 14.5 \pm 3.5$ cm^{-1} and $\mu_s' = 7.2 \pm 3.7$ cm^{-1} at 543 nm, and $\mu_a = 4.7 \pm 1.7$ cm^{-1} and $\mu_s' = 6.7 \pm 3.4$ cm^{-1} at 633 nm, are favorably compared with the limited and varied data in the literature.

One more example of the back-reflectance method is tissue probing with an oblique laser beam. A simple analytical formula for the linear shift of the center of maximum diffuse reflection from the point of beam incidence Δx has been suggested to facilitate the evaluation of the optical parameters of the medium as[670,671,736]

$$\Delta x = \frac{\sin \alpha_i}{n(\mu_s' + 0.35\mu_a)}, \tag{2.19}$$

where α_i, is the incidence angle of the beam, n is the relative mean refractive index of the scattering medium, and $\mu_s' \gg \mu_a$. The relative index of refraction is unity for a matched boundary.

It was demonstrated that spectral dependencies of the absorption and reduced scattering coefficients can be easily obtained with this method, with an accuracy of 10–17% and 5–6%, respectively.[670] Oblique-incidence reflectometry has also been implemented with optical fibers in the same way as the normal-incidence reflectometry described above.[671] White light was delivered, and the diffusely reflected light was collected with a fiber-optic probe made from black derlin and 600-μm core diameter, low-loss optical fiber. The source fiber was oriented at a 45-deg angle of incidence, and the nine collection fibers, arranged in a linear array, collected the diffusely reflected light. This probe was sensitive for the anisotropy in the absorption and reduced-scattering coefficients, which is related to the structural anisotropy in the tissue caused, for instance, by the alignment of muscle fibers. The lower absorption coefficient at a 0-deg probe orientation (with respect to the muscle fibers) than that at 90 deg was probably caused by the light-guiding effect of the muscle fibers, which are less absorbing than the space between the muscle fibers, which is occupied by blood capillaries of great absorption.[736]

Two precise optical systems, the fiber-optic spectrometer yielding spatially resolved back-reflectance spectra and the single-wavelength fiber-optic-CCD tissue imager, were used for *in vivo* measurements of anisotropy of scattering and absorption coefficients of human skin at different body locations.[692] The source-detector distances between 0.33 and 10.0 mm for 18 detecting 200-μm core diameter fibers linearly aligned with a central illuminating fiber provided a 2D mapping of reflected intensity by rotation of the detecting fiber system around the illuminating fiber. A video reflectometry system consisted of a photometric fiber-coupled CCD system in direct contact with the skin, and a central optical illumination fiber delivering 810-nm laser light from a laser diode into the tissue. The images acquired consisted of 1024^2 pixels of 24 μm^2. A 16-bit analog-to-digital converter was used with the CCD chip to provide the high dynamic range needed for reflectometry. The MC code accounting for a two-layered tissue model (skin itself and a semi-infinite subcutaneous fat layer) with two groups of scatterers, one of randomly distributed scatterers and another of infinite dielectric cylinders (dermal collagen fibers) aligned along one of the principle Cartesian axes parallel to the skin surface, was designed to evaluate scattering and absorption coefficients distributions. In the skin layer, the scattering coefficient was recalculated before each interaction event according to the current direction of photon propagation as[692]

$$\mu_s = \mu_{s0}[1 + f(0.5 - |\cos \psi|)], \tag{2.20}$$

where μ_{s0} is a base scattering coefficient, f is the fraction of scatterers oriented in the preferential direction, and ψ is the angle between the current photon direction and the cylinder axis.

Optical coherence tomography (OCT)[1,3,8,13,17,18,76,77,84,102,108–111,116,127,129, 135,139,142] is a newly developed modality that allows one to evaluate the scattering and absorption properties of tissue *in vivo* within the limits of an OCT penetration depth of 1–3 mm.[13,711–713,716–718,720,721] The principles and applications of OCT are described in detail in Chapters 4 and 9. The use of OCT to measure the single-scattering coefficient of tissues μ_s has been described by Schmitt et al. in 1993.[13] In its simplest form, this method assumes that backscattered light from a tissue decreases in intensity according to[720,737]

$$I_b \cong I_0 \exp[-2(\mu_a + \mu_s)z], \qquad (2.21)$$

where $(\mu_a + \mu_s)$ is the total attenuation coefficient and $2z$ is the round-trip distance of light backscattered at a depth z. For most tissues in the NIR, $\mu_a \ll \mu_s$; thus, μ_s can be estimated roughly as

$$\mu_s \cong \frac{1}{2z\{\ln[I_b(z)/I_0]\}} \qquad (2.22)$$

or as the gradient of a graph $\ln[I_b(z)/I_0]$ versus z. Experimental data for tissue OCT images show that the logarithmically scaled average for multiple in-depth scans' backscattered intensity, $\ln[I_b(z)]$, decays exponentially; thus, by performing a linear regression on this curve, the scattering coefficient can be determined.[13] More comprehensive algorithms accounting for multiple scattering effects and properties of a small-angle scattering phase function are available in the literature.[711–713,716–718]

Using OCT, the directional anisotropy of tissue can be studied. Thus, using an OCT system working on 1300 nm, the authors of Ref. 720, for cortical bone tissue, found changes in the scattering coefficient at about 40% for a light beam perpendicular ($\mu_s = 28$ cm^{-1}) and parallel ($\mu_s = 20$ cm^{-1}) to the main direction of tissue striations. This result is qualitatively described by Eq. (2.20).

The values of absorption and scattering coefficients and scattering anisotropy factor for many of the human tissues measured *in vitro*, *ex vivo*, or *in vivo* and calculated using the discussed and some other approaches are presented in Table 2.1.

2.7 Direct measurement of the scattering phase function

Direct measurement of the scattering phase function $p(\theta)$ is important for the choice of an adequate model for the tissue being examined.[1,58,164,630,724,725] The scattering phase function is usually determined from goniophotometric measurements in relatively thin tissue samples.[1,37,56,58,87,96,221,222,227,228,232,255,630,657,658, 665,666,669,719,724,725] A typical goniometer setup is depicted in Fig. 2.5. The scattering indicatrix measured with due regard for the geometry of the sample and

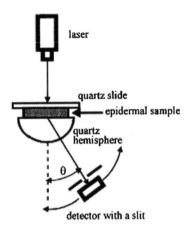

Figure 2.5 Schematic diagram of a goniometer for measurement of light scattering as a function of angle (scattering indicatrix measurement).[255]

experimental datum is approximated either by the Henyey-Greenstein phase function (HGPF)[1,31,255,724,725] [see Eq. (1.15)] or by a set of HGPFs, with each function characterizing the type of scatterers and specific contribution to the indicatrix [see Eq. (2.7)].[657] In the limiting case of a two-component model of a medium containing large and small (compared with the wavelength) scatterers, the indicatrix is represented in the form of anisotropic and isotropic components.[56,228,658] Other approximating functions are equally useful, e.g., those obtained from the Rayleigh-Gans approximation,[228] ensuing from Mie theory,[96,654,655] or a two-parameter Gegenbauer kernel phase function (GKPF) [HGPF is a special simpler case of this phase function, see Eq. (2.8)].[725] Some of these types of approximations were used to find the dependence of the scattering anisotropy factor g for dermis and epidermis on the wavelengths in the range 300 to 1300 nm, which proved to coincide fairly well with the empirical formula[37]

$$g_e \sim g_d \sim 0.62 + \lambda \times 0.29 \times 10^{-3}, \qquad (2.23)$$

on the assumption of a 10% contribution of isotropic scattering (at least in the spectral range of 300–630 nm). The wavelength λ is given in nanometers.

Analysis of scattering indicatrices measured for sequentially stripped human-skin-epidermal slices has demonstrated that the g value averaged over five epidermal slices is $g = 0.89 \pm 0.02$ at $\lambda = 633$ nm.[255] The measurements have been performed using the setup presented in Fig. 2.5. A single-mode He:Ne laser was used as a light source. The detector was a photon-counting system based on the photomultiplier. The whole system was computer controlled. The epidermal sample was placed between a quartz slide and a hemisphere in order to avoid refraction of both incident and scattered lights. The measurements were performed in the range 0–60 deg with one-degree steps. The experimental values of the anisotropy factor g obtained using direct measurements of the scattering phase function for many types of human tissues are presented in Table 2.1.

It should be noted that the correct prediction of light transport in tissues depends on the exact form of the phase function used for calculations.[49,725] Simulations performed with different forms of $p(\theta)$ (HGPF, Mie, and GKPF) with the same value of $\langle \cos(\theta) \rangle$ result in the collection of significantly different fractions of the incident photons, particularly when small numerical-aperture delivery and collection fibers (small source-detection separation) are employed.[49,725] More photons are collected for the distribution that has a higher probability of scattering events with $\theta > 125$ deg. For the clinically relevant optical parameters employed in Ref. 49, the differences in light collection were more than 60%.

Moreover, for media with high anisotropy factors, precise measurements of the scattering phase function in the total angle range from 0 to 180 deg is a difficult technical task that demands an extremely large dynamic range of measuring equipment. Most of the scattered radiation lies in the range from 0 to 30 deg, counting from the direction of the incident beam. In addition, measurements at angles close to 90 deg are strongly affected by scattering of higher orders, even for samples of moderate optical thickness.[442]

2.8 Estimates of the optical properties of human tissue

The above-discussed methods and techniques were successfully applied for estimation of optical properties of a wide number of tissues. Measurements done *in vitro*, *ex vivo*, and *in vivo* by different research groups are summarized in Table 2.1. Evidently, many types of animal and human tissues may have very close optical properties, but some specificity is expected. For example, normal bovine sclera is more pigmented, thicker, and its collagen structure makes it more sensitive to swelling than human sclera. Another example is porcine skin, whose epidermis structure may be quite different from human skin, particularly for aged skin. Therefore, in the Table 2.1 optical parameters of only human tissues are presented. On the other hand, human and animal tissues such as muscle, vessel wall tissue, and liver may have very similar optical properties. Thus, another reason to present only human tissues is not to overburden the table. Early published data on optical properties of both human and animal tissues are summarized in Refs. 40, 87, 691, and 696. More recent data can be found in Refs. 98, 129, 130, 164, 236–238, 263, 572, 655, 656, 672–689, 691–697, and 699–708.

Data presented in Table 2.1 reflect well the situation in the field of tissue optical parameters measurements. It is clearly seen that the major attention was paid to female breast and head/brain optical properties investigations because of great importance and perspectives of optical mammography, and optical monitoring and treatment of mental diseases. Skin and underlying tissues are also well studied. Nevertheless, in general, not many data for optical transport parameters are available in the literature. Moreover, these data are dependent on the tissue preparation technique, sample storage procedure, applied measuring method and inverse problem-solving algorithm, measuring instrumentation noise, and systematic errors.

The most detailed *in vitro* investigations of normal and coagulated brain tissues (gray matter, white matter, cerebellum, pons, and thalamus), as well as of native tumor tissues (astrocytoma WHO grade II and meningioma), using single-integrating-sphere spectral measurements in the spectral range from 360 to 1100 nm and IMC algorithm for data processing are described in Ref. 264 (see Table 2.1). As it follows from Table 2.1, all brain tissues under study shared qualitatively similar dependencies of the optical properties on the wavelength. The scattering coefficient decreased and the anisotropy factor increased with the wavelength, which can be explained by the lowering of the contribution of Rayleigh scattering and growing of the contribution of Mie scattering with the wavelength. The wavelength-dependent absorption coefficient behavior of all brain tissues resembled a mixture of oxy- and deoxy-hemoglobin absorption spectra. This means that in spite of careful sample preparation, it was not possible to remove all blood residuals from the tissue sections.

At the same time, the differences in the spectral characteristics of brain tissues have been observed. For example, the total attenuation coefficients ($\mu_t = \mu_a + \mu_s$) of white matter are substantially higher than those of gray matter. The two brain stem tissues (pons and thalamus) also have different optical properties. The tumors are generally macroscopically less homogeneous than any normal tissues; thus, their scattering coefficients and anisotropy factors are slightly higher than those of normal gray matter. The same tendency of scattering coefficients growing is typical for breast tumors (carcinomas, see Table 2.1 and Refs. 660 and 699).

After coagulation, the values of the absorption and scattering coefficients increased for all tissues. The extent of this increase, however, is different for each tissue type, and is characterized by factors from 2 to 5. It was shown[264] that a significant increase of both interaction coefficients is a result of substantial structure changes, caused mostly by tissue shrinkage and condensation, as well as collagen swelling and homogenization of the vessel walls. Tissue shrinkage caused by losing water at coagulation makes tissue more dense, which leads to increases of both scattering and absorption coefficients in the spectral range where water absorption is weak (up to 1100–1300 nm). The refractive index microscopic redistribution of a tissue due to cellular and fiber proteins' denaturation and homogenization at thermal action also may have a strong inclusion in alteration of scattering and absorption properties. The similar increase of both absorption (by a factor of 2–10) and scattering (by a factor of 2–4) coefficients in the wavelength range from 500 to 1100 nm was found for coagulated human blood.

The reduced scattering coefficient of skull bone is considerably less than that of brain white matter and is comparable with that of gray matter, cerebellum, and brain stem tissues. It is also comparable with scalp tissue values. At coagulation of soft brain tissues, their reduced scattering coefficient may considerably exceed that of skull bone for all tissues presented in Table 2.1. This would imply that in NIR spectroscopy on the adult head, the effect of light scattering by the skull is of the same order of magnitude as that of surrounding scalp tissue and brain.[719] A possible reason for this is the high values of scattering anisotropy factor *g* due to the specific structure of bone. For example, cortical bone consists of an underlying matrix of collagen fibers, around which calcium-bearing hydroxyapatite crystals are deposited. These crystals are the major scatterers of bone;[720] they are big in size and have a high refraction power, and therefore may be responsible for the high values of g. Actually, the optical properties of bone samples taken from pig skull and measured using the goniophotometric technique of thin bone slices over the wavelength range 650–950 nm gave values of anisotropy factor in the range from $g = 0.925 \pm 0.014$ at 650 nm to $g = 0.945 \pm 0.013$ at 950 nm, averaged for six samples.[719] The corresponding values of the absorption and of the scattering coefficients measured on 18 samples using the integrating sphere technique and IMC were: $\mu_a = 0.40 \pm 0.02$ cm^{-1} and $\mu_s = 350 \pm 7$ cm^{-1} at 650 nm to $\mu_a = 0.50 \pm 0.02$ cm^{-1} and $\mu_s = 240 \pm 6$ cm^{-1}.

Analyzing data received by different groups for the same brain tissue, the influence of the theoretical approach used or the sample preparation technique on results can be demonstrated. Because of a lack of experimental data for various brain tissues, at present, such a comparison can be done only for gray and white brain matter (see Table 2.1). The authors of Ref. 264, by using the IMC method for data processing of single-integrating sphere measurements, have obtained lower values for the absorption and scattering coefficients than the author of Ref. 698, who used an inverse δ-Eddington method. This discrepancy may be explained by limitations of the δ-Eddington model, which is principally one-dimensional and therefore could not account for the losses of light at the side edges of the samples. This might have led to an overestimation of the extinction coefficients. On the other hand, in the framework of the application of identical theoretical approaches (IMC), the usage of shock freezing and homogenization for sample preparation[697] in comparison with the usage of tissue cryosections[264] gives lower values of scattering coefficients, at least for white brain matter. The same tendency was also demonstrated for liver samples[697] and for breast tissue (compare data of Refs. 660 and 699 in Table 2.1).

The ten-sphere discrete particle model of a soft tissue indicates that the scattering coefficient decreases with the wavelength approximately as $\mu_s \sim \lambda^{2-D_f}$ for $600 \leq \lambda \leq 1400$ nm, where D_f is the limiting fractal dimension; $3 < D_f < 4$ for typical soft tissues.[156] In the model of spheres ranging from 5 nm to 30,000 nm, at an interval of 5 nm, $\mu_s \sim \lambda^{3-D_f}$ for $600 \leq \lambda \leq 1500$ nm and the range of fractal dimension is $4 < D_f < 5$.[107] Both models give the same power law for dependence of the scattering (or reduced scattering) coefficient on the wavelength $\mu_s(\mu_s') = q\lambda^{-h}$, with h in the range from 1 to 2 [see Eqs. (1.178)–(1.181)]. As it follows from the data of Tables 1.5 and 2.1, most tissues such as aorta, skin, *dura mater*, sclera, and mucosa have parameter $h = 1.16$–1.62,[569,570,703,704,706] which satisfies the model's predictions. The corresponding values of fitting parameter q are in the range from 8.9×10^4 to 4.7×10^5 cm^{-1}. An *in vitro* study of rat skin in the range from 500 to 1200 nm gave $h = 1.12$.[571] For soft tissues, Jacques modeled the reduced scattering coefficient by the same power law with q ranging from 2×10^5 cm^{-1} to 2×10^6 cm^{-1} and $h = 1.5$.[710] The experimental data for *ex vivo* skin samples of

Ref. 677 in the spectral range from 1000 to 2200 nm (with exclusion of dispersion of the strong water bands) are better modeled using a value q equal to 2×10^5 for $h = 1.5$. For the *in vivo* backscattering investigation of human skin and underlying tissues in the wavelength range from 700 to 900 nm, constants q and h were determined as 550 ± 11 and 1.11 ± 0.08, respectively.[572] The power constant h is related to an averaged size of the scatterers; thus, once h is determined, the Mie equivalent radius a_M can be derived from Eqs. (1.180) and (1.181).[572] If the relative refractive index between spheres and surrounding medium is $m = 1.037$, the measured constant $h = 1.11$ leads to an a_M value of 0.30 μm. Diffuse reflectance measurements for female breast tissues gave an a_M value of 0.17 μm for normal tissue and of 0.29 μm for malignant tissue (see Table 2.1).[699]

In contrast to the above-discussed tissues, fat and bone tissue show very low values of the power constant: $h = 0.59$ for abdominal[705] and $h = 0.79$[705] or $h = 0.68$[726] for subcutaneous fat, and $h = 0.65$ for bone.[738,739] One of the possible reasons for this is the specificity of fat and bone tissue structure. Fat consists mostly of fat cells; each fat cell contains a smooth drop of fat, which fills up a whole cell. Cells are spherically shaped and their diameters depend on fat content, and are in the range from 10 to 200 μm. For such big and rather homogeneous scatterers, a weak wavelength dependence of light scattering coefficients might be expected. It is similar for bone, where hydroxyapatite crystals, the major scatterers, are big in size and have a high refraction power.[720]

Another reason for lower h is the possible influence of dispersion of lipids and water bands (see Fig. 1.5), which should decrease the inclination of the wavelength dependence in the range around 1000–1300 nm.

A decrease in h from 1.12 to 0.52 for rat skin studied *in vitro* in the range from 500 to 1200 nm induced by glycerol application was found.[571] Because the major action of glycerol on tissue is its dehydration causes increase of tissue density, this may be a third reason for such small values of power constant h for fat and bone, being rather dense tissue and having the lowest hydration ability amongst a variety of tissues.

A low power dependence on the wavelength was also found for the scattering coefficient of leg bone of the horse (only the cortical part of equine bone taken from the shaft of the third metacarpal of 2-mm thickness) measured using a single-integrating sphere and IMC techniques.[720] In the wavelength range from 520 to 960 nm, values of the scattering coefficient were changed from 350 to 250 cm^{-1} for the constant value of $g = 0.93$ supposed in the calculations.

2.9 Determination of optical properties of blood

Fresh human blood placed in a calibrated thin cuvette (thickness from 0.01 to 0.5 mm, slab geometry) is usually used for the determination of blood optical parameters. Prior to the optical measurements, standard clinical tests are necessary to determine the concentration of red and white blood cells, concentration of platelets, hematocrit, mean corpuscular volume and hemoglobin, and the other parameters of interest. If blood sample oxygenation level is of interest, it may be controlled using a conventional blood gas analyzer.[164] In most cases, the experiments are performed with either completely oxygenated or completely deoxygenated blood.[48,164,724,729,730] To obtain complete oxygen saturation, the sample is exposed to air or O_2.[48,164] To completely deoxygenate the blood, sodium dithionite ($Na_2S_2O_4$) is added.[164] To be sure that neither the volume nor the surface area of the blood particles changes during the experiments, the pH of the samples should be maintained in the range of physiological values, at approximately 7.4.

In reality, blood is flowing through the blood vessels and it is therefore preferable to study the optical properties of flowing blood. The RBCs in flow are subject to deformation and orientation. At lower shear rates, reversible aggregation occurs; while under the higher shear rates, erythrocytes are deformed into ellipsoids. The experiments with flowing undiluted and diluted blood are reported in Refs. 48, 49 and 689. Roggan et al.[48] have assembled sophisticated equipment to analyze the influence of different hematocrit, flow velocity, osmolarity, hemolysis, and oxygen saturation on the optical properties of RBC suspensions submerged in a saline solution. Nilsson et al.[49] investigated the influence of slow heating on the optical properties of whole flowing blood. The influence of the shear stress on the optical properties of whole completely oxygenated blood was studied by Steenbergen et al.[689]

Several authors reported the values of the optical parameters of blood determined from the single scattering experiments (Table 2.2). Reynolds et al.[740] determined values of the absorption cross section, the scattering cross section, and the anisotropy factor of blood for a number of wavelengths in the visible and near-infrared spectral range, and compared the experimental values with the calculated (Mie theory) ones. In Mie calculations, they used the value of 2.79 μm for the RBC radius, and the value of 1.036 for the RBC refractive index (relative to blood plasma).[183,740]

Flock et al.[690] measured the total attenuation coefficient and the scattering phase function of a diluted whole blood sample [phosphate buffered saline solution (PBS), hematocrit (Hct) of 1%, cuvette < 100-μm thick] at a wavelength of 632.8 nm.

Steinke and Shepherd[741] determined the total attenuation coefficients, the scattering cross sections and the anisotropy factors of RBCs suspended in blood plasma and in PBS (0.9%) from the collimated transmittance and scattering phase function measurements for a wavelength of 632.8 nm, and from the calculations using Mie theory. For measurements of collimated transmittance, cuvettes with a thickness of 144 μm (slab geometry) were used. For the goniometrical measurements, an American Optical Hemoglobinometer cuvette (path length 51 μm) was employed.

Yaroslavsky et al.[164,724] measured the scattering phase functions of diluted whole blood samples; approximated the experimental scattering phase functions using Mie theory, Henyey-Greenstein (HGPF), or Gegenbauer kernel (GKPF) functions [see Eqs. (1.15), (2.7), (2.8), and (2.10)]; and determined the anisotropy factors for each approximation at a wavelength of 633 nm. For Mie calculations,

Table 2.2 Optical parameters of blood determined and approximated from the single scattering experiments (S—oxygen saturation, Hct—hematocrit, a_{RBC}—radius of RBC, m_{RBC}—relative index of refraction of RBC, l_{cuv}—cuvette thickness).[725]

λ, nm	S, %	σ_a, μm²	σ_s, μm²	σ_t, μm²	μ_t, cm⁻¹	g	Phase function	Condition	Ref.
665	100	0.060	57.20		7.47	0.9951	Mie	Comparison with Mie theory; $a_{RBC} = 2.79$ μm; $m_{RBC} = 1.036$	740
675	100	0.060	56.14		7.44	0.9950			
685	100	0.059	55.09		7.39	0.9949			
955	100	0.191	33.47		6.66	0.9925			
960	100	0.187	33.18		6.66	0.9924			
965	100	0.185	32.90		6.65	0.9924			
665	0	0.542	56.58		7.38	0.9951			
675	0	0.535	55.53		7.35	0.9950			
685	0	0.484	54.56		7.31	0.9949			
955	0	0.090	33.54		6.68	0.9925			
960	0	0.085	33.27		6.67	0.9924			
965	0	0.080	32.98		6.66	0.9924			
630	100	0.099	56.37					Experiment	
660	100	0.066	54.20						
685	100	0.063	53.53						
800	100	0.131	42.24						
632.8	100				29	0.974	HGPF	Hct = 1%; $l_{cuv} < 100$ μm	690
632.8	100						Mie	$l_{cuv} = 144$ μm and 51 μm RBC in plasma	741
	100		63.82		7.09	0.9853			
	100		66.62		7.40	0.9948			
	100		81.24		9.03	0.9818		RBC in PBS (0.9%)	
	100		79.27		8.81	0.9926			

Table 2.2 (Continued).

λ, nm	S, %	σ_a, μm^2	σ_s, μm^2	σ_t, μm^2	μ_t, cm^{-1}	g	Phase function	Condition	Ref.
632.8	100					0.982	HGPF		724
	100					0.995	GKPF	($\alpha = 1.82$)	
632.8	100					0.971	HGPF	Hct = 0.1%; pH = 7.4; l_{cuv} = 10 μm ($\alpha = 3.658$)	164
	100					0.997	GKPF		
	100					0.996	Mie	a_{RBC} = 2.995 μm, m_{RBC} = 1.04	
577	100		≈ 95			0.966	HGPF	Hct = 1%; pH = 7.4; l_{cuv} = 100 and 10 μm ($\alpha = 1.5$)	730
	100					0.997	GKPF		
	100					0.997	Mie		
	100					0.9995	Rayleigh-Gans		

the RBC radius was assumed to be equal to 2.995 μm, and the RBC refractive index equal to 1.04 (relative to PBS). The scattering phase functions were measured in the angle range from 2 to 18 deg. For the experiments, fresh samples of whole blood were collected into heparinized containers and diluted with a phosphate buffer solution (pH = 7.4) to a Hct = 0.1%. The diluted blood samples were placed into the cuvettes (10-μm thick, slab geometry).

Hammer et al.[730] presented a comprehensive study of RBC single scattering behavior. The authors measured the collimated transmittance and the scattering phase functions of the RBC suspensions in isotonic PBS (pH = 7.4, Hct = 1%) for a number of wavelengths in the visible spectral range from 458 to 660 nm. The scattering phase functions were measured for 20 scattering angles in the range between 0.75 and 14.5 deg. For the transmission measurements, a cuvette with a thickness of 100 μm (slab geometry), and for the scattering phase function measurements, a cuvette with a thickness of 10 μm (slab geometry) were used.

The optical properties of the diluted and whole human blood, determined using indirect techniques, were reported by Yaroslavsky et al.,[164,724] Nilsson et al.,[49] Roggan et al.,[48] and Steenbergen et al.[689] A summary of the optical properties of diluted and whole blood determined using indirect techniques is given in Table 2.3.

The optical parameters of completely oxygenated whole blood samples were determined on a selected wavelength of 633 nm[164] and in the near-infrared spectral range[724] from double integrating sphere measurements using an inverse Monte Carlo technique (see Table 2.3). The measured values included the diffuse reflectance, the total transmittance, and the collimated transmittance. From the measured data, the absorption coefficient, the scattering coefficient, and the anisotropy factor (under the assumption of the Henyey-Greenstein phase function) were derived. In Ref. 164, blood samples with Hct = 38% and oxygen saturation $S > 98\%$ were studied. In Ref. 724, the spectral range investigated extended from 700 to 1200 nm and blood samples with Hct = 45.5 ± 0.5% placed into calibrated cuvettes (thickness 0.1 and 0.5 mm, slab geometry) were used. The spectral dependences of the optical parameters of whole blood obtained in Ref. 409 are presented in Fig. 2.6. In addition, the effect of the scattering phase function approximation on the resulting estimates of the optical parameters was analyzed.[164,724] The Henyey-Greenstein, Gegenbauer kernel, or Mie phase functions were considered [see Eqs. (1.15), (2.7), (2.8), and (2.10)]. The calculated angular distributions of scattered light were compared with goniophotometric measurements performed at a wavelength of 633 nm. The scattering phase functions of highly diluted blood samples (Hct = 0.1%, $S > 98\%$) were also measured using a goniophotometer. To evaluate the obtained data, the angular distributions of scattered light for optically thick samples were calculated and the results were compared with goniophotometric measurements. The data presented have shown that the employed approximation of the scattering phase function can have a substantial impact on the derived values of μ_s and g, while μ_a and the reduced scattering coefficient μ'_s are much less sensitive to the exact form of the scattering phase function. It was shown that both R_d and T_t are strongly affected by the form of the phase function, and that

Table 2.3 Overview of the optical properties of blood (*data taken from the graphs of the respective reference; Hct—hematocrit, S—oxygen saturation, a_{RBC}—radius of RBC, m_{RBC}—relative index of refraction of RBC, t_b—blood temperature, v_{sh}—shear rate, l_{cuv}—cuvette thickness).[725]

λ, nm	μ_a, cm⁻¹	μ_s, cm⁻¹	μ_t, cm⁻¹	g	μ_s', cm⁻¹	Phase function	Conditions	Ref.
633	15.5	645	—	0.982	11.6	HGPF	Hct = 45%, S > 98%	724
	15.4	2239	—	0.995	11.2	GKPF	α = 1.82	
633	15.2 ± 0.6	400 ± 30	—	0.971 ± 0.001	11.7 ± 1.2	HGPF	Hct = 38%, S > 98% 7 samples	164
	16.1 ± 0.6	4130 ± 170	—	0.997 ± 0.0001	12.4 ± 0.9	GKPF	α = 3.658	
	16.3 ± 0.5	2390 ± 160	—	0.9962 ± 0.0001		Mie	a_{RBC} = 2.995 μm m_{RBC} = 1.04	
633						HGPF	Hct = 44 ± 3%, S = 100%	49*
	3.0	—	—	—	18.5		t_b = 25°C	
	3.5	—	—	—	18.2		t_b = 35°C	
	4.0	—	—	—	18.0		t_b = 42°C	
	4.5	—	—	—	21.0		t_b = 48°C	
	6.0	—	—	—	17.0		t_b = 54°C	
633						GKPF	α = 1.0; Hct = 41%	48*
	20	—	—	—	20		S = 25%	
	16	—	—	—	20		S = 50%	
	12	—	—	—	20		S = 75%	
	7	—	—	—	18		S = 100%	
							α > 0.99, Hct = 5%	
	1.25	300	—	—	—		S = 0%	
	1.10	300	—	—	—		S = 100%	
633						HGPF	Hct = 50 ± 0.5% S = 100%	689*
		—	—	0.950–0.963	—		v_{sh} = 50 s⁻¹	
		—	—	0.956–0.965	—		v_{sh} = 100 s⁻¹	

Table 2.3 (Continued).

λ, nm	μ_a, cm^{-1}	μ_s, cm^{-1}	μ_t, cm^{-1}	g	μ_s', cm^{-1}	Phase function	Conditions	Ref.
	—	—	≈1200	—	—	0.960–0.966	$v_{sh}=150$ s^{-1}	
	—	—	≈1200	—	—	0.962–0.967	$v_{sh}=200$ s^{-1}	
	—	—	≈1200	—	—	0.963–0.968	$v_{sh}=300$ s^{-1}	
	—	—	≈1200	—	—	0.963–0.970	$v_{sh}=400$ s^{-1}	
	—	—	≈1200	—	—	0.964–0.973	$v_{sh}=500$ s^{-1}	
488	102.2	134.4	—	—	—	0.91	IAD, HGPF, $l_{cuv}=90$ μm	742

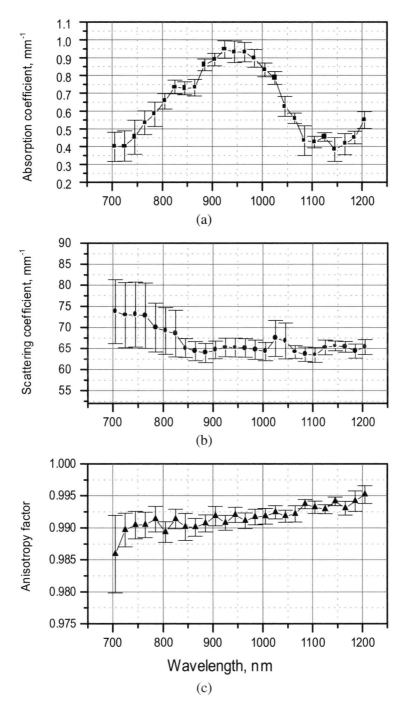

Figure 2.6 Optical properties of whole blood.[724,725] Hematocrit, Hct $= 45.5 \pm 0.5\%$; oxygen saturation, $S > 98\%$. Average of six samples. Bars are standard errors. (a) Absorption coefficient, (b) scattering coefficient, (c) anisotropy factor.

the magnitude of this influence depends on the thickness of the blood sample. The presented data prove that the variations of the employed scattering phase function approximation can cause large discrepancies in the derived optical parameters. Therefore, the exact knowledge of the scattering phase function is required for the precise determination of the blood optical constants.

Nilsson et al.[49] studied the influence of slow heating on the optical properties of completely oxygenated whole blood at a wavelength of 633 nm (Table 2.3). The diffuse reflectance, the total transmittance, and the collimated transmittance were measured at different temperatures using a double integrating sphere technique. The absorption coefficient, the scattering coefficient, and the anisotropy factor (assuming the Henyey-Greenstein phase function) were determined using an inverse adding-doubling method. For the measurements, whole blood was collected into tubes that contained ethylenediaminetetraacetic acid (EDTA) to prevent coagulation. The hematocrit of the investigated samples was $44 \pm 3\%$. During the measurements, the blood was pumped at a flow rate of 10.7 ml/min. The flow cell (length = 65 mm, height = 34 mm, total thickness = 2.5 mm) was placed between the integrating spheres. The blood sample thickness in the flow cell was 0.48 ± 0.02 mm. The blood was heated from approximately 25 to 55°C at rates between 0.2 and 1.1°C/min. While the blood was heated, the integrating sphere measurements were continuously taken. The authors found that changes in optical properties of blood due to slow heating were reversible until a temperature of 44.6–46.6°C. Coagulation of blood occurred at approximately 55°C.

One of the most extensive studies of the macroscopic optical properties of RBC suspension at different physiological and biochemical conditions (hematocrit, oxygen saturation, flow velocity, osmolarity, and hemolysis) were done by Roggan et al. (Table 2.3).[48] The authors measured the optical parameters of RBCs suspended in PBS under flow conditions using a double integrating sphere technique and determined optical coefficients using an inverse Monte Carlo method. The absorption coefficient, the scattering coefficient, and the anisotropy factor (assuming Gegenbauer kernel phase function with $\alpha = 1$) were determined for the oxygenated and deoxygenated RBC suspensions (Hct = 5%) under normal physiological conditions (see Fig. 2.7). For the experiments, erythrocytes were separated from the blood plasma and white cell fraction, washed in PBS (300 mosmol/l, pH = 7.4), and suspended in the PBS. The hematocrit was adjusted by diluting the erythrocytes with PBS. By using PBSs with different osmolarities, the osmolarity of the RBC suspension was varied. Hemolysis was induced by diluting the suspensions with distilled water. Blood oxygenation and circulation was adjusted and controlled using an extracorporal circulation unit. Blood temperature was kept constant at 20°C. The thickness of the flow-through cuvette was 97 μm.

Roggan et al.[48] have also come to the conclusion that an accurate approximation of the scattering phase function plays an important role in the correct determination of the optical properties of blood. It was found that absorption and scattering increased linearly with hematocrit (for Hct < 50%). Absorption and scattering decreased slightly with an increase of shear rate. Among the flow parameters, axial

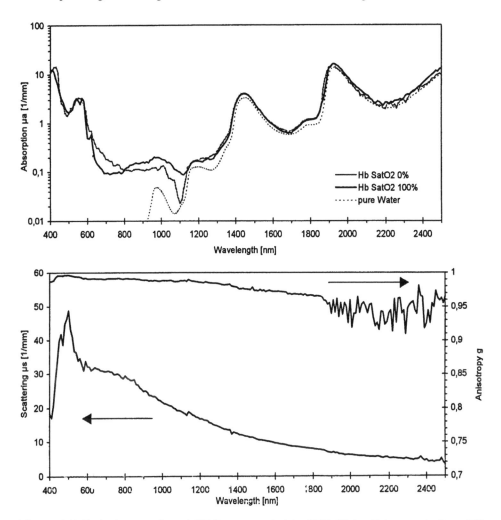

Figure 2.7 Optical properties of RBCs suspended in PBS (Hct = 5%, osmolarity = 300 mosmol/l, shear rate = 500 s^{-1}).[48]

migration was the main factor that influenced optical properties. Deformation of the erythrocytes had no impact on optical properties if the volume and hemoglobin content of the RBCs were kept constant. Hemoglobin solutions had a smaller absorption than RBC suspensions with the same concentration of hemoglobin. Obviously, the change in oxygenation of RBC suspensions induced the expected change in the absorption coefficient. The scattering coefficient was not affected by the change in the oxygenation of erythrocytes. The spectral dependences of the optical parameters of RBCs suspended in a PBS (Hct = 5%, shear rate = 500 s^{-1}, osmolarity = 300 mosmol/l) are given in Fig. 2.7.

Steenbergen et al.[689] analyzed the effect of shear rate on the optical properties of the completely oxygenated whole blood (Table 2.3). The collimated transmission and the angular distributions of light intensity were measured at 633 nm for various shear rates (from 50 to 500 s^{-1}) and blood layer thicknesses (from 20 to 100 μm). For shear rates above 150 s^{-1}, the total attenuation coefficient was determined directly from the collimated transmission measurements. The anisotropy factor was determined from the angular intensity distributions using an inverse Monte Carlo technique and assuming the Henyey-Greenstein scattering phase function. The value of the total attenuation coefficient ($\mu_t = 1200$ cm^{-1}) was determined from the collimated transmittance measurements, and the values of the absorption coefficient ($\mu_a = 7$ and 10 cm^{-1}) were taken from the literature.[48] In addition, the authors measured the anisotropy g-factor for blood layers with different thicknesses and determined the actual g-factor by extrapolating their results to the layer thickness of zero. The hematocrit of the investigated blood varied between 49.5 and 50.5%. A continuous increase of the g-factor (from 0.950 to 0.973) with an increase of shear rate was found.

The optical properties of blood-perfused tissues are significantly affected by tissue blood content. This is caused by two factors: first, the optical properties of whole blood itself are substantially different from those of soft tissues; and second, whole blood is an extremely turbid medium with an extraordinary high scattering anisotropy (see Tables 2.2 and 2.3). Thus, it has a very short optical mean free path and a very long transport mean free path compared to the majority of bloodless tissues. As a result, the presence of even a small amount of blood greatly changes the process of light propagation in tissues. This point is illustrated by Fig. 2.8, where the transport mean free path has been calculated for bloodless tissues and blood-containing brain tissues at two wavelengths.[666,725] Optical properties of other blood-containing tissues are affected in a similar manner. As a result, the optical response of tissue depends strongly on the presence of blood and on its relevant parameters such as oxygen saturation and hematocrit. This opens wide possibilities for optical diagnostics, but also makes the dosimetry of light in tissues a more difficult task.

Laser photodynamic therapy[19,26,29,35] and laser-induced interstitial thermal therapy (LITT) of deep tumors[2] are the most promising techniques among the least invasive therapies of cancer. In this case, besides the knowledge of the optical properties of tumor tissue and the surrounding substances, the knowledge of the blood content and its optical properties is essential for therapy planning and for exact dosimetry. In addition, knowledge of the optical properties of tissues and blood allows one to determine the most effective treatment wavelength, where the penetration depth of laser light is maximal. This emphasizes the need for an explicit account of the blood content in the modeling of laser-tissue interaction—for example, the planning of clinical procedures such as LITT or photodynamic therapy.

2.10 Measurements of tissue penetration depth and light dosimetry

In practice, the direct measurements of the penetration depth of various tissues at different wavelengths or at some specific wavelength are valuable. In partic-

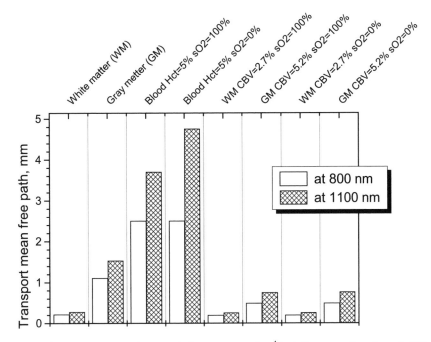

Figure 2.8 Transport mean free path $[l_t = (\mu_a + \mu'_s)^{-1}]$ at the wavelengths of 800 and 1100 nm for white brain matter (WM), gray brain matter (GM), oxygenated blood, deoxygenated blood, perfused white matter, and perfused gray matter.[725] These are based on the results of Refs. 48 and 666. A blood hematocrit of 40% was assumed in computing the data for perfused tissues. CBV—cerebral blood volume.

ular, such data allow one to provide a strategy of laser phototherapy. As shown earlier, a detailed calculation of light distribution in tissues can be very complex and frequently requires numerical solutions of the radiative transfer equation, Eq. (1.9). However, if a specific experimental arrangement is provided, i.e., a "wide" beam irradiation of "semi-infinite" samples, and light is scattered into a practically isotropic distribution very close to the irradiated surface, the one-dimensional diffusion model may be used, which gives the solution described by Eq. (1.30) valid for the depths $z \geq 2l_d = 2/\mu_{eff}$, where μ_{eff} is defined by Eq. (1.18).

Using an analog of Eq. (1.30) and providing measurements within thick tissue slabs at irradiation by a parallel laser beam 5-cm wide (at one of the wavelengths 633, 675, 780, or 835 nm) and light detecting by the measuring needle with an optic fiber inserted into a tissue sample, values of penetration depth were estimated for a number of normal and pathological tissues.[693] These data are summarized in Table 2.4. It should be noted that from the performed measurements, $l_d = 1/\mu_{eff}$ was determined. The detecting fiber tip captures an equal proportion of the fluence rate of light at every point from $z \geq 2l_d$ to greater tissue depths. Logarithmizing the detector response as a function of the position of the needle, z, and using the method of least squares, a fitted straight line was obtained, whose slope is the effective attenuation coefficient $\mu_{eff} = 1/l_d$ [see Eq. (1.30)].

Table 2.4 Optical penetration depth of tissues l_d in millimeters measured *ex vivo* for a few wavelengths. The number of samples from different bodies measured for each tissue is given in brackets ([a] standard error and [b] absolute mean deviation, for others error obtained by the method of least squares is presented).[693]

Tissue	l_d, mm $\lambda = 633$ nm	l_d, mm $\lambda = 675$ nm	l_d, mm $\lambda = 780$ nm	l_d, mm $\lambda = 835$ nm
Blood	0.19 ± 0.01^a (10)	0.28 ± 0.01^a (10)	0.42 ± 0.02^a (10)	0.51 ± 0.02^a (10)
Sarcomas	0.2–4.0 (10)	0.4–4.3 (6)	0.5–4.6 (6)	–
Liver (cirrhosis)	0.43 ± 0.06^b (5)	0.60 ± 0.02 (2)	1.04 ± 0.02 (2)	–
	–	0.58 ± 0.01	0.99 ± 0.02	–
Spleen	0.49 ± 0.07^b (5)	0.87 ± 0.02 (2)	1.21 ± 0.01 (2)	–
	–	0.94 ± 0.01	1.16 ± 0.02	–
Parotid gland	0.61 ± 0.08^b (3)	–	–	–
Bronchial ganglion metastasis	1.05 ± 0.01 (2)	–	–	–
	1.01 ± 0.01	–	–	–
Lung	0.81 ± 0.06^a (10)	1.09 ± 0.11^b (4)	1.86 ± 0.12^b (4)	2.47 ± 0.03 (1)
Bronchial cyst	1.05 ± 0.02 (2)	–	–	–
	0.97 ± 0.02	–	–	–
Cloquet ganglion metastasis	1.12 ± 0.01 (1)	–	–	–
Thyroid gland	1.23 ± 0.08^a (15)	1.42 ± 0.15^b (5)	1.70 ± 0.16^b (5)	3.04 ± 0.05 (1)
Neurilemoma	1.23 ± 0.02 (1)	–	–	–
Pelvic ganglion	1.39 ± 0.11^b (6)	1.42 ± 0.01 (2)	1.83 ± 0.02 (2)	2.32 ± 0.03 (1)
	–	1.45 ± 0.02	1.78 ± 0.02	–
Aggressive fibromatosis	1.41 ± 0.16^b (4)	1.54 ± 0.03 (2)	1.87 ± 0.02 (2)	–
	–	1.44 ± 0.03	1.77 ± 0.03	–
Hepatic metastasis	1.53 ± 0.15^b (5)	1.81 ± 0.21^b (3)	2.48 ± 0.30^b (3)	3.27 ± 0.03 (2)
	–	–	–	3.81 ± 0.03
Lung carcinoma	1.68 ± 0.15^b (7)	2.01 ± 0.27^b (3)	2.82 ± 0.31^b (3)	3.89 ± 0.03 (1)
Prelaryngeal striated muscle	1.72 ± 0.20^b (3)	–	–	–

Table 2.4 (Continued).

Tissue	l_d, mm $\lambda = 633$ nm	l_d, mm $\lambda = 675$ nm	l_d, mm $\lambda = 780$ nm	l_d, mm $\lambda = 835$ nm
Mammary fat	1.81 ± 0.09^a (10)	2.03 ± 0.18^b (6)	2.24 ± 0.19^b (6)	2.79 ± 0.28^b (3)
Mammary tissue	2.59 ± 0.18^a (14)	2.87 ± 0.30^b (5)	3.12 ± 0.32^b (5)	3.54 ± 0.40^b (3)
Mammary displasia	2.21 ± 0.20^b (9)	2.68 ± 0.29^b (3)	3.03 ± 0.33^b (3)	–
Mammary carcinoma	2.87 ± 0.22^a (10)	3.14 ± 0.36^b (3)	3.62 ± 0.41^b (3)	4.23 ± 0.04 (1)
Uterine mioma	2.74 ± 0.22^b (6)	2.93 ± 0.03 (1)	3.28 ± 0.03 (1)	–
Uterus	2.14 ± 0.18^a (15)	2.40 ± 0.22^b (4)	2.61 ± 0.25^b (4)	3.31 ± 0.02 (1)
Submaxillary gland	2.49 ± 0.23^b (3)	–	–	–
Malignant fibrous histiositoma	2.48 ± 0.03 (1)	–	–	–
Colon	2.48 ± 0.21^b (7)	2.73 ± 0.29^b (3)	2.91 ± 0.31^b (3)	–
Lipoma	2.83 ± 0.21^a (11)	3.03 ± 0.29^b (4)	3.71 ± 0.33^b (4)	4.19 ± 0.03 (1)
Mesenquinoma	4.01 ± 0.03 (1)	–	–	–
Axillar epidermoid carcinoma	2.12 ± 0.18^b (8)	2.51 ± 0.22^b (4)	2.64 ± 0.23^b (4)	3.24 ± 0.03 (1)
Liver (postmortem)	1.20 ± 0.13^a (10)	1.69 ± 0.16^a (10)	2.91 ± 0.30^a (10)	3.68 ± 0.35^a (10)
Brain (postmortem)	0.92 ± 0.08^a (10)	1.38 ± 0.13^a (10)	2.17 ± 0.16^a (10)	2.52 ± 0.19^a (10)
Muscle (postmortem)	1.47 ± 0.10^a (10)	1.63 ± 0.10^a (10)	3.46 ± 0.23^a (10)	3.72 ± 0.29^a (10)

The quantity usually measured in dosimetry is the irradiance $F(\bar{r})$ [see Eq. (1.11)], which is defined as the power per receiving area of a flat detector.[694] For this definition, light entering differently from perpendicular incidence contributes with reduced impact and light from below does not contribute at all. Light-induced tissue heating or any photobiological effect in tissue or cells depends on light absorption. For isotropic media, absorption is not sensitive to the angle of irradiation; thus, an adequate light dosimetric quantity should be the total radiant energy fluence rate $U(\bar{r})$ [see Eq. (1.12)] or the space irradiance, defined as the light power hitting a sphere divided by the sphere's cross section.[694] For an isotropic space distribution of light intensity, the space irradiance is four times the irradiance measured for the same point within the tissue $(\bar{r})$.

In Ref. 694, experimental data for the diffuse reflectance R_d and the collimated transmission T_c of an isolated bone specimen with a defined thickness d were used for the MC calculation of the transmitted irradiance $F(d)$ and its comparison with the space irradiance at the same point $U(d)$ inside a specimen of infinite thickness. Finally, the dosimetric correction factor U/F was evaluated. The results of dosimetric correction using *in vitro* experimental data and corresponding calculated data for human skull bone are presented in Table 2.5. The calculations of the absorption coefficient μ_a and the reduced scattering coefficient μ_s' from the measured R_d and T_c were performed by a simplified procedure valid for a thickness d of the bone with $\mu_{eff}d > 2$. In this case, $T_c = T_c^{eff} \exp(-\mu_{eff}d)$. As shown in Ref. 694, in good approximation, T_c^{eff}, R_d, and U/F depend only on the ratio μ_a/μ_s'. The knowledge of T_c^{eff} allows one to evaluate μ_{eff} from the equation for T_c and, furthermore, μ_a and μ_s' from Eq. (1.18) and the known ratio μ_a/μ_s'. All MC calculations were done for a tissue index of refraction $\bar{n} = 1.35$ and anisotropy factor $g = 0.8$.

2.11 Refractive index measurements

The mean refractive index $\bar{n}$ of a tissue is defined by the refractive indices of its scattering centers material n_s and ground (surrounding) matter n_0 [see Eqs. (1.150)–(1.154)]. The refractive index variation in tissues, quantified by the ratio $m \equiv n_s/n_0$, determines light scattering efficiency. For example, in a simple monodisperse tissue model, such as dielectric spheres of equal diameter $2a$, the reduced scattering coefficient is[179]

$$\mu_s' \equiv \mu_s(1 - g) = 3.28\pi a^2 \rho_s \left(\frac{2\pi a}{\lambda}\right)^{0.37} (m - 1)^{2.09}, \qquad (2.24)$$

where $\mu_s = \sigma_{sca}\rho_s$ is the scattering coefficient, σ_{sca} is the scattering cross section, ρ_s is the volume density of the spheres, g is the scattering anisotropy factor, and λ is the light wavelength in the scattering medium. This equation is valid for noninteracting Mie scatterers $g > 0.9$, $5 < 2\pi a/\lambda < 50$, and $1 < m < 1.1$.

For example, epithelial nuclei can be considered as spheroidal Mie scatters with refractive index, n_{nc}, that is higher than that of the surrounding cytoplasm, n_{cp}. Normal nuclei have a characteristic diameter of $d = 4$–7 μm. In contrast, dysplastic

Table 2.5 Optical properties and dosimetric correction factor U/F of skull bone for different wavelengths (values are presented as mean ± SEM; to obtain the space irradiance U in an intact cochlea transmitted irradiance measured for specimen slabs have to be multiplied by U/F).[694]

λ, nm	μ_a/μ_s'	T_c^{eff}	μ_a, cm^{-1}	μ_s', cm^{-1}	μ_{eff}, cm^{-1}	U/F
593	0.0135 ± 0.0048	0.585 ± 0.054	0.561 ± 0.108	47.1 ± 8.3	8.70 ± 0.91	10.0 ± 1.5
635	0.0072 ± 0.0018	0.501 ± 0.038	0.371 ± 0.022	55.7 ± 9.1	7.80 ± 0.44	12.9 ± 1.4
690	0.0035 ± 0.0008	0.398 ± 0.026	0.169 ± 0.011	51.1 ± 7.3	5.04 ± 0.32	17.7 ± 1.7
780	0.0028 ± 0.0005	0.367 ± 0.026	0.107 ± 0.009	40.0 ± 4.6	3.56 ± 0.18	19.5 ± 1.6
830	0.0028 ± 0.0005	0.367 ± 0.027	0.104 ± 0.009	38.8 ± 4.4	3.45 ± 0.16	19.4 ± 1.6

nuclei can be as large as 20 μm, occupying almost the entire cell volume.[620] In the visible range, where the wavelength $\lambda_0 \ll d$, the Van de Hulst approximation can be used to describe the elastic scattering cross section of the nuclei as[180,181]

$$\sigma_{sca}(\lambda, d) = \frac{1}{2}\pi d^2 \left[1 - \frac{2\sin\delta}{\delta} + \left(\frac{2\sin\delta}{\delta} \right)^2 \right], \qquad (2.25)$$

where $\delta = 2\pi d(n_{nc} - n_{cp})/\lambda_0$; λ_0 is the wavelength of the light in vacuum. This expression reveals a component of the scattering cross section, which varies periodically with inverse wavelength. This, in turn, gives rise to a periodic component in the tissue optical reflectance. Since the frequency of this variation (in inverse wavelength space) is proportional to particle size, the nuclear size distribution can be obtained from the Fourier transform of the periodic component.

Measuring refractive indices in tissues and their constituent components is an important focus of interest in tissue optics because the index of refraction determines light reflection and refraction at the interfaces between air and tissue, detecting fiber and tissue, and tissue layers; it also strongly influences light propagation and distribution within tissues, defines the speed of light in tissue, and governs how the photons migrate.[31,129,130,175,178,206,743,677,712,713,744–754] Although these studies have a rather long history,[87] the mean values of refractive indices for many tissues are missing in the literature. According to Ref. 87, most of them have refractive indices for visible light in the 1.335–1.620 range (e.g., 1.55 in the stratum corneum, 1.620 in enamel, and 1.386 at the lens surface). It is worthwhile noting that *in vitro* and *in vivo* measurements may differ significantly. For example, the refractive index in rat mesenteric tissue *in vitro* was found to be 1.52 compared with only 1.38 *in vivo*.[87] This difference can be accounted for by the decreased refractivity of ground matter, n_0, due to impaired hydration.

Indeed, the optical properties of tissues, including refractive indices, are known to depend on water content. The refractive indices of water over a broad wavelength range from 200 nm to 200 μm have been reported in Ref. 87. Specifically, $n_w = 1.396$ for $\lambda = 200$ nm, 1.335 for $\lambda = 500$ nm, 1.142 for $\lambda = 2,800$ nm, 1.400 for $\lambda = 3,500$ nm, 1.218 for $\lambda = 10,000$ nm, and 2.130 for $\lambda = 200$ μm. Equation (1.202) was shown to be valid for pure water in the visible and NIR wavelength ranges corresponding to the best light transmission through tissues.[630]

To model tissue by a mixture of water and a bioorganic compound of a tissue is more adequate. For instance, the refractive index of human skin can be approximated by a 70/30 mixture of water and protein.[677] Assuming that protein has a constant refractive index value of 1.5 over the entire wavelength range, the authors of Ref. 677 have suggested the following expression for estimation of skin index of refraction:

$$n_{skin}(\lambda) = 0.7(1.58 - 8.45 \times 10^{-4}\lambda + 1.10 \times 10^{-6}\lambda^2 - 7.19 \times 10^{-10}\lambda^3$$
$$+ 2.32 \times 10^{-13}\lambda^4 - 2.98 \times 10^{-17}\lambda^5) + 0.3 \times 1.5, \qquad (2.26)$$

where wavelength λ is in nanometers.

For different parts of a biological cell, values of refractive index in the NIR range can be estimated as follows: extracellular fluid, $\bar{n} = 1.35$–1.36; cytoplasm, 1.360–1.375; cell membrane, 1.46; nucleus, 1.38–1.41; mitochondria and organelles, 1.38–1.41; melanin, 1.6–1.7.[58] Scattering arises from mismatches in refractive index of the components that make up the cell. Organelles and subcomponents of organelles having indices different from their surroundings are expected to be the primary sources of cellular scattering. The cell itself may be a significant source of small-angle scatter in applications like flow cytometry in which cells are studied separately.[145,149] In contrast, in tissues where cells are surrounded by other cells or tissue structures of similar index, certain organelles become the important scatterers. For instance, the nucleus is a significant scatterer because it is often the largest organelle in the cell and its size increases relative to the rest of the cell throughout neoplastic progression.[150–153,163,166,170,180,704] Mitochondria (0.5–1.5 μm in diameter), lysosomes (0.5 μm), and peroxisomes (0.5 μm) are very important scatterers whose size relative to the wavelength of light suggests that they must make a significant contribution to backscattering. Granular melanin, traditionally thought of as an absorber, must be considered an important scatterer because of its size and high refractive index.[58] Structures consisting of membrane layers, such as the endoplasmic reticulum or Golgi apparatus, may prove significant because they contain index fluctuations of high spatial frequency and amplitude. Besides cell components, fibrous tissue structures such as collagen and elastin must be considered as important scatterers.

Refractivity measurements in a number of strongly scattering tissues at 633 nm performed with a fiber-optic refractometer are schematically shown in Fig. 2.9.[178]

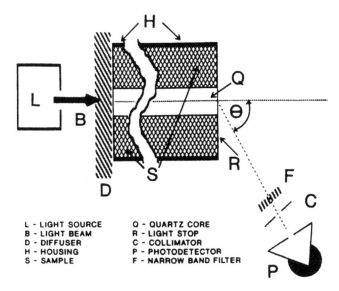

L - LIGHT SOURCE   Q - QUARTZ CORE
B - LIGHT BEAM   R - LIGHT STOP
D - DIFFUSER   C - COLLIMATOR
H - HOUSING   P - PHOTODETECTOR
S - SAMPLE   F - NARROW BAND FILTER

Figure 2.9 Schematic of experimental setup for determining the index of refraction. A bare quartz fiber is placed in a cladding of the substance to be measured. The angular light output distribution is measured, and the index is determined from Eq. (2.27).[178]

The method is based on a simple concept: that the cone of light issuing from an optical fiber is dependent on the indices of the cladding material, core material (quartz), and air into which the cone of light emerges. The cladding on a 1-mm core diameter optical fiber was stripped from the fiber, and the tissue for which the index is to be measured was substituted for the cladding. With the index for air (n_0) and the quartz fiber (n_q) known, along with the emitted angular light distribution (θ) measured at the optical fiber's output, the following equation for the determination of tissue index of refraction ($\bar{n}$) can be derived from the expression for the fiber numerical aperture:[178]

$$\bar{n} = \left\{ n_q^2 - [n_0 \sin \theta]^2 \right\}^{1/2}. \tag{2.27}$$

Using this simple and sensitive technique, it was found that fatty tissue has the largest refractive index (1.455), followed by kidney (1.418), muscular tissue (1.410), and then blood and spleen (1.400).[178] The lowest refractive indices were found in lungs and liver (1.380 and 1.368, respectively).[178] Also, it turned out that tissue homogenization does not significantly affect the refractive indices (the change does not exceed a measurement error equal to 0.006), whereas coagulated tissues have higher refractive indices than native ones (for example, for egg white, $\bar{n}$ changing from 1.321 to 1.388). Moreover, there is a tendency for refractive indices to decrease with increasing light wavelength from 390 to 700 nm (for example, for bovine muscle in the limits 1.42 to 1.39), which is characteristic of the majority of related abiological materials.

Experimental values of the mean refractive index for some tissues measured for selected wavelengths are summarized in Table 2.6.

The principle of total internal reflection at laser beam irradiation is also used for tissue and blood refraction measurements.[746,747] The schematic of a laser refractometer is shown in Fig. 2.10.[746] A thin tissue sample is sandwiched between two right-angled prisms that are made of ZF5 glass with a high refractive index,

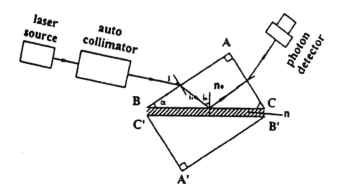

Figure 2.10 Schematic of a laser refractometer based on the principle of total internal reflection.[746]

Table 2.6 Experimental mean values of phase n or group n_g refractive indices of tissues, blood, and their compounds measured *in vitro* and *in vivo*[*]; rms. values are given in parentheses.

Tissue	λ, nm	n, n_g	Comments
Human aorta:			
Normal:			
Intima	456–1064	1.39	Ref. 691
Media	456–1064	1.38	
Adventitia	456–1064	1.36	
Calcified:			
Intima	456–1064	1.39	
Media	456–1064	1.53	
Human bladder:			
Mucous	456–1064	1.37	Ref. 691
Wall	456–1064	1.40	
Integral	456–1064	1.38	
Human brain:			
Gray matter	456–1064	1.36	Ref. 691
White matter	456–1064	1.38	
White and gray	456–1064	1.37	
Human colon:			
Muscle	456–1064	1.36	Ref. 691
Submucous	456–1064	1.36	
Mucous	456–1064	1.38	
Integral	456–1064	1.36	
Female breast tissue:			
Normal	800	1.403	Ref. 31
Malignant	800	1.431	

Table 2.6 (Continued).

Tissue	λ, nm	n, n_g	Comments
Rat breast (mammary) tissue (8 animals, 32 tumors):			OCT, titanium: sapphire laser source with a central wavelength of 800 nm and a bandwidth of ~100 nm; N-methyl-N-nitrosourea-induced rat mammary tumors (similar in pathology to human ductal carcinoma), Ref. 1275
Adipose	750–850	1.467 (0.026)	
Fibrous stroma	750–850	1.388 (0.043)	
Tumor	750–850	1.390 (0.028)	
Human esophagus:			
Mucous	456–1064	1.37	Ref. 691
Human fat:			
Subcutaneous	456–1064	1.44	Ref. 691
Abdominal	456–1064	1.46	
Human mesenteric fat	1300	1.467 (0.008)	OCT, optical path length measurements[767]
Bovine fat	633	1.455 (0.006)	Ref. 178, fiber-optic refractometer (FOR); homogenized tissue
Porcine fat	488	1.510 (0.002)	Ref. 746,
	632.8	1.492 (0.003)	laser refractometer (LR)
	1079.5	1.482 (0.002)	
	1341.4	1.478 (0.004)	
	632.8	1.493 (0.005)	Ref. 747, LR
Human heart:			
Trabecula	456–1064	1.40	Ref. 691
Myocard	456–1064	1.38	
Human left ventricular cardiac muscle	1300	1.382 (0.007)	OCT, optical path length measurements[767]
Human femoral vein	456–1064	1.39	Ref. 691
Kidney:			
Human	456–1064	1.37	Ref. 691
Human	633	1.417 (0.006)	Ref. 178, FOR

Table 2.6 (Continued).

Tissue	λ, nm	n, n_g	Comments
Canine	633	1.400 (0.006)	
Porcine	633	1.390 (0.006)	
Bovine	633	1.390 (0.006)	
Liver:			
Human	456–1064	1.38	Ref. 691
Human	633	1.367 (0.006)	Ref. 178, FOR; homogenized tissue
Canine	633	1.380 (0.006)	
Porcine	633	1.390 (0.006)	
Bovine	633	1.390 (0.006)	
Lung:			
Human	456–1064	1.38	Ref. 691
Canine	633	1.380 (0.006)	Ref. 178, FOR; homogenized tissue
Porcine	633	1.380 (0.006)	
Muscle:			
Human	456–1064	1.37	Ref. 691
Canine	633	1.400 (0.006)	Ref. 178, FOR; homogenized tissue
Bovine	633	1.412 (0.006)	
Bovine	592 (560–640)	1.382 (0.004)	Ref. 1283, fluorescence confocal microscopy
Ovine$_\parallel$	488	1.404 (0.003)	Ref. 746, LR, tissue samples labeled as $\parallel$
	632.8	1.389 (0.002)	and $\perp$ are the same sample with the tissue
	1079.5	1.378 (0.004)	fibers oriented in parallel and perpendicular
	1341.4	1.375 (0.003)	to the interface, respectively
Ovine$_\perp$	488	1.402 (0.002)	
	632.8	1.389 (0.002)	

Table 2.6 (Continued).

Tissue	λ, nm	n, n_g	Comments
Porcine$_\parallel$	1079.5	1.375 (0.003)	
	1341.4	1.373 (0.003)	
	488	1.402 (0.002)	
	632.8	1.381 (0.002)	
	1079.5	1.372 (0.003)	
	1341.4	1.370 (0.003)	
Porcine$_\perp$	488	1.399 (0.002)	
	632.8	1.379 (0.002)	
	1079.5	1.370 (0.002)	
	1341.4	1.367 (0.003)	
Porcine$_\parallel$	632.8	1.380 (0.007)	Ref. 747, LR
Porcine$_\perp$	632.8	1.460 (0.008)	
Muscle from abdominal wall of the rat (Species Wistar Han)	589	1.3980 ($m = 0.1623$ g) [*]	Abbe refractometer, refractive index and mass (m) measurements in a course of a dehydration process recurring to sample heating with hairdryer, [*] natural tissue, Ref. 1276
	589	1.3995 ($m = 0.1455$ g)	
	589	1.4105 ($m = 0.1361$ g)	
	589	1.4200 ($m = 0.1252$ g)	
	589	1.4295 ($m = 0.1144$ g)	
	589	1.4410 ($m = 0.1053$ g)	
	589	1.4525 ($m = 0.0955$ g)	
	589	1.4640 ($m = 0.0860$ g)	
	589	1.4785 ($m = 0.0747$ g)	
	589	1.4910 ($m = 0.0654$ g)	
	589	1.5035 ($m = 0.0551$ g)	
Human skin:			
Stratum corneum (SC) [*]	1300	$n_g = 1.51$ (0.02)	Ref. 767, OCT, reference mirror and focus tracking
Epidermis [*]	1300	$n_g = 1.34$ (0.01)	

Table 2.6 (Continued).

Tissue	λ, nm	n, n_g	Comments
Dermis	1300	$n_g = 1.41 (0.03)$	OCT, optical path length measurements[767]
Dermis	1300	$n_g = 1.400 (0.007)$	Ref. 712, OCT, focus tracking by moving of fiber tip/collimating lens
SC* (Palm of hand)	1300	$(nn_g)^{1/2} = 1.47 (0.01)$	
Epidermis* (Palm of hand, granular layer)	1300	$(nn_g)^{1/2} = 1.43 (0.02)$	
Epidermis* (Palm of hand, basal layer)	1300	$(nn_g)^{1/2} = 1.34 (0.02)$	
Epidermis* (Volar side of lower arm)	1300	$(nn_g)^{1/2} = 1.36 (0.01)$	
Upper dermis* (Palm of hand)	1300	$(nn_g)^{1/2} = 1.41 (0.03)$	
Upper dermis* (Volar side of lower arm)	1300	$(nn_g)^{1/2} = 1.43 (0.02)$	
SC* (Dorsal surface of a thumb)	980	$(nn_g)^{1/2} = 1.50 (0.02)$	Bifocal OCT refractometer, Ref. 770
Air/skin interface* (Volar side of a thumb)	980	$(nn_g)^{1/2} = 1.56$	Ref. 771
SC/epidermis interface* (Volar side of a thumb)	980	$(nn_g)^{1/2} = 1.34$	
Pig skin	1300	$(nn_g)^{1/2} = 1.415$	Ref. 713, OCT, focus tracking
Pig skin (treated by a detergent solution)	1300	$(nn_g)^{1/2} = 1.365$	
Human stratum corneum	400–700	1.55	Ref. 87
Rat skin	456–1064	1.42	Ref. 691
Mouse skin	456–1064	1.40	
Porcine skin (dermis)	325	1.393	Prism laser refractometer, Fresnel's equations, fresh tissue samples of thickness from 0.31 to 0.84 mm, the total uncertainty in n of the samples was estimated to be ±0.004, Refs. 1277 and 1278
	442	1.376	
	532	1.359	
	633	1.354	
	850	1.364	
	1064	1.360	
	1310	1.357	
	1557	1.361	
Human skin (epidermis) (12 female, between 27 and 63 yr; 10 are Caucasian* and 2 are African Americans**)	325 (*)	1.489 (S) 1.486 (P)	Prism laser refractometer with an incident beam of S- or P-polarization, Fresnel's equations, fresh tissue samples performed
	442 (*)(**)	1.449 (S) 1.447 (P)	
	532 (*)(**)	1.448 (S) 1.446 (P)	

Table 2.6 (Continued).

Tissue	λ, nm	n, n_g	Comments
Human skin (dermis) (12 female, between 27 and 63 yr; 10 are Caucasian* and 2 are African Americans**)	633 (*)	1.433 (S) 1.433 (P)	at the room temperature within 30 hr after the abdominoplasty procedure, the total uncertainty in n of the samples was estimated to be ±0.006, Ref. 1279
	850 (*)	1.417 (S) 1.416 (P)	
	1064 (*)	1.432 (S) 1.428 (P)	
	1310 (*)	1.425 (S) 1.421 (P)	
	1557 (*)	1.404 (S) 1.400 (P)	
	325 (*)	1.401 (s) 1.403 (p)	
	442 (*)(**)	1.395 (s) 1.400 (p)	
	532 (*)(**)	1.378 (s) 1.381 (p)	
	633 (*)	1.396 (s) 1.393 (p)	
	850 (*)	1.384 (s) 1.389 (p)	
	1064 (*)	1.375 (s) 1.385 (p)	
	1310 (*)	1.358 (s) 1.364 (p)	
	1557 (*)	1.363 (s) 1.367 (p)	
Spleen:			
Human	456–1064	1.37	Ref. 691
Canine	633	1.400 (0.006)	Ref. 178, FOR; homogenized tissue
Porcine	633	1.400 (0.006)	
Human stomach:			
Muscle	456–1064	1.39	Ref. 691
Mucous	456–1064	1.38	
Integral	456–1064	1.38	
Porcine small intestine	488	1.391 (0.002)	Ref. 746, LR
	632.8	1.373 (0.002)	
	1079.5	1.361 (0.003)	
	1341.4	1.359 (0.004)	
Human cerebral spinal fluid	400–700	1.335	Ref. 87

Table 2.6 (Continued).

Tissue	λ, nm	n, n_g	Comments
Rat mesentery	400–700	1.52 (0.01)	Ref. 87
Rat mesentery*	400–700	1.38 (0.1)	
Rat mesentery	850	1.4245 ($T = 25°C$)	Ref. 750, OCT, several pieces of rat mesenteries, mainly composed of phospholipids bilayers; gel-to-liquid phase transition in the range from 38 to 42°C
		1.4239 ($T = 30°C$)	
		1.4223 ($T = 35°C$)	
		1.4216 ($T = 38°C$)	
		1.4186 ($T = 40°C$)	
		1.4027 ($T = 42°C$)	
		1.4016 ($T = 44°C$)	
		1.4000 ($T = 46°C$)	
		1.3986 ($T = 48°C$)	
Human eye:			
Aqueous humor	400–700	1.336	Ref. 87
Cornea:			
Integral	400–700	1.376	
Fibrils	400–700	1.47	
Ground substance	400–700	1.35	
Lens:			
Surface	400–700	1.386	
Center	400–700	1.406	
Vitreous humor	400–700	1.336	
Tears	400–700	1.3361–1.3379	
Sclera	442–1064	1.47–1.36	Ref. 691
Cornea:			Abbe refractometer measurements and calculations on the basis of x-ray diffraction data, Ref. 778
Human:			
Fibrils	589	1.411 (0.004)	
Extrafibrillar material	589	1.365 (0.009)	

Table 2.6 (Continued).

Tissue	λ, nm	n, n_g	Comments
Ox:			
Fibrils	589	1.413 (0.004)	
Extrafibrillar material	589	1.357 (0.009)	
Rabbit:			
Fibrils	589	1.416 (0.004)	
Extrafibrillar material	589	1.357 (0.010)	
Trout:			
Fibrils	589	1.418 (0.004)	
Extrafibrillar material	589	1.364 (0.009)	
Bovine:			Data from Refs. 779 and 780
Stroma	589	1.375	
Hydrated fibrils	589	1.413	
Hydrated extrafibrillar matrix	589	1.359	
Dry collagen	589	1.547	
Dry extrafibrillar material	589	1.485	
Solvent (salt solution)	589	1.335	
Hydrated stroma:	589	$1.335 + 0.04/(0.22 + 0.24H)$	$H = 3$–8, $H = 3.2$—physiological hydration, Ref. 779
Calf cornea:			
Normal	820	$n_g = 1.380$ (0.001)	Ref. 772, OCT, reference mirror method;
Hydrated ($H = 1.5$–5):	820	$a = 1.324$ (0.002)	$H = 5.3 \cdot d - 0.67$, d is the corneal
$n_g(H) = a + b/(H + 1)$		$b = 0.272$ (0.009)	stroma thickness in mm
Human cornea	550	1.3771	Obstfeld, 1982, datum from Ref. 774
	589	1.380 (0.005)	Patel et al., 1995, datum from Ref. 774
	855	$n_g = 1.3817$ (0.0021)	Ref. 773, OCT
	1270	$n_g = 1.389$ (0.004)	Ref. 774, OCT, 21°C
	1270	$n_g = 1.386$	Ref. 774, extrapolation of datum for 550 nm

Table 2.6 (Continued).

Tissue	λ, nm	n, n_g	Comments
Human tooth:			
Enamel	1270	$n_g = 1.390$ (0.005)	Ref. 774, extrapolation of datum for 589 nm
Enamel	1270	$n_g = 1.3838$ (0.0021)	Ref. 774, extrapolation of datum for 855 nm
Apatite	220	1.73	Ref. 87
Enamel	400–700	1.62	
Apatite	400–700	>1.623	
Dentin matrix	Visible	1.553 (0.001)	Ref. 763, optical immersion method
Enamel	856	$n_g = 1.62$ (0.02)	Ref. 423, OCT, reference mirror method
Dentin	856	$n_g = 1.50$ (0.02)	
Enamel	850	$n_g = 1.65$	Ref. 768, OCT
Dentin	850	$n_g = 1.54$	
Human nail[*]	850	$n_g = 1.51$	Ref. 768, OCT
Human hair shaft:			
Black	850	$n_g = 1.59$ (0.08)	Ref. 766, OCT
Brown	850	$n_g = 1.58$ (0.06)	
Red	850	$n_g = 1.56$ (0.01)	
Blond	850	$n_g = 1.57$ (0.01)	
Gray	850	$n_g = 1.58$ (0.01)	
White	850	$n_g = 1.58$ (0.01)	
Human hair strands	400–600	1.45 (304 nm, 0.6%)	Ellipsometry, values depend on the
	400–600	1.46 299.5 nm, 0.1%)	parameters of the cuticle surface
	400–600	1.47 (308.7 nm, 0.8%)	roughness layer thickness (from 304 to
	400–600	1.46 (273.7 nm, 2.2%)	359.7 nm) and the air inclusion (from 0.6
	400–600	1.50 (327.5 nm, 4.7%)	to 5.7%), Ref. 1280
	400–600	1.50 (359.7 nm, 5.7%)	
Human whole blood	633	1.400 (0.006)	Ref. 178, FOR

Table 2.6 (Continued).

Tissue	λ, nm	n, n_g	Comments
Human whole blood	488	1.395 (0.003)	Ref. 746, LR
	632.8	1.373 (0.004)	
	1079.5	1.363 (0.004)	
	1341.4	1.360 (0.005)	
0%-solution in water	633	1.34	Ref. 742, the equilateral hollow prism
20%-solution in water	633	1.35	
40%-solution in water	633	1.35	
60%-solution in water	633	1.36	
Undiluted blood (extrapolated)	633	1.38	
Human blood plasma	488	1.350 (0.002)	Ref. 746, LR
	632.8	1.345 (0.002)	
	1079.5	1.332 (0.003)	
	1341.4	1.327 (0.004)	
Human red blood cells (dry):			
Healthy patients ($n = 7$, fixed RBC)	550	1.61–1.66	Ref. 754, pH = 6–8, Nomarski
Diabetic patients ($n = 9$, fixed RBC)	550	1.56–1.62	polarizing-interference microscope
Healthy patients ($n = 7$, intact RBC)	550	1.57–1.61	
Diabetic patients ($n = 9$, intact RBC)	550	1.61–1.64	
Hemoglobin:			
Oxygenated (from porcine blood)	800	1.392 (0.001)	Refs. 751, OCT, 37°C, hemoglobin of 93 g/l
Deoxygenated (from porcine blood)	800	1.388 (0.002)	
Glycated (Glucose from 40 to 400 mg/dl)	820	1.382 → 1.415	Ref. 753, OCT, hemoglobin of 140 g/l
Glycated (Glucose from 400 to 800 mg/dl)	820	1.415 → 1.385	
Hemoglobin (human, oxygenated)	250	1470 (0.03)	Data presented by the authors of Refs. 1281
	300	1.441 (0.03)	and 1282, Fresnel reflectance measurements,
	400	1.409 (0.03)	IS spectrometer, Hemoglobin of 287 g/l

Table 2.6 (Continued).

Tissue	λ, nm	n, n_g	Comments
	500	1.413 (0.03)	
	589	1.406 (0.03)	
	700	1.404 (0.03)	
	800	1.400 (0.03)	
	900	1.401 (0.03)	
	1000	1.401 (0.03)	
	1100	1.400 (0.03)	
	250	1.435 (0.03)	Data presented by the authors of Refs. 1281
	300	1.405 (0.03)	and 1282, Fresnel reflectance measurements,
	400	1.383 (0.03)	IS spectrometer, Hemoglobin of 165 g/l
	500	1.383 (0.03)	
	589	1.375 (0.03)	
	700	1.374 (0.03)	
	800	1.370 (0.03)	
	900	1.369 (0.03)	
	1000	1.370 (0.03)	
	1100	1.369 (0.03)	
	250	1.416 (0.03)	Data presented by the authors of Refs. 1281
	300	1.389 (0.03)	and 1282, Fresnel reflectance measurements,
	400	1.367 (0.03)	IS spectrometer, Hemoglobin of 104 g/l
	500	1.363 (0.03)	
	589	1.357 (0.03)	
	700	1.356 (0.03)	
	800	1.353 (0.03)	
	900	1.352 (0.03)	
	1000	1.353 (0.03)	
	1100	1.352 (0.03)	

Table 2.6 (Continued).

Tissue	λ, nm	n, n_g	Comments
	250	1.398 (0.03)	Data presented by the authors of Refs. 1281
	300	1.373 (0.03)	and 1282, Fresnel reflectance measurements,
	400	1.354 (0.03)	IS spectrometer, Hemoglobin of 46 g/l
	500	1.348 (0.03)	
	589	1.343 (0.03)	
	700	1.341 (0.03)	
	800	1.338 (0.03)	
	900	1.338 (0.03)	
	1000	1.338 (0.03)	
	1100	1.337 (0.03)	
	633	1.3750 (0.0003)	Abbe refractometer,[1282] Hemoglobin of 165 g/l
	633	1.3600 (0.0003)	Abbe refractometer,[1282] Hemoglobin of 104 g/l
Collagen (Type I)			
Dry	850	$n_g = 1.53$ (0.02)	Ref. 764, OCT
Fully hydrated	850	$n_g = 1.43$ (0.02)	
Cytoplasm	400–700	1.350–1.367	Ref. 87
Nuclei of cervical epithelium cells:		$n(\Delta n)$	Ref. 745, histology, cytometry and modeling;
Normal:			20 nuclei were analyzed for each case; Δn is
Basal/parabasal	Far visible/NIR	1.387 (0.004–0.007)	the refractive index spatial fluctuation
Intermediate	Far visible/NIR	1.372 (0.004–0.006)	
Superficial	Far visible/NIR	1.414 (0.005–0.008)	
Cervical intraepithelial neoplasia (CIN 3):			
Basal/parabasal	Far visible/NIR	1.426 (0.008–0.010)	
Intermediate	Far visible/NIR	1.404 (0.007–0.009)	
Superficial	Far visible/NIR	1.431 (0.008–0.011)	

Table 2.7 Values of Cauchy coefficients of dispersion equation (2.29).[746]

Tissue sample	A	$B \times 10^{-3}$	$C \times 10^{-9}$
Porcine muscle$_\parallel$	1.3694	0.073223	1.8317
Porcine muscle$_\perp$	1.3657	1.5123	1.5291
Porcine adipose	1.4753	4.3902	0.92385
Porcine small intestine	1.3563	4.3905	0.92379
Ovine muscle$_\parallel$	1.3716	5.8677	0.43999
Ovine muscle$_\perp$	1.3682	8.7456	−0.16532
Human whole blood	1.3587	1.4744	1.7103
Human blood plasma	1.3194	14.578	−1.7383

$n_0 = 1.70827$, and angle, $\alpha = 29°55'41.4''$. For an incident laser beam polarized in the S-plane, the following equation for the determination of the mean refractive index of tissues is valid:[746]

$$\bar{n} = \sin i_t \times \cos \alpha + \sin \alpha \times [n_0^2 - \sin^2 i_t]^{1/2}, \tag{2.28}$$

where the incident angle of total reflectance i_t is a measurable parameter.

Measurements for fresh animal tissues and human blood at four laser wavelengths of 488, 632.8, 1079.5, and 1341.4 nm and room temperature were presented in a form of Cauchy dispersion equation as[746]

$$\bar{n} = A + B\lambda^{-2} + C\lambda^{-4} \tag{2.29}$$

with λ in nanometers; values of the Cauchy coefficients are presented in Table 2.7. Measured mean values with standard deviation for four wavelengths are presented in Table 2.6. Porcine (or ovine) muscle samples labeled as $\parallel$ and $\perp$ are the same sample with the tissue fibers oriented in parallel with and perpendicular to the interface, respectively.

An expression for human blood plasma received in Ref. 746 was extrapolated to shorter wavelengths from 400 to 1000 nm as[552,748]

$$n_{bp}(\lambda) = 1.3254 + 8.4052 \times 10^3 \lambda^{-2} - 3.9572 \times 10^8 \lambda^{-4} - 2.3617 \times 10^{13} \lambda^{-6}. \tag{2.30}$$

For modeling of the behavior of refractive index of tissues, blood, and their components, one may use a remarkable property of proteins: that equal concentrations of aqueous solutions of different proteins all have approximately the same refractive index n_{pw}.[749] Moreover, the refractive index varies almost linearly with concentration C_p as

$$n_{pw}(\lambda) = n_w(\lambda) + \beta_p(\lambda)C_p, \tag{2.31}$$

where n_w is the refractive index of water and β_p is the specific refractive increment; C_p is measured in grams per 100 ml (g/dl). For example, the refractive index of human erythrocyte cytoplasm, defined by the cell-bounded hemoglobin solution, can be found from this equation at $\beta_p = 0.001942$ valid for a wavelength of 589 nm; i.e., for normal hemoglobin concentration in cytoplasm of 300–360 g/l, the RBC refractive index $n_{RBC} = 1.393–1.406$.[48] Since the scattering coefficient of blood, which is defined mostly by hemoglobin refractive index, is not significantly dependent on the wavelength in the range 580–800 nm,[48] this value of β can be used for estimation of the refractive index of a hemoglobin solution in the NIR range. Values of specific refractive increments β_p for other proteins measured by Abbe refractometer at a wavelength of 589 nm are presented in Table 2.8.[749] Other materials of specific biological interest are the carbohydrates, lipoids, and nucleic acid compounds. The first two usually have low values of β, in the region of 0.0014–0.0015, and nucleic acids have higher values, 0.0016–0.0020.[749]

Table 2.8 Values of specific refractive increment β_p measured by Abbe refractometer on the wavelength 589 nm for the proteins.[749]

Protein	β_p, dl/g
Total serum (human)	0.00179
Euglobulin	0.00183
Pseudoglobulin	0.00181
Total albumin	0.00181
Recrystallized albumin	0.00181
Lipoprotein	0.00170–0.00171
Hemocyanin *Helix*	0.00179
Octopus	0.00184
Carcinus	0.00187
Egg albumin	0.001813
Sheep CO hemoglobin	0.001945
Globin (ox)	0.00178
CO hemoglobin (ox)	0.00193–0.00195

The wavelength dependence of the specific refractive increment of the oxygenated native hemoglobin solution $\beta_{Hb}(\lambda)$ normalized to the refractive index of pure water $n_w(\lambda)$ [see Eq. (2.31)] is presented in Table 2.9.[1282] The estimated error which includes the error of the determination of the hemoglobin concentration and the refractive index is of ± 0.00003. Therefore the derivation of a mean constant normalized specific refractive increment of $(\beta_{Hb}/n_w) = 0.00199$ dl/g for the spectral regions 310–355 nm and 500–1100 nm is possible, because the standard deviation of an averaged value of (β_{Hb}/n_w) in these regions is ± 0.000036 and is in the same range as the estimated error for the determination of (β_{Hb}/n_w) for a fixed wavelength.

The spectral dependencies of refractive indices for oxy- and deoxyhemoglobin in the 450–820-nm wavelength range were obtained in Ref. 755. These and later determinations[159,730,751] are based on absorption spectral measurements (see

Table 2.9 Wavelength-dependent values of specific refractive increment of hemoglobin $\beta_{Hb}(\lambda)$ normalized to refractive index of pure water $n_w(\lambda)$ [see Eq. (2.31)] with an estimated error of ± 0.00003; oxygenated native hemoglobin solution; Fresnel reflectance measurements using a modified integrating sphere spectrometer; data from Ref. 1282 (more complete data are presented in Ref. 1282).

Wavelength, nm	$\beta_{Hb}(\lambda)/n_w(\lambda)$, dl/g	Wavelength, nm	$\beta_{Hb}(\lambda)/n_w(\lambda)$, dl/g	Wavelength, nm	$\beta_{Hb}(\lambda)/n_w(\lambda)$, dl/g	Wavelength, nm	$\beta_{Hb}(\lambda)/n_w(\lambda)$, dl/g
250	0.002210	350	0.001989	450	0.002156	620	0.001964
260	0.002105	360	0.001983	460	0.002109	640	0.001954
270	0.002048	370	0.001860	470	0.002078	680	0.001970
280	0.002044	380	0.001774	480	0.002056	760	0.001958
290	0.002047	390	0.001694	490	0.002033	800	0.001939
300	0.002020	400	0.001664	500	0.002005	840	0.001935
310	0.001998	410	0.001799	520	0.001983	900	0.001998
320	0.002007	420	0.002117	540	0.001981	980	0.002017
330	0.002021	430	0.002273	560	0.001992	1060	0.002040
340	0.002010	440	0.002210	580	0.002004	1100	0.002056

Fig. 2.11) and conversion of the received imaginary part of the complex refractive index [see Eqs. (1.165) and (1.166)] to its real part using Kramers-Kronig relationships.[159,730,751,755] These relations follow from the principle of causality, which demands that the real and imaginary parts of the complex index of refraction to be a mutual Hilbert transform as

$$n'(\tilde{v}) - 1 = Hi[n''(\tilde{v})], \quad n''(\tilde{v}) = Hi^{-1}[n'(\tilde{v}) - 1], \qquad (2.32)$$

where $\tilde{v} = 1/\lambda$.

Thus, the original formula for determination of $n'(\lambda)$ on the basis of measurements of $\mu_a(\lambda) = (4\pi/\lambda)n''(\lambda)$ has a view as

$$n'(\tilde{v}) = 1 + \frac{2}{\pi} \int_0^\infty \frac{n''(\tilde{v}')\tilde{v}'d\tilde{v}'}{(\tilde{v}')^2 - (\tilde{v})^2}. \qquad (2.33)$$

It follows from this relation that to calculate the index of refraction for a single wavelength $\lambda = 1/\tilde{v}$, one has to know absorption spectra over the whole interval $[0, \infty]$. Another problem is to provide integration in the vicinity of the wavelength of interest. To overcome these difficulties, suitable boundary conditions on the finite integral can be determined, analytical continuation of experimental data before integration, or series expansion of experimental data also can be used.[159,730,751,755] For numerical integration of Eq. (2.33), a proper step of integration and a symmetrical region around the $\tilde{v} = 1/\lambda$ of interest should be chosen.[751,755] When the series expansion method is used, the n'' spectrum may be presented as a sum of several peak functions, usually Gaussian or Lorentzian, which correspond to absorption bands within the measured spectral range.[730,751] Since the Hilbert transform is linear, the spectrum of the index of refraction is then simply the sum of

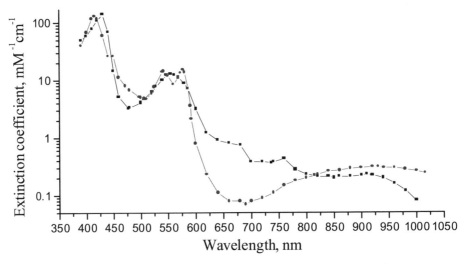

Figure 2.11 Absorption spectra of deoxy- and oxyhemoglobin. ─■─ $-\varepsilon_\lambda^d$, pH $= 5.5$–9.5; ─●─ $-\varepsilon_\lambda^o$ pH $= 5.5$–10.0[725]

the corresponding Hilbert transforms of these peak functions. Hammer et al.[730] and Borovoi et al.[159] used this approach to determine the index of refraction of RBCs in the wavelength range from 400 to 1000 nm, and Faber et al.[751] made this analysis for the wavelength range from 250 to 1000 nm for both oxygenated and deoxygenated hemoglobin. These data are presented in Fig. 2.12.

To account for the dispersion of absorbing bands in the UV and far-IR regions within the spectral range of interest (visible and NIR), absolute measurements of the refractive index for at least one wavelength chosen in the studied spectral range but far from the absorption bands should be provided. Such measurements may serve as reference data and can be done, for example, using an Abbe refractometer for hemoglobin solutions or the OCT technique for whole blood.[751–753] Another technique, which in principle allows for refractive index measurements of blood and other bioliquids at a few separate wavelengths, is shown schematically in Fig. 2.13. This conventional method uses an equilateral small-angle (10 deg) hollow prism made from thin quartz slides and the following expression for calculation of the refractive index:[742]

$$ n = \frac{\sin[(A + \delta_m)/2]}{\sin(A/2)}, \tag{2.34} $$

where A is the prism angle and δ_m is the angle of minimum deviation.

A Nomarski polarizing-interference microscope was successfully used to measure the refractive index of fixed and intact dry erythrocytes taken from healthy and

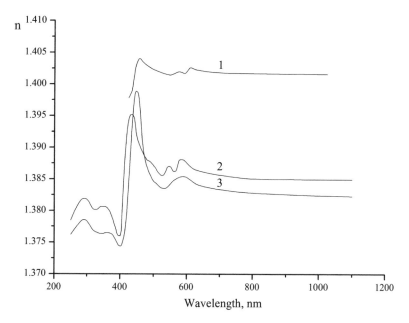

Figure 2.12 Spectral dependencies of the index of refraction (real part) for: (1) RBCs, 100% oxygenation of hemoglobin and its mean concentration in RBCs of 340 g/l;[159,730] (2) oxygenated (100%) hemoglobin; and (3) deoxygenated hemoglobin at a concentration of 140 g/l, which corresponds to the mean concentration of hemoglobin in whole blood.[751]

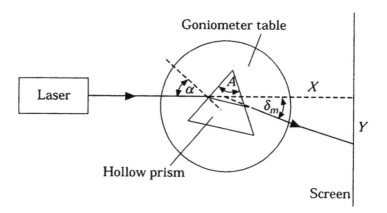

Figure 2.13 Schematic of the hollow prism refractometer for the measurement of the index of refraction of blood and other bioliquids.[742]

diabetic patients.[754] It was shown that for intact RBCs at physiological pH 7.3, hyperglycation of hemoglobin leads to a higher refractive index; at maximum it increased from 1.55 at normal to 1.65 for diabetics. The increase, followed-up saturation, and damping of the refractive index of solutions of hemoglobin or whole blood with glucose at an increased concentration of glucose were found using OCT measurements.[752,753] The results for the hemoglobin solution at concentration of 140 g/l, which is characteristic for blood at normal physiological conditions, are shown in Fig. 2.14.

According to Eq. (2.31), the initial refractive index of the hemoglobin solution of 140 g/l in water with zero concentration of glucose at 820 nm is expected as $n_{Hb140} = 1.355$. To evaluate the contribution of glucose at different concentrations to the mean refractive index of the solution supposing noninteracting hemoglobin and glucose molecules, the weighted average of refractive indexes [see Eq. (1.151)] of the glucose solution in water, n_{glw}, and hemoglobin, n_{Hb}, should be calculated as

$$n_{Hb+gl} = f_{glw}n_{glw} + (1 - f_{glw})n_{Hb}, \tag{2.35}$$

where f_{glw} is the volume fraction of the glucose solution. In experiments, the volume fraction of glucose solution was kept constant at $f_{glw} = 0.86$, which corresponds to a hemoglobin concentration of 140 g/l (14%). In this equation, the refractive index of dry hemoglobin n_{Hb} is presented. The value n_{glw} can be calculated using the expression[172,339,340]

$$n_{glw} = n_w + 1.515 \times 10^{-6} \times C_{gl}, \tag{2.36}$$

where C_{gl} is the glucose concentration in mg/dl. Since n_w can be found for 820 nm from Eq. (1.202) as $n_w = 1.328$ and C_{gl} is known, n_{glw} can be calculated for each used concentration of glucose.

The refractive index of hemoglobin n_{Hb} can be estimated from Eqs. (2.31) and (2.35) when glucose concentration is zero. From Eq. (2.31), it follows that

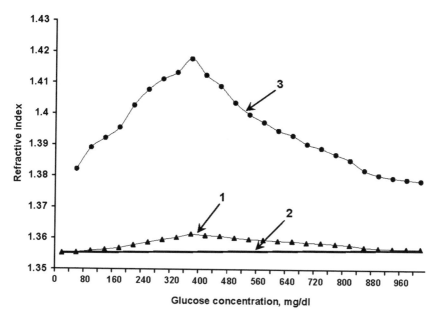

Figure 2.14 Experimental and reconstructed data for the refractive index change of human hemoglobin at glucose concentration increase in solution.[753] OCT refractometer working on 820 nm, hemoglobin concentration of 140 mg/l at pH = 7.3. (1) Raw data; (2) calculated data using Eqs. (2.35) and (2.36) for noninteracting hemoglobin and glucose; (3) reconstructed on the basis of Eq. (2.37), refractive index of the glycated hemoglobin fraction.

$n_{Hb140} = 1.355$; thus, from Eq. (2.35), $n_{Hb140} = f_w n_w + (1 - f_w)n_{Hb}$, and for $f_w = 0.86$ and $n_w = 1.328$, $n_{Hb} = 1.521$, which correlates with experimental data for the refractive index of dried RBCs of normal blood.[754] Therefore, n_{Hb+gl} can be found for solutions with different glucose concentrations and a constant concentration of hemoglobin. As it follows from Eq. (2.35), the mean refractive index for noninteracting molecules at an increase of glucose concentration of 10 times (from 40 to 400 mg/dl) causes only a slight increase of the refractive index in the range from 1.355 to 1.356 [see linear dependence (2) in Fig. 2.14].

In contrast, the experimental data show that the refractive index of a hemoglobin solution at an increase of glucose concentration from 40 to 400 mg/dl changes more effectively, from 1.355 to 1.361 [curve (1) in Fig. 2.14]. The obtained degree of refractive index increase, its saturation, and subsequent fall evidently can be explained using the concept of glucose and hemoglobin molecules interaction when different forms of glycated hemoglobin with new molecular structures and optical properties are originated.[756] The volume fraction of glycated hemoglobin (GHb) in the blood of diabetic patients linearly depends on the mean blood glucose (MBG) in the plasma, which is described by the following empirical equation:[756]

$$f_{GHb} = 2.7 \times 10^{-4} \, MBG(mg/dl) + 0.058. \tag{2.37}$$

This relation allows one to reconstruct the refractive index of the glycated portion of the total hemoglobin using the general relationship, Eq. (2.35). The final result of the reconstruction is presented by curve (3) in Fig. 2.14. To understand the behavior of the index of refraction of glycated hemoglobin, the classical theory of light dispersion in condensed matter can be used. This theory gives the following formula for the refractive index:[757]

$$n = 1 + \alpha N \frac{q^2}{M},\tag{2.38}$$

where α is the wavelength-dependent coefficient, N is the number of molecules, M is the molecule's mass, and q is the molecule's charge. From this equation, it follows that the refractive index of hemoglobin depends on molecular weight and charge only: it is a square-law function of charge and an inversely proportional function of molecular weight. Each protein has several different side groups (R), which define a molecule's charge. As it follows from Ref. 754, the charge of an R-group of hemoglobin molecules may be increased at glucose binding, but at the same time the increased mass of glycated hemoglobin molecules decreases the refractive index. These facts may explain the obtained changes of refractive index in the experiments. At glucose concentrations from 40 to 200–300 mg/dl, the increase in charge of the R-group of glycated hemoglobin molecules is higher than that of molecular weight and the refractive index increases. At glucose concentrations higher than 200–300 mg/dl due to significant increase of M and charge saturation, refractive index dependence saturates and even falls with glucose concentration.

Some other reasons may also affect the refractive index change, such as uncontrolled hemoglobin oxygen saturation (see Fig. 2.13)[750,751] and/or increase of the hemoglobin's affinity to oxygen at glucose elevation (up to 200% increase in affinity for 15–20 mM of glucose was found by the authors of Ref. 758).

Because the refractive index of tissue and blood components defines their scattering properties, measured scattering parameters may have an advantage to evaluate the refractive index of tissue and blood components and their mean values.[703,721,759–761] Let us discuss this technique in more detail.[759] For a monodisperse system of spherical scatterers, the reduced scattering coefficient can be described by the following expression, written in a more general form than Eq. (2.24):

$$\mu_s' = N_0 \pi a\, F(f_s) Q_s(n_s, n_0, a, \lambda)(1 - g),\tag{2.39}$$

where N_0 is the number of scatterers in a unit volume, a is their radius, $F(f_s)$ is the function accounting for the density of particle packing, f_s is the volume fraction of scatterers, n_s is the refractive index of the scatterers, n_s is the refractive index of the ground material, λ is the wavelength, and Q_s and g are factors of scattering efficiency and anisotropy, which are calculated from Mie theory.[129,146,148]

Determination of the reduced scattering coefficient of a tissue sample using integrating sphere or spatially resolved techniques and corresponding algorithms for extraction of the scattering coefficient, such as inverse adding-doubling or Monte Carlo, the knowledge of the refractive indices of the scatterers and the ground material at one of the wavelengths, as well as experimental or theoretical estimations for mean radius of the scatterers, allows one to solve the inverse problem and re-construct the spectral dependence of the refractive index of the scatteres for a given spectral dependence of the refractive index of the ground material.[759] Similar mea-surements and theoretical estimations done for a tissue sample before and after its prolonged bathing in saline or other biocompatible liquid with known optical char-acteristics allow one to evaluate the spectral dependencies of the refractive index of the scatterers and the ground material.

Let us consider a few examples. The major scatterers in human sclera are long collagen fibers with a wide range of diameters and a mean value of 100 nm. Fibers are arranged quasi-randomly in the bundles (see Chapter 3).[723,762] Due to the char-acteristic structure sizing and multiple crossings of bundles, this system can be approximated by a monodisperse system of spherical scatterers with similar spec-tral properties. In that case, the Mie-equivalent scatterer radius is equal to 250 nm. This value of particle radius is fitted to values of Mie-equivalent radius received for *in vivo* measurements of skin, in which the scattering properties are mostly defined by the dermis—also fibrous tissue [see Eqs. (1.180) and (1.181)]. Using experi-mental spectral dependence for the reduced scattering coefficient and accounting for a scleral sample that has been placed into a physiological solution for a long time, the interstitial fluid was therefore replaced by a physiological solution whose refractive index is close to water, the spectral dependence for refractive index of the scatterers was reconstructed.[703,760] The spectral dependence for water, described by Eq. (1.202), was used at reconstruction. The following approximated formula for the refractive index of the material of effective scatterers of scleral tissue valid within the spectral range from 400 to 800 nm was received as a final result of the reconstruction:

$$n_c(\lambda) = 1.4389 + 1.5880 \times 10^4 \lambda^{-2} - 1.4806 \times 10^9 \lambda^{-4} + 4.3917 \times 10^{13} \lambda^{-6}.$$
(2.40)

In fact, this dispersion relation should be close to the spectral dependence of the in-dex of refraction of hydrated collagen because 75% of sclera's dry weight is due to collagen.[723] The estimated value of the refractive index of normally hydrated scle-ral collagen (68% of hydration for a whole tissue) of $n = 1.474$,[172] corresponding to direct refraction measurements for whole sclera at a wavelength of 589 nm,[723] is well fitted to the value calculated from this semi-empirical relation.

The similar analysis of experimental data of the scattering properties of normal and immersed human skin in the spectral range from 400 to 700 nm allows one to reconstruct spectral dependences of both refractive indices for material of effective scatterers $n_{ss}(\lambda)$ and ground (interstitial liquid) material $n_{si}(\lambda)$ as[703]

$$n_{ss}(\lambda) = 1.4776 - 1.7488 \times 10^4 \lambda^{-2} + 6.7270 \times 10^9 \lambda^{-4} - 3.3390 \times 10^{14} \lambda^{-6},$$
(2.41)

$$n_{si}(\lambda) = 1.3510 + 2.1342 \times 10^3 \lambda^{-2} + 5.7893 \times 10^8 \lambda^{-4} - 8.1548 \times 10^{13} \lambda^{-6}.$$
(2.42)

Using the law of Gladstone and Dale [Eq. (1.150)] and these expressions, one can derive the dispersion formula for a whole skin as[703]

$$n_{skin}(\lambda) = 1.3090 - 4.3460 \times 10^2\lambda^{-2} + 1.6065 \times 10^9\lambda^{-4} - 1.2811 \times 10^{14}\lambda^{-6}.$$
(2.43)

This is a more precise formula for describing the refractive index of skin than Eq. (2.26), which was received from the simplest suppositions for a skin model as a mixture of water and proteins with a constant refractive index.

For tissue optics, this is of great importance to know the dispersion properties of melanin, which is contained in skin, hairs, eye sclera and iris, and other tissues. Melanin granules are the major back-reflecting particles in OCT and small-scale spatially resolved spectroscopy of skin. The above-described spectroscopic studies of water suspensions of natural melanin, where the mean radius of particles was determined using electronic microscopy, allow us to solve the inverse problem and to reconstruct the wavelength dependence of the refractive index of melanin particles in the range from 350 to 800 nm as[703,761]

$$n_M(\lambda) = 1.6840 - 1.8723 \times 10^4\lambda^{-2} + 1.0964 \times 10^{10}\lambda^{-4} - 8.6484 \times 10^{14}\lambda^{-6}.$$
(2.44)

An original method for measuring the refractive indices of dentine matrices, based on optical immersion and taking advantage of its tubular structure and the ability to transmit light as in a waveguide, was proposed in Ref. 763. Using this method for freshly cut teeth, n_0 was found to be 1.553 ± 0.001 for visible light.

A short-pulse time-delay technique was also successfully applied for refractive index estimation of normal breast tissue (of thickness $d = 0.8$ mm) and malignant breast tissue ($d = 0.85$ mm).[31] Using the known thickness of the sample and the measured shift Δt of the transmitted pulse peak relative to the delay time measured through a layer of air of the same thickness, the mean phase refractive index $\bar{n}$ of a tissue sample can be calculated. Very short pulses should be used in such measurements; thus, a group of different wavelengths propagates in a media and the material dispersion $(d\bar{n}/d\lambda)$ should be accounted for by introducing the group refractive index

$$\bar{n}_g = \bar{n} - \lambda\left(\frac{d\bar{n}}{d\lambda}\right).$$
(2.45)

The time delay in the pulse arrival for a tissue sample of thickness d is[31]

$$\Delta t = \left(\frac{d}{c_0}\right)(\bar{n}_{g1} - n_{g2}),$$
(2.46)

where c_0 is the light velocity in a vacuum, $\bar{n}_{g1}$ is the effective (mean) group refractive index of a tissue, and n_{g2} is the group refractive index of the homogeneous reference medium (air). The effective group refractive index of a tissue is

$$\bar{n}_{g1} = f_s n_{gs} + (1 - f_s)n_{g0},$$
(2.47)

where f_s is the volume fraction of the scatterers composing a tissue, n_{gs} is the group refractive index of the scatterers, and n_{g0} is the group refractive index of the ground material of a tissue. The values of the phase refractive index of the above-mentioned two samples were calculated to be $\bar{n} = 1.403$ for normal and 1.431 for malignant tissue.[31]

As it was already shown, OCT dynamic and spatially confined measurements of refractive index and scattering coefficients of tissue and blood are very important for the monitoring of physiological changes in living tissues.[737,711–713,716–718,720,750–753] For basic principles and applications of OCT, see Chapters 4 and 9. OCT provides simple and straightforward measurements of the index of refraction both *in vitro* and *in vivo*.[423,712,713,737,750–753,765–777] The in-depth scale of OCT images is determined by the optical path length Δz_{opt} between two points along the depth direction. Because a broadband light source is used, the optical path length is proportional to the group refractive index n_g and geometrical path length Δz as[693]

$$\Delta z_{opt} = n_g \Delta z. \tag{2.48}$$

Usually, $n_g \cong n$. This simple relation is valid for a homogeneous medium and can be used in *in vitro* studies when geometrical thickness of a tissue sample Δz is known.

Sometimes both the refractive index and thickness of a tissue sample should be measured simultaneously. In that case, a two-step procedure can be applied.[765,767,772] First, a stationary mirror is placed in the sample arm of an interferometer to get the geometric position of the mirror supposing that the group refractive index of air is $1(z_1)$. Then a tissue sample with unknown index n_g and thickness d should be placed before the mirror in the sample arm. Two peaks from the anterior (z_2) and the posterior (z_3) surfaces of the sample will appear with the distance between them equal to a sample optical thickness [see Eq. (2.48)], and the position of the mirror (z_4) will be shifted by $(n_g - 1)d$ due to the sample whose group refractive index is greater than that of air. Thus, the calculation of the geometrical thickness and the group refractive index proceeds as follows:

$$d = (z_3 - z_2) - (z_4 - z_1), \quad n_g = \frac{z_3 - z_2}{d}. \tag{2.49}$$

For *in vivo* measurements of the index of refraction, a focus-tracking method that uses OCT to track the focal-length shift that results from translating the focus of an objective along the optical axis within a tissue was introduced[767] and further developed.[712,713,768–771] For the refractive index evaluation, the coincidence of the maxima of the interference pattern and spatial focus, registered as a signal maximum, is needed. At least two points along the depth direction have to be probed to estimate a mean value of the refractive index between them. Usually a multistep measurement is provided. The geometric average refractive index for a fiber/lens focus tracking system is defined by the following expression:[712,713]

$$\tilde{n} = \sqrt{n_g n} = \frac{n_{obj}}{\sqrt{1 - \dfrac{\Delta z_{L1}}{\Delta z_{Fiber}}}}, \qquad (2.50)$$

where n_{obj} is the refractive index of the objective in the sample arm, Δz_{L1} is the change of position of the first objective lens, and Δz_{Fiber} is the fiber tip position in the sample arm. The difference between both refractive indices is usually small, only a few percent, and can be ignored in practice. For a piecewise homogeneous medium along the depth direction, the slope $\Delta z_{L1}/\Delta z_{Fiber}$ has to be evaluated at the focus tracked condition (Δz_{L1} positioned for maximum signal).

   A bifocal optical coherence refractometer, which is based on the measurements of the optical path length difference between two foci simultaneously, was recently suggested.[770,771] The main advantage of this technique is that it avoids the need to physically relocate the objective lens or the sample during an axial scan. At employment of a relatively low numerical aperture (NA) objective lens in the sample arm, the ratio of the optical path length difference between two foci, measured in the medium, Δz_{f-opt}, and in air, Δz_f, is described by the expression[771]

$$\frac{\Delta z_{f-opt}}{\Delta z_f} \approx n_g n \left[1 + \frac{1}{2}(NA)^2 \left(1 - \frac{1}{n^2} \right) \right]. \qquad (2.51)$$

For a typical value of tissue index of refraction $n = 1.4$ and $NA = 0.2$, the second term in the square parentheses is of only 1% of the magnitude of the ratio. Accounting for this estimation and that $n_g \cong n$, a much simple relation, as used in Ref. 712, can be found as

$$\Delta z_{f-opt} \approx n^2 \Delta z_f. \qquad (2.52)$$

   Received relations [see Eqs. (2.48)–(2.52)] for refractive index evaluation supposed homogeneous media under study. Tissues and blood are inhomogeneous media with a high scattering. Thus, these relations should be modified. For example, the modified Eq. (2.48) can be applied for describing dynamic OCT images for blood samples at sedimentation (see Fig. 2.15).[737] The OCT image demonstrates that in a process of blood sedimentation, the mean refractive index of a blood layer is reduced (the line, showing the reflectance of the posterior surface of a cuvette, is moving up with time). Such behavior can be understood through the mechanism of the reduction of the bulk scattering due to cell aggregation.

   When the refractive index of the scatters n_s differs little from the ground medium n_0, the scattered field $E_{sc}(r)$ at position r can be written as the following iterative series:[402]

$$E_{sc}(r) = \alpha E_1(r) + \alpha^2 E_2(r) + \cdots, \qquad (2.53)$$

where

$$\alpha = (n_s - n_0)/2\pi n_0. \qquad (2.54)$$

The first term in Eq. (2.53) accounts for single-scattering events, the Rayleigh-Gans approximation; the second term accounts for all double-scattering events. Values of $E_{sc}(r)$ in the direction of propagation of the incident light (along the positive z-axis) make up the "forward-scattered light." This portion of the scattered light adds to the incident wave, slightly changing both its phase and magnitude, which can be expressed as[402]

$$\exp\left[ik\left(z + L\frac{\Delta n}{n_0}\right)\right], \qquad (2.55)$$

where $k = 2\pi/\lambda$ is the wave number, λ is the wavelength within the medium of index n_0, and L is the thickness of the scattering medium. The real part of the quantity Δn gives a phase change of the transmitted light, so it should be interpreted as an index change of the medium due to light scattering. The imaginary part of Δn leads to an exponential decay of the transmitted wave caused by the scattered light escaping from the propagating light.

The refractive index n_Σ of the medium is[402]

$$n_\Sigma = n_0 + \Delta n = \bar{n} + \frac{\overline{n^2} - \bar{n}^2}{\bar{n}} Q(\lambda/l_c), \qquad (2.56)$$

where $\bar{n}$ is defined by the refractive indices of tissue or blood compounds [see Eq. (1.150)]; for a two-compound medium it is equal to

$$\bar{n} = f_s n_s + (1 - f_s)n_0, \qquad (2.57)$$

where f_s is the volume fraction of scattering particles; $\overline{n^2}$ is the mean-square value of refractive index fluctuations, $Q(\lambda/l_c)$ refers to the form of scatters and their aggregation, and l_c is the correlation length of randomly distributed refractive index fluctuations. $Q = 1.17$ in the limit of large correlation length, $l_c \gg \lambda$ (large particles), and $Q = 0$ in the limit of small l_c (Rayleigh limit). In the case that index fluctuations take the form of parallel cylinders, $Q = 0.67$ for the large l_c.

In the process of blood sedimentation, the two-phase system of plasma and RBCs is formed. Each phase has its own volume (thickness after separation) and refractive index. Let us define the time-dependent thickness of the RBC layer as $H(t)$, then the thickness of the upper clear plasma is $[L - H(t)]$ (see Fig. 2.15). The averaged refractive index of the layer of thickness L, containing two layers with different refractive indices, can be written in the form

$$n_{sed}(t) = \frac{[L - H(t)]}{L}\bar{n} + \frac{H(t)}{L}n_\Sigma, \qquad (2.58)$$

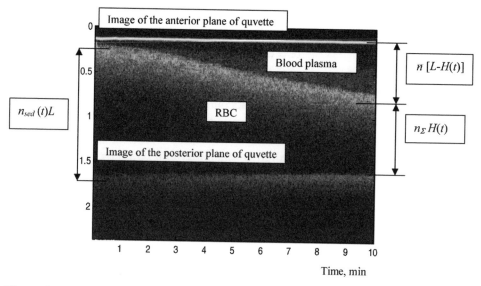

Figure 2.15 Blood sedimentation in a cuvette of $L = 1.1$ mm in thickness. Dynamic OCT in-depth image ($\lambda = 820$ nm) of whole blood sample slightly diluted by saline (13%) taken from a healthy volunteer (woman, 35 years old).[737]

where n and $\bar{n}$ are defined by Eqs. (2.56) and (2.57). Because of n_Σ always being larger than $\bar{n}$ and the sedimentation process in general is expressed as $H(t)/L \rightarrow$ Hct (blood hematocrit), then the total refractive index must go down with time.

For describing the influence of time-dependent refractive index changes on OCT images during blood sedimentation, n should be replaced by n_Σ in Eq. (2.48). The initial refractive index before sedimentation is started can be estimated from experimental the OCT image presented in Fig. 2.15 for whole blood slightly diluted by saline. The experimental value of $\Delta z_{\rm opt}$ (distance between upper and lower bright lines at zero time) is equal to 1.533 mm or for thickness of the blood vessel $\Delta z = 1.1$ mm, from relation $\Delta z_{\rm opt} \cong n_\Sigma \Delta z$ we can find $n_\Sigma = 1.394$. Accounting for the fact that the whole blood refractive index is $n_{\rm b} = 1.400$, we can estimate the expected value of the refractive index $n_\Sigma(t = 0)$ from $n_\Sigma(t = 0) = f_{\rm b} n_{\rm b} + (1 - f_{\rm b}) n_{\rm saline}$, where $f_{\rm b}$ is the volume fraction of whole blood in the sample and $n_{\rm saline}$ is the index of saline. For $f_{\rm b} = 0.87$ and $n_{\rm saline} = 1.330$, the expected value of $n_\Sigma = 1.391$ is well fitted to the measured one.

The experimental value of $\Delta z_{\rm opt}$ at 10 min is equal to 1.483 mm; thus, $n_{\rm sed}(t = 10$ min$) = 1.348$. Accounting for this, from the OCT image, where $(L - H)/L = 0.55$, $H/L = 0.45$, and $\bar{n} = f_{\rm bp} n_{\rm bp} + (1 - f_{\rm bp}) n_{\rm saline} = 0.87 \times 1.340 + 0.13 \times 1.33 = 1.339$, we can evaluate n_Σ from Eq. (2.58) as $n_\Sigma = 1.359$ and the corresponding relative index fluctuations of the RBC layer from Eq. (2.56) as $[(n^2 - \bar{n}^2)/\bar{n}] \cong 0.017$ for $Q = 1.17$.

Results of *in vitro* and *in vivo* measurements of phase and group refractive indices of tissue, blood, and their compounds using the technique discussed and some other techniques are summarized in Table 2.6.

3

Optical Properties of Eye Tissues

In this chapter, optical models of tissues with basic single and low-step scattering, with ordered and randomly distributed scatterers are analyzed. Three types of eye tissues with various structure and turbidity such as cornea, healthy or cataract lens, and sclera are presented as examples. Basic principles of transmission, reflection, and scattering spectra formation are discussed. Examples of measurements of the Mueller matrix elements for diagnostics and monitoring of biological objects are presented.

3.1 Optical models of eye tissues

3.1.1 Eye tissue structure

Healthy tissues of the anterior human eye chamber (see Fig. 3.1)[780–783] (e.g., the cornea and lens) are highly transparent for visible light because of their ordered structure and the absence of strongly absorbing chromophors. Scattering is an important feature of light propagation in eye tissues. The size of the scatterers and the distance between them are smaller than or comparable to the wavelength of visible light, and the relative refractive index of the scatterers is equally small (soft particles). Typical eye tissue models are long round dielectric cylinders (corneal and scleral collagen fibers) or spherical particles (lens protein structures) having a refractive index n_s; they are randomly (or quasi-orderly) (sclera, opaque lens) or regularly (transparent cornea and lens) distributed in the isotropic base matter with a refractive index $n_0 < n_s$.[3,10,24,61,63,64,77,129,172,397,399,402,403,432,433,435,436,439,440,722,723,762,778–799]
Light scattering analysis in eye tissue is often possible using a single scattering model owing to the small scattering cross section (soft particles).

Let us first consider the structure of the cornea and the sclera in more detail to demonstrate tissues with different size distributions and spatial ordering of scatterers.[3,129,432,722,723,762,778–787] The cornea is the frontal section of the eye's fibrous capsule; its diameter is about 10 mm. The sclera is a turbid opaque tissue that covers nearly 80% of the eye and serves as a protective membrane to provide, along with the cornea, for counteraction against internal and external forces and to retain eye shape. Both tissues are composed of collagen fibrils immersed in a ground substance.[432,722,723,762,778–780,784–787] The fibrils have a shape similar to that of a cylinder. They are packed in bundles like lamellae. Within each lamella, all of the fibers are nearly parallel with each other and with the lamella plane. Fibrils

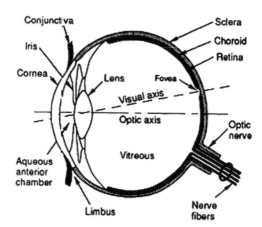

Figure 3.1 Diagram of the human eye showing the location of cornea, lens, sclera, and other eye components.[783]

and lamellar bundles are immersed within an amorphous ground (interstitial) substance containing water, glycosaminoglycans, proteins, proteoglycans, and various salts. The glycosaminoglycans play a key role in regulating the assembly of the collagen fibrils as well as in tissue permeability to water and other molecules.[786] The indices of refraction for the fibers and the ground substance differ markedly.

The structural elements that give the cornea the strength to preserve its proper curvature while withstanding intraocular pressure (14–18 mm Hg) are located within its stromal layer, which constitutes 0.9 of the cornea's thickness.[432,433,435,762,781–783] The stroma is composed of several hundred successively stacked layers of lamellae (see Fig. 3.2), which vary in width (0.5–250 µm) and thickness (0.2–0.5 µm), depending on the tissue region[762] (three sequential lamellae are shown in Fig. 3.3). A few flat cells (keratocytes) are dispersed between the lamellae, and these occupy only 0.03–0.05 of the stromal volume. Each lamella is composed of a parallel array of collagen fibrils. Human corneal thickness averages 0.52 mm.

Although the cornea fibril diameters vary from 25 to 39 nm in different mammals, the fibrils are quite uniform in diameter within each species.[762,778,786] Spacing between fibril centers is equal to 45–65 nm; intermolecular spacing within fibrils is in the range of 1.56–1.63 nm.[778] The fibrils in the human cornea have a uniform diameter of about 30.8 ± 0.8 nm with a periodicity close to two diameters, 55.3 ± 4.0 nm, and rather high regularity in the organization of fibril axes about one another (see Fig. 3.3). The intermolecular spacing is 1.63 ± 0.10 nm.[778] Thus, the stroma has at least three levels of structural organization: the lamellae that lie parallel to the cornea's surface; the fibrillar structure within each lamella that consists of small, parallel collagen fibrils with uniform diameters that have some degree of order in their spatial positions; and the collagen molecular ultrastructure.

The sclera contains three layers: the episclera, the stroma, and the lamina fusca.[723] The stroma is the thickest layer of the sclera. The thickness of the sclera and the arrangement of scleral collagen fibers show regional (limbal, equatorial,

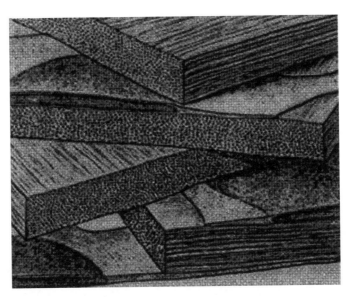

Figure 3.2 Schematic illustration of the lamellar organization of the cornea stroma. The diagram also depicts how keratocytes are interspersed between lamellae.[433]

and posterior pole region) and aging differences. In the scleral stroma, the collagen fibrils exhibit a wide range of diameters, from 25 to 230 nm (see Fig. 3.4).[762] The average diameter of the collagen fibrils increases gradually from about 65 nm in the innermost part to about 125 nm in the outermost part of the sclera;[785] the mean distance between fibril centers is about 285 nm.[787] Collagen intermolecular spacing is similar to that in the cornea; in bovine sclera, particularly, it is equal to 1.61 ± 0.02 nm.[786]

These fibrils are arranged in individual bundles in a parallel fashion, but more randomly than in the cornea; moreover, within each bundle, the groups of fibers are separated from each other by large empty lacunae randomly distributed in space.[762] Collagen bundles show a wide range of widths (1 to 50 μm) and thicknesses (0.5 to 6 μm) and tend to be wider and thicker toward the inner layers. These ribbonlike structures are multiply cross-linked; their length can be a few millimeters.[723] They cross each other in all directions, but remain parallel to the scleral surface. The episclera has a similar structure, with more randomly distributed and less compact bundles than in the stroma. The lamina fusca contains a larger amount of pigments, mainly melanin, which are generally located between the bundles. The sclera itself does not contain blood vessels, but has a number of channels that allow arteries, veins, and nerves to enter into or leave the eye.[723]

The thickness of the sclera is variable. It is thicker at the posterior pole (0.9 to 1.8 mm); it is thinnest at the equator (0.3 to 0.9 mm), and at the limbus is in the range of 0.5 to 0.8 mm.[723] Hydration of the human sclera can be estimated as 68%. About 75% of its dry weight is due to collagen, 10% is due to other proteins, and 1% to mucopolysaccharides.[723]

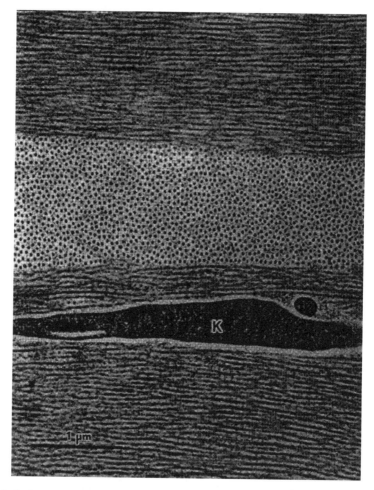

Figure 3.3 Collagen fibrils in the human cornea have a uniform diameter and are arranged in the same direction within the lamellae.[762] K is the keratocyte ($\times$32,000, scanning electron microscopy).

In designing an optical model of a tissue, in addition to form, sizes, and density of the scatterers (fibrils) and the tissue thickness, it is important to have information on the refractive indices of the tissue components. Following Refs. 172, 723, 778, and 780, we can estimate the refractive index of the corneal and scleral fibrils (hydrated collagen) n_c using Eq. (1.151), which was written for the average refractive index of the tissue, $\bar{n}_t$:

$$n_c = \frac{\bar{n}_t - (1 - f_c)n_{is}}{f_c}, \tag{3.1}$$

where f_c is the volume fraction of the hydrated collagen and n_{is} is the refractive index of the interstitial fluid. The refractive indices measured for the dry corneal collagen and for the interstitial fluid are: $n_c^{dry} = 1.547$ and $n_{is} = 1.345-$

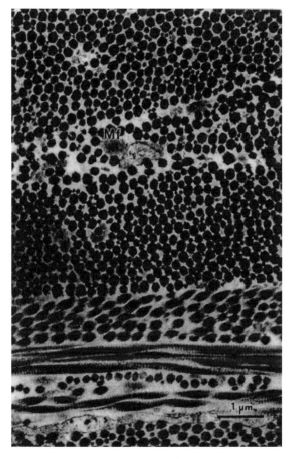

Figure 3.4 Collagen fibrils in the human sclera.[762] Scleral collagen fibrils display various diameters. They are much larger than those in the cornea. Mf is the microfibril ($\times$18,000, scanning electron microscopy).

$1.357.$[432,433,435,723,778,780] The refractive index of the corneal stroma measured for many species is $\bar{n}_t = 1.375 \pm 0.005$.[778] Therefore, for $n_{is} = 1.356$ and $f_c = 0.32$, corresponding to a tissue hydration of 76.2% and a collagen content of 61.3% of the dry weight,[778] on the basis of Eq. (3.1), it is easy to obtain the refractive index of the hydrated fibrils as $n_c = 1.415$. The direct measurement of the average refractive index of sclera using an Abbe refractometer gives $\bar{n}_t = 1.385 \pm 0.005$ for $\lambda = 589$ nm. Because of the similarly fibrous nature of the cornea and the sclera, it is expected that at equal hydration the refractive indices of scleral collagen and its interstitial fluid should be equal to these indices in the cornea. For $\bar{n}_t = 1.385$, $n_{is} = 1.345$, and $f_c = 0.31$, corresponding to a tissue hydration of 68% and a collagen content of 75% of the dry weight, it follows from Eq. (3.1) that for the refractive index of the scleral fibrils, $n_c = 1.474$. Changes of n_c and f_c with hydration can be evaluated from measurements of the refractive index and the thickness of the collagen films.[764]

Although both tissues are composed of similar molecular components, they have different microstructures and thus very different physiological functions. The cornea is transparent, allowing for more than 90% of the incident light to be transmitted. The collagen fibrils in the cornea have a much more uniform size and spacing than those in the sclera, resulting in a greater degree of spatial order in the organization of the fibrils in the cornea compared with the sclera. The sclera of the eye is opaque to light; it scatters almost all wavelengths of visible light and thus appears white.

Light propagation in a densely packed disperse system can be analyzed using the radial distribution function $g(r)$, which statistically describes the spatial arrangement of particles in the system. The function $g(r)$ is the ratio of the local number density of the fibril centers at a distance r from a reference fibril at $r = 0$ to the bulk number density of fibril centers.[433] It expresses the relative probability of finding two fibril centers separated by a distance r; thus, $g(r)$ must vanish for values of $r \leq 2a$ (a is the radius of a fibril—fibrils cannot approach each other closer than touching). The radial distribution function of scattering centers $g(r)$ for a certain tissue may be calculated on the basis of tissue electron micrographs (see Figs. 3.3 and 3.4).

The technique for the experimental determination of $g(r)$ involves counting the number of particles, placed at a specified spacing from an arbitrarily chosen initial particle, followed by statistical averaging over the whole ensemble. In a two-dimensional case, the particle number ΔN at the spacing from r to $r + \Delta r$ is related to the function $g(r)$ by the following equation:

$$\Delta N = 2\pi \rho g(r) r \Delta r, \tag{3.2}$$

where ρ is the mean number of particles for a unit area.

The radial distribution function $g(r)$ was first found for rabbit cornea by Farrell et al.[433] Figure 3.5(a) depicts a typical result for one of the cornea regions, which was obtained by determining the ratio of the local mean density of the centers as a function of radii taken from 700 fibril centers. The function $g(r) = 0$ for $r \leq 25$ nm, which is consistent with a fibril radius of 14 ± 2 nm, can be calculated from the electron micrograph.[433] The first peak in the distribution gives the most probable separation distance, which is approximately 50 nm. The value of $g(r)$ is essentially unity for $r \geq 170$ nm, indicating that the fibril positions are correlated over no more than a few of their nearest neighbors. Therefore, a short-range order exists in the system.

Similar calculations for several regions of human eye sclera[439,798] are illustrated in Fig. 3.5(b). Electron micrographs from Ref. 762, averaged for 100 fibril centers, were processed (see Fig. 3.4). The function $g(r)$ for the sclera was obtained on the basis of the spatial distribution of the fibril centers, neglecting discrepancies in their diameters. Some noise is due to the small volume of statistical averaging. The obtained results present evidence of the presence of a short-range order in the sclera, although the degree of order is less pronounced than in the

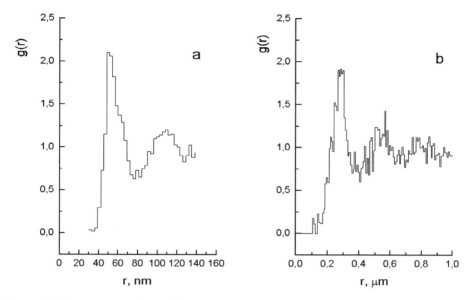

Figure 3.5 Histograms of radial distribution functions $g(r)$ obtained from electron micrographs of rabbit cornea (a)[433] and human sclera (b).[439,798]

cornea. The function $g(r) = 0$ for $r \leq 100$ nm, which is consistent with the mean fibril diameter of ≈ 100 nm derived from the electron micrograph (see Fig. 3.4).[762] The first peak in the distribution gives the most probable separation distance, which is approximately 285 nm. The value of $g(r)$ is essentially unity for $r \geq 750$ nm, indicating a short-range order in the system. The short-range order, being characterized by a ratio of this specific distance (decay of spatial correlation) to the most probable particle separation distance, $(750/285) \approx 2.7$, is smaller than the similar ratio for the cornea, $(170/50) = 3.4$.

The spatial density (refractive index) fluctuations of a tissue can also be analyzed by resolving 2D profiles of refractive index variations into Fourier components, which provides a basis for a detailed and quantitative description of the microstructure.[779,787] These Fourier components represent the predominant spatial density fluctuations and the structural ordering. A comparable study of human cornea and sclera has shown that cornea reveals much less collagen fibril spacing and greater spatial order than sclera.

The eye lens is also an example of a tissue in which the short-range spatial order is of crucial importance. Because of its high index of refraction and transparency, a lens focuses light to form an image at the retina (see Fig. 3.1). The eye lens material exhibits a certain viscosity that is capable of altering its radius of curvature and thus its focal length through the action of accommodating muscles. The healthy human lens is a coherent structure containing about 60% water and 38% protein.[789-797] The lens consists of many lens fiber cells. The predominant dry components of a mammalian lens are three kinds of structural proteins, named α-, β-, and γ-crystallins, and their combined weight accounts for about 33% of the total weight of the lens.[619] The crystalline lens grows throughout life and in addition undergoes a variety of biochemical changes as one ages. These changes include the possibility of age-related cataract formation, leading to greatly increased light scatter and coloration, and eventually to lens opacity. Photooxidation of lens proteins by chronic UV, UVA, or visible light results in oxidized forms of these proteins, which cross-link to other proteins, causing opacities or pigment formation.[800] The light scattering is caused by random fluctuations in the refractive index. These fluctuations can be density or optical anisotropy fluctuations.[64,397,401,402,409,789,791,795] Fluctuations in the refractive index due to density may arise because of (1) aggregation of lens proteins, (2) microphase separation (cold-induced cataract), or (3) syneresis (water is released from the bound state in the hydration layers of lens proteins and becomes bulk water; this increases the refractive index difference between the lens proteins and the surrounding fluid). Analyses of polarized light scattering of human cataracts have shown that 15 to 30% of the turbidity results from optical anisotropy fluctuations.

Eye lens transparency can be explained by a short-range ordering in the packing structure of the lens proteins. This idea was first suggested by Benedek.[801] The primary role among the ocular lens proteins is played by the water-soluble α-crystallin, which has a shape that is close to spherical with a diameter of about 17 nm. Studies of lens transparency, birefringence, and optical activity are of importance to the facilitation of early diagnosis of cataracts.[619,789–797,800–804]

The types of fiber cell disruption due to cataract formation include intracellular globules, clusters of globules, vacuoles with the contents wholly or partially removed, clusters of highly curved cell membranes, and odd-shaped domains of high or low density.[797] These spherical objects are variable in size (often in the range 100 to 250 nm) and occur in clusters that create potential scattering centers.

Optical models of the eye tissues have the following specific features:

- Optical inhomogeneity gives rise to light scattering.
- The mean distance between scatterers and their dimensions are less than or comparable with the wavelength.
- Scattering particles are "soft," i.e., the refractive index of their material, n_s, is close to the refractive index of the ground (interstitial) substance, n_0 ($n_s \geq n_0$).
- In the major cases, absorption is small.
- Transparent tissue has an approximately monodispersive and ordered structure.

The major structural characteristics of the human eye tissues are summarized in Table 3.1.

3.1.2 Tissue ordering

A certain correlation exists between waves scattered by adjacent particles in a densely packed medium that has characteristic dimensions on the order of a wavelength. Therefore, it is necessary to sum the amplitudes of scattered waves with

Table 3.1 Structural and optical properties of human eye tissues (the refractive index of the ground (interstitial) substance $n_0 = 1.345$).

Tissue	Model	Tissue thickness, mm	Diameter of scatterers, nm	Refractive index of scatterers, n_s	Multiplicity of scattering
Cornea	Monodispersive system of regularly distributed long dielectric cylinders	0.46–0.52	30.8 ± 0.8	1.470	Single or low-step
Sclera	Polydispersive system of randomly distributed long dielectric cylinders	0.3–1.8	25–230	1.474	Multiple
Normal lens	Monodispersive system of regularly distributed dielectric spheres	5.0	20–200	1.380	Single or low-step
Cataract lens	Two-phase system of randomly distributed dielectric spheres	5.0	200–2000	1.40–1.48	Low-step or multiple

regard to their phase relations. The interference interaction may result in an essential alteration of the total scattered intensity, of its angular dependence, or of the polarization characteristics of the scattered light as compared with similar quantities for a system of noninteracting particles.

To illustrate light scattering in a correlated disperse system, we will use a radial distribution function $g(r)$, which is a statistical characteristic of the spatial arrangement of the scatterers[129,433] (see Fig. 3.5). Let us consider N spherical particles in a finite volume. The pair distribution function $g_{ij}(r)$ is proportional to the conditional probability of finding a particle of type j at distance r from the origin, given that there is a particle of type i at the origin (Fig. 3.6).[805] In a model of mutually impenetrable (hard) spheres, the interparticle forces are zero, except for the fact that two neighbor particles cannot interpenetrate each other.

The arrangement of particles in a densely packed system is not entirely random. A short-range order can be observed that is more ordered when the density of the scattering centers is greater and their size distribution is narrower. Near the origin of the coordinates, in the region within the effective particle diameter, the function $g(r) = 0$, which points to the impenetrability of a particle. Function $g(r)$ has a few maxima whose positions correspond to distances from the chosen particle to its first, second, etc., neighbors. Nonzero values of minima are indicative of a particle distribution between various coordination spheres. It is obvious that the correlation between the pairs of particles should be degraded with r; hence, $\lim_{r \to \infty} g(r) = 1$. Function $g(r)$ is the ratio of the local number density of the scattering centers at a distance r from an arbitrary center to the bulk number density.

The medium composed of N scatterers considered here is analogous to an ensemble mixture of L types of particles in the study of statistical mechanics, by considering the dynamics and positions of the particles with regard to the interparticle forces. Studies have been made in obtaining the pair distribution functions using various approximate theories. One of the important results is based on the Percus-Yevick (PY) approximation. As applied to a model of hard spheres distributed in a three-dimensional space, there exists an analytical solution of this equation. To find the function of radial distribution, the Monte Carlo method is also used. The solution of the Ornstein-Zernice equation for the case of single species has been solved by Wertheim.[806] For the case of two species, the solution can be found in Ref. 807. For the general case of L species, the solution based on a generalized Wiener-Hopf technique is obtained by Baxter.[808] The polydispersity of the real system is approximated by an L-step distribution function.

For monodisperse systems of spherical particles with a diameter of $2a$, $g(r)$ is represented by an approximation of the hard spheres as follows:[809]

$$g(r) = 1 + \frac{1}{4\pi f} \int_0^\infty \frac{H_3^2(z)}{1 - H_3(z)} \frac{\sin zx}{zx} z^2 dz, \quad \text{for } x > 1, \qquad (3.3)$$

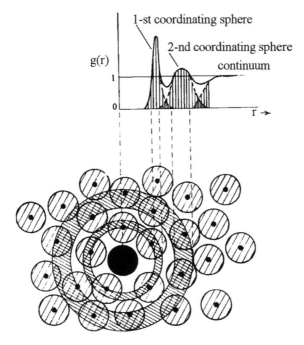

Figure 3.6 Diagram of the radial distribution function $g(r)$, which is proportional to the probability of particle displacement at a certain distance r from an arbitrarily fixed particle.[805]

where $x = r/2a$,

$$H_3(z) = 24f \int_0^1 c_3(x)\frac{\sin zx}{zx}x^2 dx, \quad c_3(x) = -\alpha - \beta x - \delta x^3, \tag{3.4}$$

$$\alpha = \frac{(1+2f)^2}{(1-f)^4}, \quad \beta = -6f\frac{(1+0.5f)^2}{(1-f)^4}, \quad \delta = \frac{1}{2}f\frac{(1+2f)^2}{(1-f)^4}, \tag{3.5}$$

where f is the volume fraction of the particles.

Let us consider light scattering by a system of N spherical particles.[442] In general, the field affecting a particle differs from the field of the incident wave E_i since the latter also contains the total field of adjacent scatterers. Within the single-scattering approximation (Born's approximation), the field that affect the particle does not essentially differ from that of the initial wave. In cases where double scattering of the field affects the particle, one needs to take the sum of the initial field plus the single-scattered field, and so on.[75] For transparent tissues composed of optically soft quasi-regularly packed particles, the use of the single-scattering approximation yields quite satisfactory results.[10,24,63,64,77,129,399,402,403,433,435,436,440,780,789,791,801,802]

A field scattered by a particle with the center defined by radius vector $\vec{r}_j$ differs from one scattered by a particle placed at the origin of the coordinates by a phase multiplier characterizing the phase shift of the waves. The phase difference is equal to $(2\pi/\lambda)(\vec{S}_0 - \vec{S}_1)\vec{r}_j$, where $\vec{S}_0$ and $\vec{S}_1$ are the unit vectors of the directions of the incident and the scattered waves (see Fig. 1.23). The difference between these vectors is called the scattering vector $\vec{q}$:

$$\vec{q} = \frac{2\pi}{\lambda}(\vec{S}_0 - \vec{S}_1). \tag{3.6}$$

Taking into account that the wave vector module is invariable with elastic scattering, the value of the scattering vector is found as follows:

$$|\vec{q}| \equiv q = \frac{4\pi}{\lambda}\sin\left(\frac{\theta}{2}\right), \tag{3.7}$$

where θ is the angle between directions $\vec{S}_0$ and $\vec{S}_1$, i.e., it is the scattering angle. The amplitude of a wave scattered by a system of N particles will be

$$E_s = \sum_{j=1}^{N} E_{sj} = \sum_{j=1}^{N} E_{0j} e^{i\vec{q}\vec{r}_j}, \tag{3.8}$$

where E_{0j} is the scattering amplitude of an isolated particle. The single-scattering intensity for the given spatial realization of the N particle arrangement is

$$I = |E_s|^2 = \sum_{j=1}^{N} E_{0j} \sum_{i=1}^{N} E_{0i}^* e^{i\vec{q}(\vec{r}_j - \vec{r}_i)}. \tag{3.9}$$

For real systems, the only mean scattering intensity of an ensemble of particles is detected; the natural averaging is caused by thermal particle motion, finite measuring time, and a finite area of a photodetector, thus

$$\langle I \rangle = \left\langle \sum_{j=1}^{N} \sum_{i=1}^{N} E_{0j} E_{0i}^* e^{i\vec{q}(\vec{r}_j - \vec{r}_i)} \right\rangle. \tag{3.10}$$

The brackets show the averaging over all possible configurations of the particle arrangement in the system. This equation represents the sum of the two contributions to the noncoherent scattered intensity. One defines the light distribution on the assumption that there is no interference of light scattered by various particles. The other term regards the interference affect on the light field structure and depends on the degree of order in the particle arrangement that is characterized by the radial distribution function $g(r)$. For an isotropic system of identical spherical particles, we may write[436]

$$\langle I \rangle = |E_0|^2 N S_3(\theta), \tag{3.11}$$

$$S_3(\theta) = \left\{ 1 + 4\pi\rho \int_0^R r^2 [g(r) - 1] \frac{\sin qr}{qr} dr \right\}, \qquad (3.12)$$

where q is defined by Eq. (3.7), ρ is the mean density of particles, and R is the distance for which $g(r) \rightarrow 1$. Quantity $S_3(\theta)$ is the 3D structure factor. This factor describes the alteration of the angle dependence of the scattered intensity that appears with a higher particle concentration (Fig. 3.7). To approximate the hard spheres used for the derivation of Eq. (3.12), the structure factor is defined as

$$S_3(\theta) = \frac{1}{1 - H_3(q)}, \qquad (3.13)$$

where $H_3(q)$ is defined by Eq. (3.4).

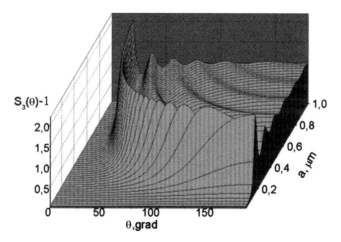

Figure 3.7 The structure factor $S_3(\theta)$ [Eq. (3.12)] as a function of the scattering angle θ and particle radius a; the wavelength 633 nm; the volume fraction $f = 0.4$; the relative refraction index $m = 1.105$ (calculated by I. L. Maksimova).

For small particle concentrations, the approximation of the excluded volume is applicable: $g(r) = 0$ for r that are shorter than the particle diameter and have unity over long distances. In this approximation, the structure factor for a system of spherical particles takes the form that was first discovered by Dirac as[442]

$$S_3(\theta) = 1 - f\Phi(qa), \qquad (3.14)$$

where a is the particle radius and $\Phi(qa)$ is the function defined by the following equation:

$$\Phi(qa) = \frac{3(\sin qa - qa \cos qa)}{(qa)^3}. \qquad (3.15)$$

Function $\Phi(qa)$ modulates the angular dependence of the scattering intensity by diminishing its value at small angles and generating a diffusion ring at 10-deg angles for particle dimensions comparable with the wavelength.

For the case of infinitely long identically aligned cylinders with a radius a and a light that is incident normally to their axes, the 2D structure factor is defined within the approximation of a single scattering as follows:

$$S_2(\theta) = \left\{ 1 + 8\pi a^2 \rho \int_0^R [g(r) - 1] J_0\left(\frac{2\pi a}{\lambda} r \sin \frac{\theta}{2} \right) dr \right\}, \qquad (3.16)$$

where R is the distance for which $g(r) \to 1$. Since the light is incident perpendicularly to the cylinder axis, the scattered light propagates only in the direction perpendicular to the axis.

For a very small concentration of particles, the structure factor is nearly a unit and the intensity of scattering by a disperse system is essentially a sum of the contributions of the independent scatterers. For systems of small soft particles, the structure factor only changes slightly as a function of the scattering angle. Therefore, the particle interaction reveals itself mainly by a uniform decrease in scattering intensity in all directions for linearly polarized and unpolarized incident light (see Figs. 3.8 and 3.9). For systems of large particles, the structure factor is noticeably less than a unit only in the region of small scattering angles (see Figs. 3.10 and 3.11). The interference interaction of scatterers in some angular bands reduces the scattering intensity and in the other bands the scattering intensity is raised as compared with that for a system of an equivalent number of independent particles (Fig. 3.11). In general, particle interaction makes the angular dependence of the scattering intensity more symmetric with less overall scattered intensity, and therefore allows much more collimated transmittance for both small and large soft particles.

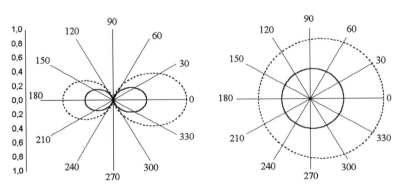

Figure 3.8 The calculated angular dependences of the scattered intensity for a system of small spherical particles, 20-nm radius; the incident wave is linearly polarized (a) parallel with or (b) perpendicular to the scattering plane; dotted line—independent particles; wavelength, 633 nm; volume fraction, $f = 0.1$; relative refraction index, $m = 1.105$ (calculated by I. L. Maksimova).

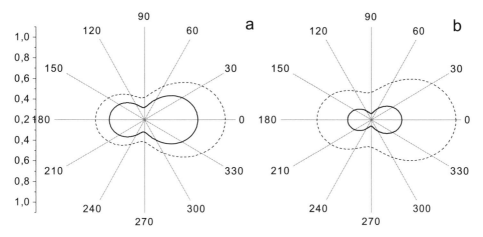

Figure 3.9 The calculated angular dependences of the scattered intensity for a system of small spherical particles, 50-nm radius; the incident wave is unpolarized; dotted line—independent particles; wavelength, 633 nm; volume fractions, (a) $f = 0.04$ and (b) $f = 0.1$; relative refraction index, $m = 1.105$.[442]

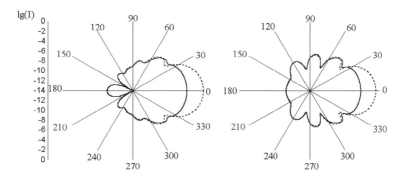

Figure 3.10 The calculated angular dependences of the scattered intensity for a system of large spherical particles, 500-nm radius; the incident wave is linearly polarized (a) parallel with or (b) perpendicular to the scattering plane; dotted line—independent particles; wavelength, 633 nm; volume fraction, $f = 0.4$; relative refraction index, $m = 1.105$ (calculated by I. L. Maksimova).

The scattering strongly deforms the spectral tissue characteristics because the extinction of transmitted light is defined not only by the absorption factor as a function of the wavelength, but also by a light fraction taken away from the beam because of the scattering. The latter process depends complexly on the wavelength, structure, and size of the particles.

The spectrum of collimated transmission of a disperse layer is interpreted as a spectral dependence of a weaker coherent component of light. Finding the coherent component of light, scattered at a system of inhomogeneities correlated in the space, is a complicated physical task exhibiting all of the difficulties inherent in the problem of light propagation through a system of many bodies.[809] Assuming that the intensity of the coherent light component I_c is reduced with a longer distance

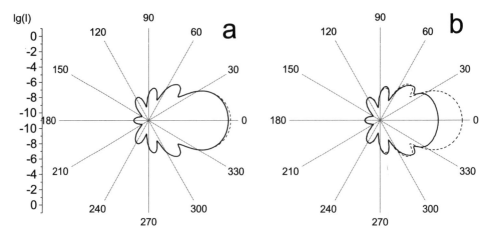

Figure 3.11 The calculated angular dependences of the scattered intensity for a system of large spherical particles, 500 nm radius; the incident wave is unpolarized; dotted line—independent particles; wavelength, 633 nm; volume fractions, (a) $f = 0.04$ and (b) $f = 0.4$; relative refraction index, $m = 1.105$.[442]

d by the exponent law due to scattering and absorption, the disperse layer collimated transmittance would be described by the Bouguer-Beer-Lambert law [see Eq. (1.1)] as

$$T_c(\lambda_0, d) \equiv [I_c(\lambda_0, d)/I_0(\lambda_0)] \propto \exp[-\rho_s \sigma_{ext}(\lambda_0)d], \qquad (3.17)$$

where σ_{ext} is the extinction cross section of an individual particle of the layer [see Eq. (1.4)]. For small volume concentrations (ρ_s), it is equivalent to the extinction cross section of an independent particle. For greater f values, the quantity σ_{ext} is determined not only by the properties of single particles, but also by their concentration. Within the assumption that the absorption cross section σ_{abs} is independent of the packing density, σ_{ext} may be calculated as a sum of σ_{abs} for the independent particle and the scattering cross section σ_{sca} obtained by taking into consideration the correlation of scatterers.

With the measuring of the scattered intensity angular distribution of the particle system, one would calculate the scattering cross section of a single particle of the system. Having integrated the scattering intensity over all directions in the space, the total energy scattered by the system can be found. The scattering cross section for the system of spherical particles is obtained similarly to Eq. (1.6); however, to calculate the scattering cross section of a single particle of the system, the scattered intensity must be divided by the particle number N and corrected by using the 3D or 2D structure factor S_3 [Eq. (3.12)] or S_2 [Eq. (3.16)].

The scattering cross section for the system of rods (cylinder particles) Σ_{sca} (cm), illuminated by a plane incident wave of intensity I_0 in the direction normal to the cylinder axis, is defined by numerically integrating over all possible scattering directions in plane perpendicular to the cylinder axis:[148]

$$\Sigma_{sca} = \frac{2\pi}{\lambda I_0} \int_0^{2\pi} I_\Sigma(\theta) d\theta, \tag{3.18}$$

where $I_\Sigma(\theta)$ is the angular distribution of the scattered intensity of a system of N particles. Dividing Σ_{sca} by the particle number N, one may find the scattering cross section σ_{sca} for a single particle of the system. For an interacting particle system, the result obtained may differ substantially from the scattering cross section of an independent particle.

Even the scattering cross section for an independent particle sized on the order of a wavelength has a very strong nonmonotonous dependence on the wavelength. Effects associated with dense packing also have a substantial dependence on the wavelength. As a result, the transmission spectra for a system of identical particles can differ highly depending on the packing density and its degree of order. Wonderful examples are the transmission spectra of the cornea in the norm and with turbidity caused by a disrupted spatial degree of order and by appearing regions denuded of fibrils, the so-called lakes.[435]

The extinction of a collimated incident beam due to scattering, even in systems of nonabsorbing particles, would result in a substantial difference in the transmittance in different spectral regions. The values of the real and imaginary part of the indices of refraction depend weakly on the wavelength far from the absorption bands and they may be assumed to be constant under calculation. In systems of small nonabsorbing particles, the interference interaction causes the shift of the short-wavelength transmission spectrum boundary to a smaller wavelength and a slightly greater steepness of the spectrum.[442] If a scattering system is formed by particles whose sizes are comparable with the light wavelength, then the spectrum of this system would be nonmonotonous, even with no absorption. In the vicinity of the absorption bands, the real and imaginary parts of the complex index of refraction of the particle substance [see Eq. (1.192)] show a pronounced spectral dependence, which determines the specificity of transmission spectra for systems of differently sized particles, with the imaginary part of refractive index usually described by the Lorentz contour.[442] The scattering deforms the symmetric contour of the absorption line and the spectra appear essentially different for systems of small and big particles with varying packing densities.

In general, this is typical for spectroscopy of tissue or blood when an absorbing band of a chromophore (hemoglobin) is detected on the background of the scattering part of the spectrum. For example, evaluation of hemoglobin saturation by oxygen in tissues is the problem that is usually solved by the exclusion of the scattering part of measured tissue spectra. The calculated transmission spectra also explain a phenomenon of substantial difference of spectra for the whole blood, where hemoglobin with a high index of refraction and strong absorption band is concentrated in erythrocytes (system of big particles with absorption), and for hemolyzed blood, where only small particles (blood residuals—cell skeletons, etc.) scatter light.

For the densely packed system of large weakly refracting particles, the following equation was obtained in Ref. 810 within the approximation of hard spheres and neglecting of mutual particle radiation for the coherent transmission of a layer with thickness d:

$$T_c = \left[1 - \frac{2b}{(1+b)} \frac{\sigma_{ext}}{\pi a^2} + \frac{b^2}{(1+b)^2} \frac{2\lambda}{\pi a^3} \sigma_{sca} I_1(0) \right]^{d/2a}, \qquad (3.19)$$

where $b = 1.5f \exp(1.5f)$ and $I_1(0)$ is the intensity of forward scattering by an individual particle of radius a. This formula is transformed into Bouguer's law [see Eq. (3.17)] for the scattering systems of noninteracting particles at the rarefaction of the scattering layer.

Not only coherent weakened light, but also a portion of noncoherently scattered light is usually recorded in real experiments owing to the finite angular aperture of the receiving unit. For this reason, a transmittance called the instrumental transparency, which is found experimentally, is somewhat different from the coherent transmission T_c.

For the first time, the approximation regarding the near-order degree of tissue arrangement has been used to describe light propagation in the cornea with calculating its transmission spectrum by the authors of Refs. 432, 433, and 435. The near order in the arrangement of scattering particles and the related interference interaction of scattered light are the course of the high transparency of the human eye's cornea and lens in their normal state.[63,64,802]

The light-scattering intensity angular dependences for systems of spherical and cylindrical particles in the single-scattering approximation are described by Eqs. (3.11), (3.12), and (3.16). The structure factor, which transforms these dependences, is defined by the spatial particle arrangement, and it is independent of the state of light polarization. Therefore, for systems of identical particles, when the single scattering approximation is valid, the angular dependences of all of the elements of the light-scattering matrix (LSM) are multiplied by the same quantity, accounting for interference interaction [see Eq. (3.11)], as

$$M_{ij}(\theta) = M_{ij}^0(\theta) N S_3(\theta), \qquad (3.20)$$

where $M_{ij}^0(\theta)$ is the LSM element for an isolated particle. Consequently, the LSM for the system of monodispersive interacting particles coincides with that of the isolated particle [see Eq. (1.72)] if normalization to the magnitude of its first element M_{11} is used.

Unlike in monodispersive systems, in differently sized densely packed particle systems, the normalization of the matrix elements to M_{11} does not eliminate the influence of the structure factor on the angular dependences of the matrix elements. In the simplest case of a bimodal system of scatterers, expressions analogous to Eqs. (3.12) and (3.16) can be found using four structural functions, $g_{11}(r)$, $g_{22}(r)$, $g_{12}(r)$, and $g_{21}(r)$, which characterize the interaction between particles of similar and different sizes.[436] A bimodal system formed by a great number of equally sized small particles, and a minor fraction of coarse ones, provides a good model of pathological tissue, e.g., a cataract eye lens.

Figure 3.12 depicts the calculated results for the LSM elements for a binary mixture of spherical particles with two different diameters, 60 and 500 nm, and corresponding volume fractions of $f_1 = 0.3$ and $f_2 = 0.02$.[436] For comparison, the LSM elements' angular dependences for the same binary mixture, neglecting cooperative effects, have also been calculated. It is seen from the figure that the normalized LSM elements of a dense binary mixture are substantially altered due to the interference interaction. As a consequence, the results of the solution of the inverse problem for the experimental LSM of a dense mixture, neglecting the co-operative effects, should yield an overestimated value for the relative fraction of large particles. The LSM variations due to cooperative effects are of a more com-plicated nature for a binary system whose two components are sized on the order of the wavelength of incident light, and they could not be interpreted as uniquely as those in the preceding case. Numerical estimates for binary systems of different compositions show[436] the considered effects to be of the most crucial importance for the LSM in the visible region for the mixtures of particles with $2a_1 < 200$ nm and $2a_2 > 250$ nm.

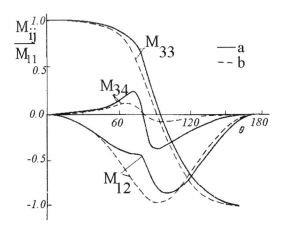

Figure 3.12 The LSM elements' angular dependences for a binary mixture of spherical particles.[436] Calculated taking into account particle interactions (solid lines), and neglecting cooperative effects (dashed lines). Particle diameters, $2a_1 = 60$ nm and $2a_2 = 500$ nm; volume fractions, $f_1 = 0.3$ and $f_2 = 0.02$; relative index of refraction, $m = 1.07$; wavelength, 633 nm.

Unlike the transmission spectra, the spectral dependences of the intensity of light scattered in different directions are poorly studied. This is related, on the one hand, to experimental difficulties due to the need for standard spectral devices to be modernized. On the other hand, an additional problem of correct comparison of different experimental results arises with examining the scattering spectra because the form of the scattering spectrum depends substantially on the macrogeometry of the sample and measuring system. Nevertheless, the scattering spectra are of great interest.[47,58,94-96,150-153,163,166,170,173,180,736,790] The authors of Ref. 736 deal with the absorption and scattering spectra of the chest muscle of a chicken in the visible range. The scattering spectra visually define the observed tissue color, and they can be employed for express estimating its state. For example, one traditional method for eye ocular lens diagnostics assumes the observation of varying color character- istics for light scattered at different angles. The theoretical background for quan- titative analysis of scattering spectra and color formation by eye lens (presented as a model of dispersive system of spherical particles with low absorption) and *in vitro* measured scattering spectra of the human eye lens are given in Ref. 811. The age-related alterations of the eye lens particle composition and correspond- ing transmittance and light-scattering spectra are modeled[173] and compared with experimental data from Ref. 790.

The spectral characteristics vary most strongly with high packing densities be- cause the volume fraction occupied by particles exceeds 50%. For these dense systems, the considered approximation of single scattering is incorrect and it is necessary to account for the effects of the reradiation of the particles.

3.2 Spectral characteristics of eye tissues

The collimated transmission spectrum of a tissue layer of thickness d with a mean density ρ_s of scattering particles with absorption is defined by Eq. (3.17), where $I_c(\lambda_0)$ is the spectrum of the transmitted intensity detected in a far field using a pinhole; the scattering cross section σ_{sca} for a given scattering model can be cal- culated using Eq. (1.6) for the corresponding angular dependence of the intensity scattered by a particle, $I(\theta)$. In the framework of Mie theory, the scattering and the absorption cross sections can be calculated using Eqs. (1.192)–(1.94). For ex- ample, for unpolarized collimated light incidence on a system of Mie particles, the scattered intensity is defined as

$$I_\Sigma(\theta, \lambda_0) \approx N\left(|S_1|^2 + |S_2|^2\right), \tag{3.21}$$

where N is the number of spherical particles and the S_1 and S_2 functions are de- fined by Eq. (2.11). Particle interaction can be accounted for using Eqs. (3.11), (3.12), and (3.16). The simpler Eq. (3.19) also can be used.

In turn, the transmission spectrum when a measuring system with a finite angle of view is used (a collimated light beam with some addition of a forward scattered light in the angle range 0 to θ is detected) is defined by

$$T_\theta(\lambda_0) = T_c(\lambda_0) + \left[\frac{1}{I_0(\lambda_0)}\right]\int_\theta I_\Sigma(\theta, \lambda_0)d\Omega, \tag{3.22}$$

where Ω is the solid angle in steradians.

The total transmission spectra $T_t(\lambda_0)$ and the spectrum of light scattered under the angle $(\theta + d\theta)$, $R_\theta(\lambda_0)$ can be calculated using the following definitions:

$$T_t(\lambda_0) = T_c(\lambda_0) + \left[\frac{1}{I_0(\lambda_0)}\right] \int_{2\pi} I_\Sigma(\theta, \lambda_0) d\Omega, \tag{3.23}$$

$$R_\theta(\lambda_0) = \left[\frac{1}{I_0(\lambda_0)}\right] \int_\theta^{\theta+d\theta} I_\Sigma(\theta, \lambda_0) d\Omega. \tag{3.24}$$

Corneal transmittance was calculated using a model monodisperse system of long dielectric nonabsorbing cylinders (fibrils) of 26 nm in diameter and with a refractive index $n_c = 1.470$. The cylinders were regularly oriented parallel to the corneal surface in the ground matter ($n_0 = 1.345$). Figure 3.13 demonstrates the transmittance anisotropy for linearly polarized radiation and the marked effect of scattering on corneal transmittance in the UV spectral region. The corneal transparence in the visible range is explained by the high degree of its fibrils' arrangement, so the diffuse light intensity decreases owing to interference along all directions (destructive interference), except the incident light direction (constructive interference). The effect of scattering is the most essential in a short-wavelength region and defines small UV radiation transmittance of the cornea, which is approximately 50% for 320 nm. It should be noted that in the UV range, light extinction is defined not only by scattering; the absorption bands of water and proteins provide a very strong extinction as well (see Figs. 1.3 and 1.5).

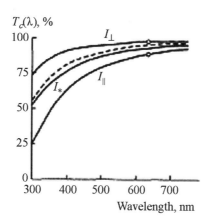

Figure 3.13 Collimated transmittance spectra of human cornea: $I_\parallel$, $I_\perp$, and I_* are calculated spectra for two orthogonal states of linear polarization and unpolarized light. Light polarization is parallel, $I_\parallel$, to the fibrils (calculations were made for the light normally incident on the corneal surface; they are valid for the peripheral conical portion where the fibrils are similarly oriented in tissue layers). The cornea is 0.46-mm thick, with a scatterer density $\rho_s = 3 \times 10^{10}$ cm^{-2}. The dotted line shows the experimental data for unpolarized light. The circles are measurements for two orthogonal states of polarization at $\lambda = 633$ nm.[63]

Disordering of the fibrils' arrangement (for example, after keratotomy) results in a decrease in corneal transmission, especially for the short wavelengths (Purkinje's effect).[63] Another essential feature of the cornea is the presence of a preferable direction of the fibrils' alignment. The results of such anisotropy are the form birefringence and dichroism of the cornea.[63] The transmission spectrum substantially depends on the orientation of the polarization vector of the linear polarized light relative to the collagen fibrils; light polarized along fibrils is scattered more effectively. As follows from calculations and measurements presented in Fig. 3.13, the peripheral corneal polarization sensitivity in the UV region (320 nm) is about fivefold higher than in the red region (633 nm). In the Rayleigh limit ($\lambda \gg 2a$), the form birefringence is defined by Eq. (1.53). The birefringence can be high for small-diameter cylinders and goes to zero for a system that consists of parallel cylinders with large diameters ($2a \geq \lambda$).[402]

The total and collimated (axial) experimental transmission spectra for the human cornea are presented in Fig. 3.14. They illustrate well that the cornea scatters light since the total and axial transmissions are not identical. Water absorption peaks are evident at 300, 980, 1180, 1450, 1900, and 2940 nm (see Fig. 1.3);[812] they provide poor transmission in the cornea in the UV and IR spectral regions.

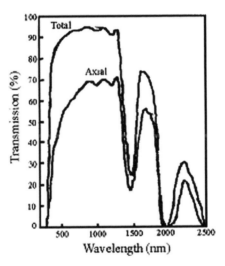

Figure 3.14 Total and axial (collimated) transmission through human cornea.[812]

No age effect was found when corneal transmittance in the spectral range 320 to 700 nm on 10 aphakis subjects (14 to 75 yr) was measured.[813] The average spectral transmittance derived from these measurements was modeled by the following functions for the total transmittance (acceptance angle close to 180 deg) and on-axis transmittance (acceptance angle on the order of 1 deg):

$$\log T_t(\lambda) = -0.016 - 21 \times 10^8 \lambda_0^{-4}, \tag{3.25}$$

$$\log T_c(\lambda) = -0.016 - 85 \times 10^8 \lambda_0^{-4}, \tag{3.26}$$

where λ_0 is the wavelength in nanometers.

The lens is less transparent than the cornea. The visible light passing through the human lens undergoes an appreciable degree of both scattering and absorption by different chromophores, including protein-bound tryptophane, 3-hydroxy-L-kynurenine-O-β-glucoside (3-HKG), and age-related protein (responsible for lens yellowing in aged subjects) (Fig. 3.15).[800] The 3-HKG content slightly decreases with age. In the single-scattering model being examined, absorption is taken into account by introducing a complex refractive index for the scatterers[24] [see Eq. (1.192)] as

$$n_s(\lambda_0) = n'_s + in''_s = n'_s + i[tn''_t(\lambda_0) + kn''_k(\lambda_0) + pn''_p(\lambda_0)], \qquad (3.27)$$

where the coefficients t, k, and p characterize the contribution of each chromophore to absorption.

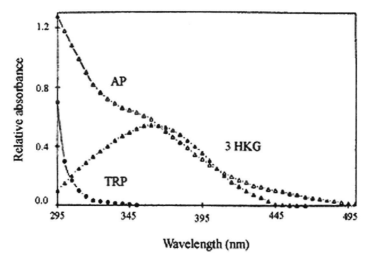

Figure 3.15 The main species in the human lens that absorb light transmitted by the cornea: protein-bounded tryptophan (TRP), 3-hydroxy-L-kynurenine-O-β-glucoside (3-HKG), and aged lens protein (AP).[800]

Age-related changes in the lens optical properties are, as a rule, due to the appearance of scatterers with increased diameters and refractive index, and also to the enhanced content of age-related protein.[24,64] Figure 3.16 presents collimated transmittance spectra calculated using "young" and "old" lens models. A remarkable difference between the short-wave portions of the two profiles is readily apparent. The total transmittance spectra experimentally obtained for senile and cataractous lenses are shown in Fig. 3.17.[24] Age-related variations in the composition of scatterers and absorbers led to significant differences in scattering spectra. There is a qualitative correlation between the experimental findings and the calculated values for both backscattering and scattering at 90 deg (see, for instance, Fig. 3.18).[24,173,790]

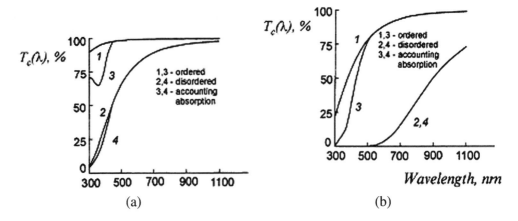

(a)   (b)

Figure 3.16 Collimated transmittance spectra of the human lens calculated for ordered (1, 3) and disordered (2, 4) scatterers. 1, 2, in the absence of absorption; 3, 4, with absorption: (a) Model of a "young" lens (diameter of scatterers $2a = 20$ nm, $n' = 1.43$, $t = 0.003$, $k = 0.005$, $p = 0$). (b) Model of an "old" lens ($2a = 40$ nm, $n' = 1.47$, $t = 0.003$, $k = 0.002$, $p = 0.015$). Volume density of scatterers $f_s = 0.3$, $n_0 = 1.345$, lens thickness 5 mm.[24,173]

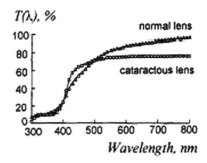

Figure 3.17 Experimental total transmittance spectra of isolated human lens for normal lens of a 56-year-old subject and a cataractous lens (88 yrs). Measurements were made on a spectrophotometer with an integrating sphere.[24]

Calculations of the scattering spectra for the eye lens model based on the first order of multiple scattering theory (see Fig. 3.19), which accounts for attenuation of a singly scattered light intensity, and *in vitro* measured experimental scattering spectra within a whole human cataractous crystallin lens for a certain scattering angle and different locations of a measuring volume also demonstrate the usefulness of scattering spectra for prediction of eye lens pathology.[811]

As discussed above, eye sclera is a nontransparent turbid medium, at least in the visible range. Figure 3.20 displays the experimental spectra obtained for three samples of human sclera with different thicknesses, showing its poor transparency for visible light and a sufficiently high one for the wide bands in the NIR region between absorption bands of water.[722,723] In addition, a dry scleral sample has a high transmittance within a very large spectral band, including visible and IR. The origin of scleral spectra formation can be understood on the basis of light scattering

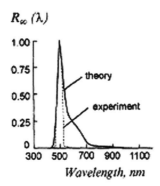

Figure 3.18 Calculated and experimental scattering spectra of the lens at 90 deg (relative units, experimental data from Ref. 790). Calculations were made for a mixture of ordered small particles (99%) having diameter $2a = 60$ nm ($t = 0.003$, $k = p = 0.03$, $n_0 = 1.345$, $n' = 1.47$) and large disordered particles (1%) ($2a = 600$ nm, $t = 0.003$, $k = 0$, $p = 0.1$).[173]

by a system of polydispersive irregularly arranged collagen cylinders immersed in the ground substance with a lower refractive index.[798,799] For natural thickness of 0.7–0.8 mm, this tissue shows multiple scattering [Figs. 3.20(a) and 3.20(b)], but the transition from multiple to low-step or even single scattering can be provided not only by tissue histological cutting, but also at dehydration of a whole tissue sample [Fig. 3.20(c)] or at its impregnation by an immersion liquid.[172,798,799] Such control of tissue scattering properties can be done *in vivo*; thus, this technology is very attractive for many biomedical applications (see Chapter 4).

3.3 Polarization properties

It has already been shown that light propagation in opaque multiply scattering tissues depends not only on the scattering and absorption coefficients and the scattering phase function, but also on the polarization properties of the tissue. The latter in turn depend on the scatterers' size, morphology, refractive index, internal structure, and the optical activity of the material.[5,6,10,43,149,181,182,814] The polarization properties of elastically scattered light are described by a 16-element LSM, each element being dependent on the wavelength, size, shape, and material of the scatterers [see Eqs. (1.69) and (1.70)].

For measurements of the LSM elements of transparent biological tissues and fluids, computer-controlled laser scattering matrix meters (LSMM) were developed.[3,5,6,10,43,64,135,149,380,450,451] The principle of operation of the LSMM[5,10,815] (Fig. 3.21), which is the modulation of the polarization of the incident laser beam followed by the scattered light demodulation (transformation of polarization modulation to intensity modulation), is described by the following matrix equation:

$$\mathbf{S} = \mathbf{AF'MFPS_0},\tag{3.28}$$

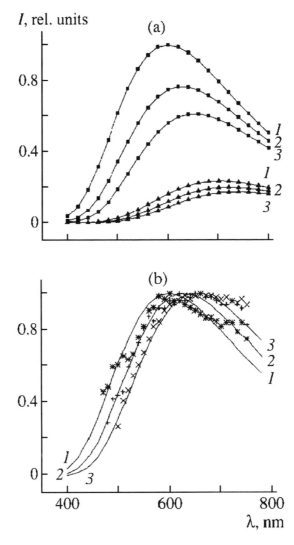

Figure 3.19 (a) The scattering spectra calculated in the first order of multiple scattering theory (accounting for attenuation of a singly scattered light intensity within a sample) for different angles: $\theta = $ (■) 149 deg and (▲) 90 deg. The particle radius is 25 nm, the radius of the system is 5 mm, and the relative volume of the particles is 0.3. The elementary scattering volume of 1 mm^2 is located at a distance $l = $ (1) 0.5 mm, (2) 0.6 mm, and (3) 0.7 mm. (b) The experimental (symbols) and corresponding calculated (1–3) scattering spectra at an angle of 149 deg for a cataractous crystallin lens of a human eye for three different locations of scattering volume: (∗, 1) in the vicinity of front surface, (+, 2) in the central part, and (×, 3) in the vicinity of a rare part of the crystallin lens.[811]

where **S** and **S**$_0$ are the Stokes vectors of the recorded and source radiation, respectively; **P** and **A**, and **F**$'$ and **F** are the Mueller matrices for the linear polarizers and the phase plates placed, respectively, ahead of and after the scattering medium. As the phase plates are rotated, the intensity recorded by a photodetector, i.e., the first element of the Stokes vector **S**, depends on time. By multiplying the matrices in

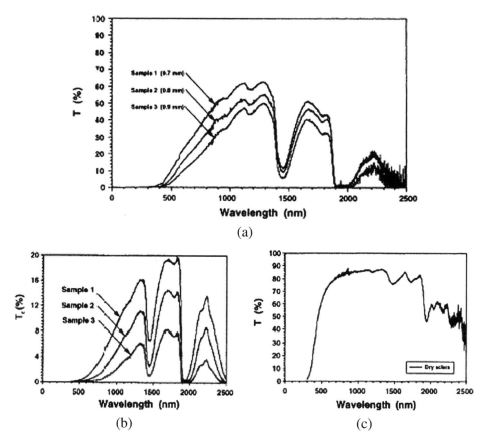

Figure 3.20 Transmittance spectra of the human sclera.[722,723] (a) Total transmittance for three samples. (b) Axial (collimated) transmittance for the same three samples. (c) Total transmittance of the dry sclera sample.

Eq. (3.28) and performing the appropriate trigonometric transformations, one can show that the output intensity can be represented as a Fourier series, namely,[816]

$$I = a_0 + \sum_{k=1}^{K}(a_{2k}\cos 2k\varphi + b_{2k}\sin 2k\varphi), \qquad (3.29)$$

where

$$a_{2k} = \sum_{i=1}^{N}I(\varphi_i)\cos 2k\varphi_i, \quad b_{2k} = \sum_{i=1}^{N}I(\varphi_i)\sin 2k\varphi_i, \qquad (3.30)$$

$I(\varphi_i)$ is the intensity of the scattered light detected by the photoreceiver for a certain orientation of the fast axis of the first retarder, φ_i, and N is the number of measurements per one rotation cycle of the first phase plate F.

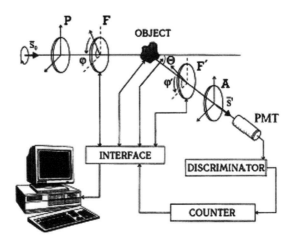

Figure 3.21 Scheme of a laser scattering matrix meter (see text for details).[5,10]

The coefficients of the series described by Eq. (3.29) are defined by the values of the matrix **M** elements of the object under study, and their measurement ensures a system of linear equations to determine the matrix **M**. The number of equations and the degree of stipulation for this system of equations are dependent on the choice of the ratio between the rotation rates of the phase plates (retarders). An optimal choice of the rotation rates' relationship at 1:5 allows an optimally stipulated system of linear equations [$K = 12$ equations to be derived to find the full matrix **M** of the object under study using Eq. (3.29)].[816]

A scheme shown in Fig. 3.21 was designed with the rotating retarders ($\lambda/4$-phase plates) that uses a comparatively simple software and allows one to avoid many of the experimental artifacts peculiar to dc measurements and to systems utilizing electrooptic modulators.[43] The LSMM has a fixed polarizer P and analyzer A, and two rotating-phase plates F and F' ahead and after the sample. The polarizer and analyzer are aligned in parallel with each other and their transmission planes are orthogonal to the scattering plane; the fast optical axis of each of the phase plates F and F′ forms an angle with the scattering planes φ and φ'; as a result, respective phase differences δ and δ' are induced. The ratio of the rotation rates of the phase plates was taken as equal to 1:5, i.e., $\varphi' = 5\varphi$, because all of 16 matrix elements are uniquely determined in this case. The computer-controlled LSMM provides the automatic scattering angle scanning in the range 0 ± 175 deg with a step of 4′ and accuracy of 5″. A single-mode stable He:Ne laser (633 nm) was used as a light source. Computer-driven retarders provided $N = 256$ indications per one rotation cycle of the first phase plate F [see Eq. (3.30)]. A photon-counting system was used with the photomultiplier tube (PMT), amplitude discriminator (clipping amplifier), and counter. The fast Fourier transform (FFT) analysis allowed one to measure and calculate all 16 S-matrix elements for the fixed scattering angle during the time of about 1 s with an accuracy of 3–5%.

The measurement of angular dependencies of LSM elements in a human lens shows their significant difference for clear and opaque (cataractous) eyes (see

Fig. 3.22). This difference may be caused by the appearance of large nonspherical scattering particles due to aggregation of high-molecular-weight proteins.

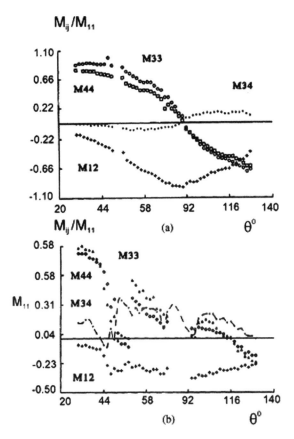

Figure 3.22 Experimental angular dependencies for LSM elements of (a) a normal lens 5 hr after the death of a 56-year-old subject and (b) a cataractous lens 5 hr after the death of an 88-year-old subject.[24]

The comparison of transmittance (see Fig. 3.17) and angular dependencies of LSM elements measured at the same wavelength indicates that the latter are more sensitive to variations in the structure of scattering media. This allows for measured LSM elements to be used for early diagnosis of structural changes in a tissue, e.g., those caused by a developing cataract.

This inference can be illustrated by the results of direct model experiments presented in Fig. 3.23.[6,10,335] The measurements were performed in an α-crystallin solutions (quasi-monodispersive particle fraction about 0.02 μm in diameter) from a freshly isolated calf lens (a contribution by J. Clauwaert, University of Antwerp, who also participated in the experiment) and in solutions of high-molecular-weight proteins (mean diameter 0.8 μm) from opaque lenses. The figure shows that measurements of the indicatrices of LSM elements permits the identification of a

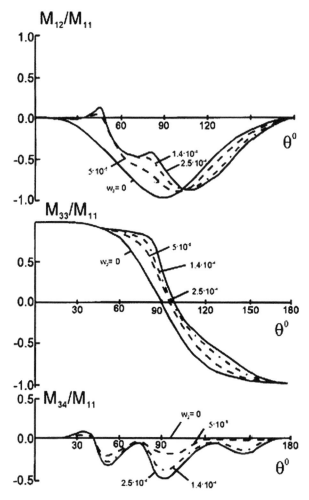

Figure 3.23 Indicatrices for LSM elements of α-crystallin solutions and a fraction of large-sized scatterers isolated from cataractous lens. The relative volume concentrations of α-crystallin $w_p = 0.3$ and the large-particle fraction $w_2 = 0$ ($\tau = 99\%$), 5×10^{-5} ($\tau = 98\%$); 1.4×10^{-4} ($\tau = 94\%$); and 2.5×10^{-4} ($\tau = 90\%$). τ is the transmittance of the 5-mm thick solution at $\lambda = 633$ nm.[24]

coarsely dispersed fraction of scatterers that is difficult to achieve by spectrophotometry because the corresponding decrease in sample transmittance does not exceed 1%.

Laser scattering matrix measurements may be employed for *in vitro* examination of various eye tissues, from cornea to retina. *In vivo* measurements in the intact eye are equally feasible, provided a fast LSMM is used to exclude a sensorimotor eye globe response. In this case, structural information about selected eye tissues can be obtained to diagnose cataract and other ophthalmologic disorders.

A survey of rabbit eye LSM has demonstrated that the aqueous humor in the anterior eye chamber is actually a transparent isotropic substance exhibiting weak light-scattering properties (the intensity of scattered light does not exceed 1.5–2% of the incident light intensity) owing to the presence of dissolved organic components. The results of an LSM study in the vitreous humor indicate that its amorphous tissue does not affect the polarization of straight-transmitting light, offering the possibility of examining the ocular fundus and imaging the optic nerve structure, which is important for early diagnosis of glaucoma.[168,377,388] On the other hand, certain pathological changes in the vitreous humor may be responsible for the alteration of LSM elements. Specifically, a minor intraocular hemorrhage is easy to identify by virtue of conspicuous light scattering from erythrocytes.

The angular dependence of LSM elements in a monolayer of disk-shaped or spheroidal erythrocytes in relation to their packing density was examined in Ref. 69. The angular dependence of the matrix element M_{11} in both cell types turned out to be influenced by the packing density in the angular scattering range of $\theta = 15$–16 deg. The angular dependencies of the elements M_{11}, M_{22}, M_{33}, and M_{21} at $\theta = 110$–170 deg were found to be affected far more by the shape of the scatterers than by their concentration. It was possible to derive the refractive indices of erythrocytes from measurements of the M_{12} magnitude at scattering angles $\theta \approx 140$–160 deg. A study[814] revealed the high susceptibility of the angular dependencies of LSM elements (M_{11} and M_{12}) to the degree of erythrocyte aggregation in blood plasma.

LSM measurements were also used to examine the formation of liposome complexes with plague capsular antigen and various particle suspensions,[10] e.g., those of spermatozoid spiral heads and different bacterial species.[43,149] The angular dependencies of the normalized element M_{34} for different bacteria turned out to be oscillating functions (similar to those in Fig. 3.23) whose maxima positions are

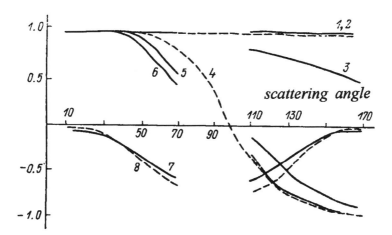

Figure 3.24 Angular distributions of the normalized (to M_{11}) LSM elements of the monolayer of erythrocytes: experimental: M_{22} (1, 3), M_{33} (5, 6), M_{12} (7), M_{21} (8); theoretical (Mie theory): M_{22} (2), M_{33} (4); for disklike erythrocytes (3, 5, 7, 8) and spherocytes (1, 2, 4, 6) (from Ref. 69 with corrections).

very sensitive to the varying size of bacteria.[817,818] This allows bacterial growth to be followed. Determination of LSM elements is equally promising for more effective differentiation between blood cells by time-of-flight cytometry.[149,819,820]

4

Coherent Effects in the Interaction of Laser Radiation with Tissues and Cell Flows

In this chapter, coherent effects that accompany the propagation of laser radiation in tissues and the interaction of laser radiation with cell flows are considered. These effects include diffraction, formation of speckle structures, interference of speckle fields, scattering from moving particles, etc. Principles of quasi-elastic light scattering (QELS) spectroscopy, diffusion wave spectroscopy (DWS), full-field speckle imaging (LASCA), confocal microscopy, optical coherence tomography (OCT), and second-harmonic generation (SHG) imaging are discussed.

4.1 Formation of speckle structures

Speckle structures are produced as a result of interference of a large number of elementary waves with random phases that arise when coherent light is reflected from a rough surface or when coherent light passes through a scattering medium.[45,76,77,82,83,112,113,129,136,139,155,157,343,396,821–837] The speckle phenomenon is a three-dimensional interference effect that exists in all points of space where the reflected or transmitted waves from an optically rough surface or volume intersect. Generally, there are two types of speckles: *subjective speckles*, which are produced in the image space of an optical system (including an eye), and *objective speckles*, which are formed in a free space and are usually observed on a screen placed at a certain distance from an object. Since the majority of bioobjects are optically nonuniform, irradiation of such objects with coherent light always gives rise to speckle structures that either distort the results of measurements and, consequently, should be eliminated in some way, or provide new information concerning the structure and the motion of a bioobject and its components. In this tutorial, we will mainly discuss the information aspects of speckle fields.

Figure 4.1 schematically illustrates the principles of the formation and propagation of speckles produced in the regime of transmission and reflection of coherent light in an optically nonuniform media; Fig. 4.2 shows a real speckle pattern formed at He:Ne laser beam transmission through a thin layer of a human epidermal sample. The average size of a speckle in the far-field zone is estimated as

$$d_{\mathrm{av}} \sim \lambda/\varphi, \tag{4.1}$$

where λ is the wavelength and φ is the angle of observation.

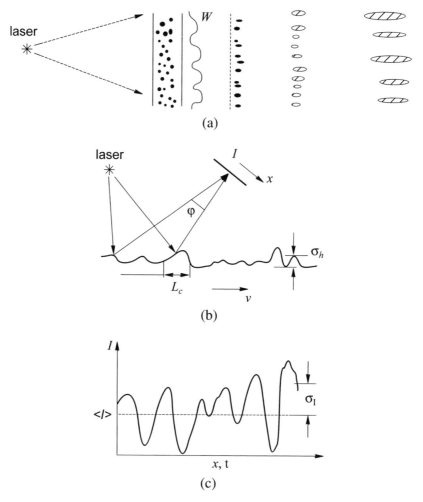

Figure 4.1 (a) Formation and propagation of speckles, (b) observation of speckles, and (c) intensity modulation; W is the scattered wave.[821]

Displacement x of the observation point over a screen or the scanning of a laser beam over an object with a certain velocity v (or an equivalent motion of the object itself with respect to the laser beam) when the observation point remains stationary gives rise to spatial or temporal fluctuations of the intensity of the scattered field. These fluctuations are characterized by the mean value of the intensity $\langle I \rangle$ and the standard deviation σ_I [see Fig. 4.1(b)]. The object itself is characterized by the standard deviation σ_h of the altitudes (depths) of inhomogeneities and the correlation length L_c of these inhomogeneities (random relief).

Since many tissues and cells are phase objects,[77,343] the propagation of coherent beams in bioobjects can be described within the framework of the model of a random phase screen (RPS).[75] The amplitude transmission coefficient of an RPS is given by

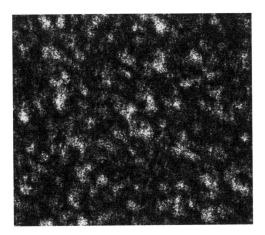

Figure 4.2 Speckle pattern produced at He:Ne laser beam transmission through a thin human skin epidermal sample (skin epidermal strip).

$$t_s(x, y) = t_0 \exp\{-i\Phi(x, y)\}, \tag{4.2}$$

where t_0 is the spatially independent amplitude transmission and $\Phi(x, y)$ is the random phase shift introduced by the RPS at the (x, y) point. Such spatial phase may be due to variations in the refractive index $n(x, y)$ or the RPS thickness $h(x, y)$ from point to point. For thin transmitting and reflecting RPSs, we have

$$\Phi(x, y) = \left(\frac{2\pi}{\lambda}\right)\{n(x, y) - 1\}h(x, y),$$

$$\Phi(x, y) = \left(\frac{4\pi}{\lambda}\right)h(x, y), \tag{4.3}$$

respectively. Phase fluctuations of the scattered field are characterized by the standard deviation σ_ϕ and the correlation length L_ϕ. Generally, there are two types of RPSs: weakly scattering RPSs ($\sigma_\phi^2 \ll 1$) and deep RPSs ($\sigma_\phi^2 \gg 1$).

The ideal conditions for the formation of speckles, when completely developed speckles arise, can be formulated in the following manner:

1. Coherent light irradiates a diffusive surface (or a transparency) characterized by Gaussian variations of optical length $\Delta L = \Delta(nh)$ with the probability density distribution

$$p(\Delta L) = \left\{2\pi\sigma_L^2\right\}^{1/2} \exp\left\{-\frac{(\Delta L)^2}{2\sigma_L^2}\right\}. \tag{4.4}$$

2. The standard deviation of relief variations is such that $\sigma_L \gg \lambda$; both the coherence length of light and sizes of the scattering area considerably exceed the differences in optical paths caused by the surface relief, and many scattering centers contribute to the resulting speckle pattern.

Statistical properties of speckles can be divided into statistics of the first and second orders. Statistics of the first order describe the properties of speckle fields at each point. Such a description usually employs the intensity probability density distribution function $p(I)$ and the contrast

$$V_I = \frac{\sigma_I}{\langle I \rangle}, \quad \sigma_I^2 = \langle I^2 \rangle - \langle I \rangle^2, \tag{4.5}$$

where $\langle I \rangle$ and σ_I^2 are the mean intensity and the variance of the intensity fluctuations, respectively. In certain cases, statistical moments of higher orders are employed. For example, in addition to contrast, generally defined as

$$V_I = \left(\frac{\mu_2}{\mu_1} \right)^{1/2}, \tag{4.6}$$

we can introduce the asymmetry parameter

$$Q_a = \frac{\mu_3}{\mu_2^{1.5}}, \tag{4.7}$$

which provides additional information concerning the scattering object. Here, the statistical moments are defined as

$$\mu_n = (N-1)^{-1} \sum_{j=1}^{N} (I_j - \mu_1)^n. \tag{4.8}$$

For ideal conditions, when the complex amplitude of scattered light has Gaussian statistics, the contrast is $V_I = 1$ (developed speckles), and the intensity probability distribution function (PDF) is represented by a negative exponential function as[157]

$$p(I) = \left(\frac{1}{\langle I \rangle} \right) \exp\left\{ -\frac{I}{\langle I \rangle} \right\}. \tag{4.9}$$

Thus, the most probable intensity value in the corresponding speckle pattern is equal to zero; i.e., destructive interference occurs with the highest probability.

Equation (4.9) is plotted as curve 1 in Fig. 4.3, and it can be seen that the most probable speckle is dark. The intensity PDF described by this equation can be produced only by the interference of light that is polarized all in the same manner, resulting in a similarly polarized speckle pattern.[828] Thus, the scattering surface can not depolarize the scattered light. Materials into which the light does not penetrate and is scattered only a single time generally produce speckle patterns that have an intensity distribution in accordance with Eq. (4.9). On the other hand, materials into which the light penetrates and is subject to multiple scattering, such as most biological tissues, tend to depolarize the interfering light.

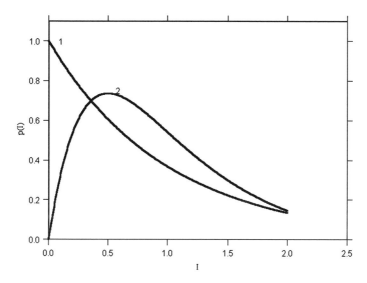

Figure 4.3 Theoretical intensity probability distribution functions $p(I)$ of a fully developed speckle pattern [curve 1, Eq. (4.9)] and the incoherent combination of two speckle fields [curve 2, Eq. (4.10)].[828]

Laser speckle patterns originating from most biological tissues are not "fully developed" in the sense that their intensity distribution does not follow a negative exponential relationship [Eq. (4.9)]. Such speckle patterns may have a distinctly different intensity PDF, one that is best thought of in terms of an incoherent combination of two speckle fields. Many speckle interferometers function by allowing two independent speckle patterns to interfere.[157,822–835] The speckle patterns can interfere either coherently or incoherently. In the case of a coherent combination, the statistical properties of the resulting third speckle pattern remain fundamentally the same as the two original patterns, typically following Eq. (4.9). However, in the case of an incoherent combination of two speckle fields, the final intensity PDF does not obey negative exponential statistics, but instead follows the equation[828]

$$p(I) = 4\left(\frac{I}{\langle I\rangle^2}\right)\exp\left\{-\frac{2I}{\langle I\rangle}\right\}. \tag{4.10}$$

The shape of this relationship is shown as curve 2 in Fig. 4.3. The intensity PDF of individual speckle patterns arising from most biological tissues obeys this equation. The reason is as follows: coherent light scattered from most biological tissues produces randomly polarized speckle patterns, and any two orthogonally polar-ized components of scattered light are incoherent with one another. Thus, single speckle patterns arising from biological tissues that randomly polarize the speckle pattern can be considered to be the incoherent combination of two or more speckle patterns. Figure 4.4 shows the measured intensity PDF of a backscattered speckle pattern arising from illuminating a sample of porcine skin with an expanded He:Ne laser (633 nm). It is clearly seen that the intensity PDF of the scattered light from the skin more or less follows that predicted by Eq. (4.10).

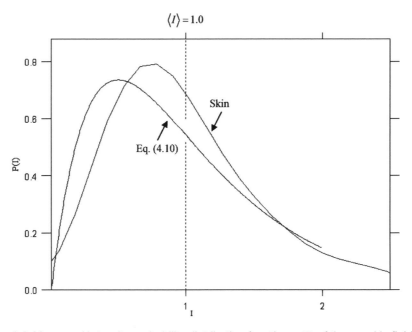

Figure 4.4 Measured intensity probability distribution function $p(I)$ of the speckle field gen-erated by illuminating a sample of porcine skin with a He:Ne laser (633 nm) compared to that predicted by an incoherent combination of two fields [Eq. (4.10)].[828]

Partially developed speckle fields are characterized by a contrast $V_I < 1$. The contrast may be lower for the following reasons:

(1) If a uniform coherent background with intensity I_b is added to the speckle field, then we have

$$V_I = \left(1 - \rho_b^2\right)^{1/2},\qquad(4.11)$$

where $\rho_b = \langle I_b \rangle / (\langle I_b \rangle + \langle I \rangle)$. For example, with a decrease in the rough-ness of a surface (or the nonuniformity degree of a solid scatterer), we have $\sigma_\phi^2 \to 0$. Under these conditions, the strong specular (nonscattered) com-ponent of the coherent beam interferes with the speckle field. In the limiting case of an ideally plane surface (a uniform medium), speckles vanish and $V_I = 0$.

(2) If a uniform incoherent background (e.g., due to lowering of the coherence of the light source or multiple scattering in the medium) arises, then we have

$$V_I = 1 - \rho_b. \tag{4.12}$$

For Gaussian statistics and a Gaussian correlation function of phase fluctuations, the propagation of intensity of the speckle field in a free space along the z-axis behind the RPS is described by the expression[75]

$$\sigma_I^2(z) = \left(\frac{\sigma_\phi^2}{2}\right)\{1 + (1 + D^2)^{-1}\}, \tag{4.13}$$

where $D = z\lambda/\pi L_\phi^2$ is the wave parameter. For a weakly scattering RPS ($\sigma_\phi^2 \ll 1$), the contrast of the speckle field is always less than unity. For a deep RPS ($\sigma_\phi^2 \gg 1$), the contrast reaches its maximum in the Fresnel zone ($D \cong 1$) when $z_{\max} = (2\pi/\lambda)(L_\phi^2/\sigma_\phi)$, $V > 1$. The fact that the contrast is higher than unity implies that dark areas predominate in the speckle pattern. The appearance of the maximum of intensity fluctuations is due to the focusing of scattered waves behind the RPS. In the Fraunhofer zone, we have $V_I \rightarrow 1$.

The intensity distribution for the light transmitted through an RPS can be represented in the following form:[75,157]

$$I_\Sigma(x, y) = I_c(x, y) + I_s(x, y). \tag{4.14}$$

Here, $I_c(x, y)$ is the intensity of light transmitted in the forward direction (the specular component) and $I_s(x, y)$ is the intensity of the scattered component. For a scattered field with Gaussian statistics, the intensity $I(0)$ at the center of the beam and the radius r_s of the scattered beam in the observation plane are determined by the following relations:

$$I(0) \cong I_0(0) \exp(-\sigma_\phi^2), \tag{4.15}$$

$$r_s \cong \frac{z\lambda}{\pi L_\phi}, \quad \sigma_\phi^2 \ll 1,$$

$$r_s \cong \left(\frac{z\lambda}{\pi L_\phi}\right)\sigma_\phi, \quad \sigma_\phi^2 \gg 1, \tag{4.16}$$

where $I_0(0)$ is the intensity of the incident beam at its axis.

For both weakly scattering and deep RPSs moving with a velocity v in the direction perpendicular to the laser beam with a radius w, the correlation time of intensity fluctuations in the scattered field is given by[823]

$$\tau_c \cong \frac{2^{1/2} w}{v}. \tag{4.17}$$

This relationship holds true for a Gaussian incident beam when the observation plane lies in the Fraunhofer zone.

For phase objects with $\sigma_\phi^2 \gg 1$ and a small number of scatterers $N = w/L_\phi$ contributing to the field at a certain point in the observation plane, the contrast of the speckle pattern is greater than unity[824]

$$V_I = \left\{ 1 - \frac{2}{N} + \left(\frac{\sigma_\phi^2}{4N} \right) \exp\left[\left(\frac{2\pi L_\phi}{\lambda \sigma_\phi} \right) \sin\theta \right]^2 \right\}^{1/2}, \tag{4.18}$$

where θ is the angle of observation (scattering angle). Note that the statistics of the speckle field in this case are non-Gaussian and nonuniform (i.e., the statistical parameters depend on the observation angle).

Statistics of the second order show how fast the intensity changes from point to point in the speckle pattern, i.e., they characterize the size and the distribution of speckle sizes in the pattern. The statistics of the second order are usually described in terms of the autocorrelation function of intensity fluctuations,

$$g_2(\Delta\xi) = \langle I(\xi + \Delta\xi) I(\xi) \rangle, \tag{4.19}$$

and its Fourier transform, representing the power spectrum of a random process; $\xi \equiv x$ or t is the spatial or temporal variable; $\Delta\xi$ is the change in variable. The angular brackets in Eq. (4.19) stand for the averaging over an ensemble or the time. To describe comparatively small intensity fluctuations, it is convenient to employ an autocorrelation function $\tilde{g}_2$ of the fluctuation intensity component and the corresponding structure function D_I,

$$\tilde{g}_2(\Delta\xi) = [\langle I(\xi + \Delta\xi) - \langle I \rangle \rangle][I(\xi) - \langle I \rangle], \tag{4.20}$$

$$D_I(\Delta\xi) = \langle [I(\xi + \Delta\xi) - I(\xi)]^2 \rangle,$$

$$D_I(\Delta\xi) = 2[\tilde{g}_2(0) - \tilde{g}_2(\Delta\xi)]. \tag{4.21}$$

Analysis is usually performed in terms of normalized autocorrelation and structure functions. An autocorrelation function is preferable for the analysis of intensity

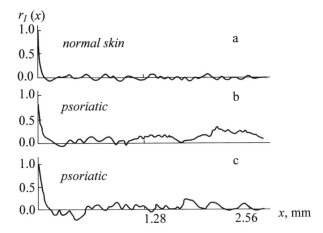

Figure 4.5 Normalized autocorrelation functions of intensity fluctuations in speckles $r_I(x)$ for thin layers of (a) normal and (b and c) psoriatic human epidermis probed with a focused laser beam.[77,343]

fluctuations caused by comparatively large inhomogeneities in the scattering object. At the same time, the structure function is more sensitive to small-scale intensity oscillations. Figures 4.5 and 4.6 display typical autocorrelation and structure functions measured for two types of normal and pathological tissues—epidermis of human skin and human tooth enamel.[77,343,834] These plots clearly illustrate the difference in the sensitivity of these functions to spatial fluctuations on different scales.

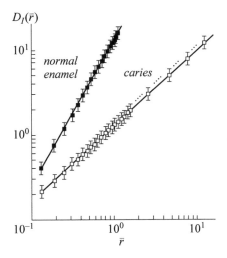

Figure 4.6 The difference between the structure functions of speckle fluctuations for the scattering of a focused laser beam from (the upper line) normal and (the lower line) pathological human tooth enamel (caries).[77,343]

4.2 Interference of speckle fields

Generally, owing to the considerable contribution of bulk scattering, the reflection of laser radiation from a biological object gives rise to the formation of partially developed speckle structures with comparatively small sizes of speckles, a contrast different from unity, and random polarization of light in individual speckles. In the elementary case when reflected light in speckle structures retains linear polarization, the intensity distribution at the output of a dual-beam interferometer can be written as[835,836]

$$I(r, t) = I_r(r) + I_s(r) + 2[I_r(r)I_s(r)]^{1/2}|\gamma_{11}(\Delta t)| \cos\{\Delta \Phi_I(r) + \Delta \Psi_I(r)$$
$$+ \Delta \Phi_I(t)\}, \tag{4.22}$$

where $I_r(r)$ and $I_s(r)$ are intensity distributions of the reference and signal fields, respectively, r is the transverse spatial coordinate, $\gamma_{11}(\Delta t)$ is the degree of temporal coherence of light, $\Delta \Psi_I(r)$ is the deterministic phase difference of the interfering waves, $\Delta \Phi_I(r) = \Phi_{Ir}(r) - \Phi_{Is}(r)$ is the random phase difference, and $\Delta \Phi_I(t)$ is the time-dependent phase difference related to the motion of an object. Specifically, for longitudinal harmonic vibrations with an amplitude l_0 and frequency Ω_v, we have

$$\Delta \Phi_I(t) = \left(\frac{4\pi}{\lambda}\right) l_0 \sin(\Omega_v t). \tag{4.23}$$

In the absence of speckle modulation, the deterministic phase difference $\Delta \Psi_I(r)$ governs the formation of regular interference fringes. On average, the output signal of a speckle interferometer reaches its maximum when the interfering fields are phase matched [$\Delta \Psi_I(r) = $ a constant within the aperture of the detector], focused laser beams are used (speckles with maximum sizes are produced), and a detector with a maximum area is employed.

For a large aperture photodetector, when it does not resolve amplitude-phase in the interference field, the modulation depth of the photoelectric signal of the interferometer with focused beams can be expressed as[837]

$$\beta = \left|\sin\frac{(u)}{u}\right|, \quad u = \frac{\pi(NA)^2 \Delta z}{\lambda}, \tag{4.24}$$

where (NA) is the numerical aperture of the objective in the subject arm of the speckle interferometer (see Fig. 4.7) and Δz is the longitudinal displacement of the object.

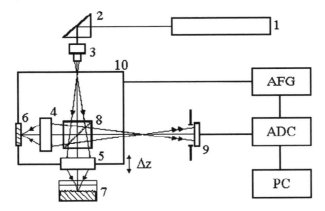

Figure 4.7 Laser wavefront matching speckle interferometer[837]: 1, He:Ne laser (633 nm); 2, prism; 3,4,5, objectives; 6, reference mirror; 7, multilayer object; 8, beamsplitter; 9, photodetector; 10, scaninng platform; AFG, audio-frequency generator; ADC, synchronized analog-to-digital converter; PC, personal computer.

4.3 Propagation of spatially modulated laser beams in a scattering medium

Objects under study are irradiated with spatially modulated laser beams (beams with regular interference) for surface microprofiling and shape diagnostics, translations of rough surfaces, laser anemometry of biological fluids, and cytometry.[5,22,76,77,343,832,838–846] These methods take advantage of a small spacing of interference fringes, $\Lambda_I = \lambda / 2\theta_I$ (θ_I is the angle between the wave vectors of the interfering fields), which is comparable to the sizes of inhomogeneities in the object. The use of modulated beams with large distances between interference fringes considerably exceeding the sizes of inhomogeneities results in the appearance of new correlation effects in the scattered field and, consequently, provides an opportunity to investigate random phase objects by means of new speckle technologies.[343,832,843–846] The interference fringes of average intensity arising in this case display a contrast varying along the direction of propagation z. If the beam diameter and the separation between the fringes are sufficiently large, the fringes modulate the speckle field, and the evolution of the contrast of average-intensity fringes along the z-axis is determined by the statistical parameters of the object and the separation between the fringes.

A spatial-temporal optical modulator ensures the formation and the motion of fringes.[343,832,843–846] Average-intensity interference fringes are registered by a photodetector with a slit oriented along the fringes. The width aperture is employed for averaging the speckle modulation of the scattered field. The modulation depth of the photoelectric signal is equal to the relative contrast of interference fringes:

$$\frac{\overline{V}_I(z)}{V_{I0}} = |\mu(z)|, \qquad (4.25)$$

where $\overline{V}_I(z)$ is the contrast of average-intensity fringes, V_{I0} is the contrast in the initial laser beam, and $|\mu(z)|$ is the modulus of the transverse correlation coefficient of the complex amplitude of the scattered field. Special phantom specklograms with smoothly varying and oscillating correlation coefficient of the boundary field have been developed for the experimental modeling of tissues and cellular structures with different statistic properties of phase inhomogeneities.[832,846]

Figure 4.8 presents theoretical and experimental dependencies for the spatial evolution of the relative contrast of the fringes obtained for phantom specklograms with nearly Gaussian correlation coefficient $K_\phi(\Delta x)$ of phase fluctuations of the boundary field. These dependencies allow us to reconstruct statistic parameters of the phase object, including the correlation coefficient $K_\phi(\Delta x)$.[343,832,843–846]

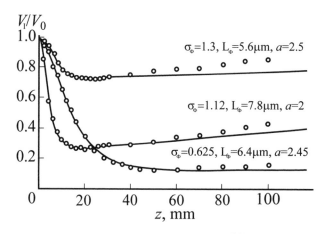

Figure 4.8 Experimental and theoretical dependencies[846] of the relative fringe contrast V_I/V_{I0} on the distance z from an object for phantom specklograms with a smoothly varying correlation coefficient of phase fluctuations of the boundary field $K_\phi(\Delta x) = \exp\{-|\Delta x|/L_\phi\}^a$.

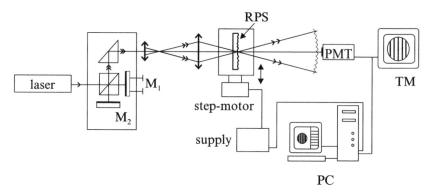

Figure 4.9 Experimental setup for the investigation of the contrast of interference fringes induced by focused, spatially modulated laser beam scattering by a random phase object.[846]

When a spatially modulated light beam is focused with the use of a diffraction-limited optical system with an aperture $D > \Lambda_I$, two spatially separated light spots are produced in the area of focusing. The optical scheme for such a system is presented in Fig. 4.9. Since two different areas of an object are irradiated, the interaction of these light spots with a scattering medium gives rise to two completely nonidentical (noncorrelated) speckle fields in the diffraction field. If the separation between the interference fringes satisfies the inequality $\Lambda_I < d_{av}$ (the average size of speckles in the observation plane), then the diameter of the beam waist meets the inequality $2w_0 > L_\phi$. In such a situation, regular interference fringes oriented in a random manner from speckle to speckle are observed within the limits of a single speckle. The contrast of fringes depends in this case only on the relation between the intensities of the interfering fields and does not depend on the statistical properties of an object. If $\Lambda_I > d_{av}$ and $2w_0 > L_\phi$, no fringes occur in the scattered field [see Fig. 4.10(b)]. However, when an object moves in the transverse direction, a set of average-intensity interference fringes arises [see Fig. 4.10(c)]. The contrast of this pattern is determined by the statistic properties of the object.

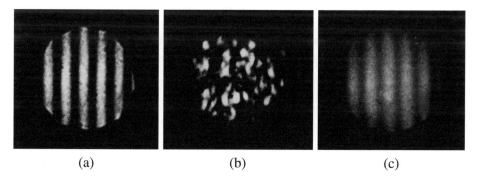

| (a) | (b) | (c) |

Figure 4.10 Interferograms observed (a) without an object, (b) with a stationary object, and (c) with a moving object (phantom specklegram).[846]

The speckle method for testing random phase objects with the use of a spatially modulated beam provides an opportunity to determine such statistical parameters of an object as the standard deviation σ_ϕ and correlation length L_ϕ of phase fluctuations.[343,832,843–846] Strictly speaking, this method can be applied to phase objects with smooth irregularities and Gaussian statistics. However, this approach can be also employed to study objects with non-Gaussian statistics or sharp inhomogeneities, but calibration is required in this case. Direct measurements using a sufficiently fast detection system make it possible to analyze objects in real time, which is especially important for the investigation of tissue and cellular structures; in particular, in creating optical topographic schemes. This technique can be employed for studying thin layers of human epidermis, thicker transparent tissues of the front segment of the human eye (cornea and crystalline lens), and sclera in

the process of optical clearing (enhanced translucence) under conditions of mechanical or osmotic stresses.[172,343,722] Along with the monitoring of statistical parameters of tissues, this approach should also be useful for the development of the
new generation of laser interferential retinometers, i.e., devices for the determining
of retinal visual acuity in the human eye.[5,832,847] Since the interference pattern is
statistically averaged as a focused spatially modulated laser beam is scanned, even
patients with a turbid (cataractous) crystalline lens can see interference fringes (see
Fig. 4.10).

4.4 Dynamic light scattering

4.4.1 Quasi-elastic light scattering

Quasi-elastic scattering of light, photon-correlation spectroscopy, spectroscopy of
intensity fluctuations, spectroscopy of intensity fluctuations, and Doppler spectroscopy are synonymous terms related to the dynamic scattering of light, which
underlies a noninvasive method for studying the dynamics of particles on a comparatively   large   time   scale.[5,78,79,112,113,343,838,]
[839–841,848,849] The implementation of the single-scattering regime and the use of
coherent light sources are of fundamental importance in this case. The spatial scale
of testing of a colloid structure (an ensemble of biological particles) is determined
by the inverse of the wave vector modulus, $|\bar{q}|^{-1}$, defined by Eq. (3.7)

$$|\bar{q}|^{-1} = \left(\frac{4\pi n}{\lambda_0}\right)\sin\left(\frac{\theta}{2}\right),$$

(4.26)

where n is the refractive index of the ground substance of the scattering medium (or
average refractive index of the ground and scatterer materials, $n = \bar{n}$) and θ is the
angle of scattering. With allowance for self-beating due to the photomixing of the
electric components of the scattered field, we can write the intensity autocorrelation
function in the following form:

$$g_2(\tau) = \langle I(t)I(t+\tau)\rangle.$$

(4.27)

For Gaussian statistics, this autocorrelation function is related to the first-order
autocorrelation function by the Siegert formula,

$$g_2(\tau) = A\left[1 + \beta_{sb}|g_1(\tau)|^2\right],$$

(4.28)

where τ is the delay time; $A = \langle i\rangle^2$ is the square of the mean value of the photocurrent, or the baseline of the autocorrelation function; β_{sb} is the parameter of
self-beating efficiency, $\beta_{sb} \approx 1$; and

$$g_1(\tau) = \frac{\langle E^*(t+\tau)E(t)\rangle}{\langle|E(t)|^2\rangle}$$

(4.29)

is the normalized autocorrelation function of the optical field.

For a monodispersive system of Brownian particles, we have

$$g_1(\tau) = \exp(-\Gamma_T \tau), \tag{4.30}$$

where $\Gamma_T = q^2 D_T$ is the relaxation parameter and $D_T = k_B T / 6\pi \eta r_h$ is the co-efficient of translation diffusion, k_B is the Boltzmann constant, T is the absolute temperature, η is the absolute viscosity of the medium, and r_h is the hydrodynamic radius of a particle. Many biological systems are characterized by a bimodal distribution of diffusion coefficients, when fast diffusion (D_{Tf}) can be separated from slow diffusion (D_{Ts}) related to the aggregation of particles.[5,849–851] In this case, the first-order autocorrelation function is written as

$$g_1(\tau) = p_1 \exp(-q^2 D_{Ts}\tau) + p_2 \exp(-q^2 D_{Ts}\tau), \tag{4.31}$$

where p_1 and p_2 are the coefficients proportional to the concentration and efficiency of scattering of small- and large-sized particles, respectively. The goal of spectroscopy of quasi-elastic scattering is to reconstruct the distribution of scattering particles in sizes, which is necessary for the diagnosis or monitoring of a disease.

4.4.2 Dynamic speckles

The specific features of the diffraction of laser beams from moving phase screens underlie speckle methods of structure diagnostics and monitoring of biological flows and motion parameters of bioobjects, including biovibrations, which are easy to implement from the technical point of view.[22,76,82,83,825–831,833–836,852–858]

The fluctuations of individual speckles can be analyzed to provide information about the movement of the scatterers producing the fluctuations. This analysis can be based either on the techniques of *photon correlation spectroscopy* or *laser Doppler velocimetry*. It is not intuitively obvious that time-varying speckle and Doppler-induced fluctuations are identical. The theory of time-varying speckle starts with the classical (though random) interference pattern produced when light beams of the same frequency interfere. The fluctuations are caused by the changes in optical path lengths of the interfering beams caused by the movement of the scatterers. Doppler fluctuations, on the other hand, are explained by the beating effect that occurs when two waves of slightly different frequency are superimposed, the difference being due to the frequency shift induced by the Doppler effect when light is scattered by a moving object. Thus, the speckle explanation is based on the superposition of waves of the *same* optical frequency, whereas in the Doppler explanation the superimposed waves have *different* frequencies. Despite these apparent differences in approach, it can be shown that mathematically the two explanations lead to identical equations linking the intensity fluctuations to the velocity distribution of the scatterers.[82,83] Thus, the two approaches are just different ways of looking at the same physical phenomenon.

In the case of diffraction of a sharply focused Gaussian beam from a moving RPS with the Gaussian statistics of phase inhomogeneities and a Gaussian correlation function, the power spectrum of intensity fluctuations in the far-field zone can be represented in the form of homodyne (I) and heterodyne (II) parts as[852]

$$S(\omega) = \left[C_1 (2b)^{0.5} \exp\left(-\frac{b\omega^2}{2}\right)\right]_I$$
$$+ \left(C_2 b^{0.5} \exp\{[-b(\omega - \omega_0)^2] + \exp[-b(\omega + \omega_0)^2]\}\right)_{II}. \quad (4.32)$$

Here, $\omega = 2\pi f \lambda / v$ is the unscaled frequency; f is the modulation frequency; v is the velocity of a moving RPS,

$$b = \frac{L_c^2 + 2M w_0^2}{4M},$$

and

$$\omega_0 = 4\pi M (w_0 / L_c)^2 (x^0 / z) / [1 + 2M (w_0 / L_c)^2],$$

where M is the parameter that depends on RPS dispersion of heights (σ_h) and irradiating wavelength (λ), w_0 is the radius of the beam waist, x^0 is a fixed point where speckles are observed in the moving frame of reference, and z is the distance between the scattering and observation planes.

For a weakly scattering RPS (e.g., a model of a thin blood vessel), we have $M = 1$ and $C_1 \ll C_2$. For a deep RPS (e.g., a model of a thick blood vessel), we have $M \sim (\sigma_h/\lambda)^2$ and $C_1 \gg C_2$. In the case of thin vessels, we should expect the appearance of a high-frequency peak in the spectrum of intensity fluctuations (the heterodyne part of the spectrum) owing to the interference interaction of the specular and scattered components. The specular component (in transmission or reflection) serves as a reference wave. The position of the peak on the frequency scale depends on the observation angle (x^0/z). Since the standard deviation of profile fluctuations is small ($\sigma_h \ll \lambda$), the spectrum $S(\omega)$ of intensity fluctuations features only high-frequency components. By contrast, in the model of a deep RPS, because of suppression of the specular component (due to scattering), interference interaction vanishes and the spectrum features only low-frequency components (the homodyne part).

The aforesaid concept is illustrated by theoretical and experimental spectra presented in Figs. 4.11 and 4.12. Thus, the statistical characteristics of transmitted (reflected) light essentially depend on the observation angle and the degree of nonuniformity of an object. Such statistics of speckles are associated with a small number of scatterers and can be classified as statistically nonuniform, non-Gaussian statistics [cf. Eq. (4.18)]. Similar to the case of spectroscopy of quasi-elastic scattering (Doppler spectroscopy), the frequency shift is a linear function of both the velocity

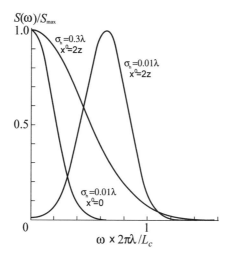

Figure 4.11 Normalized theoretical power spectra of intensity fluctuations for dynamic speckles arising from the interaction of a focused laser beam ($w_0 = 10\lambda$) with phase objects characterized by various degrees of nonuniformity (σ_h) for different observation angles (x^0).[852]

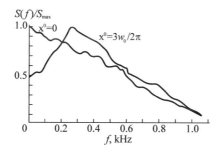

Figure 4.12 Scattering from a random flow: normalized experimental spectra of fluctuations for dynamic speckles for different observation angles (x^0); $w_0 \approx 2.3\lambda$; the spectra are averaged over 256 realizations of instantaneous spectra.[852]

of a scatterer and the observation angle of speckles only when the number of scatterers irradiated by a laser beam is sufficiently large. If the number of scatterers is small, $N = (w_0/L_c) < 5$, we should expect an additional strong dependence of the frequency shift on N in accordance with the theoretical dependence presented in Fig. 4.13.

4.4.3 Full-field speckle technique—LASCA

One problem of using the temporal statistics of time-varying speckle is that measurements are made at only one point in the speckle pattern (a single speckle). If an area needs to be analyzed, it is necessary to scan the detector over the field of view. If a map of velocity distribution is required, some method of scanning the area of interest is necessary. Such a map is of particular importance if blood

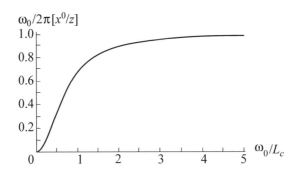

Figure 4.13 Normalized theoretical dependence of the central frequency in the spectrum of intensity fluctuations on the number of scatterers, $N_s = w_0/L_c$.[852]

flow is to be used as a diagnostic tool. A linear CCD array was used to simultaneously monitor a line of speckles, and a scanning mirror was used to extend this to a two-dimensional area.[859,860] To characterize a local blood flow, the ratio of the mean intensity to the intensity difference in the speckle pattern was utilized; a quantity called "normalized blur" was a measure of velocity. In particular, a microcirculation map of the retina of a rabbit eye was received while illuminating the retina with light from a diode laser, scanning and storing the speckle images, and then calculating the differences between successive images. These measurements showed good correlation with invasive methods.[860] Scanning has also been applied to the laser Doppler technique,[861,862] and commercial scanning Doppler systems are now on the market that can provide monitoring of capillary blood flow over quite large areas of the body.

However, nonscanning, so-called full-field, techniques for monitoring capillary blood flow are more attractive. The contrast of a speckle pattern used as a measure of time integration of a fluctuating speckle pattern can be employed as a detecting parameter to provide a full-field technique. If the integration time is comparable with the period of the intensity fluctuations caused by dynamic light scattering, it is clear that the effect will be a blurring of the recorded speckle pattern—a reduction in the speckle contrast.

The use of such *time-integrated speckle* led in the early 1980s to a technique for flow visualization that simultaneously achieves full-field operation and very simple (and cheap) data collection and processing (see Refs. 82, 83, 112, 827, 831, 863, and 865–868). Originally called "single-exposure speckle photography," it was developed primarily for the measurement of retinal blood flow. The basic technique was simply to photograph the retina under laser illumination using an exposure time that is of the same order as the decorrelation time of the intensity fluctuations. It is clear that a very short exposure time would "freeze" the speckle and result in a high-contrast speckle pattern, whereas a long exposure time would allow the speckles to average out, leading to a low contrast. In general, the velocity distribution in the field of view is mapped as variations in speckle contrast. Subsequent high-pass optical spatial filtering of the resulting photographs converted these contrast variations to more easily seen intensity variations. Later work introduced digital image processing of the speckle photographs, including a color coding of the velocities. More recently, the method has been developed into a fully digital, real-time technique for the mapping of skin capillary blood flow.[82,83,863,865] As the method is no longer photographic, it is now called laser speckle contrast analysis (LASCA). A closely related technique has been used as a remote method of sensing heartbeats;[864] a TV camera was used to record the speckle pattern produced by a vein, which was digitized frame by frame, and then the speckle contrast was computed and plotted as a function of time. A minimum in this contrast indicated the occurrence of a heartbeat.

LASCA uses only a laser with diverging optics, a CCD camera, a frame grabber, a frame grabber, and a personal computer. Specially developed software computes the local contrast and converts it to a false-color map of contrast (and hence of velocity). The contrast is quantified by the ratio of the standard variation of the intensity fluctuations to the mean intensity, $\sigma_I/\langle I \rangle$ [see Eq. (4.5)]. The image is a time-integrated exposure, but for most flow fields (including, for example, capillary blood flow), the exposure is short enough to render the technique effectively real time. Figure 4.14 shows the simplicity of the basic setup. Light from the laser is diverged by simple optics to illuminate the area under investigation. The CCD camera images the illuminated area and the image is observed on the PC monitor. On receiving an instruction from the PC, the frame grabber captures an image and the software immediately processes it to produce a false-color contrast map indicating velocity variations. This is typically accomplished in less than one second (again, making the technique effectively real time). The operator has several options at his disposal, including the number of pixels over which the local contrast is computed, the scaling of the contrast map, and the choice of contour colors. The most important of these is the choice of the number of pixels over which to compute the speckle contrast: too few, and the statistics will be questionable, too many

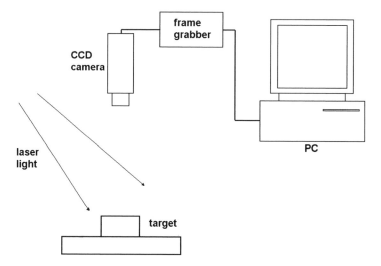

Figure 4.14 Basic setup for LASCA (laser speckle contrast analysis).[827]

and spatial resolution will be lost. In practice, a square of 7×7 or 5×5 pixels is usually a satisfactory compromise.

As indicated above, the principle of LASCA is very simple. A time-integrated image of a moving object exhibits blurring. In the case of a laser speckle pattern, this appears as a reduction in the speckle contrast, defined (and measured) as the ratio of the standard deviation of the intensity to the mean intensity. This occurs regardless of the "movement" of the speckle. For random velocity distributions, each speckle fluctuates in intensity. For lateral motion of a solid object, on the other hand, the speckles also move laterally and become "smeared" on the image— but a reduction in speckle contrast still occurs. For fluid flow, the situation might be a combination of both these types of "movement." In each case, the problem for quantitative measurements is the determination of a relationship between the speckle contrast and the velocity (or velocity distribution).

The higher the velocity, the faster are the fluctuations and the more blurring occurs in a given integration time. By making certain assumptions, the following mathematical relationship between the speckle contrast and the temporal statistics of the fluctuating speckle can be found:[827]

$$\sigma_s^2(T) = \frac{1}{T} \int_0^T \tilde{g}_2(\tau) d\tau, \tag{4.33}$$

where σ_s^2 is the *spatial* variance of the intensity in the speckle pattern, T is the integration time, $\tilde{g}_2(\tau)$ is the autocovariance of the *temporal* fluctuations in the intensity of a single speckle, and $\tilde{g}_2(\tau)$ is defined in Eq. (4.20). This equation defines the relationship between LASCA and those techniques that use the intensity fluctuations in laser light scattered from moving objects or particles. LASCA measures the quantity on the left-hand side of Eq. (4.33); photon correlation spectroscopy, laser Doppler, and time-varying speckle techniques measure the quantity on the right-hand side. It is also worth noting that LASCA uses *image speckle*, whereas most of the temporal techniques use *far-field speckle*. However, this does not detract from the fundamental equivalence of the two approaches expressed in Eq. (4.33).

All the techniques allow the correlation time τ_c to be determined. In the case of photon correlation, this parameter is measured directly. In the case of LASCA, some further assumptions must be made in order to link the measurement of speckle contrast with τ_c.

Depending on the type of motion being monitored, various models can be used to find a relation between the speckle contrast and the correlation time τ_c for a given integration time T. For example, for the case of a Lorentzian velocity distribution, this relation has a view (see also Fig. 4.15)[827]

$$\frac{\sigma_s}{\langle I \rangle} = \left[\frac{\tau_c}{2T} \left\{ 1 - \exp\left(-\frac{2T}{\tau_c} \right) \right\} \right]^{1/2}. \tag{4.34}$$

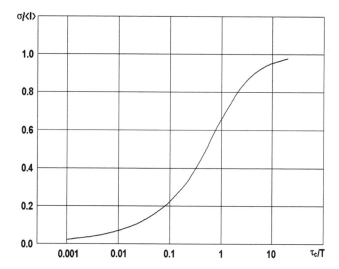

Figure 4.15 Variation of speckle contrast with the ratio of decorrelation time (τ_c) to integration time (T) for the Lorentzian model of LASCA.[827]

As all the *temporal* frequency measurement techniques (photon correlation spectroscopy, laser Doppler, and time-varying speckle), LASCA suffers on the problem of relating the correlation time τ_c to the velocity distribution of the scatterers. It is not straightforward and depends on the effects of multiple scattering, the size and the shape of the scattering particles, non-Newtonian flow, non-Gaussian statistics, non-Gaussian statistics resulting from a low number of scatterers in the measuring volume, spin of the scatterers, etc. Much work is going on regarding these effects and the question is far from being settled. Because of the uncertainties caused by these factors, it is common in all these techniques to rely mainly on calibration rather than on absolute measurements.

To measure the temporal statistics of fluctuating speckle patterns, it is necessary to monitor the intensity of a single speckle. In order to do this accurately, the aperture of the detector must be smaller than the average speckle size. Otherwise, some spatial averaging will occur and the first-order statistics will be corrupted (some accuracy loss in the second-order statistics may also take place). For LASCA, the matter is more complicated because it computes the local speckle contrast within a square of pixels, the size of the square being under the control of the operator. The larger the square sampled for each measurement the better the statistics. But it is also important to sample a large enough number of *speckles* as well as pixels: if the speckles are much larger than the pixels, as suggested above, fewer speckles are sampled. This means that the viable speckle size is more restricted. If it is too small, each pixel samples more than one speckle, leading to speckle averaging and loss of measured contrast. If it is too large, not enough speckles are sampled to ensure good statistics. Thus, speckle size needs to be carefully controlled. This can be done by fixing the aperture of the imaging optics, as this alone determines the speckle size,[822] but it removes the control on the amount of light entering the camera, as the shutter speed (the other variable available) has already been determined in order to select the range of velocities to be measured. Unless the dynamic range of the camera is very large, this can be a significant restriction and can require the use of neutral density filters to ensure usable light levels at the detector.

Another problem that has occurred with LASCA is a failure to realize the full range of contrasts that should theoretically be available. A stationary object should give a speckle contrast of unity ($\sigma_I = \langle I \rangle$, in accordance with the well-established speckle statistics theory and experiment). A fully blurred speckle pattern produced by rapidly moving scatterers should have zero contrast. The Lorentzian model [see Eq. (4.34) and Fig. 4.15], for example, suggests that for a given integration time T, the dynamic range of the technique that corresponds to contrasts between 0.1 and 0.9 should be about two and a half orders of magnitude in τ (and hence in velocity). In practice, contrasts of only 0.6 were being measured, even for stationary random diffusers.[83] One of the possible causes of this is the CCD camera dark current. By carrying out some data preprocessing, it is possible to remove the effect of the dark current and to get the measured speckle contrast for the stationary diffusing surface equal to 0.95, very close to the theoretical value of 1.0 expected for a fully developed speckle pattern.[863] Other problems of LASCA connected with the statistics owning to the Gaussian profile of the laser beam and the nonlinearity of the CCD camera also take place.[863] However, many of these problems are also characteristic of laser Doppler, photon correlation, and other time-varying speckle techniques.

To summarize, the LASCA technique offers a full-field, real-time, noninvasive, and noncontact method of mapping flow fields, such as capillary blood flow.[82,83,112,827,831,863,865–868] It uses readily available off-the-shelf equipment and the software operates in a user-friendly way using the Microsoft Windows NT interface. Laser Doppler, photon correlation spectroscopy, and time-varying speckle are related techniques, but work by analyzing the intensity fluctuations in the scattered laser light. Since they are essentially methods that operate at a single point in the flow field, some form of scanning must be used if a full-field velocity map of the flow area is required. Typical scanning laser Doppler systems take some minutes to complete this scan. LASCA achieves this goal in a single shot by utilizing the spatial statistics of time-integrated speckle. The technique produces a false-color map of blood flow in less than a second, without the need to scan. The main disadvantage of LASCA is the loss of resolution caused by the need to average over a block of pixels in order to produce the spatial statistics used in the analysis. However, the advantage of real-time operation without scanning outweighs the problem of loss of resolution, especially for biomedical applications.

4.4.4 Diffusion wave spectroscopy

Diffusion wave spectroscopy (DWS) is a new class of studies in the field of dynamic light scattering related to the investigation of the dynamics of particles

within very short time intervals.[73,80,81,343,825,829,830,869–871] A fundamental difference of this method compared with the spectroscopy of quasi-elastic light scattering is that this approach is applicable in the case of dense media with multiple
scattering, which is very important for tissues. DWS is uniquely suited for the
measurements of the average size of particles and their motion within the turbid
macroscopically homogeneous highly scattering media.

Despite the definite similarity between the experiments in DWS and conventional experimental schemes of correlation spectroscopy of optical mixing [see
Eq. (4.28)] DWS theory is based on a qualitatively different interpretation of radiation propagation in strongly scattering media. It is assumed thereby that due
to multiple scattering, each photon that has reached a given observation point
of the detector experiences a great number of scattering events N. The successive scattering acts taking place at the instant of time t at the scattering particles located in points $r_1(t), r_2(t), \ldots, r_i(t), \ldots, r_N(t)$ in a medium with wave vectors $k_1, k_2, \ldots, k_i, \ldots, k_N$, result in formation of the field $E(t)$, whose total phase
change $\Delta\phi(t)$ is determined as[869]

$$\Delta\phi(t) = \sum_{i=0}^{N} k_i(t)[r_{i+1}(t) - r_i(t)]. \tag{4.35}$$

$\Delta\phi(t)$ is dependent on the total path length s of each photon migrated from the
source r_0 to the detector r_{N+1} points (Fig. 4.16),

$$s = \sum_{i=0}^{N} |r_{i+1}(t) - r_i(t)| = \sum_{i=0}^{N} \left(\frac{k_i}{|k_i|}\right)[r_{i+1}(t) - r_i(t)]. \tag{4.36}$$

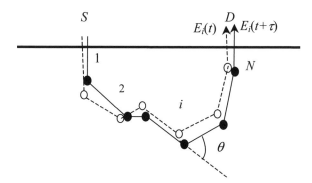

Figure 4.16 Schematic diagram of coherent radiation propagation through a randomly inhomogeneous semi-infinite medium with strong scattering, in which light passes from the
radiation source (S) toward the detector (D): (●) shows the location of scattering particles
at the instant of time ($t + \tau$) and (○) indicates the location of scattering particles at the instant
of time τ.

The quantity s is related to the number of scattering acts N by the relation $s = N l_s$, where $l_s = (\mu_s)^{-1}$. In highly scattering media, e.g., human skin, s can be considered as a statistically independent random walk. The distribution function of photon migration paths $p(s)$ in the medium is determined as the probability that light will cover the optical paths s, moving from the point r_0 to the point r_{N+1} as[869]

$$p(s) = \left(\frac{c}{4\pi s D}\right)^{3/2} \exp\left(\frac{c|r_0 - r_{N+1}|^2}{4 s D}\right). \tag{4.37}$$

Here, D is the photon diffusion coefficient [see Eqs. (1.25) and (1.26)], and c is the speed of light in the medium.

The field $E(t)$ interferes with the field $E(t + \tau)$ scattered slightly later in the same series of the scattering particles at the instant of time $t + \tau$ (see Fig. 4.16). The time it takes the photons to travel the entire optical path in the medium is much shorter than the characteristic time of changing the position of scattering particles in the medium. Thus, as a result of motion of the particles, the phase between fields $E(t)$ and $E(t + \tau)$ will be different at different instants of time, or fluctuate. This predetermines temporal fluctuations of the scattered radiation intensity recorded in the far zone. The patterns of the intensity fluctuations (speckles) can be visualized on a screen or sensed by a homodyne detector.[872]

Quantitatively, these fluctuations are described by the temporal field autocorrelation function

$$G_1(\tau) = \langle E^*(t + \tau) E(t) \rangle, \tag{4.38}$$

determined as[873]

$$G_1(\tau) = I_0 \sum_{j=0,\infty} p(s_j) \exp\left(-\frac{N}{6} \langle q^2 \rangle \langle \Delta r^2(\tau) \rangle\right), \tag{4.39}$$

where $I_0 = \langle | E(t)|^2 \rangle$, the angular brackets denote an ensemble average, and q is the change in the wave vectors k_i and k_{i+1},

$$q = |k_i - k_{i+1}| = 2k_0 \sin\frac{\theta}{2}. \tag{4.40}$$

Respectively,

$$\langle q^2 \rangle = \langle 4k_0^2(1 - \cos\theta) \rangle = 2k_0(1 - \langle \cos\theta \rangle) = 2k_0\frac{l_s}{l_t}, \tag{4.41}$$

where $k_0 = |k_i| = |k_{i+1}|$, θ is the angle between the directions $k_i = k_{i+1}$ (i.e., angle of the ith scattering act), and l_t is the transport length of the photon free path (which corresponds to the mean distance where a photon completely loses its initial direction of motion) [see Eq. (1.16)].

In an elementary situation where particles move independently of each other, their positions are represented by Gaussian random quantities, and the change in the photon momentum in each scattering event is independent of the position of a particle; the *path-dependent* normalized first-order autocorrelation function is written as[80]

$$g_1(\tau, s) = \exp\left[-\left(\frac{4\pi^2}{3\lambda^2}\right)\langle \Delta r^2(\tau)\rangle\left(\frac{s}{l_t}\right)\right]. \tag{4.42}$$

Here, s is the total photon path length.

In a dense medium, we have $s \gg l_t$. Therefore, in contrast to the case of single scattering, the correlation function $g_1(\tau, s)$ is sensitive to the motion of a particle on the length scale on the order of $\lambda[s/l_t]^{-1/2}$, which is generally much less than λ. Thus, DWS autocorrelation functions decay much faster than analogous functions employed in spectroscopy of quasi-elastic scattering.

Substituting Eq. (4.41) in Eq. (4.39), we find that the normalized temporal field autocorrelation function $g_1(\tau) = G_1(\tau)/\langle |E(t)|^2\rangle$ has the form

$$g_1(\tau) = \int_0^\infty p(s) \exp\left(-\frac{1}{3}k_0^2\langle \Delta r^2(\tau)\rangle \frac{s}{l_t}\right) ds. \tag{4.43}$$

It is seen that, similar to the conventional dynamic light scattering technique,[78,79] the change in $g_1(\tau)$ is determined in terms of their mean-square displacement $\langle \Delta r^2(\tau)\rangle$, with the difference that the slope of $g_1(\tau)$ increases in proportion to the average number of scattering particles. This has been verified directly by Yodh et al., who used a pulsed laser and gated the broadened response to select photon path lengths of a specific length.[874] For continuous wave illumination, Eq. (4.43) is valid given the assumption that the laser coherence length is much longer than the width of the photon path length distribution.

For a system that multiply scatters laser radiation, the transport of the temporal field correlation function is accurately modeled by the correlation diffusion equation,[875] i.e.,

$$\left(D\nabla^2 - c\mu_a - 2c\mu_s' D_B k_0^2 \tau\right)G_1(\bar{r}, \tau) = -cS(\bar{r}). \tag{4.44}$$

Here, $G_1(\bar{r}, \tau)$ is determined by Eq. (4.38) and is a function of position $\bar{r}$ and correlation time τ; it has units of energy per area per second; D is the photon diffusion coefficient; k_0 is the wave number of the light in the medium; c is the speed of light in the medium; $D_B \equiv D_T = k_B T/6\pi\eta r_h$ [see Eq. (4.30)]; and $S(\bar{r})$ is the distribution of light sources with units of photons per volume per second. Note that, similar to μ_a, describing losses of correlation due to photon absorption, $(2\mu_s' D_B k_0^2 \tau)$ is a loss term representing the losing of correlation due to dynamic processes. The correlation diffusion Eq. (4.44) is valid for turbid samples with the dynamics of scattering particles governed by Brownian motion (D_B). When $\tau = 0$, there is no "dynamical absorption" and Eq. (4.44) reduces to the steady-state photon diffusion equation, described by Eq. (1.17).

The correlation diffusion equation can be modified to account for other dynamic processes. In the cases of random flow and shear flow, the correlation diffusion equation becomes[876,877]

$$
\left(D\nabla^2 - c\mu_a - \frac{1}{3}c\mu_s'k_0^2\langle \Delta r^2(\tau)\rangle - \frac{1}{3}c\mu_s'k_0^2\langle V^2\rangle\tau^2 \right.
$$
$$
\left. - \frac{1}{15}c\mu_s'^{-1}\Gamma_{\text{eff}}^2 k_0^2\tau^2 \right) G_1(\bar{r},\tau) = -cS(\bar{r}). \tag{4.45}
$$

Here, the forth and fifth terms on the left-hand side arise from random and shear flows, respectively, $\langle V^2\rangle$ is the second moment of the particle velocity distribution (assuming the velocity distribution is isotropic and Gaussian), and Γ_{eff} is the effective shear rate. Notice that the "dynamical absorption" for flow in Eq. (4.45) increases with τ^2, compared to the τ increase for Brownian motion, because particles in flows travel ballistically; also, D_B, $\langle V^2\rangle$, and Γ_{eff} appear separately because the different dynamical processes are uncorrelated. The form of the "dynamical absorption" term for random flow is related to that for Brownian motion. Both are of the form $(1/3)c\mu_s'k_0^2\langle \Delta r^2(\tau)\rangle$, where $\langle \Delta r^2(\tau)\rangle$ is the mean square displacement of a scattering particle. For Brownian motion, $\langle \Delta r^2(\tau)\rangle = D_B$, and for random flow, $\langle \Delta r^2(\tau)\rangle = \langle V^2\rangle\tau^2$.

A schematic diagram of a DWS experimental arrangement is presented in Fig. 4.17. It may consist of a multimode optical fiber that transports a laser beam with an adequate coherence length (larger than or equal to the total photon path length s owing to multiple scattering). Laser radiation diffusely scattered within the sample is then collected by means of a single-mode optical fiber, which allows the fluctuations of the light intensity within the coherence area of the scattered radiation to be

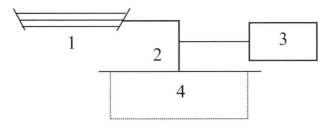

Figure 4.17 Schematic diagram of DWS experimental arrangement: 1, laser with a coherence length that is larger or equal to the total photon path length s owing to multiple scattering; 2, fiber optic probe—a multimode irradiating fiber and a single-mode detecting fiber; 3, detecting system—a photomultiplier tube (PMT) or an avalanche photodiode (APD), operated in the photon counting mode and connected with a digital multichannel autocorrelator; 4, blood perfused tissue.

recorded by the detecting system; this includes a photomultiplier tube (PMT) or an avalanche photodiode (APD), operated in the photon counting mode and connected with a digital multichannel autocorrelator. The output signal is then processed with an autocorrelator to the temporal intensity correlation function $g_2(\tau)$ [Eq. (4.27)], which is related to the normalized temporal field autocorrelation function $g_1(\tau)$ [Eq. (4.29)] by the Siegert relation [Eq. (4.28)]. Further subsequent analysis of the determined $g_1(\tau)$ can be performed similar to the conventional dynamic light scattering approach, where the autocorrelation function is evaluated by its representation in a semilogarithmic scale.

4.5 Confocal microscopy

Confocal laser scanning microscopy, which employs the confocal principle (with two optically conjugate diaphragms or small-size slits in the object and image planes) for the selection of scattered photons coming from a given volume (Fig. 4.18), is a well-developed imaging technique for medical investigations.[1,3,28,76,120, 122,614,878–898] It is from this technique that the most impressive results on three-dimensional imaging of living tissues (in particular, skin) have been recently obtained. The resolution of this technique provides an opportunity to recognize different types of cells and simultaneously observe moving blood cells in microvessels.[887]

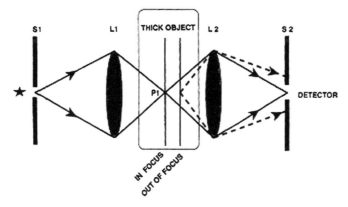

Figure 4.18 Principle of confocal microscope.[889]

In a conventional microscope, the lateral and axial resolutions are not independent. The great advantage of a confocal microscope is that the axial resolution is enhanced, which results in the "optical sectioning" capability of confocal microscopes.[614,878–881] The lateral resolution of a confocal microscope is inversely proportional to the NA of the microscope objective lens,[887]

$$\Delta x = \frac{0.46\lambda}{\mathrm{NA}}.$$

(4.46)

The predicted resolution Δx is 0.4 μm with a 1.2-NA water-immersion objective lens at wavelength $\lambda = 1064$ nm. The axial resolution is more sensitive to the numerical aperture of the microscope objective lens. Therefore, to obtain the maximum axial resolution (and, hence, the best degree of optical sectioning), it is preferred to use microscope objectives with the largest numerical aperture. The full width at half-maximum of the axial irradiance distribution defines the axial resolution or optical section thickness,[887]

$$\Delta z = \frac{1.4n\lambda}{(\text{NA})^2},\qquad(4.47)$$

where n is the refractive index of the objective lens immersion medium. The predicted axial resolution Δz is 1.4 μm with a 1.2-NA water-immersion objective lens at wavelength $\lambda = 1064$ nm and $n = 1.35$. The lateral Δx and axial Δz resolution of the confocal microscope measured for the scattering medium with $n = 1.35$ at $\lambda = 1064$ nm for a 1.2-NA objective lens were 0.7 and 3 μm, respectively.[887] The differences in predicted and measured resolution can be attributed to spherical aberration. For an oil-immersion microscope objective with a numerical aperture of 1.4 and blue light of wavelength 442 nm, the lateral resolution is 0.14 μm and the axial or depth resolution is 0.23 μm.[614]

The lateral resolution of a conventional (conv) and a confocal (conf) microscope can be compared.[614,880] If the image of a single point specimen is viewed in reflected light by conventional microscopy, the image intensity distribution is given by

$$I_{\text{conv}}(\tilde{r}) = \left(\frac{2J_1(\tilde{r})}{\tilde{r}}\right)^2,\qquad(4.48)$$

where J_1 is the first-order Bessel function, $\tilde{r} = (2\pi/\lambda)(\text{NA})r$, and r is the lateral distance in the focal plane. For the confocal case in the presence of the pinhole, the image is now given by

$$I_{\text{conf}}(\tilde{r}) = \left(\frac{2J_1(\tilde{r})}{\tilde{r}}\right)^4.\qquad(4.49)$$

For the confocal case, the image is sharpened by a factor of 1.4 relative to the conventional microscope. With a confocal microscope, the resolution is about 40% better than in a conventional microscope.

Let us consider axial resolution in a confocal microscope for imaging both points and planes.[614,880,881] If a confocal microscope is scanned axially so that the intensity of light reflected from a plane mirror is detected as a function of the distance that the mirror moves toward the focal plane, the intensity of the reflected light is given by simple paraxial theory as[881]

$$I_{\text{conf}}(z) = \left[\frac{\sin(\upsilon(z)/2)}{\upsilon(z)/2}\right]^2.\qquad(4.50)$$

The symbol $\upsilon(z)$ is a normalized axial coordinate related to the real axial distance z by

$$\upsilon = \frac{8\pi}{\lambda} n z \sin^2 \left(\frac{\alpha}{2} \right), \tag{4.51}$$

where $n \sin \alpha = NA$. At the focal plane, the intensity of the reflected signal is maximal. These equations are valid for the imaging of plane reflectors. For point or line reflectors, Eq. (4.50) becomes

$$I_{\mathrm{conf}}(z) = \left[\frac{\sin(\upsilon(z)/2)}{\upsilon(z)/2} \right]^4. \tag{4.52}$$

The optical sectioning is weaker for a point or a line than for a plane. All of these equations refer only to bright field imaging in the reflection mode. For fluorescence imaging, which is incoherent light imaging, all of the equations are different.[614] Image quality is not only dependent on resolution, but also is very dependent on the contrast of the image.

The principle of the out-of-focal-plane rejection in a confocal microscope is shown in Figs. 4.18 and 4.19. The reflected light from the focal plane passes through the pinhole and reaches the detector. In the case of an unfocused system,

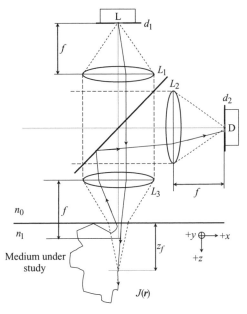

Figure 4.19 Schematic of the confocal probing technique: $L_1, L_2,$ and L_3, short-focus lenses ($f = 8$ mm) forming in pairs a small-aperture collimator; d_1 and d_2, limiting diaphragms with diameters of 10 μm; z_f, depth of focal point immersion into the medium under study; L, laser source; D, detector of optical radiation; and n_0 and n_1, refractive indices of the external and studied media.[896]

the reflected light is spread out over a region larger than the pinhole; only a very small amount of the light from the outside of the focal plane passes the pinhole and is detected. An important problem in confocal microscopy is the optical aberrations that are introduced by the specimen and/or the instrument itself.[614]

A high image contrast and a high spatial resolution of reflection confocal microscopy (RCM) are achieved due to probing a small (10–100 μm^2) volume of the tissue. The localization of a desired signal within the measured volume of such small dimensions becomes possible as a result of mutual optical matching between the laser radiation source, the measured volume, and the photodetector. The field of view of the light source and photodetector are limited by pinholes, which are mounted in the planes of object and image (Fig. 4.19).[896] If the penetration depth z_f of the lens focus into the tissue does not exceed three to four lengths of the photon mean free path l_{ph} [see Eq. (1.8)], then such pinholes ensure that photons reflected strictly back by the tissue and cell components within the probed volume (so-called ballistic photons) dominate in the detected signal. Just these photons carry valid information that allows one to reconstruct the internal structure of the medium under study.

As z_f increases, i.e., when the focus penetrates deeper into the scattering medium, the fraction of ballistic photons in the detected signal decreases, while the fraction of photons scattered by the medium increases. Under typical conditions of experiments with biological tissues, RCM allows one to distinguish ballistic photons against a background of the totality of the medium-scattered photons, until z_f becomes higher than l_{ph} by a factor of 5–8. In other words, because of an intense multiple light scattering characteristic of most of tissues, RCM makes it possible to obtain an image of the cellular structure of skin, for example, located at a depth of at most 300–400 μm.[878,885–887]

Figure 4.20 shows the results of Monte Carlo simulation of spatial distribution $J(\bar{r})$ of the probability density of the effective photon optical paths performed for a confocal probing scheme with a focus of the objective lens immersed into a homogeneous scattering medium to a depth of $z_f = 300$ μm. The parameters of RCM are presented in Fig. 4.19. As is expected, when the immersion depth z_f does not exceed 3–4 MFPs ($\mu_s \leq 10$ mm^{-1} or, equivalently, $l_{ph} \geq 100$ μm), clearly pronounced photon focusing at a depth of 300 μm is observed in the spatial distribution of the density of effective optical photon paths [Fig. 4.20(a)].

If z_f amounts to 8–20 MFPs ($\mu_s = 26.6$–40.0 mm^{-1} and, correspondingly, $l_{ph} = 25$–37.5 μm), then the tendency of probing-radiation focusing in the tissue is still held [Fig. 4.20(b)]. However, the central focal spot region is much larger than in the case of a less scattering medium [Fig. 4.20(a)]. With a further increase in the medium scattering coefficient ($\mu_s \geq 100$ mm^{-1}) and the corresponding shortening of photon MFP ($l_{ph} \leq 10$ μm), the incident radiation turns out to be defocused, although its narrow directivity remains unaltered [Fig. 4.20(c)].

These data (Fig. 4.20) clearly illustrate the possibility of localizing the focused probing laser radiation inside a homogeneous, multiply and anisotropically scattering ($g = 0.9$) and weakly absorbing ($\mu_a = 0.01$ mm^{-1}) medium at its probing by RCM.

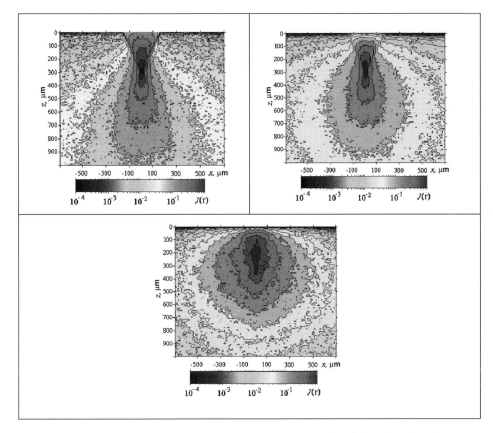

Figure 4.20 Spatial distribution $J(r)$ of the probability density of the effective photon optical paths calculated for a homogeneous ($n_1 = 1.4$), multiply [$\mu_s = 10$ (a), 26.6 (b), and 100 mm^{-1} (c)], and anisotropically ($g = 0.9$) scattering, and weakly absorbing ($\mu_a = 0.01$ mm^{-1}) medium at its probing by the reflection confocal microscopy in the geometry presented in Fig. 4.19 and $z_f = 300$ µm.[896]

4.6 Optical coherence tomography (OCT)

Methods of interferometry and tomography of tissues and organs with the use of partially coherent light sources have progressed rapidly in recent years,[1,3,8,17,18,28, 45,76,77,84,102,108–111,116,126,127,129,135,136,138,139,142,343,412–424,620,711–713,716–718,737, 750–753,764–776,899–939] which provided the grounds for organizing a special international conference[8,45,116] and special issues of the *Journal of Biomedical Optics* on this subject.[17,18] OCT was first demonstrated in 1991.[899] Imaging was performed *in vitro* in human retina and in atherosclerotic plaque as examples of imaging in transparent weakly scattering media as well as highly scattering media. A brief historical review and analysis of the fundamentals of low-coherence interferometry and tomography are presented by Fercher and coworkers,[84,142,901,902] who also discussed ophthalmologic applications of these methods. An overview of the early development of optical low-coherence reflectometry and some recent biomedical applications is given by Masters.[931]

Different terms are employed in the literature to specify this method of investigations: dual-beam coherent interferometry or laser Doppler interferometry, optical coherence tomography (OCT) or optical coherence reflectometry. The tomographic scheme differs from the interferometric one by additional transverse scanning, which allows one to obtain topograms of various tissue layers.

OCT is analogous to ultrasonic imaging, which measures the intensity of reflected infrared light rather than reflected sound waves from the sample. Time gating is employed so that the time for the light to be reflected back, or echo delay time, is used to assess the intensity of back-reflection as a function of depth. Unlike ultrasound, the echo time delay on the order of femtoseconds cannot be measured electronically due to the high speed associated with the propagation of light. Therefore, a time-of-flight technique has to be engaged to measure such an ultrashort time delay of light back-reflected from the different depth of a sample. OCT uses an optical interferometer illuminated by a low-coherent-light source to solve this problem.

This technique is conventionally implemented with the use of a dual-beam Michelson interferometer. If the path length of light in the reference arm is changed with a constant linear speed v, then the signal arising from the interference between the light scattered in a backward direction (reflected) from a sample and light in the reference arm is modulated at the Doppler frequency

$$f_D = \frac{2v}{\lambda}. \tag{4.53}$$

Owing to the small coherence length of a light source,

$$l_c = \frac{2\ln(2)}{\pi} \frac{\lambda^2}{\Delta\lambda}, \tag{4.54}$$

where $\Delta\lambda$ is the bandwidth of the light source with a Gaussian line profile, the Doppler signal is produced by backscattered light only within a very small region (on the order of the coherence length l_c) that corresponds to the current optical path length in the reference arm. If a multimode diode laser or a superluminescent diode (SLD) with a bandwidth of 15–60 nm ($\lambda \sim 800$–860 nm) is employed, the longitudinal resolution falls within the range of 5–20 µm. For a titanium sapphire laser with a wavelength of 820 nm, the bandwidth may reach 140 nm. Correspondingly, the resolution is 2.1 µm.[45,84]

A typical scheme of a dual-beam Michelson interferometer with a low-coherence source and the principle of operation of such a device are shown in Fig. 4.21, which illustrates ophthalmologic applications of this technique.[901,902] Let us consider the interference of light reflected from the front surface of eye cornea (1) and pigment epithelium of retina (2). Under these conditions, each of the two beams E' and E'' is split into two beams, E'_1, E'_2 and E''_1, E''_2. Suppose that d is

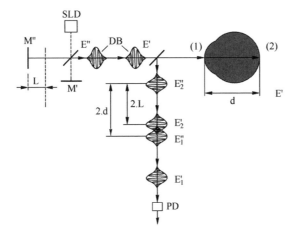

Figure 4.21 Dual-beam Michelson interferometer with a partially coherent source of excitation for ophthalmologic applications:[901,902] SLD, superluminescent diode; M' and M", interferometer mirrors; DB, dual beam; and PD, photodetector.

the geometric distance between the reflective surfaces of the eye. Then, the components of the field are characterized by additional delay times and the total field of light beams reflected from the eye is written as

$$E(t) = E_1(t) + E_2(t-\tau) = E_1'(t) + E_1''(t-\delta) + E_2'(t-\tau) + E_2''(t-\delta-\tau), \quad (4.55)$$

where $\tau = 2nd/c_0$ and n is the refractive index of a medium between two reflective surfaces. When quasi-monochromatic sources are used, the interfering beams consist of groups of waves, and n should be replaced by the group refractive index

$$n_g = n - \lambda \frac{dn}{d\lambda}. \quad (4.56)$$

We should take into account that the coherence length of light increases in a dispersive medium, and spatial resolution lowers. This is especially noticeable for broadband laser systems. Specifically, for a titanium sapphire laser with a bandwidth of 140 nm, the coherence length is equal to 2.1 μm for air (in the absence of dispersion) and 60 μm for water (in a layer with a thickness of 24 mm).[917] According to Ref. 917, the coherence length in a medium is

$$l_c' = \left\{ l_c^2 + \left[\frac{dn_g}{d\lambda} d\Delta\lambda \right]^2 \right\}^{1/2}, \quad (4.57)$$

where d is the thickness of the medium. Hence, we find that if the thickness of a tissue being probed is not large (on the order of 1 mm), the additive to the coherence length due to dispersion may remain small. For example, for a titanium sapphire laser with the largest bandwidth, this addition is the same order of magnitude as the coherence length in free space.

Figure 4.22 presents a typical waveform of the interference signal corresponding to *in vivo* probing of the fundus of the human eye with the use of partially coherent beams of the interferometer shown schematically in Fig. 4.21. By analyzing such a signal, one can very accurately determine the thickness of the layer of nerve fibers (the distance between ILM and GCL, 75 μm). Along with geometric parameters, partially coherent interferometry provides an opportunity to determine optical parameters of tissues, such as scattering and absorption coefficients and the refractive index. The dependence of these parameters on the physiological state of a tissue allows one to obtain reliable diagnostic data in both ophthalmology and other fields of medicine. It was demonstrated that the spatial resolution of the interference technique is approximately an order of magnitude higher than the spatial resolution provided by conventionally employed ultrasonic diagnosis. In addition, owing to its contactless character, the interference technique does not require eye anesthesia. The results of measurements obtained with the use of the interference technique are characterized by a high reproducibility and can be easily interpreted, even by nonexperts.[901,902] In addition to the determination of geometric and optical parameters of the rear segment of the human eye (the thickness of the fundus and its components), low-coherence interferometry can be successfully used to measure the thickness of the cornea with a resolution on the order of 1.6–3.5 μm, which is necessary for monitoring during conventional and laser surgical operations aimed at changing the refraction of the cornea; for assessing various corneal pathologies, including edema; and for measuring the depth of the front eye chamber and the axial length of an eye. The latter possibility is especially important when cataracts are treated surgically, because an error of 0.2–0.3 mm in determining the axial length of an eye gives rise to an error in eye refraction of about one diopter.[901,902]

OCT can also be described on the basis of the principles of the heterodyne technique.[939] Figure 4.23 shows a typical fiber-optical scheme, where two beams

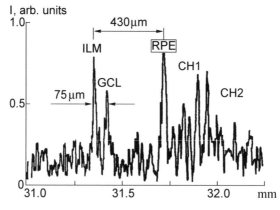

Figure 4.22 Interference signal (in arbitrary units) obtained by *in vivo* probing of the fundus of the human eye. The wavelength of the radiation of a superluminescent diode is 825 nm, and its coherence length is 12 μm[901,902]; ILM, inner boundary layer; GCL, ganglion layer; RPE, retinal pigment epithelium; and CH1 and CH2, choroid layers. The distance is measured relative to the cornea.

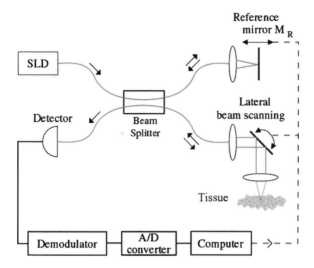

Figure 4.23 A typical fiber-optic OCT system. Light from the superluminescent diode (SLD) is split up by a beam splitter into a local oscillator (LO) beam and a signal beam that is incident on to the medium (tissue) under investigation. The reflected field is superposed with the LO beam reflected from the longitudinally scanned reference mirror; the superposed field is measured by a detecting-demodulating system.[939]

(signal and local oscillator beam) are generated from a broadband source such as an SLD. The signal beam is incident on the sample; the transmitted or scattered light is then superposed with the local oscillator beam in the balanced detector. Due to the broad spectrum of the light (and, therefore, small longitudinal coherence length), the light coming from the sample and the local oscillator beam only interfere if their path lengths are matched within the coherence length of the light. By increasing the path length of the local oscillator beam Δl with the reference mirror M_R, the local oscillator beam interferes only with those parts of the signal field that have traveled the same distance Δl in the medium. Therefore, signal field contributions from different photon path lengths in the sample can be selected. In practice, the reference mirror is moved at a fixed speed, and the heterodyne beat signal resulting from the Doppler shift of the local oscillator beam reflected from the moving mirror is recorded at the same time [see Eq. (4.53)]. By moving the laser beam in a two-dimensional raster and taking vertical scans for each point, a three-dimensional image can be obtained.

Figure 4.24(a) shows an example of a time-modulated interference signal detected by the photodetector. If the detected ac signal is band-pass filtered with respect to the central Doppler frequency (as the center frequency) it is then rectified and low-pass filtered. The output of the low-pass filter is the envelope of the time-modulated ac interference signal, which is equivalent to the cross-correlation amplitude. Figure 4.24(b) gives an example of the detected envelope corresponding to Fig. 4.24(a).

OCT performs cross-sectional imaging by measuring the time delay and magnitude of optical echoes at different transverse positions, essentially by the use

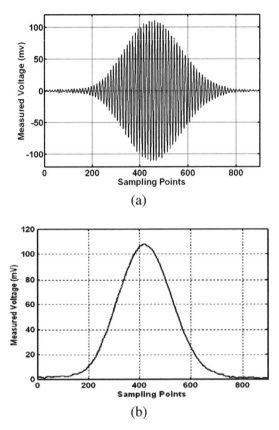

Figure 4.24 Low-coherence interferometer output signals: (a) time-modulated ac term of interference signal, (b) corresponding signal after demodulation (cross-correlation amplitude, i.e., envelope).[932]

of low-coherence interferometry. A cross-sectional image is acquired by performing successive rapid axial measurements while transversely scanning the incident sample beam onto the sample (see Fig. 4.25). The result is a two-dimensional data set, which represents the optical reflection or backscattering strength in a cross-sectional plane through a biological tissue. The system implemented by the optic-fiber couplers, matured in the telecommunication industry, offers the greatest advantage for the OCT imaging of biological tissues because it can be integrated into almost all the currently available medical imaging modalities, for example, endoscope and microscope.[108,109,111,717,775] Figure 4.23 gives an example of the fiber-optic versions of OCT.

Numerous fiber-optical OCT systems are described in the literature (see, for example, Refs. 1, 108, 109, 111, 127, 136, and 142). In these systems, light from a low-coherence light source is coupled to a single-mode fiber coupler where half of the light power is conducted through the single-mode fiber to the reference mirror. The remaining half enters the sample via proper focusing optics. The distal end of the fiber in the sample arm serves a dual role as a coherent light receiver

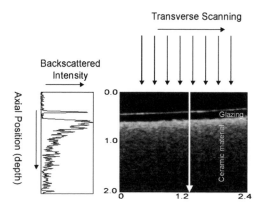

Figure 4.25 OCT image (right-hand lower) is generated by performing measurements of the reflected signal time delay and magnitude of backscattered light intensity (left) over a range of transverse positions (upper). As an example, the OCT image of a ceramic material with glazing that models a hard tissue (tooth or bone) is presented.[932]

and spatial filter analogous to a confocal pinhole. Because the dc signal and intensity noise generated by the light from the reference arm add to the interference signal, it makes the system prone to excess photon noise. One way to reduce this type of noise is to use a balanced detection configuration that would cancel the background noise components by subtracting the photocurrents generated by two photodetectors.[932,939] The interference signals at the output of the detectors add because they vary out of phase.

OCT has the advantage that it can achieve extremely high axial image resolution independently of the transverse image resolution. The axial resolution is determined by the coherence length of light source used, i.e., Eq. (4.54), which is independent of the sampling beam focusing conditions. The lateral or transverse resolution achieved with an OCT imaging system is determined by the focused spot size limited by the numerical aperture of the lens used to deliver the light onto the sample, and the wavelength, as in conventional or confocal microscopy [see Eqs. (4.48) and (4.49)].

4.7 Second-harmonic generation

Second-harmonic generation (SHG) is a new high-resolution nonlinear optical imaging modality for study of intact tissues and cellular membranes.[940–948] SHG is a second-order nonlinear optical process that can only arise from media lacking a center of symmetry, e.g., an anisotropic crystal or at an interface such as membrane. It can be used to image highly ordered structural proteins without any exogenous labels,[940,941,943–948] as well as biological membrane probes with high membrane specificity.[942]

Collagen as a main component of connective tissues has an appreciable nonlinear susceptibility for SHG.[940,941,943–948] The helix of the collagen secondary structure is noncentrosymmetric, satisfying a condition for SHG, which self-assembles into higher-order structures. Collagen has been shown to have a dominant uniaxial second-order nonlinear susceptibility component aligned along the fiber axis. In such multicomponent tissues as skin, SHG light is generated mostly within dermis, not in cellular layers like epidermis or subcutaneous fat. The SHG technique has a number of advantages connected with the incident wavelength dividing and selectivity to tissue structure, which allow one to easily reject surface reflection and multiple scattering of the incident light in the epidermis layer without any gating technique. In addition, SHG polarimetry is an effective tool to probe collagen orientation in tissues.[944–947]

In general, the nonlinear polarization for a material can be expressed as[942]

$$P = \chi^{(1)}\vec{E} + \chi^{(2)}\vec{E}\vec{E} + \chi^{(3)}\vec{E}\vec{E}\vec{E} + \cdots, \qquad (4.58)$$

where P is the induced polarization, $\chi^{(n)}$ is the nth order nonlinear susceptibility, and $\vec{E}$ is the electric field vector of the incident light. The first term describes normal absorption and reflection of light; the second, SHG, sum, and difference frequency generation; and the third, both two- and three-photon absorption, as well as third-harmonic generation.

SHG, by contrast to two-photon fluorescence (see Section 1.7.2), does not arise from an absorptive process. Instead, an intense laser field induces a nonlinear second-order polarization in the assembly of molecules, resulting in the production of a coherent wave at exactly twice the incident frequency (or half the wavelength). The spectral and temporal profiles of two-photon excited fluorescence and SHG are also different. For two-photon fluorescence, the width of the emission spectrum is determined by the relative geometries of the ground and excited molecular state, and the emission lifetime is related to the oscillator strength of the transition and is typically on the order of a few nanoseconds. In SHG, by contrast, both the spectral and temporal characteristics are derived from the laser source: the bandwidth scales as $1/\sqrt{2}$ of the bandwidth of the excitation laser and, due to the coherence of the process, the SHG pulse is temporally synchronous with the excitation pulse.

A simplified expression for the SHG signal intensity has the form[942]

$$I(2\omega) \propto \left[\chi^{(2)}\frac{E(\omega)}{\tau_p} \right]^2 \tau_p, \qquad (4.59)$$

where $\chi^{(2)}$ is the second-order nonlinear susceptibility, and $E(\omega)$ and τ_p are the laser pulse energy and width, respectively. As in two-photon fluorescence [see Eq. (1.189)], the signal is quadratic with peak power, but since SHG is an instantaneous process, a signal is generated only during the duration of the laser pulse. The macroscopic value $\chi^{(2)}$ can be expressed in terms of the first molecular hyperpolarizability β as

$$\chi^{(2)} = \rho_M \langle \beta \rangle, \qquad (4.60)$$

where ρ_M is the density of molecules and the brackets denote an orientational average. This underscores the need for a noncentrosymmetric region, since $\langle \beta \rangle$ would vanish for an isotropic distribution of dipole moments. As it follows from Eqs. (4.59) and (4.60), the SHG signal depends on the square of the molecular surface density, whereas two-photon fluorescence intensity is linear with the density of fluorophores [see Eq. (1.189)].

Within the two-level system model, the first molecular hyperpolarizability β is given by[942]

$$\beta = \frac{3e^2}{2\hbar^3} \frac{\omega_{ge} f_{ge} \Delta\mu_{ge}}{[\omega_{ge}^2 - \omega^2][\omega_{ge}^2 - 4\omega^2]}, \tag{4.61}$$

where e is electron charge, ω_{ge}, f_{ge}, and μ_{ge} are the energy difference, oscillator strength, and change in dipole moment between the ground and excited states, respectively. While SHG is not an absorptive process, the magnitude of the SHG wave can be resonance enhanced when the energy of the second-harmonic signal overlaps with an electronic absorption band. It follows from Eq. (4.61) that β becomes large when the laser fundamental frequency approaches the electronic transition, and then the total second-order response is a sum of the nonresonant and resonant contributions,

$$\chi_{total}^{(2)} = \chi_{nonres}^{(2)} + \chi_{res}^{(2)}. \tag{4.62}$$

Depending on the specific properties of the molecule and the excitation wavelength, the resonant contribution can dominate, resulting in enhancement of an order of magnitude or more.

5

Controlling of the Optical Properties of Tissues

This chapter describes the fundamentals and advances in controlling tissue optical properties. As a major technology, the optical immersion method at usage of exogenous optical clearing agents (OCAs) is discussed. Water transport in a tissue, tissue swelling, and hydration at its interaction with an OCA are considered. Optical clearing properties of fibrous and cell-structured tissues are analyzed using spectrophotometry, frequency-domain, fluorescence, and polarization measurements; confocal microscopy and OCT; as well as nonlinear spectroscopy techniques such as two-photon fluorescence and SHG. *In vitro*, *ex vivo*, and *in vivo* studies of a variety of human and animal tissues such as eye sclera, skin, cerebral membrane (*dura mater*), gastric tissue, tendon, blood vessels, and blood are presented. OCA delivery, tissue permeation, and skin reservoir function are discussed. Cell and cell flow imaging at optical clearing are also discussed. Some important applications of the tissue immersion technique, such as glucose sensing, precision tissue laser photodisruption, as well as other techniques of tissue optical properties control, such as tissue compression and stretching, noncoagulating and coagulating temperature action, and tissue whitening, are described.

5.1 Fundamentals of tissue optical properties controlling and a brief review

Reflection, absorption, scattering, and fluorescence in living tissues and blood can be effectively controlled by various methods.[1–6,9,10,24,26,29,48,49,54,57,61,62,76,77,90,91, 95,96,129,139,155,172,266,267,324,335,339–341,343,396,409,410,442,453,534,549–552,558,569–571,575, 630–633,667,668,681,703,704,717,723,737,748–754,759,760,777,788,798,799,812,831,850,866,867,896, 897,916,932,946,947,949–1065] Staining (sensitization) of biological materials is extensively used to study mechanisms of interaction between light and their constituent components, and also for diagnostic purposes, and selective photodestruction of individual components of living tissues. This approach underlies the diagnosis and photodynamic therapy (PDT) of malignant neoplasm, UV-A photochemotherapy of psoriasis and other proliferative disorders, angiography in ophthalmology, and many other applications in medicine.

In the visible and NIR regions, tissues and biological liquids are low absorbing, but highly scattering media (see Table 2.1). Scattering defines spectral and angular characteristics of light interacting with living objects as well as its penetration depth; thus, optical properties of tissues and blood may be effectively controlled by changes of scattering properties. Living tissue allows one to control its optical (scattering) properties using various physical and chemical actions such as compression, stretching, dehydration, coagulation, UV irradiation, exposure to low temperature, and impregnation by chemical solutions, gels, and oils. All these phenomena can be understood if we consider tissue as a scattering medium that shows all optical effects that are characteristic to turbid physical systems. It is well known that the turbidity of a dispersive physical system can be effectively controlled by providing matching refractive indices of the scatterers and the ground material. This is a so-called optical immersion technique. Another possibility to control optical properties of a disperse system is to change its packing parameter and/or scatterer sizing (see Chapters 1–3).

In vivo control of tissue optical properties is very important for many medical applications. A number of laser surgery, therapy, and diagnostic technologies include tissue compression and stretching, which is used for better transportation of a laser beam to underlying layers of tissue. The human eye compression technique allows one to perform transscleral laser coagulation of the ciliary body and retina/choroid.[266,667,723] The possibility of selective translucence of the upper tissue layers should be very useful for development of the eye globe imaging techniques and for detecting local inhomogeneities hidden by a highly scattering medium in functional tomography. Results on control of human sclera optical properties by tissue impregnation with optical clearing agents (OCA), which are typically hyperosmotic chemical agents, such as x-ray contrast (trazograph or hypaque), glucose, and polyethylene glycol (PEG), were also reported.[6,24,61,77,155,172,788,812,949,958–964,1022,1023,1033]

In general, the scattering coefficient μ_s and scattering anisotropy factor g of a tissue is dependent on refractive index mismatch between cellular tissue components: cell membranes, cytoplasma, cell nucleus, cell organelles, melanin granules, and the extracellular fluid. For fibrous (connective) tissue (eye scleral stroma, corneal stroma, skin dermis, cerebral membrane, muscle, vessel wall noncellular matrix, female breast fibrous component, cartilage, tendon, etc.), index mismatch of the interstitial medium and long strands of scleroprotein (collagen-, elastin-, or reticulin-forming fibers) is important. The refractive index matching is manifested in the reduction of the scattering coefficient ($\mu_s \rightarrow 0$) and increase of single-scattering directness ($g \rightarrow 1$). For skin dermis and eye sclera, μ_s reduction can be very high.[172,571,722,788,965] For hematous tissue like the liver, its impregnation by solutes with different osmolarity also leads to refractive index matching and reduction of the scattering coefficient, but the effect is not as pronounced as for skin and sclera due to cells changing size as a result of osmotic stress.[956,957]

Soft tissue is composed of closely packed groups of cells entrapped in a network of fibers through which interstitial liquid percolates. At a microscopic scale, the tissue components have no pronounced boundaries; thus, tissue can be considered as a continuous structure with spatial variations in the refractive index. As it was already discussed, to model such a complicated structure as a collection of particles, it is necessary to resort to a statistical approach (see Chapter 1). The tissue components that contribute most to the local refractive index variations are the connective tissue fibers (collagen-, elastin-, or reticulin-forming), which form part of the noncellular tissue matrix around and among cells and cell membranes, cytoplasmic organelles (mitochondria, lysosoms, and peroxisomes), cell nuclei, and melanin granules.[63,64,96,156,558,781–783,956,957] Figure 1.45 shows a hypothetical index profile formed by measuring the refractive index along a line in an arbitrary direction through a volume of tissue and the corresponding statistical mean index profile. The average background index $\bar{n}_0$ is defined as the weighted average of refractive indices of the cytoplasm and the interstitial fluid, n_{cp} and n_{is} [see Eq. (1.151)]. The refractive index of a particle can be defined as the sum of the background index and the mean index variation, $\langle \Delta n \rangle$, described by Eqs. (1.152)–(1.154).

For a two-component model, the mean refractive index of a tissue $\bar{n}$ is defined by the refractive indices of its scattering center's material n_s and ground matter n_0, $\bar{n} = f_s n_s + (1 - f_s)n_0$ [see Eq. (2.57)]. The $n_s/n_0 \equiv m$ ratio determines the scattering coefficient. For example, in a simple monodisperse model of scattering dielectric spheres (Mie theory), the reduced scattering coefficient μ_s' is defined by Eq. (2.24), where $\mu_s' \sim (m - 1)^2$. It follows from Eq. (2.24) that only a 5% increase in the refractive index of the ground matter ($n_0 = 1.35 \rightarrow 1.42$), when that of the scattering centers is $n_s = 1.47$, will cause a sevenfold decrease of μ_s'. In the limit of equal refractive indices for nonabsorbing particles and background material, $m = 1$ and $\mu_s' \rightarrow 0$. In a living tissue, the relative refractive index is a function of the tissue physiological or pathological state. Independence of the specificity of the tissue state refractive index of the scatterers and/or the background may be changed (increased or decreased); therefore, light scattering may correspondingly increase or decrease.

Light scattering and absorption of particles that compose tissue or blood can be calculated by Mie theory. The relevant parameters are the size (radius a) of the particles, their complex refractive index [see Eq. (1.192)], the complex refractive index of the dielectric host (ground material in tissues, or plasma in blood) n_0, and the relative refractive index of the scatterers and the ground materials, $m = n_s'/n_0$. The imaginary part of the complex refractive indices is responsible for light losses due to absorption. Mie theory yields the absorption and scattering efficiencies and the phase function from which the absorption and scattering coefficients $\mu_s = \rho \sigma_{sca}$ and $\mu_a = \rho \sigma_{abs}$ and the scattering anisotropy g are calculated; ρ is the scatterers' (particles) density. The corresponding scattering and absorption cross sections σ_{sca} and σ_{abs}, and g-factor are described by Eqs. (1.193), (1.194), and (1.195), respectively.

The transport scattering coefficient increases strongly with the ratio of the real part of the scaterer index and the background medium index, n_s'/n_0, especially for 0.1–1 μm-sized particles (see Fig. 1.56).[632,633] For fully matched refractive indices of scatterers and background material, the scattering coefficient goes to zero and the scattering anisotropy factor is maximal and approaches 1 for particles with sizes above 1 μm.

However, in practice, the total index matching cannot always be provided; thus, other mechanisms of tissue clearing may be essential. Sometimes, action of hyperosmotic chemical agents or strong mechanical compression may lead to a reversible or irreversible change in the scatterers' size. The wavelength dependencies of the scattering parameters for systems of partially matched refractive indices of scatterers and background ($n'_s/n_0 = 1.07$) are shown in Fig. 1.57. Such a level of matching is typical for many normal connective and cell-structured tissues. The spectral variation of the relative index has been neglected in calculations, but may be relevant in practice. If the particle size and ratio of refractive indices are fixed, the wavelength dependencies are caused by the spectral variation of the ratio of the wavelength to the particle size. For particles with a refractive index close to that of the host (see Fig. 1.57), the scattering coefficient of the particle systems with very small or very big diameters of particles is almost independent of the wavelength in the range from 400 to 800 nm, while that of the system with intermediate diameters of particles decreases with wavelength. The same tendency in the wavelength dependence (no dependence for very small and very big scatterers, and decreasing for intermediate diameters) is expected for the scattering anisotropy factor.

It follows from this consideration that reduction of scattering may be associated not only with the refractive index matching, but also with the changes of the scattering system sizing. Both aggregation to big-sized particles and disaggregation to small-sized particles leads to scattering damping, but the scattering anisotropy properties of the newly formed system should be quite different. The latter can be used in the understanding of the tissue clearing mechanisms associated with the particle sizing and the refractive index matching. Conceptually, for many situations, the leading mechanism of tissue clearing might be a refractive index match because the equalizing of the refractive indices of scatterers and surrounding media always takes place at tissue immersion, dehydration, or compression, and the sensitivity of the scattering properties to refractive index matching is very high.

As a particle system, whole blood shows pronounced clearing effects that may be accompanied by induced or spontaneous aggregation and disaggregation processes as well as RBC swelling or shrinkage at application of biocompatible clearing agents with certain osmotic properties.[737,748,981–985,932,1036,1037,1042,1043]

It is possible to achieve a marked impairment of scattering by means of intratissue administration of appropriate OCAs. Conspicuous experimental optical clearing in human and animal sclera; human, animal, and artificial skin; human gastrointestinal tissues; and human and animal cartilage and tendon in the visible and NIR wavelength range induced by administration of x-ray contrast agents (verografin, trazograph, and hypaque), glucose, propylene glycol, polypropylene glycol-based polymers (PPG), polyethylene glycol (PEG), PEG-based polymers, glycerol, and other solutions has been described in Refs. 6, 24, 61, 77, 155, 172, 343, 339–341, 409, 410, 453, 571, 704, 717, 777, 788, 798, 799, 812, 831, 866, 867, 916, 932, 946, 949, 958–975, 977–980, 986, 987, 997, 1008, 1009, 1011, 1012, 1021–1034, 1038–1041, 1044–1047, and 1052–1065.

Coordination between refractive indices in multicomponent transparent tissues showing polarization anisotropy (e.g., cornea) leads to its decrease.[5,10] In contrast, for a highly scattering tissue with a hidden linear birefringence or optical activity, its impregnation by immersion agents may significantly improve the detection ability of polarization anisotropy due to reduction of the background scattering.[409,410,1033,1034]

Concentration-dependent variations in scattering and transmission profiles in α-crystallin suspensions isolated from calf lenses are believed to be related to osmotic phenomenon.[952] Osmotic and diffusive processes that occur in tissues treated with verografin, trazograph, glucose, glycerol, and other solutions are also important.[172] Osmotic phenomena appear to be involved when optical properties of biological materials (cells and tissues) are modulated by sugar, alcohol, and electrolyte solutions. This may interfere with the evaluation of hemoglobin saturation with oxygen or identification of such absorbers as cytochrome oxidase in tissues by optical methods.[956,957]

Experimental studies on optical clearing of normal and pathological skin and its components (epidermis and dermis) and the management of reflectance and transmittance spectra using water, glycerol, glycerol-water solutions, glucose, sunscreen creams, cosmetic lotions, gels, and pharmaceutical products were carried out in Refs. 57, 213, 255, 341, 343, 453, 571, 777, 916, 932, 946, 961–967, 969, 970, 973, 975, 978, 980, 988, 1027, 1031, 1038, 1039, 1044–1047, 1049, 1052, 1053, 1055–1063, and 1065. The control of skin optical properties was related to the immersion of refractive indices of scatterers (keratinocytes components in epidermis, collagen, and elastic fibers in dermis) and ground matter, and/or reversible collagen dissociation.[946] In addition, some of the observed effects appear to have been caused by the introduction of additional scatterers or absorbers into the tissue or, conversely, to their washing out.

A marked clearing effect through hamster,[571] porcine,[1058] and human[932,965,967,973] skin, human and rabbit eye sclera,[61,960] and rabbit *dura matter*[831] occurred for an *in vivo* tissue within a few minutes of topical application (eye, *dura matter*, skin) or intratissue injection (skin) of glycerol, glucose, propylene glycol, trazograph, and PEG and PPG polymers.

Albumin, a useful protein for index matching in phase contrast microscopy experiments,[749,953–955] can be used as the immersion medium for tissue study and imaging.[58,96] Proteins smaller than albumin may offer a potential alternative because of the relatively high scattering of albumin. Sometimes, medical diagnosis or contrasting of a lesion image can be provided by the enhancement of tissue scattering properties by applying, for instance, acetic acid, which has been successfully used as a contrast agent in optical diagnostics of cervical tissue.[58,96,998–1003] It has been suggested that the whitening effect caused by acetic acid seen in cervical tissue is due to coagulation of nuclear proteins. Therefore, an acetic acid probe may also prove extremely significant in quantitative optical diagnosis of precancerous conditions because of its ability to selectively enhance nuclear scatter.[58,96]

Evidently, the loss of water by tissue seriously influences its optical properties. One of the major reasons for tissue dehydration *in vivo* is the action of endogenous or exogenous osmotic liquids. In *in vitro* conditions, spontaneous water evaporation from tissue, tissue sample heating at noncoagulating temperatures, or its freezing in a refrigerator cause tissue to loose water. Typically in the visible and NIR regions, far from water absorption bands, the absorption coefficient increases by a few dozens of percent and the scattering coefficient by a few percent due to closer packing of tissue components caused by its shrinkage. However, the overall optical transmittance of a tissue sample increases due to decrease of its thickness at dehydration.[569,570] Specifically, in the vicinity of the strong water absorption bands, the tissue absorption coefficient decreases due to less concentration of water in spite of a higher density of tissue at its dehydration.

It is possible to significantly increase transmission through a soft tissue by squeezing (compressing) or stretching it.[951] The optical clarity of living tissue is due to its optical homogeneity, which is achieved through the removal of blood and interstitial liquor (water) from the compressed site. This results in a higher refractive index of the ground matter, whose value becomes close to that of the scatterers (cell membrane, muscle, or collagen fibers) [see Eq. (2.24)]. Closer packing of tissue components at compression makes the tissue a less chaotic, but more organized, system, which may give less scattering due to cooperative (interference) effects.[442,950] Indeed, the absence of blood in the compressed area also contributes to altered tissue absorption and refraction properties. Certain mechanisms underlying the effects of optical clearing and changing of light reflection by tissues at compression and stretching were proposed in Refs. 61, 62, 442, 667, 722, 723, 950, and 1013.

Long-pulsed laser heating induces reversible and irreversible changes in the optical properties of tissue.[569,570,997] In general, the total transmittance decreases and the diffuse reflectance increases, showing nonlinear behavior during pulsed laser heating. Many types of tissues slowly coagulated (from 10 min to 2 hr) in a hot water or saline bath (70–85°C) exhibit an increase of their scattering and absorption coefficients (see Table 2.1).

UV irradiation causes erythema (skin reddening), stimulates melanin synthesis, and can induce edema and tissue proliferation if the radiation dose is sufficiently large.[54,575,991,992] All these photobiological effects may be responsible for variations in the optical properties of skin and need to be taken into consideration when prescribing phototherapy. Also, UV treatment is known to cause color development in the human lens.[800]

Natural physiological changes in cells and tissues are also responsible for their altered optical properties, which may be detectable and thus used as a measure of these changes. For example, measurements of the scattering coefficient allow one to monitor glucose[339–341,534,549–551,1018,1019] or edema[1017] in the human body, as well as blood parameters.[568] A nearly parabolic dependence between the scattering coefficient and hematocrit values (Hct) in thin blood layers was demonstrated [see Eq. (1.172)].[568] Many papers report optical characteristics of blood as a function of hemoglobin saturation with oxygen. The alterations of the optical properties of blood caused by changes of hematocrit value, temperature, and parameters of flow can be found in Tables 2.1–2.4 and 2.6.

5.2 Tissue optical immersion by exogenous chemical agents

5.2.1 Principles of the optical immersion technique

Let us consider the principles of the optical immersion technique based on the impregnation of a tissue or dilution of blood by a biocompatible chemical agent, which also may have some hyperosmotic properties. Any connective (fibrous) tissue can be effectively impregnated by a liquid agent or its solution. As an example of fibrous tissue, human sclera will be analyzed.

A model of human sclera in a local region can be represented as a slab with a thickness d that is filled by thin and long dielectric cylinders (collagen fibers) with average diameter $\sim$100 nm and refractive index $n_c = 1.474$ (see Fig. 5.1).[172,798,799] The cylinders are located in planes that are in parallel to the slab surface, but within each plane their orientations are random (see Fig. 3.4). The space between collagen fibers is filled by a homogeneous ground substance with refractive index $n_0 = 1.345$. Considerable refractive indices are mismatched between collagen fibers, and a ground substance causes the system to become turbid, i.e., causes multiple scattering and poor transmittance of propagating light. The refractive index of the background is a controlled parameter and may be changed in the range of 1.345 to 1.474, which transits the system from multiple to low-step and even

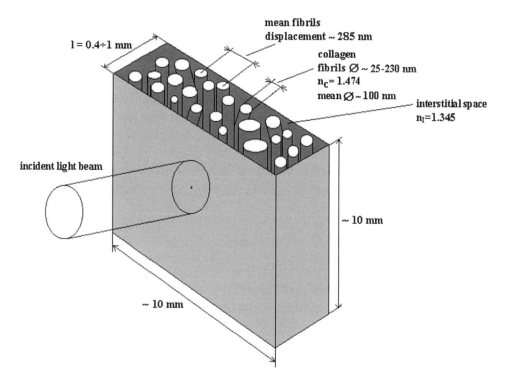

Figure 5.1 Schematic representation of a human scleral sample and the geometry of light irradiation.[172]

single-scattering mode. For $n_c = n_0 = 1.474$, the medium becomes totally homogeneous and optically transparent if absorption of scatterers is small.

The described model of tissue is applicable to any fibrous tissue including skin dermis and muscle. Indeed, refractive indices and fibers' diameters and their spacing should be changed. The transmission of collimated light by a tissue layer of thickness d is defined by the Bouguer-Beer-Lambert law [see Eq. (1.1)] as

$$T_c = \frac{I(d)}{I_0} = \exp(-\mu_t d), \tag{5.1}$$

where I_0 and $I(d)$ are the intensities of the incident and detected light, respectively, and $\mu_t = \mu_a + \mu_s$ is the attenuation coefficient. As it follows from Table 2.1, for the human sclera at wavelength $\lambda = 800$ nm, the absorption coefficient is $\mu_a \cong 1.6$ cm^{-1} and reduced scattering coefficient is $\mu_s' = \mu_s(1 - g) \cong 38$ cm^{-1}. For $g = 0.9$, $\mu_s \cong 380$ cm^{-1}.

Owing to the fibrous structure of the sclera, it is quite reasonable to assume that the dynamics of fluid diffusion within the tissue could be approximated by free diffusion.[172,1021,1066] Therefore, to describe the dynamics of the refractive index change and the corresponding decrease of the scattering coefficient when a chemical agent diffuses within the interfibrillar substance of a tissue, we used the model of free diffusion with the approximate solution of the diffusion equation[172,1066]

$$\frac{\partial C_f(x,t)}{\partial t} = D_f \frac{\partial^2 C_f(x,t)}{\partial x^2}, \tag{5.2}$$

where $C_f(x,t)$ is the fluid concentration, D_f is the coefficient of diffusion, and x is the spatial coordinate. This equation is applicable in cases where the rate of the process is not limited by membranes, such as the diffusion of substances in the interfibrillar space or when a substance in solution has a high rate of permeation through membranes.[1066] For a plane slab with a thickness d that is placed at the moment $t = 0$ in a solution with the initial concentration of the agent C_{a0} (the initial concentration of the agent within the slab is equal to 0; i.e., $t = 0$; $0 \leq x \leq d$; $C_a(x,0) = 0$; the boundary conditions are $C_a(0,t) = C_a(d,t) = C_{a0}$), Eq. (5.2) has the following solution describing the time-dependent distribution of agent concentration within a sample:[172,1066]

$$C_a(x,t) = C_{a0}\left\{1 - \frac{4}{\pi}\left[\exp\left(-\frac{t}{\tau}\right)\sin\left(\frac{\pi x}{d}\right)\right.\right.$$
$$+ \frac{1}{3}\exp\left(-\frac{9t}{\tau}\right)\sin\left(\frac{3\pi x}{d}\right)$$
$$\left.\left.+ \frac{1}{5}\exp\left(-\frac{25t}{\tau}\right)\sin\left(\frac{5\pi x}{d}\right) + \cdots\right]\right\}, \tag{5.3}$$

where

$$\tau = \frac{d^2}{\pi^2 D_a},\qquad(5.4)$$

and D_a is the agent diffusion coefficient.

The ratio of the amount of dissolved matter m_t at the moment t to its equilibrium value m_∞ is defined as[1066]

$$\frac{m_t}{m_\infty} = \frac{\int_0^d C_a(x,t)dx}{C_{a0}d}$$

$$= 1 - \frac{8}{\pi^2}\left[\exp\left(-\frac{t}{\tau}\right) + \frac{1}{9}\exp\left(-\frac{9t}{\tau}\right) + \frac{1}{25}\exp\left(-\frac{25t}{\tau}\right) + \cdots\right].\quad(5.5)$$

This ratio in its turn defines the volume-averaged concentration of an agent $C_a(t)$, which in the first-order approximation has the form[172,987,1021]

$$C_a(t) = \frac{1}{2}\int_0^d C_a(x,t)dx \cong C_{a0}\left[1 - \exp\left(-\frac{t}{\tau}\right)\right].\qquad(5.6)$$

Equations (5.3)–(5.6) allow one to find the time-dependent concentration of chemical agents with a relatively low molecular weight at a depth x within a tissue sample, or time variations of the total amount of these agents in the sample if the diffusion coefficient D_a of these molecules in the tissue is known. On the other hand, measurements of $C_a(t)$ make it possible to estimate the D_a value of implanted molecules in the interstitial fluid of the tissue. For low molecular weight compounds, the values of their diffusion coefficients in their own media are about 10^{-5} cm^2 s^{-1}, for water, $D_a = 2.5 \times 10^{-5}$ cm^2 s^{-1}, and $D_a = 0.5 \times 10^{-5}$ cm^2 s^{-1} for saccharose.[1066]

When the agent is administrated through only one sample surface (such a situation also may take place for *in vivo* topical agent application), Eq. (5.6) is still valid, but with another expression for the characteristic diffusion time:[1038]

$$\tau = \frac{d^2}{D_a}.\qquad(5.7)$$

Equations (5.3)–(5.7) were received for diffusion through a homogeneous slab. Due to its fibrous structure, a tissue can be presented as a porous material, which leads to modification of the chemical agent diffusion coefficient as

$$D_a = \frac{D_{ai}}{p}.\qquad(5.8)$$

Here, D_{ai} is the chemical agent diffusion coefficient within the interstitial fluid and p is the porosity coefficient defined as

$$p = \frac{V - V_C}{V},$$ (5.9)

where V is the volume of the tissue sample and V_C is the volume of collagen fibers.

To describe the bigger molecules' diffusion, the theory of hindered diffusion through a permeable membrane should be used.[172,1021,1066] Based on Fick's law, which limits the flux of matter J (mol/s/cm^2) to a gradient of its concentration,

$$J = -D_a \frac{dC}{dx}.$$ (5.10)

For stationary transport of matter through a thin membrane, we have[1066]

$$J = P_a(C_1 - C_2),$$ (5.11)

where $P_a = D_a/d$ is the coefficient of permeability, and C_1 and C_2 are the concentrations of molecules in two spaces separated by a membrane.

Using Eqs. (5.10) and (5.11), it is possible to find the variation in concentration of molecules inside a closed space with a volume V surrounded by a permeable membrane with an area S by using the following equation:[1066]

$$\frac{dC_2}{dt} = \frac{P_a S}{V}(C_1 - C_2).$$ (5.12)

For a large external volume, where C_1 can be considered as a constant, Eq. (5.12) has an approximate exponential solution in a similar form to Eq. (5.6),[172,1021,1066] with $C_2 = C_a$, $C_1 = C_{a0}$, and

$$\tau = \frac{d^2}{D_a}.$$ (5.13)

Equation (5.13) indicates that in experiments with tissue plane slabs (see Fig. 5.2), $V = Sd$, where S and d are the area and thickness of the sample. The form of this equation is the same as that for free diffusion, but the values of the diffusion coefficient for free and hindered diffusion can be significantly different.

At tissue impregnation by a chemical agent, the refractive index of the background (interfibrillar) media n_0 is a time-dependent function of the agent concentration, which penetrates into a sample $C_a(t)$ and is defined by Eq. (5.6). The time-dependent volume fraction of the agent within the tissue sample f_a is proportional to its concentration C_a; thus, using the law of Gladstone and Dale [see Eq. (1.150)], we can write

$$n_0(t) = n_0(t) f_0(t) + n_a f_a(t),$$ (5.14)

where $f_0(t) + f_a(t) = 1$. For application of nonosmotic or low-osmotic agents, the initial refractive index of the interfibrillar space can be considered as being independent of time, $n_0(t) \cong n_0(t = 0)$.

The expression for the scattering coefficient, derived for a system of noninteracting thin cylinders with a number of fibrils per unit area ρ_s, has the form[172,1021]

$$\mu_s \cong \rho_s \left(\frac{\pi^5 a^4 n_0^3}{\lambda_0^3} \right)(m^2 - 1)^2 \left[1 + \frac{2}{(m^2 + 1)^2} \right], \qquad (5.15)$$

where $\rho_s = f_{cyl}/\pi a^2$, f_{cyl} is the surface fraction of the cylinders' faces, a is the cylinder radius, $m = n_s/n_0$ is the relative index of refraction of cylinders (scatterers) to the background (interfibrillar space), and λ_0 is the wavelength in vacuum.

As a first approximation, it is reasonable to assume that the radii of the scatterers (fibrils) and their density cannot be significantly changed by chemicals (no tissue swelling or shrinkage take place), the absolute changes of n_0 are not very high, and variations in μ_s are caused only by the change in the refractive index of the interstitial (interfibrillar) space in respect to the refractive index of the scatterers. Then, accounting for the fact that a majority of tissues has $m \approx 1$, the ratio of the scattering coefficients at a particular wavelength as a function of the refractive index ratio m can be written in the following form:[172,1021]

$$\mu_{s2} \cong \mu_{s1} \left(\frac{m_2 - 1}{m_1 - 1} \right)^2. \qquad (5.16)$$

Indeed, this relation describes tissue scattering properties' change due to refractive index match or mismatch caused by changes of refractive indices of the scatterers or the background, or both. The similar equation for Mie spherical particle systems follows from Eq. (2.24). Due to square dependence, the sensitivity to indices matching is very high, for instance, for $m_1 = 1.1$ and $m_2 = 1.01$, $\mu_{s2} \cong 0.01\mu_{s1}$.

For the immersion technique, the refractive index of the scatterers n_s is usually kept constant during tissue impregnation by an agent. Thus, we can use Eq. (5.14) to rewrite Eq. (5.16) in a form that is specific for the tissue impregnation by an agent with a weak osmotic strength as

$$\mu_s(t) = \mu_s(t = 0) \times \frac{\{[n_s/n_0(t)] - 1\}^2}{\{[n_s/n_0(t = 0)] - 1\}^2}. \qquad (5.17)$$

It should be noted that a more rigorous approach to calculating the scattering coefficient must be based on consideration of light scattering by densely packed systems of thin dielectric cylinders or spherical particles with a particular size distribution (see Chapters 1–3).

To estimate changes of tissue collimated transmittance caused by agent diffusion into a sample (see Fig. 5.2), Eqs. (5.1), (5.6), (5.14), and (5.17) should be used together. Usually, immersion agents do not have strong absorption bands within the

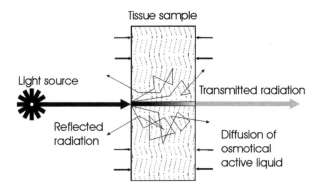

Figure 5.2 Schematic representation of the diffusion of the immersion agent into a tissue sample and light transmittance and scattering.[987]

wavelength range of interest; thus, the absorption coefficient often may be considered as a constant value. Indeed, the diffuse transmittance and reflectance as well as differential scattering characteristics (angular dependent scattering) for a tissue sample can be calculated if the behavior of the scattering anisotropy factor g at optical immersion is known. For Mie particles, the analysis of the g-factor behavior due to refractive index matching can be done using Eq. (1.195); corresponding calculations are presented in Figs. 1.54 and 1.55, and Eqs. (5.6), (5.14), and (5.17).

For *in vivo* studies, the back-reflectance geometry of the measurements is principle; thus, Eqs. (5.6), (5.14), and (5.17) should be used together with Eqs. (1.27) or (2.17), or their analogous equations received for the interacting particles (see Chapters 1–3).

5.2.2 Water transport

A water balance in living tissues is one of the important features of tissue condition. At tissue interaction with external or internal molecules' diffusion (proteins, sugars, alcohols, polymers, etc.), tissue water should be involved in molecular displacement processes.[172] Water may be transported through a membrane (a certain tissue layer) by an increased concentration of dissolved substance in one of two parts of the system. This happens for membranes more permeable for water than for dissolved material and is called osmosis.[1066] The simplest case of water transport is when a membrane is permeable for water and totally unpermeable for molecules of dissolved substances. However, in general, biological membranes are permeable for both water and dissolved substances, but the degree of permeability for them can be quite different. This is the most complicated case to describe, but the situation becomes simpler when water and dissolved substance permeate by the same paths inside a membrane [such as interfibrillar spaces (pores) in fibrous tissues, which are filled by the interstitial fluid containing water]. In that case, fluxes of water and dissolved substance interact and each flux is dependent on the degree of interaction. Such interaction between the stationary fluxes can be well described within the framework of irreversible thermodynamics.[1066]

Assuming that in a system there is only one type of dissolved molecule (i.e., two fluxes move through a membrane: the water flux J_W and a dissolved matter flux J_S, which are proportional to the gradients of the chemical potential of water and dissolved matter), we can find the volumetric flux defined as[1066]

$$J_V = J_W \overline{V}_W + J_S \overline{V}_S, \tag{5.18}$$

where $\overline{V}_W$ and $\overline{V}_S$ are the partial mole volumes, in the form

$$J_V = L_p(\Delta p - \sigma RT \Delta C_S). \tag{5.19}$$

The flux of dissolved matter can be expressed as[1066]

$$J_S = RT \omega \Delta C_S + \overline{C}_S(1 - \sigma)J_V. \tag{5.20}$$

Here, in Eqs. (5.19) and (5.20), L_p is the phenomenological coefficient indicating that the volumetric flux can be induced by rising hydrostatic pressure Δp; σ is the reflection coefficient [$\sigma = -(L_{pd}/L_p)$, where L_{pd} is the phenomenological coefficient indicating on the one hand that the volumetric flux that can be induced for the membrane by the osmotic pressure $RT \Delta C_S$, and on the other, the efficiency of the separation of water molecules and dissolved matter]; $\omega = (L_D - L_p\sigma^2)\overline{C}_S$, where L_D is the phenomenological coefficient characterizing the interchange flux induced by osmotic pressure $RT \Delta C_S$; and $\overline{C}_S$ is the average concentration of dissolved matter in two interacting solutions.

For the ideal partially permeable membrane, $\sigma = 1$. For membranes that are permeable for molecules of dissolved matter, $0 < \sigma < 1$. Equations (5.19) and (5.20) are valid for solutions with a low concentration. It should be noted that the volumetric flux for a partially permeable membrane described by Eq. (5.19) has the same mechanism of creation for both hydrostatic and osmotic pressure. So for porous (fibrous) materials (such as sclera, derma, muscle, *dura mater*), it is expected that osmotic pressure induces the flux of water due to increasing hydrostatic pressure, but not through independent diffusion of water molecules caused by their concentration gradient, because this entails considerably more resistance.

5.2.3 Tissue swelling and hydration

When applying a chemical agent, a change of environmental pH level is very important because swelling or shrinkage of tissue is expected.[1067] The swelling or shrinkage of a fibrous tissue is caused not only by the increase (decrease) of collagen (elastin) fibril size, but also by the increase (decrease) of the sample volume due to the rise (diminution) of the mean distance between fibrils. It is well known that the change of the environmental pH to the more acid or more alkaline side from a colloid isoelectric point increases the degree of swelling. It is explained by the appearance of a positive or negative charge of colloid particles and, therefore, by the increase of hydration degree. In general, the initial pH condition of the tissue under study and the acid or alkaline nature of the impregnated solution may lead to different dependencies of tissue thickness or volume on chemical agent concentration (or time of impregnation) due to changes of pH. Such behavior of a tissue sample should be taken into account when optical measurements are used for estimation of tissue properties. For example, the swelling or shrinkage was watched for different initial conditions of scleral tissue sample preparation and solutions used.[172,343,960,963,1022,1023]

A detailed study of the swelling of bovine sclera and cornea as a function of pH and ionic strength of the bathing medium, using an equilibration technique that prevents the loss of proteoglycans during swelling, is presented in Ref. 786. X-ray diffraction was used to measure the intermolecular spacings (IMS), fibril diameters and D-periodicity, and interfibrillar spacings (IFS) of collagen as functions of pH, ionic strength, and tissue hydration. Hydration H was defined as

$$H = \frac{\text{Weight}_{\text{wet}} - \text{Weight}_{\text{dry}}}{\text{Weight}_{\text{dry}}}. \tag{5.21}$$

It was found that both tissues swelled least near pH 4 (the isoelectric point), that higher hydrations were achieved at low ionic strengths, and that sclera swelled about one-third as much as cornea under most conditions. The IMS in both tissues decreased as the ionic strength was increased; for sclera, hydration $H \cong 2.5$ and pH 7.0 IMS changed from 1.71 to 1.61 nm at a 33-fold increase of ionic strength. The IMS has virtually no change on hydration when $H > 1$, $H = 3.2$ is physiological hydration; the corresponding mean value for the cornea was 1.75 ± 0.04 nm ($n = 12$), and for the sclera it was 1.65 ± 0.02 nm ($n = 9$) at pH 7.4. For dehydrated tissues ($H = 0$), the mean spacing was 1.25 ± 0.02 nm ($n = 2$) for the cornea and 1.27 ± 0.01 nm for the sclera.

The packing of fibrils, defined as IFS^2, is another important parameter, which determines control of tissue light scattering. For bovine cornea at physiological pH 7.4, the squared IFS decreased linearly from approximately 9.2×10^3 nm^2 for a highly hydrated tissue ($H = 9.7$) to approximately 2.1×10^3 nm^2 at tenfold less hydration, and was equal to 4.2×10^3 nm^2 at physiological hydration, $H = 3.2$. Both fibril diameters [mean value 39.0 ± 1.1 nm ($n = 6$)] and the D-periodicity [mean value 64.50 ± 0.35 nm ($n = 6$)] of corneal collagen were essentially independent of hydration and pH when hydration was above unity. This means that the fibrils preferentially absorb the initial water and then remain at a relatively constant diameter. The remaining unchanged value of the D-periodicity with hydration indicates no significant changes in the dimensions along the axis of the fibrils during swelling. The same tendencies are expected for sclera as a collagen-based media. The volume of a tissue at a given hydration may be expressed in terms of the dry volume. The corresponding expression that describes the volume of the cornea at its hydration can be written as[786]

$$V_H = V_T(1 + 1.066H). \tag{5.22}$$

This equation should apply equally to any volume of the tissue, i.e., to the volume associated with each fibril.

The swelling of scleral tissue follows similar principles as for cornea with the same isoelectrical point around pH 4, but at a lower level of swelling. As it was noted in Ref. 786, there are several reasons for the low hydrations of the sclera: the low concentration of proteoglycans; a high collagen content and larger fibrils with a smaller combined surface area than in the cornea; and structural peculiarities connected with the fibrils arranged in bands, which may branch and interweave with each other.

It was found by the authors of Ref. 786 that the high light scattering (low transmittance) of bovine cornea increased more rapidly with hydration (even below physiological hydrations) at pH values around the isoelectric point. For example, at pH 5, transmittance was approximately 98% for $H = 2$, 87% for $H = 3.2$, and only 12% for $H = 6$. In contrast, the light scattering at higher pH values (6–8) changed slowly with hydration: transmittance was higher than 90% for each level of hydration from 1 to 7 with the local maximum of transmittance of 98% for $H = 4$. According to current models, discussed in detail in Chapter 2, corneal transparency at a given wavelength depends on certain structural parameters such as fibril diameters, the density of fibril packing, the position of each fibril relative to its neighbors, and the refractive indices of the collagen and the interfibrillar matrix, and changes in one or more of these parameters may be sufficient to decrease or increase light scattering.

From these studies, it follows that to improve corneal transparency caused by stromal edema, hypertonic drops extracting enough water from tissue may be used. As it was shown in Ref. 786, sodium chloride could be better than other hypertonic preparations for the treatment of corneal edema because it may also reduce the swelling pressure in the stroma and decrease the fibril diameter if used frequently.

The connection between the hydration H (milligrams water per milligrams dry tissue weight) and corneal thickness d (in millimeters) is described by the following empirical formulas:[772,1024,1025]

for rabbit cornea

$$H = 10d - 0.42, \tag{5.23}$$

and for bovine cornea

$$H = 5.3d - 0.67. \tag{5.24}$$

5.3 Optical clearing of fibrous tissues

5.3.1 Spectral properties of immersed sclera

Normally, eye sclera (see Section 3.1 and Fig. 3.20) is a turbid medium that is nontransparent in the visible range.[722,723] The origin of scleral spectra formation can be understood on the basis of light scattering by a system of polydispersive irregularly arranged collagen cylinders immersed in the ground substance with a lower refractive index (see Chapter 3)[798] and strong absorption bands.[722,723,788] With a natural thickness of 0.6–0.8 mm, this tissue shows multiple scattering and looks like white matter. The transition from a multiple to a low-step/single scattering can be provided by the drying of a tissue sample[722,723] [Fig. 3.20(c)] or its impregnation by an immersion liquid.[172,788,798,1021]

Figure 5.1 is a schematic representation of the human scleral sample structure and geometry of light irradiation. Analytical approaches for describing the propagation of light in the sclera are valid only when strongly simplifying assumptions are used, which make the model substantially less adequate. Thus, the direct simulation of photon migration in a medium using a Monte Carlo simulation was used for calculating spectral characteristics and photon statistics.[172,798] The Monte Carlo simulation of the sclera transmission and reflection spectra was carried out using the probability function for the free photon path l (see Section 1.1.3). The ordering of scatterers (thin dielectric cylinders) was taken into account, using the experimental radial distribution function $g(r)$ obtained from electron micrographs of the human sclera [762,798] (Fig. 3.5). It was assumed that the ordering affects only each individual event of the interaction between a photon and a particle. As the angular dependence of the scattered light intensity by a particle it was taken the scattering indicatrix for a fiber with a diameter corresponding to the modal value of the size distribution, 120 nm. The effect of the multiple scattering is included automatically in the procedure of simulation of the photon path by the Monte Carlo method, in that part of simulations the spatial distribution of scattering centers being assumed completely arbitrary. This approximation is valid if the dimension of the region of local ordering of scattering particles is far smaller than the mean free path of a photon in the medium, which takes place for the sclera.

The results of such modeling for a scleral sample (1-mm thickness, 120-nm mean fibril diameter, and 285-nm mean separation between collagen fibrils; their refractive index $n_c = 1.474$; and initial refractive index of interfibrillar space $n_0 = 1.345$) are presented in Figs. 5.3–5.6. The collimated transmittance represents a fraction of photons leaving a tissue layer in the direction that differs from the direction of the incident radiation no more than by ± 0.5 deg, which corresponds to their entering into the aperture of a spectrometer. Total transmittance and diffuse reflectance spectra accounting for a real geometry (losing of some amount of the scattered light) of the integrating spheres used in experiments were also calculated. The calculations were performed for different values of the refractive index of the background substance, from 1.345 to 1.450, corresponding to different levels of indices matching. It is clearly seen that the model describes the major features of normal and immersed tissue spectra in the visible range. A comparison of calculated and experimental spectra (see Fig. 5.7) shows that refractive index matching can be considered as the main mechanism responsible for tissue-enhanced translucence.

The Monte Carlo simulation technique allows one to describe the transition of the tissue scattering mode from complete diffusion to a coherent (ballistic photons

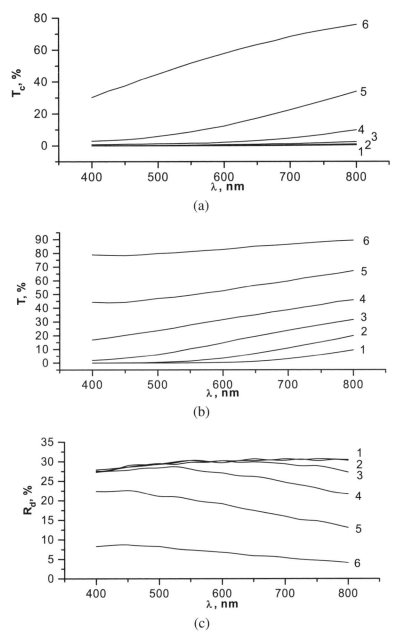

Figure 5.3 Collimated (a) and total (b) transmittance spectra as well as diffuse reflectance (c) spectra of human sclera of 1-mm thickness calculated by the Monte Carlo method for different refractive indices matching with a geometry very close to the experimental one (see Fig. 5.7); refractive index of collagen fibrils $n_c = 1.47$ and interfibrillar material $n_0 = 1.35$, 1.37, 1.39, 1.41, 1.43, and 1.45.[439,798]

dominate) caused by refractive index matching. Such transition is well illustrated by the histograms in Figs. 5.4–5.6. The numbers of back- and forward-scattered photons collected by integrating spheres were calculated. These histograms show

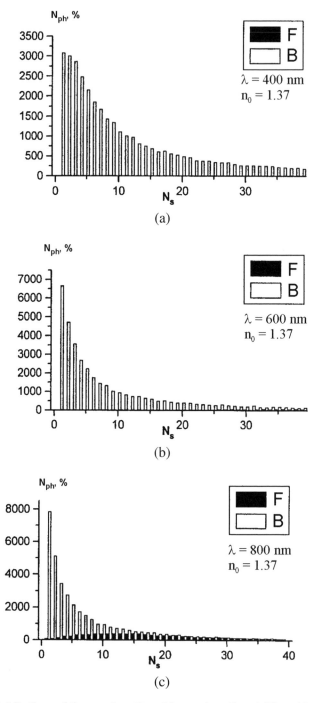

Figure 5.4 Distributions of the number N_{ph} of forward-scattered (F) and backscattered (B) photons calculated by the Monte Carlo method that undertake a definite number of collisions N_s before escaping a human scleral slab of 1-mm thickness (two integrating sphere geometry) for slightly matched refractive indices of collagen fibrils and interfibrillar material ($n_c = 1.474$, $n_0 = 1.370$): (a) $\lambda = 400$ nm; (b) $\lambda = 600$ nm; (c) $\lambda = 800$ nm.[439,798]

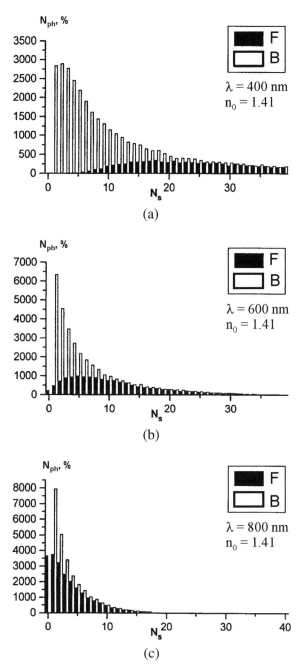

Figure 5.5 Distributions of the number N_{ph} of forward-scattered (F) and backscattered (B) photons calculated by the Monte Carlo method that undertake a definite number of collisions N_s before escaping a human scleral slab of 1-mm thickness (two integrating sphere geometry) for partly matched (midlevel) refractive indices of collagen fibrils and interfibrillar material ($n_c = 1.474$, $n_0 = 1.410$): (a) $\lambda = 400$ nm; (b) $\lambda = 600$ nm; (c) $\lambda = 800$ nm.[439,798]

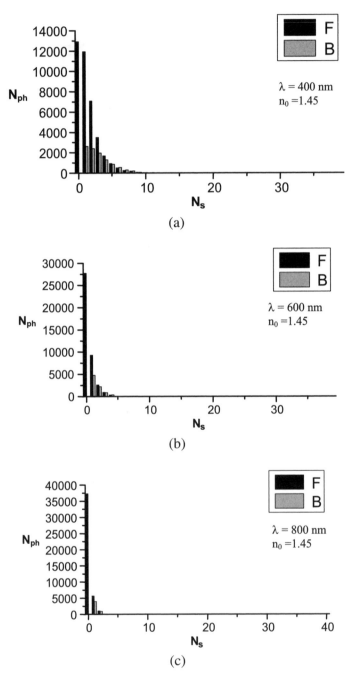

Figure 5.6 Distributions of the number N_{ph} of forward-scattered (F) and backscattered (B) photons calculated by the Monte Carlo method that undertake a definite number of collisions N_s before escaping a human scleral slab of 1-mm thickness (two integrating sphere geometry) for strongly matched refractive indices of collagen fibrils and interfibrillar material ($n_c = 1.474$, $n_0 = 1.450$): (a) $\lambda = 400$ nm; (b) $\lambda = 600$ nm; (c) $\lambda = 800$ nm.[439,798]

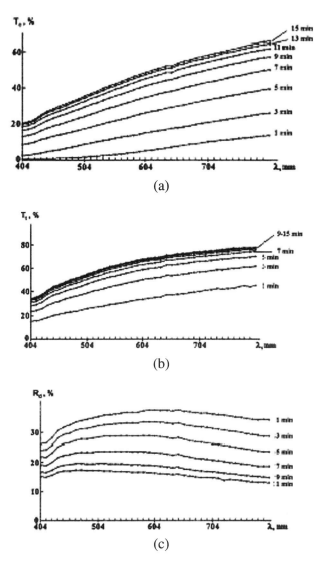

(a)

(b)

(c)

Figure 5.7 Experimental spectra of human scleral samples measured for different time intervals of administration of trazograph-60. Spectra were measured 1 min after the sample was immersed in solution and then at 2-min intervals. The measurement time for an individual spectrum, scanning from higher to lower wavelengths, was about 85 s. (a) Collimated transmittance T_c; sample thickness, 0.6 mm. (b) Total transmittance T_t; sample thickness, 0.7 mm. (c) Diffusion reflection R_d; sample thickness, 0.7 mm (heavily pigmented tissue).[172,1021]

that for sclera with unmatched or slightly matched refractive indices ($n_0 = 1.370$), there is a broad distribution of the number of scattering events (with the mean value of 25–30 collisions for the NIR region) that forward-traveling photons undergo; no ballistic photons (the coherent part of transmitted light) are seen. For fairly matched refractive indices, there are ballistic photons that come into being. In particular, for moderately matched refractive indices ($n_0 = 1.410$), the unscattered and low-step scattered photons dominate in both directions, forward and back, with the mean number of collisions for the forward-traveling NIR photons of 3–4 and a rather big ballistic component. For strongly matched indices ($n_0 = 1.450$), the ballistic component dominates and both scattering components in the forward and backward directions are small. In the NIR region, the optical clearing of tissue and transformation of scattering mode from multiple to low or even single steps begins much earlier than for visible light. A strong ballistic component formed at tissue clearing gives perspectives to coherent-domain diagnostic methods to be more widely used in biomedicine.

The total transmittance, diffuse reflectance, and collimated transmittance were measured in the 200–2200-nm wavelength range using a commercially available Varian Cary 5E, 500, or 2415 spectrophotometers with an internal integrating sphere.[172,571,971,972,1021] To reconstruct the absorption and reduced scattering coefficients of a tissue from such measurements, the inverse adding-doubling (IAD) method[680] or inverse Monte Carlo (IMC) method was applied.[960]

For *in vitro*, and especially *in vivo*, studies of tissue optical clearing, fiber-optic grating-array spectrometers such as the LESA-5, 6, and 7 (BioSpec, Russia), and the PC1000, PC2000, and USB2000 (Ocean Optics Inc., USA) are suitable due to their fast spectra collection in a course of immersion agent action.[575,704,960,965,978,980,986,987,831,1031,1034] Typically, the spectral range of interest is from 400 to 1000 nm and the spectrometer fiber probe consists of seven optical fibers. One fiber transmits light to the object and six fibers collect the reflected radiation. The mean distance between the irradiating and receiving fibers is about 200 µm for the PC1000 and LESA-6, and about 2 mm for the LESA-5. The spectrometers are calibrated using white slab of $BaSO_4$ with a smooth surface.

Spectra were measured *in vitro* with human sclera samples.[172,1021] The sclera was carefully purified from ciliary body and retina, washed, and cut into pieces of area 10×10 mm. The sclera sample was placed into a cell of volume 1 ml filled with osmotic liquid or physiological solution. Three different types of chemical agents were used for scleral optical clearing in Refs. 172 and 1021. The main parts of the experiments were performed using the x-ray contrast agent trazograph (a derivative of 2,4,6-triiodobenzene acid) with a molecular weight of about 500; 60% and 76% solutions in water. Some measurements were performed for two OCAs with quite different molecular weights, such as glucose (~180) and PEG (6000 or 20,000). At room temperature and measured by the Abbe refractometer, refractive indices of some of the used agents were the following: trazograpth-60, $n = 1.437$; trazograph-76, $n = 1.460$; PEG (6000) solutions, $n = 1.368$ (0.4 g/ml), 1.394 (0.6 g/ml), 1.403 (0.8 g/ml), and 1.469 (1.0 g/ml); glucose solutions, $n = 1.363$ (0.2 g/ml), 1.378 (0.3 g/ml), 1.391 (0.4 g/ml), and 1.415 (0.54 g/ml). For the glucose-water solutions, the refractive index at any wavelength in the visible and NIR regions, where glucose has no strong absorption bands, can be estimated using Eqs. (1.202) and (2.36).

The typical transmission spectra $T_c(\lambda)$ and $T_t(\lambda)$, and diffusion reflection spectra $R_d(\lambda)$ measured by the integrating sphere spectrophotometer for different time intervals of trazograph-60 administration, are presented in Fig. 5.7.[172,1021] It is easily seen that the untreated sclera is poorly transparent for visible and NIR light. Trazograph administration makes this tissue highly transparent—up to 70–75% at 600–800 nm for the sample kept in solution for 7–10 min. In addition, its spectral reflectivity decreased from 35–40% to 13–15% in this wavelength range.

In general, for many of measured samples, it can be concluded that for untreated scleral samples transmittance was less than 1–2% in the range of 400 to 500 nm and increased up to 6–30% for NIR wavelengths, depending on the sample thickness and pigmentation. Trazograph or other agent administration not only leads to increased transmittance but changes the form of the spectral curve: on average, for the short wavelengths, collimated transmittance increased from 1–2 to 20% (10–20 times) and for the long wavelengths from 20–30 to 50–80% (~2.5 times).

For optically cleared sclera, the collimated light makes the main contribution to transmittance. Direct measurements performed for a scleral sample of 0.75-mm thickness treated with trazograph-60 for 40 min showed that transmittance for the detector acceptance angle of 30 deg $T_{30} \cong 35\%$ at 400 nm and $\cong 85\%$ at 840 nm, $T_c \cong 27\%$ at 400 nm and $\cong 85\%$ at 840 nm. It also follows from the CCD image of a laser beam transmitted through the sclera at different levels of optical clearing (see Fig. 5.8), that showing the process of formation of a ballistic group of photons (see the center of the pattern) at reduction of scattering multiplicity. These images also qualitatively support the calculated statistics of photon interactions at tissue clearing (Figs. 5.4–5.6).

The efficiency of tissue clearing depends on the concentration and temperature of the solutions used. For bovine sclera at room temperature (18.5°C), the maximum collimated transmittance at 450 nm is in the range $T_{c\,max} = 13\%$ (trazograph-60), 22% (glucose, 45%), 39% (trazograph-76), and 46% [(PEG (6000), 80%]; and at 700 nm $T_{c\,max} = 73\%$ (glucose, 45%), 76% (trazograph-60), and 99% [trazograph-76 and PEGs (6000 and 20,000), 80%].[1028] The maximal transmittance is achieved at 15–30 min. At physiological temperature, this time interval is considerably shortened. For example, for a PEG 20,000 solution (80%), the time interval for maximal tissue clearing changed from 27 min at 18.5°C to 12 min at 38°C.

The time-dependent collimated transmittance of scleral sample measured at 633 nm concurrently with trazograph-60 administration is presented in Fig. 5.9. It shows the dynamics of tissue clearing. Similar characteristics were measured for glucose and PEG administration. The registration of the dynamic response of the intensity of transmission can be used to estimate diffusion coefficients of the interacting fluids: water and agent (trazograph, glucose, glycerol, PEG, etc.). Based on the theoretical background given earlier, we can estimate the coefficient of diffusion of the agent assuming that water and agent have the same paths for diffusion. The following set of equations gives the simple algorithm for diffusion coefficient determination: Eqs. (5.1), (5.4), (5.6), (5.14), and (5.17). More sophisticated algorithms accounting for tissue swelling and shrinkage and appropriate to the measuring procedure of inverse optical problem solving (IAD, IMC) are also available.[960,986,987,1020,1022]

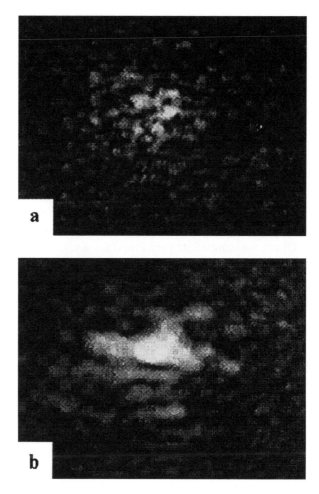

Figure 5.8 Specklegrams recorded at two different moments of time in the far-field zone for a sample of translucent human eye sclera irradiated with a focused beam of an He:Ne laser (633 nm). Enhanced translucence was provided by trazograph-60 in a cuvette during (a) 2.5 and (b) 10 min.[343]

Data for the diffusion coefficient values of different samples of human sclera are collected in Table 2 of Ref. 949. The estimated values of D_T calculated using about 30 magnitudes of T_c measured for different time intervals for each sample have quite reasonable rms errors and differences in mean values from sample to sample. As can be seen from Fig. 5.9, the rms values include the low-frequency oscillations of $T_c(t)$, which can be caused by spatial-temporal fluctuations of the agent diffusivity at interacting with tissue structure. On average, the D_T values are not far from the values of D_a for diffusion of low-weight molecules in water.[1066]

It should be noted that for the hyperosmotic agents, fluid transport within tissue is more complicated because there are at least two interacting fluxes, so the model for describing these processes should be more complicated and should include monitoring additional measurement parameters such as the refractive index of the

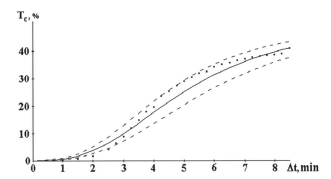

Figure 5.9 The time-dependent collimated transmittance (dots) of a 0.5-mm-thick scleral sample measured at 633 nm concurrently with the administration of trazograph-60.[172] The solid and dashed lines represent the mean value and the upper and lower limits of T_c obtained by a calculation of T_c using experimental data: $D_T = (1.46 \pm 0.19) \times 10^{-5}$ cm^2/s.

chemical agent, tissue weight and/or thickness, and osmotic pressure in a process of tissue clearing. Such monitoring of the refractive index of a trazograph-60 in a bath during a process of scleral clearing gave 1.4370 ($t = 0$), 1.4321 (12 min), 1.4222 (20 min), and 1.4025 (40 min). Measurements of tissue samples' weights before and after administration of the agents gave the following values: trazograph-60 (sample 5 × 8 × 0.6 mm), 54 mg ($t = 0$) and 51 mg (34 min); glucose (40%, pH 3.5) (sample 10 × 11 × 0.5 mm), 82 mg ($t = 0$) and 66 mg (20 min); and PEG (6000) (1 g/ml) (sample 8 × 10 × 0.5 mm), 65 mg ($t = 0$) and 48 mg (60 min). Thus, the relative decrease of the sample weight is: 5.5% for trazograph-60, 15.5% for 40%-glucose, and 28% for PEG (6000). Both experiments with refractive index and weighting show differences in osmotic properties of the used agents and their tissue dehydration abilities, which are in the range: low (trazograph-60), midlevel (40%-glucose), and high [PEG (6000)]. It follows from the experiment that in optical clearing of the sclera, trazograth-60 dominates the process of the replacement of the interfibrillar fluid (mostly water) by trazograph-60, which has a refractive index higher than water. The rather large reduction of refractive index in the bath with the sample means that water effectively escapes tissue and small loss of sample weight indicates that water is replaced by trazograph-60. Thus, we may assume that in the system there are two approximately equal fluxes moving through a tissue layer: the water flux J_W directed out of a layer and a dissolved matter flux J_S into a layer, which are proportional to the gradients of the chemical potential of water and dissolved matter [see Eq. (5.19)].[1066] For glucose, and especially for PEG, dehydration plays an important role due to the unequality of two fluxes: the water flux J_W out of a tissue layer is stronger than a dissolved matter flux J_S into a layer. Thus, structural changes of collagen fibrils and interfibrillar spacings caused by tissue dehydration and described in Section 5.2.3[786] should be accounted for in the tissue-clearing model based on tissue dehydration.

The interaction of the OCA penetrated inside a tissue with collagen fibrils may be responsible for a quasi-periodic low-frequency (3–4 min of period) oscillations of the light transmittance that are well seen in Fig. 5.9. The oscillating character of tissue response may be explained as a multistep origin of fluid diffusion.[172,343] The first step, OCA penetration into the tissue, leads to refractive index matching of interstitial fluid and hydrated fibril collagen—the significant translucence of tissue growth. The second step is characterized by the interaction of the OCA, contained within the renovated interfibrillar liquid with fibril collagen, which leads to collagen dehydration and consequent growth of its refractive index that slightly breaks down optical matching and causes a slight decrease of transmittance. The subsequent imbalance of water-OCA concentrations leads in turn to penetration of an additional amount of OCA into the sample, which causes reestablishment of the refractive index matching and a corresponding light transmittance—this is the origin of the third step. The inertia of each of the considered processes may cause the establishing of a quasi-periodic oscillation with the period and amplitude, depending on parameters of the nonlinear system. Rather regular oscillations of OCT image depth of hamster and rat skin with the period close to 2.5 and 3.5 min, respectively, was also found at tissue immersion by glycerol.[1059]

Measured values of osmotic pressure for trazograph-60 were equal to 4.3 MPa, and 7.1 MPa for trazograph-76.[172] For untreated sclera, the value of osmotic pressure was equal to 0.74 MPa, and it increased after administration of trazograpth-60 for 30 min—up to 5.02 MPa. On one hand, the osmotic pressure causes the flows generation and their intensities [see Section 5.2.2 and Eqs. (5.19) and (5.20)]; but on the other hand, rather strong osmotic pressure may destroy tissue structure. A direct histological study showed that there were no serious irreversible changes in the cellular and fibrous structure of human sclera for a rather long period of OCA administration.[1029] For example, for a trazograph-60, the time is at least about 30 min, and rather minor changes of tissue structure, which are characterized by a moderate tissue swelling, were seen.

The reversibility of tissue structure change at an OCA administration is also demonstrated by the data in Fig. 5.10,[343,1030] which show that the multiple-single scattering transition (i.e., optical translucence, improvement of linear polarization) is reversible when the OCA bath is replaced by a physiological solution and vice versa when the OCA is administrated again.

The theoretical and experimental results show that administration of OCAs to the sclera affects the refractive index matching of the collagen fibrils and interfibrillar fluid, leading to dramatic changes (a reduction) in the scattering properties of the sclera. For different OCAs, refractive index matching can be implemented in different ways: (1) water can leave the interfibrillar space and exit the sample (dehydration); (2) the administered fluid can enter the tissue and fill up the interfibrillar space, and water can partly leave the interfibrillar space and partly exit the sample. The first mechanism is characteristic only for highly hyperosmotic agents. For fibrous tissue similar to sclera, the second mechanism is preferable for all tested chemical agents because their molecule sizes are much less than the mean cross section of interfibrillar space, which is about 185 nm, whereas the diameter of the biggest molecule of PEG (20,000) should be less than 5 nm. Indeed, the

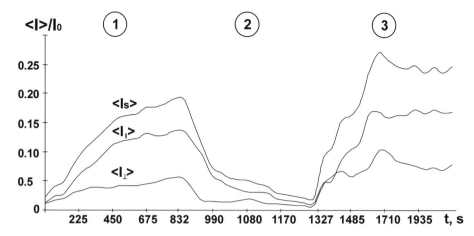

Figure 5.10 Temporal dependencies for the values of mean speckle intensity $\langle I_s \rangle$ and its polarization components $\langle I_\perp \rangle$ and $\langle I_\parallel \rangle$ measured in the paraxial region of a sample of human sclera with a thickness of 0.4 mm and averaged over the scanning trajectory (1.5 mm): 1, 2, 3, sequential measurements with a sample that was first placed in trazograph-60, then in physiological solution (0.9% NaCl), and then again in trazograph-60; $\lambda = 633$ nm.[1030]

structure of the interfibrillar matrix and molecular structural properties may also have their influence on diffusion; thus, the diffusivity of foreign molecules and the corresponding strength of the water flux is different for the various agents used. A stronger water flux in the sclera was induced by PEGs, a midlevel one by 40%-glucose, and a small one by trazograph-60 (see weight measurements).[172]

The dynamics of tissue optical clearing using OCA is defined by a characteristic time response of about 3 to 10 min. This is in good agreement with results obtained by Rol,[723] but he used a pointwise mechanical stress or local heating induced by a laser beam. Actually, as follows from Eq. (5.19), osmotic pressure and hydrostatic pressure caused, for example, by mechanical stress, have the same mechanism for inducing the fluid flux, and the time response is defined by water diffusion through the interfibrillar space. Therefore, optical clearing using local mechanical stress should be somewhat equivalent to the action of a hyperosmotic agent because a local stress picks up water from the compressed site and diminishes the tissue layer thickness. In practice, optical clearing with OCAs may be preferable over a mechanical stress because there are more possibilities to control the time/spatial response and efficiency using various chemical agents; in addition, the function of these agents may be combined (tissue optical clearing and treatment).

These results are general and can be used to describe many other fibrous tissues. It should be noted that human sclera can be considered a living scattering etalon in the visible range, like a white glass (see diffuse reflectance spectra in Fig. 5.7). For example, due to the simpler structure and stable and controllable parameters of sclera in comparison with skin, light-scattering technologies of glucose monitoring designed for skin measurements[339–341,534,549–551] may be more effective in the application to sclera. In this connection, it is interesting to analyze a change in the sclera color during its clarification.[410,798] The quantitative estimation of this change from transmission and reflection spectra in Fig. 5.7 was done by calculating the chromaticity coordinates for the CIE 1964 color system. From the calculated color triangles follows that the native sclera has a reddish tint in the transmitted light; however, this does not appreciably change the visual perception because of a very low transmission coefficient. During sclera clarification, its color becomes whiter. In diffuse reflectance, the native sclera is white, as is visually observed. Upon clarification, the sclera color in the reflected light slightly shifts from white to bluish.

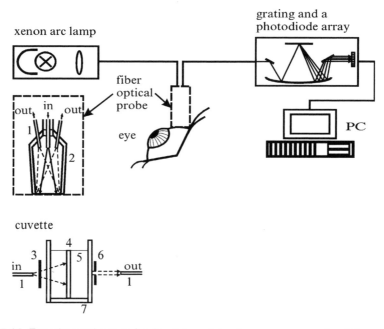

Figure 5.11 Experimental setup for *in vitro* and *in vivo* measurements of the collimated light transmittance and the reflectance spectra.[960] *In vitro* measurements: 1, optical fiber; 2, aluminum jacket; 3, neutral filters; 4, sclera sample; 5, OCA; 6, 0.5 mm pinhole; 7, cuvette.

To study more precisely the time-dependent transmittance and reflectance of a tissue, a fiber-optic photodiode array or CCD spectrometer that provides a fast collection of spectra should be used. This is especially important for diffusion coefficient determination in *in vitro* studies and in *in vivo* monitoring of tissue clarification. A fiber-optic photodiode array spectrometer, as shown in Fig. 5.11, detailed *in vitro* measurements for human sclera at tissue impregnation by various solutions such as glucose, trazograph, verografin, and propylene glycol, which do not have strong absorbing bands within the spectral range of interest, 400–800 nm.[986] In the *in vitro* study, the conjunctiva and ciliary body, as well as the retina with choroid were removed. The mean thickness of samples was about 0.5 mm. They were fixed on a plastic plate with a square aperture 5 × 5 mm (effective impregnation by a chemical agent via both surfaces of the sample was provided) and placed in a 5-ml cuvette filled with the solution under study.

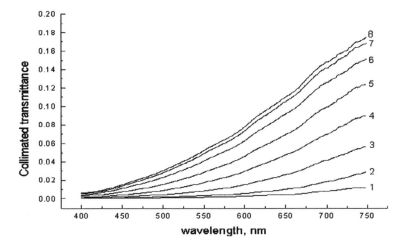

Figure 5.12 The time-dependent collimated transmittance spectra of a human sclera sample impregnated by 40%-glucose: (1) 10 sec; (2) 1 min; (3) 2 min; (4) 3 min; (5) 4 min; (6) 5 min; (7) 6.5 min; and (8) 8.5 min after the scleral sample was immersed in 40%-glucose.[960]

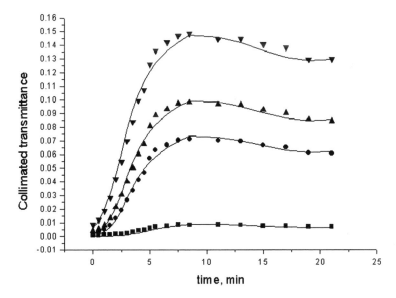

Figure 5.13 The time-dependent collimated transmittance of a human sclera sample measured at 420 nm (squares); 589 nm (circles); 630 nm (up triangles); and 700 nm (down triangles) concurrently with administration of 40%-glucose.[960]

To understand the mechanisms of scleral tissue optical clearing, the collimated transmittance spectra and change of the scleral sample weight were measured concurrently with the administration of glucose solution. Figures 5.12, 5.13, and 5.14 illustrate the dynamics of the transmittance spectra and typical weight change. It is easily seen that the untreated sclera is a poorly transparent media for the visible

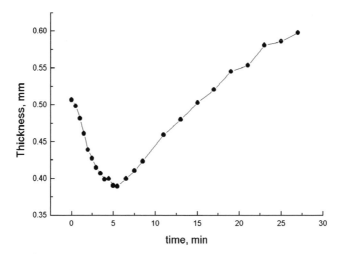

Figure 5.14 The calculated time-dependent thickness of a human sclera sample (Monte Carlo simulation as the best fit to the experimental data for the collimated transmittance shown in Figs. 5.12 and 5.13).[703]

light. Glucose administration makes this tissue highly transparent. As it follows from Fig. 5.13, the characteristic time response of sclera optical clearing is about 5 min.

Based on these measurements and accounting for the fact that a commercially available 40%-glucose from the drug store, which has a low pH of 3.5, was used, the following model of action of an osmotically active liquid on a fibrous tissue seems to be adequate. At the first stage, which takes place approximately 5 min after a sample is placed in glucose solution, the substantial optical clearing was accompanied by the sample thickness decrease. Thus, we may suppose that optical clearing occurs due to two main mechanisms: (1) refractive index matching between collagen fibers and penetrated glucose, and (2) glucose osmotic action that dehydrates tissue, resulting in up to 25% decrease of thickness. In the late stage of glucose administration, to the seventh minute, the optical clearing process saturates due to equilibration of fluid (glucose, water, proteins, salts, etc.) concentrations in the system and the thickness increases somewhat. From the seventh to the fifteenth minute, the inclusion of the thickness change (increase to its initial thickness) in optical clearing is well seen on the background of the inclusion of the saturated molecular fluxes—collimated transmittance is slightly reduced, but is still very high. The further tissue swelling with time up to 20% of the initial thickness to the twenty-first minute does not seriously influence tissue transmittance. It is important that in spite of the complex behavior of tissue thickness at administration of this specific chemical agent (40%-glucose with pH 3.5), thickness variations do not strongly affect the optical clearing. Such nonmonotonous behavior of tissue thickness (first shrinkage and later swelling) can be explained using the results of Ref. 786, where it was experimentally shown that for bovine sclera, hydration (swelling) may change from $H = 2.48$ for pH 7, close to physiological, to $H = 7.15$ for pH 3. In our case, this means that at the first stage when the tissue pH, which is close to the physiological one, is not seriously affected by glucose (a small amount penetrated into the sclera), the dehydration of tissue dominates due to osmotic action of glucose; but in the late stages of glucose administration, due to a large amount of glucose penetrating and in the bath, the pH of the whole system (tissue/glucose bath) is reducing and swelling takes place.

It should be stressed again that the discussed effects with tissue shrinkage and swelling are important but do not dominate at glucose action; thus, the experimental data for the collimated transmittance (Figs. 5.12 and 5.13) and the time-dependent measurements of tissue sample thickness changes under OCA action (Fig. 5.14) can be used to estimate the glucose diffusion coefficient in sclera.[442,703] The detailed model of glucose transport in fibrous tissue is described in Ref. 987. Equations (5.1), (5.6), (5.14), and (5.17) are the basis for this model, which can be used for reconstruction of the diffusion constant. The estimated average value of the diffusion coefficient of 40%-glucose transport in the scleral sample is $D_G = (3.45 \pm 0.46) \times 10^{-6}$ cm^2 s^{-1} at a temperature of 20°C. This value is not far from the values of D_a for diffusion of low-weight molecules (such as sucrose, glucose, etc.) in water at zero concentration $(3.6\text{--}5.2) \times 10^{-6}$ cm^2 s^{-1} at 12–15°C.[1066,1068,1069] When hyperosmotic agents are used, the diffusion coefficient should be close to that of water diffusion in a tissue because this is the main flux in the system. Depending on the tissue structure, this value should be equal to or above the value of the diffusion coefficient of water in water, $D_W = 2.5 \times 10^{-5}$ cm^2 s^{-1}.

The diffusion coefficient is a function of the dimension and form of the diffusing molecule,[1066]

$$D_a = \text{const} \times M^{-S}. \tag{5.25}$$

For small molecules, $S = 1/2$, and for spherical molecules diffusing in water (large proteins), $S = 1/3$. In general, the parameter S for diffusion in water is in the range 0.3–0.5, and for diffusion through a biological membrane, it is about 3.5. For example, changing of the molecule weight M from 45 to 122 at diffusion in water changes the diffusion coefficient from 1.6×10^{-5} cm^2 s^{-1} to 0.8×10^{-5} cm^2 s^{-1} (twofold); and for the same molecules' diffusion through the plasmatic membrane, from 1.4×10^{-8} cm^2 s^{-1} to 2.0×10^{-10} cm^2 s^{-1} (70-fold).[1066]

5.3.2 Scleral *in vitro* frequency-domain measurements

The dynamic response of optical properties (modulation depth and phase shift of intensity modulation of the backscattered light) of human eye sclera in respect to the interval of an OCA administration can be measured using a photon-density wave (frequency-domain) technique.[961] When the intensity of the light source is modulated at a frequency ω, a photon-density wave is induced in a scattering medium as[1-4,129]

$$A(r) = A_{dc} + A_{ac} \exp[-i(\omega t - \theta)], \qquad (5.26)$$

where A_{dc}, A_{ac}, and $(\omega t - \theta)$ are the dc and ac components of the amplitude of the photon-density wave and its phase, respectively.

Photon-diffusion theory provides independent determination of the absorption and reduced scattering coefficients from the measurements at a single modulation frequency. The expressions for the measured quantities phase delay θ and ac amplitude A_{ac} have been presented elsewhere[1-4,129] (see Sections 1.3 and 7.2). These expressions depend on the source-detector separation r_{sd}, reduced scattering coefficient μ_s', and absorption coefficients μ_a.

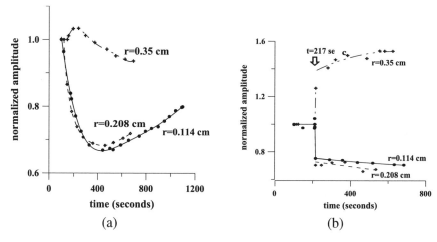

Figure 5.15 Frequency-domain measurements. The time-dependent changes in the amplitude of an optical signal from a human eyeball *in situ* after (a) trazograph-60 injection and (b) trazograph-60 drops in the vicinity of the detector fiber tip.[961]

Data shown in Fig. 5.15 are the temporal changes of ac amplitude during trazograph-60 administration for three different source-detector separations and two different techniques of immersion solution administration, by injection and by drops. The intensity and phase of photon-density waves generated by the NIR optical source were measured at several source-detector separations. The light source was a laser diode with a wavelength of 786 nm and 4-mW power at the end of a coupled multimode fiber (core diameter of 62.5 μm).[961] The intensity modulation depth of approximately 80% at a frequency of 140 MHz was provided by modulation of the injection current of the laser diode. The experimental setup was designed at the University of Pennsylvania. A multifiber detection system with small source-detector separations together with a Dicon multichannel fiber-optic switcher was used for the immersion experiment on human sclera *in situ* for a whole eyeball. The clearing of scleral tissue was observed during the first 3 min of trazograph-60 administration by injection. For small source-detector separations (about 1–2 mm) and a relatively large one (3.5 mm), the temporal dependencies are quite different. Keeping in mind that in the first 3 min after injection of the OCA the positive time scale corresponds to a decrease of scattering due to tissue immersion, the opposite tendencies of considered dependencies can be understood as follows. For the small source-detector separation close to the back-reflectance geometry, the intensity of reflected light decreases along with scattering decrease; and for rather large separations, where lateral photon diffusion effects are important, the intensity at first goes up with decreased scattering, but if scattering continues to decrease, intensity will lessen. That is why a local maximum on a curve for a separation of 3.5 mm was observed. At the third minute after OCA injection, due to its diffusion into neighboring tissue regions, amplitudes for all separations have a tendency to go to the initial values. Another technique of OCA administration by drops shows the same tendencies for small and large separations as for injection, but essential changes of the amplitudes happen momentarily after chemical agent drops are applied, and then amplitudes slowly change in opposite directions. Such behavior depends on the specific features of an OCA application, which are (1) superficial impregnation (underlines the importance of surface immersion effect) and (2) continuous renovation of the OCA on the tissue surface (many drops during the measurement interval).

This study, which was performed under circumstances that are very close to *in vivo* measurements, also shows that the impregnation of eye sclera by a hyperosmotic OCA affects the reversible refractive indices matching the collagen fibrils and interstitial media that leads to dramatic reduction of the tissue scattering ability, up to 60% in ac signal change for 10–12 min at trazograph-60 application.

5.3.3 Scleral *in vivo* measurements

In vivo measurements were done for rabbit eye using the experimental setup presented in Fig. 5.11. Experimental spectra and dynamic response on selected wavelengths are shown in Figs. 5.16 and 5.17. The surface temperature of the rabbit eye was ~38°C. 40%-glucose was used as a chemical agent for the scleral optical clearing, administered in the form of eye drops. A significant decrease of the reflectance during the first 5 min of glucose administration is seen. Dips appearing at 420, 530, and 570 nm are caused by blood perfusion. The lower reflectance at 420 nm is caused by the strong absorption of blood. Evidently, faster decay at this wavelength reflects blood perfusion dynamics due to eye conjuctiva and sclera inflammation induced by light irradiation and the osmotic action of glucose. Because blood absorption has less influence at 630 to 700 nm, measured dynamic responses can be used for *in vivo* estimation of diffusion coefficient for glucose in scleral tissue.

From the experimental data presented in Figs. 5.16 and 5.17, one can see that for *in vivo* measurements reflectance decreases up to twofold; such a value of decrease is comparable with *in vitro* studies for trazograph-60 immersion [see Fig. 5.7(c)]. Transmittance measurements are difficult to provide in *in vivo* experiments; thus, to estimate translucent efficiency at optical immersion, we may

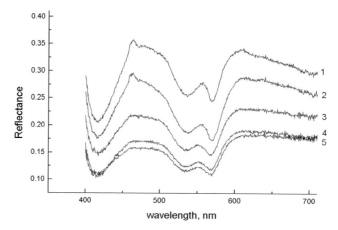

Figure 5.16 The *in vivo* time-dependent reflectance spectra of rabbit eye sclera measured concurrently with administration of 40%-glucose solution: 1, 1 min; 2, 4 min; 3, 21 min; (4) 25 min; and (5) 30 min after drop of glucose into the rabbit eye.[960]

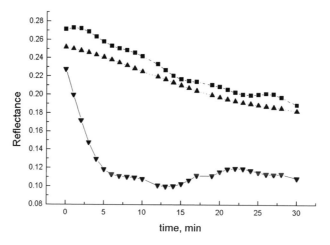

Figure 5.17 The *in vivo* time-dependent reflectance of rabbit eye sclera measured concurrently with administration of 40%-glucose at 420 nm (▼), 630 nm (■), and 700 nm (▲).[960]

use results of *in vitro* measurements of collimated transmittance that show up to a 26-fold increase in transmittance. Using Monte Carlo modeling based on experimental data and the arrangement used for *in vivo* and *in vitro* measurements, a correct comparison of *in vivo* and *in vitro* clearing efficiency can be done.[1032] The calculated ratios of maximal (untreated tissue) to minimal (well-treated tissue) diffuse reflectance R_d for *in vitro* and *in vivo* measurements show the same tendency of their change with the wavelength. Differences in the absolute values of this ratio ($\cong 1.2$ for *in vitro* and $\cong 2$ for *in vivo* at 700 nm), which are higher for the *in vivo* case, can be explained by a multilayered structure of the living tissue (consisting of the conjunctiva, the Tenon's capsule, the sclera itself, the ciliary muscle, and the ciliary pigmented epithelium)—some of which are extremely absorbing. The living tissue seems to be more effectively controlled by an immersion phenomenon due to the stronger influence of absorbing layers that reduce the fluence rate of the backscattered photons as the light penetrates more deeply inside the tissue (due to reduction of the scattering coefficient), where absorption is maximal for this specific tissue. Less scattering causes shorter photon migration paths and less probability for photons to be absorbed.

Other reasons for more effective control are the blood perfusion and metabolic activity of leaving tissue, which cause more effective impregnation of tissue at physiological temperatures in spite of the fact that the agent was applied only to the exterior surface of the sclera. In general, the rate of agent diffusion in a tissue increases from the minimal rate for the fixed tissue samples, where additional bonds between the protein molecules hindering the agent transport are formed, to the midlevel for fresh tissue samples, and the highest for *in vivo* immersion.[949]

It is also important that the total transmittance for the *in vivo* case is threefold to sixfold more effectively controlled by tissue immersion than that for separated scleral samples measured *in vitro*. The total transmittance of anterior eye layers measured at the posterior interface of the sclera determines the laser energy applied to the ciliary body, when its coagulation is needed. The collimated transmittance in its turn determines the efficiency of laser irradiation through the sclera at some local area of the eye bottom to destroy a tumor, for example.

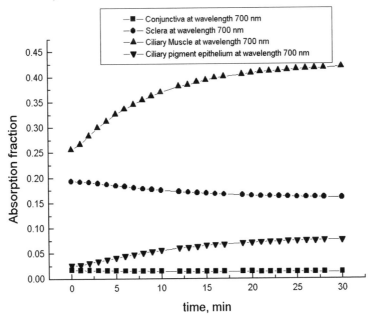

Figure 5.18 The time-dependent light absorption fractions for different layers of a rabbit eye at 700 nm, calculated using Monte Carlo simulation for tissue impregnated by 40%-glucose. Squares correspond to conjunctiva, circles to sclera, up triangles to ciliary muscle, and down triangles to ciliary pigment epithelium.[1032]

The time-dependent light absorption fractions for different layers of rabbit eye at 700 nm, calculated using Monte Carlo simulation for tissue impregnated by a

40%-glucose is shown in Fig. 5.18. The initial values of the scattering and absorption coefficients for various tissue layers were taken from Refs. 266 and 267. The time-dependent diffuse reflectance, the total transmittance, and the light absorbed fractions at tissue immersion were calculated using the *in vivo* studies discussed above. From the graphs of Fig. 5.18, it follows that due to a significant translucence of the upper layers of the rabbit eye, the lower absorbing layers of the eye membrane, such as ciliary body components, are well irradiated, and thus absorb light well. It is found that as far as the light absorption fraction in the conjunctiva and the sclera is decreased, in the ciliary body, it is considerably increased. This confirms the declared possibility of using OCAs for the transcleral selective phodestruction of the ciliary body.[61,723,788]

It is shown that administration of OCAs to a fibrous tissue allows one to effectively control its optical characteristics. The dynamics of scleral tissue optical clearing is characterized by a time response of about 5–10 min, which is defined by the diffusivity of an immersion agent in a tissue, tissue condition (intact or fixed), and tissue thickness. The tissue shrinkage and swelling may play an important role in the tissue clearing process. At a prolonged time of some OCAs' administration (for example, glucose at pH 3.5), tissue shrinkage at the first step of clearing may be replaced by a swelling, which in its turn may cause saturation or even slight reduction of tissue optical transmittance.

Dynamic optical characteristics can be used for the determination of the diffusion coefficient of endogenous (metabolic) and exogenous (chemical agent) fluids in human tissues. Obtained values for diffusion coefficient of glucose, trazograph, and PEG (6000) in intact human sclera correspond well to values of the diffusion coefficient for small molecules diffusing in water.[949]

5.3.4 *Dura mater* immersion and agent diffusion rate

Optical clearing of human *dura mater* is important for cerebral optical diagnostics, phototherapy, and laser surgery. *Dura mater* is a typical fibrous tissue and demonstrates the same behavior of optical clearing as eye sclera, cornea, or skin dermis and muscle, but has its own diffusion coefficient, characteristic time, and degree of clearing, defined by its structure. The first results from an *in vitro* experimental study of human and rabbit *dura mater* optical clearing under the action of mannitol, glucose, and glycerol solutions at various concentrations are presented in Refs. 704, 831, 969, 987, and 1024.

Figure 5.19 illustrates the dynamic changes in rabbit *dura mater* turbidity after application of glycerol.[831] A resolution target was placed under a sample. After the treatment of glycerol for 1 min, the target, which was not visible under the native *dura mater* [Fig. 5.19(a)], was seen through the specimen [Fig. 5.19(b)]. Results of the measurement of the optical properties [Fig. 5.19(c)] confirm the visually observed reduction in scattering. Figure 5.19(c) shows the increase in transmittance within the wavelength range of 400–750 nm as a function of the time the sample was soaked in glycerol. The hemoglobin absorption became much more prominent after application of glycerol [Fig. 5.19(c)]. This indicates that the quality of images received by techniques based on the detection of hemoglobin absorption spectra can be significantly improved at reduction of scattering of the tissue upper layers. *In vivo* studies of glucose and glycerol action on rabbit *dura mater* at the open cranium and with epidural agent application also confirm the concept of effective optical clearing of fibrous tissue.[831] Total optical clearing was achieved very fast in 1950s after tissue treatment by glycerol.

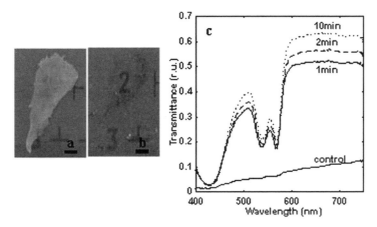

Figure 5.19 Visual changes in *in vitro* turbid rabbit *dura mater* and the measured optical changes before and after epidural application of glycerol. (a) Native *dura mater* placed over the resolution target, bar = 1 mm. (b) One-minute application of glycerol, bar = 1 mm. (c) Transmittance spectra for native *dura mater* measured at application of glycerol for 1, 2, and 10 min.[831]

Figure 5.20 presents the collimated transmittance spectra and temporal dependencies of the spectral components for human *dura mater* samples impregnated by glucose solution. It is well seen that glucose is also a very effective agent for *dura mater* clearing. Using such measurements for glucose and mannitol, and the algorithm described in Refs. 960 and 987, the diffusion coefficients for 40%-glucose and mannitol solution (0.16 g/ml) were found: $D_G = (5.43 \pm 0.88) \times 10^{-6}$ cm^2 s^{-1} and $D_M = (1.67 \pm 0.21) \times 10^{-6}$ cm^2 s^{-1}.[949,987]

5.4 Skin

5.4.1 Introduction

Skin has a very complicated structure, which is schematically presented in Fig. 5.21. It possesses a protective function that prevents penetration of pollutions and microorganisms inside the body. The outermost cellular layer of skin is the epidermis, which consists of stratum corneum (SC) (mostly dead cells) and four layers of living cells. Stratum corneum is a lipid-protein biphasic structure that has a thickness of only 10–20 μm on most surfaces of the body. Due to cell membrane

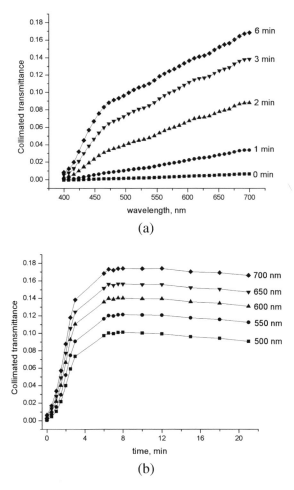

Figure 5.20 (a) The collimated transmittance spectra and (b) corresponding temporal dependencies measured for a human *dura mater* sample in a course of administration of 40%-glucose solution in a bath.[969,987]

keratinization, tight packing of cells, and lipid bridges between them, SC is a dense medium with a poor penetration for foreign molecules.[1070,1071] The excellent diffusional resistance of the SC makes the transdermal delivery of immersion agents and water lost by skin difficult. To understand the transport and barrier functions of the skin, it is important to have knowledge of the water and ion distribution within the different layers.[1072,1073] Water content is known to influence various physical characteristics, such as brittleness, elasticity, tensile strength, and viscoelasticity; barrier characteristics; electrical resistance; thermal conductivity; and appearance. The SC receives water from within the body, but water may also be taken up from the environment. From within the body, water reaches this tissue from the sweat glands and by diffusion from underlying tissues. *In vivo* diffusion of water across the SC is a passive process that can be modified at application of hyperosmotic agents. The water content of the innermost layer of the SC is in equilibrium with the adjacent moist granular layer. The outside cell layer, however, is in equilibrium with the environment and it is certainly drier than the innermost cornified layer. Thus, there exists a concentration gradient causing transepidermal water lost (TEWL).

No significant difference was found for the diffusion across epidermis and SC. The diffusion coefficient D of the flow in water through a stationary macromolecular gel (the tissue) corresponds to viscose flow through a very fine porous medium. As has been determined in strongly hydrated SC, D is about four orders of magnitude less than the water self-diffusion coefficient.[1072] The diffusivity (D) of water in SC increases from $\sim 3 \times 10^{-10}$ to 10^{-9} cm^2/s as humidity H increases from 46 to 81%. It should be noted that the hydration of the dermis is not significantly different from that of the viable cell layers of the epidermis.[1073] The average water content of the SC as measured in Ref. 1073 is 54%, while other authors arrived at a water content as low as 15 to 40% in the same layer. The rate of diffusion of molecules with a molecular weight of 119 in the SC of volunteers is in the range from $\sim 10^{-10}$ to 3.5×10^{-10} cm^2/s.[1071]

Dermis is the next thicker layer of the skin, which is mostly fibrous tissue well supplied by blood and thus can be easily impregnated by exogenous or endogenous liquids (immersion agents). Subcutaneous tissue contains a big portion of a fat cellular layer, which is much less penetrative for diffusing molecules than dermis. Such a specific structure of skin defines the methodology of its effective optical clearing, which is related to the immersion of refractive indices of scatterers (keratinocyte components in epidermis, collagen and elastin fibers in dermis) and ground matter.[57,213,571,946,965,1065] Experimental studies of optical clearing of skin using water, glycerol, glycerol-water solutions, glucose, propylene glycol, oleic acid, DMSO, sunscreen creams, cosmetic lotions, gels, and pharmaceutical products were carried out in Refs. 57, 213, 255, 343, 571, 704, 777, 946, 947, 949, 953, 961–965, 969, 973, 975, 1027, 1030, 1039, 1047–1049, 1052, and 1055–1065.

5.4.2 *In vitro* spectral measurements

Table 5.1 illustrates the efficiency of the different immersion agents' action on the transmittance of the human skin stripped samples (30–40 μm in thickness) taken from volunteers using glass substrate-glue technology.[1065] Because of the small thickness of the sample with a few layers of dried and living keratinocytes and

Table 5.1 The efficiency of the OCA action on the skin stripping sample of 30–40 μm in thickness, expressed as a ratio of mean transmitted intensities after (I_A) and before (I_B) lotion application; n is the index of refraction of the used lotion.[1065]

OCA	Glycerol-water-urea solutions					DMSO 50%	Ultrasound gel
n	1.449	1.380	1.356	1.354	1.348	1.396	1.337
I_A/I_B	12.8	3.7	4.9	5.9	4.1	7.9	5.3

the agent supply through the living cell layer, the rate and efficiency of immersion were very high.

An *in vitro* study of rat dorsal skin impregnated by anhydrous glycerol, when the agent was applied to the dermal side of the skin sample, showed a power wavelength dependence of the reduced scattering coefficient in the wavelength range from 500 to 1200 nm, described by Eq. (1.179), $\mu_s' \sim \lambda^{-h}$, with reduced scattering coefficient at 500 nm $\mu_s' \approx 50$ cm^{-1} and $h = 1.12$ for normal skin, and with subsequent decrease in μ_s' (500 nm) and h with increased time in glycerol (mostly due to the dehydration effect): $\mu_s' \approx 30$ cm^{-1} and $h = 1.09$ for 5 min, $\mu_s' \approx 20$ cm^{-1} and $h = 0.85$ for 10 min, $\mu_s' \approx 12$ cm^{-1} and $h = 0.52$ for 20 min, and $\mu_s' \approx 23$ cm^{-1} and $h = 0.9$ for the rehydrated sample kept in a physiological phosphate-buffered saline solution for 20 min.[571] A 60% decrease in hydration was estimated on the basis of changes in the water absorption peaks and a 21.5% corresponding decrease in thickness was found going from the native tissue to the tissue treated with glycerol for 20 min. The rehydration process caused the thickness and turbidity of the sample to go back toward the initial state, but during the course of rehydration, which lasted 20 min, the turbidity (μ_s') did not reach the initial state. Accounting for the relatively short period of time (~20 min) for the optical clearing of the skin samples of about 1 mm in thickness in this experiment and high viscosity of glycerol, its action as a hyperosmotic agent should mostly have drawn interstitial water out of the tissue and, at a slower rate, should have replaced the water and salts of the ground substance. The 20 min of rehydration are also not enough for water to reenter all of the cells and collagen fibers in the tissue; thus, the scattering coefficient and spectral power parameter h for rehydrated tissue are somewhat less than their initial values.

More prolonged administration of glucose (up to 6 hr) and glycerol (up to 45 min) into the fresh rat skin samples at room temperature in the course of tissue collimated transmittance measurements was also done.[1031,1038,1039] These studies were performed to clarify the mechanisms of the skin optical clearing and to optimize the technique. To avoid tissue damage and to provide a lower viscosity of the chemical agent, a glycerol-water solution (88%) and 40%-glucose (both are available in a drug store) were used as immersion agents. Skin samples were of 0.57–0.90 mm in thickness and 1×1 cm^2 in area, some of them contained whole skin including epidermis, dermis, and hypodermic fatty layer, and for others the fatty layer was removed. Hairs were removed by tweezers and the immersion agent was applied to both sides of the sample in a bath. Figures 5.22 and 5.23 illustrate the typical collimated transmittance spectra and optical clearing dynamics. It is well seen that the untreated rat skin is poorly transparent for visible light. Both glucose and glycerol administration make this tissue highly transparent; the 15-fold increase of the collimated transmittance for glucose [Fig. 5.23(a)] and 10-fold increase for glycerol [Fig. 5.23(c)] at 700 nm for the samples with a fatty layer kept in solution for 45 min are seen. The efficiency is substantially greater with removed fatty layer [Fig. 5.23(b)]; about a 50-fold transmittance increase is seen for the glucose solution at the same wavelength during the same time interval, and a further increase of transmittance and its saturation happens for more prolonged time intervals.

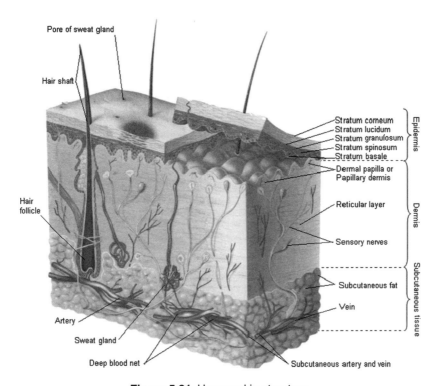

Figure 5.21 Human skin structure.

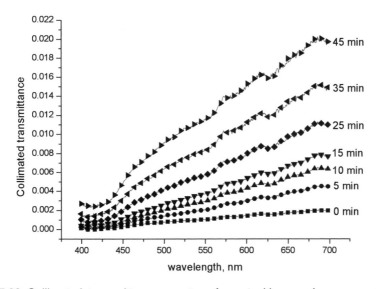

Figure 5.22 Collimated transmittance spectra of a rat skin sample measured concurrently with administration of 88%-glycerol at different time intervals (sample thickness of 0.9 mm).[1031]

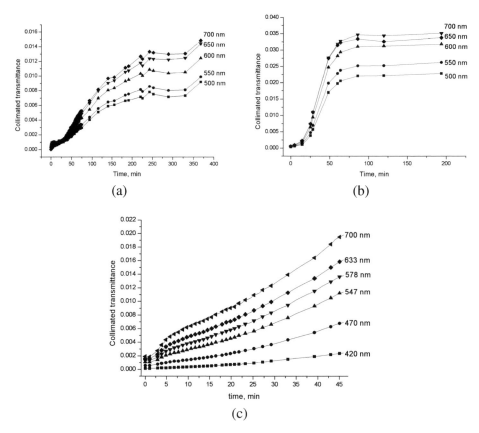

Figure 5.23 The time-dependent collimated transmittance of rat skin samples (1 hour after autopsy, hairs were removed with tweezers) measured at different wavelengths in a course of administration of immersion solution in a bath. (a) Sample thickness 0.73 mm, with hypodermic fatty layer, immersion agent 40%-glucose; (b) sample thickness 0.57 mm, with removed hypodermic fatty layer, immersion agent 40%-glucose; (c) sample thickness 0.9 mm, with hypodermic fatty layer, immersion agent glycerol-water solution (88%, vol/vol).[1038,1039]

Table 5.2 presents characteristics (refractive index and osmolality) of a variety of chemical agents with different optical clearing potential (OCP), defined as the ratio of the values of tissue reduced scattering coefficient before and after agent action, $OCP \equiv \mu'_s(\text{before})/\mu'_s(\text{after})$.[1055] OCP was measured *in vitro* at agent application to the dermis side of human skin using a Franz diffusion chamber after a 20-min application time. It follows from Table 5.2 that there is no correlation between OCP and refractive index for used agents with indices in the range from 1.43 to 1.48, as well as no correlation with osmolality in a wide range from 1,643 to 26,900 mOsm/kg, but the highest values of OCP, from 2.4 to 2.9, are provided by the agents having both the highest refractive index and osmolality, such as glycerol, 1,4-butanediol, and 1,3-butanediol.

It is evident that the penetration rate of the OCA into the skin is much slower than that for sclera or *dura mater*, which take only 8–10 min to be saturated by trazograph or glucose solutions. In comparison with sclera and *dura mater*, no sat-

Table 5.2 OCA characteristics and *in vitro* measured optical clearing potential (OCP) at agent application to dermis side of human skin using a Franz diffusion chamber; OCP is defined as the ratio of values of tissue reduced scattering coefficient before and after agent action, OCP $\equiv \mu_s'$(before)$/\mu_s'$(after), was measured after 20 min application time.[1055]

OCA	Refractive index	Osmolality (mOsm/kg)	OCP
Glycerol	1.47	14,550	2.9 ± 0.8
50% TMP (trimethylolpropanol)	1.43	6,830	2.2 ± 0.3
100% TMP	1.47	13,660	2.1 ± 0.7
1,3-butanediol	1.44	22,050	2.4 ± 0.7
1,4-butanediol	1.44	26,900	2.8 ± 0.5
Ethylene glycol	1.43	22,640	1.9 ± 0.6
MPDiol glycol (1,3-diol, 2-methyl-propane)	1.44	23,460	2.3 ± 0.2
P-0062*	1.48	1,643	2.0 ± 0.5

*P-0062 is a polyethylene glycol based prepolymer developed at University of California, Irvine.

uration of the clearing process was seen up to 6 hr if the fatty layer is not removed. This phenomenon can be connected with the low permeability of the epidermal and fat tissue cellular layers for any molecules, which slows down both fluxes— the water flux from the tissue and immersion agent flux from the outside into the tissue. Saturation of the optical transmittance can be expected when the equilibrium state in the immersion agent/water diffusion process will be achieved, i.e., when concentrations of water and immersion agent inside and outside tissue will be approximately equal. For skin with epidermis and fatty layer, such saturation was not reached even for 6 hr of glucose administration; but with removed fatty layer, saturation was achieved in 1 hr.

Using the algorithm described by Eqs. (5.1), (5.6), (5.14), and (5.17) and experimental data (see Fig. 5.23) discussed earlier, the diffusion coefficient of water in the skin at glycerol action can be estimated. Such estimation is valid for the agents with a strong osmotic strength because the water flux dominates in the system. The mean value of the diffusion coefficient averaged for the six rat skin samples at 20°C for glycerol-water solution penetration, mostly from the dermal side of the skin, is equal to $(5.12 \pm 2.27) \times 10^{-7}$ cm^2 s^{-1}, which is about two orders less than the diffusion coefficient of water in water, $D_W \cong 10^{-5}$ cm^2 s^{-1} (see Ref. 1069), or one order less than water diffusion in an intact human lens, $D_W \cong 3.0 \times 10^{-6}$ cm^2 s^{-1} (see Ref. 1020). For a subcutaneous fat free sample, a 40%-glucose action is characterized by a higher diffusion rate,[949] $D = (3.1 \pm 0.1) \times 10^{-6}$ cm^2 s^{-1} that may be due to more effective penetration of glucose into a tissue.

Using near-infrared spectroscopy (800–2200 nm), mass and water loss measurements, and transdermal skin resistance measurements, such enhancers of skin permeability as dimethyl sulfoxide (DMSO) and oleic acid, a monounsaturated fatty acid, were compared at propylene glycol (PG) application onto the epidermal surface of samples of fresh porcine skin with a thickness of 1.52 ± 0.18 mm.[1027] It was shown that when compared with DMSO as an enhancer, oleic acid has a similar synergetic optical clearing effect. Accounting for clinical safety reasons, oleic acid could be an optimal choice as an enhancer for optical clearing of skin because it is recognized as safe and free-of-side-effects agent, whereas DMSO has some potential toxicity. After application of oleic acid solution (0.1 M of oleic acid and PG-40), the total transmittance measured on the wavelength 1278 nm of the skin sample increased by 41 and 58%, respectively, for 30 and 60 min treatment, while diffuse reflectance decreased by 39 and 47%, respectively.

The difference in apparent absorbance (diffuse reflectance spectra were transformed into apparent absorbance, $A = \log(1/R_d)$) between two wavelengths of 1936 and 1100 nm was adopted to monitor the change in water content.[932,971,972,1011,1026,1027] It is important that the oleic acid solution provided the greatest water loss in comparison with the other tested solutions, 37 and 46% after 30 and 60 min treatment, respectively. As for DMSO-50, water loss was of 15 and 20%, PG-80 was 20 and 29%, and PG-80 + DMSO-50 was 34 and 44% after 30 and 60 min treatment, respectively. But the mass loss at oleic acid solution application was the minimal among the tested solutions; after 30 min PG-80 provided 10.9% of mass loss, PG-80 + DMSO-50 provided 6.4%, and oleic acid (0.1 M) + PG-40 provided 6.3%. More mass loss was obtained after 60 min of these agents' application: PG-80, 14.2%; PG-80 + DMSO-50, 9.9%; and oleic acid (0.1 M) + PG-40, 8.3%. The comparison of water and mass loss data give a nice confirmation of the basic conception of the optical clearing that refractive index matching is achieved by two main diffusing processes: water flux from tissue (dehydration) and agent flux into tissue (replacement of interstitial water by the agent).

A method of accelerating penetration of the index-matching compounds by enhancing skin permeability by creating a lattice of microzones (islets) of limited thermal damage in the SC was recently proposed.[1056,1057] A combination of a flashlamp system (EsteLux, Palomar Medical Technologies, Inc.) and a specially designed appliqué with a pattern of absorbing centers (center size ~75 μm, lattice pitch ~450 μm) has been used to create a lattice of islets of damage (LID).[1074] Several index-matching agents, including glucose and glycerol, have been tested. A high degree of optical clearance of full-thickness pig, rat, chicken, and human skin *in vitro* and *in vivo* has been demonstrated with 40%-glucose and 88%-glycerol solutions after creating a LID with a few optical pulses (fluence 14–36 J/cm^2, 20-ms pulse duration).

5.4.3 *In vivo* spectral reflectance measurements

In vivo topical application of glycerol, glucose, x-ray contrasts, propylene glycol, cosmetic lotions, and gels also made human skin more translucent, within a time period from a few minutes to a few hours.[916,961,963,964,1044,1046] Water loss or increase by means of moisturizing substances seriously influences the optical properties of skin.[622,1045–1048,1071–1073] NIR reflectance spectroscopy is used as a method to directly determine changes in free, bulk, and protein-bound water, and to assess scattering effects in skin for the evaluation of skin care products.[1046] The following spectral bands are associated with water: free water, 1879 nm; bulk water, 1890 nm; and protein-bound water, 1909 and 1927 nm. The effect of increases in ambient humidity is associated with increased levels of free water in the skin, while moisturizers containing hydroxyethyl cellulose, propylene glycol, dipropylene glycol, and glycerol contribute to a decrease in light scattering.[1046] The water observed in such experiments is primarily in the SC, since only a small part of the reflected light comes from the epidermis or below.

Noninvasive measurement of the SC hydration can be performed using attenuated total reflectance Fourier transform infrared (ATR FTIR) spectroscopy.[622,1047,1071] Three absorption bands are relevant for determining water content in the SC: 3300 cm^{-1} (3030 nm), O-H and N-H vibrations; 1645 cm^{-1} (6079 nm), amide I band; and 1545 cm^{-1} (6472 nm), amide II band. The amide I band intensity is pronounced in the presence of water due to the strong absorption of water at 1645 cm^{-1} and the changes in carbonyl absorption under the influence of water, while the amide II band intensity is due to protein alone. The intensity ratio of the amide I to amide II bands, also called the moisture factor, is assumed to be a relative measure of C hydration.[1047] Various SC moisturizers based on glycerol, propylene glycol, sodium lactate, natural moisturizing vegetal, liposomes, butylene glycol, polyglycerylmethacrylate, and urea were used for an *in vivo* SC hydration study.[1047] Depending on the composition and concentration, maximal SC hydration could be reached in 0.5–2 hr after application of the substance on the skin surface. For some substances, a considerable moisturizing effect was detectable up to 8 hr following application. Dual-wavelength (1300 and 1450 nm) optical coherence reflectance measurement is a prospective technique for depth profiling of water absorption within the skin.[1048]

To enhance OCA permeation through SC, a number of specific procedures such as heating, electrophoresis, and sonophoresis are usually applied.[1039,1044,1070] To increase efficiency of the topical application of the OCAs, gelatin gels that contain clearing agents (verografin, glycerol, or glucose) were designed.[1044] The diffusion rate of the agents within the gel layer can be rather high, and this along with the comparatively large volume of the gel provided the constant concentration of OCA, equal to agent content in the gel, at the skin surface. For intact skin of a volunteer, the best dynamics, i.e., the rate and the degree of clearing (17%), was observed in the case of verografin-gel [Fig. 5.24(a)] where after 40 min of observation, clearing still proceeds at a marked rate, while for glycerol-gel after 27 min, the curve flattens out; no clearing was observed in 40 min of glucose-gel application.

Because a barrier function of the skin is associated mainly with SC, the measurement was carried out on the skin after 30–50 μm epidermal glue stripping [Fig. 5.24(b)]. Application of glucose-gel to the skin without upper epidermis gave a rapid 10% drop of reflected light intensity. Glycerol-gel gave better results; over the time of observation, the decrease of reflected signal ranged up to ~20%, which was twice what was attained for intact skin. Surprisingly, no clearing effect of verografin-gel was observed.

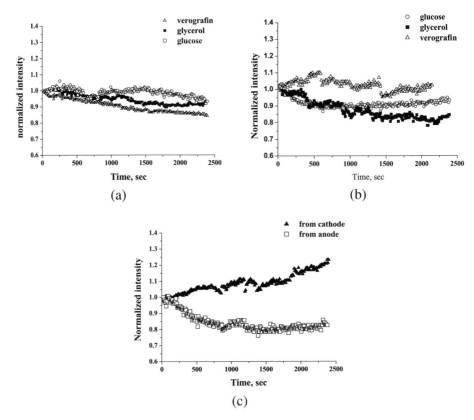

Figure 5.24 Back reflectance at 830 nm measured by a fiber-optic probe ($r_{sd} = 1.2$ mm, source fiber of 0.2 mm, and detector fiber of 1 mm in diameter) perpendicular to the skin surface at clearing gel (glucose: 3.9 ml 40%-glucose and 0.2 g gelatin; glycerol: 1.3 ml glycerol, 0.1 g gelatin, and 2.6 ml distillate water; verografin: 2.6 ml verografin-60, 0.1 g gelatin, and 1.3 ml distillate water) application on (a) intact skin; (b) on skin after glue epidermal stripping; (c) at electrophoretic application of gelatin gel with glycerol (1.3 ml glycerol, 0.2 g gelatin, and 2.5 ml distillate water).[1044]

The electrophoretic applicator and gel with twice the content of gelatin were also applied to human skin optical clearing.[1044] In Fig. 5.24(c), the results for glycerol-gel are shown. When the active electrode was connected as an anode, a reduction of optical signal by ~20% was attained. This value is comparable to the results with stripping, but the time of attainment of minimum signal is nearly halved. When the active electrode was connected as a cathode, an increase of back-reflectance was observed over the whole duration of measurement. The effect was attributed to the development of erythema.

It may be concluded that for the topical application of glycerol-gel and glucose-gel, the employment of epidermal stripping and the electrophoresis technique does lead to the enhancement of the dynamics of *in vivo* optical clearing of human skin. The best characteristics were obtained with electrophoretic administration of glycerol from an anode. In the case of glucose, stripping and electrophoresis from a cathode give similar results, but the application of glucose should be terminated after 10–12 min because of the risk of deterioration of clearing by erythema development.

The administration of glucose or glycerol by intradermal injection into rat or hamster skin causes a decrease of reflectance and the corresponding increase of tissue transmittance.[571,969,978,980,1031,1038,1039,1058] This effect was observed at all wavelengths during a 15–18 min period after glucose injection.[978,980] The highest degree of tissue reflectance change is found at wavelengths from 580 to 750 nm, where scattering dominates. At the sixteenth minute, the reflectance of the skin was minimal (maximal transmittance); it decreased by about 3.5-fold at 700 nm, then the tissue went slowly back to its normal state. At the seventy-sixth minute, a reduction of reflectance of only twofold was observed. It was shown that a glycerol injection causes a more prolonged effect of tissue optical clearing, but reflectance decreased a little bit less than for glucose injection. This can be explained by the higher viscosity of glycerol and by its mostly indirect action through tissue dehydration. The reaction of the rat skin upon injection of distillate water, as a model of a nonosmotic agent, was also studied. The reduction of reflectance was observed only for a short period (the first minute) after injection. It happened due to a much higher transmittance of the injected water with respect to the surrounding tissues. At the second minute, water diffuses into the bulk tissue and the transparency of the tissue was decreased; the reflectance spectrum was elevated gradually to its initial value. Injection of water does not cause immersion clearing of the skin.

The virtual transparent window (VTW) with a diameter of ∼4 mm in the skin is created with the living time period of ∼30 min for 40%-glucose and more than 60 min for 75%-glycerol. Such a window allows one to clearly identify blood microvessels in the skin visually by the naked eye.[978,980] The swelling white ring (edema) appears around the VTW after agent injection. The images of skin after intradermal injection of glucose, glycerol, and water were recorded by a digital video camera. The diameters of swelling area (D_S) and VTW (D_T), and their ratio (D_S/D_T) were measured (Fig. 5.25).[978] For a glucose injection, the diameter of the VTW was registered at the first minute after injection. At the second minute, the diameter was slightly decreased. For the next 15 min, this diameter and the diameter of the swelling area were not changed. After the twentieth minute, significant reduction of the VTW was observed. For glycerol injection, the diameter of the VTW was approximately the same, but the swelling ring was bigger, and both transmittance and swelling were seen for longer times than at glucose injection [Fig. 5.25(b)]. The injection of distillate water causes only the appearance of swelling at the site of the injection. The diameter of the swelling area is decreased gradually and swelling disappears by the thirtieth minute after injection.

Figure 5.26 shows the reflectance spectra and the corresponding time-dependent reflectance for a few spectral components measured for a human healthy volunteer at intradermal 40%-glucose solution.[965] The reflectance spectra show a scattering background determined by the diffusion reflection of the skin layers with the well-pronounced bands caused by blood optical absorption. Within one hour after glucose injection, the skin reflection coefficient decreases on average by a factor

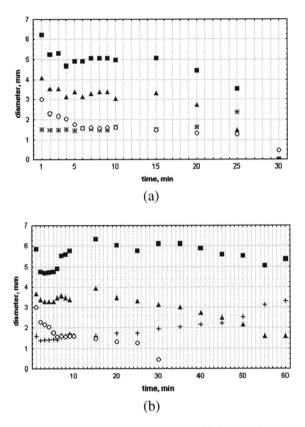

Figure 5.25 The changes of skin reaction on injection of (a) 40%-glucose and (b) 75%-glycerol: ▲, the diameter of the virtual transparent window (VTW) (D_T); ■, the diameter of swelling area around the VTW (D_S); ∗ and +, the ratio D_S/D_T; ○, the diameter of swelling area at injection of distillate water.[978,980]

of 3.8 and then exhibits a slow increase, which indicates that glucose is eliminated from the observation area and the skin reflectance tends to restore itself to the initial level. Based on these results and the proposed skin clearing model, we may suggest that the main contribution to clearing in the first stage (first hour) is due to the refractive index matching between collagen fibrils of the dermis ($n = 1.46$) and the interstitial space (initially $n = 1.36$) to which glucose ($n = 1.39$) diffuses. Estimated from the experimental data [Fig. 5.26(b)], the diffusion coefficient of glucose in dermis is $D_G = (2.56 \pm 0.13) \times 10^{-6}$ cm^2/s; this value is 3.6-fold less than for glucose diffusion in water at $37°$, $D_G \approx 9.2 \times 10^{-6}$ cm^2/s, and reflects the character of dermis permeability for glucose.

For applications, it is important that skin preserves transparency (low reflectance) for a few hours after injection, which is defined by glucose diffusion along the skin surface, because the upper and lower layers of the skin—epidermis and fat—have much lower permeability than dermis. For the optical clearing effect to be still seen, glucose should diffuse at least at the distance $l = 1.25$–1.75 mm for the fiber probe used in experiments (Fig. 5.11), i.e., the diffusing (optical

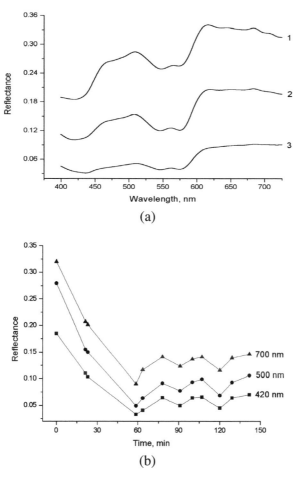

Figure 5.26 (a) The reflectance spectra and (b) the time-dependent reflectance at three wavelengths (420, 500, and 700 nm) of human skin measured at hyperdermal injection of 0.1 ml of 40%-glucose into the internal side of the forearm of a male volunteer for different time intervals: (1) intact skin, (2) at 23 min, and (3) at 60 min after injection.[965]

clearing) time $\tau \approx l^2/D_G \approx 1.7$–3.3 hr (corresponds well to experimental data) [Fig. 5.26(b)].

As is well seen from Fig. 5.26(a), at dermis clearing (reduction of scattering), the contrast of hemoglobin absorption bands is significantly higher than that for the control; but for prolonged immersion (curve 3), contrast is again not very high. This result is very important for contrasting of tissue abnormalities (tumors) associated with hemoglobin or other probe absorbers' concentration (for instance, indocyanine green dye). Therefore, there is an optimal immersion time interval (for human skin at glucose injection, it is on the order of 60 min) that allows one to see skin absorbers and localize them more precisely at reduced scattering. Indeed, for prolonged immersion, contrast goes down due to fewer light interactions with absorption at low-step scattering.

5.4.4 *In vivo* frequency-domain measurements

The dynamical response of optical properties of human skin treated by a chemical agent can be measured using a photon-density wave (frequency-domain) technique.[961] The intensity and phase of photon-density waves generated by the NIR optical source (786 nm) were measured at several source-detector separations.[961,963] For the small (1–3 mm) source-detection separation measurements that allow for thin tissue layer examination, a special multichannel fiber-optic probe was designed. It was used together with the Dicon multichannel fiber-optic switcher. Dynamical response of optical properties (modulation depth and phase shift of intensity modulation of the backscattered light) was measured for human skin via intervals of a chemical agent administration. The measurement for each separation was done during 10 s and averaged, corresponding to one point in Fig. 5.27. The relative amplitude (normalized to the initial amplitude) and phase changes (the current phase minus the initial phase) during 20 min of glycerol topical application are shown in Fig. 5.27. Only scattering changes must be considered due to the extremely low absorption of glycerol at the measuring wavelength. The observed amplitude and phase changes are small, reflecting minor permeation of epidermal cell layers to any chemical agent. Nevertheless, these measurements show enough sensitivity of the frequency-domain method to small changes of the scattering coefficient of the skin.

For large (2.5 cm) source-detector separation studies, the source and detector fiber tips were mounted in a rubber pad and fastened to the surface of the human forearm to avoid random moving artifacts. The cosmetic gel with refractive index $n = 1.403$ was placed on the surface of the arm and the phase and ac amplitude

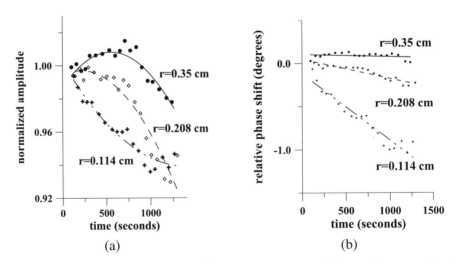

(a)   (b)

Figure 5.27 Frequency-domain back-reflectance measurements for small source-detector separations.[961,963] The time-dependent changes of the (a) amplitude and (b) phase shift of the signal for several source-detector separations (1.14, 2.08, and 3.5 mm) for *in vivo* study of a human arm under glycerol administration of 20 min.

measurements were provided continuously. One sampling point corresponded to one second. The results of measurement during 30 min of gel administration are shown in Fig. 5.28(a). The observed temporal quasi-periodic fluctuations in the phase and amplitude of the optical signal are caused mainly by heartbeats.

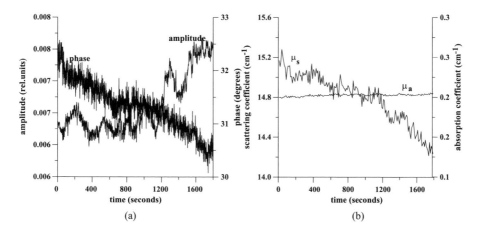

(a)   (b)

Figure 5.28 Frequency-domain back-reflectance measurements for the large source-detector separation (2.5 cm).[961,963] (a) The raw experimental data of the phase and ac amplitude of the optical signal and (b) calculation of the absorption and the scattering coefficients. A cosmetic gel with refractive index $n = 1.403$ has been used.

Results of reconstruction of tissue optical parameters are shown in Fig. 5.28(b). The initial values of μ_s' and μ_a for human skin were taken from Table 2.1, and relative changes of these parameters were calculated with a continual averaging procedure for every 5-s interval in order to exclude the influence of heartbeats. Corresponding temporal evolutions of the scattering and absorption coefficients have been received. This study shows that there are no noticeable changes in the absorption during the gel administration trial. A slight increase in the absorption can probably be explained by the increase of the water content in the skin due to the moisture effect of the applied gel. The selected source-detector separation (2.5 cm) and corresponding measuring volume are too large to make the matching effect a useful procedure for topical application of the gel. Only about 6% reduction of the scattering coefficient averaged over the large measuring volume was observed. This means that the scattering coefficient of the upper (superficial) layers of the skin changed more effectively. Refractive index matching of fiber tips and tissue surface is also important.

In vivo frequency-domain measurements for immersed tissues show that the refractive index matching technique provided by the appropriate chemical agent or cosmetic preparation application can be successfully used in tissue spectroscopy and imaging when reduction of scattering properties is needed.

5.4.5 OCT imaging

The typical optical coherence tomography (OCT) fiber-optic system employs a broadband light source (a superluminescence diode) delivering light at the central wavelength of 820 nm or 1300 nm with a bandwidth of 25–50 nm. Such an OCT system provides 10–20 μm of axial and transverse resolution in free space with a signal-to-noise ratio up to 100 dB (see Section 4.6).[127,136]

The result of the OCT study is the measurement of optical backscattering or reflectance, $R(z)$, from the tissue versus axial ranging distance, or depth, z. The reflectance depends on the optical properties of tissue, i.e., the absorption μ_a and scattering μ_s coefficients, or total attenuation coefficient $\mu_t = \mu_a + \mu_s$. The relationship between $R(z)$ and μ_t is, however, highly complicated because of the high and anisotropic scattering of tissue. But for optical depths of less than 4, reflected power can be approximately proportional to $-\mu_t z$ in an exponential scale according to the single-scattering model,[932] i.e.,

$$R(z) = I_0 \alpha(z) \exp(-2\mu_t z), \tag{5.27}$$

where I_0 is the optical power launched into the tissue sample and $\alpha(z)$ is the reflectivity of the sample at the depth z. The factor of 2 in the exponential accounts for the light passing through the sample twice after it is backscattered. Optical depth is a measure in terms of the number of mean free path lengths, i.e., $\mu_s z$. $\alpha(z)$ is linked to the local refractive index and the backscattering property of the blood sample. If $\alpha(z)$ is kept constant, μ_t can be obtained theoretically from the reflectance measurements at two different depths, z_1 and z_2, as

$$\mu_t = \frac{1}{2(\Delta z)} \ln\left[\frac{R(z_1)}{R(z_2)}\right], \tag{5.28}$$

where $\Delta z = |z_1 - z_2|$. Because noise is inevitable in the measurement, a final result should thus be obtained by use of a least-squares fitting technique to improve the accuracy of the determined value of μ_t.

Optical clearing (enhancement of transmittance) ΔT by an agent application can be estimated using the following expression:

$$\Delta T = \left[\frac{R_a - R_s}{R_s}\right] \times 100\%, \tag{5.29}$$

where R_a is the reflectance from the backward surface of the sample impregnated by an agent, and R_s is that from a control sample.

Multiple scattering is a detrimental factor that limits OCT imaging performances: imaging resolution, depth, and localization. To improve the imaging capabilities, the multiple scattering of tissue must be reduced. The immersion technique at application of biocompatible agents is expected to be a prospective technique for OCT because the depth of OCT images and their contrast can be essentially improved very easily at immersion.[136,139,573,717,896,916,932,949,958,959,966,968,971,973, 1008,1012,1059]

OCT imaging combined with OCA immersion is a useful technology for skin disease diagnosis and monitoring. To illustrate the dynamics of skin optical clearing after the application of glycerol, a set of OCT images (820 nm) of a rat skin sample was recorded at regular time intervals over a period of 40 min (Fig. 5.29).[966] Both the index-matching effect, leading to the enhanced depth capability, and the localized dehydration effect, leading to the improvement of imaging contrast, are clearly evident. Analogous results were received for fresh porcine and chicken skin at imaging on 1300 nm by 50%- and 80%-glycerol solutions by Wang. The OCT image of human skin with psoriatic erythrodermia acquired sometime after application of glycerol [Fig. 5.30(b)] differs from the initial image [Fig. 5.30(a)] in

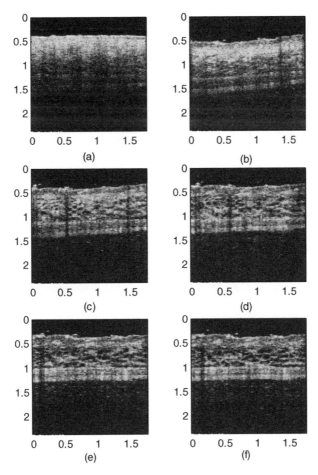

Figure 5.29 Dynamic OCT images ($\lambda = 820$ nm) at (a) 0, (b) 3, (c) 10, (d) 15, (e) 20, and (f) 40 min after a topical application of 80%-glycerol solution onto rat skin. Images were prepared right after the rat was sacrificed; all the units presented are millimeters, and the vertical axis presents the imaging depth.[966]

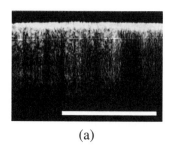   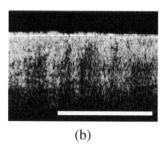

(a)   (b)

Figure 5.30 OCT images of skin with psoriatic erythrodermia: (a) before topical application of glycerol; (b) 60 min after application of glycerol.[717]

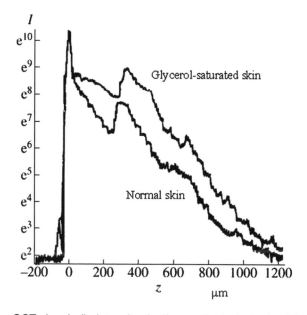

Figure 5.31 The OCT signals (in intensity-depth coordinates) obtained for *in vivo* probing of human finger-tip skin. The upper curve corresponds to skin saturated with glycerol. The scattering coefficient for the skin with glycerol is reduced: for the SC by a factor of two; for epidermis and upper dermis by 20%; and for deeper dermis layers only by 5%.[916]

greater penetration depth and better contrast. These image improvements facilitate identification of important morphological phenomenon of acanthosis.[717]

The possibility of *in vivo* diagnostics of malignant melanoma, observation of subepidermal blisters, and control of the scattering properties of skin through the saturation of skin with glycerol by its topical application was demonstrated on the basis of OCT imaging of human skin both *in vitro* and *in vivo*.[916] According to the estimates done by the authors of Ref. 916, the scattering coefficient for the SC with glycerol is reduced by a factor of two (Fig. 5.31). For epidermis and upper dermis, the coefficient of scattering decreases by 20%. For deeper dermis layers, the coefficient of scattering lowers only by 5%. The effect on enhancement of both the imaging depth and contrast was found in *in vivo* studies of human skin optical clearing at topical application of the 50% propylene glycol solution.[967]

The OCT images captured from the skin site of the volunteer at hyperdermal injection of 40%-glucose allowed one to estimate the total attenuation coefficient [see Eq. (5.28)].[967] The attenuation initially goes down and then goes up within the time course. Such behavior well correlates with the spectral measurements shown in Fig. 5.26 and also reflects the index matching induced by the glucose injection. The light-beam attenuation in tissue, $I/I_0 \sim \exp(-\mu_t)$, for intact skin (0 min) was found from OCT measurements as $I/I_0 \cong 0.14$, and for immersed skin at 13 min $I/I_0 \cong 0.30$, i.e., the intensity of transmitted light increased 2.1-fold. That value also correlates well with the spectral measurements.

It should be noted that high sensitivity of the OCT signal to immersion of living tissue by glucose allows one to monitor its concentration in the skin at a physiological level.[534,549,550]

Although glycerol and glucose are effective OCAs when injected into the dermis,[571,967,980] they normally do not penetrate so well into intact skin. In recent OCT experiments with human skin *in vivo* at topical application during 90–120 min of combined lipophilic polypropylene glycol-based polymers (PPG) and hydrophilic polyethylene glycol (PEG)-based polymers, both with refraction indices of 1.47 that closely match that of skin scattering components in SC, epidermis, and dermis, it was shown that a polymer mixture can penetrate intact skin and improve OCT images, allowing one to see dermal vasculature and hair follicles more clearly.[973] This composition may have some advantages in skin optical clearing due to a hydrophilic component, which may be more effectively diffuse within living epidermis and dermis; less osmotic strength may also have some advantages, but the optical clearing depth could not be improved radically in comparison with topical application of other clearing agents, such as glycerol, glucose, x-ray contrast, and propylene glycol, because of the principle limitations of chemical agent diffusion through intact cell layers (see Table 5.2). Thus, to provide fast and effective optical clearing of skin, the appropriate well-known or newly developed methods of enhanced agent delivery should be applied. Some of them are discussed above.

5.4.6 OCA delivery, skin permeation, and reservoir function

The general principles of designing cosmetic preparations that allow one to provide deep permeation within skin for the improvement of its physiological properties are discussed elsewhere.[1075] As it was shown earlier, the same cosmetic preparations with or even without any corrections may serve as optical immersion compositions. This is the best solution when the immersion composition improves both physiological and optical properties of the skin. However, the excellent diffusional resistance of the SC makes the transdermal delivery of an immersion agent difficult.[1070]

Lipids define a high permeability of creams and lotions in upper layers of epidermis and hair follicles.[1075] Ethers of fat acids with single-atom spirits like isopropyl myristate, isopropyl palmitate, and isopropyl laurate are very important chemicals as components of deep-penetrating creams and lotions.

Technical lecithin [60% natural phospholipids (major phosphatidylcholine), 30–35% plant oil, glycerol, etc.] is a basis for many nourishing (nutritive) creams due to its possibility to penetrate deep into the skin.

Silicon wax and oils easily penetrate into hair follicles via friction (rubbing) and, due to low surface tension, do not induce inflammation, and do not influence the thermal balance of the skin.

Emulsions are oils in water and water in oils, with sizes of particles more than 0.1 μm. Emulsions like oils in water are widespread in cosmetics for deep penetration into the skin, as providers of biologically active substances, etc.

Nourishing (nutritive) creams easily penetrate to the deep layers of epidermis and prevent transepidermal water loss (TEWL). Skin hydration can be provided by two mechanisms—osmotic or physiological. As the hydrating substances, sodium lactate, pyrrolidonecarboxylic acid, derivatives of amino acids and sugars, proteins, and mucopolysaccharides are usually used. As a hygroscopic component, glycerol is often used (usually less than 10% in composition). At present, glycerol is usually replaced by a propylene glycol.

Currently in the market of cosmetic products, numerous creams and lotions providing enough deep impregnation of the skin are available. Many cosmetic emulsions, gels, and lotions for skin hydration use gyaluronic acid (the best for TEWL), sea collagen (also good for TEWL), liposomes, and nanospheres (fat particles) for transportation of biologically active substances to the deep layers of epidermis and hair follicles. As a rule, creams based on liposomes and nanospheres are used after application of peeling creams; for example, creams containing α-hydroxy acids (AHAs) or abrasive creams that make skin relief more smooth and penetrative for liposomes and nanospheres.

Liposomes have been suggested as a vehicle for dermal and transdermal drug delivery, but the knowledge about the interaction between lipid vesicles and human skin is still poor. In Ref. 1076, the visualization of liposome penetration into human skin *in vitro* using a confocal microscope was done. Liposomes were prepared from phospholipids in different compositions and labeled with a fluorescent lipid bilayer marker. Liposome compositions containing dioleylphosphatidylethanolamine (DOPE) were able to penetrate deeper into the SC than that from liposomes without DOPE; the liposomes containing DOPE may fuse or mix with skin lipids *in vitro* and loosen the SC lipid bilayers. Among the factors not affecting SC penetration were: negative charge, cholesterol inclusion, and acyl chain length of the phospholipids. Fusogenicity of the liposome composition appears to be a prerequisite for skin penetration. The liposome sizes determined by quasi-elastic light-scattering method were in the range 40–76 nm. The penetration depth into skin in 72 hr was in the 2–38 μm range. It should be noted that effective mixing of liposomes containing DOPE with SC lipid bilayers happens in a few minutes.[1076]

Occlusion enhances the percutaneous absorption of a variety of compounds.[1070] The effect is relatively independent of the structure of the compound. For example, hydration of the SC appears to enhance diffusion of water as well the percutaneous absorption of a homologous series of alcohols, phenols, and steroids. Occlusion leads to a threefold increase in the percutaneous absorption of several steroids applied from acetone vehicles. Occlusion reduces or blocks TEWL and the evaporation of volatile solvents or compounds from the skin surface. In turn, this results in a profound (300–400%) increase in the water content of the SC. Most transdermal preparations are partially or completely occlusive. Partial occlusion may also be obtained with formulations based on petrolatum, ointments, or creams, though lotions offer little occlusive activity. In addition, baths act to increase the water content of the SC and enhance percutaneous absorption. The effect of occlusion on the water content of the SC is relatively transitory, and typically returns to "normal" levels within 15 min after removal of an impermeable wrap. Since TEWL also returns to a normal level, it is likely that the reduction in barrier activity is also transitory.

Water uptake by the SC under occlusive conditions is primarily localized in the corneocytes. Hydration appears to have very little influence on the structure or properties of the intercellular lipids. Full hydration of the SC by occlusion appears to provoke the formation of water pools associated with rough structures. These structures can be considered as small water channels that reduce the diffusional path length and resistance for hydrophilic compounds. However, lipophilic as well as amphiphilic drugs may also profit from such shortened pathways.

A possible mechanism of occlusion action is that the swelling of the corneocytes directly alters the skin barrier function. Swelling of the corneocytes may provide an alternative penetration pathway, i.e., by facilitating entry into the corneocytes, increasing the diffusivity of compounds through the corneocytes, or altering the structure of a minor lipid component.

In general, skin permeation enhancers act at the level of the SC.[1070] The molecular basis of their activity can be attributed to: (1) an increase in the partitioning of compounds into the SC; (2) an increase in the diffusivity of the compound through the SC; and (3) a change in the penetration pathway.

The *in vitro* studies of passive transport of polar molecules, such as urea, mannitol, sucrose, and raffinose, across intact and two-hour ethanol pretreated human epidermal membrane (HEM) and theoretical analysis of the hindered diffusion showed that permeation pathways of HEM can be characterized by membrane porosity.[1077] Effective pore radii estimates for intact HEM fell between 1.5 to 2.5 nm, while similar estimates fell compactly between 1.5 to 2.0 nm for ethanol-pretreated HEM. Thus, approximately a 100-fold increase in permeability for ethanol-pretreated HEM relative to intact HEM was explained by increased porosity of HEM at extraction of HEM lipids by ethanol pretreatment, while creating pores with effective radii that are quite small.

Up to three orders of permeation decrease was found for large molecules (8000 Da) in comparison with the small ones (~200 Da).[1078] The examination of macromolecules' (up to 18 kDa) permeation through ethanol-pretreated (2 hr) HEM yielded estimates of effective pore sizes for this biological membrane in the range 2.2–5.4 nm.[1078] Approximately twice as large pore radii at studies with larger molecular size may reflect the existence of a distribution of pore sizes; probe permeants of larger molecular size would then yield a larger average pore size than those determined with smaller molecular permeants.

Such behavior was also observed in skin penetration studies where ethanol was topically applied.[1079–1082] In these studies, ethanol reduced the barrier of the SC due to its interaction with the intercellular lipids that resulted in enhanced SC permeation of topically applied substances, including aspirin. Effects of ethanol/propylene glycol composition on macroscopic barrier properties of skin were also analyzed.[1080]

Recently, ethanol evaporation through skin was measured after oral intake of ethanol (0.30 to 0.52 g/kg of body weight) at skin sites differing in the thickness of the SC and the density of follicles and sweat glands.[1083] The selective sealing of skin appendages had no significant influence on ethanol evaporation; this indicates that the evaporation of orally ingested ethanol occurs mostly through the SC lipid layers. Thus, an influence of ethanol on the penetration of topically applied products can be expected. However, in the study of Ref. 1083, orally administered ethanol had no effect on the penetration of a topically applied UV filter substance. Presumably, the available concentration of ethanol within the SC was too small (a theoretical maximum of 1.7 mg per 1 cm^2 skin surface) to influence its permeation significantly. Therefore, the effect of topically applied substances should not be influenced by a single ethanol dose of 31.2 g as used in the study.[1083]

Permeability of biological membranes may be induced not only by ethanol; a number of various chemical agents may serve as enhancers of membrane permeation.[1066,1070] For example, such a polyenic antibiotic as Amphotericin B provides a twofold increase in water permeation through a cell membrane, more than 44-fold for glycerol, and more than 200-fold for urea.[1066]

Dimethylsulfoxide (DMSO), a polar aprotic solvent, is also a good enhancer. This is a natural substance derived from wood pulp that has a unique capability to penetrate living tissues; to associate with water, proteins, carbohydrates, nucleic acid, ionic substances, and other constituents of living systems; possesses hygroscopic and antiinflammatory properties; and is FDA approved as a preservative of transplanting organs and for interstitial cystitis treatment.[1084]

A concentration of approximately 60% is required for activity of DMSO to disrupt the human skin barrier function, and enhancement ratios of 20–200 have been reported.[1070] DMSO provides irreversible disruption of the SC, perhaps due to solubilizing of the intercellular lipids and/or denaturing of proteins. Unfortunately, DMSO has some side effects such as skin irritation, chemical instability, the degree of damage to the SC, and the characteristic taste/odor of its oxidation products. Some other polar aprotic solvents also have been used experimentally as enhancers, but only one of them, decylmethylsulfoxide, has found its way into practice.[1070]

There are a great variety of surfactants that reduce the skin barrier function, classified as nonionic, anionic, and cationic based on the dependence of their charge at physiological pH.[1070] Certain unsaturated fatty acids increase percutaneous agent absorption by reducing the skin barrier function as well as by increasing the thermodynamic activity of compounds in some formulations.[1070] Monounsaturated fatty acid oleic acid (C18) is frequently chosen as a good enhancer for a wide variety of polar and moderately lipophilic compounds.[1027,1070] Oleic acid increases TEWL *in vivo* by approximately 1.5–2 times, consistent with a general decrease in the skin barrier function. There is a well-established synergy between the enhancer activity of oleic acid and propylene glycol vehicles.[1027,1070]

The stripping of the SC represents the simplest approach to physically enhancing the percutaneous absorption of a compound across skin [see Fig. 5.24(b)].[1044,1070] Although it is not always suitable for therapeutic applications because of irritation responses, skin stripping is a very useful scientific tool for evaluating the maximum amount of percutaneous agent absorption that can be expected from a topical application.[1085,1086]

The ultrasound or phonophoresis (sonophoresis) technique provides enhanced absorption of low-molecular-weight compounds as well as proteins such as insulin.[1070] A continuous or pulsed exposure of ultrasound of frequency from 20 kHz to 10 MHz at an intensity of up to 3 W/cm^2 can be applied during a period of up to 10 min. The intensity is limited by heat production in the tissue. The enhancement activity of high-frequency ultrasound (5–10 MHz) is connected with the induction of convective pathways through hair follicles and disruption of the intercellular lipid lamellae; the cavitation phenomenon when small air bubbles are formed within the SC plays an important role in its permeation.

A low-frequency ultrasound may be particularly suitable for enhancement.[1070] *In vivo* application of ultrasound of 20 kHz to the skin of hairless rats for 1 hr resulted in a 100-fold increase in TEWL and sufficient delivery of insulin through the skin to reduce the blood glucose levels of rats.

Iontophoresis refers to the enhancement of agent percutaneous absorption by the application of moderate (0.5 V/cm^2) voltages across the skin [see Fig. 5.24(c)].[1044,1070] Iontophoresis is not restricted to charged ions, and the flux of uncharged molecules across the skin is also enhanced in a process termed electroosmosis. This results from the combination of a reduced SC barrier and an induced solvent convective flow. Iontophoresis appears to drive molecules through discrete sites located in the SC such as hair follicles and sweat glands. A quantitative comparison of the flux of ions through appendages and through the intercellular lipid domain is estimated to be between 50 and 95% during iontophoresis.[1070] After a clinically relevant exposure of 0.16 mA/cm^2 for 1 hr, the subsequent permeability of human skin *in vitro* was reduced tenfold. The effect exists during and after application of the current and is fully reversible after approximately 24 hr. Enhancement of percutaneous absorption by iontophoresis has been studied for a wide variety of agents.[1070] At higher voltages (5–200 V/cm^2) and short pulse exposure, electroporation of biological membranes may occur,[1070] which also provides agent permeation into a tissue.

It was shown recently that laser-generated stress waves (photomechanical waves) can also permeabilize the SC.[1088–1091] Permeabilization of the SC was first demonstrated with δ-aminolevulenic acid (ALA) as a probe. The permeability of the SC depends on the peak stress. The onset of the permeability of the SC is observed at ~380 bar and increases with increasing peak stress. The efficiency of ALA transport through the SC is nonlinear. A small increase of the peak stress, from 440 to 500 bar (14% increase in peak pressure), caused the fluorescence intensity (protoporphyrin IX concentration induced by ALA application) to increase by ~200%. The application of stress waves does not cause any pain and discomfort and does not appear to affect the structure and viability of the skin. The change of the permeability of the SC is transient and its barrier function recovers within a few minutes. The increased permeability allows macromolecules to diffuse through the SC to epidermis and dermis. The maximum size of particles that has been transported through the SC is 100 nm in diameter.[1088] Thus, laser-generated stress waves can facilitate the transdermal delivery of large particles and molecules such as novel probes (carbon, gold, melanin nanoparticles, quantum dots, and encapsulated molecular probes), encapsulated drugs, or plasmid DNA. The combined action of laser-stress waves and anionic surfactant, such as sodium lauryl sulfate (2% of w/v), enhanced the delivery of nanoparticles through the SC.[1088] The application of sodium lauryl sulfate increases the size of the channels in the biomembrane as well as delays the recovery of the SC barrier function. The synergism of light and surfactant action was manifested as a significant reduction of time interval for providing the similar SC permeation: only 5 min of the application of sodium lauryl sulfate was enough at laser single pulse action (~7 J/cm^2), providing a peak pressure of ~600 bar and stress pulse duration of ~250 ns instead of a few hours without laser pulse.

It was also shown that laser-generated stress waves increase the permeability of the cell plasma membrane. The increase of the skin structures' permeability allows the introduction of macromolecules into the SC, the cytoplasm of living epidermal cells, and fibrous dermis. Thus, stress waves have the potential to deliver chemicals topically and noninvasively into the deep layers of the skin.

As a possible mechanism of the recently proposed method of enhancing skin permeability by creating a lattice of microzones of limited thermal damage in the SC by applying of a few consequent optical pulses,[1056,1057] the phase transition of SC intercellular lipids from the gel phase to the liquid crystalline phase due to local heating can be considered.[750,1092]

Alternative techniques of clearing agent delivery based on injection of an agent into the skin with a needle-free injection gun and laser skin surface ablation, and their combinations, are also under development.[1058,1059] A diode laser source with a 980 nm wavelength in conjunction with an artificial absorber on the skin surface was used to facilitate enhanced penetration of the topically applied skin clearing agent glycerol into *in vivo* hamster and rat skin.[1059] Such a technique provides a sufficient skin surface heating, which leads to keratinocyte disruption and possibly skin surface ablation of less than 20 μm with a treatment site of 16 mm^2 at laser beam scanning. Results indicate an improvement of the ability to deliver NIR light of 1290 nm up to 36% deeper into *in vivo* rodent skin using a laser fluence of less than 96 J/cm^2. Higher fluences caused unwanted thermal denaturation of skin tissue.

SC ablation can be provided directly by application of pulsed erbium lasers with wavelengths of 2790–2940 nm, corresponding to the strong water absorption band.[1093,1094] Laser ablation of 12.6% of the surface area of porcine SC produced a 2.8- and 2.1-fold increase in permeability constant (P_a) for ^{3}H-hydrocortisone and ^{125}I-γ-interferon, respectively.[1093] These studies demonstrate that a pulsed (250-μs pulse width) laser with a wavelength of 2790 nm and 1 J/cm^2 of fluence density can reliably and precisely remove the SC at 10–14 laser pulses, facilitating penetration of large molecules such as ^{125}I-γ-interferon, which cannot penetrate intact skin.

Among such modalities as skin microdermabrasion, iontophoreses, electroporation, and Erb:YAG ($\lambda = 2940$ nm) ablation, tested by the authors of Ref. 1094, laser ablation showed the greatest enhancement of ALA permeation through pig skin samples. Laser fluence was found to play an important role in controlling the drug flux, producing enhancement ratios from fourfold to 246-fold relative to the control. The skin permeation of ALA across microdermabrasion-treated skin was approximately fivefold to 15-fold higher than that across intact skin. The application of iontophoresis or electroporation alone also increased the ALA permeation by approximately 15-fold and twofold, respectively. The incorporation of iontophoresis or electroporation with the resurfacing techniques (laser ablation or microdermabrasion) caused a profound synergistic effect on ALA permeation.

The SC is functioning not only as a barrier against clearing agent penetration into skin, but also as a reservoir for topically applied substances.[1095,1096] Skin appendages, in particular sebaceous glands, also serve as reservoirs for clearing agents.[988–990,1085,1097]

For the development of technologies for topical application of clearing agents, the knowledge of the reservoir function is of fundamental interest. The long-term reservoir functioning of the SC in human skin was investigated in vivo.[1095,1096] Using laser confocal scanning microscopy and the tape stripping method, the long-term reservoir of the SC was determined both qualitatively and quantitatively, depending on the polarity of the applied formulation. Formulations with different physicochemical properties were studied. A follicular long-term reservoir was only observed for hydrophilic sodium fluorescein after application in propylene glycol. A follicular penetration of dyes was also reported for the application in emulsions,[1085] solvents such as ethanol and glycerol,[988–990] and 5-μm microspheres containing dye and suspended in silicon oil at w/w concentration of 4%.[1097] The penetration depth and reservoir properties of human skin in vivo for methylene blue (MB) and indocyanine green (ICG) dissolved in ethanol/glycerol solvents were recently reported.[988–990] These studies were applied for the improvement of sebaceous glands functioning at photodynamic acne treatment; the most intensive sebaceous gland staining was just after the 15–20 min massage and heating procedure. It was also shown that highly porous nylon microspheres suspended in silicon oil provide a penetration depth of MB into hairless rat skin in vivo up to 150 μm in 2 hr and 400 μm in 26 hr.[1097]

The results of the study described in Refs. 988–990 and 1095–1097 led to the assumption that the better the penetration into the SC and the follicles, the longer the reservoir will remain there. Two pathways of release of the dyes from the reservoir are possible: (1) the desquamation of the SC and, the release of sebum, respectively, or (2) the penetration into the viable tissue.

In conclusion it should be noted that for topically applied UV skin filters their efficiency may be significantly reduced, if not, appropriate cosmetic composition will be used as a ground material for such a filter. Two main effects can be important: (1) reduction of light scattering in SC due to optical immersion and (2) inhomogeneous distribution of the topically applied substances.[1087] Both effects lead to reduction of UV filters' efficiency: the first because of a fewer number of interactions of migrating photons in skin with sunscreen material at less scattering, and the second because of the formation of islands free of sunscreen that are not blocking UV radiations. The second problem is analyzed in detail in Ref. 1087.

5.5 Optical clearing of gastric tissue

5.5.1 Spectral measurements

Transmittance and diffuse reflectance measurements were performed over a range from 800 to 2200 nm for frozen-thawed and fresh native porcine stomach cardiac and pyloric mucosa sections of 1.2–1.6 mm in thickness.[932,971,972,1011,1026,1027] Mucosa consists of moist epithelium and the connective tissue immediately beneath it. Mucosal structure is somewhat identical to skin, with cell epidermal and fibrous dermal layers. The absence of the dead cell layer, such as SC of skin, makes normal mucosa more permeable for chemical agents. Immersion solutions (glycerol/DMSO/water) of different concentrations were topically applied onto the epithelium surface of the sample and then spectra were acquired at time intervals of 5, 10, 20, and 30 min. The difference in apparent absorbance (extracted from the diffuse reflectance) between two wavelengths, 1936 and 1100 nm, was used to estimate water content. Some results are presented in Fig. 5.32. It can be seen from Figs. 5.32(a) and 5.32(b) that over the whole wavelength range investigated, the transmittance was increased with time and diffuse reflectance was decreased over the range of 800–1370 nm. The greatest increase in transmittance was at 1278 nm, and the greatest decrease in reflectance was at 1066 nm.

A strong correlation has been found between optical clearing and water desorption.[971,972,1011,1026,1027] At 30 min after the treatment, 80%-glycerol caused 15% water loss, whereas 50% glycerol and 50% DMSO caused 9% and 7% water loss, respectively. The patterns of optical clearing are similar to those of water desorption. The water loss was maximal (~19%) and optical transmittance at 1278 nm was also maximal (~30%) for the mixture of 50% glycerol and 30% DMSO (synergetic effect).

Reduction of scattering and water absorption allows one to get more pronounced signatures of absorbing bands of tissue components. In particular, this is

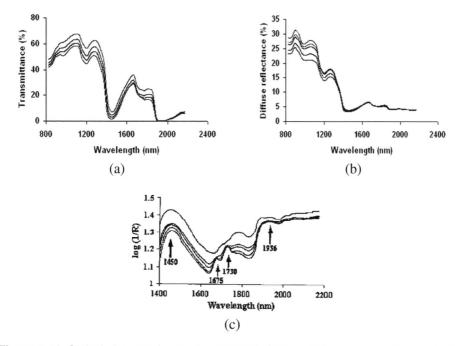

Figure 5.32 Optical changes for porcine stomach fresh pyloric mucosa before and after application of an immersion solution, measured by spectrophotometer with an integrating sphere at the time intervals of 0, 5, 10, 20, and 30 min [(a) from bottom to top, (b) and (c) from top to bottom], respectively. (a) Total transmittance, and (b) diffuse reflectance over the range of 800–2200 nm after topical application of 80%-glycerol onto the epithelium surface of a sample of thickness 1.6 ± 0.2 mm.[932,971] (c) Apparent absorbance spectra calculated from diffuse reflectance measurements over the range of 1400–2200 nm after application of 50%-DMSO, a sample of thickness 1.15 ± 0.12 mm.[972]

demonstrated by the apparent absorbance spectra (1400–2200 nm) in Fig. 5.32(c) measured at 50% DMSO solution application. The major features of these spectra are the bands near 1450 and 1936 nm, corresponding to the first overtone of OH stretch in water and the combination mode of OH stretch and HOH bend in water, respectively. DMSO application significantly changes the absorbance spectrum of the tissue. The peaks of 1730 and 1675 nm appeared at 5 min after DMSO administration, i.e., with the water loss (scattering and water absorption reduction) and possibly corresponding to resolvable CH groups in lipids and proteins.

5.5.2 OCT imaging

In vitro studies of optical clearing of gastrointestinal tissues, such as stomach, esophagus, and colonic mucosa, were also performed using the OCT imaging technique.[967,968,971,1012] Figure 5.33 shows two OCT images of intact and normal fresh human stomach tissue (fundus) treated by 80% propylene glycol solution. A more cleared image with excellent differentiation of epithelium, isthmus, lamina propia, and muscular tissue is achieved at the agent action.[967,968]

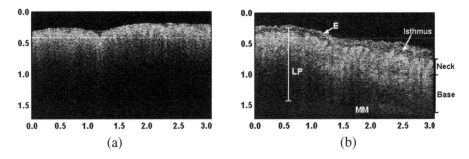

(a)   (b)

Figure 5.33 OCT images of normal fresh human stomach tissue (fundus): (a) without and (b) with topical application of 80%-propylene glycol solution. E, epithelium; LP, lamina propia; MM, muscularis mucusae.[967]

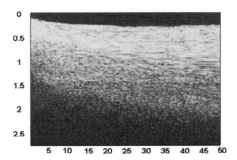

Figure 5.34 The time course of repeated OCT A-scans of porcine stomach tissue with the application of glycerol. The horizontal and vertical axes represent the time (min) and the imaging depth (mm), respectively; the registration of the OCT signal starts at time ~0.5 min after the agent application.[1012]

Figure 5.34 illustrates the M-mode OCT images obtained from repeated A-scans of porcine stomach with the application of glycerol.[1012] From the image, it is clearly seen that the penetration depth increases gradually with the increase of time duration. There is a slope of the surface of the tissue. The downward trend of the tissue surface is attributed to tissue dehydration induced by the chemical agent.

It should be pointed out that the experiments mentioned above were performed on *in vitro* biological tissues. The dynamic optical clearing effect induced by the chemical agent would differ from that of the *in vivo* case. Because of cell self-regulation and blood circulation, the living tissues would have less dehydration after the application of a hyperosmotic chemical agent.

5.6 Other prospective optical techniques

5.6.1 Polarization measurements

Dynamics of the polarization structure of a tissue image at immersion can be easily observed using an optical scheme with a "white" light source and a tissue sample placed between two in-parallel or crossed polarizers. Figure 5.35 illustrates the evolution of polarization images during scleral optical clearing.[442,1065] In such experiments, a tissue layer "works" as a phase plate (or number of phase plates[441,1034]) in which linear birefringence is spatially and temporally dependent. As scattering decreases with time due to refractive index matching, the birefringence of the fibrillar structure of the sclera affects the transmittance of the optical system. The spatial inhomogeneities of images may be due to spatial variations of the sample thickness and structure, both of which may influence the efficiency of the OCA impregnation and corresponding phase shift between the orthogonal optical field components (see Section 1.4).[410]

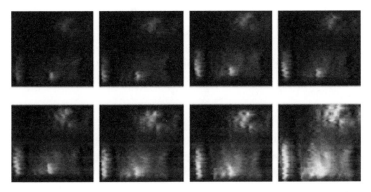

Figure 5.35 Polarization images of a sclera sample (white light source, crossed polarizers). Images from left to the right correspond to 4, 5, 6, 7, 8, 9, 9.5, and 10 min of tissue impregnation by trazograph-60. The supporting wires of the sample are seen for the translucent tissue.[442,1065]

At reduced scattering, the degree of linearly polarized light propagating in sclera improves. This is clearly seen from the experimental graphs in Figs. 5.10 and 5.36.[1033] As far as immersed tissue, the number of scattering events decreases and the residual polarization degree of transmitted linearly polarized light increases. As a result, the dynamics of tissue average transmittance and polarization degree are similar (see Fig. 5.10). It follows from Figs. 5.10 and 5.36 that tissue optical clearing leads to increasing depolarization length.[36,135,138,383,438,1098] Due to less scattering of the longer wavelengths, the initial polarization degree is the highest for these wavelengths. The polarization imaging is a useful tool for detection of subsurface lesions, but it is effective only at depths smaller than the depolarization length.[36,382,383] Optical clearing may give a possibility to substantially increase the depth of polarization imaging.

The image contrast $C(t) = B(t)/B_{max}$, where $B(t)$ is the current sample brightness and B_{max} is the maximal one, characterizing transmittance of linear polarized light through a tissue sample, was used for a quantitative evaluation of the diffusion process of an agent in a tissue. A white-light video-digital polarization microscope is suitable for the measurements.[409] Sections of the various connective and vascular tissues of a thickness of 0.1–1.5 mm were studied. The immersion solution was

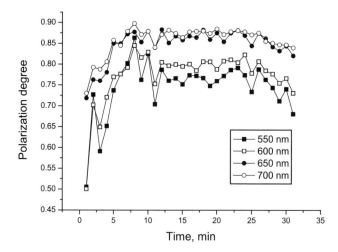

Figure 5.36 The time-dependent polarization degree, $(I_\parallel - I_\perp)/(I_\parallel - I_\perp)$, of collimated transmittance measured *in vitro* at different wavelengths for rabbit eye sclera at administration of 40%-glucose.[1033]

heated to 36–40°C and simply dropped on the tissue sample surface. Figure 5.37 shows different rates of tissue optical clearing for vein and aorta samples caused by the different interaction of these tissues with the immersion agent—the denser aorta is less penetrative for the agent than vein; therefore, its action on aorta can be seen only in a few hours, whereas for the vein sample about 10 min is enough to complete clearing. However, both tissues finally turn from an initially turbid (multiple scattering mode) at $t = 0$ to a less depolarized and more transparent state (less scattering mode), $C(t) \to 1$.

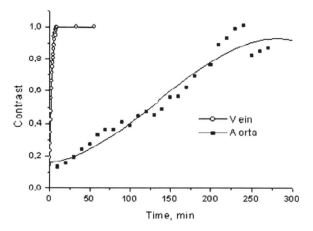

Figure 5.37 Experimental temporal dependencies for image contrast of linear polarized light transmitted through vascular tissue sections (aorta and vein-*vena cava inferior*) measured by a white-light video-digital polarization microscope at the application of trazograph-60.[409]

Reduced scattering at optical immersion makes it possible to detect the polarization anisotropy of tissues more easily and to separate the effects of light scattering and intrinsic birefringence on the tissue polarization properties. It is also possible to study birefringence of form with optical immersion; but when the immersion is strong, the average refractive index of the tissue structure is close to the index of the ground media, and the birefringence of form may be too small to see because both phenomena are based on the refractive index mismatch—scattering due to irregular refractive index variations, and birefringence due to regular ones [see Eqs. (1.53) and (1.54)].

At reduced scattering, tissue birefringence can be measured more precisely; in particular, birefringence of form and material can be separated. For example, for the translucent human scleral sample by its impregnation with a highly concentrated glucose solution (about 70%), the measured optical anisotropy[410] $\Delta n = (n_e - n_o)$ was $\approx 10^{-3}$. This is 1.5-fold to 4.5-fold less than for other birefringent tissues described in Section 1.4, and is mostly explained by a reduction of inclusion of birefringence of form at optical immersion. The additional measurements of the collimated transmittance allows one to estimate the refractive index of the ground substance of the translucent tissue n_2 using the expressions from radiative transfer and Mie theories [see Eqs. (5.1) and (5.16)]. For a human scleral sample impregnated by 70% glucose solution, n_2 was evaluated as 1.39. Using this value and the value of the refractive index of hydrated collagen, $n_1 = 1.47$, and $\Delta n = 10^{-3}$, the collagen volume fraction f_1 was calculated from Eq. (1.53) as $f_1 \cong 0.32$, which correlates well with an estimation made in Section 3.1.

Figure 5.10 illustrates the reversibility of the polarization immersion effect. A polarization-speckle microscope working in transmittance mode was used to carry out these measurements.[343,1030] The sample was irradiated by a linear polarized focused laser beam that was scanned along the trace of 1.5 mm on the sample surface to average the speckle modulation in the far zone, where the analyzer and photodetector were placed. Two orthogonal linear polarized components of the transmitted light were detected. It can be seen that the sample initially had poor transmittance with the equal intensity components $\langle I_\parallel \rangle = \langle I_\perp \rangle$ and that multiple scattering takes place. When the immersion agent acts in the fourteenth minute, $\langle I_\parallel \rangle$ prevails substantially over $\langle I_\perp \rangle$, and the tissue becomes less scattering. The subsequent action of the physiological solution, which washes out the immersion agent, returns the tissue to its normal state, and it becomes turbid again in the twenty-second minute with no measured difference between the intensities of the orthogonally polarized components. The secondary application of the immersion agent again makes the tissue less scattering and more polarization sensitive with a maximum reached at the twenty-eighth minute.

Figure 5.38 shows the reversible loss of turbidity and birefringence in rodent tail tendon observed at glycerol (13 M) application.[946] The dark background in each of the images demonstrates the extinction of illuminating light at the crossed polarizers in the polarized light microscope used in the measurements. Characteristic banding patterns observed in the tendon sample indicate ordered fibril organization. The distribution of pattern brightness corresponds to the distribution of

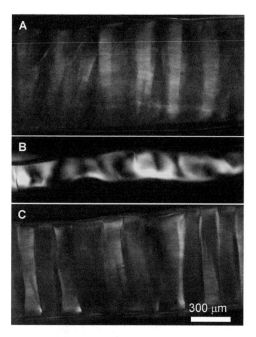

Figure 5.38 Reversible loss of turbidity and birefringence in rodent tail tendon following glycerol (13 M) application observed by polarized light microscopy at crossed polarizers. (A) Before glycerol application: banding patterns observed in the tendon indicate ordered fibril organization. (B) At glycerol application: loss of transmittance at the sample edges and bright spots in the middle indicate refractive index matching of collagen fibers; the complete refractive index matching at the edge region causes the tissue to lose scattering and birefringence, whereas in the middle sample region the refractive index is not completed and mostly scattering is reduced (loss of turbidity). (C) The tissue sample after rehydration in saline (figure was kindly presented by Alvin T. Yeh and Bernard Choi).

a phase shift between orthogonal optical field components [see Eq. (1.52)], and the smooth background brightness corresponds to light scattering. Loss of transmittance at the sample edges and the appearance of bright spots in the middle of the sample in the course of glycerol action indicate refractive index matching of collagen fibers (not seen in the image due to their small diameter). The complete refractive index matching at the edge region happens earlier than in the middle of the sample, and causes tissue to lose scattering and birefringence completely in this region. In the middle region of the sample, refractive index matching is not completed and scattering is mostly reduced (loss of turbidity); thus, bright and dark areas that correspond to a certain phase shift are well seen. Tissue shrinkage at the glycerol action due to tissue dehydration, and hypothesized by the authors of Ref. 946, the reversible dissociation of collagen fibers may have influence on the pattern formation. The rehydration of the tissue sample in saline makes its banding structure fully visible in the crossed polarizers due to resumption of the tissue birefringence and turbidity approximately to the initial states.

Practically all healthy connective and vascular tissues show the strong or weak optical anisotropy typical of either uniaxial or biaxial crystals.[409,410,441,1034] Pathological tissues show isotropic optical properties.[29,382,383]

5.6.2 Confocal microscopy

Increasing of the upper tissue layers' transparency can improve the penetration depth, image contrast, and spatial resolution in confocal microscopy as well.[896,897] By Monte Carlo simulations of the point-spread function, it was shown that the signal spatial localization offered by a confocal probe in the skin tissues during their clearing is potentially useable for *reticular dermis* monitoring (Fig. 4.20).[759] The results of the simulation predict that after 20 min of the chemical agent diffusion after intradermal glycerol or glucose injection, a signal from the tissues located twice as deep in skin can be detected.

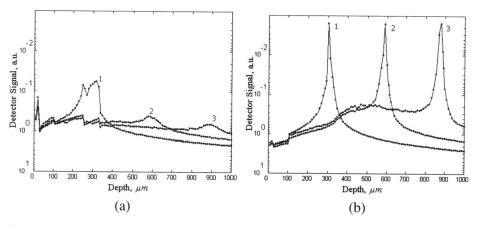

(a)   (b)

Figure 5.39 The axial profile of a detector signal distribution (a) before and (b) 20 min after glycerol administration (intradermal injection) predicted by numerical Monte Carlo simulation for a confocal microscope focusing at (1) 300 μm, (2) 600 μm, and (3) 900 μm into the skin. Confocal probe parameters are: lens diameter 5 mm and focal length 10 mm; pinhole diameter is 10 μm; the height of the lens above the surface is 9.7 mm (see Fig. 4.19).[897]

A significant improvement of the confocal microscopy signal at glycerol administration is well seen from theoretical axial profiles of a detected signal calculated for three different in-depth focusings (Fig. 5.39).[897]

5.6.3 Fluorescence detection

Recently, the improvement of the detected fluorescence signal traveling through skin in *in vitro* and *in vivo* experiments at topical application of hyperosmotic OCAs, such as anhydrous glycerol (13 M, index $n = 1.47$) and pure DMSO (14 M, index $n = 1.47$), and a highly concentrated glucose (7 M, index $n = 1.46$), was demonstrated.[777] Fluorescence measurements were performed for hamster dorsal skin with OCA applied to the subdermal side of the skin and rhodamine fluorescent film placed against the same skin side. Fluorescence was induced by a dye laser pulse at 542 nm delivered to the skin epidermal side by a fiber bundle and was detected by a collection fiber bundle from the epidermal surface at wavelengths longer than 565 nm. A skin flap window preparation in an area void of blood vessels was used for *in vivo* studies. Approximately equal enhancement of transmitted fluorescence was achieved for *in vitro* and *in vivo* measurements (Fig. 5.40). On average, up to 100% increase in fluorescence intensity is seen for 20-min glucose and glycerol applications, and up to 250% for DMSO. The significantly larger increase in the case of DMSO is associated with its twice greater osmolarity than for the glycerol and glucose concentrations used.

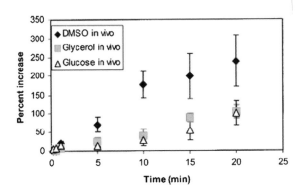

Figure 5.40 Comparison of the percent increase in fluorescent signal due to 100%-glycerol, 100%-DMSO, and 7M glucose *in vivo*.[777]

A significant enhancement of both the sensitivity (~fivefold) and the spatial resolution (~threefold) for low-level light-emitting probes (a broadband violet-blue chemiluminescence with a center wavelength of 425 nm) was demonstrated in *in vitro* experiments with a 3-mm-thick fresh porcine skin sample at topical application of 50%-glycerol during 30 min.[977] A higher efficiency of luminescent light transportation through the skin at immersion in that case is connected with a higher initial scattering and absorption of skin at the shorter wavelengths. Refractive index matching effectively damps light scattering, and thus absorption of light also occurs due to the lower number of photons circulating within a tissue.

In a recent theoretical study,[976] it was shown that by refractive index matching at the skin interface and with a fiber-optical fluorescence probe, one can improve the contrast and spatial resolution of the shallow sampling volume.

Both model experiments described above well demonstrated changes of tissue layer transmittance at optical immersion for light from a fluorescent source placed behind a tissue layer. However, fluorophores are more often distributed within a tissue layer or even a multilayered tissue structure and may contain a number of different fluorophores. In that case, the behavior of a fluorescence signal at tissue immersion is not so evident because the cross section for fluorescence emission depends on the amount of the absorbed light by fluorescent centers. Such a cross section decreases as multiple scattering decreases. Thus, at tissue optical clearing, instead of an enhanced fluorescence signal, one can see its damping. Evidently, that depends on the depth, where the fluorophore is, and what layer of a tissue is optically cleared.

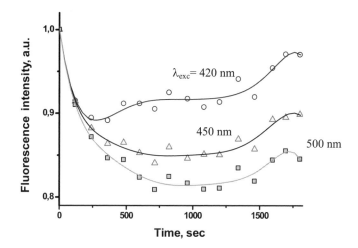

Figure 5.41 *In vivo* dynamics of human skin autofluorescence intensity ($\lambda_{exc} = 337$ nm) after intradermal injection of 0.1 ml of trazograph-76. Intensity values at different emission wavelengths are normalized by correspondent initial values.[975]

Figure 5.41 illustrates that fluorescence can be damped at tissue scattering reduction due to refractive index matching.[975] These data were received *in vivo* for human skin at intradermal injection of the immersion liquid, trazograth-76. Such behavior of the autofluorescence signal means that the main fluorophore (collagen) is in the dermis, where the immersion agent was inserted. However, with time, due to more in-depth penetration of the exciting light and less attenuation of the induced fluorescence by the upper layers of skin, fluorescence intensity is going up. Tissue optical clearing can be a helpful technology in looking for endogenous or exogenous fluorophore distribution within a tissue, and their differentiation.

5.6.4 Two-photon scanning fluorescence microscopy

One of the new directions in tissue spectroscopy is associated with multiphoton fluorescence scanning microscopy (see Section 1.7.2).[114,122,131,137,609–618,1099–1102] However, it has been shown that the effect of light scattering in multiphoton fluorescence scanning microscopy is to drastically reduce the penetration depth to less than that of the equivalent single-photon fluorescence while largely leaving the resolution unchanged.[618,1099] This happens mostly due to excitation beam defocusing (distortion) in the scattering media. Although some improvement in the penetration depth of two-photon microscopy can be obtained by optimizing the pulse shape and repetition rate for the sample under investigation,[1100] reduction of scattering is believed to be more effective with penetration-depth and image-contrast improvement.[1063] Two-photon fluorescence microscopy provides high-resolution images of human skin *in vivo*.[1101,1102] Evidently, the technique is applicable for many other tissues, but its penetration depth is normally limited to 20–30 μm.

The first demonstration of two-photon in-depth signal improvement using the optical immersion technique with hyperosmotic agents, such as glycerol, propylene glycol, and glucose, was done by the authors of Ref. 1063 in *ex vivo* experiments with human dermis. Thick (150 μm) slices of dermis excised during plastic surgery were imaged within the same day. Images were collected in stacks, each comprising four images of a 100 μm² area taken at depths of 20, 40, 60, and 80 μm from the surface of the sample. Before data acquisition, the sample was immersed in 0.1 ml of phosphate buffered saline (PBS) in order to prevent drying and shrinkage. The sample was then immersed in 0.5 ml of an OCA and one image stack was acquired every 30 s for 6–7 min. The OCA was finally removed and the sample was immersed again in 0.1 ml of PBS in order to observe the reversibility of the clearing process. Glycerol and propylene glycol were both used in anhydrous form, and glucose as a concentrated aqueous solution (5M). The upper limit of tissue shrinkage was estimated as 2% in the course of 6–7 min of OCA application.

The average contrast in each image and relative contrast (RC) were defined as[1063]

$$\text{contrast} = \sum_{i,j=1}^{N_{\text{lines}}} |I_{ij} - \langle I_{ij} \rangle|, \quad \text{RC}(\%) = 100 \frac{\text{contrast[OCA]} - \text{contrast[PBS]}}{\text{contrast[PBS]}},$$

where $\langle I_{ij} \rangle$ is the mean intensity of the nearest eight pixels and $N_{\text{lines}} = N - 2$, with $N = 500$; contrast [OCA] and contrast [PBS] are calculated for OCA and PBS immersion, respectively. Contrast, as defined here, is linearly dependent on the fluorescence intensity and varies according to structures in the image. Hence, its usefulness is primarily to enable comparison between images of the same sample at the same depth, maintaining the same field of view. Normalization to the total intensity would be required in order to compare different images. The relative contrast RC also serves for the purpose of comparison.

Figure 5.42(a) shows two typical images stacks: the first received for a sample immersed in PBS and the second received 7 min after application of glycerol. The images show connective tissue in human dermis, which is primarily composed of collagen and elastin fibers. The enhancement of contrast as well as the increase of penetration depth (from 40 to 80 μm) and total intensity [i.e., the intensity summed over all pixels, Fig. 5.42(b)] are clearly seen from the images. The corresponding absolute and relative contrast levels are plotted in Figs. 5.42(a) and 5.42(d). RC has a value of 215% at 40 μm and dramatically increases with increasing depth.

The effect on deeper layers is greater because of the cumulative effect of the reduction in scattering in the superficial layers of the tissue sample, which provides less attenuation of the incident and detected fluorescent light. The contrast is also dependent on fluorescence intensity, which is proportional to the squared intensity of the excitation intensity and mostly dependent on the excitation beam focusing ability. The better focus (less focused beam distortion) is achieved in a less scattering media.

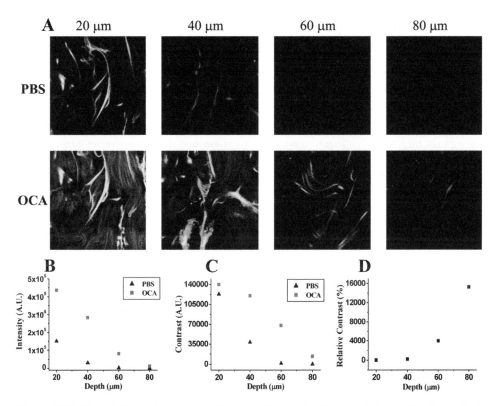

Figure 5.42 Two-photon microscopy of human skin *ex vivo* by use of glycerol as the optical clearing agent.[1063] (a) Image stacks for a skin dermis sample immersed in PBS (upper) and after immersion for 7 min in glycerol (lower). The corresponding total intensity, contrast, and relative contrast are plotted in (b), (c), and (d), respectively.

It was shown experimentally that application of each OCA among glycerol, propylene glycol, and glucose resulted in contrast enhancement with varying degrees of efficiency and saturation. The dynamics and the final contrast level attained depend on the OCA and on the tissue depth. Saturation of contrast occurs most rapidly in superficial layers of the sample. This is consistent with a diffusion model for the penetration of the agent from the surface into the tissue [see Eqs. (5.2), (5.6), and (5.7)], i.e., if the contrast is proportional to agent concentration, then the saturation time at a given depth will be proportional to the depth. As it follows from data of Ref. 1063, glycerol is the most efficient with respect to saturation level (RC = 49.7% at 20 μm depth, ~304% at 40 μm depth, ~1900% at 60 μm depth, and ~9260% at 80 μm depth), but also the slowest. Propylene glycol provides RC ~ 64% at 20 μm depth, ~1090% at 40 μm depth, ~5640% at

60 μm depth, and ~447% at 80 μm depth. Whereas, glucose (5M) is the worst with RC = 10.9% at 20 μm depth, ~134% at 40 μm depth, ~471% at 60 μm depth, and ~406% at 80 μm depth, but diffuses three times faster than glycerol and five times faster than propylene glycol. Diluted agents gave similar tendencies in contrast enhancement and increase of penetration depth, providing higher efficiency in both characteristics with OCA concentration increase.

These data illustrate that, as well as in linear spectroscopy, the refractive index matching is the leading mechanism in reduction of tissue scattering and two-photon signal improvement. In contrast to *in vivo* single-photon fluorescence spectroscopy (see Fig. 5.41), where fluorescence intensity may decrease at multiple scattering decrease, a two-photon tomography signal is always increased due to less distortion of the focused beam and less attenuation of a two-photon fluorescence signal by superficial optically cleared tissue layers. However, there was found some specificity in action of the three different OCAs. Results presented in Ref. 1063 show for propylene glycol and glucose a slowing in the rate of contrast increase following addition of PBS rather than a decrease as it is seen for glycerol. Such behavior may be associated with a lesser inclusion of the dehydration mechanism in optical clearing for propylene glycol and glucose, and a greater amount of these agents diffused into a tissue in comparison with glycerol.

5.6.5 Second-harmonic generation

Optical clearing seems to be a promising technique for improvement of detected signals in multiphoton microscopy and nonlinear spectroscopy, and imaging of tissues.[946,947] On the other hand, these techniques might be useful in the understanding of molecular mechanisms of tissue optical clearing at immersion and dehydration.

In skin, second harmonic generation (SHG) (see Section 4.6) is provided mostly within dermis due to its main component, which is collagen that has an appreciable nonlinear susceptibility. Evidently, due to optical clearing, less scattering in the epidermis for the incident long wavelength light (800 nm), and especially for the backward SHG short wavelength light (400 nm), may improve SHG images of dermis collagen structures.

At 100%-glycerol application to rodent skin dermis and tendon samples, as well as to engineered tissue model (raft), a high efficiency of tissue optical clearing was achieved in the wavelength range from 400 to 700 nm, but the SHG signal was significantly degraded in the course of glycerol application and it was returned back to the initial state after tissue rehydration by application of saline.[946] The loss of the SHG signal in Ref. 946 is associated with the collagen fibers' reversible dissociation and corresponding loss of fibril organization at glycerol action. Such an explanation is somewhat contradictory because less organization of collagen fibers will lead to less transmittance.[442] Since the significant effect of optical clearing at glycerol application is tissue dehydration, the following explanation of data from Ref. 947 seems to be more adequate. Using reflective-type SHG polarimetry, it was shown in Ref. 947 that the SHG polarization signal (SHG radar graphs) for chicken skin dermis was almost unchanged (Fig. 5.43) and the SHG intensity was decreased to about a fourth at tissue dehydration. The authors have hypothesized that the decrease of the SHG intensity results in a change of linear optical properties, i.e., scattering efficiency, rather than that of the efficiency of SHG radiation in the tissues. As it follows from Fig. 5.43, the tissue fixation process also indicates almost unchanged SHG polarization radar graphs while SHG intensity was slightly increased. Since formalin fixing induces cross-linking of collagen in tissues, this result may imply that the cross-linking does not affect collagen orientation but essentially contributes to the efficiency of the SHG signal.[947] These two examples illustrate the dependence of the SHG signal on light scattering of the sample, which was decreased at tissue dehydration and increased at tissue fixation. Thus, to study tissue structure (collagen orientation) using SHG, one of the methods that provides light-scattering suppression may be applied, such as SHG polarimetry[947] or the optical immersion technique.

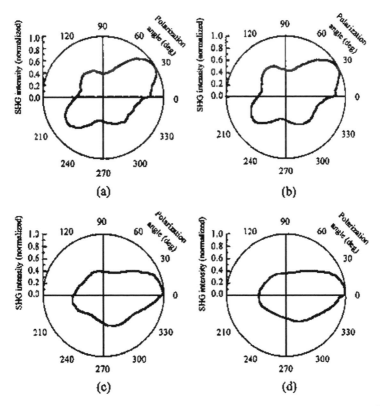

Figure 5.43 SHG radar graphs received for native samples of chicken dermis.[947] SHG signal distributions (a) before and (b) 5 hr after formalin fixation, (c) before and (d) 13 hr after air drying.

5.7 Cell and cell flows imaging

5.7.1 Blood flow imaging

Small blood microvessels can be clearly identified visually by the naked eye in *in vivo* study of hamster[571,979] and rat[980] skin, where a transparent window in the skin was created by glycerol drops to the subdermal side of a native hamster dorsal skin flap window preparation,[979] or by intradermal injection of glycerol[571,980] or 40%-glucose[980] (see Fig. 5.25). In an *in vitro* study of fresh human fat tissue at topical application of a propylene glycol (PG) solution (50–80% with pure water), blood vessels were also seen.[1008]

Besides more precise visualization of the vessel network, immersion agents may have influence on blood microvessel functioning[571,831,866,867,979,980] that gives the possibility of controlling the functioning tissue within the area of agent action. Functioning of microvessels of rat mesentery under the topical action of glycerol and glucose was described.[980] A topical application of 75%-glycerol during the initial period of 1–3 s led to a slowing down of blood flow in all microvessels (arterioles, venules, and capillaries). After 20–25 s, the stasis appeared and vessels were dilated by 30% on average, intravascular hemolysis took place to 1 min after agent application diameters of vessels were increased still more, to 40%. To the sixth minute, stasis was maintained in all vessels, but the diameters of vessels were slightly decreased. Such changes of microcirculation were exactly local within the area of glycerol application. The topical application of glucose also decreased blood flow velocity in microvessels. For example, at an action of 40% glucose on a venule with a diameter of 11 μm and with initial flow rate of 1075 μm/s, the flow rate decreased to 510 μm/s at 3 s after glucose application and to 202 μm/s at 5 s. Similarly with the action of glycerol, there were dilation and stasis of blood flow in all vessels (arterioles, venules, capillaries, and shunts) within 20–30 s, but no intravascular hemolysis was found, and only RBC aggregates in the lumen of microvessels were seen. The strength of vessel dilation was more than that for glycerol; the mean diameter increased by 30% to the thirtieth second after glucose application, but to the fourth minute, it rose on average by 2.5 times. From the third to the fifth minute, blood flow appeared again in a few microvessels and the velocity of reflow was markedly slower than in the control. The changes in blood flow were also local, but with a larger area than for glycerol, approximately 1 × 1 cm, and there were no any disturbances in the functioning of blood microvessels in the other parts of the mesentery. Evidently, a decrease in glucose concentration and corresponding loss of the agent hyperosmotic property led to softer glucose action on blood circulation; in particular, no blood stasis were observed for 20%-glucose, and after 3–4 min of glucose application, blood flow in all vessels was not significantly different from the initial one.

The vasculature under the *dura mater* also became visible after the treatment of glycerol in an *in vivo* experiment with rabbit.[831,866,867] The reflectance decreased as a function of time of glycerol action, which proved the visual observation. The *dura mater* nearly recovered to the native condition after 1 min. Velocity images of *in vivo* cerebral blood flow (CBF) under the effect of glycerol are shown in Fig. 5.44. Glycerol was applied around the exposed area. When glycerol diffused in brain tissue and influenced CBF under the *dura mater*, the CBF in the exposed area would also change. Figure 5.45 illustrates the spatiotemporal characteristics of CBF changes under the treatment of glycerol. Under the action of glycerol, blood flow first decreased while the blood vessels underneath the *dura mater* became increasingly visible. The blood flow then increased to near baseline; at the same time, the turbidity of the *dura mater* returned. Figure 5.45 gives the time course of changes in four different vessels (Fig. 5.44), which is expressed as the ratio of the measured velocity in the conditions of treatment with glycerol to that of the control condition. Vessel 2 is an arteriole. Vessels 1, 3, and 4 are veinules. Blood flow in vessel 2 (arteriole) began to decrease after the twenty-second application of glycerol, while that in the other vessels (veinules) decreased immediately after application with glycerol. The blood flow in vessel 1 decreased slower than that in the other vessels, which suggested that blood flow in the arteriole had a different response from that in the veinules. Blood flow in all vessels decreased to 70–80% of baseline after treatment with glycerol.

An example of the subdermal side of native hamster dorsal skin flap window preparation is shown in Fig. 5.46(a). The main arteriole (A) is 97 ± 18 μm in diameter (lumen) and the main venule (V) is 188 ± 21 μm in diameter. The diameters of the branches, a and v, are 92 ± 18 μm and 181 ± 21 μm, respectively. Figure 5.46(b) shows the blood vessels in the same window preparation ten minutes after the application of 100%-glycerol. The smallest branches of the arterioles and venules can now be seen in the image. This is likely due to the increased clearing of the tissue overlying the vessels and could also occur with vasodilation. The venule branch, v, is dilated to 259 ± 19 μm. The main vessels and the arteriole branch (a), however, are not noticeably dilated. After twenty minutes, the main venule branch in the window preparation appears very dark and is occluded [Fig. 5.46(c)]. The diameters of the main vessels are 97 ± 18 mm (A), and 189 ± 20 mm (V), and the diameters of the branches are 141 ± 17 mm (a) and 259 ± 21 mm (v).

Optical clearing of vascularized tissue may have some important biomedical applications connected with the investigation of vascular system structure and function, including the relation of the diameters of arterioles and venules, capillary density, bifurcation angles, etc. These parameters can be important in physiology and therapy for the diagnosis and treatment of some diseases (vascular disease, cancer, etc.). On the other hand, the optical clearing effect coupled with temporary and local cessation of blood flow in microvessels in the area of treatment may help vascular photothermal therapy significantly.[979]

5.7.2 Optical clearing of blood

Refractive index mismatch between erythrocyte cytoplasm and blood plasma causes strong scattering of blood that, for example, prevents getting high-quality

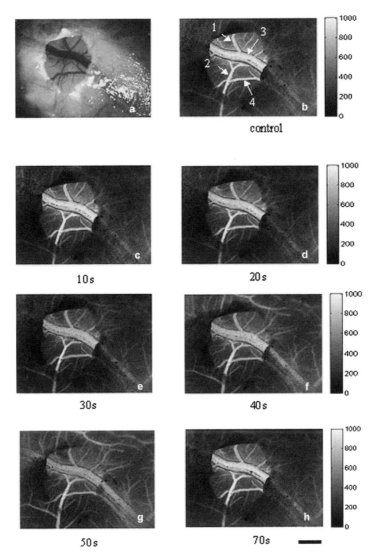

Figure 5.44 Blood flow images following the epidural application of glycerol around the exposed area of *in vivo dura mater*. (a) The white-light image of the area of interest. (b)–(h) Blood flow maps expressed as measured velocity, which is proportional to the blood flow velocity, during the treatment with glycerol and represented by images at the time points shown in Fig. 5.45. (b) Imaged blood flow before the application of glycerol (control); four vessels are indicated. (c) Ten-second application of glycerol, no obvious change in blood flow was observed. (d) Twenty-second application of glycerol, blood flow began to decrease. (e) Thirty-second application of glycerol, the blood vessels underneath the *dura mater* began to be clear. (f) Forty-second application of glycerol, blood flow decreased and the transparency of the surrounding *dura mater* increased. (g) Fifty-second application of glycerol, more blood vessels could be seen through the *dura mater* and the blood flow decreased significantly. (h) Seventy-second application of glycerol, the blood flow increased and the *dura mater* became turbid again. Bar = 1 mm.[831]

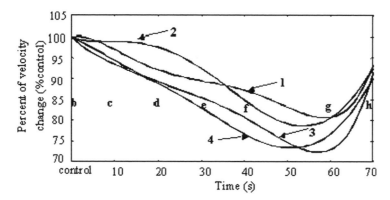

Figure 5.45 The time course of change in relative blood flow in vessels 1, 2, 3, and 4, which are indicated in Fig. 5.44(b), before and after the application of glycerol epidurally. After 20 s, the blood flow in vessel 2 (arteriole) began to decrease, while blood flow in the other vessels (veinules) decreased immediately after the application of glycerol. Decreases of blood flow in these vessels were 20–30% of the baseline. The letters b, c, d, e, f, g, and h denote the time points of corresponding images in Figs. 5.44 (b)–(h).[831]

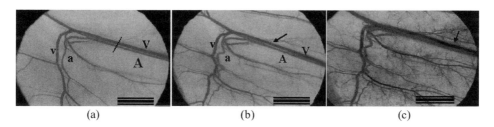

(a)   (b)   (c)

Figure 5.46 Images of the subdermal side of *in vivo* hamster dorsal skin flap window preparation.[979] (a) Native, the main arteriole (A) is 97 ± 18 μm in diameter (lumen) and the main venule (V) is 188 ± 21 μm in diameter; the diameters of the branches, a and v, are 92 ± 18 μm and 181 ± 21 μm, respectively. (b) Ten minutes after the application of glycerol (100%); (c) 20 min after the application of glycerol, the diameters of the main vessels are 97 ± 18 mm (A), and 189 ± 20 mm (V), and the diameters of the branches are 141 ± 17 mm (a) and 259 ± 21 mm (v). Scale bar: 0.25 cm.

images of intravascular structures through whole blood. The refractive index of erythrocyte cytoplasm is mostly defined by hemoglobin concentration.[48] Hemoglobin oxygenation[751] and glycation may have some role in refractive index mismatch (see Section 2.9).[752,753] The scattering properties of blood are also dependent on erythrocyte volume and shape, which are defined by blood plasma osmolarity[48,1035] and aggregation or disaggregation ability.[737,982,1036,1037,1103–1105]

Recently, the feasibility of index matching as a method to overcome the limited penetration through blood to obtain OCT tissue images has been demonstrated for circulating, steady-state, or sedimenting blood.[737,981,982,1036,1037] Glucose, low- and high-molecular dextrans, x-ray contrast, glycerol, and some other biocompatible agents were used to increase the refractive index of blood plasma closer to that of the erythrocyte cytoplasm to improve the penetration depth of OCT images. OCT and other noninvasive imaging techniques, such as back-reflectance spectrophotometry, polarization-sensitive, fluorescence, multiphoton, and Raman spectroscopies, which already have witnessed widespread and exciting application in biomedical diagnostics,[126–144] may have additional advantages in the early diagnostics of vascular disease through optically clarified blood.

Normal human blood is a scattering system that consists of about 43% by volume of scattering particles [99% red blood cells (RBC), 1% leukocytes and thrombocytes) and the about 57% by volume of plasma.[48,725] Under normal physiological conditions, hematocrit (Hct), defined as the volume fraction of cells within whole blood, ranges from 36.8 to 49.2%.[48] Propagation of light in such a medium can be studied within the model of light scattering and absorption by an individual particle, taking into account the interparticle correlation effects and polydispersity.

As it was noted, the blood plasma osmolarity is an important factor in changes in the scattering properties of blood.[48,552,737] The effects of glucose, glycerol, trazograph, and propylene glycol, which are hyperosmotic agents, led to significant change of blood plasma osmolarity. The change in osmolarity induces a variation of the RBC volume due to water exchange and therefore has an impact on the hemoglobin concentration within the RBC and consequently on their refractive index. It was demonstrated that a glucose solution with a concentration less than 20% led to an increase of blood scattering due to the osmotic dehydration of erythrocytes.[552] Significant optical clearing was obtained at a glucose concentration higher than 40%, but such a concentration can cause erythrocyte aggregation.[737]

The result of the OCT study is the measurement of optical backscattering or reflectance $R(z)$ from the RBCs versus axial ranging distance, or depth z. The reflectance depends on the optical properties of blood, i.e., the absorption μ_a and scattering μ_s coefficients, or total attenuation coefficient $\mu_t = \mu_a + \mu_s$. The relationship between $R(z)$ and μ_t is, however, highly complicated because of the high and anisotropic scattering of blood. But for optical depths less than 4, the reflected power can be approximately described by Eq. (5.27). Optical depth is a measure of depth in terms of the number of mean free path lengths, i.e., $\mu_s z$. $\alpha(z)$ is linked to the local refractive index and the backscattering property of the blood sample. If $\alpha(z)$ is kept constant, for which at least a laminar blood flow for circulating blood or measurements before the sedimentation process begins for uncirculating blood should be provided, μ_t can be obtained theoretically from the reflectance measurements at two different depths, z_1 and z_2 [see Eq. (5.28)]. Optical clearing (enhancement of transmittance) ΔT by an agent application can be estimated using Eq. (5.29), where R_a is the reflectance from the backward surface of the vessel within a blood sample with an agent, and R_s is that with a control blood sample (whole blood with saline).

A 1300-nm OCT system was used for taking images of the reflector through circulated blood *in vitro*.[981] As immersion substances, dextran (group refractive index, 1.52) and IV contrast (group refractive index, 1.46) were taken. The system allows the blood to be circulated *in vitro* through transparent tubing to reproduce coronary flow. Blood with Hct ~ 35% was pumped through a closed system of tubing by a perfusion pump. The flow rate was 200 ml/min, which is approximately the peak flow in the coronary artery. The diameter of the tubing was 6 mm, approximately the diameter of a normal adult coronary artery. A reflector was placed in the tubing; the section of the reflector imaged is approximately 2 mm below the inner surface of the tubing. Once blood was introduced into the system and circulated, OCT imaging of the reflector was performed. The total intensity of the signal off the reflector is used to represent penetration [see Eq. (5.29)]. The more light that is scattered by blood the smaller the signal off the reflector.

After baseline data had been obtained with blood, test substances were added to the blood. The test substances were dextran (0.25 g/ml in normal saline), IV contrast, or normal saline.[981] Hematocrit and RBC concentrations were measured before and after the experiments. All substances added had a volume of 40 mls, which was added to a total volume of 260 ml. For the saline control, a $7 \pm 3\%$ increase in signal intensity was noted, which was not a statistically significant effect. A $69 \pm 12\%$ increase in ΔT was noted for dextran, which was statistically different from the saline control ($p < 0.005$). For the IV contrast, a $45 \pm 4\%$ increase was noted, which was also significantly different from the control ($p < 0.001$).

By OCT imaging in the presence of saline, blood (Hct 35%), or lysed blood (Hct < 1%), it was directly demonstrated that RBC intracellular/extracellular mismatch, and not membrane or hemoglobin absorption, is the main source of near-infrared attenuation by blood. In the presence of blood, the reflector was difficult to locate. However, when the RBCs were lysed, signal intensity returned to values not significantly different from saline. The fact that the cell membrane is not the major source of scattering is not surprising since it is too small relative to the wavelength to significantly scatter (see Figs. 1.54 and 1.55).

In the case of dextran, the effect was consistent with index matching. With the IV contrast, a small but significant decrease in RBC volume was noted by a decrease in hematocrit but not the RBC number relative to the saline control. Therefore, some improvement in penetration may be due to a reduction in cell volume. The lack of improved penetration with the addition of normal saline (40 ml) is consistent with data of Ref. 48 that suggested dilution of the hematocrit to below 10% was necessary before significant improvement in penetration was seen.

Studies of blood scattering reduction by the immersion technique using various osmotically active solutions that are biocompatible with blood, such as saline, glucose, glycerol, propylene glycol, trazograph, and dextrans, were also described.[737,982,1036,1037] The 820- and 1310-nm OCT systems were applied for, taking images of the reflector through a layer of uncirculating fresh whole blood. The OCT system used yields 12-μm axial resolution in free space. This determines the imaging axial resolution that is comparable with the dimensions of RBCs or small aggregates. It was shown that for uncirculating blood, the sedimentation may play an important role in blood clearing using the immersion technique and OCT allows for precise monitoring of blood sedimentation and aggregation.

Venous blood was drawn from healthy volunteers and stabilized by 9NC coagulation sodium citrate 3.2% or by K2E EDTA K2. The major blood samples were prepared immediately after blood was taken by gently mixing blood and agent (for agents in liquid state) or agent-saline solution (for agents in solid state) with low rate manual rotation for 1 min before each OCT measurement. A few samples were stored before measurements up to 24 hr after blood taking. Four groups of the blood samples with various hematocrit values were investigated in the study.[737,982,1036,1037]

A few different glass vessels from 0.2- to 2-mm thick were used as blood sample holders. For some holders to enhance reflection from the bottom interface, a metal reflector was used. The sample holder was mounted on a translation stage at the sample arm and was placed perpendicular to the probing beam. The amplitude of reflected light as a function of depth at one spatial point within the sample was obtained. The result is the measurement of optical backscattering or reflectance $R(z)$ from the RBCs versus axial ranging distance, or depth z, described by Eq. (5.27). The total attenuation coefficient μ_t and enhancement of transmittance (optical clearing) ΔT by an agent application were estimated using Eqs. (5.28) and (5.29), respectively. Averaging for a few tenths of z-scans was employed.

The scattering μ_s and reduced scattering coefficient μ_s' of blood depend on mismatch of averaged refractive indices of blood plasma and erythrocyte cytoplasm. The ratio $n_{RBC}/n_{bp} \equiv m$ determines the scattering coefficient, n_{RBC} is the mean refractive index of erythrocyte cytoplasm, and n_{bp} is the mean refractive index of the blood plasma. For the model of RBC ensemble as a monodisperse system of noninteracting scattering dielectric spheres of radius a irradiated at a NIR wavelength λ, when $5 < 2\pi a/\lambda < 50$, anisotropy scattering factor $g > 0.9$, and $1 < m < 1.1$, the reduced scattering coefficient μ_s' is described by Eq. (2.24).

Blood plasma contains up to 91% water, 6.5–8% (about 70 g/l) various proteins, and about 2% low molecular compounds. Because of the low concentration and relatively low refractive index of low molecular chemical compounds, the mean blood plasma (background) index can be estimated as the weighted average of the refractive indices of water (92%) n_w and proteins (8%) n_p as

$$n_{bp} = f_w n_w + (1 - f_w)n_p, \qquad (5.30)$$

where f_w is the volume fraction of water contained in plasma, $n_w = 1.329$ at 800 nm, and the index of proteins can be taken as $n_p = 1.470$.[749] Since approximately 92% of the total plasma is water, it follows from Eq. (5.30) that $n_{bp} = 1.340$. The empirical formula, described by Eq. (2.30), can be used to estimate the blood plasma index in the wavelength range from 400 to 1000 nm. The refractive index of erythrocyte cytoplasm, defined by the cell-bounded hemoglobin solution, can be found from Eq. (2.31). As it follows from Eq. (2.24), about a tenfold reduction of the scattering coefficient μ_s' is expected when the refractive index of the blood plasma is changed from $n_{bp} = 1.340$ to 1.388 and the refractive index of RBC cytoplasm is kept constant at $n_{RBC} = 1.412$ (for hemoglobin concentration in cytoplasm of 400 g/l).[48]

For slightly diluted blood (Hct $\sim$ 35%), optical clearing was found only for dextran of molecular weight M $= 500,000$ with concentration in a blood sample of

0.325 g/dl and glycerol with a volume fraction of 13%. Values of ΔT, characterizing optical clearing, were from 20.2 to 78.4% for dextran and from 13.7 to 95% for glycerol, depending on time of blood sample storage (Table 5.3). The minimal and maximal values have been found for blood samples that were stored after taking the blood for a short (1–3 hr) and for a long (24 hr) time interval, respectively. For the time interval of 4–6 hr of blood storage, $\Delta T = 46.5\%$ for dextran and 74.5% for glycerol. Evidently, at high concentrations of RBC in a sample, interaction of used agents with blood significantly depends on the physicochemical parameters of blood, which may be changed at prolonged storage (hemolysis). Thus, all other measurements were done as fast as possible after taking the blood.

For 56.5%-diluted blood by saline, the blood samples with trazograph-60, propylene glycol, and glycerol had a lower total attenuation coefficient than the control. Optical clearing ΔT was from 45.3 to 117.1% as measured immediately after mixture, when sedimentation is not critical for the optical properties of the blood layer (Table 5.3). The minimal attenuation (approximately half of that for the control) and the maximal enhancement of transmittance ($\Delta T = 117.1\%$) were found for application of glycerol. Propylene glycol is also a good enhancer of blood transmittance ($\Delta T = 77.2\%$).

Similar effects of increase in transmittance and decrease in scattering were demonstrated by use of dextrans of various molecular weights. Table 5.3 shows that all three dextrans used, A, B, and C, reduced the amount of the attenuation (scattering) coefficient in blood with respect to saline. Optical clearing ΔT was in the range from 52.1 to 150.5%. The dextran with the highest molecular weight appeared to have a much stronger effect on the increase in transmittance immediately after mixing. A blood sample mixed with an agent of higher refractive index, for example, dextran C, had a higher reflectivity from the metal surface than did agents such as saline (control) and dextran A with lower refractive indices. The results support the hypothesis that the refractive index matching effect is important for clearing of 50%-diluted blood.

It can be seen from Table 5.3 that dextrans C and B at concentration of 2.43 g/dl in 35%-diluted blood are effective agents for decreasing the light attenuation of blood compared to the saline control, with the total attenuation coefficient decreased from 37.1 cm^{-1} for the saline control to 31.2 cm^{-1} and 29.7 cm^{-1}, respectively. The optical clearing capability ΔT was approximately 90% and 100% for dextran C and B, respectively. It is interesting that dextran C, providing a higher refraction, had less effect than that of dextran B at the same concentration. Moreover, the increase in concentration (refraction power) cannot always achieve higher optical clearance: 0.5 g/dl dextran C had a stronger effect than 5 g/dl in samples with 20% blood and 80% saline.

The changes in scattering property brought about by the addition of a dextran solution may first be explained by the refractive index matching hypothesis. It can be seen that scattering can be reduced when the refractive index of plasma is increased. The refractive index of the dextran saline solution was increased with concentration in all molecular weight groups. The measured indices of blood samples with dextrans were in good agreement with the theoretical values calculated

Table 5.3 The total attenuation coefficient and enhanced transmittance ΔT (%) of blood samples diluted by saline and added agents; pH for all solutions was approximately 7.5; dextran A (M = 10,500); dextran B (M = 65,500), and dextran C (M = 473,000).

Agent	Concentration (vol.% or g/dl)	Hct (%)	μ_t (cm^{-1})	ΔT (%)	Comments
Saline	13% (control)	35	61(3)	–	From 1 to 24 hr
Glycerol	13%	35	51(5)	13.7–95.0	after taking blood;
Dextran	0.325 g/dl	35	55(5)	20.2–78.4	dextran sulfate, $M \approx 500,000$[1036]
Saline	35% (control)	26	37.1(1.3)	–	Male volunteer,
Dextran A	2.43 g/dl	26	38.2(2.4)	11.9(8.3)	24 yr old[982]
Dextran B	2.43 g/dl	26	29.7(3.6)	100.1(20.2)	
Dextran C	2.43 g/dl	26	31.2(1.8)	86.7(29.1)	
Saline	56.5% (control)	17.4	42	–	Female volunteer, 35 yr old[737,1036]
Trazograph-60	6.5% + 50% saline	17.4	26	45.3	
Propylene glycol	6.5% + 50% saline	17.4 / 17.4	26	77.2	
Glycerol	6.5% + 50% saline	17.4	20	117.1	
Glucose	1.62 g/dl	17.4	57	45.3	
Dextran A	1.62 g/dl	17.4	43	47	
Dextran B	1.62 g/dl	17.4	54	44.6	
Dextran C	1.62 g/dl	17.4	58	20.5	
Saline	56.5% (control)	17.4	36.5	–	Male volunteer, 35 yr old[737]
Dextran A	1.62 g/dl	17.4	29.5	52.1	
Dextran B	1.62 g/dl	17.4	30.0	110.6	
Dextran C	1.62 g/dl	17.4	32.5	150.5	
Saline	56.5% (control)	17.4	25.6(1.6)	–	Male volunteer, 23 yr old[982]
Dextran A	1.62 g/dl	17.4	22.5(2.4)	20.5(4.2)	
Dextran B	1.62 g/dl	17.4	19.0(3.8)	44.5(3.4)	
Dextran C	1.62 g/dl	17.4	14.3(4.3)	47.0(9.7)	
Saline	80% (control)	8	13.5	–	Male volunteer,
Dextran A	1 g/dl	8	17.5(0.9)	11.4(6.2)	36 yr old,
Dextran A	5 g/dl	8	14.3(1.2)	11.3(3.3)	hemoglobin:
Dextran A	10 g/dl	8	12.2(1.8)	49.4(12.1)	initial—175 g/l,
Dextran B	1 g/dl	8	14.2(1.5)	21.1(5.4)	diluted—37 g/l,
Dextran B	5 g/dl	8	13.0(2.8)	49.0(26.2)	Ref. 982.
Dextran B	10 g/dl	8	11.5(1.3)	76.8(21.2)	At the beginning of blood sedimentation

Table 5.3 (Continued).

Agent	Concentration (vol.% or g/dl)	Hct (%)	μ_t (cm^{-1})	ΔT (%)	Comments
Dextran C	0.5 g/dl	8	10.0(1.6)	106.3(39)	
Dextran C	5 g/dl	8	13.3(0.7)	67.0(5.8)	
Dextran A	1 g/dl	8	–	90	Compared to that of the
Dextran A	5 g/dl	8	–	61	saline control on light
Dextran A	10 g/dl	8	–	32	transmission after
Dextran B	1 g/dl	8	–	144	10 min sedimentation,
Dextran B	5 g/dl	8	–	126	$(\Delta T_{dext}/\Delta T_{saline})\%$
Dextran B	10 g/dl	8	–	18	
Dextran C	0.5 g/dl	8	–	285	
Dextran C	2 g/dl	8	–	133	
Dextran C	5 g/dl	8	–	15	

according to the equation $n = c_b n_b + (1 - c_b)n_{saline}$, where c_b is the volume fraction (20%) of whole blood in the diluted sample and n_{saline} is the index of saline with or without dextrans. As expected, the refractive index of blood with dextran increases as the concentration of the added dextran increases due to an increase of the index of the ground matter of the sample.

It should be noted that the total attenuation coefficient for glucose and dextrans was not changed significantly with respect to the control; nevertheless, transmittance enhancements of 45% for glucose and of 52–150% for dextrans were found. The concurrent increase of attenuation and transmittance by dextran B and C relative to A shows not only that refractive index matching is important for blood layer optical clearing, but also that RBC aggregation, which defines the scattering indicatrix, may be substantial. Dextran macromolecules are neutral polymers. The high molecular weight dextrans are used artificially to induce RBC aggregation by bridging surfaces of adjacent cells after adsorption on their surfaces. The low molecular weight dextrans prevent normal blood aggregation. From blood smear microscopy, it can be seen that rouleaux occurred in the blood diluted with dextran C, but no aggregates were produced in the blood mixed with low molecular weight dextran A.[1018,1019,1036,1037] The lower sedimentation rate of blood with dextrans B and C and the higher sedimentation rate of blood with dextran A relative to the rates for whole blood or for blood diluted with saline also reflect the aggregation abilities of various dextrans.[737] The high molecular weight dextran C has greatly changed the scatter (RBCs and aggregates) morphology and size. Normal RBCs are biconcave disks of 8-μm diameter and 2-μm thickness when they are in an isotonic solution. It is known that the RBCs' sizes, shapes, and orientations contribute to the properties of blood backscattering.[1103–1105] Aggregation results in a decrease in diffusing surfaces, which in turn leads to a decrease of the backscattered signal.[1104] It can be concluded that the greater transmittance enhancement of dextran C is governed strongly by the scattering changes (refractive index matching) accompanied by RBC aggregation.

Some discrepancy between μ_t and ΔT can be also explained by the fact that different algorithms are used to estimate them: μ_t is defined as a single-scattering parameter and ΔT is defined as an experimental value that accounts for multiple scattering, which is why it is more sensitive for the reduction of scattering. It has been shown that immersion leads at first to a reduction in the number of scattering events and only then to the appearance of ballistic photons (see Figs. 5.4–5.6).[798] For example, for the scattering system described in Ref. 798, which normally has for unmatched indices of scatterers $n_s = 1.47$ and ground material $n_0 = 1.35$ a total transmittance at 800 nm of 10%, after index matching ($n_0 = 1.41$) the total transmittance rises to 45%, but the number of scattering events (as many as 10–15) remains high [see Fig. 5.5(c)].

It should be noted that for fresh erythrocyte concentrates flowing at a physiological velocity at an oxygen saturation of 98%, the change of Hct from 0.4 to 0.2 causes a reduction of the transport scattering coefficient μ_s' from 16.8 to 8.8 cm^{-1} at 633 nm, measured by an integrating sphere technique.[48] The corresponding changes in scattering coefficient μ_s and anisotropy factor g are: μ_s from 850 to 800 cm^{-1} and g from 0.980 to 0.989. A largely reduced value (by more than ten times) of the total attenuation coefficient measured by OCT (see Table 5.3) relative to the value of the scattering coefficient measured by an integrating sphere technique for blood samples with approximately equal hematocrit also shows the limitations of a single-scattering algorithm to extract a proper value of the total attenuation coefficient. Another reason for such strong discrepancy between μ_t and ΔT data may be the spatial variations of the reflectivity of the blood sample $\alpha(z)$ associated with the variations of the local refractive index and the backscattering property of the blood sample.

Sedimentation increases the transparency of a blood layer because there is less bulk scattering as the RBCs fall. As expected, the undiluted blood sample has the lowest reflectance from the metal plate because it has a higher concentration of scatters (RBCs) and a lower sedimentation rate.[737,1036,1037] For blood slightly diluted by a saline and at addition of the low molecular weight dextran A, reflectance from the metal plate in the depth of the blood sample increases because both the dilution by saline and addition of dextran A cause more intense sedimentation. Dextran B, which has a mean molecular weight, permits higher reflectance than the control (i.e., blood diluted by saline) only during the first 4 min; this result reflects the competition between two processes: refractive index matching, which is important at the beginning, especially for dextran, and sedimentation, which is more important for the control sample after some time has elapsed. The high molecular weight dextran C permits an increase in metal plate reflectance compared with that of the control for only a short period at the beginning of sedimentation, when only the refractive index matching effect dominates. Such behavior shows that, after some time, interval RBC sedimentation may be more important for increasing reflectance than the refractive index matching effect, which is provided by dextrans with higher molecular weight. This result is clearly seen from the in-depth reflectance profiles presented in Fig. 5.47, which show the three main evolution peaks in time: the first peak is independent of time and is induced by reflectance at the glass-blood interface; the second peak, which is broad and has some structure, is caused by reflectance at the RBC-plasma interface (within this peak, aggregates can be seen); and the third peak is caused by the metal reflector. Qualitatively, the height difference between the first and the third peaks shows changes in the blood layer's transmittance, and the second broad peak is related to the attenuation coefficient of this layer.

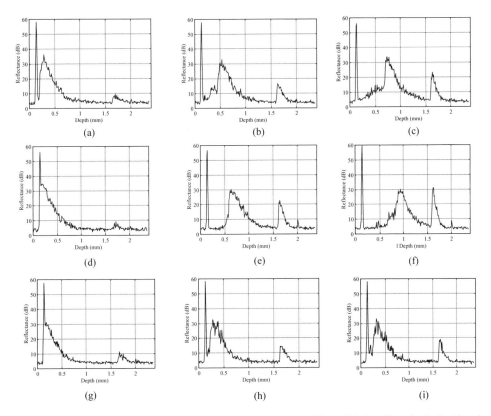

Figure 5.47 OCT in-depth reflectance profiles measured for slightly diluted whole blood (13% volume fraction of saline, hematocrit ~35%, concentration of dextran 3.25 g/dl in the blood sample). (a), (d), and (g), at the beginning of the sedimentation process; (b), (e), and (h), at 5 min; and (c), (f), and (i), at 10 min for (a)–(c) saline only, (d)–(f) dextran A added, and (g)–(i) dextran C added. The first peak is induced by reflectance at the glass-blood interface; the second peak, which is broad and has some structures, is caused by reflectance at the RBC-plasma interface; and the third peak is caused by the metal reflector.[737]

To clarify the role of RBC aggregation on optical clearing and accounting for the fact that the aggregation process is time dependent, the blood sample was allowed to sediment after the addition of dextrans and before measurements were done. Table 5.3 shows a summary of the effect of dextrans compared to the saline

control on light transmission for the sample with 20% blood and 80% saline after 10 min sedimentation. It can be seen that the influence of dextran on the light
transmission was different compared to that at the beginning of mixing dextrans
in blood (corresponding upper rows). The lower concentration (0.5 g/dl) dextran C
still had the strongest effect on reducing the scattering of light in the blood, with
a 2.8-fold stronger effect than that of the saline control. However, enhancement by
the highest concentration of dextran C (5 g/dl) and dextran B (10 g/dl) was dramatically lower than that of the saline control. At the beginning, they both had a very
high blood optical clearing capability with 67.5 and 76.8% of ΔT, respectively. In
addition, the effect was decreased with the increase of dextran in the blood within
all three groups, contrary to the expectation of the refractive index matching hypothesis.

The decreased aggregation capability of dextran with concentration explained
well that light transmission decreased less with the increase of dextran for both
types (midmolecular and large molecular). Over a range of concentrations, dextran C and B induced RBC aggregation. However, dextrans have been known to
exert a biphasic effect on RBC aggregation; they induce aggregation at low concentration, and disaggregation at high concentration.[1106] For example, with dextran B,
the maximal aggregation size is obtained at approximately 3%, above which the
size decreases. In OCT measurements of Ref. 982, 2 g/dl dextran C and 5 g/dl dextran B in 20% blood with 80% saline appeared to be the critical concentration to
affect RBC aggregation. Their aggregation parameters became smaller than those
of 0.5 g/dl dextran C and 1 g/dl dextran B. When the concentration increased to
5 g/dl for dextran C and 10 g/dl for dextran B, they played a role of disaggregation. That is the reason why the cells are much less packed than with the saline
control, accounting for the reduced light transmission. Although refractive index
matching suggested a higher light transmission, it can be seen that the aggregation-
disaggregation effects are now dominant.

The behavior of RBC in flow is dependent on the processes of aggregation-
disaggregation, orientation, and deformation. For normal blood, rouleaux are easily decomposed to their individual cell constituents as blood flow (shear) increases.
In some pathological cases, however, the capillary circulation is seriously affected
because nonseparable rouleaux are formed. Increased RBC aggregability has been
observed in various pathological states, such as diabetes and myocardial infarction, or following trauma.[1107] The aggregation and disaggregation properties of
human blood can be used for the characterization of the hemorheological status of
patients suffering from different diseases.[1105] In this connection, optical clearing
methodology for controlling of optical properties of blood using molecules with a
specific action on the RBCs and plasma may be useful in the monitoring of blood
parameters in flow.

It is obvious that refractive index matching is not the only factor to affect transmittance in these experiments. The amount of the aggregation certainly has an
effect, but other factors, such as the hematocrit, the manner in which RBCs are
packed, the shape of the aggregates, the variance in size of these aggregates, and
the fluctuation of all these parameters in time and space, may all contribute.

It should be noted that the blood plasma's osmolarity is also an important factor in changes in the scattering properties of blood and, therefore, in the control of blood clearing and the improvement of the contrast of OCT images obtained within or behind a layer of blood. In the discussed experiments, the osmolarity of the plasma was different for each of the added agents. Variation in plasma osmolarity leads to changes in the shape of the erythrocytes: RBC shrinking (acanthocytes) when the plasma is hyperosmotic and swelling (spherocytes) when it is hypoosmotic. For the diluted blood samples (Hct of 7.5%), the scattering coefficient μ_s shows a slight decrease ($\sim$10%) with increasing osmolarity in the range from 225 to 450 milliosmol/l; also, the anisotropy factor g decreases from 0.995 to 0.991, and the reduced (transport) scattering coefficient μ'_s correspondingly increases linearly with osmolarity up to 70%.[48] Such a strong effect on the scattering properties of the blood solution is caused not only by changes in cell shape, but also by the variation with osmolarity of the refractive index of the cell-bounded hemoglobin solution. The refractive index of the cell-bounded hemoglobin solution can be estimated from Eq. (2.31). Assuming a mean erythrocyte volume of 90 μm^3 and an inner cell hemoglobin concentration of 350 g/l for isotonic conditions, the following values of refractive indices and sphere equivalent diameters were calculated. Table 5.4 shows this data and that the osmolarity of the blood solution can substantially change the scattering properties of the blood layer. Refractive index matching is easier to achieve in conditions of low osmolarity, but for OCT imaging of RBCs or their aggregates, the hypertonic conditions are preferable.

Table 5.4 RBC parameters found from osmolarity of the blood solution.[48]

Osmolarity, milliosmol/l	Hct, %	RBC volume, μm^3	RBC hemoglobin concentration, g/l	Refractive index at 589 nm	Equivalent sphere diameter, μm
250 (hypotonic)	8.1	96.7	325	1.397	5.70
300 (isotonic)	7.5	90.0	350	1.402	5.56
400 (hypertonic)	6.6	78.6	400	1.412	5.32

From the above analysis of experimental data follows that to theoretically describe light transport in the immersed blood, we have to consider blood as a turbid medium with multiple scattering, defined by the scattering and absorption properties of individual particles (erythrocytes) and by the concentration effects and polidispersity of the cell suspension. The erythrocyte size and complex refractive indices ($n' + in''$) of erythrocytes and blood plasma define the absorption μ_a and scattering μ_s coefficients, and scattering anisotropy factor g. The size, shape, and optical parameters of blood cells as well as the optical properties of a blood suspension are presented in Section 2.9 and Tables 2.2, 2.3, and 5.4. The erythrocyte mean volume at isotonic medium is 94 $\pm$ 14 μm^3, and the volume distribution is in the range from 30 to 200 μm^3 (see Refs. 48, 725, 730, 1108, and 1109). The hemoglobin concentration in hemolized blood is between 134 and 173 g/l. Each erythrocyte contains approximately 29 pg of hemoglobin. The hemoglobin concentration within an erythrocyte ranges from 300 to 360 g/l. The real part of the refractive index of the red blood cell is very close to 1.4 in the wavelength range from 400 nm to 1200 nm.[183,730,755,1108]

The phase function and scattering cross section of an individual erythrocyte depend on its orientation.[159] However, the light-scattering characteristics of a large number of randomly distributed nonspherical particles is very close to the light-scattering characteristics of a system of randomly distributed spherical particles with an equal volume.[48,1110] Therefore, calculations can be done for a model of homogeneous spheres with the volume equal to the volume of real erythrocytes. Such a model provides simpler calculations than that for a rigorous theory accounting for particle nonsphericity[145] and allows one to account for particle polydispersity in the simplest way; in particular, on the basis of the data presented in Ref. 730 (see Fig. 5.48). The presence of big particles in the distribution can be associated with small aggregates of RBCs.

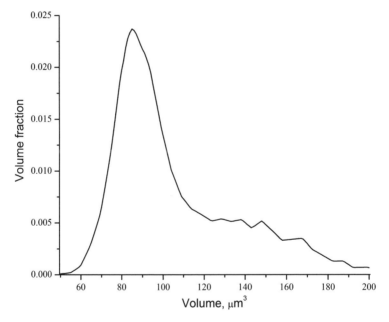

Figure 5.48 Size distribution function of spherical particles modeling erythrocytes in blood.[730] The volume fraction of erythrocytes in the blood (hematocrit) is 45%, which corresponds to venous blood of an adult male.

Evidently, the hemoglobin concentration C_{Hb} in an erythrocyte correlates with its volume V_{RBC}. In accordance with data of Ref. 1108, such dependence is defined by

$$C_{Hb} = 0.72313 - 0.00451 V_{RBC},\qquad(5.31)$$

were C_{Hb} is the hemoglobin concentration in g/ml and V_{RBC} is the RBC volume in μm^3.

The spectral dependence for the real part of the RBC refractive index is presented in Fig. 2.12,[159,730] and the spectral dependence for the imaginary part can be calculated using data presented in Fig. 2.11. Both refractive index components are proportional to hemoglobin concentration in RBCs; the real part is defined by Eq. (2.31) with $\beta_{Hb} = 0.001942$ dl/g at 589 nm[48] and $\beta_{Hb} = 0.00284$ dl/g at 640 nm,[159] and the imaginary part is defined by the following expression:

$$n'' = \alpha_{Hb}C_{Hb}, \tag{5.32}$$

where α_{Hb} is the spectrally dependent coefficient equal to 1.477×10^{-6} dl/g at 640 nm.[159]

Since the concentration of salts, sugars, and other organic components in RBC cytoplasm is negligible, hemoglobin can be dissolved in water only [see Eq. (2.31)]; thus, the spectral dependence of the refractive index of the medium in which hemoglobin is dissolved is defined by water. For a more precise description of the refractive index of this medium $n_0(\lambda)$ when organic components are accounted for, instead of $n_w(\lambda)$, $n_0(\lambda) = n_w(\lambda) + 0.007$ may be used.[1042]

The spectral dependence of the real part of the refractive index of blood plasma can be described by the empirical Eq. (2.30) and, because blood plasma contains up to 91% of water, only 6.5–8% (about 70 g/l) proteins (hemoglobin, albumin, and globulin), and about 2% of low-molecular compounds, its imaginary part is negligible and can be ignored in calculations.

For further calculation of the scattering and absorption coefficients and the scattering anisotropy factor, the Mie theory valid for a homogeneous spherical particle is used. The corresponding equations for scattering and absorption cross sections and anisotropy factor are given by Eqs (1.193)–(1.195). For a densely packed polydisperse particle system, which whole blood is, the absorption and scattering coefficients and the scattering anisotropy factor are defined by [see Eqs. (1.173) and (1.176)][156]

$$\mu_a = \sum_{i=1}^{N_{RBC}} N_i \sigma_{a_i}, \tag{5.33}$$

$$\mu_s = F(\text{Hct}) \sum_{i=1}^{N_{RBC}} N_i \sigma_{s_i}, \tag{5.34}$$

$$g = \frac{\sum_{i=1}^{N_{RBC}} \mu_{s_i} g_i}{\sum_{i=1}^{N_{RBC}} \mu_{s_i}}, \tag{5.35}$$

where $F(\text{Hct})$ is the packing function of RBCs [see Eqs. (1.170)–(1.172)],[183,567,568] which accounts for the interparticle correlation effects; Hct is the hematocrit; N_{RBC} is the number of RBC diameters (volume fractions); and $N_i = f_{\text{RBC}i}/V_{\text{RBC}i}$ is a number of RBCs in a unit volume of blood; $f_{\text{RBC}i}$ is the volume fraction of RBCs with volume $V_{\text{RBC}i} = (4/3)\pi a_i^3$ (see Fig. 5.48), where a_i is the radius of an individual equivalent volume spherical particle.

At glucose application as an immersion agent, the spectral dependence of the index of refraction of blood plasma corrected by the added glucose-water solution should be accounted for [see Eqs. (2.36) and (1.202)] as

$$n_{\text{bp}+\text{gl}}(\lambda) = n_{\text{bp}}(\lambda) + 0.1515 C_{\text{gl}}, \tag{5.36}$$

where $n_{\text{bp}}(\lambda)$ is the refractive index of blood plasma defined by Eq. (2.30), and C_{gl} is the concentration of glucose in g/ml. Because glucose has no strong absorption bands within the spectral range from 400 to 1000 nm, its absorption may be neglected. It can also be hypothesized that glucose molecules do not bound with proteins in blood plasma and hemoglobin in RBCs during the limited time (a few minutes maximum) of their interaction.

As we already discussed, the RBC is very sensitive to changes in blood plasma osmolarity (see Table 5.4). At osmolarity increase due to cell dehydration, the RBC volume decreases, hemoglobin concentration within the cell increases, and the index of refraction increases. Glucose injection in blood causes the linear increase of plasma osmolarity with glucose concentration, up to 6000 mOsm/l at glucose concentration in blood plasma of 1.0 g/ml. Indeed, for patients, such large glucose concentrations may be applied only locally in the vicinity of a vessel wall site under spectroscopic study or optical imaging. Using data of Ref. 48, the following empirical relation was suggested to describe RBC volume change with osmolarity:[552]

$$V_{\text{RBC}}(osm) = V_{\text{RBC}}(300)\left(0.463 + 1.19\exp\left\{-\frac{osm}{376.2}\right\}\right), \tag{5.37}$$

where $V_{\text{RBC}}(osm)$ is the RBC volume in μm^3 at a given osmolarity expressed in mOsm/l and $V_{\text{RBC}}(300)$ is the RBC volume at isotonic osmolarity $osm = 300$ mOsm/l. At glucose injection the local Hct decreases. If Hct before injection of glucose was 45% at $osm = 300$ mOsm/l, then at $C_{\text{gl}} = 0.05$ g/ml, $osm = 580$ mOsm/l and Hct $= 32\%$; at $C_{\text{gl}} = 0.1$ g/ml, $osm = 850$ mOsm/l and Hct $= 26\%$; and at $C_{\text{gl}} = 0.2$ g/ml, $osm = 1400$ mOsm/l and Hct $= 22\%$. At further increase of glucose concentration (0.3–1.0 g/ml), osm is constant and Hct $\cong 21\%$, in spite of the linear increase of blood plasma osmolarity (2000–6000 mOsm/l).

Results of modeling of the scattering properties' control for whole blood at its immersion (local intravessel injection) by a glucose solution at different concentrations accounting for the RBC packing function in the form $F(\text{Hct}) = (1 - \text{Hct})$ [see Eq. (1.170)], polidispersity [150 volume fractions of volume (size) distribution, Fig. 5.48], osmolarity, and hematocrit effects are presented in Fig. 5.49. The scattering coefficient and scattering anisotropy factor were calculated. The scattering coefficient behavior with concentration and the wavelength [Fig. 5.49(a)] is defined by: (1) the change in blood plasma osmolarity (increase of scattering for all wavelengths far from the Soret band caused by RBC shrinkage and increase of refractive index for low concentrations of glucose, see Table 5.4); (2) reduction of blood hematocrit (plays some role in the scattering decrease for glucose concentration less than 0.3 g/ml); (3) refractive index matching, the main effect (a significant reduction of scattering for glucose concentration from 0.5 to 0.7 g/ml dependent on the wavelength); and (4) dispersion of hemoglobin absorbing bands [within a strong Soret band (415 nm), it does not allow a significant reduction of scattering and slightly modifies the position of the dip and the depth of scatter damping for other lower-absorbing hemoglobin bands, 542 and 575 nm].

The maximal damping of the scattering corresponds to 900 nm, where the influence of hemoglobin band dispersion is minimal, but the highest glucose concentration of 0.7 g/ml is needed in that case. The scattering coefficient increase at higher glucose concentrations is caused by refractive index mismatch, where the refractive index of the RBCs becomes less than that for blood plasma modified by adding glucose. The same factors define the behavior of the scattering anisotropy parameter [Fig. 5.49(b)]: RBC shrinkage causes a decrease of the g-factor for small glucose concentrations, refractive index matching causes its increase for moderate concentrations, and further refractive index mismatch causes its reduction. For applications, especially when OCT endoscopy is used, concurrent reduction of scattering and increase of the g-factor at immersion agent administration is important. The transport scattering coefficient, $\mu'_s = (1 - g)\mu$, decreases and transport free path length for a photon, $l_t \cong 1/\mu'_s$, increases dramatically; thus, a greater amount of photons, which carry information about the hidden object (for example, thin-wall plaques in the coronary arteries), can be detected. From data in Fig. 5.49, it follows that for the wavelength 900 nm, the scattering coefficient of blood is changed from 1200 cm^{-1} to approximately 50 cm^{-1} and the g-factor from 0.991 to 0.994 at glucose immersion; thus, the transport free path length increases more than 35 times. Correspondingly, the depolarization depth of blood,[348,371,438] which is proportional to l_t, should be much bigger at optical clearing.

The described method for immersed blood modeling is applicable for any other biocompatible immersion agent administration, such as dextrans, glycerol, and trazograph (Table 5.3). At blood clearing, there also exists another possibility of blood immersion: using the local blood hemolysis, which can be provided in the vicinity of the fiber-optic endoscopic probe.[748] In that method, free hemoglobin is the immersion agent. To model optical properties, all effects discussed earlier should be taken into account. A local increase of hemoglobin concentration in plasma can lead to a local change of plasma osmolarity,[552]

$$osm' = osm + \frac{C_{bpHe}}{M_{Hb}},\qquad(5.38)$$

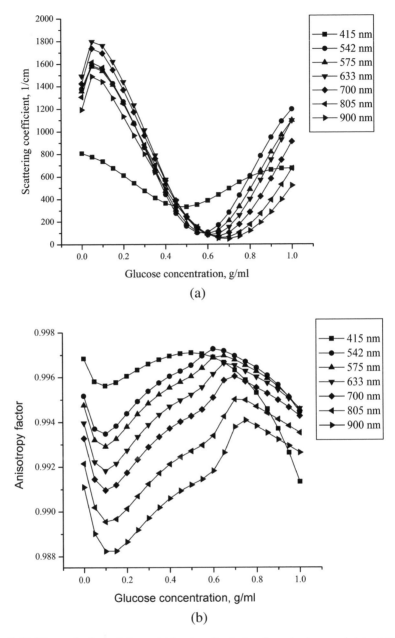

Figure 5.49 Theoretical modeling of blood optical clearing at glucose intravessel injection. The calculated curves for the scattering coefficient (a) and scattering anisotropy factor (b) at glucose concentration in blood.[1042] The initial blood hematocrit of 45% and RBC hemoglobin concentration of 322 g/l; 150 volume fractions of RBCs with different volume (size) in accordance with the RBC volume distribution function, which is presented in Fig. 5.48, were used in the modeling.

where *osm* is the plasma osmolarity under physiological condition (280–300 mOsm/l); C_{bpHb} is the concentration of plasma hemoglobin, g/l; and M_{Hb} is the molar mass of hemoglobin ($M_{Hb} = 66500$ g/M). The expected change of RBC volume calculated using empirical Eq. (5.37) is not more than 0.1%; at hemolysis, less than 20%. For simplicity, the polydispersity of RBCs can be taken into account on the basis of the six-fraction blood model given in Table 5.5,[1111] which correlates with a more complete distribution given in Fig. 5.48.

Table 5.5 Size distribution of the equivalent spherical particles modeling RBC.[1111]

Volume fraction, %	4	14	30	32	14	6
Radius, μm		1.2 ± 0.2	1.7 ± 0.3	2.2 ± 0.2	2.7 ± 0.3	3.4 ± 0.4 4.3 ± 0.5

Calculations of the absorption coefficient, scattering coefficient, and anisotropy factor of whole blood at normal conditions and at local hemolysis have been performed using Eqs. (5.33)–(5.35) with the packing function $F(\text{Hct}) = (1 - \text{Hct})(1.4 - \text{Hct})$. In contrast with the small changes of the absorption coefficient, more significant changes of the scattering properties of blood have been observed at an increase of free hemoglobin concentration in plasma. A rather spectrally smooth decrease of scattering coefficient for all wavelengths with free hemoglobin release at hemolysis was found.[748] At a hemolysis rate of 20%, decrease of the scattering coefficient for both wavelengths 633 and 820 nm was calculated as 40%, while the anisotropy factor increases from 0.9940 to 0.9952 at 633 nm and from 0.9919 to 0.9929 at 820 nm.

The described method can be realized not only at blood hemolysis, but also at local free hemoglobin injection. Hemoglobin administration may also serve as a clearing agent for tissue clearing when clearing is needed in the spectral range far from the strong absorption bands of hemoglobin. On the other hand, the sensitivity of the scattering properties of blood to RBC hemolysis may be used for designing an effective optical technology for *in vivo* monitoring of blood hemolysis in vessels.

5.7.3 Cell studies

The optical immersion method is a valuable technique for studying refractive and scattering properties of living cells.[150,175,749,953–955,1035,1112] For cellular refraction measurements, this technique has been in use since the 1950s.[749,953,954] It has been successfully used in combination with phase refractometry to study water and solids distribution in animal cells (mechanisms of cell cornification); mechanisms of animal cell motility connected with water redistributions; cell permeability, damage, and death; and the vitality and growth cycles of bacteria, fungi, yeasts, and spores. Some of the hematological applications of the immersion technique in cell suspensions studies are discussed earlier in Section 5.7.2.

In cell examination, the requirements of immersion agents should be somewhat different than in tissue optical clearing, where for many applications only cell damage is critical and the hyperosmotic property of agents provides one of the leading mechanisms for tissue clearing. In general, an immersion substance (IS) to be used for the refractometry of living cells should fulfill the following requirements:[749,954]

(1) The IS should be nontoxic and not affect the structure or function of living cells, i.e., chemically inert and not affecting any chemical components of a cell.

(2) It should be isotonic, i.e., not cause any changes of cell volume. Cell shrinkage or swelling induced by water displacement from a cell into the surrounding medium or vice versa are accompanied by the corresponding changes of cell refractive index; thus, the measured refractive index will not be a true value. The isotonic property is a biological character of a cell in solution that is connected with such physical characteristics of a solution as its isoosmotic property, but may not be similar. To provide isoosmotic and isotonic conditions, the IS should exert a low osmotic pressure; that is, it should consist of dissolved particles with high molecular weight and dimensions. For example, a water solution of bovine serum albumin (BSA) with an osmotic pressure of 10% is equivalent to a water solution of sodium chloride (NaCl) with a pressure of 0.08%.

(3) The IS should not penetrate the cell when the refractive index of a whole cell under study. Otherwise, at cell immersion in a medium with the higher refractive index, this substance diffuses inside the cell and equalizes the refractive indices inside and outside the cell, making the measured cell refractive index value far from a true value. Thus, for many cases, the IS should have a macromolecular structure to prevent cell permeability. However, for some specific cases, when intracellular organelles are under investigation, immersion agents with a controllable permeation can be used.

(4) The IS should be freely soluble in water so that the refractive index of the solution can be equal or exceed that of the part of the cell to be measured. As for animal cells, the refractive index range is from 1.350 to 1.426 (see Table 2.6); and for bacterial cells, from 1.360 to 1.420.[954] The IS refractive index values must be variable in these ranges with a step of 0.002–0.005. The best decision is to find two well-mixing solutions, one with the minimal index and another with the maximal index of the range under study. It is very important that for each of mixed solutions, the IS keeps its isotonic properties. Evidently, this condition can be satisfied if both solutions have a low osmotic pressure and their mixing is not accompanied by a specific chemical reaction causing increase of osmotic pressure.

(5) The IS should be optically transparent and isotropic, i.e., conditions of less absorption and scattering in the measuring wavelength range as well as less linear birefringence and chirality should be provided.

(6) The IS should be stable in the range from room temperature to physiological temperatures, and their optical properties should not change during prolonged storage.

Such requirements are fulfilled most completely for water solutions of albumin and water-glycerol gelatinous gels.[749,954] The fifth fraction of bovine or human serum albumin contains a total mass of serum albumin and about 3% of α-globulin, and less than 0.5% of β-globulin,[954] and its index of refraction has a linear dependence on concentration with an increment of $\beta_p = 0.00185$ [Eq. (2.31)]. For high concentrations, some discrepancy from linearity is seen that is possibly connected with their relatively high viscosity. For microbiological studies, protein solutions are usually prepared with the refractive index range from 1.360 to 1.420 with the interval of 0.002 on the basis a 0.5–0.6% solution of NaCl in a distilled water.[954]

The water-glycerol gelatinous gels are applicable when cell motility does not allow one to provide precise measurements using protein solutions.[954] Such gels fix and immobilize cells, preserving their vitality; they are optically transparent with low birefringence and high stability of optical properties, if correctly exploited, and have low osmotic pressure. Isotonic gel kits for studies are prepared by the dilution of concentrated salt-free and purified gelatinous gels with a turbidity of 0.5×10^{-3} cm^{-1} in a 0.2% sterile solution of glycerol in a 0.5% solution of NaCl with pH 7.0–7.2; other compositions with 1%-glycerol, 1%-glycerol, and 0.5%-glucose, or 10%-saccharose can also be used. Using protein solutions and gelatinous gels as immersion substances and phase-contrast microscopy with effective suppression of the background light, refractive indices of numerous bacteria of such families as *Coccaceae*, *Bacteriaceae*, *Bacillaceae*, *Spirillaceae*, and *Proactinomycetaceae* have been measured.[954] On the basis of refraction measurements, the concentration of dry materials and water in bacterial cells, their density, and bacterial growth cycle, as well as rehydration of lyophilized bacterial cells and hydration of spores, were studied. The differentiation between vital and dead cells in lyophilized cell preparations and percentage of vital spores were also determined.

The optical clearing effect can be most easily demonstrated by analyzing phase microscope images of bacterial cells that contain only a cytoplasm and a membrane.[954] If a biological object is homogenous, matching its refractive index value with that of the host medium will make it optically invisible. In the case of a bacteria containing only a cytoplasm and a membrane, matching the refractive index of the cytoplasm with that of the extracellular fluid will make the image of the cytoplasm disappear and sharply enhance the brightness of the optical image of the membrane. In a case where the refractive index of the extracellular fluid is externally controlled by the administration of an appropriate chemical agent, the disappearing cytoplasm and the sharp enhancement of the membrane brightness can be used as an efficient method of measuring of the refractive index of the cytoplasm and monitoring of cell vitality. Figure 5.50 illustrates the optical clearing effect.

The finite-difference time-domain (FDTD) approach was recently suggested as a promising tool for a more detailed study of the optical clearing effect in cells and its possible applications.[1053,1054] In Refs. 1053 and 1054, the 3D and 2D FDTD simulation results of light transmission through a biological cell that contain only

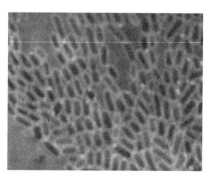

Figure 5.50 Effect of the extracellular fluid on cytoplasm refractive index matching on a phase-contrast microscope image of dysentery bacteria cells. There is a sharp enhancement of the membrane brightness. (Ref. 954, p. 70)

cytoplasm and membrane are presented. The calculated 2D distributions and two cross sections of phase of the E_z component of the forward-scattered light through a biological cell in the near field are shown in Fig. 5.51. It is clearly seen that refractive index matching (graphs on the right) significantly enhances the phase contrast of the cell membrane as it follows from the experimental data of Fig. 5.50. The intensity of phase microscope images is directly proportional to the phase accumulated by the light beam after its propagation through the cell. Calculations were done for typical parameters of a microbial cell: the diameter of the cell, 1.44 μm, and the thickness of the membrane, 0.06 μm; the refractive index of the cytoplasm, 1.36, and of the membrane, 1.47. In calculations, the FDTD cell size was taken as 0.02 μm and the extracellular fluid refractive index values were 1.33 for no refractive index matching and 1.36 for refractive index matching conditions.

Experimentally determined ratios of the scattering intensities from cells (rat fibroblast cell clone MR1, $\sim 10^5$ cells/ml) immersed in media of low and high indices of refraction are presented in Ref. 150. As a medium with a low index of refraction $n = 1.332$, phosphate buffer saline (PBS) was used in both cases. The media of higher index had $n = 1.345$ [bovine serum albumin (BSA) in PBS] and $n = 1.343$ (ovalbumin in PBS). The scattered light intensity at small angles (<20 deg) was significantly greater when the cells were immersed in PBS with a low refractive index than when they are immersed in a protein solution with a higher index. Thus, it may be concluded that there is significant scattering at small angles from cell structures that are in contact with the IS. However, at larger angles (>40 deg), the effect of increasing the index of refraction of IS on light scattering is much smaller. Following estimations of authors of Ref. 150, the percentage of light scattering from internal cellular structures can be determined. Accounting for the fact that the ratio of scattering intensity from cells suspended in IS with low and high indices for angles above 40 deg is 1.3, the fraction of scattering intensity from particles internal to the cell can be estimated. The scattering intensity in IS with low refraction is given by $I_{nc} + I_c$, where I_{nc} and I_c are the intensities of scattering from structures not in contact with and in contact with the IS, respectively. In the IS with high refraction, the scattering from the particles in contact with the IS

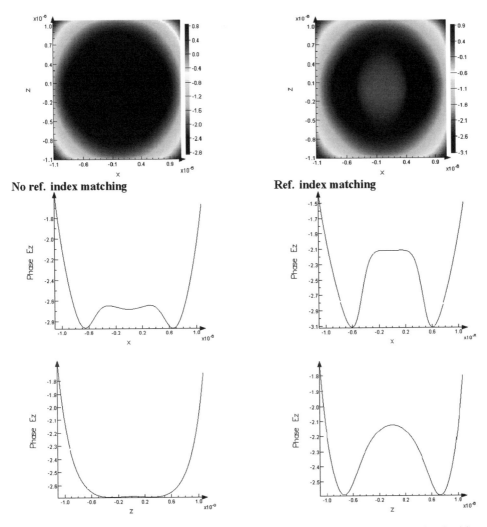

Figure 5.51 The finite-difference time-domain (FDTD) modeling of light scattering by biological cells in controlled extracellular media.[1054] The calculated 2D distributions and two cross sections of phase of the E_z light component in the near field of a biological cell containing only cytoplasm and membrane. It is clearly seen that refractive index matching (graphs on the right) significantly enhances the phase contrast of the cell membrane. Cell radius 0.72 μm, membrane thickness 0.06 μm, cytoplasm refractive index 1.36, membrane refractive index 1.47. Asymmetry is due to the z-polarization of the incident light. The simulations were performed by the FDTD solutions software, which is commercially available from Lumerical Solutions Inc., Vancouver, BC, Canada.

is reduced by about a factor of 2.1 and the scattering is given by $I_{nc} + 0.48I_c$. Thus, the relative light scattering from internal cell components when the cells are immersed in PBS, $I_{nc}/(I_{nc} + I_c) \approx 0.55$, because $(I_{nc} + I_c)/(I_{nc} + 0.48I_c) \approx 1.3$.

5.8 Applications of the tissue immersion technique

5.8.1 Glucose sensing

Noninvasive and continuous monitoring of glucose concentration in blood and tissues is one of the most challenging and exciting applications of optics in medicine. The major difficulty preventing development and clinical application of a noninvasive blood glucose sensor is associated with the very low signal produced by glucose molecules. This results in low sensitivity and specificity of glucose monitoring.[105,138]

The concept of noninvasive blood glucose sensing using the scattering properties of blood as an alternative to spectral absorption and polarization methods[105,534] for monitoring physiological glucose concentrations in the blood of diabetic patients is under intensive discussion.[339–341,534,549–551,631,752–754,957,985,1018, 1019,1113–1115] Many of the effects considered in Section 5.7.2, such as RBC size, refractive index, packing, and aggregation, changed under glucose variation are important for glucose monitoring in diabetic patients. Indeed, at physiological concentrations of glucose ranging from 40 to 400 mg/dl, the role of some of the effects may be changed, and some other effects, such as the rate of glucose penetration inside the RBCs and the followed hemoglobin glycation, may be important[752–754,985,1116] (see Section 2.11 and Fig. 2.14).

Noninvasive determination of glucose was attempted using light scattering of skin tissue components measured by a spatially resolved diffuse reflectance[341,1114] or NIR frequency-domain reflectance techniques.[339] Both approaches are based on change in glucose concentration, which affects the refractive index mismatch between the interstitial fluid and tissue fibers, and hence μ_s'. A glucose clamp experiment (the concentrations of injected glucose and insulin are manipulated to result in a steady concentration of glucose ever a period of time[534]) showed that $\delta\mu_s'$ at 650 nm qualitatively tracked changes in blood glucose concentration for the volunteer with diabetes studied (Fig. 5.52).[341] The distances between the source and detector fibers were in the range $r_{sd} = 1$–10 mm, which corresponds to the approximate 0.5–5 mm in tissue upon which μ_s' is determined. Drift in μ_s' that was independent of glucose prevented statistical analysis and was attributed by the authors to other physiological processes contributing to $\delta\mu_s'$.[341] Changes in μ_s' did not exclusively result from changes in the refractive index of the interstitial fluid caused by increased glucose concentration. The spatially resolved reflectance measurements (at 800 nm and $r_{sd} = 0.8$–10 mm) and oral glucose tolerance test were done to study five healthy volunteers and 13 volunteers with type 2 diabetes using a probe continuously attached to the abdomen.[1114] For volunteers without diabetes, 80% of the measurements showed tracking between $\delta\mu_s'$ and blood glucose concentration, and the other 20% showed no correlation. For volunteers without diabetes, 73% of the measurements resulted in calibration models for μ_s' versus blood glucose concentration. A poor correlation between measured $\delta\mu_s'$ and glucose concentration in these experiments may be connected with a sensitivity to the probe used having a large probing depth on the vascular effect of glucose that induces temporal variations of the blood flow in the skin and subcutaneous tissue.[534]

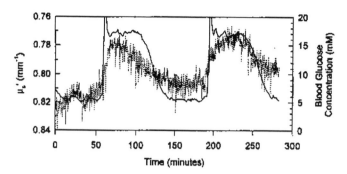

Figure 5.52 Reduced scattering coefficient at 650 nm (dots) and blood glucose concentration (solid curve) measured on a volunteer with insulin-dependent diabetes mellitus during a double clamping experiment.[341] A multichannel CCD-based spatially resolved fiber-optic back-reflectance spectrometer and neural network software were used to measure and extract the optical properties. Reflectance measurements were collected at 15-s intervals for ~5 h, and skin and room temperature were monitored throughout the course of the experiment; the volunteer remained as still as possible, and food and drink were not permitted.

The response of a nondiabetic male subject to a glucose load of 1.75 g/kg body weight, as a standard glucose tolerance test, was determined while continuously monitoring the product of $n\mu_s'$ measured on muscle tissue of the subject's thigh using a portable frequency-domain spectrometer (Fig. 5.53).[339] The refractive index n of the interstitial fluid modified by glucose is defined by Eq. (2.36). As the subject's blood glucose rose, $n\mu_s'$ decreased. Figure 5.53(b) shows the correlation plot obtained from the data of Fig. 5.53(a). The correlation plot fits well to a simple physical model based on the Rayleigh-Gans approximation and accounts for the refractive index matching concept. Key factors for the success of this approach are the precision of the measurements of the reduced scattering coefficient and the separation of the scattering changes from absorption changes, as obtained with the NIR frequency-domain spectrometer.[339] Evidently, other physiological effects related to glucose concentration could account for the observed variations of μ_s' and, as it was mentioned earlier, the effect of glucose on the blood flow in the tissue may be one of the sources of the errors at μ_s' measurements.

So-called occlusion spectroscopy is an approach that is based on light scattering from RBCs.[534,1018,1019] This method suggests a controlled occlusion of finger blood vessels to slow blood flow in order to provide the shear forces of blood flow to be minimal and thus to allow RBCs to aggregate. Change in light scattering upon occlusion is measured. Occlusion will not affect the rest of the tissue components, while the scattering properties of aggregated RBCs differ from those of the nonaggregated ones and from the rest of the tissue. As it was already discussed, a change in glucose concentration affects the refractive index of blood plasma and hence affects blood light scattering at occlusion due to refractive index

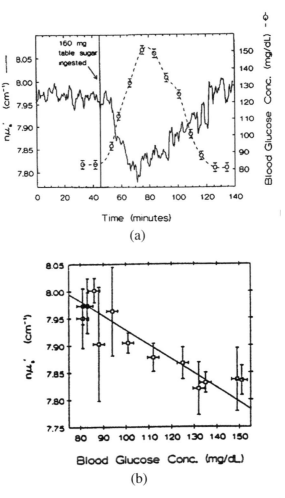

Figure 5.53 Glucose tolerance test performed on a human subject with a portable frequency-domain (120 MHz) NIR (850 nm) spectrometer.[339] (a) At time $t = 45$ min, the subject ingested a glucose load of 160 g of table sugar (1.75 g/kg body weight); the solid curve is the measurements of $n\mu'_s$ on the thigh of the subject, n is defined by Eq. (2.36); the open circles indicate blood glucose concentration as determined by a home blood glucose monitor; the data acquired every 30 s were averaged in sets of five to produce the plot. (b) The correlation corresponding to (a) between the measured blood glucose and product $n\mu'_s$ averaged over a time of 2.5 min centered on the time the finger was lanced for the measurement. The error in $n\mu'_s$ is the standard deviations of the five measurements averaged to get a single point. The error in the blood glucose concentration is estimated to be ± 2.5 mg/dl. The solid line is the theoretical result according to the Rayleigh-Gans model.

match/mismatch between aggregates and plasma. Occlusion spectroscopy differs from that of spatially resolved reflectance and frequency-domain measurements in that it proposes measurements of glucose in blood rather than in the interstitial fluid. The occlusion spectroscopy method was tested in a human study using a hyperinsulinemic-hypoglycemic clamp.[1019] This technique offers the potential of directly measuring the change in the refractive index of blood plasma; but in clinical studies, many other factors affecting the scattering of RBCs and their aggregates should be accounted for: (1) the complexity of the RBC aggregation phenomenon and its dependence on glucose concentration and other pathological conditions and diseases;[534,1103,1105] (2) the effect of glucose on the shape and structure of RBCs.

OCT can be proposed for noninvasive assessment of glucose concentration in tissues.[534,549–551,1113,1115,1117] The high resolution of the OCT technique may allow high sensitivity, accuracy, and specificity of glucose concentration monitoring due to the precise measurements of glucose-induced changes in the tissue optical properties from the layer of interest (dermis). Unlike the diffuse reflectance method, OCT allows one to provide depth-resolved qualitative and quantitative information about tissue optical properties of the three major layers of human skin: the dead keratinized layer of squames (stratum corneum of epidermis); the prickle cells layer (epidermis); and the connective tissue of dermis. Dermis is the only layer of the skin that contains a developed blood microvessel network. Since glucose concentration in the interstitial fluid is closely related to the blood glucose concentration, one can expect glucose-induced changes in the OCT signal detected from the dermis area of the skin. Two methods of OCT-based measurement and monitoring of tissue glucose concentration were proposed: (1) monitoring of the tissue scattering coefficient μ_s as a function of the blood glucose concentration using standard OCT;[549–551] (2) measurement of glucose-induced changes in the refractive index Δn using a novel polarization-maintaining fiber-based dual-channel phase-sensitive optical low-coherence reflectometer (PS-OLCR).[1113]

Experiments were performed with a portable OCT system with the central wavelength of 1300 nm, power of 0.5 mW, and coherence length and lateral resolution of approximately 14 μm and 12 μm, respectively.[549–551,1117] The authors reported results obtained from phantom (aqueous suspension of polystyrene microspheres and milk), animal (27 New Zealand rabbits and 13 hairless Yucatan micropigs), and human (20 healthy volunteers in 24 experiments) studies. OCT images were obtained from skin (ear of the rabbits, dorsal area of the micropigs, and arm of the volunteers). The slopes of the OCT signals were calculated at a depth of 150–900 μm. Glucose administration was performed using: (1) intravenous bolus injections for rapid increase of blood glucose concentration and (2) an intravenous clamping technique for slow, controlled changes of the blood glucose concentration in animal studies; and (3) the standard oral glucose tolerance test (OGTT) in human studies. Blood samples were analyzed using OneTouch (Lifescan Inc., Milpitas, CA), HemoCue (Ryan Diagnostic, Inc., Naperville, IL), and Vitros 950 (Ortho-Clinical Diagnostics, Inc., Raritan, NJ) blood glucose analyzers.

First, an OCT image of the layers of skin is taken and the OCT signal as a function of depth is evaluated. The slope of the portion of the plot in the dermis layer is used to calculate μ_s. In an anesthetized animal skin experiment, OCT images demonstrate that glucose affects the refractive index mismatch in skin and decreases μ_s.[1117] The slope of the OCT signal versus depth line is determined and is correlated with the concentration of blood glucose (Fig. 5.54).

Typical results obtained in the clinical studies are shown in Fig. 5.55. OCT images and blood samples were taken from the left and right forearm, respectively.

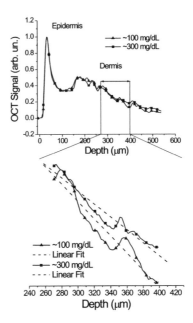

Figure 5.54 Representative OCT signals obtained from Yucatan micropig skin during a glucose clamping experiment at low and high blood glucose concentration (top) and a part of the OCT signal in the dermis area with the linear fit of the OCT signals in this layer (bottom).[551]

Good correlation between the increase of the blood glucose concentration and decrease of the smoothed OCT signal slope has been observed at the depth of 200–600 μm during OGTT. Measurements performed in layers of epidermis and upper dermis either did not show changes in the OCT signal slope at variations of blood glucose concentration or the changes were very weak. Most likely, it is due to a gradient of glucose concentration from dermal blood microvessels to the SC. Thus, the sensitivity and accuracy of the OCT measurements of blood glucose concentration would be maximal in the regions of a developed blood microvessel network (that is, the dermis area).

A comparison of results obtained from the skin of rabbit ear during bolus glucose injection experiments and the skin of a micropig during glucose clamping showed that the OCT signal slope changed approximately 8%/mM during the bolus glucose injection experiment and 2%/mM during glucose clamping. That suggests the possibility of a tissue physiological response to the sharp increase of analyte concentration in the interstitial fluid during bolus glucose injection experiments.

The results obtained in phantoms, animals, and clinical studies demonstrated the potential of the OCT technique to detect small glucose-induced changes in scattering coefficient of the turbid media with high accuracy and sensitivity. However, additional studies should be performed on: (1) the reduction of noise associated with speckles and tissue inhomogeneity, (2) development of algorithms and methods for compensation of motion artifacts, and (3) approbation of the system in clinical studies involving diabetic patients. Although OCT-based glucose sensors most

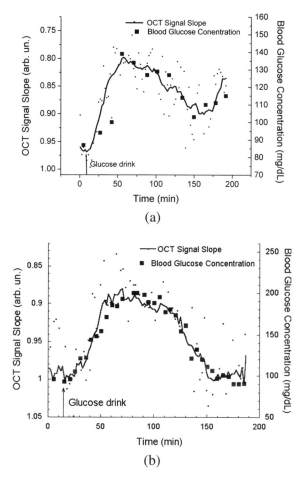

Figure 5.55 Slope of OCT signal and blood glucose concentration versus time. OCT images and blood samples were taken from the human skin of the (a) left and (b) right forearm during an OGTT.[550]

likely may need calibration with invasive glucose sensors, they may dramatically reduce the number of invasive measurements and provide continuous monitoring of the blood glucose concentration.

A question of the specificity of the OCT technique to monitor blood glucose concentration in tissues has been addressed.[551] Experimental and theoretical analyses of the influence of several physical and physiological parameters (such as altering the refractive index mismatch between the interstitial fluid and scattering centers, and structural modifications in tissue due to changes in glucose concentration) on the OCT signal slope were performed. Results obtained demonstrate that: (1) several body osmolytes may change the refractive index mismatch between the interstitial fluid and scattering centers in tissue (however, the effect of the glucose is approximately one to two orders of magnitude higher); (2) an increase of the interstitial fluid glucose concentration in the physiological range (3–30 mM) may decrease the scattering coefficient by 0.22%/mM due to cell volume change;

(3) the stability of the OCT signal slope is dependent on tissue heterogeneity and motion artifacts; and (4) moderate skin temperature fluctuations ($\pm 1°C$) do not decrease the accuracy and specificity of the OCT-based glucose sensor [however, substantial skin heating or cooling (several degrees) significantly change the OCT signal slope]. These results suggest that the OCT technique may provide blood glucose concentration monitoring with sufficient specificity under normal physiological conditions.

A new differential phase-contrast OCT-based method (PS-OLCR) of monitoring glucose-induced changes in tissue optical properties has been also proposed.[1113] While conventional OCT uses the detection and the analysis of intensity of backscattered optical radiation, phase-sensitive OCT utilizes the phase information obtained by probing a sample simultaneously with two common-path low-coherence beams. Variations in the sample refractive index are exhibited in the phase difference $\Delta\varphi$ between these two beams. The PS-OLCR technique is capable of measuring angstrom/nanometer-scale path length changes between the beams [associated with the phase difference $(\lambda/4\pi)\Delta\varphi$] in clear and scattering media. The theoretical and experimental pilot studies on the application of PS-OLCR for noninvasive, sensitive, and accurate monitoring of analyte concentration were reported by the authors of Ref. 1113. They studied concentration-dependent changes of phase, $d\varphi/dC$, and refractive index dn/dC in aqueous solutions of glucose, $CaCl_2$, $MgCl_2$, NaCl, KCl, $KHCO_3$, urea, bovine serum albumin (BSA), and globulin in clear and turbid tissuelike media. The obtained results demonstrate: (1) good agreement between refractive indices measured with the PS-OLCR technique and the conventional white-light refractometer, as previously reported in the literature for the visible spectral range; (2) the effect of glucose on dn/dC is approximately one to four orders of magnitude greater than that of other analytes at the physiological concentrations; (3) good agreement between results obtained in translucent and scattering media, suggesting PS-OLCR could be applied for *in vivo* measurements; and (4) high sub-mM sensitivity of PS-OLCR for measurement of glucose concentration.

Like other scattering techniques, the detected phenomenon in OCT is the effect of glucose on the refractive index of the interstitial fluid. However, it does not allow for blood circulation and temperature changes. Unlike the spatially resolved back-reflectance and frequency-domain methods that use larger measuring volumes and span multiple layers in tissues,[339–341,534,1114] OCT offers a certain advantage because it limits the sampling depth to the upper dermis without unwanted signals from other layers. Precise sampling is very important at glucose monitoring in tissue because glucose uptake is different in different tissue layers, being the lowest in connective tissue and smooth muscle, and highest in adipose tissue and skeletal muscle.[1118] Besides, when blood glucose changes rapidly, there is a time lag of 10–25 min, resulting in a transient difference between the blood and subcutaneous glucose concentrations, which should be accounted for.[1118]

It is important that blood glucose concentrations alter thermally modulated optical signals from skin.[534,996] This is due to some physiologic and physical effects induced in temperature-modulated skin—the temperature modulation affecting mostly cutaneous vascular circulation (physiological effect), and the change of glucose concentration affecting mostly cutaneous light scattering (physical effect). A device based on the thermo-optical response of human skin was used to collect signals from the forearm of volunteers.[681,996] Glucose concentrations were correlated with temperature-modulated localized reflectance signals at wavelengths between 590 and 935 nm. There are no known NIR glucose absorption bands in this range; thus, μ_a is mostly defined by blood absorption, reflecting hemodynamic changes in cutaneous tissue. Evidently, μ_s' is a measure of the refractive index mismatch between the interstitial fluid (ISF) and tissue connective fibers.

Localized reflectance data were collected continuously over a 90-min period of probe–skin contact as temperature was repetitively stepped between 22 and 38°C for 15 temperature modulation cycles.[534,996] Each cycle comprised the following steps: skin was equilibrated for 2 min at a probe temperature of 22°C, and the temperature was raised to 38°C over the course of 1 min, maintained for 2 min, and then lowered to 22°C over a 1-min period. At each temperature limit (during the 2-min window), four optical data packets were collected and values of μ_a and μ_s' were determined. Temperature modulation between 38 and 22°C caused a periodic set of cutaneous refractive index and vascular changes, leading to periodic changes in skin reflectance.[534,996] A four-term linear least-squares fitting of glucose to the reflectance data was used,

$$[\text{glucose}] = a_0 + \Sigma_i a_i [R_i'(r, \lambda, T)]. \qquad (5.39)$$

The reflectance parameter $R'(r, \lambda, T)$, as defined by Eq. (5.39), is equal to $\log_e R(r, \lambda, T)$, where $R(r, \lambda, T)$ is the measured localized reflectance at temperature T. Thirty-two sequences of R' (at $T_{22°C}) = \log_e R(r, \lambda, T_{22°C})$ and R' (at $T_{38°C}) = \log_e R(r, \lambda, T_{38°C})$ were used in the linear least-squares correlation. For each meal tolerance test (MTT) over the 2-hr period, the temperature sequences encompassed 20 data points.[534,996] The correlation between glucose values and optical signals in this spectral range was attributed to the effect of glucose on the refractive index and on the cutaneous hemodynamic response; the correlation coefficient was in the range from 0.69 to 0.94 for two volunteers tested for six days each.

The thermo-optical response method offers certain compartmentalization advantages over localized reflectance measurements that use large source-detector separations[339–341,1114] because it limits the sampling depth to the dermis by virtue of the probe design (short source-detector separations) and the use of temperature control.

5.8.2 Precision tissue photodisruption

Femtosecond laser pulses can generate high-precision subsurface photodisruption in transparent tissues such as cornea.[788] The strong optical intensities required for photodisruption can be achieved at the focus of a high peak power laser beam. The location of optical breakdown can be controlled to occur only at the focus of the beam, where the intensity exceeds the threshold level of breakdown. If the laser is focused beneath the surface of a tissue, subsurface breakdown occurs only at the focus. No damage takes place in the tissue layers that the beam was focused through. In contrast to transparent tissues, turbid tissues scatter light, spreading the pulse in both space and time, and making it difficult to maintain the tight focus and short pulse duration needed for well-confined photodisruption.[788] The same problems are characteristic for nonlinear spectroscopy, including multiphoton fluorescence microscopy and SHG imaging.[609–618,945–947,997,1119]

The ability to focus light through turbid tissue is limited, especially at wavelengths less than 1300 nm. Tissue optical clearing technology using an appropriate immersion agent can be applied for a temporal reduction of scattering needed for providing an effective nonlinear study or underlying tissue photodisruption. In particular, a femtosecond laser technology was used to demonstrate early proof of a concept for high-precision subsurface photodisruption in the translucent human sclera.[788] Approximately 5-mJ femtosecond pulses from two laser sources, 1060 nm (500 fs) and 775 nm (150 fs) with a repetition rate of 1 kHz, were used to make subsurface incisions in sclera *in vitro*. The beam was focused to a 1.5 (775 nm) or 5 μm (1060 nm) spot size and scanned below the tissue surface at various depths to produce incision patterns.

Tissue samples were impregnated by hypaque-76 (x-ray contrast) to make them transparent, usually within 15 min. The measured axial transmission spectra of normal scleral tissue and treated with hypaque-76 (the light forward-scattered in a small cone angle around the incident beam was detected), as well as saline and hypaque-76 spectra, are presented in Fig. 5.56. As it seen, transmission of normal sclera is never greater than 10%, with a broad maximum at 1600–1800 nm. For sclera treated by hypaque-76, the transmittance greatly increases across the entire spectrum, especially for wavelengths in the NIR region from 800 to 1350 nm. A transparent window is also created between two strong water-absorption bands, from 1500 to 1800 nm. Transmission at 775 and 1060 nm is above 60%.

The difference in transmission is not expected to affect the results of photodisruption itself because photodisruption depends on the intensity of the pulse and not the linear absorption. Thus, spectral windows with less scattering and absorption allow for a focused beam to penetrate into a tissue with less attenuation and distortion, and do not influence photodisruption efficiency.

As expected, at 775 nm, the size of the intensity distribution emerging from the normal sclera did not change on the position of the focusing lens, since scattering is very strong. The emergent beam is many times larger than the unscattered spot and is strongly speckle modulated (see Fig. 5.8).[343] At a longer wavelength, 1060 nm, due to less scattering, the distribution is smaller, but still heavily scattered. Therefore, focusing to the back surface of the tissue is not possible using these wavelengths; thus, for the normal scleral, tissue breakdown was only possible at the front surface first.[788] After treating the tissue with hypaque-76, the spot size decreases to almost that of the unscattered beam for both wavelengths; thus,

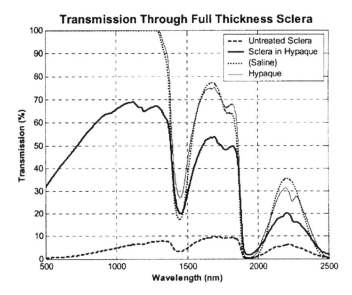

Figure 5.56 Transmission spectra of normal and human scleral samples treated by hypaque-76 along with saline and hypaque-76.[788] All samples were approximately 0.5-mm thick.

the strong focusing of the beam should permit controlled back-surface photodisruption. Several types of intrascleral incisions were experimentally demonstrated using optical clearing technology, such as: partial thickness channel creation that could be used to perform a transscleral procedure analogous to deep sclerotomy, where a block of inner surface sclera is removed with minimal disruption to overlying layers, or in altering the mechanical properties of the sclera for the treatment of presbyopia; full thickness channel creation that may be useful for draining aqueous for the treatment of glaucoma; creation of a grid of tissue pores that may be useful in changing the bulk properties of the tissue, including the tissue's hydraulic conductivity; and scleral pocket creation that may be useful for inserting implants to treat presbyopia.[788]

5.9 Other techniques of tissue optical properties control

5.9.1 Tissue compression and stretching

As it was already mentioned in Section 5.1, squeezing (compressing) or stretching of a soft tissue produces a significant increase in its optical transmission.[951] The major reasons for that are the following: (1) increased optical tissue homogeneity due to removal of blood and interstitial fluid from the compressed site [see Eq. (2.24)], (2) closer packing of tissue components causes less scattering due to cooperative (interference) effects (see Chapters 1 and 3),[442,950] and (3) less tissue thickness. Mechanisms underlying the effects of optical clearing and changing of light reflection by soft tissues at compression and stretching were proposed in a number of theoretical and experimental studies.[61,62,442,575,580,667,692, 722,723,950,992,1005,1013]

It should be emphasized, however, that squeezing-induced effects in tissues that contain little blood, such as sclera, are characterized by a marked inertia (for a few minutes) because of the relatively slow diffusion of water from the compressed region.[723] It was suggested that compression of sclera may displace water from the interspace of collagen fibrils, increasing the protein and mucopolysaccharide concentrations. Since these proteins and sugars have refractive indexes closer to that of the collagen fibrils, a more index-matched environment can be created. On the other hand, compression reduces specimen thickness d, which might increase the effective scatterer concentration inside the tissue.[667] Therefore, compression may also give rise to an increase in tissue scattering coefficient μ_s. However, the total effect on the change of optical properties, which is proportional to the product of $\mu_s d$, is characterized by less scattering.

Sometimes the increase in scatterer concentration is likely to be more dominant than the reduction in index mismatch.[667] In addition, reduction of tissue thickness causes an increase in local chromophore concentration (for bloodless tissue, or tissue specimens that have aggregated and/or coagulated blood), i.e., the absorption coefficient increases. The authors of Ref. 667 observed that compression caused leaking around the specimen. Some of the extracellular fluids along the edge of the tissue sample were forced out upon compression. Unless sufficient pressure was applied to rupture the cell walls, the intracellular fluids would be retained by the cells at the bulk of the sample. When compressed, the tissue thickness was reduced and so the volumetric water concentration was increased. This may explain the increase of the absorption coefficient at the wavelengths of water bands with compression. The authors of Ref. 667 have studied the optical properties *in vitro* of human skin, bovine aorta, bovine sclera, and porcine sclera in the spectral range from 400 to 1800 nm, using the integrating sphere technique and inverse adding-doubling method for the convolution of absorption and reduced scattering coefficients. The diffuse reflectance and transmittance of these tissue samples of about 2×2 cm were measured at no pressure and at pressures of 0.1, 1, and 2 kg/cm^2 uniformly distributed over the sample surface. They generally observed a decrease in reflectance, while the transmittance, absorption, and scattering coefficients increased owing to compression. Some of these data for human skin are presented in Table 2.1. As was explained earlier, the amount of scattering depends on the refractive index mismatch, as well as on scatterer concentration and spacing. Along the load direction, the spacing between tissue components is reduced and, due to water escaping from the compression site, refractive index matching should occur; both effects decrease the averaged light scattering (transmittance increases and reflectance decreases). On the other hand, compression reduces specimen thickness, which might increase the effective scatter and chromophore concentration inside the tissue. In experiments with a uniformly distributed compression, the scatter concentration increase was likely more dominant than the reduction in index mismatch and scatterer packing affect. It should be noted that the relative balance of the contributions of the listed mechanisms is expected to be changed if a point-wise compression is applied.[266,267,723] To understand the optical properties of compressed tissue, time-resolved studies in the range of minutes are important.[723]

Spectral properties of skin can be effectively controlled by applying an external localized pressure in *in vivo* experiments when UV-induced erythema (skin redness) is developed.[575,580,991] Figure 5.57 shows the apparent optical density (OD) evaluated from the *in vivo* measured back-reflectance spectra of erythematous human skin for different values of external localized mechanical pressure. On the third day after UV irradiation, erythema develops and is exhibited as increased absorbance (OD) in the 520–580 nm spectral range due to increased blood volume blood volume in the skin. Blood hemoglobin blocks the backscattered intensity from the deep skin layers. For the longer wavelengths from 600 to 700 nm, increased blood volume causes an increase in light scattering from tissue, which is seen as an increase of the apparent OD. At pressures of $(8.4–14) \times 10^5$ Pa, blood is leaving the compressed area of the skin; thus, OD spectral dependence becomes smoother due to less absorption in the range 520–580 nm and less scattering in the range 600–700 nm.

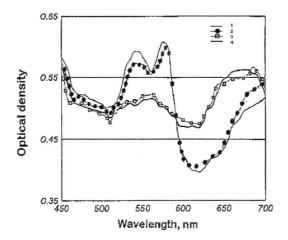

Figure 5.57 The apparent optical density (OD) spectral distridutions of erythematous human skin (three days after UV irradiation) for different values of external mechanical pressure: (1) without pressure; (2) 5.6×10^4 Pa; (3) 8.4×10^4 Pa; (4) 1.4×10^5 Pa.[575,991]

The intensity of skin autofluorescence is also well controlled at external localized pressure applied to the skin site. As it follows from Fig. 5.58, the external localized pressure in the range from 0 to 1.4×10^5 Pa changes the fluorescence output considerably with the wavelength of 460 nm at induced erythema. Due to more effective fluorescence light attenuation by blood hemoglobin at more intensive erythema (14 days after UV irradiation), skin compression more effectively controls (increase) fluorescence output.

As it was also shown, the application of a pressure cuff to the upper arm of healthy volunteers at levels of 0-, 20-, 30-, 40-, and 60-mm Hg did not signifi-

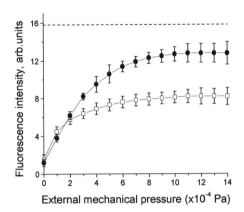

Figure 5.58 Autofluorescence (AF) intensity of erythematous human skin ($\lambda_f = 460$ nm) with dependence on external mechanical pressure: (□) 7 days after UV rradiation (less developed erythema); (●) 14 days after UV irradiation (more developed erythema). The AF intensity of human skin without erythema and compression (dotted line) is marked as a reference value.[575,580]

cantly alter the levels of oxyhemoglobin or melanin of preliminary UV-irradiated volar forearm skin (induced erythema and melanin pigmentation).[1005] In contrast, deoxyhemoglobin significantly contributes to the skin color appearance. Blood pooling, expressed as increased deoxyhemoglobin, can contribute to what is visually perceived as pigmentation. Oxyhemoglobin values increased to a maximum on the first day after UV irradiation, correlating well with the clinical evaluation of erythema, and then decreased exponentially to baseline. Melanin contents showed a significant increase on the seventh day and remained relatively constant for the next three weeks, correlating well with the clinical evaluation of pigmentation (tanning). Deoxyhemoglobin increased slightly on the first day and remained elevated for the next two weeks. Thus, it correlated moderately well with the clinical erythema scoring on day 1 only, while it contributed significantly to what is clinically perceived as skin tanning on days 7 and 14. Application of pressure below the diastolic level increased the deoxyhemoglobin concentration as measured by diffuse reflectance spectroscopy. This increase corresponded to a decrease of a "pigmentation" parameter in a similar fashion to that which has been documented for increases in melanin concentration. Topical application of H_2O_2 reduced deoxyhemoglobin levels as measured by reflectance spectroscopy. This reduction coincided kinetically with a visible skin blanching.

The light propagation in human skin at mechanical tension was studied *in vivo* using a steady-state diffuse reflectometry with a variable source-detector separation r_{sd}.[692] To examine the effect of skin tension on the optical properties, the skin was maintained in a stretched position by pulling it mechanically in a defined direction and then fixing it to an aluminum ring with double-sided adhesive tape. For medium and far distances of the detector from the light source ($r_{sd} = 2$ and 7 mm), it was found that anisotropy of light propagation followed the stretching direction. The direction of stretching complies with that of the maximal reflectance signal for a given distance greater than about 2 mm. Thus, the scattering coefficient is minimal when measured along the direction of stretching because the intensity is maximal for the distant detector. MC modeling that accounts for the anisotropy of the scattering coefficient, caused by different photon interaction with the medium when it was traveling along the tissue fibers and across them and described by Eq. (2.20) with the fraction of scatterers (cylinders) oriented in the preferential direction, $f = 0.35$, was also done.[692] As it follows from Eq. (2.20), the scattering cross section varies with the direction cosine of the incident photon with respect to the axis of the cylinder. It is maximal for perpendicular incidence and is minimal for parallel incidence. The MC modeling has demonstrated that for short source-detector separations, the detected signal is much higher (scattering coefficients are also higher) for the perpendicular direction regarding the preferential direction of the collagen fibers. For farther detectors, the signal is higher in the parallel direction (scattering coefficient is lower). Such correlated or anticorrelated dependences between the intensity back-reflectance and the scattering coefficient, respectively, for short and long source-detector separations also follow from the data in Fig. 5.27.

From this analysis it follows that at skin stretching, the scattering coefficient and corresponding light back-reflectance and transmittance can be effectively controlled. On the other hand, intact skin has its own anisotropy, which is believed to be caused by the preferential orientation of collagen fibers in the dermis, as described by Langer's skin tension lines.[692] Thus, the human skin's reduced scattering coefficient varies by a factor of two between different directions of light propagation at the same position (see Table 2.1). At external forced tension, more significant damping of scattering along the direction of mechanical stress is expected.

The measurements of the deformations and applied loads, along with the estimating of the biomechanical properties of tissue, are critical to many areas of the health sciences, including monitoring of the tension in wound closures, skin flaps, and tissue expanders.[1013] Such measurements, which can be provided by detection of the polarized light reflectivity, will allow surgeons to treat wounds more successfully by minimizing scar tissue and maximizing the speed of treatment by letting them know how much the skin can be stretched at each treatment step. *In vivo* human experiments showed that the specular reflection from skin changes with stretch.[1013] For small values of stretch, the specular reflectivity measured for a He-Ne laser ($\lambda = 633$ nm) beam with a 45-deg angle of incidence increases linearly with strain. The linear relationship between applied stretch and polarized reflectivity can be understood if the skin surface is approximated by a sinusoidal profile in the resting stage. Stretching reduces the amplitude and increases the spatial scale of the skin profile, thereby making it smoother and flatter, resulting in a corresponding increase of reflectivity. For ten tested subjects with various skin complexions, the slope of the dependence of the reflectivity (normalized to a maximal value) on strain (expressed in percents) is in the range from 0.0074 to 0.0391 (1/%) with the linear correlation coefficient R^2 from 0.88 to 0.99. For larger stretches [for strains above 8.8% (5-mm stretch)] for the human subject tested, the dependence is saturated and even goes down. The stretches in two perpendicular directions (parallel and perpendicular to the long axis of the forearm) yield good correlation between stretch and reflected light intensity and show that skin has anisotropic properties that can be detected by light reflection. For example, the slope measured in a parallel direction to the long axis of the forearm was 0.0095 ± 0.0002 (1/%), and in a perpendicular direction, 0.0065 ± 0.0008 (1/%).[1013]

5.9.2 Temperature effects and tissue coagulation

A reproducible effect of temperature between 25 and 40°C on the reduced scattering coefficient of human dermis and subdermis was found in an *ex vivo* study in the NIR region.[236,237] For dermis, the relative change in the reduced scattering coefficient showed an increase [$(4.7 \pm 0.5) \times 10^{-3} °C^{-1}$], and for subdermis, a decrease [$(-1.4 \pm 0.28) \times 10^{-3} °C^{-1}$]. The absolute values of the coefficients are presented in Table 2.1. It was hypothesized that the observed positive and negative temperature coefficients of scattering for dermis and subdermis are connected with differences in their structural components. The main scattering components of subdermis were assumed to be lipids in membranes and vacuoles. It is known that lipids undergo phase changes at certain temperatures, which alter their orientation, mobility, and packing order.[750,1070,1071] Glycolipids found in human cell membranes undergo phase transitions in the temperature range from 25 to 45°C, namely, a transition from a gel phase through a stable crystalline phase to a liquid-crystalline phase with increasing temperature. The decrease in the scattering coefficient seen experimentally with increasing temperature is therefore consistent with an increase in fluidity known to occur in lipids with increasing temperature. Modifications of the collagen fiber structure of dermis caused by increasing temperature, possibly through changes in hydration, is the most plausible explanation of the increased scattering properties.[236,237] As claimed by the authors of Refs. 236 and 237, a tissue that is largely protein has a positive temperature coefficient and a tissue that is largely lipid has a negative temperature coefficient leads to interesting possibilities in tissues where the protein/lipid ratio is intermediate, such as brain tissue.

The temperature change of absorption, μ_a, and the reduced scattering, μ_s', coefficients of human forearm skin have also been determined in the course of *in vivo* studies for two skin surface temperatures, 22 and 38°C[681] (see data in Table 2.1). A rather high increase of 16–21% for μ_a and much smaller increase of 2.7–4.6% for μ_s' coefficient values were found with temperature change from 22 to 38°C for the wavelengths 950–590 nm.

Low-intensity laser radiation, when used for spectroscopy (diagnostics) or therapy, may heat tissue and therefore distort results of tissue optical properties measurements or may induce an uncontrolled change in a photobiological response of a tissue caused by a local heating. Human skin temperature increase at CW laser irradiation can be estimated on the basis of experimental and theoretical studies presented in Refs. 261, 262, and 995. It was found experimentally that for near-infrared laser radiation (789 nm) guided to the skin surface of the fore-arm of an awake human volunteer by a 1-mm optical fiber, the temperature in-creased linearly with power level as $0.101 \pm 0.001°$C/mW at the depth of 0.5 mm, as $0.038 \pm 0.001°$C/mW at the depth of 1 mm, and as $0.029 \pm 0.0005°$C/mW at the depth of 1.5 mm in the range of illuminating power up to 10 mW.[995]

The combination of the MC technique to calculate the fluence rate distribution of light and the adaptive finite element method to solve the heat transfer equation was applied to investigate the process of hyperthermia induced by transskin irradi-ation with a He-Ne laser (633 nm).[261,262] It was shown that the overheated tissue volume, heating depth, and temperature can be effectively controlled by chang-ing the free convention boundary conditions on the tissue surface and varying the power, radius, and shape of the incident laser beam. The four-layer model of human skin (epidermis, upper dermis, blood plexus, and lower dermis) with optical and thermal properties of the tissue layers taken from the literature was used for mod-eling. The modeling was done for Gaussian and rectangular incident light beams at noncoagulating intensities. By variation of the value of the heat transfer coeffi-cient A, corresponding to free convection at initial skin surface temperature equal to 34°C ($A = 0.009$ W/cm^2 K), to weak isolation ($A = 0.004$ W/cm^2 K), and to strong isolation ($A = 0.0005$ W/cm^2 K), the effect of thermal insulation on tissue temperature distributions was studied. For a 25-mW Gaussian incident beam of a 1 mm in diameter, the subsurface temperature maxima at the depths of 0.20 mm, 0.18 mm, and 0.10 mm and equal to 36.7°C, 41.3°C, and 42.8°C were found as isolation increased. At the depth of 1 mm, the calculated temperature was 37.7°C, 38.1°C, and 38.5°C as the degree of isolation increased. It should be noted that the above-mentioned experimental data[995] are well fit to the modeled ones for free con-vention boundary conditions on the skin surface. From experiments, it follows that for light power of 25 mW, temperature increase at the depth of 1 mm is expected to be $0.038°$C/mW $\times$ 25 mW $= 0.95°$C. In its turn, calculations showed the tempera-ture increasing from the initial value without radiation of 36.4°C to 37.7°C at laser action, i.e., by 1.3°C. The somewhat higher temperature increase than expected in theory from the experimental estimation may be explained by the shorter wave-length of light used, which is more effectively absorbed by tissue chromophores.

The loss of water by tissue due to temperature effects (freezing in a refrig-erator or noncoagulating heating) seriously influences its optical properties. For instance, in an *in vitro* study of human aorta, the absorption coefficient increased by 20–50%, especially in the visible range, when an average 46.4% of total tis-sue weight was lost as a result of a dehydrated tissue sample prolonged freezing in a refrigerator.[569,570] The weight loss was accompanied by an average shrinkage in thickness of 19.5%. Primarily because of shrinkage (denser packing of tissue components), the absorption coefficient was increased in the spectral range 400–1300 nm. There was only a slight increase of 2–15% in the reduced scattering coefficient in the visible range, again due to closer packing of tissue components.

The slope of the wavelength dependence of the reduced scattering coeffi-cient μ_s', which is proportional to λ^{-h} [see Eq. (1.178)], is a good test for the alteration of tissue morphology at heating or freezing. Data summarized in Table 1.5 demonstrate experimental values of parameter h for normal, dehydrated, and coagulated human aorta received at an *in vitro* study in the spectral range 400–1300 nm.[569,570] Tissue dehydration (by its slow freezing) increases the slope (h) from 1.15 (control) to 1.22, which reflects denser scatterers' packing at tissue shrinkage. Sample heating during 5 min in a saline bath at temperatures in the vicinity of the tissue coagulation threshold may increase h [e.g., for 60°C, from 1.21 (control) to 1.28 (possibly due to a local protein coagulation)] or decrease h [e.g., for 70°C, from 1.30 (control) to 1.10 (possibly due to more extensive protein coagulation)]. This result reflects the fact that collagen denaturation starts dominating tissue behavior between 55 and 70°C.[569] Due to aorta tissue's heterogeneity, its components may have reached different end points at the end of the 5-min heating period. At 100°C heating of the samples in a saline bath, h was reduced from 1.38 for the normal tissue samples to 1.06 for the heated ones, and for the samples preliminarily wrapped in aluminum foil, h was reduced from 1.26 to 1.03.

As tissue heats in a bath, the absorption coefficients may increase up to 28% (60°C) or decrease up to 22% (70°C) on selected wavelengths. At the same time, the values of the reduced scattering coefficient were increased for all used heating temperatures in a wide range from 1.1 to 76%, depending on the wavelength in the range from 350 to 1320 nm and heating temperature. At a temperature of 60°C, the increase was rather smooth (16–19%) in this wavelength range. At 70°C, the increase of μ_s' was not as smooth, being changed from 1.1 to 24.8%. Heating up to 100°C gave an increase in in reduced scattering coefficient of 22–76%, but tissue wrapping decreased these values to 15–54%. Such complex behavior of scattering and absorption properties of precoagulated and coagulated tissues reflects tissue heterogeneity and the specificity of the protein denaturation process leading to the appearance of coarse and small thermally coagulated granular cellular proteins and some tissue chromophore damage, as well as interactions of heated saline with tissue resulting in saline and chromophore diffusion.[569]

Following Ref. 569, it may be verified that tissue progresses from normal to denaturated states between 60°C and 70°C, and that at ~60°C some changes in the optical properties caused by thermal damage are still reversible, even though the thermal threshold for protein coagulation is exceeded. In general, the complex behavior of tissue optical properties at heating can be explained by particular changes in tissue morphology. To model the optical properties of heated tissues, the modified morphology should be expressed in such terms as scatterer size distribution, particle and interstitial fluid refractive index mismatch, particle packing, and chromophore concentrations.

Long-pulsed laser heating may induce reversible and irreversible changes in the optical properties of tissue.[570,997] The total transmittance decreased and the diffuse reflectance increased in both fresh and precoagulated human skin and canine aorta samples when it was irradiated by a 0.2-ms pulsed Nd:YAG laser emitting at 1064 nm with the a repetition rate of 10 Hz (20 pulses of 0.9 J/pulse) and a 1.5-mm light spot.[570] The existence of nonlinear behavior in the optics of biological media was indicated.[570] Possible mechanisms responsible for this nonlinear optical response are listed in Table 5.6. The *in vitro* skin-equivalent raft tissue irradiated with one pulse from a perovskite laser ($\lambda = 1341$ nm) with a fluence of 20 J/cm^2 and pulse duration of 20 ms showed thermal injury areas characterized by less scattering as seen on the OCT images and loss of the SHG signal.[997] Such behavior was interpreted by the authors of Ref. 997 as collagen fiber disintegration at thermal tissue protein denaturation, which can be rejuvenated at tissue healing.

Laser ablation or coagulation is usually accompanied by a change in the normal optical properties of the tissue.[570,1050] For example, ablation of aortal tissue using an eximer laser (308 nm) results in a 2.3-fold to 3.7-fold increase in its optical density compared with the untreated material.[1050] Published results on optical properties of coagulated tissues are presented in Table 2.1. In spite of some variations in the dependence on tissue type, wavelength studied, and sample preparation technique, the general tendency at tissue coagulation is the increase of both the absorption and scattering coefficients, from a few dozens to two- or three-hundred percent.

Low temperatures ($+12°C$) sometimes result in the so-called cold cataract, i.e., a sharp rise in the scattering coefficient due to protein aggregation.[850,1016] This process is reversed with an increase in temperature.

Cryogenic temperatures used in cryosurgery may also change scattering properties of tissues due to local variations in the refractive index, such as the boundary between liquid and frozen water in tissue.[1004] The corresponding subsurface morphological changes were evident during freezing ($-80°C$) of *in vivo* hamster skin.

Table 5.6 Possible mechanisms responsible for inducing reversible changes in tissue optical response on laser long-pulsed irradiation.[570]

Mechanism	Description	Optical response
Thermal lensing, $n(T) = n(273 \text{ K}) + \Delta T(r, z, t)(dn/dT)$	Gradient in the index of refraction caused by nonuniform heating	Decrease in T_t and increase in R_d
Temperature dependence of the reduced scattering coefficient: $\mu'_s(T) = \mu_s(T)[1 - g(T)]$	Change in the size and/or shape of scatterers due to temperature rise	Increase in T_t and decrease in R_d (as μ'_s decreases)
Water transport	Temporary local dehydration during laser heating	Increase in T_t and decrease in R_d
Thermal expansion	Decrease in tissue density and increase in tissue thickness caused by thermal expansion of tissue	Decrease in T_t and increase in R_d

5.9.3 Tissue whitening

Sometimes, to provide higher-contrast images of intracellular components of the epithelial tissues, instead of optical clearing, the usage of induced tissue turbidity (whitening) is more preferable.[998–1006,1014] For example, a fundamental part of the colposcopic exam is the use of acetic acid, which when applied to the cervix induces transient whitening changes in the epithelial tissues.[1003] The spatial and temporal changes of "acetowhitening" are the major visual diagnostic indicators in the determination of the location of the most severe dysplastic regions. The acetowhitening effect causes a differential brightening of dysplastic tissue relative to normal tissue, and besides cervical disorders, is used for skin and other epithelial disease screening.

The brightening of nuclei enhances the contrast and significantly improves the detectability of nuclear morphology in basal cell cancers.[1006] Under normal conditions, the nucleous contains a diffuse network of thin chromatin filaments that are typically 30–100 nm in diameter and occupy a small volume. Because of the small dimensions and difference between the refractive index of the chromatin, which is not high and can be estimated as 1.39, and surrounding tissue components (cell cytoplasm and interstitial fluid) of about 1.35, its backscattering is low. The acetic acid causes assembling of the chromatin into thick fibers that are 1–5 μm in diameter; the compacted chromatin fills a large fraction of the intranuclear volume,[1006] and some increase in its refractive index is also expected;[1003] thus, the backscattering signal from the nuclei is increased and they appear bright. After washing *ex vivo* samples of human epidermis with 5% acetic acid for three minutes, the epidermal cell nuclei appear bright as seen in the confocal reflectance images.[1006]

The temporal kinetics of the acetowhitening process as measured by the reflected light maximizes the first 1–2 min and decays over several minutes (5–10 min) thereafter, allowing one to clearly distinguish high-grade cervical intraepithelial neoplasia (CIN 2/3) from normal cervical epithelium when the ratio of green to red light intensities of the backscattered light was analyzed.[1003] Normalizing the green light by the red light preserves kinetics in the reflected signal, indicating that the reflected light has a spectral change. Roughly, acetowhitening in the CIN 2/3 cervical tissue *in vivo* causes a 20–80% rise of the original reflectance. In contrast, mature squamous epithelium appears to increase in reflectance only by approximately 5%; moreover, reflectance is constant in time after acetic acid application.

5.10 Conclusion

This chapter shows that optical immersion technology allows one to effectively control the optical properties of tissues and blood. Such control leads to the essential reduction of scattering and therefore causes much higher transmittance (optical clearing) and the appearance of a large amount of least-scattered (snake) and ballistic photons, allowing for successful application of coherent-domain and polarization imaging techniques. The dynamics of tissue optical clearing, defined by the dynamics of refractive index matching, is characterized by a time response of about 5–30 min, which in its turn depends on the diffusivity of the immersion agent in a tissue layer, water diffusion rate, and tissue layer thickness. The swelling or shrinkage of the tissue and cells may play an important role in the tissue clearing process at application of osmotically active agents.

In vivo reflectance spectrophotometry and frequency-domain measurements for immersed tissues show that the refractive index matching technique provided by the appropriate chemical agent can be successfully used in tissue spectroscopy and imaging when radical reduction of scattering properties is needed. Hyperdermal injection of glucose causes the essential clearing of human skin. For such tissues as sclera or cornea, the application of some drops of glucose is sufficient to make up very high and rather prolonged tissue clearing. In *in vivo* experiments, the impregnation of a tissue by an agent is more effective than in *in vitro* studies due to the higher diffusivity of an agent at physiological temperature and by involvement of blood and lymph microvessels into the process of agent distribution. However, some physiological reactions of living tissue on osmotically active solutions may influence the measured spectra.

Dynamic optical characteristics can be used for the determination of the diffusion coefficient and concentration of endogenous (metabolic) and exogenous (chemical agent) fluids in human sclera, skin, and other tissues.

The immersion technique has great potential for noninvasive medical diagnostics using OCT due to the rather small thickness of tissue layers usually examined by OCT, which allows for fast impregnation of a target tissue at a topical application of an immersion liquid. It has been demonstrated that the body's interior tissues such as the blood vessel wall, esophagus, stomach, cervix, and colon can usually be imaged at a depth of about 1–2 mm. For more effective diagnosis using OCT, a higher penetration depth can be provided by the applying of immersion substances.

The method of tissue clearing is convenient, inexpensive, and simple for diagnostic purposes; in particular, it can be applied for *in vivo* monitoring of microcirculation. It may be useful for the study of the structure and function of blood microvessels—diameters of arterioles and venules, capillary density, bifurcation angles, etc.

Optical clearing might be a fruitful technique for various methods of tissue spectroscopy, microscopy, and imaging (Raman, fluorescence, confocal, laser scanning, near field, multiphoton, SHG, etc.) where scattering is a serious limitation. Encouraging results were recently received for the enhancement of a fluorescence signal at tissue optical immersion. It is important to note that reduction of light scattering may help in the differentiation of various fluorophores in the depth of a tissue, for instance of skin.

The concept that index matching could improve the optical penetration depth of whole blood is proved experimentally in *in vitro* studies. It should be accounted for that blood optical clearing is defined not only by the refractive index matching effect, but also by changes in the size of red blood cells and their aggregation ability when chemicals are added.

Many of the tested agents and the methods of their delivery have both advantages and disadvantages. The main disadvantages are the osmotic stress, which occurs at high concentration of the hyperosmotic agent applied, and low permeability of tissue cell structures for the clearing agents. Therefore, the finding of new agents and delivery techniques are important.

The immersion optical clearing concept and technology is applicable not only to soft tissues and blood, but also to hard tissues. At present, tendon[409,410,946] (see Fig. 5.38), cranial bones,[738] and tooth enamel[1041] have been tested.

Part II

Light Scattering Methods and Instruments for Medical Diagnosis

6

Continuous Wave and Time-Resolved Spectrometry

The specificity of optical spectral diffusion techniques is discussed in this chapter. As usual for this tutorial, two types of instruments and measuring techniques are presented: spectroscopic, used for tissue local parameters monitoring, and tomographic, used for tissue pathology imaging. Some of them are based on CW light source tissue probing. A few examples of CW measuring and imaging instruments and results of clinical studies are presented. Time-resolved techniques and instruments, which are the most promising for an accurate *in vivo* measurement, are also analyzed. In accordance with the basic principles discussed in Chapter 1, three types of time-resolved techniques and instruments are considered: the time-domain technique, which uses ultrashort laser pulses; the frequency-domain technique, which exploits an intensity-modulated light and narrowband heterodyne detection; and the phased array technique, which utilizes an interference of photon diffusion waves.

6.1 Continuous wave spectrophotometry

6.1.1 Techniques and instruments for *in vivo* spectroscopy and imaging of tissues

For the *in vivo* study of thick tissue (for example, the female breast), the collimated light transmittance can be described by an exponential law such as Eq. (1.1), taking into account that due to multiple scattering, the effective migration path of a photon before it is absorbed should be larger than the thickness of the tissue.[288] For a slab of thickness d, the diffusion equation can be used to calculate a mean path length L of the photons as[272]

$$L = \frac{\mu_{\text{eff}}}{2\mu_a \mu_s'} \frac{(\mu_s' d - 1)\exp(2\mu_{\text{eff}}/\mu_s') - (\mu_s' d + 1)}{\exp(2\mu_{\text{eff}}/\mu_s') - 1}, \quad (6.1)$$

where μ_{eff} is defined by Eq. (1.18). Using Eq. (1.1) for the matched boundaries ($n = 1$), the collimated transmittance can be written in the form[288]

$$T_c(\lambda) = x_1 \exp[-\mu_a(\lambda)L(\lambda)x_2], \quad (6.2)$$

where $L(\lambda)$ reflects the wavelength dependence of $\mu_a(\lambda)$ and $\mu_s'(\lambda)$; x_1 takes into account multiply scattered but not absorbed photons, which do not arrive at the

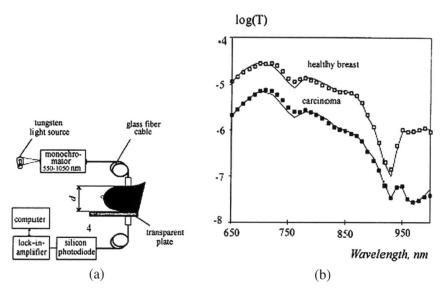

(a)   (b)

Figure 6.1 (a) Schematic setup of a spectrophotometer system used for *in vivo* measurements of breast tissue spectra.[288] (b) Spectra and respective fits of a breast cancer patient (56 yrs., breast thickness of 60 mm) within the area of carcinoma and for a healthy breast and the similar localization as carcinoma.

detector, and the measurement geometry; and x_2 compensates for measurement error of the thickness d and inaccuracies in the reduced scattering coefficient μ_s'.

The semiempirical Eq. (6.2) was successfully used for fitting the *in vivo* measurement spectra of the female breast and estimation of the concentrations of the following absorbers: water (H_2O), fat (f), deoxyhemoglobin (Hb), and oxyhemoglobin (HbO_2) as[288]

$$\mu_a = c_{H_2O}\sigma_{H_2O} + c_f\sigma_f + c_{Hb}\sigma_{Hb} + c_{HbO_2}\sigma_{HbO_2}, \qquad (6.3)$$

where σ_i is the cross section of the absorption of the ith component.

By varying the concentrations of the four tissue components, the measurement spectra could be fitted well by Eq. (6.2); the correlation coefficients were better than 0.99 in all cases.[288] Figure 6.1. shows the spectrometer for *in vivo* measurement of the collimated transmittance spectra of a female breast and some examples of measured and fitted spectra for normal and pathological (cancer tumor) tissues. Typically, most carcinoma spectra exhibit a lower transmittance than the reference spectrum (for the same breast thickness). The fits show that this is generally due to an increased blood perfusion (higher Hb/HbO_2 values of the carcinoma curve). In the wavelength region between about 900 and 1000 nm, spectra are quite different; this is clearly due to the altered water and fat content of carcinomas compared with that of the healthy breast. The majority of mastopathies and carcinomas show a higher water concentration and a higher blood volume at the lesion site. A comparison of healthy and cancerous sites yields a slightly lower concentration of oxyhemoglobin for the tumor. Unfortunately, the specificity is not good enough because it is not possible to discriminate between benign mastopathies and malignant carcinomas by means of water content, blood volume, and oxygenation.[288]

Transmittance NIR spectrometry for measuring oxygenation has had the most success to date in the newborn infant head, largely because of the small size of the head, the thin overlying surface tissues and skull, and the lower scattering coefficient of the infant brain.[55] The development of the cooled CCD and time-resolved and spatially resolved techniques and instruments has proceeded rapidly, and they are increasing the area of NIR spectroscopy investigations and applications. At present, there are more than 500 commercial clinical NIR spectroscopy instruments for monitoring and imaging the degree of oxygenation in tissues, the concentration of oxidized cytochrome, and tissue hemodynamics.

For many tissues, *in vivo* measurements are possible only in the geometry of the backscattering. The corresponding relations can be written on the basis of a diffusion approximation. For a semi-infinite medium and source and detector probes separated by a distance r_{sd}, normal to the sample surface (see Fig. 6.2), and optically matched (so that specular reflectance at the surface can be neglected), the reflecting flux is given by Eq. (2.17).[685] A more general expression valid for refractive index mismatch conditions on the boundary is given by Eq. (1.27).[205,206]

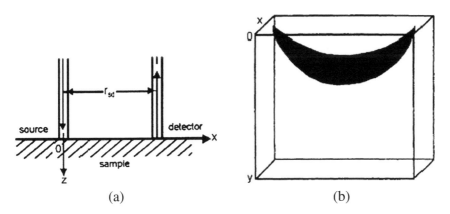

(a)   (b)

Figure 6.2 Geometry of a fiber backscattering experiment for investigation of (a) a semi-infinite medium, and (b) a "banana" shape region of photon path distribution.[1120,1121]

For backscattering optical spectroscopy and tomography, in addition to the measured coefficient of reflection defined by Eqs. (1.27) and (2.17), we have to know from what depth the optical signal is coming. That depth is defined by the photon-path-distribution function for the photons migrating from a source to a detector.[1120,1121] This spatial distribution function for a homogeneous scattering medium has a "banana" shape [see Fig. 6.2(b)]. In the weak absorption limit, the modal line of the banana region (the curve of the most probable direction of a photon migration) is given by[1120,1121]

$$z \approx \left[\frac{1}{8} \left(\left\{ \left[x^2 + (r_{sd} - x)^2 \right]^2 + 32s^2 (r_{sd} - x)^2 \right\}^{1/2} - x^2 - (r_{sd} - x)^2 \right) \right]^{1/2}, \quad (6.4)$$

where $0 \leq x \leq r_{sd}$. At $x = r_{sd}/2$, the modal line of the banana region reaches a maximum depth,

$$z^{max} \approx \frac{r_{sd}}{2\sqrt{2}}. \quad (6.5)$$

Instead of Eq. (6.2), used for *in vivo* study in transillumination experiments, using Eqs. (2.17) and (6.4), we can write a modified Beer-Lambert law to describe the optical attenuation in the following form:[1120,1121]

$$\frac{I}{I_0} = \exp(-\varepsilon_{ab} c_{ab} r_{sd} DPF - G_s), \quad (6.6)$$

where I_0 is the intensity of the incident light, I is the intensity of the detected light, ε_{ab} is the absorption coefficient measured in $\mu mol^{-1} cm^{-1}$, c_{ab} is the concentration of absorber in μmol, r_{sd} is the distance between the light source and detector, DPF is the differential path length factor accounting for the increase in the photons' migration paths due to scattering, and G_s is the attenuation factor accounting for scattering and geometry of the tissue.

When r_{sd}, DPF, and G are kept constant (for example, during the estimation of the total hemoglobin or degree of oxygenation), then the changes in the absorbing medium concentration can be calculated using measurements of the changes in the optical density (OD), $\Delta(OD) = \Delta[\log(I_0/I)]$ as

$$\Delta c_{ab} = \frac{\Delta(OD)}{\varepsilon_{ab} r_{sd} DPF}. \quad (6.7)$$

In optical imaging, the changes in optical density are measured as[1120,1121]

$$\Delta(OD) = \log\left(\frac{I_0}{I_{test}} \right) - \log\left(\frac{I_0}{I_{rest}} \right) = \log(I_{rest}) - \log(I_{test}), \quad (6.8)$$

where I_{rest} and I_{test} represent the light intensity detected when the object is at rest (brain tissue, skeletal muscle, etc.) and being tested (induced brain activity, cold or visual test, training, etc.), respectively. For example, based on the OD changes at wavelengths of 760 and 850 nm, one can get either the absorption images for these two wavelengths or functional images (oxygenation or blood volume) within the detection region of study as

$$\Delta(OD)_{oxy} = \Delta(OD)_{850} - \Delta(OD)_{760}, \quad (6.9)$$

$$\Delta(OD)_{total} = \Delta(OD)_{850} + k_{bvo} \Delta(OD)_{760}, \quad (6.10)$$

where $(OD)_{850}$ and $(OD)_{760}$ are the optical densities measured at the wavelengths 850 and 760 nm, respectively, and k_{bvo} is the modification factor for reducing the cross talk between changes of blood volume and oxygenation. This factor is determined by calibration on a blood model.

NIR absorption spectra of oxy- and deoxyhemoglobin and water are presented in Fig. 6.3.[4] The water band at about 980 nm can be used as an internal standard for the evaluation of the absolute concentrations of the blood components in tissue *in vivo*.[1122]

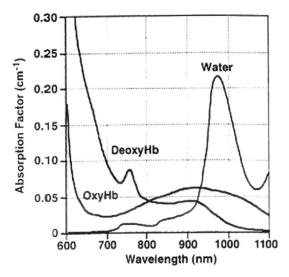

Figure 6.3 Near-infrared attenuation $[\log_{10}]$ for 1-cm depth deoxyhemoglobin (DeoxyHb), oxyhemoglobin (OxyHb), and water; hemoglobin concentration, 210 μM in water.[4]

6.1.2 Example of a CW imaging system

The whole-spectrum NIR spectroscopy system described in Ref. 1123 uses illumination of the subject's head with light from a halogen lamp emitting a continuous spectrum [see Fig. 6.4(a)]. The back-reflected light is detected and spectrally analyzed by a commercial grating spectrograph equipped with a liquid nitrogen cooled CCD detector. The system provides a spectral resolution of 5 nm in the range 700–1000 nm; spectra were collected every 100 ms. Figure 6.4(b) illustrates the image received using this optical instrument and the testing algorithm described [see Eqs. (6.9) and (6.10)]. It shows a focal increase in total Hb in response to stimulation with a stationary multicolored dodecahedron. The area of the peak response is clearly focused and it is about 0.5×0.5 cm in size.

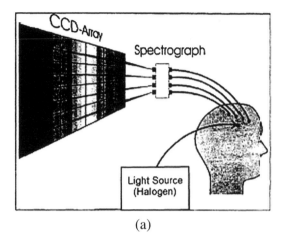

(a)

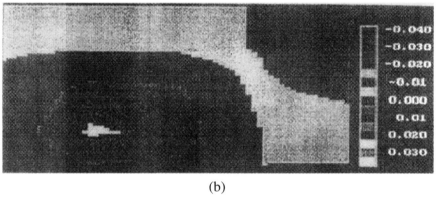

(b)

Figure 6.4 A CCD-NIR spectroscopy system.[1123] (a) Scheme. (b) Functional image, changes in blood volume (total hemoglobin) [see Eqs. (6.9) and (6.10)] during visual simulation (a stationary dodecahedron) as detected over the occipital cortex.

6.1.3 Example of a tissue spectroscopy system

A typical experimental system for *in vivo* backscattering spectroscopy and the corresponding spectra for normal and pathological tissues are shown in Fig. 6.5.[47,94,95] Figure 6.5(b) is an example of spectra taken from the colon of one patient. The absorption bands are of oxyhemoglobin (the Soret band and Q bands are clearly evident). The 400–440-nm segment encloses the hemoglobin Soret band, but also encompasses some absorption from compounds such as flavin mononucleotide, beta-carotene, bilirubin, and cytochrome. The 540–580-nm segment covers the hemoglobin Q band, with minor absorption from cytochrome and other components. On the basis of measurement of the spectral differences of normal and pathological tissue, the corresponding spectral signature "identifiers" can be created. Such spectral "identifiers" for *in vivo* medical diagnostics usually use the ratios of the reflection coefficients integrated within selected spectral bands or the measurement of the spectrum slope for the spectral bands selected.

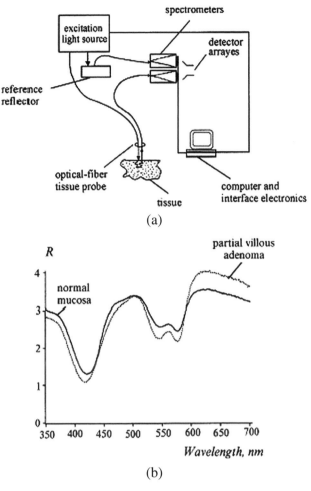

Figure 6.5 (a) Schematic diagram of an experimental system for *in vivo* measurements of spectral reflectance of internal organs.[47] (b) Typical tissue spectra, shown as examples, for two measurements made in the colon of one patient (the spectra have been normalized to the same total integrated signal between 350 and 700 nm); normal mucosa and partial villous adenoma.

A more analytic and quantitative study, provided in Ref. 1124, might yield more insight into the sensitivity of CW reflection spectroscopy. Three different detecting probes were used in the measurements within the spectral range from 400 to 1700 nm. Authors have paid attention to a proper calibration of the probes using a reflection standard (SRS-99-010, LabSphere, North Sutton, UK). For the precise recognition of the absorptions peaks of the tissue, the first derivative of the NIR spectra was computed using the method of Savitzky and Golay. It was shown that CW NIR spectroscopy can detect the presence of lipid in atherosclerotic plaque of the aorta with good sensitivity.

6.2 Time-domain and frequency-domain spectroscopy and tomography of tissues

6.2.1 Time-domain techniques and instruments

One of the designed time-resolved laser systems for *in vivo* measurements of optical properties of the human breast is presented in Fig. 6.6.[288] This system consists of a mode-locked Ti:sapphire laser at a wavelength of 800 nm with a pulse duration of 80 fs and a repetition frequency of 82 MHz. The probe laser beam transilluminates the female breast and the forward-scattered light reaches the detection side of the synchroscan streak camera (S1 photocathode, Hamamatsu C3681). For the enhancement of tissue transmittance, making it more homogeneous and providing stable boundary conditions, the breast was slightly compressed between two transparent plates. Such compression was much less than in a conventional x-ray mammography in order to avoid any influence of changed blood perfusion on the absorption properties. The scattered light is imaged onto the slit of the streak camera with a 1:1 magnification. The dimensions of the slit are 50 μm × 6 mm and the numerical aperture of the camera optics is 0.22. To provide a temporal reference, the reference laser beam was optically delayed and imaged on the streak camera slit; a trigger beam synchronized the streak camera. The working principles of a streak camera and other instrumentation used in time-resolved techniques are described in detail in Refs. 301, 302, 303.

The temporal profile of the light intensity incident on the camera was recorded with a time resolution of about 10 ps and displayed as a spatial profile. A pre-

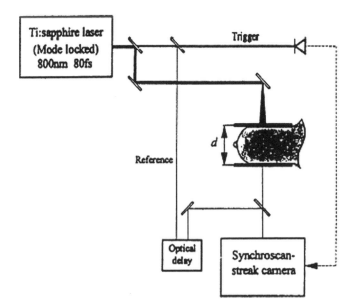

Figure 6.6 Schematic setup for time-resolved transillumination of female breast tissue *in vivo*.[288]

cise shading correction and dark count subtraction were performed for each measurement of the dispersion curve. For *in vivo* measurements, the probe laser beam with a total power of 100 to 150 mW was expanded to a diameter of 10 mm to keep the power density below the maximum permissible exposure of 200 mW/cm^2.

Normalized dispersion curves for three volunteers T_1, T_2, and T_3 and the corresponding results of the theoretical fit according to the diffusion model [see Eq. (1.36)] are shown in Fig. 6.7. The dispersion curves range over a typical period of 6 ns with a mean time of flight of more than 2 ns. Owing to the strong scattering and low absorption, most photons travel ten times the geometrical distance through the compressed breast. The signals T_1 and T_2 ($d = 45$ mm) overcome the background noise for a time of flight of about 510 ps, which is more than twice the minimum time of flight of a ballistic photon (refractive index of tissue 1.4). For a thicker tissue layer T_3 ($d = 59$ mm), this time shifts to 830 ps, which is about three times longer than for ballistic photons.

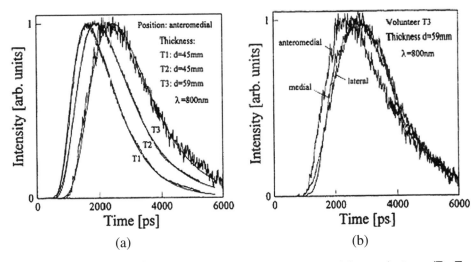

Figure 6.7 Normalized *in vivo* dispersion curves of the breasts of three volunteers (T_1, T_2, and T_3; thickness d) and corresponding theoretical fit curves: (a) three breasts in one position; (b) one breast in three positions.[288]

Measurements at different positions of the breast reflect the influence of physiological alterations within different areas of the organ (different types of tissue, different blood volumes, and oxygenation) and serves as a basis for diffuse optical mammography [see Fig. 6.7(b)]. It should be noted that the slightly different boundary conditions and degree of compression, as well as the inhomogeneity of superficial tissue pigmentation, can be critical for obtaining reliable mammograms. Table 2.1 presents the results of *in vitro*, *ex vivo*, and *in vivo* measurements of optical parameters of the human female breast and some other thick tissues carried out by the methods discussed as well as some other optical techniques.

Algorithms for the solving of the inverse problem on determination of μ_a and μ'_s using Eqs. (1.35) and (1.36) can be successfully used not only for tissue spectroscopy but also for tomography. For tomography purposes, we are not able to provide measurements of the absolute concentrations of absorbers and absolute values of the scattering coefficients (although this is desirable), which allow one to implement these algorithms faster. Generally, the imaging is aimed at the detection of pathology or at the localization of lesions. The detection of a lesion is achieved by recording a 2D image with sufficient contrast, while localization needs optical slicing and tomographic reconstruction to obtain the 3D images by which the size, shape, and position of the hidden object can be determined.[287]

Imaging systems usually use 2D or 3D scanning of a narrow laser beam or a translation optical stage with the object attached. Nonscanning systems are more robust and correspondingly fit medical applications much better. Such nonscanning systems use a multichannel fiber-optical arrangement with fixed positions of light sources and detectors, or low-noise, high-sensitivity, and fast CCD cameras with multichannel plate optical amplification. In any case, the measurement procedure is completed by sampling the intensity of each pixel as a function of time to obtain a time-space intensity mapping. The image is numerically reconstructed by attributing to each pixel the intensity measured over the selected integration time.[287]

A multichannel NIR imager/spectrometer based on the time-correlated single-photon counting technique was designed for breast imaging in clinics [see Fig. 6.8(a)].[1125] The instrument uses two NIR wavelengths, 780 and 830 nm, the mean power of each laser diode is about 40 μW, and they pulse at 5 MHz with a pulse width of about 50 ps. A highly sensitive R5600U-50 GaAs photomultiplier has been chosen for breast examination. For enhancement of the contrast of carcinoma images, intravenous administration of Infracyanine 25 (IC25), an NIR contrast agent, was used. Optical absorption changes were calculated using the following relation:

$$\Delta\mu_a = -\frac{2}{c\Delta t^2}\int_{t_1}^{t_2}\ln\frac{J_2(r,t)}{J_1(r,t)}dt, \qquad (6.11)$$

where c is the speed of light in the medium; Δt is the time resolution of the pulse-height analysis (PHA, Hamamatsu Inc.) of the multichannel analyzer (MCA, Hamamatsu Inc.); J_1 and J_2 are the photon current measurement pre- and post-IC25 injection, respectively, and t_1, t_2 are the width of the J_1 time-resolved curve. Equation (6.11) gives accurate values of $\Delta\mu_a$ for small absorption changes.

The relative displacement of the light sources and detectors, and the positions of the projection plane and pathology (carcinoma, black sphere) are shown in Fig. 6.8(b). The calculations of the absorption coefficient differences along the straight lines connecting those source-detector pairs in space that have comparable separations [shown as diamonds in Fig. 6.8(b)] allow for estimation of the IC25 distribution in tissue. Tests with patients were done simultaneously with the standard MR imaging (MRI) examination protocol.

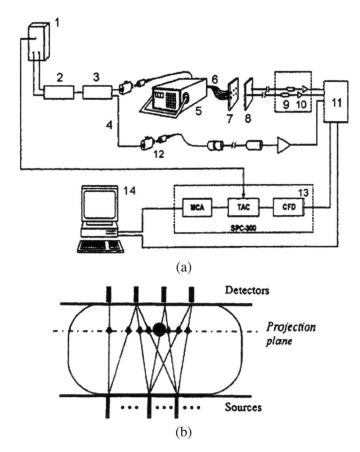

(a)

(b)

Figure 6.8 Multichannel, time-correlated single-photon counting NIR imager/spectrometer: (a) 1, two laser diodes; 2, a wavelength coupler; 3, 19:1 signal splitter; 4, the reference branch; 5, 1 × 24 optical DiCon fiber-optics switch; 6, graded index, 10-m-long optical fibers; 7, compression plates; 8, 8-step index, 10-m-long fiber bundles; 9, PMT; 10, amplification unit; 11, router; 12, attenuator; 13, SPC-300 photon counting system using an SRT-8 8-channel multiplexer; 14, Intel Pentium PC; CFD, constant-fraction discriminator; MCA, multichannel analyzer; TAC, time-to-amplitude converter. (b) Relative displacement of the light sources and detectors, and the positions of the projection plane and pathology (carcinoma, black sphere).[1125]

Figure 6.9 illustrates the possibilities of time-resolved optical diffusion mammography in comparison with MRI study. Measurements were done for a patient (70-year-old Caucasian) diagnosed with an infiltrating ductal carcinoma approximately 10 mm in diameter. For the presented image, six sources and eight detectors were employed. A good correspondence between the MRI and the NIR images is easily seen. In the 780-nm light image, two objects are resolved, either due to measurement noise or due to actual physiology of the tissue. Owing to more absorption (12%) of IC25 at 780 nm than at 830 nm, expected differences should be enhanced more.

A much more comprehensive time-resolved optical tomography system employing 32 channels and designed for imaging of the neonatal brain and the hu-

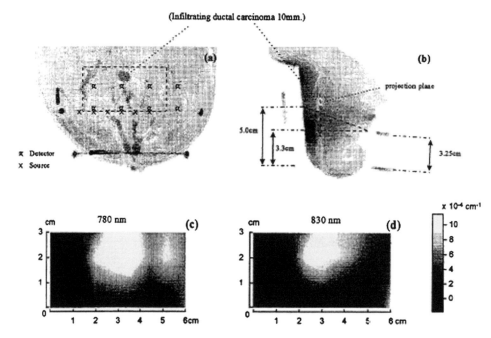

Figure 6.9 MRI and NIR image coregistration. (a) Saggital fast spin echo (FSE) MRI slice from a 70-yr-old patient with infiltrating ductal carcinoma. (b) Spin echo (SE) MRI axial image of the same patient. (c) NIR projection image at 780 nm. (d) NIR projection image at 830 nm.[1125]

man breast is shown in Fig. 6.10.[1126] This is the multichannel optoelectronic near-infrared system for time-resolved image reconstruction (MONSTIR). Light from a pulsed high-power picosecond laser source is switched sequentially into one of 32 fibers that are attached to the surface of an object under study. The detection system is used to record the temporal distribution of light exiting the tissue at certain positions around the object with a temporal resolution of about 80 ps and a rate of photon counting up to a few 10^5 per second per channel. This is accomplished by utilizing 32 fully simplex ultrafast photon-counting detectors. The scattered photons are collected by 32 low-dispersion, large-diameter (2.5-mm) fiber bundles that are coupled to 32-stepper motor-driven variable optical attenuators (VOAs). Because of the large dynamic range of light intensities around the object, the VOAs are required to ensure that the detectors are not saturated or damaged and that the system operates within the single-photon counting mode. Light transmitted via VOA is collected by a short 3.0-mm diameter single polymer fiber and then is transmitted via a visible blocking filter to the photocathodes of four ultrafast eight-anode multichannel plate-photomultiplier tubes (MCP-PMTs). The resulting electronic pulse is preamplified and converted into a logic pulse, and a histogram of the photon flight times is recorded and transfered to the control computer. A dedicated image reconstruction software package, TOAST (time-resolved optical absorption and scattering tomography, http://www.medphys.ucl.ac.uk/toast/index.html),

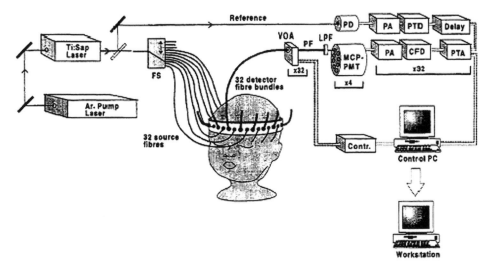

Figure 6.10 Schematic diagram of the MONSTIR imaging system: FS, fiber switch; VOA, variable optical attenuator; PF, polymer fiber; LPF, long-pass filter; MCP-PMT, multichannel plate-photomultiplier tube; PA, preamplifier; CFD, constant fraction discriminator; PTA, picosecond time analyzer; PD, photodiode; PTD, picotiming discriminator.[1126]

is used for the reconstruction of the tomographic images of the absorption and scattering profiles.

A portable three-wavelength NIR time-resolved spectroscopic (TRS) system (TRS-10, Hamamatsu Photonics K.K., Japan) is available on the market.[1127] In the TRS system, a time-correlated single-photon-counting technique is used for detection. The system is controlled by a computer through a digital I/O interface consisting of a three-wavelength (761, 795, and 835 nm) picosecond (about 100 ps) pulsed light source, a photon-counting head for single-photon detection, and signal-processing circuits for time-resolved measurement. The average power of the light source is at least 150 µW at each wavelength at a repetition rate of 5 MHz. The instrumental response of the TRS system, which included a 3-m length light source fiber (graded index type single fiber with a core diameter of 200 µm) and a 3-m length light detector fiber (a bundle fiber of 3-mm diameter), was around 150 ps full width at half maximum (FWHM) at each wavelength. This system was used for estimating the absorption and reduced scattering coefficients of the head in a piglet hypoxia model.[1127] Measurements of absolute values of the absorption coefficient at three wavelengths enable estimation of the hemoglobin concentration and its oxygen saturation in the head.

6.2.2 Frequency-domain techniques and instruments

Considerable progress in the investigation of tissues and molecules of biological importance with the use of the modulation technique provided the foundation for the development and commercial production of spectrometers of a new type (for example, ISS Fluorescence & Analytical Instrumentation). A typical scheme of the frequency-domain spectrometer for tissue study is shown in Fig. 6.11.[1–4,6,301–303,311,312] Such systems for phase measurements use a heterodyning principle (two photomultipliers with heterodyning in one of the first dynodes) to transfer a measuring signal to a low-frequency range (100 Hz for the shown system), where phase measurement can be done much more precisely.

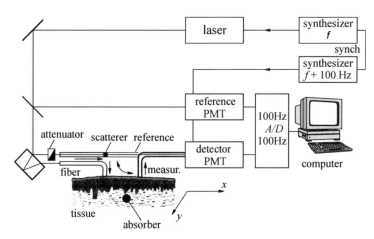

Figure 6.11 A typical scheme of a frequency-domain light-scattering spectrometer or photon-density wave imaging system (if 2D scanning of irradiating and receiving fibers is provided).[1,3]

We should also mention models of compact and comparatively cheap devices—modulation spectrometers—for noninvasive quantitative determination of oxygen saturation of blood hemoglobin, monitoring of optical parameters of tissues, and localization of absorbing or scattering inhomogeneities inside a tissue. Such spectrometers include diode lasers as radiation sources at one or two wavelengths and a photomultiplier with heterodyning in one of the first dynodes or a fast semiconductor photodetector with a high-frequency amplifier.[303,325,326] Specifically, NIM Incorporated produces a PMD 3000b two-wavelength spectrometer (with $\lambda = 760$ and 810 nm and a fixed modulation frequency of 200 MHz) for noninvasive quantitative determination of oxygen saturation of hemoglobin.[1128] Carl Zeiss Jena is the manufacturer of a more sophisticated and universal system, which operates at the wavelength of 685 nm with two fixed modulation frequencies equal to 110 and 220 MHz. This system also includes a computer-controlled optical table, which ensures the regime of tissue transillumination.[325,326] A much simpler and more universal research system has been developed and manufactured at Saratov University.[1129] This system includes quantum-well lasers ($\lambda = 790$ and 840 nm), which ensure a highly efficient low-noise modulation of laser radiation within the range of 100–1000 MHz; a set of optical fibers; and a computer-controlled optical table, which allows one to implement different geometric schemes for an experiment. The detection unit employs an avalanche photodiode with a high-frequency amplifier (20 dB). The total dynamic range of the detection unit along with a spectrum analyzer or a network analyzer is 70 dB.

From the point of view of medical devices, the requirements of a phase-measuring system are very high (better than 0.03 deg in a 2-Hz bandwidth) and close to that imposed to multifrequency, multiwavelength optical-fiber communication systems [time division multiplex (TDM) and wavelength division multiplex (WDM)].[4] Communication systems work at much higher modulation frequencies than medical ones and are well developed in their usage of digital equipment, and have a high degree of multiplexing. The last two features should be very useful for the designing of a new generation of medical equipment. While requirements for medical systems are currently quite modest (three wavelengths and two modulation frequencies), the appearance of the first generation of optical tomographs with a spatial resolution of about 1 cm^{-3} increases the need for multiplexing up to 16/32 channels. In the near future, for providing of a resolution much less than 1 cm^{-3}, the use of 10^3 source-detection combinations is expected.[4]

Phase systems are divided into homodyne and heterodyne groups, which means that, respectively, they do not and they do convert the radio frequency (RF) prior to phase measurements. Heterodyne systems have been termed "cross-correlation" or phase-delay measurement devices (PDMDs). These devices are intended to measure tissue optical properties (μ_a and μ_s') to an accuracy of 5% and hemoglobin saturation to an accuracy of 3% in the 40–80% range, requiring phase and amplitude precision as follows[4]:

- Phase and amplitude noise in a 2-Hz bandwidth should be less than 0.03 deg and 0.1% of the total signal at a carrier frequency of 50–200 MHz.
- Source-to-detector attenuation may be more than 100 dB, with radio RF coupling causing less than 0.03 drg phase error.
- Amplitude-phase cross talk should be limited—a signal attenuation of 10 dB should not cause more than a 0.03 deg phase error.
- Multifrequency operation should not cause more than 0.03 deg phase inter-channel cross talk (at 50 dB attenuation).
- Optical multiplexing employing light sources of different wavelengths should cause less than 0.03 deg phase interchannel cross talk.
- Bandwidth signal output should be variable from 0.2 to 2 Hz, or in special cases of brain study, 40 Hz.
- Sufficient information from multiple RF or multiwavelength operation should be available.

Four types of PDMDs adapted to study tissue optical characteristics study are presented in Fig. 6.12.[4] Two are homodyne [(a) and (b)] and two are heterodyne [(c) and (d)]. The system in (a) uses an in-phase quadrature (IQ) demodulator;

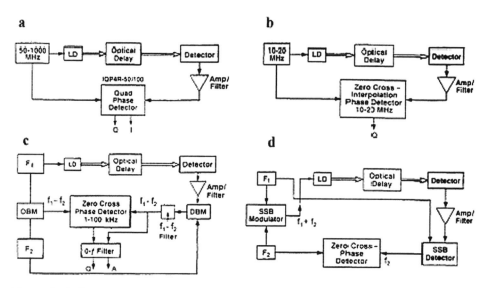

Figure 6.12 Four types of optical propagation delay measurement devices for tissue study: (a) and (b) homodyne systems; (a) has IQ demodulation, (b) a zero-crossing phase detector. (c) and (d) heterodyne systems; (c) is amplitude modulated and (d) is single sideband (SSB) with F_1 as the RF oscillator and F_2 as the local oscillator (audio); the upper sideband $f_1 + f_2$ is used.[4] LD, laser diode; DBM, double-balanced mixer.

(b) uses a zero cross-phase detector. The system in (c) uses amplitude modulation at two close RF, f_1 and f_2, and (d) uses single sideband (SSB) modulation; f_1 is a RF and f_2 is an audio frequency; both systems with zero cross-phase detectors.

A number of phase-measurement systems are described in Refs. 1 and 4. The amplitude measurements are relatively simple, but sometimes they do not provide the accuracy needed because, for example, of the influence of stray light. Phase measurements are amplitude independent and can be carried out with acceptable accuracy. Moreover, multiwavelength phase measurements alone are sufficient to estimate such important quantities as hemoglobin concentration and its degree of oxygenation. Simultaneous amplitude and phase measurements are used for the determination of absolute values of absorption coefficients.

The basic form of a homodyne system with an IQ demodulator is presented in Fig. 6.12(a). Determining the phase shift path (the phase difference between the reference oscillator and the signal pathway) involves a laser diode, an optical detector, an amplifier, and a narrowband filter. The working principle of an IQ demodulator is shown in Fig. 6.13. It includes a 90-deg splitter (hybrid), two double-balanced mixers (DBMs), and a 0-deg splitter. In the demodulator, the carrier (as reference signal) is recovered from an incoming modulated signal and fed to the 90-deg hybrid and the modulated signal (as the signal under test) is fed to the 0-deg hybrids.

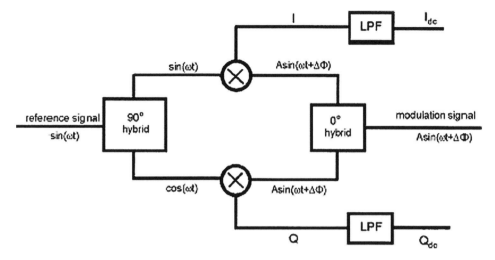

Figure 6.13 Diagram of IQ demodulator as a phase and amplitude detector;[1130] LPF, low-pass filter.

Functioning as a multiplier, the in-phase mixer produces an output of[4,1130]

$$I(t) = \sin(\omega t)2A\sin(\omega t + \Delta\Phi) = A\cos\Delta\Phi - A\cos(2\omega t + \Delta\Phi), \quad (6.12)$$

where $\sin(\omega t)$ is the carrier signal, $2A\sin(\omega t + \Delta\Phi)$ is the modulated signal, and the phase delay $\Delta\Phi$ is caused by the scattering medium.

The quadrature mixer produces an output of

$$Q(t) = \cos(\omega t)2A\sin(\omega t + \Delta\Phi) = A\sin\Delta\Phi + A\sin(2\omega t + \Delta\Phi), \quad (6.13)$$

where $A\sin\Delta\Phi$ and $A\cos\Delta\Phi$ are dc signals that carry the information on amplitude (A) and phase ($\Delta\Phi$) caused by light interaction with the scattering medium. $A\sin(2\omega t + \Delta\Phi)$ and $A\cos(2\omega t + \Delta\Phi)$ are high-frequency components that are blocked by using low-pass filters (LPFs); therefore, after filtration, such signals as I_{dc} and Q_{dc} are registered. The phase and amplitude caused by a medium can be found from the equations

$$\Delta\Phi = \tan^{-1}\left(\frac{Q_{dc}}{I_{dc}}\right), \quad A = \{Q_{dc}^2 + I_{dc}^2\}^{1/2}. \quad (6.14)$$

For backscattering geometry, such as that presented in Fig. 6.2, the analytical expressions for the phase shift $\Delta\Phi$ and modulation amplitude A in the diffusion approximation are defined as follows:[4,325,326]

$$\Delta\Phi = r_{sd}\left\{\frac{[(\mu_a c)^2 + \omega^2]^{1/2} - \mu_a c}{D}\right\}^{1/2} + \Delta\Phi_0, \quad (6.15)$$

$$A = \left(\frac{A_0}{4\pi D r_{sd}}\right) \exp\left(-r_{sd}\left\{\frac{[(\mu_a c)^2 + \omega^2]^{1/2} + \mu_a c}{2D}\right\}^{1/2}\right), \quad (6.16)$$

where r_{sd} is the source-detector separation, $\Delta\Phi_0$ is the initial phase due to the instrumental response, A_0 is the initial amplitude due to the instrumental response, $D \approx c/(3\mu_s')$, and c is the speed of light in the medium.

For relatively small modulation frequencies, when $\omega < \mu_a c$, the phase shift is a linear function of frequency,

$$\Delta\Phi = \left(\frac{r_{sd}\omega}{2}\right)(D\mu_a c)^{1/2} + \Delta\Phi_0 \approx \left(\frac{r_{sd}\omega}{2c}\right)\left(\frac{3\mu_s'}{\mu_a}\right)^{1/2} + \Delta\Phi_0. \quad (6.17)$$

For relatively large frequencies, when $\omega > \mu_a c$ ($\omega/2\pi \le 500$ MHz),

$$\Delta\Phi = r_{sd}(\omega/2D)^{1/2} + \Delta\Phi_0 \approx r_{sd}(3\omega\mu_s'/2c)^{1/2} + \Delta\Phi_0. \quad (6.18)$$

A_0 and $\Delta\Phi_0$ can be calibrated by using a standard model (phantom) with known μ_s' and μ_a. Then, after calibration of the experimental setup, optical parameters of the tissue under study can be calculated from the measured amplitude and phase shift on the basis of Eqs. (6.10) and (6.11) using the following iteration formulas:

$$\mu_a = [r_{sd}^4\omega^2 - 4D^2(\Delta\Phi - \Delta\Phi_0)^4]/4cD(\Delta\Phi - \Delta\Phi_0)^2 r_{sd}^2,$$
$$\mu_s' = c/3D - \mu_a, \quad (6.19)$$
$$D = -r_{sd}^2\omega/2(\Delta\Phi - \Delta\Phi_0)[\ln(A/A_0) + \ln(4\pi D r_{sd})].$$

Therefore, the homodyne system measures the phase difference between the reference oscillator and the signal pathway. The analogue IQ detector (see Fig. 6.13) allows one to reach an accuracy of ~0.2 deg in phase and ~0.5 dB in amplitude with carrier frequencies of 140 MHz.[4,1130]

The heterodyne principle is characteristic for many communication systems. Since the error of the phase measurements decreases when oscillator frequency slows down and the bandwidth of a detector is constant, instruments designed for a low-frequency range may give higher accuracy. The nonlinear mixing of two signals with different frequencies, f_1 and f_2, gives signals with the sum and difference frequencies, one of which, namely, $(f_1 - f_2)$, is selected, amplified, filtered, and coupled to a phase detector as a reference signal [see Fig. 6.12(c)]. Propagation of the modulation signal f_1 through the optical system, the biological tissue, the optical detector, and the amplifier/filter leads to phase and amplitude changes. The signal on an intermediate frequency [$(f_1 - f_2)$, 1–100 kHz] is obtained from a second mixer and serves as the measuring signal for the phase detector. The intermediate frequency should be high enough to avoid a $1/f$ noise problem and low enough to exclude high-frequency errors in zero-crossing phase detection. The drawback of the heterodyne system is that the oscillators F_1 and F_2 must have a phase coherence equal to the required system accuracy.

The SSB system [see Fig. 6.12(d)] provides both efficient light modulation and efficient signal detection. It has important advantages: (1) the carrier modulation and the laser diode modulation are present only when the local oscillator (F_2) activates the sideband selected (thus, convenient control of RF light modulation is available); (2) the local oscillator frequency can be in the convenient audio range; and (3) all of the RF power is in a single narrow band of frequencies set by the low-frequency oscillation.

As an example, let us consider in more detail the functioning of a two-wavelength heterodyne IQ detection system, presented in Fig. 6.14.[4,1130] The two-wavelength NIR systems are usually used to detect the hemoglobin saturation of living tissue. Two RF signal sources are used and operate at slightly different frequencies, namely, 140.00 and 140.01 MHz, which provide the driving signals for two laser diodes with different wavelengths. The two laser beams are combined and directed simultaneously with the fiber coupler to the tissue under study. The optical signals collected from the tissue are fiber coupled to the PMT (or a number of PMTs). After passing an amplifier, the two-wavelength optical signals go into each IQ demodulator at the same time (the signal differentiation is due to different RF frequencies).

If channel 1 is characterized by the RF signal $\sin(\omega_1 t)$ and the detected signal is characterized by $2A_1 \sin(\omega_1 t + \Delta\Phi_1)$, and channel 2 by $\sin(\omega_2 t)$ and $2A_2 \sin(\omega_2 t + \Delta\Phi_2)$, then the IQ signals for each channel can be expressed as

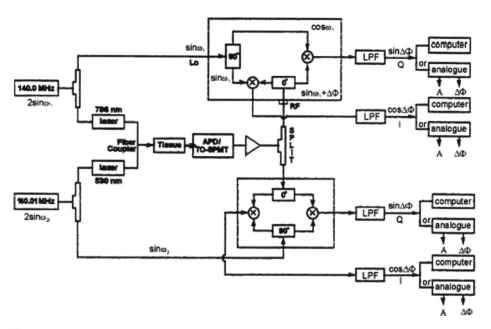

Figure 6.14 A two-wavelength phase-modulated spectroscopy system operating at 140 MHz and using analog IQ demodulation (see text for details).[4]

the following:[1130]

$$I_1(t) = [2A_1 \sin(\omega_1 t + \Delta\Phi_1) + 2A_2 \sin(\omega_2 t + \Delta\Phi_2)] \sin(\omega_1 t)$$
$$= \underline{A_1 \cos\Delta\Phi_1} - A_1 \cos(2\omega_1 t + \Delta\Phi_1) + A_2 \cos[(\omega_1 - \omega_2)t + \Delta\Phi_2]$$
$$- A_2 \cos[(\omega_1 + \omega_2)t + \Delta\Phi_2],$$

$$Q_1(t) = [2A_1 \sin(\omega_1 t + \Delta\Phi_1) + 2A_2 \sin(\omega_2 t + \Delta\Phi_2)] \cos(\omega_1 t)$$
$$= \underline{A_1 \sin\Delta\Phi_1} + A_1 \sin(2\omega_1 t + \Delta\Phi_1) + A_2 \sin[(\omega_1 - \omega_2)t + \Delta\Phi_2]$$
$$+ A_2 \sin[(\omega_1 + \omega_2)t + \Delta\Phi_2], \tag{6.20}$$

$$I_2(t) = [2A_1 \sin(\omega_1 t + \Delta\Phi_1) + 2A_2 \sin(\omega_2 t + \Delta\Phi_2)] \sin(\omega_2 t)$$
$$= \underline{A_2 \cos\Delta\Phi_2} - A_2 \cos(2\omega_2 t + \Delta\Phi_2) + A_1 \cos[(\omega_1 - \omega_2)t + \Delta\Phi_1]$$
$$- A_1 \cos[(\omega_1 + \omega_2)t + \Delta\Phi_1],$$

$$Q_2(t) = [2A_1 \sin(\omega_1 t + \Delta\Phi_1) + 2A_2 \sin(\omega_2 t + \Delta\Phi_2)] \cos(\omega_2 t)$$
$$= \underline{A_2 \sin\Delta\Phi_2} + A_2 \sin(2\omega_2 t + \Delta\Phi_2) + A_1 \sin[(\omega_1 - \omega_2)t + \Delta\Phi_1]$$
$$+ A_1 \sin[(\omega_1 + \omega_2)t + \Delta\Phi_1].$$

This system uses two low-pass filters (LPF): one is a dc 1.9-MHz band to reject the high-frequency components ($2\omega_1$, $2\omega_2$, $\omega_1 + \omega_2$) in each channel; another is a dc 10-kHz band to block the low-frequency component ($\omega_1 - \omega_2 = 10$ kHz). According to Eqs. (6.20), such filtration allows one to separate the combined signal into two signals for each wavelength, and each channel itself contains only I and Q signals [see underlined terms in Eqs. (6.20)]. However, it was shown experimentally that the third-order mixing effects influence the low-frequency cross-correlation between channels. The interchannel cross talk for a phase is less than 1.4 deg/dB, and for amplitude is less than 3.8 mV/dB (phase or amplitude changes in one channel caused by changes of amplitude in another one).

For more effective separation of signals, a fast Fourier transform analysis can be used. A much simpler solution is to use time-share control of the system. The computer-controlled time share ensures that at any one time only one wavelength optical signal may pass through the whole system. In this way, the interchannel cross talk can be reduced for phase up to 0.1 deg/dB and for amplitudes up to 0.5 mV/dB.[4]

6.2.3 Phased-array technique

In the NIR region, the wavelengths of diffusive photon-density waves in tissues are equal to 5–14 cm for modulation frequencies from 500 to 100 MHz [see Eqs. (1.47) and (1.48)]. This means that there is low resolution of imaging with the usual source and detection combination in spite of the high accuracy of phase and amplitude measurements. The photon-density waves interference method described for the first time in Ref. 331 (phase and amplitude cancellation method, or phased-array method) is very promising for the improvement of the spatial resolution of the modulation technique.[4,53,342]

The concept of this method is illustrated in Fig. 6.15. It is based on the use of either duplicate sources and a single detector or duplicate detectors and a single source so that the amplitude and phase characteristics can be nulled and the system becomes a differential. If equal amplitude at the 0- and 180-deg phases are used as sources, appropriate positioning of the detector can lead to null in the amplitude signal and a crossover between the 0- and 180-deg phase shifts, i.e., at 90 deg:

$$A\sin(\omega t + 0) + A\sin(\omega t + 180) = 2A\cos(90)\sin(\omega t + 90), \qquad (6.21)$$

where ω is the light modulation frequency.

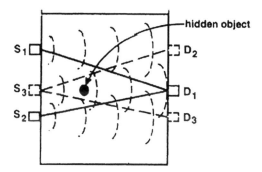

Figure 6.15 The geometry of the amplitude and phase cancellation technique; two sources (S_1 and S_2) and a single detector (D_1), or two detectors (D_2 and D_3) and a single source (S_3).[1133]

In a heterogeneous medium, the apparent amplitude's null and the phase's crossover may be displaced from the geometric midline (see Fig. 6.16). This method is extremely sensitive to perturbation by an absorber or scatterer. A spatial resolution of about 1 mm for the inspection of an absorbing inhomogeneity has been achieved and the similar resolution is expected for the scattering inhomogeneity. Another good feature of the technique is that at the null condition, the measuring system is relatively insensitive to amplitude fluctuations common to both light sources. On the other hand, inhomogeneities, which affect a large tissue volume common to the two optical paths, cannot be detected. The amplitude signal is less useful in imaging since the indication of position is ambiguous (see Fig. 6.16). Although this can be accounted for by further encoding, the phase signal is robust and a phase noise less than 0.1 deg (signal-to-noise ratio is more than 400) for a 1-Hz bandwidth can be obtained.[4]

The phase modulation system requires, for optimal results, SSB measuring technology [see Fig. 6.12(d)]. Nine sources and four detectors are used in the 50-MHz single-wavelength (780 nm) phase-array imaging system presented in Fig. 6.17.[1131] The number of sources and detectors can readily be increased;

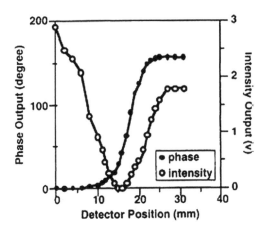

Figure 6.16 Demonstration of the existence of amplitude null and phase crossover for a phased-array measuring system used to study an adult human brain. The detector is scanned between two sources placed at 4 cm apart and excited by 0-deg and 180-deg phase-shifted RF signals at 200 MHz.[1131]

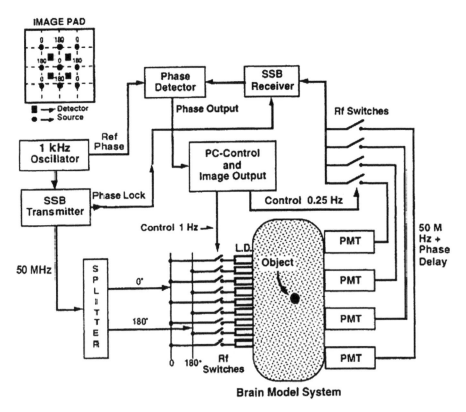

Figure 6.17 Single-wavelength (780 nm), 50-MHz phased-array, single sideband (SSB) phase modulation imaging system.[1131]

furthermore, the number of source and detector combinations can be increased simply by moving the source detector pad in two dimensions with respect to its original position by half the minimal distance between source and detector, equal to 2.5 cm. The image pad dimensions are 9 × 4 cm (see the upper left part of Fig. 6.17).

A local oscillator at 1 kHz modulates a 50 MHz SSB transmitter, the RF output of which is connected to a 0/180-deg phase splitter/inverter and then to nine switches appropriate to the nine light sources, which are sequenced at 0- and 180-deg phases by 1-Hz switches. The four PMTs are sequentially connected to the 50-MHz SSB receiver (0.5 mV sensitivity), and the audio output at 1 kHz is coupled to a zero-crossing phase detector to give the phase signals in sequence. The phase detector is coupled via a controlling computer to a computer for image computation and display (not shown). The transmitter and receiver are phase locked by RF coupling. The phase noise of the system is less than 0.1 deg (1-Hz bandwidth). A complete set of data from 16 source and detector combinations is obtained every 16 s.

Figure 6.18 illustrates a single-wavelength (780 nm), 50-MHz phased-array image test of neurovascular coupling in human brain. The image represents the increment in phase shift caused by touching the contralateral finger. Calibration with models verifies that this signal is due to an increase in hemoglobin concentration.[1131]

A more universal and comprehensive phased-array imaging system that can be used for testing the brain function of neonates is described in Ref. 1132. Single-wavelength laser diode light sources were replaced by a set of two laser diodes (750 and 830 nm, total of 18 lasers) with a 20-mW power source. The wavelength of 780 nm was shifted to 750 nm because at 750 nm the signal gain is more than

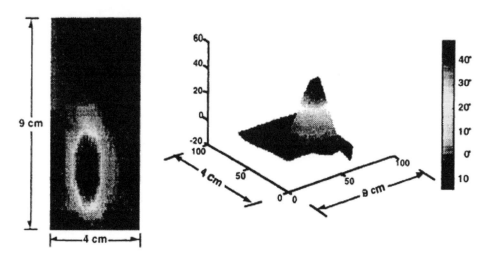

Figure 6.18 The image test for an adult human brain (blonde hair) using the 50-MHz phased-array system presented in Fig. 6.17. Parietal stimulation for 48 s by touching a contralateral finger was provided.[1131,1133]

double, owing to the respective extinction coefficients. Detection of the optical signals was provided by four PMTs (TO8, Hamamatsu). Two independent phasemeters and two SSB radio transmitters/receivers were used with 50- and 52-MHz frequencies. The size of the optical probe is slightly larger (10×5 cm) because two lasers are located in a point, but the source-detection separation was the same, 2.5 cm (see Fig. 6.17). A dual-wavelength phased-array imaging system can be used for testing the brain function of neonates and its relationship with some neurological disorders by monitoring metabolic activity, which is indicated by oxygen concentration or glucose intake to the brain cells.

Another dual-wavelength imaging system (750 and 830 nm) that uses a simple amplitude-cancellation technique (see Fig. 6.16) was used to image a human breast.[1133] The optical probe of the imager consists of 9 laser diode light sources and 21 silicon photodetectors. The imager sequences through all sources and detectors in a millisecond and gives high-quality breast tumor images every 8 s. As an example, in Fig. 6.19, four *in vivo* images of diseased and healthy breasts are presented. Since the difference image between the right and left breast is obtained, many of the background signals are eliminated and strong signals congruent with the expected position of the tumor are displayed (no evidence of the nipple is presented and two shapes for blood volume and for deoxygenation are clear).

The detection limit in the localizing of macroinhomogeneities hidden in a highly scattering tissue using phased-array imaging systems is discussed in Ref. 304.

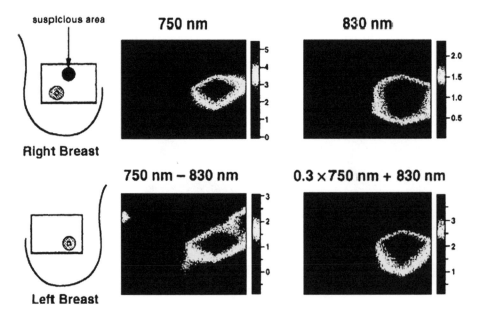

Figure 6.19 Four *in vivo* images of a diseased (with tumor) right breast with reference to the contralateral breast (left, healthy) at 750 nm and 830 nm, and two calculated images: 750–830 nm (deoxygenation image) and 0.3×750 nm + 830 nm (blood volume image).[1133]

6.2.4 *In vivo* measurements, detection limits, and examples of clinical study

Let us consider briefly a few spectroscopy and imaging frequency-domain systems that demonstrate the achievements in the field of optical *in vivo* diagnostics and that have been applied for clinical studies. It was shown previously that for the accurate evaluation of the absolute absorption and reduced scattering coefficients for a single source-detection position, frequency-dependent measurements of the amplitude and phase of photon-density waves should be provided. Therefore, to obtain quantitative measurements of the absolute optical parameters of various types of tissue, a portable, high-bandwidth (0.3–1000 MHz), multiwavelength (674, 811, 849, and 956 nm) frequency-domain photon migration (FDPM) instrument was designed[306,308] (see Fig. 6.20). The key component of an FDPM system is a network analyzer (8753C, Hewlett Packard) that is used to produce modulation sweep in the range of 0.3–1000 MHz. The RF from the network analyzer is superimposed on the direct current of four different diode lasers using individual bias tees and an RF switch. Four 100-μm diameter gradient-index fibers are used to couple each light source to an 8 × 8 optical multiplexer (GP700, DiCon Instruments). Dynamic phase reference and real-time compensation for source fluctuations were provided by an optical tap, which diverts a portion of the source output (5%) to a 1-GHz PIN diode coupled to the network analyzer channel B.

   Light is launched onto the tissue under study using up to eight source fibers corresponding to eight source positions. An avalanche photodetector (APD) (C5658, Hamamatsu) is used to detect the diffuse optical signal. Both the APD and probe

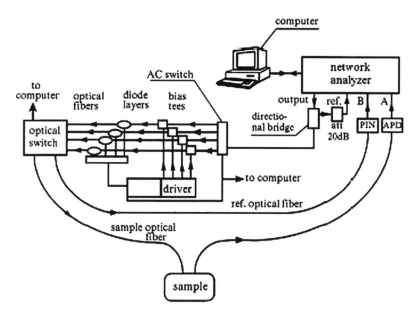

Figure 6.20 A multiwavelength, multifrequency, and multichannel frequency-domain spectrometer.[306,308]

end of the source optical fiber are in direct contact with the patient's skin surface. The optical power coupled into the tissue averages approximately 10–30 mW, roughly a factor of ten below thermal damage threshold levels for used fibers and wavelengths. Up to eight separate sources can be directed onto up to eight unique measurement positions using the 8 × 8 optical multiplexer. Measurement time depends on the precision required, the number of sweeps performed, and the RF/optical switch time. For studies in human subjects, about 0.5 s is used to sweep over the entire 1-GHz range of modulation frequencies. However, total elapsed time for four laser diodes (two sweeps per laser), data transfer, display, and source switching is about 40 s. The source-detector separation used for human subject measurements was fixed and equal to 1.7, 2.2, or 2.7 cm.

The results of experimental study for three patients using the developed FD spectrometer are presented in Tables 2.1 and 6.1. Table 6.1 also shows the calculated physiological parameters of a living tissue, such as absolute concentrations of deoxy- and oxyhemoglobin, total hemoglobin, and water. It was assumed that the chromophores contributing to the absorption coefficient μ_a in the human subject are principally oxy- and deoxyhemoglobin, and water. Therefore, the concentration of each component in the tissue is determined from the FDPM measurements of μ_a at three different wavelengths (674, 811, and 956 nm) in accordance with the following system of three equations:

$$\varepsilon_{Hb}(\lambda_i)c_{Hb} + \varepsilon_{HbO_2}(\lambda_i)c_{HbO_2} + \varepsilon_{H_2O}(\lambda_i)c_{H_2O} = \mu_a(\lambda_i), \qquad (6.22)$$

where $\varepsilon_{chrom}(\lambda_i)$ is the extinction coefficient in units of $cm^{-1} mol^{-1}$ of a given chromophore at the wavelength λ_i (674, 811, and 956 nm) defined by the matrix.

$$\begin{bmatrix} 6578300 & 740100 & 0.0748 \\ 1833100 & 2153900 & 0.427 \\ 1500600 & 3048600 & 7.24 \end{bmatrix} \begin{bmatrix} c_{Hb} \\ c_{HbO_2} \\ c_{H_2O} \end{bmatrix} = \begin{bmatrix} \mu_a(674) \\ \mu_a(811) \\ \mu_a(956) \end{bmatrix}. \qquad (6.23)$$

Each column of this matrix contains values of extinction coefficients for each of the chromophores considered at three chosen wavelengths. The values of an absorption coefficient at each wavelength were determined from experimental study.

The spectroscopy system discussed can be used as an imaging system as well. Many FD imaging systems are described in the literature (see Refs. 1, 3, 4, 301–303, and 338). One of them was designed by the University of Pennsylvania and NIM Inc. for regional imaging of brain tissue.[1134] The system can operate at selectable RFs ranging from 50 to 400 MHz. A dual-wavelength light source (two laser diodes at 779 and 834 nm), APD photodetection, and SSB modulation/demodulation electronics are the main features of the imager. It was successfully used for a preliminary clinical study, i.e., the positions of the shunt components were defined on the basis of reconstructed images (at a depth of 1.2 cm) of brain tissue of a patient with hydrocephalus [abnormal increase in the amount of cerebrospinal fluid (CSF)] who was undergoing surgery to have a shunt replaced.

Table 6.1 Results of *in vivo* measurements of optical and physiological parameters of healthy and diseased tissues of patients (source-detector separation is equal to 2.2 cm, in the brackets given r.m.s. values)[306,308]

Tissue	λ, nm	μ_a, cm⁻¹	C_{Hb}, μM	C_{HbO_2}, μM	C_{Hb+HbO_2}, μM	C_{H_2O}, M
Female breast (56 yr):						
Normal	674	0.04				
	811	0.035	4.96	10.6	15.56	6.39
	849	0.035				
	956	0.085				
Fibroadenoma with ductal hyperplasia	674	0.055				
	811	0.06	5.65	22	27.65	6.02
	849	0.055				
	956	0.12				
Female breast (27 yr):						
Normal	674	0.035				
	811	0.03	4.1	8.13	12.23	9.4
	849	0.038				
	956	0.09				
Fluid-filled cyst	674	0.07				
	811	0.07	8.1	23.6	31.7	11.3
	849	0.08				
	956	0.16				
Multiple subcutaneous large-cell adenocarcinoma(male 62 yr): Abdominal:						
Normal tissue	674	0.0589 (0.0036)				
	811	0.0645 (0.0032)	6.22 (0.64)	23.9 (1.9)	30.1 (2.0)	4.09 (2.23)
	849	0.0690 (0.0025)				
	956	0.1110 (0.015)				

Table 6.1 (Continued).

Tissue	λ, nm	μ_a, cm^{-1}	C_{Hb}, μM	C_{HbO_2}, μM	C_{Hb+HbO_2}, μM	C_{H_2O}, M
Tumor	674	0.169 (0.02)	17.4 (3.6)	73.4 (8.3)	90.8 (9.0)	—
	811	0.190 (0.015)				
	849	0.276 (0.03)				
	956	—				
Back:						
Normal tissue	674	0.0883 (0.006)	9.68 (1.04)	33.2 (2.7)	42.9 (2.9)	—
	811	0.0892 (0.005)				
	849	0.0915 (0.0030)				
	956	0.127 (0.03)				
Tumor	674	0.174 (0.02)	19.1 (3.7)	66.0 (7.4)	85.1 (8.2)	—
	811	0.177 (0.013)				
	849	0.190 (0.01)				
	956	0.186 (0.16)				

A very stable and fast scanning and imaging system that uses the diffraction of diffuse photon density waves is described in Ref. 319. The system consists of an RF-modulated (100 MHz), low-power (about 3 mW) diode laser (786 nm). The source light is fiber guided to the tissue. A detection fiber couples the detected diffuse wave to a fast APD. SSB IQ demodulation electronics were used. The dynamic range of the system is about 2500. The source position was fixed, and a single detection fiber was scanned over a square region 9.3 × 9.3 cm; the amplitude and phase of the photon density wave were recorded at each position for a total of 1024 points. To obtain projection images of hidden macroinhomogeneities in a highly scattering tissue, imaging algorithms based on K-space spectral and fast Fourier transform (FFT) analysis were developed and tested clinically. The FFT approach has yielded clinical projection images with processing times much smaller than current collection times. It was shown that boundary effects present important problems. Matching substances might be used to reduce the boundary effects; nevertheless, the boundary effects may be incorporated in the reconstruction algorithm.

A schematic diagram of an FD optical mammography apparatus (LIMA), developed at Carl Zeiss is shown in Fig. 6.21.[325,326] It uses two diode lasers at 690 and 810 nm and the lasers' intensities are sinusoidally modulated at 110.0010 and 110.008 MHz, respectively. The average power is about 10 mW. Both laser beams (2 mm in diameter) are collimated, made collinear, and directed to the object. An optical fiber (5 mm in diameter) located on the opposite side of the breast delivers light to the detector. A PMT with modulated gain at 110 MHz is used as a detector. The differences in frequencies of light and gain modulation are $\Delta f_1 = 1$ kHz (relative to the signal at 690 nm) and $\Delta f_2 = 0.8$ kHz (relative to the signal at 810 nm), and are called cross-correlation frequencies. Appropriate electronic filtering allows separation of signals at these frequencies, i.e., at the two wavelengths.

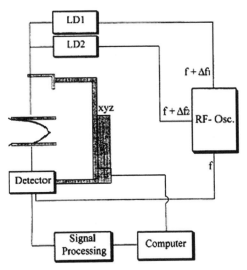

Figure 6.21 Schematic diagram of a frequency-domain mammograph (LIMA).[325,326]

The breast is slightly compressed between two parallel glass plates. The dual-wavelength laser beam and the detector fiber are scanned in tandem along the upper and lower plane, respectively, so that source-detection separation is fixed. The entire compression assembly with the two glass plates can be rotated by 90 deg to allow data to be acquired in craniocaudal and mediolateral projections. The extension of the scanning step (the image pixel size) can be set by software, but it is generally defined by the spatial resolution needed, the total acquisition time, and the signal-to-noise ratio. For this system, a scanning step of 1.5 mm in both directions requires a total acquisition time of about 3 min for a whole mammogram and has noise of about 2 deg for phase and 0.1% for amplitude measurements. The boundary effects were overcome using an appropriate algorithm [$N(x, y)$ function] based on the idea of exploring the phase information in a given pixel (x, y) to obtain an estimate of the breast thickness at that pixel. As a second step, the dependence of the amplitude signal on tissue thickness is modeled using the empirically determined dependence on the thickness in the optically homogeneous case. The LIMA system was clinically tested on 15 patients affected by breast cancer.

Two mammograms, x ray and optical (810 nm), for a female left breast with a tumor are presented in Fig. 6.22. A comparison of these mammograms clearly shows that this optical technique has good contrast and tumor detectability, rather than high spatial resolution, which is intrinsically limited by the diffusive nature of light propagation in tissue. The promise of optical imaging methods lies in high contrast, detectability, and specificity, which provide diagnostic capabilities. Further enhancement in contrast can be achieved by introducing additional light sources, wavelengths, modulation frequencies, and/or multiple detectors (see above discussion). In addition to contrast enhancement, FD and TD methods have the potential to provide an *in situ* optical biopsy by measuring localized optical properties.[306,308]

One of the first phase-imaging systems for *in vivo* studies was designed at the University of Illinois, Urbana-Champaign.[328] The optical signal at 760 nm from a mode-locked titanium:sapphire laser (Mira 900, Coherent) was modulated at 160 MHz. Heterodyne mixing at the dynode chain of the PMT produces a cross-correlation signal (1.25 kHz) carrying the same phase and amplitude information as the original signal. The imaging system provides subsecond data integration times per pixel (10^4 total pixels, 8 × 8 cm grid in a gradation of 101 steps of 0.8 mm each), resulting in a total measurement time of about 10 min. To partially compensate for limits on the detector's dynamic range and reduce the influence of boundary effects, the human hand under investigation was immersed in a highly scattering aqueous solution of Liposyn III (20%) (an intravenous fat emulsion) with the scattering and absorption properties approximately matched to those of the hand by diluting the emulsion with water and serial additions of black India ink.

An FD tissue spectrometer described in Ref. 305 uses an arc lamp as a light source that is intensity modulated at 135 MHz by a Pockel's cell and the heterodyne mixing at the dynode chain of the PMT with a cross-correlation signal at

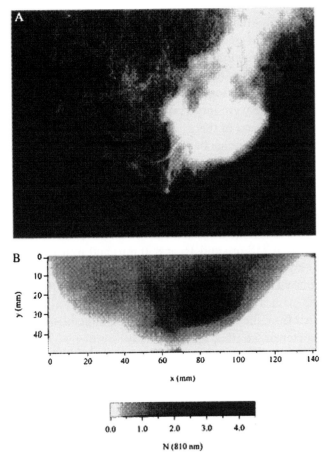

Figure 6.22 (a) X-ray and (b) optical craniocaudal mammograms of a female left breast with a tumor (55-yr-old Caucasian woman with an invasive ductal breast cancer—lateral lower quadrant; the major tumor is 3.0 cm in diameter). The x-ray and optical images cannot be compared point by point because the degree of compression and the compression geometry are different in the x-ray and optical measurements.[325,326]

100 Hz. For typical signal levels, the noise in this system is dominated by photon shot noise. The effects of the noise can be minimized by using a phased-array configuration with two detectors. For best results, signals from the two detectors should be equalized so that noise in the weaker signal is not dominant. The system can provide, at best, about 4% uncertainty in μ_a and μ'_s if the signals at the two detectors are equalized. Increasing the modulation depth and frequency allows random errors to be further reduced up to about 1%.

Systematic errors caused by finite tissue volumes and curved surfaces can be much larger than random errors induced by shot noise. As discussed earlier, these systematic errors can presumably be reduced if appropriate scattering and absorbing immersion surrounding a substance is applied or enough information about the tissue geometry is available to justify the use of a more corrected algorithm.[325,326,328] *In vivo* measurements made on the femoral biceps muscle of rabbits show that it is difficult to achieve shot noise limits in practice. The rms values for μ_a and μ_s' are typically 20% for a 15-s measurement time because the shot noise contribution is estimated to be about 8% in μ_a and 4% in μ_s'. This means that other sources of variation (tissue blood content or oxygenation, tissue inhomogeneity when scanning, finite source and detection size, uncertainty in their relative positions, etc.) with time were more important than the inherent instrument noise in determining the precision of the μ_a and μ_s' estimates.

The results of measurements of absorption and reduced scattering coefficients through the forehead on 30 adult volunteers using a multidistance FD NIR spectrometer (Imagent, ISS, Champaign, IL) were reported.[1135] The spectrometer employs laser diodes modulated at the frequency of 110 MHz and PMTs whose gain is modulated at a slightly offset frequency of 110.005 MHz to heterodyne the high frequency down to the frequency of 5 kHz. In studies described in Ref. 1135, 33 laser diodes (16 at 758 nm and 16 at 830 nm) and four PMTs were used. The laser diodes were multiplexed so that two lasers with the same wavelength and at the same location were on simultaneously. The light from the lasers was guided by optical fibers with a core diameter of 400 µm to the tissue surface and the photons reemitted from the tissue were collected simultaneously by the fiber bundles with a diameter of 5.6 mm, placed several centimeters apart from the source fibers. The collected light was carried to the PMTs and then the signals from the PMTs were digitally processed to yield the average intensity, modulation amplitude, and phase difference. These data were used for accurate estimation of the absolute absorption and reduced scattering coefficients of the adult brain. It was found that the adult head can be reasonably described by a two-layer model and the nonlinear regression for this model can be used to accurately retrieve the absolute absorption and reduced scattering coefficients of both layers if the thickness of the scalp/skull is known. For example, optical coefficients of the brain were estimated at 830 nm as $\mu_a = 0.145 \pm 0.005$ cm^{-1} and $\mu_s' = 4.1 \pm 0.1$ cm^{-1}. The hemoglobin concentration and oxygen saturation of the adult brain were also calculated with sufficiently good accuracy to provide monitoring of cerebral oxygen saturation and hemodynamics in order to assess cerebral health related to tissue oxygen perfusion.

A portable, multiwavelength, FD, NIR spectroscopy instrument similar to that shown in Fig. 6.14 was used for investigation of the optical properties of the brain in 23 neonates *in vivo*.[1136] It was found that the absorption coefficients of the infant forehead are lower than the values reported for adults and, being averaged for 23 infants, were equal to $\mu_a = 0.078 \pm 0.014$ cm^{-1} at 788 nm and $\mu_a = 0.089 \pm 0.019$ cm^{-1} at 832 nm. A large intersubject variation in μ_s' was also demonstrated, $\mu_s' = 9.16 \pm 1.22$ cm^{-1} at 788 nm and $\mu_s' = 8.42 \pm 1.23$ cm^{-1} at 832 nm. Physiological parameters derived from the absorption coefficients at two wavelengths were determined as the following: the mean total hemoglobin concentration was 39.7 ± 9.8 µM and the mean cerebral blood oxygen saturation was $58.7 \pm 11.2\%$. Therefore, it was shown that the bedside FD, NIR spectroscopy could provide quantitative optical measurement of the infant brain.

6.3 Light-scattering spectroscopy

Novel techniques capable of identifing and characterizing pathological changes in human tissues at the cellular and subcellular levels and based on light scattering were recently described.[47,61,94,95,129,130,150,170,180,450,452,620,731–735,798,811,1137] Light-scattering spectroscopy (LSS) provides structural and functional information of a tissue. This information, in turn, can be used to diagnose and monitor disease. One important application of biomedical spectroscopy is the noninvasive early detection of cancer in human epithelium.[180,452,620,732–734,1137] The enlarging, crowding, and hyperchromaticity of epithelium cell nuclei are the common features to all types of precancerous and early cancerous conditions. LSS can be used for detection of early cancerous changes and other diseases in a variety of organs such as esophagus, colon, uterine cervix, oral cavity, lungs, and urinary bladder.[452,620,733,734,1137] Eye lens cataract and other ophthalmic diseases can also be diagnosed using LSS.[811]

Cells and tissues have complex structures with very a broad range of the scatterers' sizes: from a few nanometers, the size of a macromolecule, to 7–10 μm, the size of a nucleus, and to 20–50 μm, the size of a cell itself. Most subcellular organelles are not uniform and have complex shapes and structures; nevertheless, they can be referred to as scattering "particles" (see Chapter 1). A great variety of cell organelle structures are small compared to the wavelength. Light scattering by such particles is known as Rayleigh scattering and is characterized by a broad angular distribution and a scattering cross-sectional dependence on the particle's linear dimension a as a^6 and on light wavelength λ as λ^{-4}. When the particle is not small enough, the coupled dipole theory or another approach such as the Rayleigh-Gans approximation (RGA) can be used. The RGA is particularly applicable to particles with sizes comparable to the wavelength and may be useful to study light scattering by small organelles such as mitochondria, lysosomes, etc. For RGA, the scattering in the forward direction prevails, and the total scattering intensity increases with the increase of the particle relative refractive index m as $(m - 1)^2$ and with its size as a^6.

The scattering by a particle with dimensions much larger than the wavelength, such as a cell nucleus, can be described within the framework of van de Hulst approximation that enables obtaining scattering amplitudes in the near-forward direction [see Eq. (2.25)]. For large particles, the scattered intensity is highly forward directed and the width of the first scattering lobe is about λ/a; the larger the particle, the stronger and narrower the first lobe. The intensity of the forward scattering, exhibits oscillations with the wavelength change. The origin of these oscillations is interference between the light ray passing through the center of the particle and one not interacting with it. The frequency of these oscillations is proportional to $a(m - 1)$, so it increases with the particle size and refractive index. The intensity of scattered light also peaks in the near-backward direction, but this peak is significantly smaller than the forward-scattering peak.

These results agree well with the rigorous scattering theory developed for the spherical particles (Mie theory).[148] To discriminate cell structure peculiarities, originated by the pathology, the difference in light scattering can be used. Structures with large dimensions and high refractive index produce a scattered field that peaks in the forward and near-backward directions in contrast to smaller and more optically "soft" structures, which scatter light more uniformly. Perelman et al.[150,180,620,732] studied elastic light scattering from densely packed layers of normal and T84 tumor human intestinal cells affixed to glass slides in a buffer solution (see Fig. 1.2). The diameters of the normal cell nuclei ranged from 5 to 7 µm, and those of the tumor cells from 7 to 16 µm. The reflectance from the samples exhibits distinct spectral features. The predictions of Mie theory were fit to the observed spectra. The fitting procedure used three parameters, average size of the nucleus, standard deviation in size (a Gaussian size distribution was assumed), and relative refractive index. The solid line of Fig. 6.23 is the distribution extracted from the data, and the dashed line shows the corresponding size distributions measured by light microscopy. The extracted and measured distributions for both normal and T84 cell samples were in good agreement, indicating the validity of the physical picture and the accuracy of the method of extracting information.

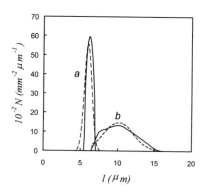

Figure 6.23 Nuclear size distributions of the samples presented in Fig. 1.2. (a) Normal intestinal cells; (b) T84 cells. In each case, the solid line is the distribution extracted from the data using Mie theory, and the dashed line is the distribution measured using light microscopy (from Ref. 180).

In tissues, the photons returned after a single scattering in the backward or near-backward directions produce a so-called single-scattering component. The photons returned after multiple scattering events produce diffuse reflectance. The spectra of both single-scattering and diffusive signals contain valuable information about tissue properties. However, the type of information is different. The single-scattering component is sensitive to the morphology of the upper tissue layer, which in the case of any mucosal tissue almost always includes or is limited by the epithelium. Its spectroscopic features are related to the microarchitecture of the epithelial cells, and the sizes, shapes, and refractive indices of their organelles, inclusions, and suborganellar components and inhomogeneities. Thus, analysis of this component might be useful in diagnosing diseases limited to the epithelium, such as preinvasive stages of epithelial cancers, dysplasias, and carcinomas *in situ* (CIS).[180,620,732,733,1137] The diffusive component contains information about tissue scatterers and absorbers as well, and its diagnostical possibilities and instrumentation are discussed early in this chapter.

The single-scattering component is more important in diagnosing the initial stages of epithelial precancerous lesions, while the diffusive component carries valuable information about more advanced stages of the disease. However, single-scattering events cannot be directly observed in *in vivo* tissues, because only a small portion of the light incident on the tissue is directly backscattered.

Several methods to distinguish single scattering have been proposed. Field-based light-scattering spectroscopy[735] and spectroscopic optical coherence tomography (OCT)[142] were developed for performing cross-sectional tomographic and spectroscopic imaging. In these extensions of conventional OCT, information on the spectral content of backscattered light is obtained by detection and processing of the interferometric OCT signal. These methods allow the spectrum of backscattered light to be measured either for several discreet wavelengths[734] or over the entire available optical bandwidth from 650 to 1000 nm simultaneously in a single measurement.[142]

A much simpler polarization-sensitive technique based on the fact that initially polarized light loses its polarization when traversing a turbid tissue is also available.[150] The conventional spatially resolved backscattering technique with enough small source-detector separation can be used as well.[180] In that case, the single-scattering component (2–5%) should be subtracted from the total reflectance spectra, which can be done using the diffusion approximation-based model by fitting to the coarse features of the diffusive component.

Zonios et al. studied the capability of diffuse reflectance spectroscopy to diagnose colonic precancerous lesions and adenomatous polyps *in vivo*.[735] Figure 6.24 shows typical diffuse reflectance spectra from one adenomatous polyp site and one normal mucosa site. Significant spectral differences are readily observed, particularly in the short-wavelength region of the spectrum, where the hemoglobin absorption valley around 420 nm stands out as the prominent spectral feature. This valley is much more prominent in the spectrum of the adenomatous polyp. This feature, as well as more prominent dips around 542 and 577 nm, which are characteristic of hemoglobin absorption as well, are all indicative of the increased hemoglobin presence in the adenomatous tissue.

Apparently, the differences between these spectra are due to changes in the scattering and absorption properties of the tissues. Both the absorption dips and the slopes of the spectra are sensitive functions of the absorption and scattering coefficients, providing a natural way to introduce an inverse algorithm that is sensitive to such features. The authors quantified the absorption and scattering properties using the diffusion-based model discussed in Section 1.1.2. The equation[735] analog to Eq. (1.27) was fit to the data using the Levenberg-Marquardt minimization method. Thus, the total hemoglobin concentration c_{Hb} and hemoglobin oxygen saturation

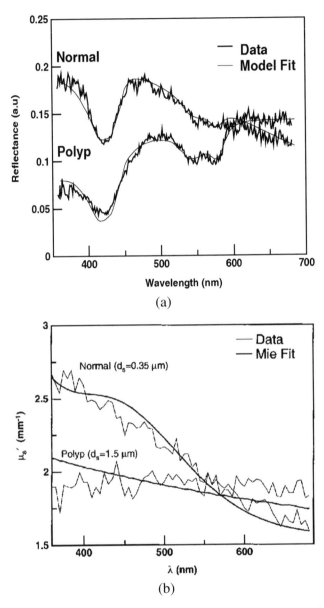

Figure 6.24 Diffuse reflectance analysis: (a) measured reflectance spectra (noisy lines) and modeled fits (smooth lines); (b) scattering spectra obtained from the reflectance measurements (noisy curves) and corresponding Mie theory spectra (smooth curves). The effective scatterer sizes d_s are indicated (from Refs. 732 and 735).

α were obtained. Also, the optimal reduced scattering coefficient $\mu'_s(\lambda)$ was found for each wavelength λ, ranging from 360 to 685 nm. It was found that $\mu'_s(\lambda)$ has a spectral dependence that resembles a straight line declining with wavelength λ. The slope of $\mu'_s(\lambda)$ decreases with an increasing effective size of the scatterers, d_s [Fig. 6.24(b)]. This allows the effective scatterer size to be determined from known $\mu'_s(\lambda)$. The model fits shown in Fig. 6.24(a) are in very good agreement with the experimental data.

The promise of LSS to diagnose dysplasia and CIS was tested in *in vivo* human studies in four different organs and in three different types of epithelium: columnar epithelia of the colon and Barrett's esophagus, transitional epithelium of the urinary bladder, and stratified squamous epithelium of the oral cavity.[733] All clinical studies were performed during routine endoscopic screening or surveillance procedures. In all of the studies, an optical fiber probe delivered white light from a xenon arc lamp to the tissue surface and collected the returned light. The probe tip was brought into gentle contact with the tissue to be studied. Immediately after the measurement, a biopsy was taken from the same tissue site. The spectrum of the reflected light was analyzed and the nuclear size distribution determined. Both dysplasia and CIS have a higher percentage of enlarged nuclei and, on average, a higher population density, which can be used as the basis for spectroscopic tissue diagnosis.

7

Polarization-Sensitive Techniques

In this chapter, polarization-sensitive techniques for imaging and functional diagnosis of biological tissue are considered. Methods based on the polarization discrimination of a probe-polarized light that is scattered by, or transmitted through, a tissue or a cell structure are described. The advantages of polarization methods for tissue imaging and functional diagnostics are discussed. It is shown that polarization-spectral selection of scattered radiation used with the polarization-fluorescence method significantly improves the diagnostic potential of the method.

7.1 Polarization imaging

7.1.1 Transillumination polarization technique

The polarization discrimination of light transmitted through a multiply scattering medium may provide high-quality images of inhomogeneities embedded in the scattering medium. Principles of transillumination polarization diaphanography of a heterogeneous scattering object are described in the literature.[1138] This technique makes it possible to locate and to image absorbing objects hidden in a strongly scattering medium. The method uses modulation of the polarization azimuth of a linearly polarized laser beam and lock-in detection of polarization properties of light transmitted through the object. The scattering sample was probed by an Ar-ion laser beam. The orientation of the polarization plane of the probe beam was modulated by a Pockel's cell as follows: during the first half-period of the modulating signal it was not changed, and during the second half-period it was rotated by 90 deg. Transmitted (depolarized) and forward-scattered (polarized) components of the probe light were collimated by two diaphragms and divided into two channels by a polarizing beamsplitter. It was found that in comparison with conventional diaphanography, polarization diaphanography allows one to get shadow images of a hidden object in a scattering medium that is characterized by up to approximately 30 scattering events on average.[1138]

A comparison of polarization and conventional transillumination imaging was carried out in Refs. 353–355 and 1139. The absorbing inhomogeneity, such as an absorbing plate placed in a scattering slab, was probed by a linearly polarized laser beam (Fig. 7.1). The shadow images were reconstructed from the profiles of the intensity and the degree of polarization P of the transmitted light (Fig. 7.2). Note that the dependencies of the degree of linear polarization on the edge position exhibit an increase in P in the vicinity of the edge. The explanation of this peculiarity is similar to that proposed by Jacques et al.[383] for the polarization-sensitive detection of backscattered light (see Section 7.1.2) and is connected with that near the absorber edge; the degree of polarization may be approximately doubled in value (for a highly scattering media) because no $I_\perp$ photons are scattered into the shadow-edge pixels by the shadow region, while $I_\parallel$ photons are directly scattered into these pixels. Better quality of the shadow images of the object is obtained with the use of the polarization imaging technique in comparison with conventional transillumination.

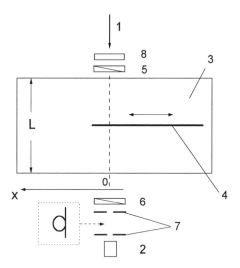

Figure 7.1 Scheme of the experimental setup for transillumination polarization imaging.[1139] 1, Linearly polarized beam of He:Ne laser (633 nm); 2, detector; 3, glass tank filled by scattering medium (diluted milk); 4, absorbing half-plane; 5, polarizer; 6, analyzer; 7, collimating diaphragms or light-collecting optical fiber; 8, chopper.

7.1.2 Backscattering polarization imaging

The principle of polarization discrimination of multiply scattered light has been fruitfully explored by many research groups in morphological analysis and visualization of subsurface layers in strongly scattering tissues.[129,135,136,138,376,378,379,382,383,1139–1143,1147] One of the most popular approaches to polarization imaging in heterogeneous tissues is based on using linearly polarized light to irradiate the object (the chosen area of the tissue surface) and to reject the backscattered light with the same polarization state (copolarized radiation) by the imaging system. Typically, such polarization discrimination is achieved simply by placing a polarizer between the imaging lens and the object. The optical axis of the polarizer is oriented perpendicularly to the polarization plane of the incident light. Thus, only the cross-polarized component of the scattered light contributes to the formation of the object image. Despite its simplicity, this technique has been demonstrated to be an adequately effective tool for functional diagnostics and for the imaging of

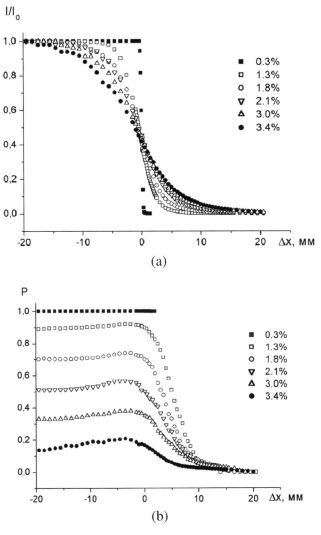

Figure 7.2 Experimental dependencies of (a) the normalized intensity and (b) degree of linear polarization of transmitted light on the absorbing half-plane edge position at different concentrations of the background scattering medium (diluted milk).[1139]

subcutaneous tissue layers. Moreover, the separate imaging of an object with copolarized and cross-polarized light permits separation of the structural features of the shallow tissue layers (such as skin wrinkles, the papillary net, etc.) and the deep layers (such as the capillaries in derma). The elegant simplicity of this approach has stimulated its widespread application in both laboratory and clinical medical diagnostics.

A typical scheme of instrumentation for polarization imaging using the approach discussed above is presented in Fig. 7.3. In the imaging system developed by Demos et al.,[1141] a dye laser with Nd:YAG laser pumping is used as the illumination source. The probe beam diameter is 10 cm and the average intensity is

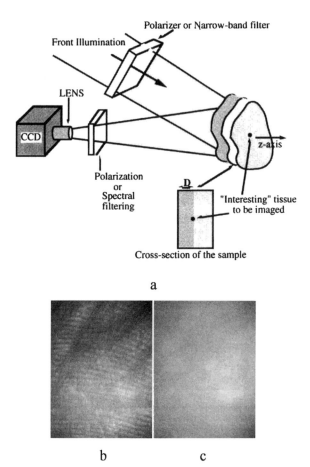

Figure 7.3 (a) An instrument for selective polarization or spectral imaging of subsurface tissue layers; (b) copolarized and (c) cross-polarized images of the human palm at 580-nm polarized laser light illumination.[1141]

approximately equal to 5 mW/cm^2. A cooled CCD camera with a 50-mm focal length lens is used to detect back-reflected light and to capture the image. The first polarizer, placed after the beam expander, is used to ensure illumination with linearly polarized light. A second polarizer is positioned in front of the CCD camera with its polarization orientation perpendicular or parallel to that of the illumination.

The efficiency of selective polarization imaging is illustrated in Fig. 7.3, where the copolarized and cross-polarized images of a human palm are presented. Figure 7.3(b) illustrates surface imaging (copolarized), where the superficial skin papillary pattern is clearly seen. Figure 7.3(c) illustrates subsurface skin imaging (cross-polarized image).

A similar camera system, but one that uses an incoherent white light source such as a xenon lamp, is described in Refs. 36, 383, and 1144, where results of a pilot clinical study of various skin pathologies using polarized light are presented. The image-processing algorithm used is based on the evaluation of the degree of polarization, which is then considered to be the imaging parameter. Two images are acquired: one "parallel," I_{par}, and one "perpendicular," I_{per}. These images are algebraically combined to yield a polarization image as

$$PI = \frac{I_{par} - I_{per}}{I_{par} + I_{per}}. \qquad (7.1)$$

It is important to note that in the polarization image, the numerator rejects randomly polarized diffuse reflectance; therefore, PI may be used to monitor tissue birefringence. Normalization by the denominator makes the expression for PI less sensitive to attenuation, which is common to the individual polarization components and is due to tissue absorption, i.e., melanin pigmentation for skin.

The polarization images of pigmented skin sites (freckles, tattoos, and pigmented nevi) and unpigmented skin sites [nonpigmented intradermal nevi, neurofibromas, actinic keratosis, malignant basal cell carcinomas, squamous cell carcinomas, vascular abnormalities (venous lakes), and burn scars] are analyzed to find the differences caused by various skin pathologies (see some examples in Fig. 7.5).[383] Also, the point-spread function of the backscattered polarized light is analyzed for images of a shadow cast from a razor blade onto a forearm skin site. This function describes the behavior of the degree of polarization at the imaging parameter near the shadow edge. It was discovered that near the shadow edge, the degree of polarization approximately doubles in value because no I_{per} photons are superficially scattered into the shadow-edge pixels by the shadow region, while I_{par} photons are directly backscattered from the superficial layer of these pixels. This result suggests that the point-spread function in skin for cross talk between pixels of the polarization image has a half width at half maximum (HWHM) of about 390 μm.

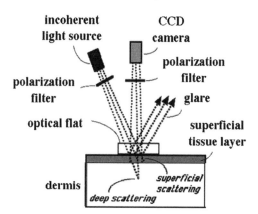

Figure 7.4 A prototype of a polarization camera for skin examination.[383] The incident light is linearly polarized parallel to the scattering plane. An optical flat enforces a uniform skin-glass interface for the reflection of glare away from the camera. The polarized scattered light and the diffusely scattered light reach the camera after passing through a linear polarizer that can be oriented parallel with or perpendicular to the scattering plane.

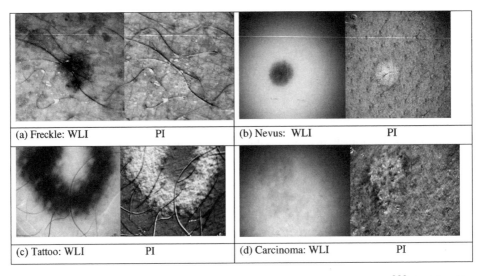

Figure 7.5 Comparison of white light (WLI) versus polarization (PI) images.[383] (a) A freckle; the polarization image removes the melanin from a freckle. (b) A benign pigmented nevus; the polarization image removes the melanin and shows apparent scatter, the drop of polarized light reflectance from epidermis lining the hair follicles is seen. (c) Tattoo; the polarization image lightens the "blackness" of the tattoo, specular reflectance of polarized light off the carbon particles yields a strong image. (d) Malignant basal cell carcinoma; the white light image underestimates the extent of the skin cancer.

Comparative analysis of polarization images of normal and diseased human skin has shown the ability of the above approach to emphasize image contrast based on light scattering in the superficial layers of the skin. The polarization images can visualize disruption of the normal texture of the papillary and upper reticular layers caused by skin pathology. Polarization imaging can be considered as an adequately effective tool for identifying skin cancer margins and for guiding surgical excision of skin cancer [see Fig. 7.5(d)]. Various modalities of polarization imaging are also considered in Ref. 1145.

The evaluation of the quality of the polarization images is based on the presentation of multiply scattered light as a superposition of partial contributions characterized by different values of the optical paths s in the scattering medium.[135,1143] The statistical properties of the ensemble of partial contributions are described by the probability density function of the optical paths $\rho(s)$, whereas the statistical moments of the scattered light are represented by the integral transforms of $\rho(s)$ with the properly chosen kernels. The degree of polarization of multiply scattered radiation with initial linear polarization can be approximately represented in the form of the Laplace transform of $\rho(s)$ as

$$P_L = \frac{I_{II} - I_{\perp}}{I_{II} + I_{\perp}} \approx \frac{3}{2} \int_0^{\infty} \exp\left(-\frac{s}{\xi_L}\right)\rho(s)ds, \tag{7.2}$$

where I_{II} and $I_{\perp}$ are, respectively, the intensities of the copolarized and cross-polarized components of the scattered light. The parameter ξ_L is the depolarization length for linearly polarized light.

By considering the polarization visualization of the absorbing macrohetero-geneity, along with the degree of polarization of backscattered light as the visualization parameter, the contrast of the polarization image can be defined as[135]

$$V_P = \frac{P_L^{in} - P_L^{back}}{P_L^{in} + P_L^{back}}, \qquad (7.3)$$

where P_L^{in} is the degree of residual linear polarization of the backscattered light detected in the region of the localization of the heterogeneity and P_L^{back} is the analogous quantity determined far from the region of localization. The contrast V_P of the reconstructed polarization image can be represented as a function of the scattering layer thickness l, the depth of inhomogeneity position h, the transport mean free path l_t of the scattering medium, the scattering anisotropy factor g, and the depolarization length ξ_L.[135] The probability density function of the optical paths $\rho(s)$ can be obtained by a Monte Carlo simulation.

To compare the efficiency of the various polarization imaging modalities, the experimental setup shown in Fig. 7.6 was used.[1139] The total normalized intensity (the intensity of the copolarized and cross-polarized components) or the degree of residual linear polarization of the backscattered light were taken as the visualization parameters. A scattering medium (a water-milk emulsion) in a rectangular glass tank ($18 \times 26 \times 26$ cm) was used as a tissue model. The side and rear walls of the tank were blackened. The absorbing object (a rectangular plate with blackened rough surfaces) was positioned in the central part of the tank at different distances h (1 to 4 cm) from the transparent front wall. The white light probe was linearly polarized perpendicular to the plane of incidence. To avoid specular reflection from the front wall of the tank, the illuminating beam was directed at an angle of 30 deg relative to the normal to the wall.

The capture of the object images for each of three chromatic coordinates (R, G, and B) was done using a color CCD camera (Panasonic NV-RX70EN) and a Miro DC20 frame grabber (MiroVideo, Germany). The color 8-bit images of the object were captured with 647×485 resolution with the use of copolarized and cross-polarized backscattered light. The brightness distributions for each of the R, G, and B image components along an arbitrarily chosen line of the image [Fig. 7.6(b)] are applied to reconstruct the images of the absorbing heterogeneity with different visualization parameters [Fig. 7.6(c)]. In the absence of a scattering medium and, hence, the backscattered radiation, the image contrast is equal to zero. An increase in the milk concentration results first in a sharp increase in the image contrast up to the maximum value, with the subsequent monotonic decrease caused by the increase of scattering multiplicity.

Comparison of the experimental data and the MC simulations[135,1139,1143] allows one to conclude that maximal contrast in the polarization image is obtained at

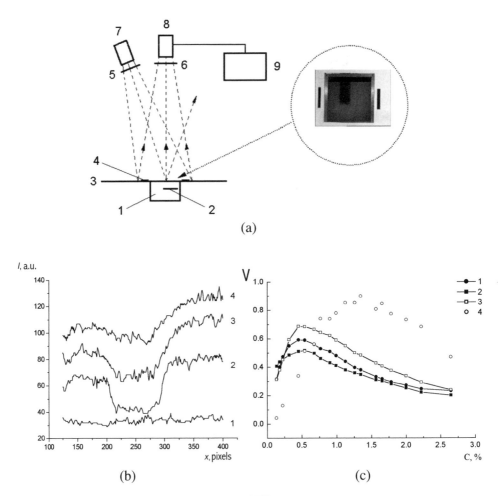

Figure 7.6 Polarization imaging experiment.[1139] (a) Schematic diagram: 1, a cell with a scattering medium; 2, absorbing plate; 3, white marker; 4, black markers; 5, polarizer; 6, analyzer; 7, a halogen lamp; 8, CCD camera; and 9, PC. (b) Distributions of backscattered radiation intensity along an arbitrarily chosen line of the image for different volume concentrations of milk emulsion: 1, 0%; 2, 0.66%; 3, 1.96%; and 4, 5.51% (R-component of the color image). (c) Dependencies of the polarization image contrast on the volume concentration of the milk emulsion when the normalized intensity of the (1) unpolarized light, (2) copolarized components, (3) cross-polarized components, and (4) the degree of polarization of backscattered radiation are used as the visualization parameter.

the depth of an inhomogeneity position on the order of (0.25–0.6) ξ_L (depending on the degree of residual polarization in the backscattered background component detected outside the region of the inhomogeneity localization). In particular, this conclusion agrees with data on polarization imaging of skin, which points to the efficiency of polarization imaging for epidermis and upper layers of papillary derma (100–150 μm).[1144]

7.2 Polarized reflectance spectroscopy of tissues

7.2.1 In-depth polarization spectroscopy

Imaging and monitoring of the morphological and functional state of biological tissues may be provided on the basis of spectral analysis of the polarization properties of the backscattering light.[1146] Tissue probing by a linear polarized white light and measuring of the spectral response of the copolarized and cross-polarized components of the backscattered light allow one not only to quantify chromophore tissue content, but also to estimate in-depth chromophore distribution.

In the visible wavelength range, skin may have a reduced scattering coefficient $\mu_s' \sim 30\text{--}90$ cm^{-1} and absorption coefficient $\mu_a \sim 0.2\text{--}5$ cm^{-1} (see Table 2.1); therefore, the expected transport mean free path of a photon $l_t = (\mu_a + \mu_s')^{-1}$ [see Eq. (1.22)] is in the range 100–300 μm. Because of the dominating of scatterers with sizes, characterized by a diffraction parameter $ka > 1$ [see Eqs. (1.99) and (1.100) and Figs. 1.27 and 1.28], the depolarization length ξ_L in skin is comparable with the transport scattering length l_t, and exceeds the skin epidermis thickness. On the other hand, such absorbers as melanin in epidermis and hemoglobin in dermis must increase the degree of the residual polarization of the backscattered light in the spectral ranges that correspond to the absorbing bands of the dominating chromophores. Moreover, these chromophores are placed at different depths; thus, their localization may be estimated owing to the characteristic absorbing bands on the differential polarization spectra.[135,1146]

Figure 7.7 shows the experimental setup for the backscattering polarization spectral measurements. Light from a white light source (halogen lamp of 200 W) is guided to the object by a fiber bundle with an attached wideband linear polarization filter. The diameter of the irradiated skin surface is approximately 8 mm. The backscattered light from the skin is collected by another fiber bundle to the input of which a polarized filter is attached. This filter is variable and may change its orientation, being parallel with or perpendicular to the optical axis of the first polarization filter. Fiber bundles are used to exclude some polarization sensitivity that may take place at the use of monofibers. To exclude specular reflection from

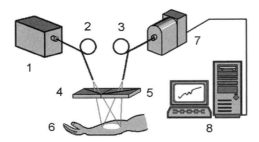

Figure 7.7 Scheme of the experimental setup for the backscattering polarization spectral measurements:[1146] 1, a white light source (halogen lamp, 200 W); 2 and 3, fiber bundles; 4 and 5, polarization filters; 6, object under study; 7, photodiode-array grating spectrometer; 8, PC.

the skin surface, the detecting fiber bundle was placed at an angle of ∼20 deg with respect to the normal to the skin surface. A distal end of the fiber was connected with the spectrometer.

This instrument is able to measure reflectance spectra at both parallel and perpendicular orientations of filters $R_{II}(\lambda)$ and $R_{\perp}(\lambda)$. From these spectra, the differential residual polarization spectra $\Delta R^r(\lambda)$ or residual polarization degree spectra $P_L^r(\lambda)$ are calculated as

$$\Delta R^r(\lambda) = R_{II}(\lambda) - R_{\perp}(\lambda), \qquad (7.4)$$

$$P_L^r(\lambda) = \frac{R_{II}(\lambda) - R_{\perp}(\lambda)}{R_{II}(\lambda) + R_{\perp}(\lambda)}. \qquad (7.5)$$

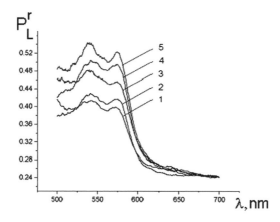

Figure 7.8 *In vivo* measured residual polarization degree spectra for a volunteer with UV-induced erythema of different degrees (erythema index, EI): 1, EI = 157; 2, EI = 223; 3, EI = 249; 4, EI = 275; and 5, EI = 290.[1146] Erythema index was measured using the erythema-melanin meter described in Ref. 1147.

Two examples of *in vivo* human skin studies using polarization spectroscopy are presented in Figs. 7.8 and 7.9.[1146] Figure 7.8 demonstrates spectral distributions of the residual polarization degree $P_L^r(\lambda)$ of the backscattered light for different values of the index of erythema induced by UV light. For a higher erythema index (EI) or skin redness (increased blood volume), $P_L^r(\lambda)$ is improved within the absorption Q-bands of the blood. This happens owing to the reduction of multiplicity of scattering for the photons with wavelengths that fall down to the absorption bands because of more intensive absorption of such photons.

Figure 7.9 presents differential polarization spectra, which are also sensitive to the absorption properties of skin that was controlled using a tape stripping technology. Less epidermal thickness corresponds to a higher blood volume within the measuring volume (higher hemoglobin absorption). Therefore, in spite of the

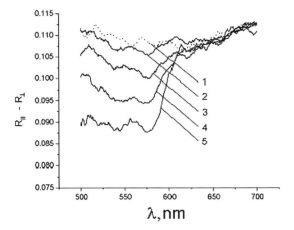

Figure 7.9 *In vivo* measured differential residual polarization spectra for a volunteer at epidermal stripping of different thicknesses:[1146] 1, normal skin; 2, thickness of the removed skin layer is 40 μm; 3, 50 μm; 4, 60 μm; and 5, 70 μm.

$[R_{II}(\lambda) - R_{\perp}(\lambda)]$ value reduction within the blood absorption bands (545 and 575 nm) due to the attenuation of both polarization components, its difference from the values measured far from the blood absorption bands, i.e., in the range 650–750 nm, is significant to providing in-depth profiling of epidermal thickness and blood vessels in skin.

As a criteria of epidermal thickness, the following parameters can be used:[1146]

$$V_{545} = \frac{\Delta R^r_{(650-700)} - \Delta R^r_{545}}{\Delta R^r_{(650-700)} + \Delta R^r_{545}} \quad \text{or} \quad V_{575} = \frac{\Delta R^r_{(650-700)} - \Delta R^r_{575}}{\Delta R^r_{(650-700)} + \Delta R^r_{575}}. \quad (7.6)$$

In these equations, indices 545 and 575 denote the differential residual polarization backscattering coefficients at the wavelengths of the hemoglobin absorption bands' centers ($\lambda = 545$–575 nm) and (650–700) at the wavelength range, where hemoglobin absorption is small ($\lambda = 650$–700 nm).

This method is still simple and, owing to the spectral information received, may provide information about living tissue that is more valuable than the nonspectral polarization methods described in Section 7.1.2. The experimental system is shown in Fig. 7.10. Monochrome images of the skin are captured by a video system, VS-CTT 60-075 (Videoscan Ltd., Russia). To get smoother white light irradiation of the skin surface and to avoid specular light detection, four halogen lamps of 50 W were positioned with their irradiation directed from four different sides at an angle ∼30 deg with respect to the normal to the skin surface. The output of each light source was filtered by identical linear polarized filters, and a rotatable polarization filter-analyzer was placed in front of the monochrome CCD camera. Figure 7.11 shows an example of skin burn lesion polarization-spectral imaging at the wavelength of hemoglobin absorption (∼550 nm). It is well seen that the maximal image contrast of ∼0.49 is provided for the polarization degree as a visualization parameter.

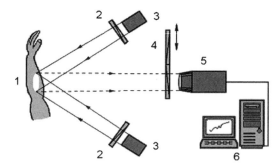

Figure 7.10 Experimental setup for polarization-spectral imaging of *in vivo* tissues:[1146] 1, tissue; 2, polarization filters; 4, polarization and interferential filters; 3, light sources; 5, monochrom CCD camera; 6, PC.

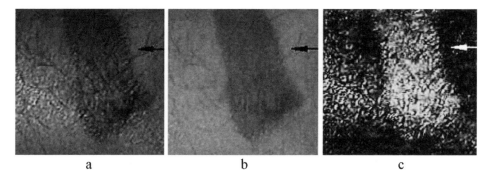

a   b   c

Figure 7.11 Polarization-spectral ($\lambda = 550$ nm) images of a skin burn lesion of the volunteer:[1146] (a) a copolarized image; (b) a crossed-polarized image; (c) degree of polarization image, P_L^r.

7.2.2 Superficial epithelial layer polarization spectroscopy

One of the promising approaches to early cancer diagnosis is based on the analysis of a single scattered component of light perturbed by tissue structure (see Section 6.3). The wavelength dependence of the intensity of the light elastically scattered by the tissue structure appears sensitive to changes in tissue morphology that are typical of precancerous lesions. In particular, it has been established that specific features of malignant cells, such as increased nuclear size, increased nuclear/cytoplasmic ratio, pleomorphism, etc., are markedly manifested in the elastic light scattering spectra of probed tissue. A specific fine periodic structure in the wavelength of backscattered light has been observed for mucosal tissue.[180] This oscillatory component of light scattering spectra is attributable to a single scattering from surface epithelial cell nuclei and can be interpreted within the framework of Mie theory. Analysis of the amplitude and frequency of the intensity spectrum's fine structure allows one to estimate the density and size distributions of these nuclei. However, the extraction of a single-scattered component from the masking multiple scattering background is a problem. Also, as it was shown in Section 7.2.1, absorption of stroma related to hemoglobin distorts the single-scattering spectrum of the epithelial cells. Both of these factors should be taken into account when interpreting the measured spectral dependencies of the backscattered light.

The negative effects of a diffuse background and hemoglobin absorption can be significantly reduced by the application of a polarization discrimination technique in the form of the illumination of the probed tissue with linearly polarized light followed by the separate detection of the elastic scattered light at the parallel and perpendicular polarization states (i.e., the copolarized and cross-polarized components of the backscattered light).[150,163] This approach, called polarized elastic light scattering spectroscopy or polarized reflectance spectroscopy (PRS), will potentially provide a quantitative estimate not only of the size distributions of cell nuclei, but also of the relative refractive index of the nucleus. These potentialities, which have been demonstrated in a series of experimental works with tissue phantoms and *in vivo* epithelial tissues,[150,163,166,180] allow one to classify the PRS technique as a new step in the development of noninvasive optical devices for real-time diagnostics of tissue morphology and, consequently, for improved early detection of precancers *in vivo*. An important step in the further development of the PRS method will be the design of portable and flexible instrumentation applicable to *in situ* tissue diagnostics. In particular, fiber-optic probes are expected to "bridge the gap between benchtop studies and clinical applications of polarized reflectance spectroscopy."[1148]

7.3 Polarization microscopy

Polarized light microscopy has been used in biomedicine for more than a century to study optically anisotropic biological structures that may be difficult, or even impossible, to observe using a conventional light microscope. A number of commercial microscopes are available on the market, and numerous investigations of biological objects have been made using polarization microscopy. However, modern approaches in polarization microscopy have the potential to enable one to acquire new and more detailed information about biological cells and tissue structures. At present, it is possible to detect optical path differences of even less than 0.1 nm.[168,388,754,1149–1151] Such sensitivity as well as the capability to examine scattering samples are due to recent achievements in video, interferential, and multispectral polarization microscopy. Full Mueller matrix measurements and other combined techniques, such as polarization/confocal and polarization/OCT microscopy, promise new capabilities for polarization microscopy including *in vivo* measurements.

In addition to that discussed in Sections 1.4, 3.3, and 5.7.1, in this section, we will discuss only a few of the recent studies and novel techniques that have the potential to examine the anisotropic properties of scattering samples. One of the examples is the multispectral imaging micropolarimeter (MIM), which can detect the birefringence of the peripapillary retinal nerve fiber layer (RNFL) in glaucoma diagnosis.[168,388] The optical scheme of the MIM is presented in Fig. 7.12.

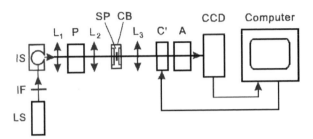

Figure 7.12 Optical scheme of the multispectral imaging micropolarimeter used in transmission mode.[388] LS, light source; IF, interference filter; IS, integrating sphere; P, linear polarizer; SP, specimen; CB, chamber; L_1, L_2, and L_3, lenses; C', linear retarder; A, linear analyzer; CCD, charge-coupled device.

Light from a tungsten-halogen lamp, followed by an interference filter (band of 10 nm), provides monochromatic illumination to an integrating sphere (IS). Lens L_1 ($F = 56$ mm) collimates the beam incident onto a polarizer (P). The use of an integrating sphere assures that the output intensity of the polarizer varies less than 0.2% as it rotates 360 deg. Lens L_2 ($F = 40.5$ mm, NA $= 0.13$) focuses the image of the exit aperture of the integrating sphere onto a specimen (SP) in a chamber (CB) with a flat entrance and exit windows. Lens L_3 ($F = 60$ mm, NA $= 0.07$) focuses the specimen image onto a cooled CCD camera that provides a pixel size of about 4 µm on a specimen in an aqueous medium (magnification ≈ 5.8). Although the lenses are achromatic, the wide spectral range (440–830 nm) requires only small changes in the detection optics' position (moving the lens L_3 and CCD together within a 0.5-mm range) to adjust the focus for each wavelength. A liquid crystal linear retarder (C'), followed by a linear analyzer (A), is used to measure the output Stokes vector of the specimen. Both polarizer and analyzer are Glan-Taylor polarization prisms. The azimuth and retardance of the retarder are set for a few discrete values, and the azimuth of the analyzer is always fixed at 45 deg. Each setting of the retarder (respectively, azimuth and retardance)—(1) 0, 90 deg; (2) 0, 200 deg; (3) 22.5, 207 deg; (4) −22.5, 207 deg)—is characterized by a 1×4 measurement vector. The four retarder/analyzer settings together are characterized by a 4×4 matrix **D**, with each row corresponding to one measured vector.

A Stokes vector $\overline{S}$ can be calculated as

$$\overline{S} = D^{-1}\overline{R}, \tag{7.7}$$

where D^{-1} is the inverse of the measurement matrix and $\overline{R}$ is a 4×1 response vector corresponding to the four retarder/analyzer settings.[816] To evaluate the linear retardance of a specimen, the Mueller matrix should be found from the measurements of the incident $\overline{S}_{inc}$ and the output $\overline{S}$ Stokes vectors (see Section 1.4) as

$$\overline{S} = K\mathrm{M}(\rho, \delta)\overline{S}_{inc}, \tag{7.8}$$

where the factor K accounts for the losses of intensity in transmission and ρ and δ are, respectively, the azimuth and retardance of the specimen. This expression includes four equations for the three unknowns, K, ρ, and δ. In most cases, it is useful to overdetermine the system of equations in Eq. (7.8) by using more than one $\overline{S}_{inc}$.

The retardance and azimuth of a living and fixed rat's RNFLs were measured over a wide spectral range.[388] It was found that the RNFL behaves as a linear retarder and that the retardance is approximately constant in a wavelength range from 440 to 830 nm. The average birefringence measured for a few unfixed rat RNFLs, with an average thickness of 13.9 ± 0.4 μm, is 0.23 ± 0.01 (nm/μm) $\equiv$ 2.3×10^{-4}. The influence of the polarization properties of the retina on the measured RNFLs' anisotropic properties was found. Images presented in Fig. 7.13 illustrate the importance of correcting for the polarization properties of the retina and for the distributions of retardance and azimuth within the sample.

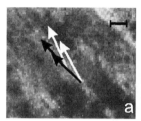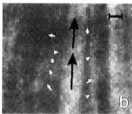

Figure 7.13 Estimated retardances (arrows' lengths) and slow axes (arrows' directions) of the bundle and gap areas of rat RNFLs.[388] The images are at the wavelength 440 nm. Images sizes: (a) 222×199 μm; (b) 187×177 μm. Nerve fiber bundles appear as brighter bands. Each arrow starts in the center of the area measured. The calibration bar is 1 nm of retardance. (a) The white arrows represent measurements that are not corrected for retinal polarization ability, and the black arrows are corrected ones. (b) The black arrows are corrected bundle retardances; the small white arrows in the gaps show the variation of residual retardances, also after correction.

Another technique, which is related to quantitative polarized light microscopy, is based on a video microscopy technique that is applied to measure variations in the orientations of the collagenous fibers arranged in lamellae within eye corneal tissue.[1149] The lamellar structure of the cornea and sclera is very visible in Figs. 3.2, 3.3, and 3.4. Within a lamella, the fibrils are parallel, but the fibrils of adjacent lamellae do not, in general, run in the same direction. They may have a relative orientation at any angle between 0 and 180 deg.

As was discussed in Section 3.1.1, in corneal stroma, the fibrils have a diameter of 25–39 nm while the mean diameter of scleral fibrils is equal to 100 nm. Therefore, the individual fibrils cannot be resolved with light microscopy; but due to the intrinsic birefringence of collagen fibrils and its dependence on the angle of their orientation from lamella to lamella, they can be recognized. Along its fiber axis, collagen is highly birefringent, so those lamellae that are cut parallel to the fiber axes [$\theta = 0$ deg, see Fig. 7.14(a)] appear brighter under polarized light when the polarizer and analyzer are crossed and the length of the tissue section is oriented at 45 deg to the polarizer/analyzer axis [see Fig. 7.14(b)]. Collagen is not birefringent perpendicular to its fiber axis [$\theta = 90$ deg, see Fig. 7.14(a)], so those lamellae that are cut perpendicular to their fibril direction appear completely dark in this section [see Fig. 7.14(b)]. The variation of intensity along the transect $X–Y$ across the cornea section [see Fig. 7.14(b)] is caused by the different angular orientation of the particular lamella (totally, about 15 lamellae are seen) and presented in Fig. 7.14(c).

Because of the regular arrangement of the lamellae, the angle θ is all that is necessary to define the three-dimensional orientation of the fibrils in sections of normal cornea. Nevertheless, to find this angle distribution for a specific tissue section, the lamellar birefringence of form that contributes about 67% to the total birefringence should be accounted for.[1149] For sections of disrupted pathological cornea and for sections of sclera and limbus (the region where the cornea and sclera fuse), the situation is more complicated because the lamellae have a much less ordered "wavy" arrangement [see Fig. 3.5(b) for sclera].

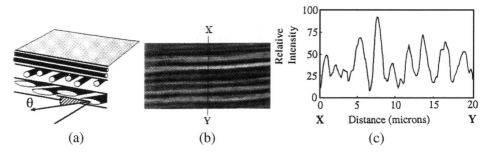

(a)   (b)   (c)

Figure 7.14 Polarization microscopy of a collagenous tissue structure.[1149] (a) Schematic diagram of a tissue section containing three lamellae (the number of fibrils is greatly reduced and the relative fibril diameter greatly exaggerated; an actual electronic micrograph is shown in Fig. 3.2); angle θ is the angle of inclination of the fibrils relative to the plane of sectioning. (b) Digital photomicrograph of a section through part of a rabbit cornea viewed under polarized light ($\times 500$). (c) The variation in intensity along the transect X–Y across the cornea section of photomicrograph (b).

Many tissues possess very complex patterns of alignment of the structure-forming elements. Some polarization microscopic methods that show promise for generating alignment maps for such tissues have been developed (see, for example, Refs. 1152–1154). The method presented in Refs. 1152 and 1153, as well as the method used in Ref. 1149, is a useful tool in cases where the tissue structure along the direction of the probing light propagation can be considered to be a uniform one. In Refs. 1152 and 1153, a microscopic polarimetry method for generating fiber alignment maps, which can be used for characterization of the structure of fibrous tissues, tissue phantoms, and other fibrillar materials, is considered. This method is based on probing the sample with elliptically polarized light from a rotated quarter-wave plate and an effective circular analyzer. Nonlinear regression techniques are implemented for estimating the optical parameters of the optic train and the sample. The processing of the sequence of images obtained with different mutual orientations of the rotated quarter-wave plate and the analyzer, which is based on fast harmonic analysis, permits the recovery of an alignment direction map and a retardation map. These maps describe a spatial distribution of a sample's local linear birefringence and, therefore, can be used for morphological analysis of tissues with an expressed structural anisotropy that have linear birefringence as their dominant optical property. The potential of this method for accurately generating alignment maps for samples that act as linear retarders to within a few degrees of retardation has been demonstrated in experiments with an *in vitro* sample of a porcine heart valve leaflet.

The method proposed in Ref. 1154 can also be used in more general situations when the orientation of the structure-forming elements (for instance, the collagen fibers) varies along the probing direction. Such variation should be taken into account when thick (>50 μm) tissue layers (e.g., dermis) are analyzed. In the method discussed,[1154] a standard polarization microscope arranged with a CCD camera can be used. The measurements are usually carried out with wide-spectral-range color filters and without a quarter-wave plate. The following expression describes the dependence of the detected signal at any detection point on the angles of orientation of the polarizer (ϑ) and the analyzer (ϑ') of the microscope:

$$i_C \approx B_0 + B_1 \cos\eta + B_2 \cos\varsigma + B_3 \sin\eta + B_4 \sin\varsigma,$$
$$\eta = 2(\vartheta - \vartheta'), \quad \varsigma = 2(\vartheta + \vartheta'),$$

(7.9)

where B_i ($i = 0, 1, 2, 3,$ and 4) are the coefficients, which depend on the local optical properties of the sample in the probed region and the spectral properties of incident light. As was shown in Ref. 1154, the measured values of B_i are capable of providing important information about the sample structure. They can also be used for characterization of specific features of light propagation in the sample; in particular, they allow us to recognize the so-called adiabatic regime of light propagation in the studied medium. This means that in the adiabatic regime, the orientation of the local optical axis changes smoothly in the probed region of the tissue. Note that for fibrous tissues, the direction of the local optical axis typically coincides with the local preferred direction of fiber orientation. If the adiabatic regime is realized, then the angles υ and ϕ, which are calculated from the obtained values of B_i as $\upsilon = (1/4)\arctan(B_2/B_4)$ and $\phi = (1/2)\arctan(B_1/B_3)$, provide information about the structure of the sample. The angle ϕ is equal to the angle between the azimuthal projections of the local optical axes of the medium at the upper and lower boundaries of the sample, and the angle υ defines the orientation of the bisector of the angle between these projections. Analysis of the experimentally obtained "B_i-maps," as well as the spatial distributions of υ and ϕ, can be proposed as an effective tool for tissue structure characterization.[1154] In particular, the B_0-map (this coefficient characterizes the local transmittance of the sample for nonpolarized light), the υ-map, and the ϕ-map for the *in vitro* sample of human epidermis (stratum corneum) are presented in Ref. 1154.

The study of collagen structure and function is important for understanding a wide range of pathophysiological conditions, including aging. One of the prospective laser techniques, which can provide *in vivo* microscopic monitoring of collagen structure, is polarized second-harmonic generation (SHG) microscopy (see Sections 4.7 and 5.75).[941,944] The backscattered SHG signal induced by a 100-fs titanium:sapphire laser, with a mean wavelength of 800 nm, a maximum energy of 10 nJ, and a pulse repetition rate of 82 MHz, was measured by a polarized SHG scanning confocal microscope.[944] The microscope objective has a transverse resolution of about 1.5 µm and an axial resolution of about 10 µm. It should be noted that inside the scattering media, both numbers increase. The maximum intensity in the sample was about 4×10^{11} W/cm^2. To avoid sample damage, a continuous scanning technique was used. A systematic analysis of type I collagen in a rat-tail tendon fascicle was conducted using this microscope. Type I collagen from the fascicles provides one of the strongest SHG signals of all of the various tissues analyzed by the authors in Ref. 944. They hypothesize that such high SHG efficiency is due to the highly ordered architecture of collagen. The polarization properties of collagen are also defined by its ordering. It was shown experimentally that the second-harmonic signal intensity varies by about a factor of two across a single cross section of the rat-tail tendon fascicle.[944] The signal intensity depends both on the collagen organization and the backscattering efficiency. To characterize collagen structure, both intensity- and polarization-dependent SHG signals should be detected. Actually, axial and transverse scans for different linear polarization angles of the input beam show that SHG in the rat-tail tendon depends strongly on the polarization of the input laser beam. In contrast to SHG signal intensity, the functional form of the polarization dependence does not change significantly over a single cross section of the sample, and it is not affected by the backscattering efficiency.

The measured data were in good agreement with an analytical model developed for a SHG signal at linear polarized excitation and were used to determine the fibril orientation and the ratio between the only two nonzero, independent elements in the second-order nonlinear susceptibility tensor, $\gamma \approx -(0.7-0.8)$.[944] The small range of values observed for γ in a tendon fascicle suggests that there is structural homogeneity. This parameter might, therefore, be useful in characterizing different collagen structures noninvasively.

The main problem encountered in the *in situ* microscopy of tissues is multiple scattering, which randomizes the direction, coherence, and polarization state of incident light. A number of optical-gating methods have been proposed to filtrate ballistic and least-scattering photons, which carry information about the object structure. One of these is the polarization-gating method and its modifications, which are described in this chapter and Sections 1.4, 3.3, and 5.7.1. The fundamental limitation of all optical-gating methods, including the polarization one, is the fact that only a small number of ballistic and least-scattering photons take part in the formation of an object image. Therefore, polarization-gating techniques in combination with image reconstruction methods can be useful for improving the image resolution in the case of a highly scattering object.[1155,1156] Both reflection-mode and transmission-mode polarization-gating scanning microscopes have been analyzed.[1155,1156]

An optical immersion technique, based on matching the refractive index of the tissue scatterers and the surrounding ground (interstitial) medium, allows one to essentially control the scattering properties of a tissue (see Chapter 5). Usually, the refractive index of the ground medium is controlled. This is accomplished by impregnating the tissue with a biocompatible agent, such as glucose, glycerol, propylene glycol, or x-ray contrasting agents. Due to the fact that the refractive index of the applied agent is higher than that of the tissue ground substance, which is close to the index of water, the refractive index of the ground increases and scattering decreases. Most of the applied agents are hyperosmotic; therefore, they can produce a temporal and local dehydration of the tissue that also leads to an increase in the refractive index of the interstitial space. Figures from 5.35 to 5.38 show experimental results on the temporal transmittance of linear polarized light through tissue sections measured by a white-light video-digital polarization microscope or polarization spectrometer on the application of an immersion agent (x-ray contrasting agent, trazograph-60, or glycerol).[409,410,442,946,1033,1065]

Reduction of the scattering at optical immersion makes it possible to detect the polarization anisotropy of a tissue more easily and to separate the effects of light scattering and intrinsic birefringence on tissue polarization properties. It is also possible to study birefringence of form with optical immersion, but when the immersion is strong and the refractive index of tissue birefringent structure is close to the index of the ground media, the birefringence of form may be too small to be detected [see Fig. 5.36 (the tendency of polarization degree to decay at a later time of tissue impregnation by the OCA) and Fig. 5.38(b) (the complete match of refractive index at the edge region causes tissue to lose not only scattering, but also the birefringence)]. The dynamics of tissue optical clearing and the manifestation of tissue anisotropy at the reduction of scattering are characteristic features, which correlate with clinical data.[343,409,410] Figure 5.10 illustrates the reversibility of the optical immersion effect in the controlling of the polarization properties of a turbid tissue.[343] Practically all healthy connective and vascular tissues show the strong or weak optical anisotropy typical of either uniaxial or biaxial crystals.[409,410] Pathological tissues show isotropic optical properties.

Polarization microscopy is also helpful for investigating individual cells; in particular, for evaluating the amount of glycated hemoglobin in erythrocytes that could be an early diagnostic marker of hyperglycemia in diabetic patients.[754] Hemoglobin glycation causes changes in the cell's refraction index. By using polarizing-interference microscopy, it is possible to measure the light refractive index in an individual erythrocyte. The refractive index of hemoglobin or a red blood cell, containing about 95% hemoglobin, varies approximately linearly with a change in glucose concentration—it saturates only under strong hyperglycemic conditions.[752,753] A Nomarsky polarizing-interference microscope, MPI-5 (Poland), was used for measurements of light phase retardation.[754] Using a Wollaston prism mounted on an object, the erythrocyte images for ordinary and extraordinary light beams were completely separated. In the thickest erythrocyte region, the first interference maxima were visually adjusted to the eye-sensitive purple color for ordinary and extraordinary images by shifting the second Wollaston prism placed in the rear focus of the object. For each erythrocyte measured, the Wollaston prism displacement rendered a second value. From the whole interference bandwidth h and the measured Wollaston prism displacement $2d$, the phase retardation Φ and the refractive index n were calculated for each erythrocyte as[754]

$$n = n_v + \frac{\Phi}{t} = n_v + \frac{d\lambda}{ht},\qquad(7.10)$$

where $n_v = 1.5133 \pm 0.0001$ is the refractive index of the embedding media, t is the thickness of the erythrocyte, and $\lambda = 550$ nm. Separate measurements of the erythrocyte thickness using two embedded media with different refractive indices gives $t = 0.89$ μm. Using this value, the refractive index is calculated with a standard deviation of ± 0.0005.

A robust z-polarized confocal microscope employing only one or two binary phase plates with a polarizer has been suggested by Huse et al.[1157] The major advantage of the microscope having a significant longitudinal field component is that it is then possible to image the z-polarized features in randomly oriented agglomerations of molecules of biomedical interest.

7.4 Digital photoelasticity measurements

Photoelasticity is an established experimental technique that has been applied to study the biomechanics of hard tissues like bone and tooth.[1158,1159] The photoelastic measuring technique is based on the stress-induced optical birefringence effect, which for plane stress analysis is described by the following stress-optic law:[1158,1159]

$$\sigma_1 - \sigma_2 = \frac{\theta}{2\pi}\frac{f_\sigma}{h} = \frac{Nf_\sigma}{h},\qquad(7.11)$$

where $(\sigma_1 - \sigma_2)$ is the difference in the in-plane principle stress, θ is the resultant optical phase generated due to stress-induced birefringence in the sample, f_σ is the material fringe value, and h is the thickness of the specimen. Since the values of f_σ and h are constants for the mechanical stresses, recording the optical phase (θ) or fringe order ($N = \theta/2\pi$) at every point of interest on the fringe pattern allows for analysis of the stress distribution.[1158,1159]

As an example, we will consider the results of photomechanical studies of post-endodontically rehabilitated teeth, using a conventional circular polariscope and an image processing system, which were the basis for the digital phase shift photoelastic technique described in Refs. 1158 and 1159. A special loading device that applies loads along the long axis (0 deg) and 60-deg lingual to the long axis of the tooth was employed. Using the polariscope, four phase-stepped images were obtained for the sample at each load by rotating the analyzer at 0-, 45-, 90-, and 135-deg angles with respect to the polarizer. The fringe patterns obtained were acquired using a CCD camera, and stored and processed by a computer. The four images were evaluated using a phase-stepping algorithm to obtain a wrapped phase map.[1158] Phase unwrapping was done on selected lines to make the fringe modulation continuous and to get information on the nature of the stress distribution.

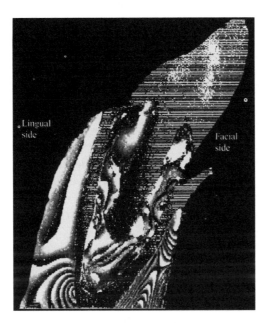

Figure 7.15 Phase-wrapped image obtained from four-phase shifted images in a rehabilitated tooth model, loaded at 125 N, 60 deg lingual to the long axis of the tooth.[1159]

Figure 7.15 shows a phase-wrapped image of the rehabilitated tooth model, loaded at 125 N at an angle of 60 deg in the direction of the long axis of the tooth. It was found that there is a significant (up to threefold) increase in the magnitude of the stress within the rehabilitated tooth model in comparison with the model of the intact tooth. Increased bending stress is identified in the cervical region and in the middle region of the root. This results in higher compressive stress in the cervical region (facial side) and higher tensile stress in the midregion (lingual side). The designed digital phase-shift photoelastic technique is of importance for the investigation of hard tissue elasticity distributions; here, for instance, it highlighted the behavior of a postcore rehabilitated tooth to functional forces.

7.5 Fluorescence polarization measurements

Fluorescence polarization measurements are used to estimate various parameters of the fluorophore environment.[573] They therefore have a potential role to play in biomedical diagnosis; in particular, in discriminating between normal and malignant tissues.[1160–1163] At polarized light excitation, the emission from a fluorophore in a nonscattering media becomes depolarized because of the random orientation of the fluorophore molecules and the angular displacement between the absorption and emission dipoles of the molecules.[573] These intrinsic molecular processes that result in additional angular displacement of the emission dipoles are sensitive to the local environment of the fluorophore. As was already shown in preceding chapters, light depolarization in tissues is determined by multiple scattering; therefore, both excitation and emission radiations should be depolarized in scattering media.[573,1160–1163] Polarization state transformation in scattering media depends on the optical parameters of the medium: the absorption coefficient μ_a, the scattering coefficient μ_s, and the scattering anisotropy factor g. Because of the different structural and functional properties of normal and malignant tissues, the contribution of multiple scattering to depolarization may be different for these tissues. The reduced (transport) scattering coefficient μ_s', or the transport mean free path (MFP) l_t, in particular, determines the characteristic depolarization depth for different tissues. Thus, fluorescence polarization measurements may be sensitive to tissue structural or functional changes, which are caused, for instance, by tissue malignancy at the molecular level (the sensitivity of excited molecules to the environmental molecules) or at the macrostructural level (the sensitivity of propagating radiation to tissue scattering properties).

Mohanty et al.[1162] have considered a fluorophore located at a distance z from the surface of a turbid medium. The homogeneous distribution of the fluorophores and the validity of the diffusion approximation for light transport in a scattering medium were assumed. The average number of scattering events experienced by the excitation light before it reached the fluorophore, and by the emitted light before it exited the medium, are described, respectively, as

$$N_1(z) = z \times \mu_s^{ex}, \tag{7.12}$$

and

$$N_2(z) = z \times \mu_s^{em}. \tag{7.13}$$

The fluorescence polarization ability is characterized by polarization anisotropy r, which is a dimensionless quantity independent of the total fluorescence intensity of the object,[573]

$$r = \frac{I_\parallel - I_\perp}{I_\parallel + 2I_\perp}. \tag{7.14}$$

It is defined as the ratio of the polarized component to the total intensity and is connected with the light polarization value P,

$$r = \frac{2P}{3 - P}. \tag{7.15}$$

The polarization, measured as

$$P = \frac{I_\| - I_\perp}{I_\| + I_\perp}, \tag{7.16}$$

is an appropriate parameter for describing a light source when a light ray is directed along a particular axis. The polarization of this light is defined as the fraction of light that is linearly polarized. In contrast, the radiation emitted by a fluorophore is symmetrically distributed around this axis, and the total intensity is not given by $I_\| + I_\perp$, but rather by $I_\| + 2I_\perp$ (see Section 10.4 of Ref. 573).

Assuming that each scattering event reduces the fluorescence polarization anisotropy r by a factor of A ($A = 0$–1), the anisotropy of fluorescence that is due to a fluorophore embedded at a depth z can be written as

$$r(z) = r_0 \times A^{[N_1(z)+N_2(z)]}, \tag{7.17}$$

where r_0 is the value of the fluorescence anisotropy without any scattering. For a homogeneous distribution of fluorophores in a tissue of thickness d, the observed value of the fluorescence anisotropy is defined by each ith tissue layer as

$$r_{\text{obs}} = \sum_i (I_i^f r_i) / \sum_i I_i^f, \tag{7.18}$$

where I_i^f is the contribution to the observed fluorescence intensity from the ith layer of thickness dz at a depth z, and r_i is the value of the fluorescence anisotropy for this layer.

For the broad-beam illumination of a flat tissue surface, the propagation of excitation (ex) light beyond a few MFPs [MFP $\equiv l_{\text{ph}} = \mu_t^{-1}$, $\mu_t = \mu_a + \mu_s$, see Eq. (1.8)] is well described by one-dimensional diffusion theory. In this approximation, and taking into account $\mu_t^{\text{ex}} \gg \mu_{\text{eff}}^{\text{ex}}$ [see Eq. (1.18)], which is valid for many tissues, the excitation intensity reaching depth z is expressed as

$$I(z) \cong C_{\text{ex}} \exp(-\mu_{\text{eff}}^{\text{ex}} z), \tag{7.19}$$

where C_{ex} is proportional to the excitation intensity and is the function of the tissue optical parameters at the wavelength of the excitation light.

The fluorescence from the fluorophores, embedded at depth z from the tissue surface, reaching the same surface will therefore be

$$I^f(z) \approx \left[C_{\text{ex}} \exp(-\mu_{\text{eff}}^{\text{ex}} z) \right] \{ \varphi [C_{\text{em}} \exp(-\mu_{\text{eff}}^{\text{em}} z)] \}, \tag{7.20}$$

where C_{em} and $\mu_{\text{eff}}^{\text{ex}}$ for the emission wavelength are defined similarly as C_{ex} and $\mu_{\text{eff}}^{\text{ex}}$ for the excitation wavelength, and φ is the fluorescence yield.

By substituting the values I_i^f from Eq. (7.20) and r_i from Eq. (7.17) into Eq. (7.18), the observed fluorescence anisotropy is expressed as

$$r_{obs} = r_0 \frac{\int_0^d \exp(-\mu_{eff}^{tot} z) \times A^{[N_1(z)+N_2(z)]} dz}{\int_0^d \exp(-\mu_{eff}^{tot} z) dz}, \tag{7.21}$$

where

$$\mu_{eff}^{tot} = \mu_{eff}^{ex} + \mu_{eff}^{em}, \tag{7.22}$$

$$\mu_s^{tot} = \mu_s^{ex} + \mu_s^{em}. \tag{7.23}$$

Integration of Eq. (7.21) gives

$$r_{obs} = r_0 \frac{\mu_{eff}^{tot}}{\mu_{eff}^{tot} - \ln(A) \times (\mu_s^{tot})} \frac{1 - \exp(-\mu_{eff}^{tot} d) \times (A)^{\mu_s^{tot} d}}{1 - \exp(-\mu_{eff}^{tot} d)}. \tag{7.24}$$

Fluorescence anisotropy measurements are usually provided by commercially available spectrometers, the sensitivity of which is different for two orthogonal polarization states. Therefore, all measured fluorescence spectra should be corrected for the system response as[573]

$$r = \frac{I_\parallel - G I_\perp}{I_\parallel + 2 G I_\perp}, \tag{7.25}$$

where G is the ratio of the sensitivity of the instrument to the vertically and the horizontally polarized light.

Typical G-corrected polarized fluorescence spectra at 340-nm excitation from malignant and normal breast tissue with thickness ≈ 2 mm are shown in Fig. 7.16.[1162] Collagen, elastin, coenzymes (NADH/NADPH), and flavins contribute to these spectra and the spectra received at a longer wavelength of 460 nm.[1162,1163] The contribution of the NADH dominates with excitation at 340 nm, and different forms of flavins dominate with excitation at 460 nm. In Fig. 7.16, a blue shift in the polarized fluorescence spectra maximum is clearly seen in the malignant, as compared to the normal, tissue. A similar shift of 5–10 nm was also observed for 460-nm excited fluorescence. This shift is associated with the accumulation of positively charged ions in the intracellular environment of the malignant cell.[1160] Some differences, in particular, a spectral shift of the maximum, between the parallel and cross-polarized fluorescence spectra observed for rather thick tissue layers (≈ 2 mm) may be associated with wavelength-dependent scattering and the absorption properties of the tissue.

The mean fluorescence anisotropy values for normal and malignant human breast samples of tissue varying from 10 μm to 2 mm in thickness, determined

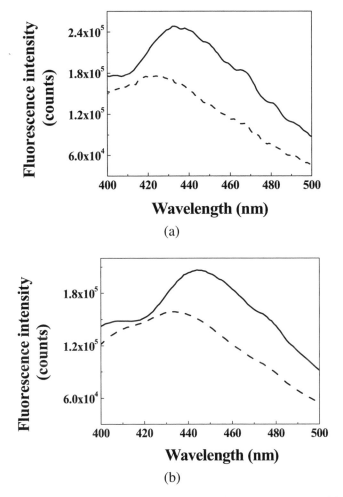

Figure 7.16 Typical polarized fluorescence spectra at 340-nm excitation of human breast tissue samples of 2-mm thickness.[1162] Solid curves, spectra with excitation and emission polarizers oriented vertically ($I_\parallel$); dashed curves, spectra with crossed excitation and emission polarizers ($I_\perp$). (a) Malignant tissue; (b) normal tissue.

with 440-nm emission and 340-nm excitation, are presented in Fig. 7.17.[1162] The theoretical fit to experimental data using Eq. (7.24) and the parameter of single-scattering anisotropy reduction $A = 0.7$ gives the following data for the anisotropy and optical parameters: $r_0 = 0.34$, $\mu_s^{tot} = 590$ cm^{-1}, $\mu_{eff}^{tot} = 53.5$ cm^{-1} for malignant tissue, and $r_0 \approx 0.25$, $\mu_s^{tot} = 470$ cm^{-1}, $\mu_{eff}^{tot} = 34.5$ cm^{-1} for normal tissue. The anisotropy values are higher for malignant tissues as compared to normal for very thin tissue sections, where $d \leq 30$ μm. By contrast, in thicker sections, the malignant tissue shows smaller fluorescence anisotropy than the normal tissue.

The fact that fluorescence anisotropy varies with tissue thickness is associated with the manifestation of various mechanisms of fluorescence depolarization that are caused by energy transfer and rotational diffusion in the fluorophores and by

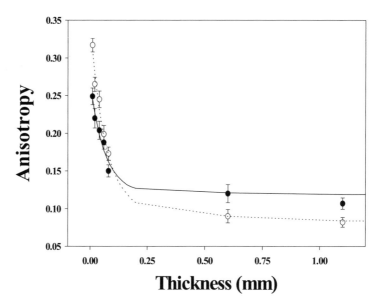

Figure 7.17 Polarized fluorescence anisotropy measured at 440 nm for excitation at 340 nm for malignant (open circles) and normal (filled circles) human breast tissues as a function of tissue thickness.[1162] The error bars represent the standard deviation. The solid and dashed curves show theoretical fits for normal and malignant tissues, respectively [Eq. (7.24)].

the scattering of excitation and emission light. Energy transfer and/or rotational diffusion of the fluorophores dominate in thin tissue sections, and these processes are faster in normal tissues than in malignant ones. In thicker sections, light scattering dominates with more contribution to depolarization during light transport within the malignant tissues.

As was already mentioned in the beginning of this section, the light scattering anisotropy factor g and, correspondingly, the reduced scattering coefficient μ_s' or the transport MFP l_t determine the characteristic depolarization depth in a scattering medium. Parameter A, characterizing the reduction of the fluorescence anisotropy per scattering event in the described model, depends on the value of the g-factor.[1162] The theoretical analysis done by the authors of Ref. 1162 has shown that, for an anisotropy parameter g ranging between 0.7 and 0.9, the value for A varies between 0.7 and 0.8. These results suggest that fluorescence anisotropy measurements may be used for discriminating malignant sites from normal ones and may be especially useful for epithelial cancer diagnostics where superficial tissue layers are typically examined.[1163]

7.6 Conclusion

As it follows from the presented analysis, polarization-sensitive methods are promising tools for optical medical diagnostics and imaging, especially for *in vivo* and *in situ* morphological analysis of living tissue. Polarization discrimination of scattered probe light, which may be easily integrated in traditional optical diagnostical techniques such as diffuse reflectance spectroscopy and imaging, offers a possibility for improving the diagnostic potential of these techniques. Another novel contribution to optical medical diagnostics should emerge from the morphological study of tissues with expressed structural anisotropy. Typically, almost all of the polarization-sensitive techniques that we considered in this chapter can be realized with inexpensive commercially available instrumentation. Neither do they require sophisticated data processing algorithms. In other words, these methods are completely suitable for widespread implementation in clinical diagnostic practice. Fluorescence polarization measurements that can provide additional information at the molecular level may be useful for discriminating malignant sites from normal ones.

8

Coherence-Domain Methods and Instruments for Biomedical Diagnostics and Imaging

In this chapter, we discuss coherent optical methods that hold much promise for applications in biomedicine, such as photon-correlation and diffusion wave spectroscopies; speckle interferometry; full-field speckle imaging; coherent topography and tomography; phase, confocal, and Doppler microscopy; as well as interferential measurements of retinal visual acuity and blood sedimentation.

8.1 Photon-correlation spectroscopy of transparent tissues and cell flows

8.1.1 Introduction

The physical fundamentals of photon-correlation spectroscopy were discussed in Chapter 4. The description of the principles and characteristics of the main modifications of homodyne and heterodyne photon-correlation spectrometers, the laser Doppler anemometers (LDAs), differential LDA schemes, and laser Doppler microscopes (LDMs) can be found in Refs. 5, 6, 22, 76–79, 82, 343, 825–827, 829, 830, 833, 838, 842, 848, and 849. A review of medical applications, mainly limited to the investigation of eye tissues (crystalline lens, cataract diagnosis), hemodynamics in isolated vessels (vessels of eye fundus or any other vessels) with the use of fiber optic catheters, and blood microcirculation in tissues, is provided in Refs. 5, 6, 22, 67, 76–79, 82, 83, 343, 825–827, 829, 830, 833, 835, 838–842, 848–850, 853, 859, and 1164–1201. In this section, we will discuss the photon-correlation technique in application to early cataract diagnostics and to measurement of blood and lymph flow in microvessels.

8.1.2 Cataract diagnostics

The photon-correlation spectroscopy or quasi-elastic light scattering (QELS) technique was originally developed to study small colloidal particles in fluids.[1170] Three decades ago, Tanaka and Benedek[1171,1172] proposed to use this technique to study the onset of cataract in the ocular lens; however, it did not find a wide-scale commercial acceptance in ophthalmology. Owing to innovations since then in the field of optoelectronics, QELS is now emerging as a potential ophthalmic tool, making the study of virtually every tissue and fluid comprising the eye possible.[849] The ability of QELS in the early detection of the molecular morphology has the potential to help develop new drugs to combat not just the diseases of the eye, such as cataract, but to diagnose and study those of the body, such as diabetes and possibly Alzheimer's, as was recently claimed by Ansari. [849,1169]

The coherent fiber-optic photon-correlation spectrometers for study of cataractogenesis and potentially useful for early diagnosis of cataract were designed about a decade ago.[850,1173] The instrument described in Ref. 850 includes two optical fibers. The first, a single-mode fiber, transmits a Gaussian beam of an He:Ne or diode laser to an object. The second, multimode or single-mode fiber is employed to collect backscattered radiation at a certain angle and to transmit this radiation to a photodetector [see Fig. 8.1(a)]. The power of the He:Ne laser radiation (at 633 nm) is on the order of 1 mW. The size of the laser beam on the crystalline lens is about 150 μm. Scattered radiation is detected at angles of 155 deg (detector 1) and 143 deg (detector 2). Figure 8.1(b) shows typical autocorrelation functions measured for bovine crystalline lens under conditions of temperature-induced cataract (reversible cold cataract). The results of the solution of the relevant inverse problem (determination of the sizes of scatterers in human crystalline lenses as functions of age), taking into account Eqs. (4.28), (4.30), and (4.31), are presented in Fig. 8.1(c). These data demonstrate that the method under consideration is sufficiently sensitive for the monitoring of age changes in the structure of the crystalline lens caused by growth in the sizes of aggregated protein components.

In Ref. 850, a clinical modification of the measuring system for the early diagnosis of cataract is presented. According to the estimates, the expected power density incident on a retina that is sufficient to measure the autocorrelation function of intensity fluctuations within a time interval of about 2 min is no higher than $0.05 \, \mathrm{mW/mm^2}$, which is almost three orders of magnitude lower than the threshold of retinal damage.

The fiber-optic QELS probe, shown in Fig. 8.2, combines the unique attributes of small size, low laser power, and high sensitivity.[849,1169] The system is easy to use because it does not require sensitive optical alignment nor vibration isolation devices. A low-power (50–100-μW) light from a semiconductor laser, interfaced with a monomode optical fiber, is tightly focused in a 20-μm diameter focal point in the tissue of interest via a GRIN (gradient index) lens. On the detection side, the scattered light is collected through another GRIN lens and guided onto an avalanche photodiode (APD) detector built into a photon-counting module. APD processed signals are then passed on to a digital correlator for analysis. The probe provides quantitative measurements of the pathologies of cornea, aqueous, lens, vitreous, and the retina. By suitable choice of optical filters, it can be converted into a device for spectral measurements (autofluoresence and Raman spectroscopy) and laser-Doppler flowmetry/velocimetry, providing measurements of oxidative stress and blood flow in the ocular tissues. The device also can easily be integrated into many conventional ophthalmic instruments such as slit lamps, Scheimpflug cameras, videokeratoscopes, and fluorometers.

This compact probe (Fig. 8.2) was used for the monitoring of cataractogenesis in mice *in vivo* by examination of the measured autocorrelation function (AF)

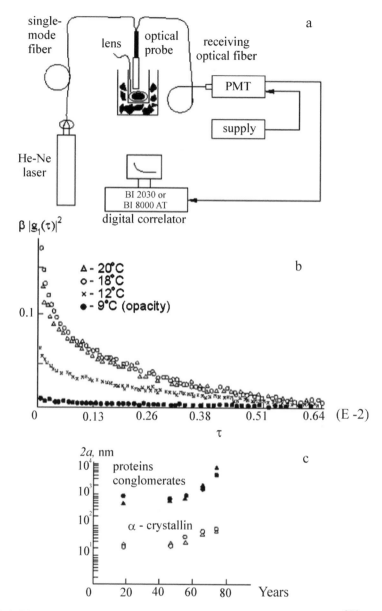

Figure 8.1 Photon-correlation spectrometer for early diagnosis of cataract.[850] (a) Diagram of the spectrometer. (b) Autocorrelation functions for temperature-dependent cataract of bovine eye. (c) Age-dependent changes of scatterers' diameters for the human lens. Two fractions, finely dispersed (α-crystallin, hollow symbols) and coarsely dispersed (protein conglomerates, filled symbols) are excluded from the empirical autocorrelation functions [see Eq. (4.31)]. Triangles and squares represent measurements made with different types of coherent fiber probes.

profiles [see Eqs. (4.28) and (4.30)] at different time lines.[849,1169] As an example, Philly mice were studied. This animal develops cataract spontaneously between day 26 and 33 after birth. The data include a 45-day-old normal mouse of the con-

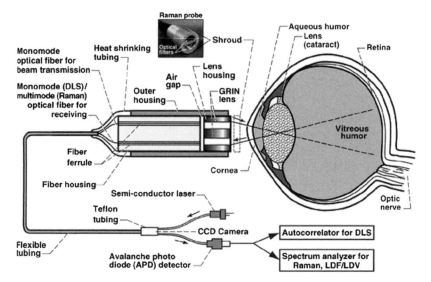

Figure 8.2 Schematic diagram of the sensitive, vibration protected, universal, and easy to use QELS fiber-optic probe.[1169] The probe was originally developed at NASA to conduct fluid physics experiments in the absence of gravity onboard a space shuttle or space station orbiter.

trol FVB/N strain, which does not develop a cataract, and two Philly mice roughly 26–29 days old. Each measurement took 5 s at a laser power of 100 μW. The changing AF slope is an indication of cataractogenesis because the lens crystallins aggregate to form high molecular weight clumps and complexes. The QELS autocorrelation data is converted into particle size distributions using an exponential sampling program and is shown in Fig. 8.3. Although conversion of the QELS data into particle size distributions requires certain assumptions regarding the viscosity of the lens fluid, these size values do indicate a trend as the cataract progress. These measurements suggest that a developing cataract can be monitored quantitatively with reasonable reliability, reproducibility (5–10%), and accuracy.

Besides cataract monitoring, the QELS probe has been proposed and experimentally tested for early, noninvasive, and quantitative detection and monitoring of such disease and abnormalities as vitreopathy, pigmentary glaucoma, diabetic retinopathy, and corneal evaluation of wound healing after laser refractive surgery.[849,1169]

A portable fiber-optic photon-correlation spectrometer based on an He:Ne laser (633-nm), single-mode fibers, a photomultiplier operating in the regime of a photon counting mode, and a 288-channel real-time correlator with a sampling time of 200 ns is described in Ref. 851. This spectrometer allows *in vivo* studies of crystalline lenses of patients. These investigations also confirmed the bimodal character of the distribution of scatterers in the tissue of a human crystalline lens. Specifically, for healthy eyes of patients aged between 39 and 43 (six eyes, three female patients), the finely dispersed fraction has a mean radius of 4.25 ± 1.7 nm, whereas the mean radius of the coarsely dispersed fraction is 497 ± 142 nm. For cataractous

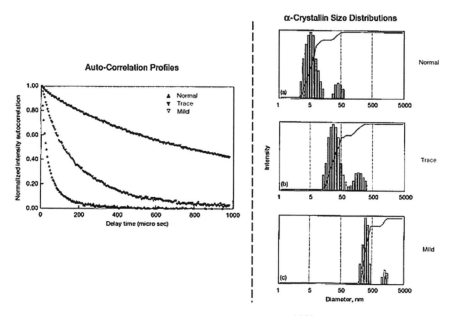

Figure 8.3 *In vivo* cataract measurements in Philly mice.[1169] (a) Autocorrelation profiles. (b) Particle size distribution for the normal eye, control mouse. (c) Particle size distribution for a mouse with trace cataract. (d) Particle size distribution for a mouse with mild cataract.

crystalline lenses, the mean radius of the finely dispersed fraction tends to 160 nm, whereas the mean radius of the coarsely dispersed fraction tends to 1000 nm. The spectrometer permits one to determine the size distribution of species for various localizations of the volume of the measurements. The bimodal size distributions of scatterers measured under conditions when the volume of measurements is shifted along the axis of a cataractous crystalline lens are presented in Fig. 8.4.

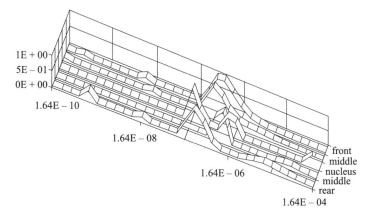

Figure 8.4 Bimodal distribution of the radii of scattering particles for a cataractous crystalline lens (female patient at the age of 76, *in vivo* measurements) with different localizations of the volume of measurements along the axis of the crystalline lens: the front part of the cortical layer, the middle part of the cortical layer, nucleus, the middle part of the rear cortical layer, and the rear part of the cortical layer.[851]

8.1.3 Blood and lymph flow monitoring in microvessels

Parameters of blood or lymph flows in individual vessels can be measured with the use of a technique based on the diffraction of a focused laser beam by moving scatterers (see Section 4.4.2).[77,343,826,833,853,854] A diagram of the relevant speckle microscope is presented in Fig. 8.5. Laser radiation focused into a spot of a small diameter on the order of 4.6λ is projected onto a segment of the microvessel under study. A photodetector whose entrance aperture is much smaller than the mean speckle size registers intensity fluctuations in the scattered light. The intensity fluctuations detected are analyzed with a low-frequency digital spectrum analyzer or converted into a digital signal for subsequent computer analysis. The typical spectra for blood and lymph flows in superficial vessels of rat mesentery averaged over 128 realizations of a random signal are displayed in Fig. 8.6.

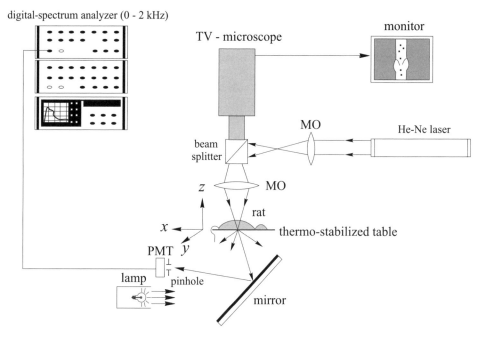

Figure 8.5 Diagram of a speckle microscope for the investigation of blood and lymph flows in microvessels.[853,854]

For a blood microvessel, the spectrum of intensity fluctuations in the scattered field has a nearly Gaussian shape in the low-frequency range. The spectra of intensity fluctuations for lymphatic vessels are rather complicated, which indicates that the motion of lymph in microvessels is much more complex than the motion of blood. For example, lymph may be involved in a characteristic shuttlelike motion, be nonmovable near the vessel wall, or move in a direction opposite to the flow in the central part of a vessel. Such a behavior of lymph is associated with a complex

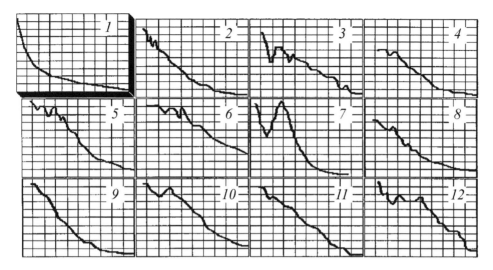

Figure 8.6 Spectra of intensity fluctuations in the scattered light (averaged over 128 realizations) for the diffraction of a focused laser beam on rat mesentery: 1, blood vessel (12 μm in diameter); 2–12, lymphatic vessels of various diameters for different rats. Measurements were performed within the frequency range of 30–1500 Hz. [853,854]

contraction dynamics of smooth-muscle cells in vessel walls, governed by a local rhythm driver (pacemaker) and the behavior of the valves of lymphatic vessels.

To estimate the parameters of blood and lymph flows in microvessels, we introduce the following quantities:[853,854]

$$V_V = \frac{\Delta F}{D_V},$$

(8.1)

$$\Sigma_V = \frac{\int_0^{\Delta F} |S(f) - G(f)|^4 df}{[\int_0^{\Delta F} |S(f) - G(f)|^2 df]^2 / \Delta F}.$$

Here, ΔF is the width of the averaged spectrum, D_V is the diameter of a microvessel, $S(f)$ is the power spectrum of the intensity fluctuations for the speckle field studied, and $G(f)$ is the spectrum with a Gaussian envelope. The spectra $S(f)$ and $G(f)$ have equal bandwidths and powers. Parameter V_V is directly proportional to the flow velocity, and Σ_V provides the information concerning spatial and temporal variations of the flow rate in the studied area of a vessel.

The characteristics given above have been employed to analyze the influence of a lymphotropic agent (*Staphylococcus* toxin, ST) on the dynamics of lymph flow in mesentery microvessels of experimental animals (rats).[853,854] It was found that even at the fifth minute of ST action, all the vessels studied showed variations in the spectra of intensity fluctuations in scattered light, which indicates that the velocity characteristics of the flow change: 59% of the 17 vessels studied displayed a decrease in the mean velocity V_V of lymph flow by $41 \pm 8\%$ and a growth in the

Σ_V parameter by $33 \pm 7\%$. The remaining 41% of the vessels displayed an increase in the mean rate of lymph flow by $63 \pm 22\%$ and a decrease in the Σ_V parameter by $35 \pm 9\%$. In later stages (between the fifth and twentieth minutes), vasoconstriction progresses and the number of vessels contracting in phase decreases, which leads to changes in lymph dynamics. After the twentieth minute, lymph flow stopped in all the vessels studied.

The optical scheme of the setup providing detection of cell flow direction and velocities in the range from 10 µm/s to 10 mm/s with a temporal resolution up to 50 ms is shown in Fig. 8.7.[833,858] Radiation from a uniphase He:Ne laser (633 nm) is delivered through the illuminator channel and focused by the objective of the microscope into a spot of a diameter of about 2 µm in a plane apart at a distance $z = 100$ µm from the axis of the microvessel. The radius of curvature of the wavefront of the beam illuminating the microvessel is quite small to ensure the acceptable translation length of biospeckles. The measuring volume is formed by the intersection of the diverging laser beam with the microvessel and has the shape of a truncated cone (whose elements have a slope of 10 deg and a mean diameter on the order of 30 µm). The laser radiation scattered by the cell flow is directed with the help of the beamsplitter to the photodetector placed at a distance of 300 mm from the objective plane of the microscope. The diameter of each photodetector is 3 mm, which corresponds to the mean speckle diameter in the observation plane. The distance between the centers of the photodetectors is about 7 mm. Signals from the photodetectors are amplified by the photocurrent transducers and digitized with the help of a two-channel 16-bit analogue-to-digital converter with a sampling frequency of 44.1 kHz. A PC is used to determine the cross-correlation function of the photodetector signals as well as the positions of its peaks.

Depending on the time resolution, the processing of the realization of photodetector signals of duration 60 s takes between 90 and 300 s. A digital video camera combined with a transmission microscope is used for analysis of microvessels' functions *in vivo* in real time: estimate the mean flow velocity and its direction, measure the diameter of a microvessel, and register the appearance of phasic contraction in the investigated lymphatics. Dynamic digital images were processed with specially developed software. The cell velocity was determined as the ratio of the difference in cell coordinates in two consecutive frames to the time interval between the two frames. The mean flow velocity was calculated by averaging the velocities of four to six cells. Dynamic digital microscopy allows one to record cell flow velocity in the range from 25 µm/s to 2–2.5 mm/s with a time resolution of 40 ms.

The described setup was tested for *in vivo* measurements of lymph flow velocity in the mesentery vessels of narcotized white rats. Animals were placed on a thermostabilized stage (37.7°C) of the microscope (see Fig. 8.7) and the mesentery and intestine was kept moist with Ringer's solution at 37°C (pH $\sim$ 7.4). The images of microvessels were evaluated by transmission microscopy and laser speckle-velocimeter simultaneously. Figure 8.8 shows the temporal dependences of the flow velocity in the investigated microlymphatic with mean diameter 170 ± 5 µm

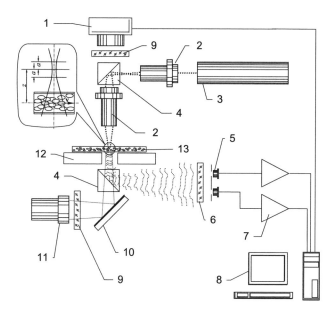

Figure 8.7 Scheme of the experimental setup of a laser speckle velocimeter integrated with dynamic digital microscopy providing measurements of absolute values of cell flow velocity and its direction: 1, digital video camera; 2, microobjective; 3, He:Ne laser (633 nm); 4, beamsplitter; 5, photodiodes; 6, red light filter; 7, photocurrent converters; 8, PC; 9, green light filters; 10, mirror; 11, illuminator; 12, thermally stabilized table; 13, lymph microvessel of mesentery. The inset shows the illumination of a lymphatic vessel by a focused Gaussian laser beam (a is the length of the laser beam waist and z is the separation between the flow axis and the waist plane of the laser beam).[858]

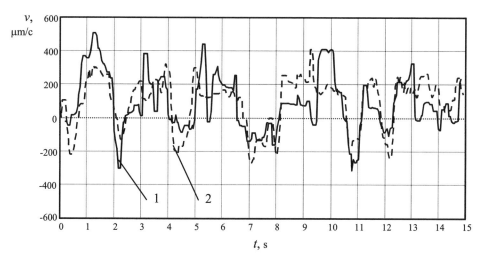

Figure 8.8 Time dependence of the lymph flow velocity in a lymphatic vessel of mean diameter 170 ± 5 μm of white rat mesentery: 1, recorded with a speckle velocimeter; and 2, with dynamic digital microscopy (see Fig. 8.7).[858]

and mean lymph flow velocity 169 ± 4.6 μm/s.[833,858] These dependences were obtained concurrently by laser speckle velocimeter and by processing of the video images. A laser speckle velocimeter allows one to measure the lymphocyte velocity in relative units only. The proportionality coefficient between the data of laser speckle velocimetry and the mean flow velocity, measured by dynamic digital microscopy, was determined from the slope of the line of linear regression between the velocities (measured by these two methods). The correlation coefficient of linear regression was equal to 0.723 for measurements in the lymph vessel and 0.966 for calibration measurements in the glass capillary.

8.2 Diffusion-wave spectroscopy and interferometry: measurement of blood microcirculation

Experimental implementation of diffusion-wave spectroscopy is very simple: a measuring system should irradiate the scattering object under investigation with a light beam produced by a continuous wave laser and measure intensity fluctuations in scattered radiation within a single speckle with the use of a photomultiplier and an electronic correlator. A typical setup employed for model experiments is presented in Fig. 8.9.[80,81,875,1174,1175] Radiation (with a wavelength of 514 nm and a power on the order of 2 W) produced by an argon laser with an intracavity etalon passes through a multimode fiber-optic cable and irradiates the surface of a solid-state bulk sample (finely dispersed TiO_2 powder suspended in resin). The sizes of the sample are $15 \times 15 \times 8$ cm. A spherical cavity 2.5 cm in diameter filled with a 0.2% aqueous suspension of polystyrene spheres 0.296 μm in diameter at the temperature of 25°C is placed at the center of the sample 1.8 cm below its upper surface. The transport MFP lengths of photons for the suspension and the sample are $l_t = 0.15$ and 0.22 cm, respectively. The absorption coefficients of these media are equal to each other, $\mu_a = 0.002$ cm^{-1}. The diffusion coefficient of Brownian motion in suspension is $D_B = 1.5 \times 10^{-8}$ cm^2/s. The single-mode fiber collects light emerging from a certain area of the object and transmits it to the photomultiplier. The output signal of the photomultiplier is fed to a digital autocorrelator, which reconstructs the time-domain autocorrelation function (AF) of the intensity fluctuations. This AF is related to the time-domain autocorrelation function of the field by the Siegert formula [see Eq. (4.28)]. Optical fibers were designed in such a manner as to pick up radiation from any area at the surface of the sample.

Figure 8.10 displays the experimental results for the normalized time-domain AF of the field for three different arrangements of optical fibers connected to a source of radiation and the detector, and compares these experimental data with theoretical predictions. Since the origin of the $x-y$ coordinate frame lies on the surface of the sample above the center of the dynamic cavity, the source of radiation and the detector were placed along the y-axis in such a manner that the coordinate of the source was $y = 1.0$ cm, and the coordinate of the detector was $y = -0.75$ cm. Measurements were performed for $x = 0.0, 1.0$, and 2.0 cm. The distance between the source and the detector remained constant. The error of these

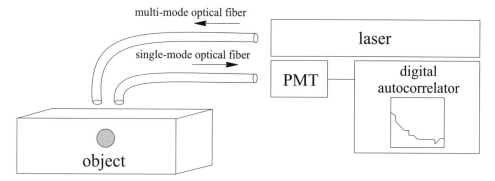

Figure 8.9 Typical experimental setup for diffusion-wave (correlation) spectroscopy of scattering media.[1175]

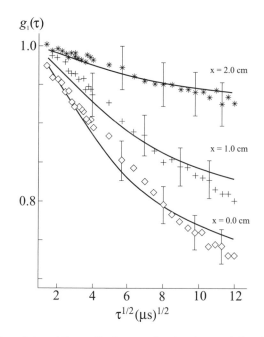

Figure 8.10 Experimental and theoretical normalized autocorrelation functions of intensity fluctuations in light scattered from a TiO$_2$ sample with a spherical cavity filled with a suspension of polystyrene spheres (see the text for the details).[1175]

measurements was estimated as 3%. The main source of errors was associated with uncertainties in the positioning of the optical fibers. Theoretical curves represent the results of simulations based on the diffusion theory of autocorrelation with allowance for the experimental data.[875,1174,1175] It can be easily seen that the AF decays faster when the source of radiation and the detector are located close to the dynamic sphere, which gives rise to fluctuations in the time domain. It is in this area that most of the detected photons pass through the dynamic volume. Such a behavior of AFs allows one to employ the variation in their slopes (decay rates) as a parameter for the imaging of dynamic inhomogeneities in a medium. This model corresponds to a situation where the microcirculation rate of blood locally increases near by, e.g., a growing tumor. Using a similar approach, one can also model a directed blood flow. For this purpose, a through hole should be drilled in a solid sample at a certain depth, and scattering fluid (e.g., Intralipid) should be circulated through this hole with a definite flow rate.[1174,1175]

To determine the AF of the field on nanosecond and subnanosecond time scales, we should replace an electronic correlator by a Michelson interferometer with a large difference in arm lengths, which should be on the order of 3 m.[80,1176] In this case, the intensity $\langle I(\tau) \rangle$ averaged in time depends on the delay time τ between the interfering fields in the interferometer, the carrier frequency ω of the optical signal, the average intensity I_{ave} of speckles, and the time-domain AF $g_1(\tau)$ of the field as

$$\langle I(\tau) \rangle = I_{ave} \frac{1 + g_1(\tau)\cos(\omega\tau)}{2}. \tag{8.2}$$

A diagram of the experimental setup and the results of model experiments are presented in Fig. 8.11. Radiation of a continuous-wave laser scattered in the forward direction by an object within a single speckle is coupled into a long Michelson interferometer. The difference between arm lengths of this interferometer can be smoothly adjusted by variation of air pressure in the short arm. Effects arising due to a finite correlation length of laser radiation and geometric factors were excluded through the calibration of the measuring system with the use of diluted samples whose AFs do not decay on the time scales studied.

The possibilities of the DWS technique for medical applications have been demonstrated in Ref. 1177. The experimental setup employed in this study is shown in Fig. 8.12(a). The experimental system was based on a titanium:sapphire laser with a power of about 100 mW and a wavelength of 800 nm. Laser radiation was transmitted onto an object through a multimode optical fiber with a core 200 μm in diameter. Radiation was detected within a single speckle with the use of a single-mode fiber 5 μm in diameter. The distance between the optical fibers on the surface of an object remained constant and was equal to 6 mm. The rate of blood flow in the bulk of a tissue from a human forearm was adjusted with the use of a medical tonometer. A digital autocorrelator coupled with a photomultiplier in the regime of a photon counter was used to measure the time-domain AF of intensity fluctuations and the dependence of the AF shape on the pressure P produced by the tonometer. Such dependences for the AF of the field, which is related to the intensity AF by the Siegert formula, are presented in the logarithmic scale in Fig. 8.12(b). These dependencies show a sufficiently high sensitivity of the AF slope to variations in the applied pressure, i.e., changes in the rate of volume blood flow. In accordance with Eqs. (4.30) and (4.43), the normalized AF of field fluctuations can be represented in terms of two components related to the Brownian and directed motion of

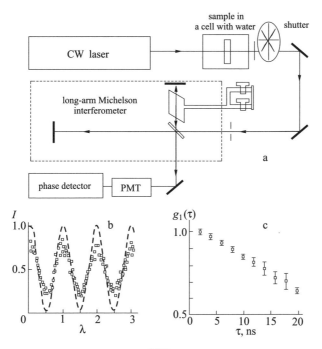

Figure 8.11 Diffusion-wave interferometry:[1176] (a) Experimental setup. (b) Normalized output signal (interference fringes) for (dots) $\tau = 0$ and (squares) 20 ns for two-phase aqueous suspensions of polystyrene spheres 0.0385 and 0.299 μm in diameter. (c) The relevant autocorrelation function of the field $g_1(\tau)$.

scatterers as[1177]

$$g_1(\tau) = \int_0^\infty p(s) \exp\left\{ -2\left[\frac{\tau}{\tau_B} + \left(\frac{\tau}{\tau_S} \right)^2 \right] \frac{s}{l_t} \right\} ds, \qquad (8.3)$$

where $\tau_B^{-1} \equiv \Gamma_T$ is defined in Eq. (4.30), $\tau_S^{-1} \cong 0.18 G_V |\bar{q}| l_t$ characterizes the directed flow, and G_V is the gradient of the flow rate. The other quantities involved in Eq. (8.3) are defined in Eqs. (4.26) and (4.43). The above relationship allows one to express the slope of the AF in terms of the diffusion coefficient and the gradient of the directed velocity of scatterers. When shear flow significantly dominates under Brownian motion, a semilogarithmic plot of $g_1(\tau)$ versus $\tau^{1/2}$ gives a straight line with a slope proportional to the velocity of the scattering particles flow.

Figure 8.12(c) displays the measured velocity of blood flow as a function of the applied pressure. If we neglect the Brownian component, this dependence is characterized by the variation in the AF slope [see Eq. (8.3)]. Since measurements were performed at the wavelength close to the isosbestic point (805 nm), changes in the degree of oxygenation of the blood due to the variation in the applied pressure only slightly influence the AF slope (the velocity of blood flow). This circumstance allows us to find the correlation between the velocity of blood flow and variations in the diameter of vessels by means of simultaneous and independent measurements

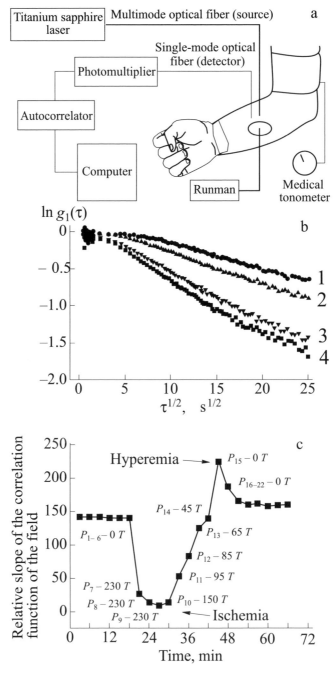

Figure 8.12 *In vivo* measurements of blood flow velocity by means of the DWS technique:[1177] (a) Experimental setup. (b) Experimental AFs of field fluctuations in backward scattering for different pressures applied to an arm (the pressure increases from 1 to 4). (c) Dynamics of the relative slope of the AFs for various pressures applied to an arm, *P* is the tonometer pressure. The arrows indicate the moments of time that correspond to the narrowing (ischemia) and broadening (hyperemia) of the vessels.

of the oxygenation degree and the volume of blood in a tissue with the use of a two-frequency Runman spectrometer (NIM Inc., Philadelphia). These measurements provide a pictorial illustration of the high efficiency of the DWS technique for *in vivo* studies of blood flow in bulk tissues.

We should also note that if the parameters of blood flow remain constant, the measured AFs provide information concerning the static optical parameters of a multiply scattering medium, i.e., l_t or μ_s', μ_a, and g [see Eq. (4.43)]. Indeed, as shown in Ref. 1178, the half-width of the spectrum of time-domain intensity fluctuations under conditions of multiple scattering depends not only on dynamic and geometric parameters of scattering particles, but also on the absorptivity of erythrocytes in blood, which allows us to estimate the degree of blood oxygenation from the results of measurements performed far from the isobestic wavelength.

The hybrid instrument and measuring protocol based on diffuse correlation spectroscopy (blood flow information) and diffuse reflectance spectroscopy (blood oxygenation information) described in Ref. 1179 provide the evaluation of microcirculation and muscle metabolism in patients with vascular diseases. A CW laser (800 nm) with a long coherence length and an avalanche photodiode were used for correlation measurements; source-detector separations ranged from 0.5 to 3 cm and the sampling time was 1.5 s. A complete frame of data, cycling through all source-detector pairs, was acquired in 2.5 s. Ten healthy subjects and one patient with peripheral arterial disease were studied during 3-min arterial cuff occlusions of the arm and leg, and during 1-min plantar flexion exercises. Signals from different layers (cutaneous tissues and muscles) during cuff occlusion were differentiated, revealing strong hemodynamic responses from muscle layers. During exercise in healthy legs, the observed approximately 4.7-fold increase in relative blood flow was significantly lower than the corresponding increase in relative muscle oxygen consumption, which was approximately sevenfold. In the diseased patient, during exercise the magnitudes of both these physiological parameters were $\sim 1/2$ of the healthy controls, and the oxygen saturation recovery time was twice that of the controls.

8.3 Blood flow imaging

It can be easily shown that the methods of Doppler flowmetry, which have been extensively developed within the past three decades, are, in general, identical to comparatively new speckle methods (which were proposed in the 1980s) in their applications to the analysis of the parameters of blood microcirculation because these two approaches provide an opportunity to determine the velocity of blood flow at a certain point.[82] The review of Doppler methods for the monitoring of blood microcirculation in tissues is provided in Refs. 5, 22, 112, 826, 827, 831, 833, 838, 841, 842, and 1180–1182 and in several original papers, e.g., Refs. 67, 839, 840, and 1183–1193. Note that the extension of the Doppler method to the investigation of blood microcirculation in thick tissues has stimulated the development of the theory of Doppler signals and the methods of simulations and detection of such signals in multiply scattering media.[247,930,1186–1190] Speckle methods of investigation of blood microcirculation are described in Refs. 3, 5, 76, 82, 83, 112, 821, 827, 829–831, 853, 854, 859, 863, 865, 1164, 1165, and 1194–1204.

The diagnosis of many diseases associated with blood microcirculation disorders requires a monitoring of microcirculation within large areas of a tissue, i.e., imaging of the field of blood flow velocity.[83,112,827,851,861–863,865,1164] Since the methods under study are characterized by a high spatial locality one ensures mechanical scanning or sequential analysis of the intensity fluctuations within a separate pixel of a CCD camera, or implements both mechanical scanning and sequential analysis. Such scanning systems for the imaging of blood circulation have been implemented and developed up to the stage of commercial production.[861,862] One such system is shown in Fig. 8.13.[862] A system for the imaging of blood circulation should be useful for diagnosis and therapy support in cases associated with diseases of the peripheral vascular system and for the medical treatment of wounds and burns. However, mechanical scanning of a laser beam or the necessity to collect and process large data arrays in systems involving CCD cameras prevented designers from creating simple and high-performance imaging systems. Apparently, the only exception was a speckle system based on a 100×100-pixel matrix photodetector, which was designed specifically for the analysis of retinal blood flow. The total time of data analysis in this system for a 0.42×0.42-mm field was 15 s.[860]

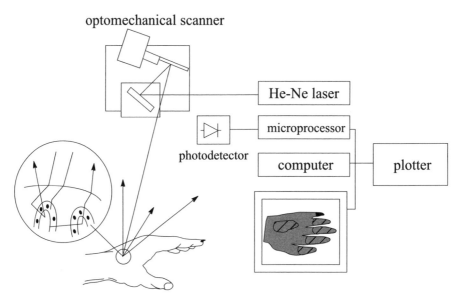

Figure 8.13 Diagram of a scanning Doppler system for the imaging of blood microcirculation in tissues.[862]

The potential exists to build a robust blood-flow imager in tissue with multiple scattering based on focused-laser-beam probing and detection of spatial cross-correlation of the scattered field using a CCD camera.[1196] The method is based on the concept that the region of single scattering within the tissue (volume occupied by a focused laser beam) will produce large correlated areas (speckles) in a transverse dimension, whereas the comparably large halo of multiple scattered photons produced by this beam will give rise to small speckles. Thus, the cross-correlation function of the intensity fluctuations in two spatial points (CCD camera pixels) with the separation Δx larger than the size of the multiscattered speckles will reflect the form of single-scattered AF. The profile of a single-scattering AF will provide information about blood or lymph flow in a volume occupied by a focused laser beam. The attractiveness of this approach is defined by its applicability to the intermediate scattering regimes, whereas QELS provides accurate information only for a single scattering regime and DWS can be applied only for a case of diffusive photon propagation.

A typical approach to improve the performance of blood flow imagers, particularly to increase the imaging speed, is to parallelize measurements by using 1D or 2D arrays of photodetectors. A new generation of high-speed instruments for full-field blood flow laser Doppler imaging (LDI) was recently developed on the basis of CMOS image sensors.[1191–1193] The LDI system employing an integrating CMOS image sensor delivers high-resolution blood flow images every 0.7–11 s, depending on the number of points in the acquired time-domain signal (32–512 points) and the image resolution (256 × 256 or 512 × 512 pixels). For the integrating imager, a digital CMOS camera based on the VCA1281 monochrome CMOS image sensor from Symagery (Canada) was utilized. This sensor operates in a rolling shutter mode; it has 280 horizontal × 1024 vertical resolution, a 7 × 7-µm pixel size, a 40-MHz sampling rate, and an 8-bit amplitude digital converter (ADC). The sensor has a specified flat spectral response in the range between 500 and 750 nm. The camera was connected to the host PC via a fast LVDS (low-voltage differential signaling) interface providing for a high-speed transfer of the obtained frames.

For the object illumination, a solid-state-diode-pumped laser of 250-mW output optical power emitting at 671 nm was used. The laser beam was coupled to a 1.5-mm diameter plastic optical fiber. A GRIN (gradient index) lens of 1.8-mm diameter was placed at the distal end of the fiber. This configuration produced a uniform illumination of the object. The illuminated area was up to a 170-mm diameter. The backscattered light was collected with an objective ($f = 6$ mm) with a low f-number (1.2), providing the system with the superior photon collection efficiency that becomes critical for short integration times (in the range of a few tens of milliseconds). Typically, the imager head was placed at a distance of 150–250 mm from the investigated tissue surface (see Fig. 8.14).

The specially developed software allows for changing the sensor parameters for control of the data acquisition mode, for acquisition of the data, and for display of the flow-related (perfusion, concentration, speed) maps. A photographic image of the sample and flow-related maps displayed on the monitor are obtained with the same image sensor; therefore, the obtained flow maps can be easily associated with an area of interest on the sample. The signal sampling frequency is inversely

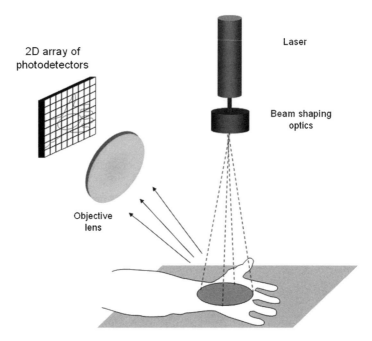

Figure 8.14 Schematic of a high-speed full-field laser Doppler imaging system on the basis of a CMOS image sensor.[1193]

proportional to the time to acquire one subframe. The subframe sampling rate of the sensor depends on its size and the pixel clock frequency. The clock frequency was fixed at 40 MHz for optimum performance speed and quality. The size of the sampled subframe finally defines the signal sampling frequency of the imager. For the 256 × 4-pixels subframe, the frame sampling frequency was 30 kHz, and at 256 × 6 pixels it was 20 kHz, at 256 × 8 pixels it was 14 kHz, etc.

To obtain one flow map over a region of interest (ROI), which was 256 × 256 or 512 × 512 pixels, the ROI must be subdivided into smaller regions (e.g., into 32 subframes of 256 × 8 pixels) and scanned electronically. From 32 to 512, sampled points were obtained for the acquired time-domain signal for each pixel of the subframe; thus, the intensity fluctuation history was recorded for each of the pixels of the ROI.

The signal processing comprises the calculation of the zero moment (M_0) and the first moment (M_1) of the power density spectrum $S(v)$ of the intensity fluctuations $I(t)$ for each pixel. The zero moment is related to the average concentration $\langle C \rangle$ of the moving particles in the sampling volume. The first moment (flux or perfusion) is proportional to the root-mean-square (rms) speed of the moving particles, V_{rms}, times the average concentration.[1205] The governing expressions are

$$\text{concentration} = \langle C \rangle \propto M_0 = \int_0^\infty S(v)dv, \qquad (8.4)$$

$$\text{perfusion} = \langle C \rangle V_{\text{rms}} \propto M_1 = \int_0^\infty \nu S(\nu) d\nu, \qquad (8.5)$$

$$S(\nu) = \left| \int_0^\infty I(t) \exp(-i 2\pi \nu t) dt \right|^2. \qquad (8.6)$$

Here, the variable ν is the frequency of the intensity fluctuations induced by the Doppler-shifted photons. To calculate the power density spectrum, an FFT algorithm, optimized for the speed performance and applied to the recorded signal variations at each sampled pixel of the ROI, was used. Noise subtraction was performed on the calculated spectra by setting a threshold level on the amplitude of the spectral components. This filtering is applied to reduce the white noise (e.g., thermal and readout noises) contribution to the signal. Thereafter, the perfusion, concentration, and speed maps were calculated and displayed on a computer monitor. The total imaging time (including data acquisition, processing, and display) depends on the number of samples obtained for each pixel and the ROI size. For the 256×256-pixel ROI, the imaging time is 0.9 s for 64 samples, 1.2 s for 128 samples, 1.7 s for 256 samples, and 2.9 s for 512 samples.

In Fig. 8.15, flow-related maps obtained on finger skin of a healthy person are shown. The images were obtained for the imager settings for the bandwidth from dc to 4000 Hz with 66 Hz resolution; the integration time was 130 μs. The total imaging time was around 5 s. A smoothing filter was applied to the row images: the value of each pixel shown was obtained by averaging the row values of eight neighboring pixels. The flow maps (perfusion, concentration, speed) are false coded with nine colors (not shown). The images clearly show the difference in the speed and concentration distributions measured on the fingers. The lower value for the concentration signal measured on the nail is caused by the higher amount of non-Doppler-shifted photons reemitted from the relatively thick statically scattering nail tissue compared to the thin statically scattering epidermis of the skin. The signal measured on the nail shows a higher speed of the moving blood cells in the undernail tissue. However, it could not be definitely predicted whether this is because the blood speed was really higher under the nail, or because the measured values were obtained due to a multiple scattering influence (see AF presented in Fig. 8.27). This ambiguity is a common problem for all laser Doppler or laser speckle imagers. The black-and-white photographic image of the object of interest is obtained with the same CMOS camera. This image is useful for determining the anatomical boundaries associated with the perfusion regions presented in the blood flow maps.

The imaging time of the this high-speed LDI system approaches the imaging time of laser speckle imaging (LSI) systems,[82,83,112,827,831,863,865–868,1197–1203] which are currently accepted as the fastest.[1200] The LSI systems obtain flow-related information by measuring the contrast of the image speckles (see Section 4.4.3). Effectively, the contrast values measured by LSI are directly proportional to the

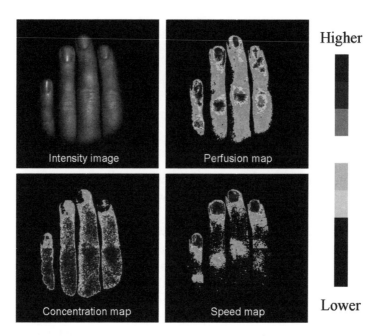

Higher

Lower

Figure 8.15 Flow-related maps obtained with a CMOS integrated imager on finger skin (ROI = 512 × 512 pixels): image of the object (intensity image); perfusion map (lower is 200 a.u. and higher is 700 a.u.); blood concentration map (lower is 140 a.u. and higher is 310 a.u.); flow speed map (lower is 400 a.u. and higher is 1500 a.u.). The imaging area is 11 × 11 cm. The imaging time is 5 s total.[1193]

normalized M_0 value that is measured by laser Doppler with integrating photodetectors. The images shown in Fig. 8.15 demonstrate a difference between the perfusion (M_1) and concentration (M_0) maps. It looks like LDI provides more objective information rather that the LSI method because with the LDI technique, the concentration and speed signals can be measured independently. In LSI, these two signals are typically mixed and it can thus be hard to attribute an exact cause for the changes in the contrast signal.[1204] However, a good correlation ($R^2 = 0.98$) between LDI and LSI measurements of the same area of regional cerebral blood flow (CBF) for different animals (male Wistar rats) was found.[1197] A detailed comparison of the laser-Doppler and speckle contrast methods of blood flow imaging can be found in Ref. 1199. It follows from this analysis that the speckle contrast technique can provide an image of tissue vascular structure with the relative distribution of blood velocity [correspondingly to a nonlinear response, described by Eq. (4.34)], but it does not provide a linear measurement of perfusion in comparison with LDI.

However, the speckle-contrast technique LASCA, whose fundamentals are discussed in Section 4.4.3, is a conceptually simple high-performance technique for blood flow imaging.[82,83,112,821,827,829–831,863,865–868,1194–1201] The measuring system employs a CCD camera, a frame grabber, and dedicated software for the computation of the local contrast of a speckle pattern and conversion of the contrast into a color map (which gives a map of flow velocities). The resulting image represents the contrast of the speckle field averaged in time. However, such an averaging is performed rather quickly (the averaging time is usually 5–30 ms) in order to permit real-time measurements.

Equation (4.34) gives an expression for the speckle contrast in the time-averaged speckle pattern as a function of the exposure time T and the correlation time,

$$\tau_c = \frac{1}{ak_0v},\tag{8.7}$$

where v is the mean velocity of the scatterers, k_0 is the lightwave number, and a is a factor that depends on the Lorentzian width and scattering properties of the tissue.[1205] As in LDI, it is theoretically possible to relate the correlation times, τ_c, to the absolute velocities of the red blood cells, but this is difficult to do in practice because the number of moving particles that light interacted with and their orientations are unknown.[1205] However, relative spatial and temporal measurements of velocity can be obtained from the ratios of $2T/\tau_c$, which is proportional to the velocity and defined as the measured velocity.[831,866,867]

The schematic diagram of the experimental setup is shown in Fig. 4.14. A He:Ne laser beam ($\lambda = 633$ nm, 3 mW) was coupled into an 8-mm diameter fiber bundle, which was adjusted to illuminate the area of interest evenly.[831,866,867] The illuminated area was imaged through a zoom stereo microscope (SZ6045TR, Olympus, Japan) onto a CCD camera (PIXELFLY, PCO Computer Optics, Germany) with 480×640 pixels, yielding an image of 0.8 to 7 mm, depending on the magnification; the exposure time T of the CCD was 20 ms. Images were acquired through easily controlled software (PCO Computer Optics, Germany) at 40 Hz.

The raw speckle images were acquired to compute the speckle contrast image. The number of pixels used to compute the local speckle contrast can be selected by the user: lower numbers reduce the validity of the statistics, whereas higher numbers limit the spatial resolution of the technique. To ensure proper sampling of the speckle pattern, the size of a single speckle should be approximately equal to the size of a single pixel in the image, which is equal to the width of the diffraction-limited spot size and is given by 2.44 $\lambda f/D$, where λ is the wavelength and f/D is the f-number of the system. In the system, the pixel size was 9.9 μm. With a magnification of unity, the required f/D is 6.4 at a wavelength of 633 nm. Squares of 5×5 pixels were used according to the theoretical studies.[83] The software calculated the speckle contrast for any given square of 5×5 pixels and assigned this value to the central pixel of the square. This process was then repeated to obtain a speckle contrast map. To each pixel in the speckle contrast map, the measured velocity ($2T/\tau_c$) was obtained through Eq. (4.34) that describes the relationship between correlation time and velocity and therefore measures the velocity map.

To compute the relative blood flows in vessels of interest, first a threshold was set in a region of interest from the measured velocity image and then the vessels of interest were identified by the pixels with values above this threshold. The mean values of the measured velocity in those pixels were computed at each time point.

The relative velocity in the vessel of interest was expressed as the ratio of the measured velocity in the condition of stimuli to that of the control condition.

LSI is a noninvasive full-field optical imaging method with high spatial and temporal resolution, which is a convenient technique in measuring the dynamics of CBF.[831,866,867,1197,1198,1201,1203,1206] In particular, in Ref. 831, the LSI method was used to monitor the dynamics of CBF in several animal models during sciatic stimulation. Stimulation of the sciatic nerve was similar to that used in conventional physiological studies. Blood flow was monitored in the somatosensory cortex in a total of 16 rats under electrical stimulation of the sciatic nerve, and the activated blood flow distribution was obtained at different levels of arteries/veins and at the change of activated areas. One example of the results is shown in Fig. 8.16, in which the brighter areas correspond to the area of increased blood flow. In comparison with LDI, an area of 1 mm^2 ROI in Fig. 8.16(a) was chosen to evaluate its mean velocity (Fig. 8.17): the evoked CBF started to increase at 0.7 ± 0.1 s, peaked at 3.1 ± 0.2 s, and then returned to the baseline level. It is consistent with the conclusions obtained from the LDI technique.[1208,1209] In order to differentiate the response patterns of artery/vein under the same stimulus, six distinct levels of vessels were labeled in Fig. 8.16(a) and their changes of blood flow displayed. The results clearly showed that the response patterns of arteries and veins in the somatosensory cortex were totally different: vein 1 (V-1, ~140 µm in diameter) remained almost unaffected, and arteriole 1 (A-1, ~35 µm in diameter) responded slowly; arteriole 2 (A-2, ~35 µm in diameter) peaked at 3.5 ± 0.5 s after the onset of stimulation and then reached the steady-state plateau; vein 2 (V-2, ~70 µm in diameter) presented a delay and mild response; blood flow in the capillaries (A-3 and V-3, ~ 10 µm in diameter) surged readily and increased significantly. The changes in arteries and veins with different diameters were also measured.[831] The activation pattern of cerebral blood flow was discrete in spatial distribution and highly localized in the evoked cortex with the temporal evolution. This is consistent with the hypothesis of Roy and Sherrington.[1207–1209]

The influence of epidurally applied hyperosmotic glycerol on *in vivo* the resting CBF was also investigated using the LSI technique (see Section 5.81).[831] The skull was removed, and intact *dura mater* was exposed. To study the influence of glycerol on *in vivo* CBF, a small area of *dura mater* was removed. Warm dehydration glycerol was administrated near the exposed area. Velocity images of CBF under the effect of glycerol are shown in Fig. 5.44. When glycerol diffused in brain tissue and influenced CBF under the *dura mater*, the CBF in the exposed area would also change. Figure 5.45 gives the time course of changes in four different vessels.

As described above, LSI is based on the first-order spatial statistics of time-integrated speckle. The main disadvantage of LASCA is the loss of resolution caused by the need to average over a block of pixels to produce the spatial statistics used in the analysis, although it actually has higher resolution than other techniques such as scanning laser Doppler. A modified LSI method utilizing the temporal statistics of time-integrated speckle was recently suggested.[1210] In this method, each pixel in the speckle image can be viewed as the single-point area.

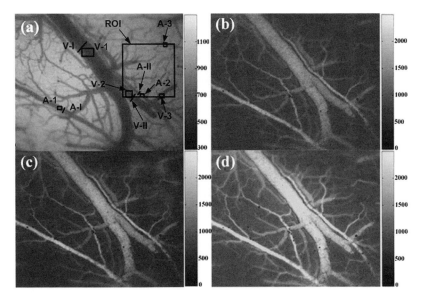

Figure 8.16 Blood flow change in the contralateral somatosensory cortex of rats under unilateral sciatic nerve stimulation.[1207] (a) A vascular topography illuminated with green light (540 ± 20 nm); (b) blood activation map at prestimulus; (c) 1 s and (d) 3 s after the onset of stimulation. The relative blood flow images are shown and converted from the speckle-contrast images, in which the brighter areas correspond to the area of increased blood flow. A-1, A-2, A-3 and V-1, V-2, V-3 represent the arbitrarily selected regions of interest (ROI) for monitoring changes in blood flow. A-I, A-II and V-I, V-II represent the selected loci on the vessel whose diameters are measured in the experiment.

Then, the signal processing consists of calculating the temporal statistics of the intensity of each pixel in the image as

$$N_{i,j} = \frac{\langle I_{i,j,t}^2 \rangle_t - \langle I_{i,j,t} \rangle_t^2}{\langle I_{i,j,t} \rangle_t^2},$$
$$i = 1\text{--}480, \quad j = 1\text{--}640, \quad t = 1 - m, \tag{8.8}$$

where $I_{i,j,t}$ is the instantaneous intensity of the ith and jth pixels at the t frame of raw speckle images, and $\langle I_{i,j,t} \rangle_t$ is the average intensity of the ith and jth pixels over the consecutive m frames. $N_{i,j}$ is inversely proportional to the velocity of the scattering particles. The value $N_{i,j}$ of each pixel in the consecutive m frames $(I_{i,j,t})$ of the raw speckle pattern is computed according to Eq. (8.8). The process is then repeated for the next group of m frames. The results are given as 2D grayscale (65,536 shades) or false-color (65,536 colors) coded maps that describe the spatial variation of the velocity distribution in the area examined.

Other approaches of LASCA technique improvement, in particular noise reduction, based on an active speckle averaging scheme that ensures perfect ensemble averaging are also described.[1199,1202] These approaches can use various methods to generate speckle images in reduced processing time, such as the use of sec-

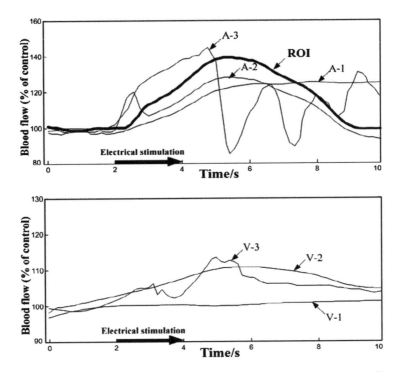

Figure 8.17 The relative change of blood flow in the six areas indicated in Fig. 8.16(a) (divided by the values of the prestimuli).[1207]

ondary low-coherence light sources (illumination with a dispersed laser beam that has passed a rotating diffuser) or vibration techniques.

8.4 Interferometric and speckle-interferometric methods for the measurement of biovibrations

A large number of optical methods have been proposed to date for the monitoring of biovibrations. Specifically, a fiber-optic sensor based on a single-mode x-coupler was successfully employed for the monitoring of heartbeats of patients examined with the use of a magnetic resonance tomograph.[1211] Contactless biovibrometers with an ultrahigh sensitivity based on heterodyne laser interferometers with a high automation degree and well-developed software were described in detail by Khanna et al.[1212,1213] Their investigations have been devoted to the measurement of vibrations of different components in the inner ear of animals. The confocal scheme of the heterodyne interference microscope employed in these studies made it possible to investigate vibrations of various layers of the tissue. This approach provided a record sensitivity with respect to small displacements of objects with low reflectivities (on the order of 10^{-4}–10^{-5}). The sensitivity achieved in these experiments within the range of vibration frequencies from 50 to 2000 Hz was 10^{-11} m. A conceptually similar but much simpler laser system for the investigation of biovibrations was described in Ref. 1214. This system also employs a heterodyne interferometer and is referred to as a laser Doppler vibrometer. This instrument, which operates within a frequency range up to 10 kHz, was used to monitor vibration spectra of a tympanic membrane under various disorders of the inner ear. Holographic analysis of vibrations of a tympanic membrane is also described in the literature (e.g., see Ref. 1215). An optical system for remote monitoring of cardiovibrations is presented in Ref. 864. An optical interferometer with a 633-nm He:Ne laser was utilized to detect micrometer displacements (sensitivity of 366.2 μm/s) of the skin surface.[1216] The detected velocity of skin movement is related to the time derivative of the blood pressure. Motion velocity profiles of the skin surface, near each superficial artery and auscultation point on a chest for the two heart valve sounds, exhibited distinctive profiles. The designed optical cardiovascular vibrometer has the potential to become a simple noninvasive approach to cardiovascular screening.

A laser Doppler technique based on the self-mixing effect in the diode laser[840,841] was used for cardiovascular pulse measurements above the radial artery in the wrist.[1217,1218] The developed self-mixing interferometer was used to measure the skin displacement, which was induced by a cardiovascular pulse. The reconstructed Doppler spectrograms followed the first derivative of the corresponding blood pressure pulse for both normal and abnormal pulse conditions. The correlation coefficient between the shapes of the Doppler spectrograms and the first derivative of the blood pressure pulse for ten investigated volunteers (738 cardiovascular pulsegrams) was found as 0.95 with a standard deviation of 0.05. A self-mixing interferometer was also used to measure the baroreflex effect and the elastic modulus of the arterial wall.

The fact that the interaction of laser radiation with tissues gives rise to the formation of speckle structures did not receive an adequate consideration in biovibrometry. The interference between speckle-modulated (reflected from a tissue) and reference fields has many specific features in this case. In designing biovibrometers, one should take into account these specific features and sometimes even make use of them[76,836,1219–1222] (see Chapter 4). The development of coherent optical contactless biovibrometers for the purpose of medical diagnostics is closely related to the solution of the problem of diffraction of laser beams propagating in nonstationary, randomly nonuniform media.[76] Several speckle techniques have been developed thus far for medical applications.[76,836,1219–1222] A diagnostic probe based on a miniature speckle/electronic-interference system, including a fiber-optic speckle interferometer and a matrix photodetector, was described in Ref. 1221. Sequential frame-by-frame analysis of the distribution of electron speckles makes it possible to image vibrations in three dimensions with a high quality. The probe was designed for the quantitative analysis of vibrations of the tympanic membrane and vocal chords.

The possibility of applying a Michelson speckle interferometer to the investigation of cardiovibrations and the detection of pulse waves was substantiated in Refs. 836, 1219, and 1220. Here, we briefly consider the main results of these studies and present some results on the detection of pulse waves with the use of the speckle technique based on the diffraction of focused laser beams. Medical diagnostics require simple and noise-resistant optical systems. The homodyne speckle interferometer shown in Fig. 8.18 meets these requirements. The output signal of this interferometer reaches its maximum when the speckle fields are matched (see Section 4.2). For focused laser beams, such matching can be easily achieved by the equalization of the arms of the interferometer. The speckle vibrometer can operate in two regimes: with comparatively large vibration amplitudes ($l_0 > \lambda/4$, the regime of fringe counting) and with small vibration amplitudes ($l_0 < \lambda/4$, when the random amplitude of the output signal displays an additional dependence on the initial phase). If the number of speckles within the receiving aperture satisfies the condition $N_{sp} > 4$, then the output signal of the interferometer has Gaussian statistics of the first order, i.e., the amplitude of this signal is characterized by a Rayleigh distribution.[836] The relevant experimental and theoretical dependencies of the averaged amplitude $\langle U \rangle$ and variance σ_U^2 of the output signal on the number of speckles within the aperture of the photodetector show a way to improve the signal-to-noise ratio in homodyne interferometers (see Fig. 8.19). It can be demonstrated that in the case of vibrations with large amplitudes, we have

$$\langle U \rangle \cong d_{av}^2 (N_{sp})^{0.5}, \qquad \sigma_U^2 \approx N_{sp}, \tag{8.9}$$

where d_{av} is the mean transverse size of a speckle and $N_{sp} = (2R_a/d_{av})^2$ for a circular aperture with a diameter $2R_a$. In writing Eq. (8.9), we assume that variations in speckle sizes do not change the intensities of the interfering beams.

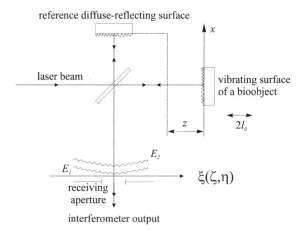

Figure 8.18 Diagram of a homodyne speckle interferometer for the investigation of biovibrations.[836]

Thus, to increase the amplitude of the output signal of a speckle interferometer, one should choose schemes that would ensure the detection of a large number of speckles with a maximum mean size, i.e., employ focused beams and a photodetector with a wide aperture. Considerable longitudinal displacements are usually accompanied by transverse and angular shifts of an object surface. As demonstrated

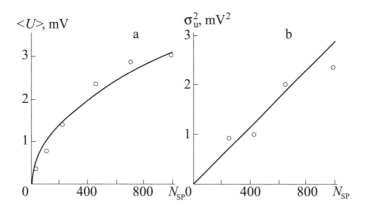

Figure 8.19 Experimental and theoretical dependencies of (a) the averaged amplitude $\langle U \rangle$ of the output signal of a speckle interferometer and (b) its variance σ_U^2 on the number of speckles N_{sp} within the receiving aperture (the rough surface is characterized by a considerable amplitude of vibrations, $l_0 \sim \lambda$; the sizes of speckles remain unchanged, and averaging is performed over 300 realizations of the reference speckle field).[836]

in Ref. 836, these shifts give rise to low-frequency modulation of the output signal of an interferometer. The depth of this modulation varies within a broad range from 0 to 100%, depending on specific realizations of the signal and reference speckle fields. Since it was demonstrated that such a modulation is caused by intensity fluctuations in a group of closely located speckles, one can considerably weaken spurious modulation by blocking the relevant group of speckles with a small opaque screen.

For vibrations with small amplitudes, the output signal of an interferometer has substantially different statistics. The modulus of the output signal in this case has an exponential distribution function with a maximum probable value equal to zero. However, the mean value of the modulus of the signal and its variance are characterized by the same dependencies on N_{sp} as in the case of vibrations with large amplitudes[836] [see Eq. (8.9)].

Taking into account the aforesaid and using Eqs. (4.22) and (4.23), we can represent the output signal of a homodyne interferometer in the following form:

$$U_i(t) = A_i \sin[\phi_i + A_L H(t)], \qquad (8.10)$$

where $H(t)$ is the normalized signal with a variance equal to unity that describes the waveform of vibrations on the surface of a bioobject, A_i and ϕ_i are random quantities determined by the conditions of detection of speckle interferograms and the chosen realization of the surface with an index i, and A_L is the amplitude of vibrations. Equation (8.10) also holds true for a differential interferometer if the quantity A_L is defined as the difference of the vibration amplitudes at two points. A laser differential speckle interferometer with two beams focused onto the surface of an object has been successfully employed for the detection of the human pulse at various points of skin surface in the wrist area.[836] As demonstrated in

Ref. 1222, the investigation of pulse waves through the analysis of phase portraits of the output signal of a differential speckle interferometer holds much promise for cardiodiagnostics. However, an appropriate filtration of the signal should be carried out in order to efficiently eliminate the influence of lateral shifts of skin surface caused by the pulse wave.

Basing on the speckle technology developed, a robust vibrometer for medical applications can be designed[1220] (see Fig. 8.20). However, the simplicity of the instrument is achieved at the cost of a nontrivial description of the response function of the vibrometer. Intensity fluctuations in scattered light in the case of diffraction of a focused Gaussian beam are related to vibrations of an object by some nonlinear random function. Nevertheless, due to regular variations in the speckle field (displacement and decorrelation of speckles) caused by vibrations of the scattering surface, the signal at the output of the photodetector contains spectral components that correspond to vibrations of the surface. The complex motion of the surface gives rise to additional nonlinearities in the response function. For example, a periodic motion of skin surface caused by a pulse wave can be considered as a superposition of at least three displacements: displacement normal to the surface, angular displacement, and transverse displacement (along the surface). For the measuring system shown in Fig. 8.20, normal vibrations do not contribute to the output signal. Comparatively small angular vibrations are responsible for transverse oscillations of speckles in the observation plane (without decorrelation of speckles), whereas the small transverse surface shifts lead to a partial decorrelation of the speckle field. Thus, time-domain intensity fluctuations of the scattered field in the case of periodic vibrations of a surface also involve a periodic component. In such a situation, the nonlinear random operator that relates intensity fluctuations to the displacement of the scattering surface depends on the sizes of the irradiated surface area, conditions of speckle observation, and the specific realization of the surface under study. However, numerical analysis of the diffraction of a focused Gaussian beam from a moving rough surface with Gaussian statistics within the framework of the Kirchhoff approximation shows that when the amplitudes of transverse shifts are less than the surface correlation length (for example, for human skin, $L_c \sim 60–80$ μm) and the amplitudes of angular vibrations are less than one degree, statistical and nonlinear properties of the signal do not exert a considerable influence on the detection of the motion law of a rough surface.[1220]

A fiber-optic sensor based on these principles is shown in Fig. 8.20(a). This sensor transforms skin vibrations caused by a pulse wave into the corresponding motion of speckles, which is detected in the observation plane. To standardize the reflective properties of the surface and exclude bulk scattering in tissues, the device employs a thin rubber membrane, which is attached to the surface of the skin in such manner that it does not perturb the motion of the skin surface. Various thin backscattering films produced by the spraying of a substance on the skin surface can also be employed as standard reflectors. It should be noted that this method also provides a sufficient efficiency in the case of an open skin surface, because the contribution of bulk scattering is suppressed to a considerable extent due to a

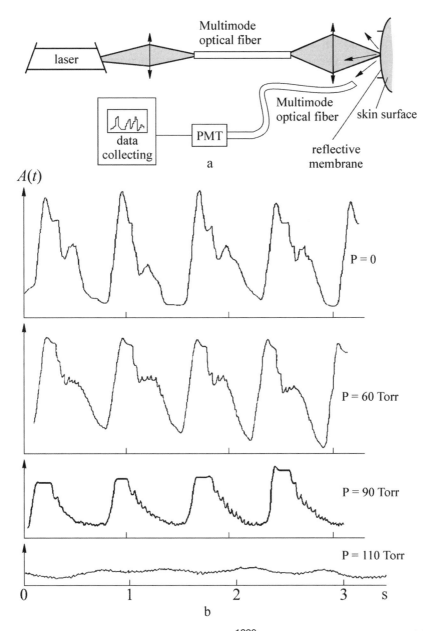

Figure 8.20 Fiber-optic laser speckle vibrometer.[1220] (a) Diagram of the instrument. (b) Pulsograms detected in the wrist area of a young man (24 yr) for various pressures P in the arm cuff of a tonometer.

sharp focusing of radiation onto the skin surface, and the skin surface itself can be satisfactorily described in terms of Gaussian statistics. Figures 8.20(b)–(e) present typical pulsograms measured with the use of a fiber-optic speckle vibrometer in the wrist area of a healthy young man for different external pressures in the forearm area (as before, a medical tonometer was used for these measurements). Obviously,

this device can be considered an advanced prototype of a compact, simple, and reliable remote probe of biovibrations with a high spatial resolution, which can be
assembled with the use of a diode laser and a photodiode integrated with segments
of multimode optical fibers. Such a probe would be useful in cardiology, for a diagnosis of vascular diseases, and in sport medicine (monitoring of self-contractions
of muscles and other tissues).

8.5 Optical speckle topography and tomography of tissues

Methods of speckle topography and tomography are rapidly progressing at
the moment.[76,135,136,138,139,155,343,395,396,566,799,825,827–832,834,835,843–846,1196,1202,
1223–1228,1239] Local statistical and correlation analysis offers much promise as a
method for topographic mapping and structure monitoring of scattering objects.
Local estimates of correlation characteristics [correlation or structure functions
or their parameters, see Eqs. (4.20) and (4.21), and Figs. 4.5 and 4.6] and normalized statistical moments [the contrast V_I and asymmetry coefficient Q_a are
usually employed, see Eqs. (4.5)–(4.7)] are highly sensitive to the structure parameters of an object, such as the correlation length L_c and the standard deviation σ_L of optical altitudes (thicknesses) of inhomogeneities or the relevant
correlation length L_ϕ and the standard deviation σ_ϕ of phase fluctuations of the
boundary field (see Section 4.1) in the case of the diffraction of focused laser
beams.[76,155,343,825,827,829,830,834,835,1224–1233] An object under study can be considered as an irregular system of lenslets with definite statistical characteristics that
display intensity fluctuations similar to those observed when a focused laser beam
is scanned over the surface of an object.[835]

Intensity fluctuations include two components (see Fig. 8.21). The first component is a background with a relatively small and comparatively smooth varying amplitude. The second component is represented by infrequent high-intensity pulses
related to matched inhomogeneities (the distances between the plane of the waist of
the incident laser beam and the object, and between the object and the photodetector are matched with the effective focal length of the inhomogeneity, which ensures
effective reimaging of the waist of the laser beam into the observation plane).

We can classify the inhomogeneities by analyzing the contrast V_I and the asymmetry coefficient Q_a as functions of the distance between the waist plane of the
laser beam and the surface of an object. Using this approach, we can reconstruct
statistical distributions of fluctuations of the refractive index of a medium.[77] The
fact that V_I and Q_a abruptly increase when the ratio of the radius of the laser beam
to the correlation length satisfies the condition $w/L_\phi \sim 1$ is a direct manifestation of the microfocusing effect in the far-field diffraction zone[835,1229] (see Fig.
8.22 for V_I, $\Delta z = \pm 0.4$ mm). The growth in the ratio $w/L_\phi(|z| > 0.4$ mm) is
accompanied by a decrease in the quantities V_I and Q_a, which reach values corresponding to completely developed speckles. These effects can occur in the case of
weakly scattering objects, such as thin tissue layers or cellular monolayers, when
$L_c \sim L_\phi \sim d$ (where d is the thickness of the sample), $L_c \gg \lambda$, and the standard

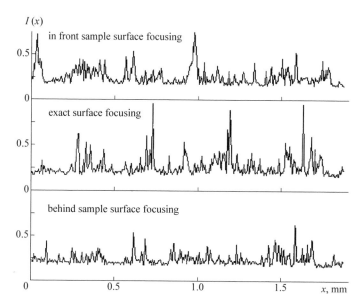

Figure 8.21 Realizations of speckle intensity fluctuations obtained with a focused laser beam scanned over an epidermis sample of psoriatic human skin (epidermal stripping).[343] The upper and lower realizations were obtained with a laser beam focused in front of and behind the sample surface, respectively. The middle realization corresponds to a laser beam focused exactly on the surface.

deviation σ_ϕ related to phase fluctuations of the field is completely determined by fluctuations of the refractive index δn.

Multiple scattering is characteristic of optically thick tissue layers. In this case, the spatial distribution of scattered light has a broad angular spectrum, and depolarization effects play an important role. The spatial distribution of the correlation properties of the scattered field, which is related to the structure of an object, can be considered in a manner similar to diffusion-wave spectroscopy [see Eq. (4.43)] with allowance for the fact that an object has a static structure, and a laser beam (or the object itself) is scanned over the surface of the object at a definite rate. Along with the chosen beam radius and the character of the optical inhomogeneities of the medium, the rate of scanning determines the fluctuations of the scattered field in the time domain. In such a situation, the normalized autocorrelation function of the intensity fluctuations is generally defined by Eq. (4.20) with $\xi \equiv t$ and $\Delta\xi \equiv \tau$. The behavior of the structure function [see Eq. (4.21)] near the zero value of its argument, which corresponds to the highest efficiency of the high-frequency spatial intensity fluctuations, can be conveniently characterized in this case in terms of the exponential factor ν_I as[835,1224]

$$\nu_I = \frac{\ln[D_I(\Delta\tau_2)/D_I(\Delta\tau_1)]}{\ln(|\Delta\tau_2|/|\Delta\tau_1|)}. \tag{8.11}$$

To analyze the polarization properties of speckle fields, we can employ the following time-domain first- and second-order statistical characteristics of the intensity

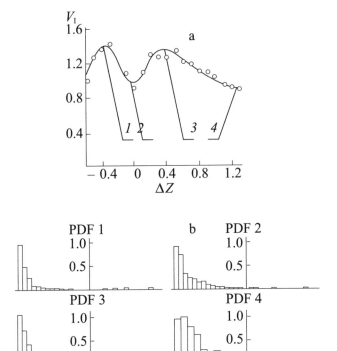

Figure 8.22 The correspondence between (a) the contrast values and (b) the shape of the distribution of speckle intensity fluctuations (PDF) as functions of the position of the waist of a focused laser beam with respect to the sample surface (an epidermal stripping of psoriatic human skin) Δz (mm); $\Delta z = 0$ corresponds to the case where the beam waist lies on the surface of the sample.[835]

fluctuations of scattered light in the paraxial region, which should be measured for two orthogonal linear polarizations (relative to the polarization of the probing beam):[343]

(1) the mean intensity of speckles,

$$\langle I_{sp} \rangle = \langle I_{||} \rangle + \langle I_\perp \rangle; \tag{8.12}$$

(2) the cross-correlation function (correlation coefficient) for two polarization states,

$$r_{\perp ||}(\tau) = \langle [I_{||}(t) - \langle I_{||} \rangle][I_\perp(t+\tau) - \langle I_\perp \rangle] \rangle, \tag{8.13}$$

where the indices ($\perp, ||$) denote combinations of polarization states, and averaging is performed over the trajectory of scanning.

Figure 8.23 presents the optical scheme of a spatial speckle correlometer intended for topography or tomography of comparatively thin samples of tissues.

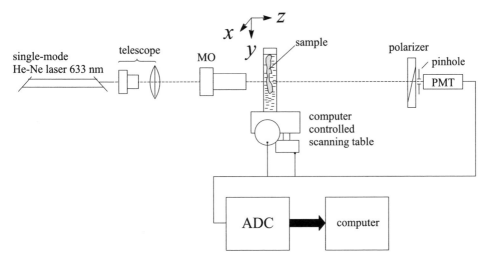

Figure 8.23 Optical scheme of a scanning polarization-sensitive spatial speckle correlometer.[155] PMT, photomultiplier tube; ADC, amplitude-digital convertor; MO, microobjective.

This device employs a focused laser beam about 5 μm in diameter produced by a single-mode uniphase He:Ne laser. Structure patterns of an object were usually reconstructed through the two-dimensional scanning of the object and an appropriate analysis of the statistical and correlation properties of the scattered light. The scanning step on both axes was 5 μm. A photodetector was placed along the direction of the axis of the incident laser beam (scattering exactly in the forward direction). The diameter of the entrance pinhole was about 25 μm, which is much less than the mean diameter of a speckle. The maximum rate of scanning was about 5 mm/s. The electronic units employed made it possible to obtain at least 20 equidistant counts per single step of scanning. An object was usually placed in the waist of the incident laser beam. The position of an object relative to the beam waist and the orientation of a polarization analyzer mounted in front of the photodetector were adjusted manually.

As was shown above, the estimation of the structure parameters of a tissue, such as the characteristic size of local inhomogeneities and spatial fluctuations of the refractive index, generally requires some assumptions concerning the scattering model. One of the simplest models of scattering is the model of a random phase screen with Gaussian statistics of inhomogeneities (see Section 4.1).[157,822,824,835,1230] In many cases, statistical models for living structures are much more complicated. In particular, some of these models are nonlinear and may take into account multiple scattering. In spite of the lack of well-developed models for the structure of many tissues, any empirical information concerning statistical properties of scattered light is useful for the analysis of structure images of tissues. Such information may be also useful for the development of structure models themselves.

Human skin is one of the most natural objects for the application of optical speckle correlometry.[76,834,835,1224,1225] All the structural specific features of skin surface are manifested in the statistical and correlation properties of the speckle field produced in the far-field diffraction zone when skin samples or skin replicas are probed with a focused laser beam. The technology that permits one to obtain thin slices (strippings) of epidermis with the use of medical glues and quartz (or glass, or metal) substrates is very convenient for *in vitro* structure studies of epidermis by means of speckle-correlation optics.[834,835] The thickness of the slices in this case usually ranges from 30 to 50 μm. This technology allows one to obtain from 5 to 7 sequential strippings from the same place. As an example, Fig. 8.21 presents three realizations for the intensity fluctuations obtained by scanning a skin epidermis sample from an area of psoriasis focus of a patient for three different positions of the waist of the laser beam. The thin layers of normal and psoriatic epidermis studied demonstrated that such samples can be described within the framework of a model of single or low-step multiple scattering, because only insignificant depolarization effects were observed in the far-field zone.

The contrast V_I and the asymmetry coefficient Q_a of intensity fluctuations in the far-field zone as functions of the variation in the defocusing parameter Δz for normal and psoriatic epidermis display two maxima near the area of exact focusing ($\Delta z = 0$).[835] Figure 8.24 shows such a dependence for a sample of psoriatic epidermis, along with the relevant probability density functions for the intensity

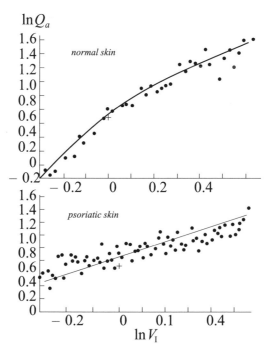

Figure 8.24 Statistical dependencies $\ln Q_a$ and $\ln V_I$ for normal and psoriatic skin samples (strippings of human epidermis); + indicates the values of Q_a and V_I for developed speckles.[1231]

fluctuations. The behavior of the first-order statistical characteristics confirms the validity of the lenslet approach for the description of the scattering properties of epidermis. Normal epidermis (where scatterers have smaller sizes and more uniform distribution) is characterized by a partial overlapping of the maxima mentioned above. The symmetry in the arrangement of V_I and Q_a peaks with respect to the plane of the beam waist allows us to assume that the statistical weights of the negative and positive lenslets in an ensemble of scatterers are equal to each other.

The differences between the curves $V_I(\Delta z)$ and $Q_a(\Delta z)$ for samples of normal and psoriatic epidermis are due to the changes in the structure of a tissue caused by the disease. These changes are associated with the appearance of parakeratotic foci (the structure of cells near such a focus is substantially disordered) and the saturation of the surrounding tissues with interstitial fluids (which decrease the efficiency of scattering, similar to immersion fluids). Later stages of the disease are characterized by the appearance of microspaces filled with air and the scaling in the formation of inhomogeneities, which increases scattering and changes its character.[835,1231] For a small Δz, the quantity V_I is greater than 1, reaching the values of 1.6–1.7 for certain samples. As a rule, samples of normal skin display a higher contrast than samples of psoriatic skin. Parametric dependencies for $\ln Q_a$ and $\ln V_I$ plotted for various Δz illustrate the differences in the statistical properties of samples of normal and psoriatic skin (see Fig. 8.24). For normal skin, the first derivative of the function $\ln Q_a = f(\ln V_I)$ is greater than that for psoriatic skin. This derivative has a negative slope in the case of normal skin and positive slope for pathological skin. For developed speckle fields with $V_I = 1$ and a negative exponential probability density function of intensity fluctuations [see Eq. (4.9)], we have $Q_a = 2$ (these points are indicated by a plus sign in Fig. 8.24).

Thus, the first-order statistics can be used as a simple and efficient criterion for the recognition of structurally specific features of tissue samples. Investigations of special skin replicas demonstrated that this technique is also efficient for the semiquantitative determination of the dryness and fatness of skin.[1227,1232]

Second-order statistical characteristics of intensity fluctuations are also highly sensitive to structural changes in tissues.[834] For normal skin, normalized 1D autocorrelation functions of the intensity fluctuations are characterized by comparatively small values of the correlation length, $L_I \sim 60$–80 μm, and the absence of considerable fluctuations of the correlation coefficient on large scales (see Fig. 4.5). As a psoriatic plaque arises, the AFs display a nearly twofold increase in the correlation length, $L_I \sim 95$–180 μm, and the appearance of large-scale aperiodic oscillations with a comparatively large amplitude. The effective sizes of structure inhomogeneities giving rise to such oscillations correlate with the sizes characteristic of an ensemble of parakeratotic foci. Detailed analysis of oscillatory components of the AF should allow one to estimate the surface density of parakeratotic foci and their mean size.

In the range of high spatial frequencies of about 1 μm^{-1} and higher, the structure function or its exponential factor ν_I [see Eqs. (4.21) and (8.11)] are preferable for the description of intensity fluctuations. Local estimates of the exponential factor permit one to determine the contribution of high-frequency structure components of a tissue and to find their spatial distribution in the form of topograms. Figure 8.25 presents topograms obtained with the use of this technique for samples of normal and psoriatic epidermis.[155,1226,1233] The topograms and the corresponding distributions of the exponential factor (see Fig. 8.26) display structure changes related to different stages of pathology development. The values of ν_I were averaged along the direction of the x-axis with an averaging gate containing no less than 10^3 counts. The epidermis of normal skin with comparatively small-scale inhomogeneities is characterized by a somewhat smaller mean value and a greater variance of the parameter ν_I than the early and middle stages of the formation of a psoriatic plaque (see Figs. 8.25 and 8.26). Large-scale structure features, such as fragments of a skin pattern, are clearly seen in the topogram of normal skin. The middle stage of pathology is characterized by a small variance and a relatively large mean value of the parameter considered. In the later stage of the process, the variance grows, the mean value of the parameter ν_I slightly decreases, and the symmetry of the distribution function lowers. The stages of the formation of a psoriatic plaque, clearly distinguished by means of correlation spectroscopy, are consistent with the results of clinical observations.

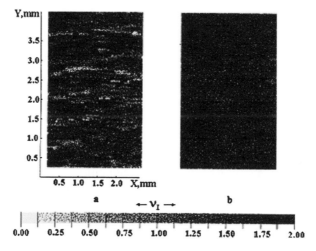

Figure 8.25 Topograms of the exponential factor ν_I obtained for samples of epidermal strippings of human skin: (a) normal skin and (b) psoriatic skin (the middle stage of the disease).[155]

The control of the optical properties of tissues, in particular the possibility of considerably decreasing the scattering coefficient, may become a key point in optical tomography of tissues in the process of searching for small tumors at early stages of their formation (see Chapter 5). Figure 5.8 presents two recorded fragments that correspond to the early and later stages of tissue clearing. The characteristic changes in speckle structures in the far-field zone were visually observed on a screen located in the plane of a photodetector and were recorded in reflected

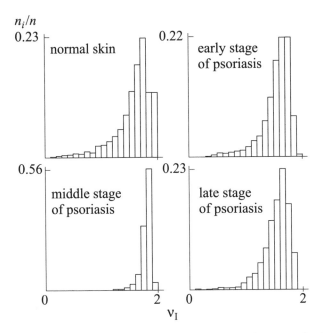

Figure 8.26 Evolution of the distributions of the exponential factor ν_I in the progress of psoriasis:[155] normal skin [corresponding to Fig. 8.25(a)], early stage of psoriasis, middle stage of psoriasis [corresponding to Fig. 8.25(b)], and late stage of psoriasis.

light by means of a CCD camera.[155,172,742] The evolution of typical normalized AFs of intensity fluctuations for sclera in the process of sclera clearing measured with the use of a speckle correlometer (see Fig. 8.23) is shown in Fig. 8.27. Within small time intervals (1–2 min), the time evolution of the shape of the autocorrelation peak, which is associated with the transition of a tissue from one scattering regime to another, can be approximated by an exponential curve; whereas for large

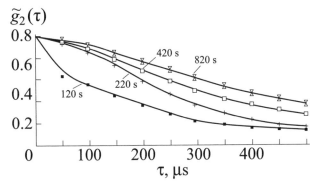

Figure 8.27 Evolution of the normalized autocorrelation function of intensity fluctuations in the speckle field produced by light scattered from a sample of human sclera in the process of scleral enhanced translucence in trazograph-60; the thickness of the sample is 0.6 mm; the measurements were performed with a sample processed in the solution during 120, 220, 420, and 820 s.[155]

time intervals, this process can be approximately described by a Gaussian curve. The initial stage of the process is characterized by the existence of many scales of intensity fluctuations (the AF displays at least three distinguishable values of its slope). At later stages of clearing, the half-width of the AF peak tends to a value of $(0.3–0.4) \times 10^{-3}$ s, which is close to the ratio of the waist radius of the incident beam to the scanning rate, w/v. This effect can be employed as a criterion of the completion of the transition from multiple scattering to single scattering. The time evolution of the exponential factor ν_I [see Eq. (8.11) and Fig. 8.28] characterizes the behavior of the high-frequency components of the intensity fluctuations.

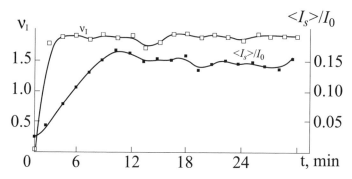

Figure 8.28 Typical time dependencies of the exponential factor ν_I and the normalized mean intensity $\langle I_s \rangle / I_0$ measured at the observation point for a scleral sample placed in trazograph-60; $\lambda = 633$ nm.[155]

We should note that the exponential factor and the relative fluctuations of the mean intensity of transmitted light have substantially different rates of response to the action of hyperosmotic optical clearing agents (OCAs): ν_I is especially sensitive to the action of OCAs at the early stages of clearing (within ~1.5 min for trazograph-60), whereas transmission reaches its maximum only by the tenth minute. This difference in response rates can be accounted for by the fact that the correlation properties of the field, characterized by transition from uniform to nonuniform speckle distributions, substantially change at the initial stages of matching of the refractive indices. By contrast, maximum collimated transmission is achieved only when the refractive indices are completely matched.

Straightforward modeling of the transport of initially collimated photons with a wavelength of 600 nm through a fibrous tissue consisting of collagen fibers with a mean diameter of 100 nm and a refractive index $n_c = 1.474$ surrounded by a ground substance whose refractive index varies within the range $n_0 = 1.345–1.474$ shows that, even with partial matching of refractive indices, $n_0 = 1.450$, nonscattered (~67%) and singly scattered (~24%) photons dominate in transmitted light (see Fig. 5.6).[798] This prediction agrees well with the measured transmission and reflection spectra of sclera and the data on correlation measurements (see Section 5.3).[798,799]

Another specific feature of scleral clearing is the appearance of quasi-periodic oscillations of mean-intensity transmission, which are also manifested in the correlation characteristics. These oscillations have small amplitude and can be clearly seen at later stages of translucence, when the main dynamic process associated with the directed diffusion of the substance from the solution into the tissue and of water from the tissue to the solution is close to its completion. The characteristic oscillation time is ∼ 1.5–2.0 min. Apparently a process with such a characteristic time can be attributed to the nonuniformity of the diffusion of substances inside a tissue in space and time. This effect may be accounted for by the multistage character of the diffusion process. At the first stage, the diffusion of the OCA into a tissue and the flow of water out of the tissue partially equalize the refractive indices of the hydrated collagen and the intercollagen substance. Under these conditions, the optical transmission of a tissue grows until the dependence under study saturates. However, at the second stage, a relatively weak process of the interaction of the new ground substance with collagen is manifested. The ground substance somewhat lowers its refractive index through the dehydration of the collagen, whereas the refractive index of collagen increases. The resulting mismatch of the refractive indices slightly decreases the optical transmission. At the next stage, a certain violation of the balance between the pressures of water and the OCA in the solution and tissue gives rise to the diffusion of water from the tissue and the OCA into the tissue, which leads to the more exact equalization of the refractive indices, and transmission grows again. Then, the process described above is repeated, and transmission oscillates in the time domain. Such oscillations are observed within the entire period of time when a hyperosmotic agent acts on a tissue up to 40–60 min in this particular experiment.[155,172,343] Probably, oscillations of a similar nature with the time period of ∼2.5–3.5 min were registered for *in vivo* hamster skin at topical application of glycerol as an OCA using an OCT system as a detector.[1059]

As it was shown earlier (see Section 5.7.1), the transition of a scattering object from the regime of multiple scattering to the regime of single scattering should change the polarization properties of scattered radiation, which can be described in terms of the first- and second-order statistical characteristics [see Eqs. (8.12) and (8.13)]. At the early stage of sclera optical clearing, both of the polarization components of transmitted light have approximately equal intensities. However, in the process of clearing, the component polarized along the polarization of the incident beam begins to dominate over the other component (see Fig. 5.10).[343] These experimental data demonstrate the reversibility of the optical clearing process, which is important for living systems, and reveal a high sensitivity of the polarization characteristics to structural changes in a tissue.

Note that translucent sclera features large-scale spatial inhomogeneities of scattering and polarization properties in the form of a domain structure, with domain areas on the order of 0.1–1 mm^2. Such a structure is associated with a spatially nonuniform distribution of the diffusion rate of substances and is clearly manifested in both time-domain realizations of intensity fluctuations for separate polarization components and the behavior of the cross-correlation function for these components (see Fig. 8.29) measured with a laser beam scanned over a sample.[155] It is obvious that, similar to the correlation characteristics of speckle fields, polarization and cross-correlation characteristics can be employed for the imaging of the structure of tissues, as well as for tissue topography and tomography.

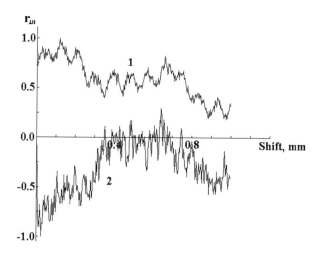

Figure 8.29 Evolution of the cross-correlation coefficient for two orthogonal polarizations of intensity fluctuations in the speckle field produced in the observation plane by a laser beam scanned over a scleral sample processed in trazograph-60 during (1) 200 s and (2) 400 s. The scanning rate was 5 mm/s.[155]

8.6 Methods of coherent microscopy

Modern methods of microscopy are developing toward *in vivo* structural investigations of individual cells without fixation of these cells, with simultaneous monitoring of intracellular dynamic processes caused by the vital activity of the cell. The above-mentioned laser Doppler microscope[5,24,841,1183] and a high-performance phase microscope with an ultrahigh spatial resolution[175,1112,1240–1242] are good examples of such devices. Another tendency in the development of microscopy is *in vivo* layer-by-layer analysis of tissues with a high spatial resolution. Confocal microscopy[1,3,28,76,120,122,614,878–898,1243] is a prominent example of this direction in microscopy (see Sections 4 and 5.7.2). Holographic microscopy[1244–1247] also offers much promise for numerous applications.

A phase microscope described in Refs. 175, 1112, and 1242 is a Linnik-Tolansky interferometer with a computer-controlled piezodriver with a mirror in the reference channel and a dissector (coordinate-sensitive detector) that registers an interference pattern (see Fig. 8.30). In fact, such a microscope is a microprofilometer with a spatial resolution up to 10 nm at a wavelength of 633 nm. The temporal resolution provided by this microscope in the investigation of dynamic processes is on the order of 1 ms. The resolution in height for this device is 0.5 nm,

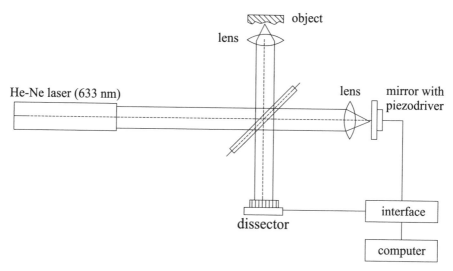

Figure 8.30 Diagram of a phase microscope.[1240]

the imaging area includes from 64×64 up to 256×256 pixels, the total gain is 10^5–10^6, the minimum pixel size is 5 nm, and the time of data processing is 4–20 s. The information concerning the structure of an object is represented in the form of altitude (optical path length) topograms, cross sections, three-dimensional images, etc. When dynamic processes are studied at an arbitrarily chosen point of an object, the results of the investigations are represented in the form of time-domain realizations, Fourier spectra, or histograms. A phase microscope was employed for structural investigations of living and dried fibroblast cells (L 929) and mitochondria extracted from cells of rat liver in the normal and condensed states.[175,1112] The phase images of L 929 cells obtained in these studies are characterized by the mean optical path length of light on the order of 600 nm for a living cell and about 50 nm for a dried cell. These findings indicate the possibility of the efficient monitoring of this type of cell metabolism. Analogous images of mitochondria demonstrate that the optical length of a normal mitochondrion with respect to the environment is about 15 nm. For the condensed state, the optical length is 3 nm. A microscope of this type was also successfully employed for structural investigations of the wall of fungi cells and erythrocytes with a high spatial resolution, for the study of intracellular motility with a high temporal resolution,[1240] and for human carcinoma cells in different physiological states induced by hyperosmotic agents.[1242]

Confocal laser scanning microscopy, the principles of which are discussed in Section 4.4, is a well-developed imaging technique for biomedical investigations.[1,3,28,76,120,122,614,878,879,780–782,883–888,890–898] In *in vivo* morphometry using real-time confocal microscopy of human epidermis, a spatial resolution better than 1 μm and depth profiling up to 150–250 μm, depending on the anatomical site and skin optical characteristics (color, transparency), were shown.[1243] Some of these results on the estimation of the nuclear size and number of keratinocytes for different layers of the living human epidermis are presented in Table 8.1. The resolution

Table 8.1 Estimation of nuclear size and number of keratinocytes in horizontal optical sections of the living epidermis.[1243]

Epidermal nuclei	Diameter, μm	Density, number/mm^2
Stratum granulosum	12–15	1500
Stratum spinosum	9–12	4000
Stratum basale	6–8	7000

achieved in structural studies of tooth dentine is comparable with the resolution characteristic of scanning electron microscopy, and additional subsurface tissue imaging with a resolution of 1 μm for depths up to 30–50 μm is also provided.[882]

Three-dimensional imaging of cells in different layers of corneal epithelium made it possible to reveal the character of mitosis in such cells.[890,891] Figure 8.31 displays a typical scheme of a confocal microscope where scanning is performed along the z-axis (along the light beam) (see Ref. 1, pp. 555–575). Such a microscope is intended for the layer-by-layer analysis of eye structure. Radiation is delivered to the microscope by means of an optical fiber. The microscope is based on two optically conjugate slits. One of these slits is imaged onto an object, whereas the second slit is placed in front of a photodetector. An objective is scanned along the z-axis by a computer-controlled piezodriver. An immersion liquid provides optical matching between the objective and the eye under study.

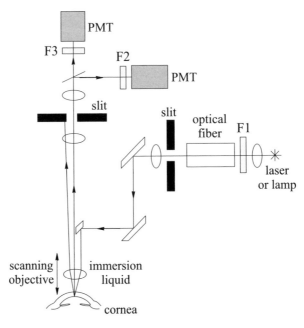

Figure 8.31 Diagram of a confocal microscope with optically conjugate slits and scanning along the z-axis.[1,879] F1, F2 , and F3, filters; PMT, photomultiplier tube.

Figure 8.32 shows a slit-scanning confocal microscope of another type. Such a microscope allows one to obtain images of an object at different depths.[883,884, 888–891] This microscope operates in real time and can be employed for *in vivo* studies of eye tissues. The main element of the microscope is a two-sided mirror, which implements transverse scanning without shifting the axis of the reflected beam (such a scheme was proposed for the first time by Svishchev in 1969 for the investigation of transparent scattering objects, including living nerve tissues). The lowering of the image quality due to the motion of the patient's eyes was excluded with the use of an electronic scheme, which ensured the required scanning frequency and phase synchronization between all the elements of the system. As an example, Fig. 8.33 presents an image of endothelium cells of human cornea obtained with the use of the confocal microscope shown in Fig. 8.32.[888] High-quality layer-by-layer images of cellular structures of eye tissues and skin in the normal and pathological states as well as the dentin structure of human teeth are presented in Refs. 1, 3, 76, 120, 122, 879–882,893, 898, and 1243.

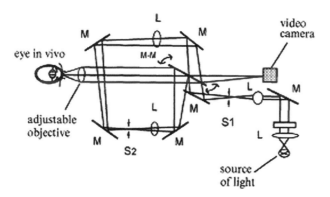

Figure 8.32 Diagram of a slit-scanning confocal microscope operating in real time.[883] M, mirrors; L, lenses; S1 and S2, conjugate slits; and M-M, scanning two-sided mirror.

Depending on the source of light employed, the detecting system, and the type of tissue under investigation, averaging over several expositions (frames) may be necessary to achieve a satisfactory signal-to-noise ratio. For example, for weakly reflecting eye tissues (usually, less than 1%), four to eight frames may be necessary. However, if a highly sensitive video camera in combination with a broadband video tape recorder is employed as a detector, averaging over frames is not necessary, and real-time *in vivo* measurements can be carried out.[883,884] Although confocal microscopes can operate with mercury or xenon arc or halogen lamps, monochromatic laser radiation provides images with a higher quality owing to the absence of chromatic aberrations introduced by the optical system. However, the type of laser should be chosen with allowance for the depth of penetration of the laser radiation into a tissue and the transmission of the optical system of the microscope.

Comparative analysis of confocal and heterodyne scanning microscopes and their applications for the investigation of scattering objects have demonstrated that

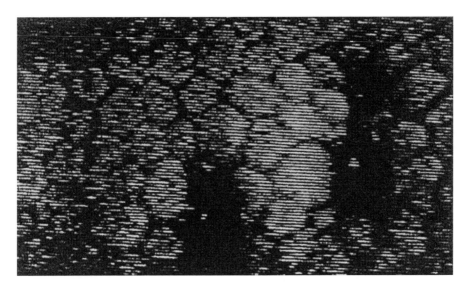

Figure 8.33 Optical map of human cornea *in vivo*. The image shows endothelial cells on the rear surface of cornea. Optical mapping is performed at a depth of 500 μm with respect to the cornea surface. Dark areas in the image correspond to pathological endothelium.[888]

in many cases the limitations of the confocal technique are mainly associated with the small level of the signal rather than with the degradation of an image due to scattered light.[894,895] Indeed, a satisfactory resolution in depth (selection of photons reflected from a definite layer and elimination of the influence of scattered light) can be achieved when a confocal system has conjugate pinholes with a radius (in optical units) of

$$\nu_p \leq 2, \quad \nu_p = \frac{2\pi r_p a_1}{\lambda f_1}, \tag{8.14}$$

where r_p is the radius of the pinhole and a_1 and f_1 are the radius and the focal length of a lens that focuses light on the pinhole. Such pinholes do not transmit much light. For example, with $\nu_p = 2$, a pinhole transmits only 40% of radiation incident on this pinhole within the limits of its aperture. At the same time, the heterodyne (interference) scheme involving a narrowband light source eliminates, to a considerable extent, this restriction due to optical amplification. Eventually, the interference scheme allows one to obtain images of an object with the same signal-to-noise ratio as in confocal microscopy within time intervals shorter than those required in confocal microscopy. Additional advantages of the interference scheme, which stem from the coherence of light and the use of the amplitude response of an object under study, are associated with the appearance of a new mechanism of suppression of scattered light and the possibility of detecting smaller differences in the reflectivities of various tissue layers. It is expected that the integration of the approaches considered above in one microscope and the use of broadband (low-coherence) sources of light (see Chapter 9) may considerably improve the selectivity of the system, which is important for the investigation of nearly uniform tissues.[894,895]

Speckle interferometry using sharply focused laser beams and spatial averaging of optical signals also has advantages in the depth profiling of scattering objects. Using a speckle interferometer (see Fig. 4.7), glue-strippings of human skin attached to metal plates were investigated. Depth profiling of thin tissue layers with a subcellular resolution was obtained (see Fig. 8.34). This method allows one to estimate the thickness of tissue layers and the depth distribution of the refractive index. Appropriate transverse scanning of the object will give tomograms with a spatial resolution of about $3 \times 3 \times 3$ µm. The optical gain of this scheme and the possibility of using powerful lasers may allow one to obtain high values of signal-to-noise ratio.

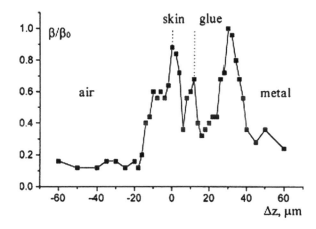

Figure 8.34 Depth profiling for glue-stripped human skin attached to a metal plate (dependence of the normalized modulation factor of the photoelectric signal β/β_0 on the longitudinal displacement of the sample).[837]

Technical developments in the different fields of optical microscopy are increasingly focusing on the *in vivo* and *in situ* imaging of metabolic functions and dysfunctions. The observation of the dynamics of biological processes on a microscale and a nanoscale is required for a more detailed understanding of both cellular physiology and pathology.

8.7 Interferential retinometry and blood sedimentation study

Laser interferential retinometers used for the monitoring of human retinal visual acuity are based on an optical dual-beam interferometer that forms two coherent beams that are focused onto the nodal plane N of the eye and form a spatially modulated laser beam (SMLB) with parallel interferential fringes on the retina (see Figs. 4.9 and 8.35).[5,832,847] The period L of the fringes and their orientation

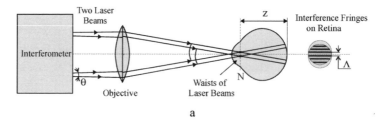

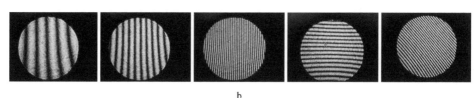

b

Figure 8.35 (a) Scheme of a laser interferential retinometer and (b) interference fringes of various spacings and orientations on a retina.[832]

depend on corresponding parameters of the incident SMLB[5] as

$$L = \frac{D\lambda}{2l},$$ (8.15)

where D is the mean distance between the eye nodal plane and retina, λ is the wavelength, and $2l$ is the separation between two point light sources formed in the nodal plane.

Normal retinal visual acuity is defined as an angular resolving power of the eye and is characterized by the density of interferential fringes per a degree of the view angle[5] as

$$N_{\text{int}} = \left[\arcsin\left(\frac{\lambda}{2l}\right) \right]^{-1}.$$ (8.16)

For the ideal conditions of the front media of the eyes, the fringe pattern contrast at the retina is very high, practically equal to unity because of the high degree of mutual coherence of the laser beams.

The procedure of estimation of retinal visual acuity is simple. First, a fringe pattern with a large period at the patient's retina is formed. The patient lets the doctor know that he/she is able to see a fringe pattern. Then, the period of the fringes is decreased and the patient must indicate his/her ability to see the pattern. This procedure is repeated until the patient is unable to see the pattern. To avoid false patient response, fringes can be rotated on an arbitrary angle [see Fig. 8.35(b)].

For patients with cataractous (turbid) lenses, the scattering of a spatially modulated laser beam by a turbid media prevents the creation of the fringe pattern [see Fig. 8.36(c)]. However, averaging of the interferential pattern may improve the visibility of the initial fringes (see Section 4.3) and, therefore, with this technique some limits may be applicable for retinal acuity estimations in eyes with cataract. The optical scheme presented in Fig. 8.36(a), where the SMLB is moving periodically by a deflector but fringes on the retina are unmovable, provides such an averaging. Some other averaging schemes are also available.[832]

Another example of SMLB application in medicine is the monitoring of the erythrocyte sedimentation rate (ESR). Usually, the test uses the measurement of the distance that erythrocytes have fallen after one hour in a vertical column of anticoagulated blood under the influence of gravity. The test is helpful in the specific diagnosis of several types of cases, including diabetes mellitus and myocardial infarction. The SMLB technique allows one to detect the temporal changes of the scattering properties of a blood suspension at its sedimentation. This method was used to investigate a highly diluted blood, i.e., to monitor the sedimentation of individual and weakly interacting erythrocytes, and was tested in clinical studies.

The experimental setup is presented in Fig. 8.37. A 633-nm He:Ne laser beam was expanded to a diameter of 10 mm; the interferometer created the parallel fringes in the illuminating beam. The piezodeflector was used to make dynamic fringes. The SMLB was positioned in order to incident vertically on a horizontally placed glass vessel with blood samples. The fringe contrast in the course of blood sedimentation was measured. At blood sedimentation, the scattering medium transits from a highly scattering to a low-scattering one due to a high degree of packing

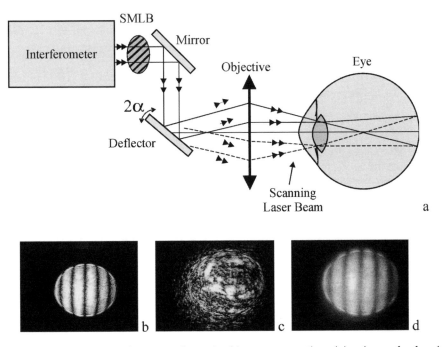

Figure 8.36 Observation of average intensity fringes on a retina: (a) scheme for forming average intensity fringes on a retina; (b) fringes for a clear lens; (c) pattern for a turbid lens; (d) average intensity fringes.[1248]

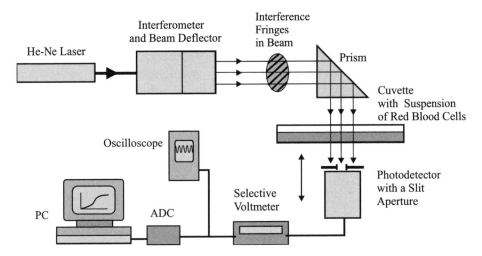

Figure 8.37 Laser system with a spatially modulated laser beam for the study of the dynamic scattering properties of a suspension of red blood cells during their spontaneous aggregation and sedimentation.[1249]

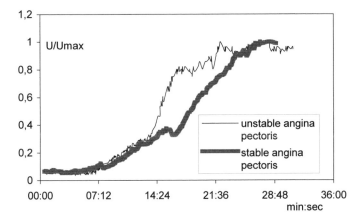

Figure 8.38 Temporal scattering characteristics of erythrocyte suspensions (whole blood diluted by saline as 1:200) at sedimentation process. Blood was taken from the patients with stable and unstable angina pectoris.[1249]

of the fallen erythrocytes; therefore, the contrast improves (see Fig. 8.38). Owing to the different properties of blood samples taken from patients with different stages of disease, the dynamic characteristics of contrast are different; therefore, contrast may serve as a diagnostic parameter.

9

Optical Coherence Tomography and Heterodyning Imaging

9.1 OCT

9.1.1 Introduction

A description of the fundamentals and basic principles of optical coherence tomography (OCT) can be found in Section 4.5. In Section 2.6, OCT is discussed as a method for tissue optical properties' measurements. Methods and data of measured absorption and scattering coefficients and refractive index are presented (see Table 2.1). The enhancement of OCT penetration depth and image contrast owing to the action of hyperosmotic optical clearing agents is given in Section 5.5.5 for skin, in Section 5.6.2 for gastric tissues, and in Section 5.8.2 for blood samples; and in Section 5.9.1, OCT glucose sensing is discussed. In this section, we will briefly give an overview of some typical OCT schemes and illustrate their biomedical applications.

9.1.2 Conventional (time-domain) OCT

A large number of schemes of coherent optical tomography for the investigation of tissues have been described in the literature, with overviews given.[1,3,8,13,17,18,28,45,76,77,84,102,108–111,116,126,127,129,135,136,138,139,141,142,343,717,775,865,901,902,909,931–939,1246,1247] Figure 9.1 presents one of the typical time-domain tomographic schemes based on a superluminescent diode (SLD) ($\lambda = 830$ nm, $\Delta\lambda = 30$ nm) and a single-mode fiber-optic Michelson interferometer.[717,904] The power of IR radiation on tissue surface is about 30 μW. The interference signal at the Doppler frequency, which is determined by the scanning rate of a mirror in the reference arm [see Eq. (4.53)], is proportional to the coefficient of reflection of the nonscattered component from an optical inhomogeneity inside the tissue. One can localize an inhomogeneity in the longitudinal direction by equalizing the lengths of the signal and reference arms of the interferometer within the limits of the coherence length of the light source (~ 10 μm) [see Eq. (4.54)]. The transverse resolution of a beam scanning along the surface of a sample is determined by the radius w_0 of the focal spot of the probing radiation (usually $w_0 \leq 20$ μm, which should be consistent with the required length of the probed area in the longitudinal direction, and is determined by the length

565

of the beam waist, $2n\pi w_0^2/\lambda_0$). Figure 5.30 displays OCT tomograms of human skin with psoriatic erythrodermia before and after topical application of glycerol.[717]

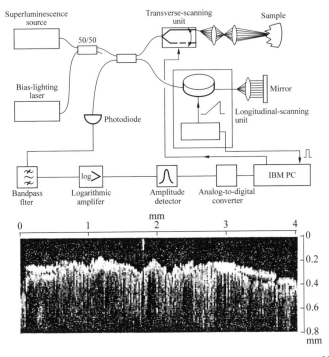

Figure 9.1 Diagram of a fiber-optic coherent optical tomograph.[904]

A scanning velocity of 50 cm/s is required to acquire images with a size of 2.5 × 4 mm (axial size × lateral size), resolution of 20 × 20 μm, and acquisition rate of 1 image/second.[717] The scanning velocity should be maintained constant with an accuracy of at least of 1% to confine the Doppler frequency signal within the detection band. Resonance properties of currently available mechanical scanning systems cannot guarantee constant velocity with the required accuracy throughout the modulation period. For OCT systems developed at the Institute of Applied Physics of the Russian Academy of Sciences, a longitudinal-scanning system is based on a fiber-optical piezoelectric converter (see Fig. 9.1).[717,904] This converter is capable of scanning the path length difference between the interferometer arms at the rate of 50 cm/s and up to 4 mm in depth. Its practically inertia-free response within the range of the amplitudes and modulation frequencies used substantially simplifies the detection of the informative signal at the Doppler frequency.

9.1.3 Two-wavelength fiber OCT

Sometimes multiwavelength images are very helpful in detecting an abnormality within the optically sampled tissue. The sensitivity and recognition range of such systems may be very high because the scattering and absorption properties of normal tissue and pathological inclusions may depend on the probing wavelength in different ways. It is very important to provide the acquiring of OCT images at different wavelengths simultaneously using the same interferometer and focusing system.[1250]

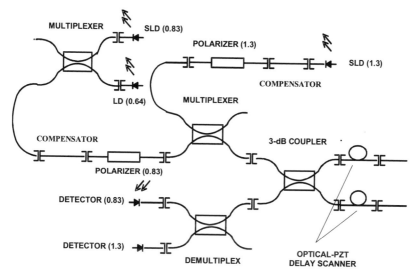

Figure 9.2 Schematic of a two-wavelength OCT.[1250]

The schematic of a two-wavelength fiber OCT system is shown in Fig. 9.2.[717,1250] Two SLDs with central wavelengths of 0.83 μm and 1.3 μm, spectral bandwidths of 25 nm and 50 nm (corresponding axial coherence lengths of 13 μm and 19 μm), and power of 1.5 and 0.5 mW, respectively, were used as light sources. The light from both SLDs was coupled to a Michelson interferometer. The incident radiation was split into two equal parts between the sample and reference arms by a fiber coupler with 3 dB of light separation at both wavelengths. The path length difference between the interferometer arms was modulated by a piezoelectric converter (see Fig. 9.1) providing in-depth scanning up to 3 mm. The most challenging problem of simultaneously compensating the wave dispersion for two different wavelengths in the interferometer arms was solved by inserting into one of the arms of the interferometer an additional piece of fiber whose dispersion properties were quite different from those of the principal fiber. The attained in-depth spatial resolution for the wavelengths 0.83 and 1.3 μm was 15 and 34 μm, respectively.

9.1.4 Ultrahigh resolution fiber OCT

The typical axial resolution of OCT imaging systems with such universally adopted broadband light sources as SLDs or mode-locked lasers varies from 10–15 μm

(SLD) to 4–5 µm (short-pulse laser sources such as organic-dye and Ti:sapphire lasers).[109,116,127,142] To provide significantly higher axial resolution (e.g., on the subcellular level), the broadband light sources covering a few hundred nanometers in the visible and NIR ranges are required. Such an ultrahigh-resolution OCT instrument for *in vivo* imaging is described in Ref. 1251. The optical scheme is presented in Fig. 9.3. A longitudinal resolution on the order of 1 µm was demonstrated for such a system; that is the highest OCT resolution achieved to date. A Kerr-lens mode-locked femtosecond Ti:sapphire laser was used as an illuminating source; it emitted sub-two-cycle pulses corresponding to bandwidths of up to 350 nm, with a center wavelength at 800 nm. Such high performance was achieved with specially designed double-chirped mirrors with a high-reflectivity bandwidth and controlled dispersion response, in combination with low-dispersion calcium fluoride prisms for intracavity dispersion compensation. A pair of fused-silica prisms and razor blades were used to spectrally disperse the laser beam and spectrally shape the laser output. The optical scheme of the low-coherence interferometer was optimized for the ultrabroad bandwidth of the illuminating source. Specially designed lenses with a 10-mm focal length and a numerical aperture of 0.30 in combination with single-mode fibers and special broadband fiber couplers were used. Polarization controllers were also used to exclude the broadening of the shape of the interference envelope due to polarization mismatch. Dispersion was matched by use of variable-thickness fused-silica and BK7 prism in order to reach a uniform group-delay dispersion. The ultrahigh-resolution OCT system was optimized to support optical spectra of up to 260 nm (FWHM), and a 1.5-µm longitudinal resolution in free space, corresponding to 1-µm resolution in tissue, was achieved.

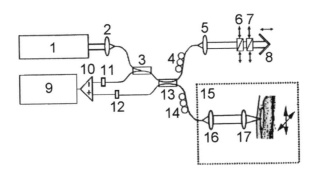

Figure 9.3 Ultrahigh resolution fiber OCT system with a Kerr-lens mode-locked Ti:sapphire laser:[1251] 1, KLM Ti:sapphire laser; 2, 5, 16, and 17, specially designed lenses; 3 and 13, special broadband fiber couplers; 4 and 14, polarization controllers; 6 and 7, dispersion-matching elements; 8, reference mirror; 9, computer-based data processing unit; 10, 11, and 12, dual balanced detector; 15, scanning system.

In vivo subcellular level resolution (1×3 µm; longitudinal $\times$ transverse) tomograms of an African frog tadpole (*Xenopus laevis*) were obtained to demonstrate the potential of the ultrahigh-resolution OCT instrument described above. The obtained images clearly depict multiple mesanchymal cells of various sizes and nuclear-to-cytoplasmatic ratios, the olfactory tract and intracellular morphology, as well as mitosis of several cells. It should be noted that high lateral resolution throughout the different depths has also been achieved.

9.1.5 Frequency-domain OCT

Frequency-domain, or Fourier-domain, OCT methods are based on backscattering spectral interferometry and, therefore, are also called spectral OCT.[109,116,127,142,919,934] One of the main advantages of this technique is that it does not require scanning in the depth of a sample. However, for a long time after the first demonstrations, it did not play a significant role among OCT methods. As it was noted in Ref. 934, this probably happened because sufficiently fast and sensitive CCD cameras were not available at the time. At present, it is clear that this technique has a great potential in terms of speed and sensitivity.[109,116,127,142,934,1252,1253] It demonstrates sensitivities that are two to three orders of magnitude greater than its time-domain counterpart.[1253,1254]

One of the first demonstrations of Fourier-domain OCT is described in Ref. 919. Figure 9.4 shows a diagram of the relevant experimental setup based on a Michelson interferometer and a high-resolution spectrometer (a spectral radar device), and the optogram of skin in a human arm measured *in vitro*. Since the spectral radar measures the amplitude of scattering $E(z)$ along the axis from the surface toward the inside of an object during a single exposition of a detector without longitudinal scanning of the beam, the time span of a tomogram recording may be very small. With allowance for the superposition of the object and reference fields on the detector, we can write the intensity of light in the following form:[919]

$$I(k) = |S(k)|^2 \int_0^\infty E(z)\cos(2kz)dz + \cdots, \qquad (9.1)$$

where k is the wave vector and $S(k)$ is the spectral distribution of the amplitude of the light source. Performing an inverse Fourier transform, we can find the dependence $a(z)$ of the scattering amplitude on the depth. Higher frequencies in the detected signal correspond to larger depths. We can estimate the maximum depth of probing based on the spectral resolution of the spectrograph. Specifically, for a spectrometer with a resolution of $\Delta\lambda = 0.05$ nm, we have $z_{max} = (1/4n)(\lambda_0^2/\Delta\lambda) \cong 2.4$ mm ($n = 1.5$, $\lambda_0 = 853$ nm). To ensure a signal-to-noise ratio at the level of 10^4, one should employ a highly sensitive CCD or CMOS camera at the output of the spectrometer.

Fourier-domain OCT can be also realized using a swept-laser source—a rapidly tunable laser over a broad optical bandwidth.[1254] In swept-source OCT, instead of CCD or photodiode arrays, a single photodiode in the detection path of the interferometer is employed, which allows the spectral interferometric signal to be encoded with a characteristic heterodyne beat frequency. It was shown that heterodyne de-

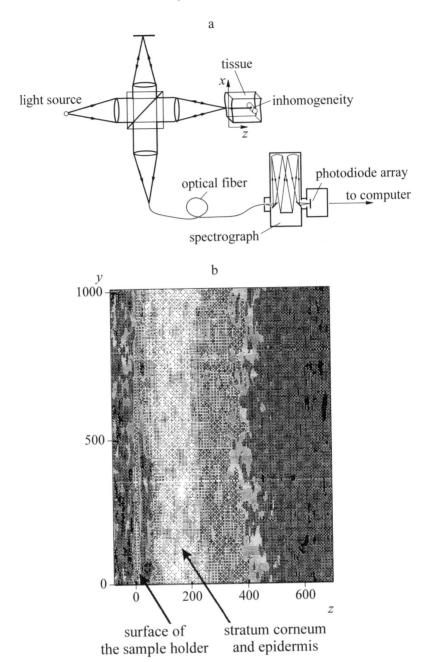

Figure 9.4 (a) Basic scheme of a spectral radar (spectral OCT) device with a source of light with a small coherence length.[919] (b) Optogram of skin in a human arm *in vitro*. The ordinate axis represents the lateral displacement over the arm surface in micrometers. The abscissa axis shows the depth of a tissue in micrometers.

tection in swept-source OCT allows for the resolution of complex conjugate am- biguity and the removal of spectral and autocorrelation artifacts, characteristic of spectral OCT.[1255]

9.1.6 Doppler OCT

Doppler OCT combines the Doppler principle with OCT to obtain high-resolution tomographic images of static and moving constituents in highly scattering biological tissues.[937] When light backscattered from a moving particle interferes with the reference beam, a Doppler frequency shift (f_{Ds}) occurs in the interference fringe,

$$f_{Ds} = \frac{2V_s n \cos \theta}{\lambda_0}, \qquad (9.2)$$

where V_s is the velocity of a moving particle, n is the refractive index of the medium that is surrounding the particles, θ is the angle between the particle flow and the sampling beam, and λ_0 is the vacuum center wavelength of the light source. The longitudinal flow velocity (velocity parallel to the probing beam) can be determined at discrete user-specified locations in a turbid sample by measurement of the Doppler shift. The transverse flow velocity can also be determined from the broadening of the spectral bandwidth due to the finite numeric aperture of the probing beam.[937]

Scanning of the reference mirror of the OCT system at velocity v produces a Doppler signal at frequency f_D, described by Eq. (4.53). Blood or lymph flow with velocity V_s produces another Doppler signal, described by Eq. (9.2). Therefore, the signal of the Doppler OCT is proportional to

$$A(t) \cos[2\pi(f_D - f_{Ds})t + \phi(t)], \qquad (9.3)$$

where $A(t)$ is the reflectivity and $\phi(t)$ is the phase shift defined by a scatterer position.

A fiber-optic Doppler OCT ($\lambda_0 = 850$ nm, $\Delta\lambda = 25$ nm, $P = 1$ mW) was employed for measurements of the blood flow velocity in a vessel located behind a strongly scattering layer and in a living object (vessel of rat mesentery).[908] This is a new approach to the investigation of directed blood flow in subsurface vessels under a layer of tissue.[908,926–930,937] Electronic data processing allows one to separate the signal that characterizes the amplitude of backward scattering, which is necessary to generate a stationary tomogram of an object from the Doppler signal, which characterizes the velocity of scatterers at a given point of an object. Figure 9.5 presents a structure image of a fragment of rat mesentery with an artery and two veins, images of the blood flow velocity in the artery and veins, and the velocity profile of the total blood flow.

9.1.7 Polarization-sensitive OCT

The specificity of conventional OCT can be improved by providing measurements of the polarization properties of the probing radiation when it propagates through a tissue. This approach was implemented in the polarization-sensitive OCT technique (PS OCT), which is described in detail in numer-

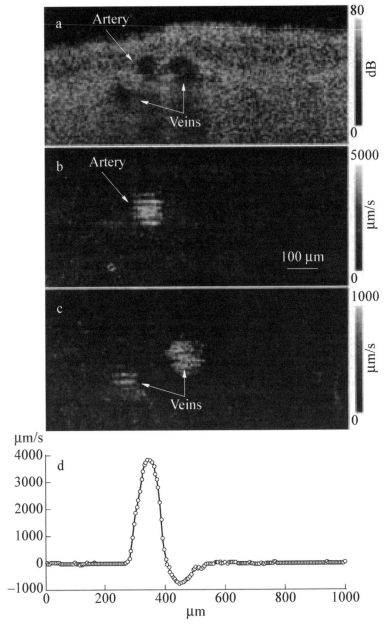

Figure 9.5 *In vivo* images of a fragment of rat mesentery: (a) Structure image (featuring an artery and two veins). (b) Image of the blood flow velocity in the artery. (c) Image of the blood flow velocity in veins. (d) Profile of the blood flow velocity measured at the depth of the artery [indicated with an arrow in Fig. 9.5(a)]. The negative peak on the right-hand side is related to the influence of the blood flow velocity in the vein.[908]

ous original papers,[412–424,913,1256–1258] and a few overview papers and book chapters.[127,135,142,717,936] Advanced PS OCT systems provide tissue imaging using Jones matrix[418] or Mueller matrix elements.[416]

In the majority of studies on PS OCT, the criterion of pathological changes in tissue is a measured decrease in tissue macroscopic birefringence. However, there is difficulty in providing correct measurements of birefringence at depths of more than 300–500 μm. For deeper layers (up to 1.5 mm), a much simpler variant of PS OCT known as cross-polarization OCT (CP OCT) can be employed.[717,913] Light depolarization caused by light scattering and tissue birefringence both lead to the appearance of a cross-polarized component in the backscattered light. Pathological processes are characterized by the changes in the amount of collagen fibers and their spatial organization. Therefore, a comparative analysis of cross-polarization backscattering properties of normal and pathological tissues may be used for early diagnosis of neoplastic processes.

The scheme of an experimental system for measuring conventional OCT and CP OCT images is shown in Fig. 9.6.[717,1256] Using a multiplexer (M), a low-coherence IR radiation from a SLD ($\lambda = 1.3$ μm and $l_c = 21$ μm) is combined with radiation from a red diode laser (RL) used for optical system alignment. One of the eigen polarization modes of a polarization maintaining (PM) 3-dB fiber coupler (FC) is selected by means of a polarization controller (CP). The PM fiber is used to transport radiation with a certain polarization state in both the signal and reference arms of the interferometer. When there is no Faraday rotator (F) in the reference arm, a copolarized component of backscattered radiation is recorded (conventional OCT is realized). The Faraday rotator performs a rotation to an arbitrary polarization state by a specified angle, and the direction of the rotation depends only on the direction of the magnetic field inside the rotator and does not depend on the propagation direction of the radiation. Therefore, in the case of the 45-deg Faraday rotator, the radiation passes through it, and being reflected by a mirror goes back through the rotator and becomes orthogonally polarized. As a result, only the cross-polarized component of the light backscattered by a

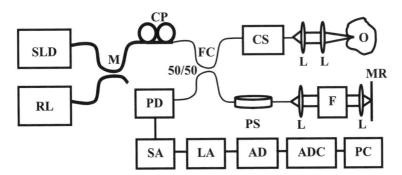

Figure 9.6 Experimental setup for cross-polarization OCT:[717,1256] SLD, superluminescence diode; RL, red diode laser; M, multiplexer; CP, polarization controller; FC, fiber coupler; CS, cross-sectional scanner; O, investigated object; PS, longitudinal piezoscanner; L, lenses; F, Faraday rotator; MR, reference mirror; PD, photodiode; SA, selective amplifier; LA, logarithmic amplifier; AD, amplitude detector; ADC, analog-to-digital converter; PC, personal computer. Bold line corresponds to single-mode fiber; thin line illustrates polarization maintaining fiber.

biological object would interfere with light from the reference arm. The acquisition time of one OCT image is 1 s. For all OCT images, a logarithmic intensity scale was used. The lateral resolution of the system, determined by the diameter of the probing beam in the focus, was chosen close to the axial (in-depth) resolution, which is determined by the coherence length and was 21 μm. Both types of images, conventional and cross-polarized, were obtained from the same tissue site.

Figure 9.7 demonstrates the facilities of the crossed-polarized imaging technique in comparison with a conventional one in the example of the imaging of *ex vivo* human esophagus scar tissue. It is well seen that in contrast to conventional OCT, the crossed-polarized image provides some additional structural information.

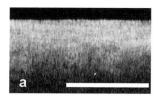 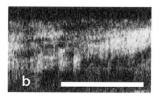

Figure 9.7 (a) Conventional OCT image of *ex vivo* human esophagus scar tissue. (b) The corresponding cross-polarized OCT image. White bar corresponds to 1 mm.[717,1256]

9.1.8 Differential phase-sensitive OCT

Differential phase-sensitive OCT (DPS OCT) provides quantitative dispersion data that are important in predicting the propagation of light through tissues, in photorefractive surgery, and in tissue and blood refractive index measurements.[142] Refractive index variations cause phase variations in the sample beam. One of the DPS OCT schemes is presented in Fig. 9.8.[1113] The probe beam is split by birefringent wedges and collimated by the sample lens. Two orthogonally oriented beams separated by x illuminate the sample. The backscattered beams are combined by the birefringent wedges and separated by the polarizing beamsplitter (Wollaston prism) in the detection arm. From the photodetector signals, three interferograms and their corresponding three images are obtained: two intensity images, and a phase difference image. Experiments have shown that measurements of angstrom/nanometer-scale path length change between the beams $[(\lambda/4\pi)\Delta\varphi]$ in clear and scattering media can be provided.[142,1113] The DPS OCT technique was demonstrated to be suitable for noninvasive, sensitive, and accurate monitoring of analyte concentrations, including glucose (see Section 5.9.1).[1113] Since DPS OCT detects phase contrast in the direction of beam separation, it detects phase gradients caused by transversal variations of the refractive index and/or the phase change on reflection at interfaces.[142]

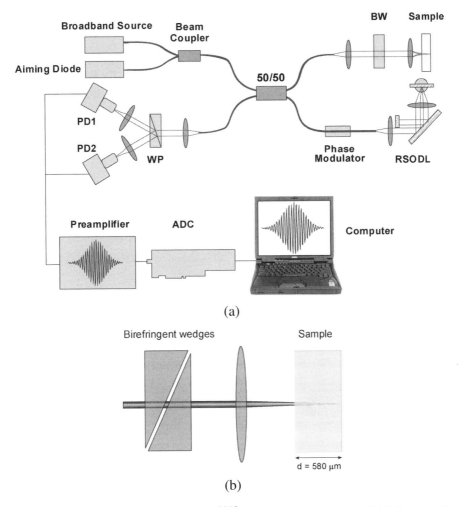

(a)

(b)

Figure 9.8 Phase-sensitive OCT system.[1113] (a) General scheme: WP, Wollaston prism; RSODL, rapid scanning optical delay line; PD, photodetectors; BW, birefringent wedges; ADC, analog-to-digital converter. (b) Sample arm.

9.1.9 Full-field OCT

Conventional time-domain OCT is a single-point detection technique. It can be used to generate two-dimensional OCT images up to video rates; however, such systems have a limited sensitivity or a limited space-bandwidth product (resolved pixels per dimension).[142] Full-field or parallel OCT uses linear or two-dimensional detector arrays of, respectively, N and N^2 single detectors. The advantage of parallel OCT is that the SNR when using linear or two-dimensional detector arrays can roughly be, respectively, $\sqrt{N}$ and N times larger, compared to the single detector signal. The disadvantages of using standard CCD sensors are connected with their time-integrating operation mode; therefore, no ac technique, mixing, or mode-lock detection are possible. To overcome these problems, synchronous illumination instead of the usual synchronous detection to obtain lock-in detection on every pixel of a CCD detector array or CMOS detector array can be used.[142] In the CMOS camera, each "smart pixel" consisting of photodetector and analog signal processing performs heterodyne detection in parallel, thus dramatically increasing the dynamic range compared to a CCD array. A corresponding two-dimensional "smart pixel detector array" that made it possible to record a data set of 58×58 pixels and 33 slices with an acquisition rate of 6 Hz is presented in Fig. 9.9.

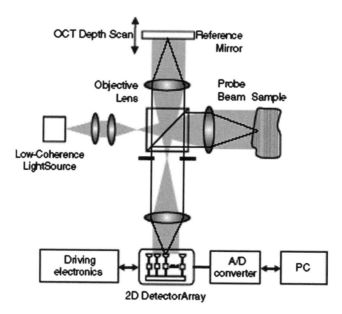

Figure 9.9 Parallel OCT setup with a two-dimensional 58×58 pixel CMOS detector array where each single detector performs heterodyne detection in parallel (Bourqin et al. 2001).[142]

To improve depth resolution, a thermal light source can be used.[142,1259,1260] A 100-W tungsten halogen thermal lamp in a modified Linnik microscope allowed a depth resolution of 1.2 μm to be obtained.[1259] Water immersion has been used to compensate dispersion; corresponding immersion-objective lenses with a NA of 0.3 provided a transverse resolution of about 1.3 μm. A three-dimensional OCT image of a *Xenopus laevis* tadpole eye has been synthesized from 300 tomographic images.

Contactless three-dimensional topology of the surface of human skin is necessary for the monitoring of wound and burn healing, observation of side effects of strong medicinal preparations, etc. Figure 9.10 shows a "coherent radar" based on a Michelson interferometer and a low-coherence light source [light-emitting diode (LED)].[919] Scanning the reference mirror in this device (with a scanning rate of 4 μm/s), one can obtain three-dimensional images of skin surface with a resolution within the limits of the coherence length of the light source. However, because the "coherent radar" has to scan the depth of the whole object with a limited velocity

(4 μm/s), the measuring time was long (about 150 s) and the field of illumination, in its turn limited by the power of the LED, was 7 × 10 mm. The influence of bulk scattering can be eliminated in this case if the skin is protected with a lightproof coating, e.g., graphite powder.[919]

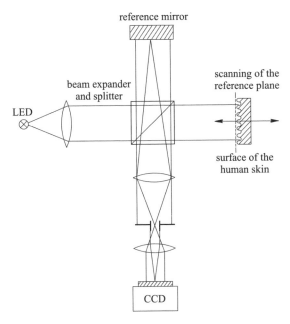

Figure 9.10 "Coherent radar" for the investigation of the three-dimensional topology of a skin surface.[919] LED, light-emitting diode; scanning of the reference plane is shown with the dashed line.

9.1.10 Optical coherence microscopy

Optical coherence microscopy (OCM) is a new biomedical modality for cross-sectional subsurface imaging of tissue combining the ultimate sectioning abilities of optical coherence tomography (OCT) and confocal microscopy (CM).[775,938] In OCM, spatial sectioning due to the tight focusing of the probing beam and pin-hole rejection provided by CM is enhanced by additional longitudinal sectioning provided by OCT coherence gating.

Figure 9.11 illustrates the results of a comparative study of imaging potential-ities of CM and full-field OCM.[1261] The significantly better quality of the recon-structed images was obtained in the latter case. The sample arm of the low-coherent interferometer consists of a high-speed scanning CM with a fast scanner (a reso-nant scanner or a rotating polygonal mirror) and a slow scanner (a galvanometric scanning mirror); the slow scanner was positioned at the image plane of the fast scanner. To exclude the mechanical scanning of the phase delay in the reference arm, a 40-MHz acoustooptic modulator (AOM) in combination with a fixed mirror was used for frequency shifting of the reference arm light due to double passage through AOM. In such a way, the reference arm length was fixed to match the optical path length of the sample arm. The setup was modified to CM by blocking the reference arm and detecting the dc centered signals from the sample arm. Both sets of images presented were recorded at eight frames per second with a polygonal mirror as a fast scanner. Each image is a single frame extracted from the video. Since the rotating polygonal mirror causes a path length change in the sample arm of the interferometer during the OCM image reconstruction, an additional frequency shift of the operating frequency of the AOM was introduced during the sample scanning. This shift was equal to 3 MHz from one side of the image to the other side. Thus, by moving the center frequency from 80 to 83 MHz, a full-field OCM image was captured.

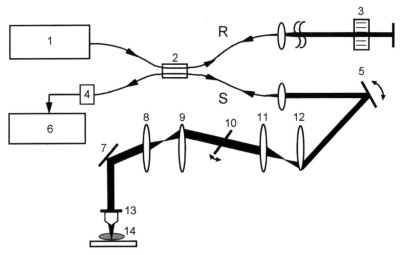

Figure 9.11 Optical scheme of a high-speed full-field optical coherence microscope:[1261] 1, low-coherence light source; 2, fiber-optical interferometer; 3, acoustooptic modulator; 4, detector; 5, resonant scanner; 6, computer-based data processing unit; 7, mirror; 8, 9, 11, and 12, lenses; 10, galvanometer; 13, microscope objective; 14, sample under study; R, reference arm; S, sample arm. By blocking the reference arm, this system can also be used as a confocal scanning microscope.

A compact OCM with a flexible sample arm and a remote optical probe for laboratory and clinical environments was developed.[775] To achieve an axial resolution of the cellular level, a light source with an effective bandwidth of 100 nm was used. The light source was comprised of two SLDs based on one-layer quantum-dimensional (GaAl)As heterostructures with shifted spectra. Radiations from both SLDs were coupled into a polarization-maintaining (PM) fiber by means of a multiplexer. The multiplexer was spectrally adjusted in order to achieve the minimum width of the autocorrelation function. The dynamic focusing was provided by scanning the output lens of the objective located at the very end of the sample arm. The lens movement was controlled by the electronic system, and aligning of the focal spot with the coherence gating during scanning up to depth of 0.5–0.8 mm into a tissue was provided. The spectral sidelobes, caused by nonuniformity of the light source spectrum, were suppressed.

9.1.11 Endoscopic OCT

Application of fiber-optical light-delivering and light-collecting cables allows one to build a flexible low-coherent imaging system providing the possibility of endoscopic analysis of human tissues and organs. In particular, an OCT system developed for endoscopic applications (high-speed *in vivo* intra-arterial imaging) is described in Ref. 907. A solid-state Cr^{+4}:Forsterite laser with Kerr lens mode locking was used as an illumination source with a median wavelength of 1280 nm and a bandwidth of 75 nm. Thus, the theoretical axial resolution of the system can be estimated as 10 μm [see Eq. (4.54)]; the actual depth resolution measured with a mirror as a standard technique for resolution evaluation gave an axial pixel size equal to 9.2 μm. The lateral resolution of this system, which depends on the spot size of the lens system used on the output tip of the light delivering fiber, was equal to 30 μm with the confocal parameter equal to 1.74 mm. Electronics allowed one to capture four frames per second for 512 transverse image pixels. The optical power incident on the imaged tissue was approximately 10 mW. The corresponding signal-to-noise ratio was 106 dB. The reference-arm phase-delay scanning device consisted of an oscillating galvanometer mirror, lens, and grating.

Various fiber-optical devices designed for endoscopic OCT imaging have been described.[717,1261] One of the examples is a fiber-optical scanning catheter used for intra-arterial imaging.[1261] Such a catheter consists of an optical coupling at its proximal end, a single-mode fiber as the light-delivering channel, and focusing and beam directing elements at the distal end. Beginning at the proximal end of the device, incident light from a fixed single-mode optical fiber is coupled through a narrow air gap into a second single-mode fiber that can rotate. The drive assembly of the catheter, located at the proximal end, uses an optical-fiber connector. A gear is attached to the connector and a shaft assembly, consisting of the connector, the fiber in the catheter, and the distal focusing elements. A dc motor is used to drive the shaft assembly through a gear mechanism. The beam is focused by a graded index lens and is directed by a microprism. The beam was scanned circumferentially by rotating the cable, fiber, and optical assembly inside the nonmovable housing. Power losses caused by suboptimal coupling and internal reflections within the catheter were 3–4 dB. For instance, an *in vivo* image of rabbit trachea, which was obtained with the described system, allows the differentiation between various tissue structures such as the pseudo-stratified epithelium, mucous, and surrounding hyaline cartilage.[1261]

A whole family of diagnostic endoscopic OCT devices suitable for studying different internal organs has been created.[1262] To probe the surface of an internal organ, a miniaturized electromechanical unit (optical probe) controlling and performing lateral scanning was developed. This probe is located at the distal end of the sample arm and its size provides fitting to the diameter and the curvature radius of standard biopsy channels of endoscopes. Figure 9.12(a) demonstrates the head of an endoscope for gastrointestinal investigations with the integrated OCT scanner.[717] A schematic diagram of the optical scanning probe and how it is positioned against a studied object is shown in Fig. 9.12(b). The probing beam is swung along the tissue surface with amplitude of 2 mm. The beam deviation system embodies the galvanometric principle, and the voltage with a maximum of 5 V is supplied to the distal end of the endoscope. The distance between the output lens and a sample varies from 5 to 7 mm; the focal spot diameter is 20 μm. The optical scanning probe and the part of the flexible sample arm that is inserted in the endoscope are both sealed; therefore, the conventional cleaning procedure and sterilization can be performed before applying the setup clinically. Implementation of an extended flexible arm of the OCT interferometer became feasible due to the use of polarization-maintaining fibers as a means for transportation of the low-coherence probing light. This allows the elimination of the polarization fading caused by polarization distortions at the sites of bending of the endoscope arm. The device features high-quality fiber polarizers and couplers. The "single-frame" dynamic range of the OCT scheme determined as the maximum variation of the reflected signal power within a single image frame attains 35–40 dB. With a scanning rate of 45 cm/s and the image depth of 3 mm (in free space units), an OCT image with 200 × 200 pixels is acquired in approximately 1 s. This acquisition rate is sufficient to eliminate the influence of moving of internal organs (moving artifact) on the image quality.

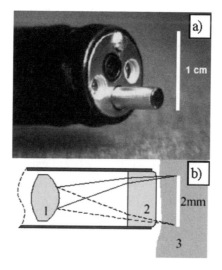

Figure 9.12 (a) Distal end of a gastroscope with OCT probe introduced through a biopsy channel.[717] (b) Schematic diagram of scanning unit: 1, output lens; 2, output glass window; 3, sample.

9.1.12 Speckle OCT

An original technique of coherent tomography that does not require transverse scanning and employs subject speckles is described in Ref. 906. Figure 9.13 shows a diagram of the experimental setup consisting of an SLD, mirror Mach-Zehnder interferometer, and a CCD camera. Radiation produced by the light source is focused onto the surface of an object. An incident light beam irradiates a surface at an angle of 45 deg. The light penetrates into the tissue and experiences scattering. Backscattered light emerges at the surface of the object. A fraction of this beam of light that propagates in the direction perpendicular to the surface of the sample is imaged by the CCD camera, where the beam is mixed with reference-wave radiation reflected from a mirror scanned with a constant rate. Observation of scattered light with an aperture of finite size gives subjective speckles in the image plane (the photosensitive surface of the CCD camera).

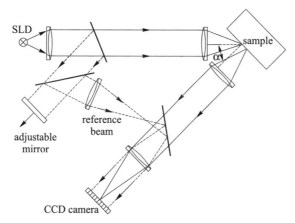

Figure 9.13 Coherent optical tomographic scheme based on subjective speckles.[906] SLD, superluminescent diode ($P = 4$ mW, $\lambda = 850$ nm, and $l_c = 30$ μm); α is the angle of radiation incidence on the surface of a sample.

In the case when partially coherent light is employed, one should consider different groups of photons passing through the image plane P_i. Each of these groups consists of photons that have traveled a definite path length $l_i \pm l_c$. Correspondingly, these photons produce their own coherent speckle pattern with intensity distribution $S_i(x, y)$. The resulting speckle pattern is produced by the incoherent superposition $\sum S_i$ of different speckle patterns. To locate regions inside an object from which photons with a definite path length $L = l_i$ come, one should superimpose a reference wave with the corresponding path length L. Then, only the photons from the chosen group P_i will ensure the required contrast V_I, which should be measured. Two sequential exposures are required to measure V_I. After the first exposition, the phase of the field in the reference beam is shifted by π, and exposure is repeated. The incoherent component remains unchanged in these two exposures and can be easily subtracted. Note that the sizes of subjective speckles should be adapted to the sizes of the pixels of the CCD camera. The maximum contrast is achieved when the coherence length l_c is as large as possible for a given resolution.

In an image processed in such a way, dark spots or speckle modulation of the surface image will be caused by the partial components of the scattered field that have run the same path length, but along different individual paths. A particular feature of the recorded image is a sharply curved edge of the impulse response, the "photon horizon." This curve defines the maximum penetration depth in the analyzed scattering system for each reference path length. Thus, different penetration depths can be visualized by a suitable adjustment of the reference path length. Figure 9.14 shows the character of these images obtained with different light sources.

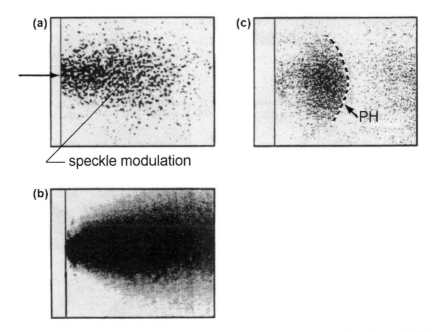

Figure 9.14 Images of the scattering process with different coherence lengths and different kinds of observation:[906] (a) Fully coherent illumination, direct observation. (b) Broadband illumination, direct observation. (c) Broadband illumination, extraction of the coherent part; dashed line shows the position of the "photon horizon" (PH).

The path-length resolution for this system is determined by the coherence length l_c of the light source used, and for a source with $l_c = 30$ μm, the resulting time resolution is about 100 fs.[906] The main advantage of this scheme is that the generation of a two-dimensional $(x - z)$ tomogram does not require transverse scanning of the beam. Being applied for the imaging of macroscopically inhomogeneous scattering phantoms and human skin *in vivo*, the "photon horizon" detection technique has demonstrated promising results.[1263] In the case of human skin, smaller exposure times are required than for a motionless scattering system because of the time integration of speckle-modulated images during the exposure. An exposure time of 40 ms is enough to provide adequate quality of "photon horizon" images of human tissues.

On the basis of the obtained results, it can be concluded that "photon horizon" detection makes it possible to get 2D surface images of strongly scattering media with a resolution better than 10 fs and in-depth range up to 350 μm. This gives the possibility to use such low-coherence imaging technique for the detection of pathological alterations of human skin (e.g., melanoma maligna).

The speckle OCT method was shown recently as an alternative to the Doppler OCT in 2D imaging of blood flow.[1186] Flow information can be extracted using speckle fluctuations in conventional amplitude OCT. Time-varying speckle is manifested as a change in OCT image spatial speckle frequencies. It was shown that over a range of velocities, the ratio of high to low OCT image spatial frequencies has a linear relation to flow velocity and that method is sensitive to blood flow of all directions without phase information needed. Using speckle OCT, 2D images of blood flow distributions for *in vivo* hamster skin were received.[1186]

9.2 Optical heterodyne imaging

Coherent heterodyne optical detection offers the following advantages over direct detection methods:[1,3,28,894,895,939,1212–1214,1264–1270]

- It has the highest sensitivity of any detection technique; the signal-to-noise ratio is several orders of magnitude better than that which can be achieved by incoherent methods.
- The extraordinary dynamic range, about 15 orders or more in magnitude of signal power for Hz-order bandwidths can be realized.
- Excellent selectivity or filtering capability in frequency domain and polarization.
- High spatial resolution, up to 60–80 lines per mm (with confocal optical arrangement).
- Substantial spatial selectivity or filtering capability due to highly directional antenna properties.
- It allows quantification of new tissue parameters by detecting the wavefront degradation within a given tissue.

The quantum limit of optical detection corresponds to the signal-limited shot noise when one employs a conventional photoelectronic detector. The minimal detectable signal power is given by[1266]

$$P_{\min} = h\nu B_{\mathrm{d}}/\eta_{\mathrm{q}}, \qquad (9.4)$$

where $h\nu$ is the photon energy, B_{d} is the detection bandwidth, and η_{q} is the quantum efficiency of the detector. In the case of the direct detection technique, this limit is impossible to reach. Only the optical heterodyning detection and photon-counting methods allow one to realize this standard quantum detection limit.

The field of view of an optical heterodyne system that has an effective aperture A for signals at wavelength λ arriving within a single main antenna lobe expressed as a solid angle is defined by[1266]

$$\Omega \cong \lambda^2 / A. \tag{9.5}$$

The antenna properties afford high spatial resolution for the detection and ranging of various bioobjects and their image formation, and excellent directionality to distinguish one specific direction from another.

Owing to these important features, which make it possible to detect and image very weak signals embedded in or hidden by appreciably large optical noise or background, the optical heterodyning technique has a good outlook for applications in tissue spectroscopy and imaging.[1,1264–1268] The coherent detection imaging (CDI) method based on the optical heterodyne detection technique was established in 1989 by Inaba (see Refs. 1 and 3). The CDI is a coherence gating method that discriminates the forward multiply scattering beam, preserving the direct geometrical correlation with the incident light beam, from the diffuse component of the transmitted light, which generally loses the properties of the incident beam, such as coherence, direction, and polarization due to multiple scattering.

The optical heterodyne detection method operates on the principle of mixing two optical waves at different frequencies [$(\omega_0 + \omega_1)$ and $(\omega_0 + \omega_2)$, where ω_0 is the optical frequency, ω_1 and ω_2 are radio modulation frequencies], on a square-law detector such as photodiode (see Fig. 9.15). The signal generated by the photodetector is the cross-product of the two optical fields as signal,

$$\sqrt{I_1(t, x, y)} \sin[(\omega_0 + \omega_1)t + \phi(t, x, y)], \tag{9.6}$$

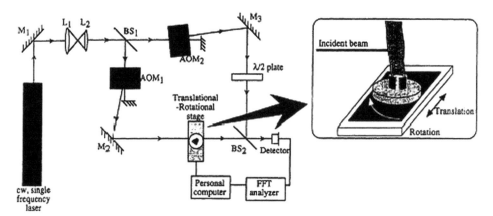

Figure 9.15 Schematic of a coherent detection imaging (CDI) system.[1267] L_1 and L_2, collimating lenses; M_1, M_2, and M_3, antireflection coated mirrors; BS_1 and BS_2, beam splitters, AOM_1 and AOM_2, acoustooptic modulators. The insert is a schematic of the finger mounted on the scanning apparatus.

and local oscillator,

$$\sqrt{I_2}\sin[(\omega_0+\omega_2)t], \qquad (9.7)$$

and can be expressed as

$$\sim\sqrt{I_1(t,x,y)}\sqrt{I_2}\cdot\sin[(\omega_1-\omega_2)t+\phi(t,x,y)], \qquad (9.8)$$

where $\sqrt{I_1(t,x,y)}$ and $\sqrt{I_2}$ are the amplitudes of the signal and local oscillator waves; t, x, and y are the temporal and spatial coordinates; and $\phi(t,x,y)$ is the spatially and time-dependent phase shift caused by the spatial and temporal fluctuations of refraction of the tissue under investigation.

The signal amplitude is subject to temporal and spatial fluctuations caused by time-dependent and spatially dependent attenuation of light by the tissue. The attenuated intensity of the signal wave by a tissue of thickness $d(t,x,y)$ can be calculated as [see Eq. (1.1)]

$$I_1(t,x,y)\approx I_{10}\exp[-\mu_t(t,x,y)d(t,x,y)], \qquad (9.9)$$

where I_{10} is the intensity of the signal wave incident at the object and $\mu_t(t,x,y)$ is the distribution of the attenuation coefficient.

The typical scheme of a CDI system is shown in Fig. 9.15. The well-collimated optical beam of a CW, single-frequency laser [Ar (514.5 nm), He:Ne (633 nm), Kr (647.1 nm), Ti:Al$_2$O$_3$ (tuned in the range 700–1000 nm) or a diode pumped Nd:YAG (1064 and 1319 nm)] with a power of about a few dozens of milliwatts is split into signal and local oscillator beams. The local oscillator beam and the signal beam are frequency shifted (modulated) by a pair of acoustooptic modulators to 80 and 80.05 MHz, respectively. The signal beam (about 0.8 mm in diameter), after passing through the object (a human finger) is mixed with the local oscillator beam at a silicon photodiode generating a signal at an intermediate frequency (IF) (the beat signal) [see Eq. (9.8)]. The IF signal is then fed to a fast Fourier transform analyzer that is interfaced to a personal computer. The dynamic range of the system, defined as P_{sat}/P_{min}, where P_{sat} is the optical power at which the detector is saturated and P_{min} is the minimal detected optical power, is about 140 dB. It should be noted that the signal power is proportional to the amplitude of the IF signal over the entire dynamic range of the heterodyne system. Very low optical power on the order of 10^{-17} W at a wavelength of 800 nm and a detection bandwidth limited to a few hertz could be detected.

Using the described CDI system, two-dimensional (projection) imaging was successfully performed for various *in vitro* and *in vivo* biological objects such as chicken legs and eggs, human tumor specimens, human teeth, animal bones, the head of an infant mouse, and a human finger.[1,1266–1268] The spatial resolution of the system is in the range 0.3 to 0.5 mm, depending on the optical and scanning arrangement. As an example, Figs. 9.15 and 9.16 illustrate the application of a CDI system for the tomographic study of a healthy human volunteer's finger. The index finger is mounted on a translational-rotational stepping motor stage (as shown in the insert of Fig. 9.15). The base of the finger was lightly bound with a silicon tube to reduce blood flow to the finger surface. This procedure was essential, especially when imaging at 715 nm, to minimize the influence of the Doppler effect on the IF signal caused by surface blood flow. The image displayed in Fig. 9.16(a) was reconstructed using 30 projections. Data for each projection consist of the averaged (32 times) amplitude of the IF signal for every 0.5-mm step of the translational scan across the finger joint. Averaging of the IF signal was necessary to minimize the speckle effect. After each translational scan, the finger was rotated by 6 deg and the translational scan was repeated. The finger was rotated by 180 deg for each data set. The data processing was carried out by the filtered back-projection method used in x-ray computed tomography (CT) image reconstruction.

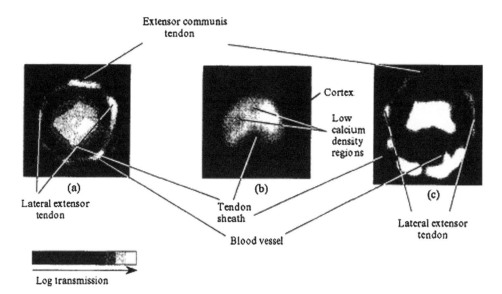

Figure 9.16 Computed tomographic images at the joint region corresponding to the head of the proximal phalanx of a healthy human index finger:[1267] (a) Laser CT image obtained with a Nd:YAG laser operating at 1064 nm. (b) Hard x-ray CT image. (c) MRI (T_1-weighted) image.

In Fig. 5.16, the CDI laser tomographic image of the finger (at the joint region corresponding to the head of the proximal phalanx) obtained at 1064 nm, as well as reference images obtained by conventional methods such as hard x-ray CT and magnetic resonance imaging (MRI), are shown. The diameter of the finger at the measurement plane was $\sim$14 mm and the incident power was $\sim$25 mW. Data for each image were collected during $\sim$25 min. The slice thickness of the x-ray and MRI images was 5 and 3 mm, respectively; whereas for the CDI images it was estimated as $\sim$0.5 mm. The use of a 2D heterodyne detector array would have helped through increased transverse resolution and reduced measurement time.[1267]

Because of the limited known data on the optical properties of human finger tissue components, it is difficult to identify all the structures in the CDI images. However, in comparison with x-ray and MRI images, some additional substructures are seen in the laser CDI images, which could correspond to ligaments, tendon sheath, etc. The usage of the ratio of images obtained at different wavelengths, as is widely employed in diffusion optical tomography, could help in identifying these substructures. A wavelength-dependent CDI should be able to provide both structural and functional information of the human finger and can be used for the early diagnosis of rheumatic arthritis, as was recently shown by utilization of another optical method.[1269] However, it should be noted that earlier optical tomographic studies of the human hand, which were done by the use of the CW[1269] and time-resolved (photon density waves)[502] imaging techniques, did not allow one to have as high a spatial resolution as that provided by the CDI method.

A method for real-time direct measuring of the mean square of the heterodyne beat amplitude (IF) and its proportionality to the overlap of the Wigner phase space distributions for a local oscillator and signal fields was demonstrated in Refs. 939 and 1270; such distributions give maximum information on the scattered field for imaging applications. A dynamic range of the experimental setup (see Fig. 9.17) of more than 13 orders of magnitude for a laser power of only 2 mW was realized. By increasing the local oscillator and input beams' power to 10 mW, a dynamic range of 15 orders is expected. The setup of the heterodyne experiments employs an He:Ne laser beam that is split into a 1-mW local oscillator (LO) and a 1-mW beam input to the sample. The beam transmitted through the sample is mixed with the LO at a 50×50 beamsplitter (BS2). Technical noise is suppressed by employing a standard balanced detection system.[939] The IF signal at 6 MHz is measured with an analog spectrum analyzer, the output signal of which was squared using a low-noise multiplier. A lock-in amplifier allows subtraction of the mean square signal

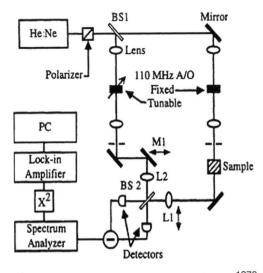

Figure 9.17 Heterodyne detection scheme.[1270]

and noise voltages with the input beam on and off. In this way, the real-time measurements of the mean square beat amplitude, $|V_B|^2$, were provided. Information about the Wigner phase space distribution of the transmitted light was obtained by measuring the beat intensity as a function of the shift in the LO center position (by translating mirror M1) and transverse momentum (angle) (by translating lens L1). The detector was in the Fourier plane of lenses L1 and L2, so that the LO position was fixed in the detection plane. The spatial resolution of the system was determined by the spatial width and diffraction angle of the LO.

The model experiments, which were performed by the authors of Ref. 939, provided a better understanding of the tomographic studies done by Inaba and coworkers for living tissues,[1266–1268] in particular, by linking the amplitude of the IF signal with tissue density and its coefficient of absorption. The beat intensity for propagation of a Gaussian beam through an Intralipid solution at fixed positions of the mirror M1 and the lens L1 corresponding to the maximal signal as a function of Intralipid solution concentration is shown in Fig. 9.18. The data clearly exhibit an initial rapid exponential decline with concentration, followed by a slower nonexponential decline. The spatial measurements showed that the fast decline corresponds to the transmission of the Gaussian beam, while the slower decline arises from a multiple scattering contribution. Using the concept of the Wigner phase space distributions, it was shown for a Gaussian input beam with a diffraction angle of about 1 mrad that at low Intralipid concentrations the amplitude of the beat signal decays exponentially due to absorption and scattering as

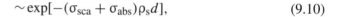

$$\sim \exp[-(\sigma_{\text{sca}} + \sigma_{\text{abs}})\rho_s d], \tag{9.10}$$

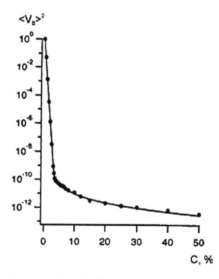

Figure 9.18 Beat intensity versus Intralipid concentration $(C \sim \rho_s)$ in percent of 10% Intralipid solution in pure water, for 0.5-μm average particle size and a sample length of 1 cm.[1270]

where σ_{sca} and σ_{abs} are the scattering and absorption cross sections, respectively, ρ_s is the particle concentration, and d is the sample thickness. At an intermediate Intralipid concentration, when a transmitted beam broadens due to multiple scattering, the beat intensity must drop as

$$\sim \rho_s^{-2} \exp(-\sigma_{abs}\rho_s d). \tag{9.11}$$

At high concentrations, the scattering light distribution becomes isotropic and the beat intensity decay is defined mainly by the absorption as

$$\sim \exp(-\sigma_{abs}\rho_s d). \tag{9.12}$$

One expects that this simple picture will break down at a sufficiently high concentration, when the diffusion photon path is substantially larger than the thickness of the sample.

9.3 Summary

Thus, a brief review of the optical schemes of coherence tomographs and topographs demonstrates the possibilities of these instruments for the investigation of tissues. Despite the continuing development of OCT and the search for advanced tomographic schemes, the area of medical applications of OCT in its present form is continually growing. Currently, this area includes analysis of damaged skin zones of patients suffering from psoriasis, erythematosus lupus, scleroderma, and malignant melanoma; investigation of postburn keloid cicatrices and vascularization of subepidermal skin layers; monitoring of laser ablation of tissues; imaging of brain tissues and fundus of the eye; imaging of hard and soft tissue of the oral cavity; investigation of the mucous membrane of inner organs, etc.[1,3,8,13,17,18,28,45,76,77,84,102,108–111,116,126,127,129,135,136,138,139,141,142,343,717,775,865,901,902,909,931–939,1246,1247]

Conclusion

This tutorial deals only with some aspects of light-tissue interactions, being focused on noncoherent and coherent light scattering by random and quasi-ordered structures. The considered methods and presented results allow us to make certain conclusions and assumptions concerning the directions of further investigations and the development of laser diagnostic and other medical systems.

Results of numerous studies on light scattering emphasize the necessity of an in-depth evaluation of the optical properties of tissues with different structural organization. At present, light propagation in tissues is fairly well described in qualitative (and sometimes in quantitative) terms, which provides a sound basis for the implementation of different diagnostic, therapeutic, and surgical modalities. At the same time, the estimation of optimal irradiation doses or the choice of correct diagnostic clues sometimes presents great difficulty because of the lack of reliable criteria for the optical parameters of tissues.

Traditional spectrophotometry or angular and polarization measurements are useful to characterize tissues, but need to be improved if more sophisticated tissue models are to be obtained and applied to biomedical studies. Such models must take into consideration the spatial distribution of scatterers and absorbers, their polydisperse nature, and optical activity, along with the birefringence properties of the materials of which scatterers and base matter consist.

It is also necessary to further develop methods for the solution of inverse scattering problems with due regard for the real geometry of the object and the laser beam, which might be equally valid for the arbitrary ratio of the scattering and absorption coefficients. The inverse MC method is sometimes useful, but the fast computations required for practical medical diagnostics and dosimetry should be based on approximate solutions of the radiative transport equations.

Extensive studies are under way to better understand the role of photon-density waves and their use in phase modulation methods to obtain optical characteristics of tissues. They are expected to bring about novel algorithms for the reconstruction of three-dimensional tissue images and practical applications of diffuse optical tomography.

The polarization properties of tissues to which this tutorial is largely devoted are of primary importance for physiological polarization optics and early skin and epithelial cancer diagnostics. The scattering matrix technique has long been used in optics and is currently applied by many authors to investigate the properties of tissues and cell suspensions. The intensity matrix (Mueller matrix) is normally employed for this purpose, but the use of two-frequency lasers (e.g., a Zeeman laser) or quadruple-channel OCT allows amplitude matrix elements to be measured, thus offering the possibility to simplify the inverse problem solution for many biological structures.

The designing of laser optoacoustic, acoustooptic, and optothermal imaging systems can be considered as a very prospective direction in biomedical optics that allows one to provide an impressive contrast and resolution in the imaging of both deep and superficial small tumors. It seems that these techniques should be optimal for the diagnosis of tissues at the middle depths (3 to 10 mm), where time-resolved diffusion and OCT methods are not effective.

Optical speckle techniques, in particular, the methods based on partially developed speckles emerging from the diffraction of focused beams, offer much promise for the investigation of the structure of tissues and the analysis of vibrations and motility (blood and lymph flow). The development of these techniques requires detailed research into the optics of speckles, speckle statistics, and the interference of light beams in dense scattering media.

Coherent optical methods are promising candidates for the development of new high-resolution and high-performance tomographic techniques allowing the imaging of subcellular structural and functional states of a tissue. Currently, investigation of superficial tissue layers with the use of optical coherent tomography (OCT) can provide important results and offer much promise for medical applications, especially for ophthalmology, early cancer detection of skin and the cervix, blood microcirculation analysis, and the endoscopic study of blood vessel wall and mucous of internal organs.

Methods based on the dynamic scattering of light are useful for the analysis of both weakly scattering and dense biological media. Many of these methods have already found their specific areas of biomedical applications. Considerable progress can be achieved with the use of the method of diffusion wave spectroscopy.

Heterodyne and homodyne interferometry, including speckle interferometry, has a wide range of biomedical applications. Laser Doppler blood flow and vibration measurements in tissues and organs are the most advanced field of applications for such techniques. The well-known advantages of confocal microscopy are very useful for the investigation of tissues and cells. Many coherent techniques and devices of medical diagnostics successfully employ the confocal principle of optical sectioning of an object under study. Two-photon and second-harmonic generation microscopies provide additional new possibilities in studying tissues and cells.

The optical immersion technique allows one to effectively control the optical properties of tissues and blood. Such control leads to an essential reduction of scattering and therefore causes much higher transmittance (optical clearing) and the appearance of a large amount of least-scattered (snake) and ballistic photons, allowing for the successful application of coherent-domain and polarization imaging techniques. It has great potentiality for noninvasive medical diagnostics using OCT due to the rather small thickness of tissue layers usually examined by OCT, which allows for fast impregnation of a target tissue at a topical application of an immersion liquid. It has been demonstrated that the body's interior tissues such as the blood vessel wall, esophagus, stomach, cervix, and colon can usually be imaged at a depth of about 1–2 mm. For more effective diagnosis using OCT, a higher penetration depth can be provided by the application of immersion substances. Evidently, reversible tissue optical clearing technology has valuable features to be applied not only to tissue spectroscopy and diagnostics, but also to a variety of laser and photothermal therapies and surgeries.

Glossary 1. Physics, Statistics, and Engineering

Abbe refractometer: an instrument for direct determination of the refractive index that uses the internal total reflection.

aberration: in optics this term is applied to certain defects in images formed in optical systems; aberration may be spherical, e.g., if the aperture of a concave spherical mirror (lens) is large, the rays at the periphery are brought to focus nearer the mirror than those rays which meet the mirror near the pole, giving a curve known as the caustic; the aberration in the case of lenses may also be **chromatic** when if the light contains more than one wavelength, e.g., white light, dispersion takes place, and since the lens is a series of small prisms the image will therefore be colored.

absolute (Kelvin) scale: a thermodynamic temperature scale in which the lower fixed point is absolute zero and the interval is identical with that on the Celsius scale.

absolute temperature: a temperature measured on an absolute scale.

absorbance: the ratio of the absorbed light intensity to the incident intensity; it is a dimensionless quantity.

absorbing medium: the medium that absorbs light at certain wavelengths or wavelength bands.

absorption: the transformation of light (radiant) energy to some other form of energy, usually heat, as the light transverses matter.

absorption band: a range of wavelengths for which a medium absorbs more strongly than at adjacent wavelengths.

absorption center: a particle or molecule that absorbs light.

absorption coefficient: in a nonscattering sample, the reciprocal of the distance d over which the light of intensity I is attenuated (due to absorption) to $I/e \approx 0.371$; the units are typically cm^{-1}.

absorption spectrum: the spectrum formed by light that has passed through a medium in which light of certain wavelengths was absorbed.

alternating current (ac): an electric current that reverses direction at regular intervals, having a magnitude that varies continuously in a sinusoidal manner.

acceptance angle: the maximum incident angle at which an optical fiber will transmit light by total internal reflection.

acoustic detector: a transducer that transforms an acoustic signal to an electrical one, such as a **microphone** or **piezoelectric transducer**; wideband piezoelectric transducers, being low-noise detectors, have proven to be most suitable for tissue spectroscopy and tomography.

acoustic (sound) waves: waves produced by a vibrating system that indexes the particles of the medium that vibrate in the same direction as the progress of the wave; successive points of high (compressions) and low (rarefactions) pressures are formed because of the regular impulses from the vibrating source; sound waves may be longitudinal progressive, longitudinal stationary, or transverse stationary; when sound is propagated through a medium (gas, liquid, or solid) it is transmitted by progressive longitudinal waves in that medium; sound waves interact with a complex and/or moving medium with their damping, refraction, diffraction, interference, and/or Doppler shift in frequency.

acoustooptical (AO) interaction (effect): the interaction of ultrasound and light beams within a homogeneous or inhomogeneous medium that occurs through a change in optical properties of the medium resulting from its compression by the ultrasound.

acoustooptical modulator: a device for intensity modulation of light at certain audio or radio frequencies using the acousto-optical effect.

acoustooptical tomography (AOT): optical tomography that is based on the acoustic [ultrasound (US)] modulation of coherent laser light traveling in tissue; an **acoustic wave** (AW) is focused into tissue and laser light is irradiating the same volume within the tissue; any light that is encoded by the ultrasound contributes to the imaging signal; axial resolution along the acoustic axis can be achieved with US-frequency sweeping and subsequent application of the Fourier transformation, whereas lateral resolution can be obtained by focusing the AW.

acquisition rate: the rate of acquiring experimental data.

acquisition time: the period of time of acquiring experimental data.

adaptive finite element method: a **finite element method**, where discretion of the underlying spatial domain (usually in two or three space dimensions) and establishment of discrete equations is done using an adaptive mesh refinement approach accounting for the complex structure of the object.

adding-doubling method: see **inverse adding-doubling (IAD) method**.

adiabatic expansion: a curve of pressure against volume, representing an adiabatic change (curves of equal **entropy**); these lines always slope more steeply than the isothermals they cross.

albedo: the ratio of scattering to the extinction cross section (or coefficient); ranges from zero for a completely absorbing medium to unity for a completely scattering medium.

algorithm: a procedure (a finite set of well-defined instructions) for accomplishing some task which, given an initial state, will terminate in a defined end-state; the computational complexity and efficient implementation of the algorithm are important in computing, and this depends on suitable data structures.

amplifier: an electronic (or optical) circuit that increases the voltage (or light power) of a signal fed into it by obtaining power from an external supply.

amplitude scattering matrix (S-matrix or Jones matrix): consists of four elements (the complex numbers) and provides a linear relationship between the incident and scattered field components; each element depends on scattering and azimuthal angles, and optical and geometrical parameters of the scatterer; both field amplitude and phase must be measured to quantify the amplitude scattering matrix.

analyzer: a **polarizer** that is placed in front of the detector.

anhydrous: having no water (for crystal, no water of crystallization).

angstrom (Å): a unit of length equal to 10^{-8} meter (m).

anisotropic crystal: a crystal for which some physical properties (mechanical, optical, magnetic, electrical, and etc.) are dependent on direction (not density and specific **heat capacity**); for example, for light propagation in transparent crystals (excluding crystals with cubic lattice) the light undertakes **birefringence** with mutually orthogonal polarization of rays propagating in different directions; for crystals with hexagonal, trigonal, and tetragonal structures (quartz, ruby, and calcite) birefringence is maximal along the direction that is perpendicular to the main axis of symmetry and is absent along this axis.

anisotropic scattering: a scattering process characterized by a clearly apparent direction of photons that may be due to the presence of large scatterers.

anode: a positive electrode that attracts anions (negative ions) during electrolysis.

antenna properties of the optical heterodyne system: the narrow field of view that provides a high spatial resolution for detection and ranging of the medium under study and its image formation.

anti-Stokes-Raman scattering: a photon interacts with a molecule in a higher vibrational level; the energy of the Raman scattered photons is higher than the energy of the incident photons.

aperture: the diameter of a circle through which light is allowed to pass; apertures may be varied and stated as fractions of the focal length, e.g., $f/6$ means that the diameter of the lens (aperture) is $1/6$ of the focal length f.

Ar (argon) laser: a laser with a lasing medium composed of ionized argon gas; the emission is mostly in the UV and visible ranges: (336.6–363.8) nm, 454.5 nm, 457.9 nm, 488 nm, 514 nm, and 528.7 nm.

arc lamp: a lamp that uses a luminous bridge formed in a gap between two conductors or terminals when they are separated.

artifact: (in microscopy) a structure that is seen in a tissue sample under a microscope but not in living tissue; may be caused by incorrect sample preparation or placement of the sample under the microscope.

A-scan: in-depth scanning perpendicular to the sample surface.

asymmetry parameter (skewness): a measure of asymmetry in a probability distribution function.

attenuated total reflectance Fourier transform infrared spectroscopy (ATR FTIR) method: based on a combination of the **total internal reflection** technique and Fourier transform infrared spectroscopy.

attenuation: a decrease in energy per unit area of a wave or beam of light: it occurs as the distance from the source increases and is caused by absorption or scattering.

attenuation (extinction) coefficient: the reciprocal of the distance over which light of intensity I is attenuated to $I/e \approx 0.37I$; the units are typically cm^{-1}.

autocorrelation: the correlation of an ordered series of observations with the same series in an altered order.

autocorrelation function: the characteristic of the second-order statistics of a random process that shows how fast the random value changes from point to point, e.g., the autocorrelation function of intensity fluctuations caused by scattering of a laser beam by a rough surface characterizes the size and the distribution of speckle sizes in the induced speckle pattern; the Fourier transform of the autocorrelation function represents the power spectrum of a random process.

autofluorescence: natural fluorescence of a tissue.

avalanche photodetector (APD): a type of silicon or germanium photodiode that uses a phenomenon of the electrical breakdown of a p-n junction, which induces collision ionization and the avalanche creation of electron-hole pairs; it increases the photocurrent up to 10^2 to 10^6.

back-projection algorithm: an approximate inverse solution to provide efficient tomographic imaging; in **x-ray** computed tomography the back-projection is reconstructed along the paths of x-ray propagation; in optical tomography the back-projection is reconstructed along the paths of **ballistic** and/or least scattering photon propagation; in **optoacoustical tomography** the back-projection is reconstructed along spherical shells that are centered at the detector and have a radius determined by the acoustic time of flight.

backscattering: the dispersion of a fraction of the incident radiation in a backward direction.

backscattering coefficient (volume-averaged): the sum of the particle cross sections weighted by their angular-scattering functions evaluated at 180 deg.

backscattering Mueller matrix: a **Mueller matrix** measured for light backscattered by a sample.

ballistic (coherent) photons: a group of unscattered and strictly straightforward scattered photons.

beam: a slender stream of light.

beat signal: the signal at the intermediate frequency produced by mixing the local and signal oscillator beams on a photodetector.

bend (bending): related to **infrared spectroscopy** that works because chemical bonds have specific frequencies at which they vibrate, corresponding to energy levels; simple diatomic molecules have only one bond, which may stretch; more complex molecules may have many bonds and vibrations can be conjugated, leading to infrared absorptions at characteristic frequencies that may be related to chemical groups; e.g., the nonlinear triatomic molecule in an H_2O atom can vibrate in three different ways: symmetrical and asymmetrical stretching and bending (scissoring); the atoms in a CH_2 group, commonly found in organic compounds, can vibrate in six different ways: symmetrical and asymmetrical stretching, bending (scissoring), rocking, wagging, and twisting.

biaxial crystal: an **anisotropic crystal** that is characterized by having two optic axes, i.e., two axes along which an incoming beam will remain collinear, and the light of both polarizations will propagate at the same speed; mica is an example.

bimodal distribution: a distribution that has two modes.

bioheat equation: describes the change in tissue temperature at a definite point in the tissue; it is defined by the thermal conductivity of tissue, the rate of metabolic heat generation, and the heat transfer caused by blood perfusion at this point.

birefringence: the phenomenon exhibited by certain crystals in which an incident ray of light is split into two rays, called an ordinary ray and an extraordinary ray, which are plane- (linear) polarized in mutually orthogonal planes.

BK7: bor-crown optical glass that is relatively hard and shows a good scratch resistance; very commonly used for manufacturing of high-quality optical components; it has the high linear optical transmission in the visible range down to 350 nm with a refractive index of $n_d = 1.51680$ (587.6 nm).

blocking filter: a filter that blocks the passage of a certain frequency (wavelength) band.

Boltzmann constant: the ratio of the universal gas constant to Avogadro's number, equal to 1.3803×10^{-16} erg per degree Celsius.

Born's approximation: the single-scattering approximation when the field affecting the particle does not essentially differ from that of the initial wave.

Bouguer-Beer-Lambert law: a exponential law describing attenuation of a collimated beam by a thin absorption layer with scattering.

boundary conditions: a stated restriction, usually in the form of an equation, that limits the possible solutions to a differential equation.

brightness: an attribute of visual perception in which a source appears to emit a given amount of light; in other words, brightness is the perception elicited by the luminance of a visual target; this is a subjective attribute/property of an object being observed.

Brownian motion: the irregular motion of particles suspended in a medium caused by the molecules of the medium bombarding these particles.

Brownian particles: small particles suspended in a liquid or a gas that undergo irregular motion caused by molecules of the medium bombarding the particles.

calcium fluoride (CaF_2): an insoluble ionic compound of calcium and fluorine; it occurs naturally as the mineral fluorite (also called fluorspar).

carbon nanoparticle: particles made of carbon with dimensions on the order of billionths of a meter; they have different physical, chemical, electrical, and optical properties than occur in bulk samples due in part to the increased surface-area-to-volume ratio at the nanoscale; carbon black is a form of amorphous carbon that has an extremely high surface-area-to-volume ratio and, as such, is one of the first nanomaterials to find common use; little is known about the interaction of carbon nanoparticles with human cells.

cathode: a negative electrode that attracts cations (positive ions) during electrolysis.

cavity-dumped mode-locked laser: a laser that produces high-energy ultrashort laser pulses by decreasing the pulse repetition rate (see mode-locked laser); the laser output mirror is replaced by an optical selector consisting of a couple of spherical mirrors and an acousto- or electrooptical deflector, which extracts a pulse from the cavity after it has passed over a few dozen cavity lengths; the pulse energy is accumulated between two sequential extractions: the pulse repetition rate can be tuned in the range from dozens of hertz to a few megahertz.

charge-coupled device (CCD): a solid-state electronic device that serves as an imaging chip and is used in video cameras and fast spectrometers.

Celsius temperature scale: a temperature scale for which the freezing point is at $0°$ and the steam point is at $100°$.

characteristic diffusion time: the reciprocal of an agent's diffusion coefficient diffused in a tissue; characterized by the time interval during which the applied agent concentration increases in the sample of ≈ 0.6 in the surrounding medium.

CH group: related to **infrared spectroscopy**, chemical bonds vibrate at the specific frequencies that correspond to energy levels; simple diatomic molecules have only one bond that may stretch; a CH group provides a stretching vibration mode.

chirality: the mirror-equal "right" or "left" modification of an object **optical activity** is one example of chirality, when the asymmetric structure of a molecule or crystal existing of two forms ("right" and "left") causes the substance (ensemble of these molecules or crystal) to rotate the plane of polarization of the incident linear polarized light: the pure "right" or "left" optically active substances have identical physical and chemical properties, but their biochemical and physiological properties can be quite different.

chromatic aberrations: the variation of either the focal length or the magnification of a lens system, with different wavelengths of light, characterized by prismatic coloring at the edges of the optical image and color distortion within it.

chromaticity coordinates: in the study of the perception of color, one of the first mathematically defined color spaces was the CIE XYZ color space (also known as CIE 1931 color space), created by the International Commission on Illumination (Commission Internationale de l'Éclairage—CIE) in 1931; the human eye has receptors for short (S), middle (M), and long (L) wavelengths, also known as blue, green, and red receptors; that means that one, in principle, needs three parameters to describe a color sensation; a specific method for associating three numbers (or tristimulus values) with each color is called a color space: the CIE XYZ color space is one of many such spaces; however, the CIE XYZ color space is special, because it is based on direct measurements of the human eye and serves as the basis from which many other color spaces are defined; the CIE1964 standard observer is based on the mean 10-deg color matching functions.

chromophore: a chemical that absorbs light with a characteristic spectral pattern.

clock frequency: in electronics and especially synchronous digital circuits, a clock signal is used to coordinate the actions of two or more circuits; for example, the clock rate (frequency) of a computer CPU is normally determined by the frequency of an oscillator crystal.

CMOS image sensors: an image sensor based on complementary metal-oxide-semiconductor (CMOS) camera that operates at lower voltages than a **CCD** camera, reducing power consumption for portable applications; analog and digital processing functions can be integrated readily onto the CMOS chip, reducing system package size and overall cost; each CMOS active pixel sensor cell has its own buffer amplifier and can be addressed and read individually—a commonly used cell has four transistors and a photoelement; all pixels on a column connect to a common amplifier.

carbon monoxide (CO) laser: a laser in which the lasing medium is CO gas with an IR emission from 5 to 6.5 μm.

carbon dioxide (CO_2) laser: a laser in which the lasing medium is CO_2 gas with an IR emission from 9.2 to 11.1 μm with the maximal efficiency at 10.6 μm.

coherence length: characterizes the degree of temporal coherence of a light source; $l_c = c\tau_c$, where c is the light speed and τ_c is the coherence time, which is approximately equal to the pulse duration of the pulsed light source or inversely proportional to the frequency bandwidth of a continuous-wave light source.

coherent detection imaging (CDI): a method based on the optical heterodyne detection technique: it is a coherence gating method that discriminates the forward multiply-scattering beam, preserving the direct geometrical correlation with the incident light beam against the diffuse component of transmitted light.

coherent light: light in which the electromagnetic waves maintain a fixed phase relationship over a period of time and in which the phase relationship remains constant for various points that are perpendicular to the direction of propagation.

collapse: catastrophic compression.

collimated beam: a beam of light in which all rays are parallel to each other.

collisional quenching rate: nonradiative relaxation of the excited molecular energy state (level) by collisions with surrounding molecules; in a condensed medium, the rate of collisional relaxation is significantly higher than the radiative one.

complex conjugation: the number corresponding to a given complex number that represents the given number's reflection with respect to the real axis.

confocal microscopy: microscopy that employs the confocal principle [two optically conjugate diaphragms (pinholes) or small-sized slits in the object and image planes] for the selection of scattered photons coming from a given volume; provides 3D imaging of living tissues.

contrast: is a distinction between two objects (or parts of an object) or colors; a large contrast is a big difference, and contrasting objects are boldly different; can refer to contrast (visibility) of regular **interference** or **speckle** patterns or the difference in color and light **intensity** between parts of an image (see **imaging contrast**).

contrast of the intensity fluctuations: the relative difference between light and dark areas of a speckle pattern.

contrasting agents: compounds used to increase the quality of x-ray, MRI, or optical tomography images.

constructive interference: the interference of two or more waves of equal frequency and phase, resulting in their mutual reinforcement and producing a single amplitude equal to the sum of the amplitudes of the individual waves.

cooled CCD: a highly sensitive CCD with the thermal noise suppressed by cooling the photosensitive chip.

correlation: the degree of co-relation between two or more attributes or measurements on the same group of elements; in probability theory and statistics, correlation indicates the strength and direction of a linear relationship between two random variables; in general statistical usage, correlation refers to the departure of two variables from independence, although correlation does not imply causation.

correlation coefficient: a number of different coefficients are used to characterize **correlation** between two random variables for different situations; the most well known is the Pearson product-moment correlation coefficient, which is obtained by dividing the covariance of the two variables by the product of their standard deviations.

correlation diffusion equation: describes the transport of temporal field correlation function in a system that multiply scatters laser radiation; may be valid for turbid samples with the dynamics of scattering particles governed by Brownian motion, and random and shear flow.

correlation length: the length within which the degree of correlation between two measurements of a spatially dependent quantity is high (close to unity); for example, L_c is the correlation length of the scattering surface of the spatial inhomogeneities (random relief).

coupler: an optical or acoustical device that interconnects optical or acoustical components with less loss of energy.

coupling gel: a gel that provides matching optical or acoustical properties from different elements of a device that minimizes the amplitude of light or acoustic reflecting signals (or both) from boundaries of the elements.

cross-correlation frequency (cross-correlation signal): a difference in the frequency of intensity modulated light at a certain wavelength and photodetector gain modulation; it carries the same phase and amplitude information as the original optical signal.

cross-correlation measurement device: a system that down converts a radio frequency prior to phase measurements.

crosstalk: the interrelations between measured signals induced by originally independent parameters (for example, by changes in blood volume and oxygenation); this factor is determined by calibration on a model (for example, a blood model).

continuous wave (CW): waves that are not intermittent or broken up into damped wave trains but, unless intentionally interrupted, follow one another without any interval of time between them.

CW laser: a laser producing CW waves.

CW RTT: the stationary radiation transfer theory that describes the intensity distribution of CW light in a scattering medium; it is based on the stationary integro-differential equation for the radiance- (or specific intensity) average power flux density at a point r in a given direction s (see **radiation transfer theory**).

dark-field illumination: used in dark-field microscopy for imaging of optically transparent nonabsorbing specimens, where illuminating light does not enter into ocular lenses and only light scattered by microparticles of the specimen creates the image; in the field of view of the microscope on the dark background, bright images of the specimen particles differing by their refractive index from the surrounding medium are seen.

decibel (dB): the engineering unit for the ratio of the input power, P_{in}, in a given device to the output power, P_{out}; it is convenient to measure the logarithm of the ratio $\log(P_{out}/P_{in})$, and the dB is a standard unit that is equal to 10 times that log: $10\log(P_{out}/P_{in})$ dB.

decorrelation of speckles: relates to statistics of the second order that characterize the size and distribution of speckle sizes and show how fast the intensity changes from point to point in the speckle pattern; decorrelation means that such changes of intensity tend to be faster.

deep RPS: a random-phase screen that induces phase fluctuations in a scattered field with a variance that is much more than unity.

deflectometry: a photorefractive technique based on the detection of refractive index gradients above and inside the sample using a laser probe beam.

deformation: in biomechanics, deformation is a change in shape due to an applied force; this can be a result of tensile (pulling) forces, compressive (pushing) forces, shear, bending, or torsion (twisting); deformation is often described in terms of strain.

0-degree hybrid (or splitter): a device that pertains to or denotes a current in one of two parallel circuits that have a single-phase current source and equal impedances and that produces currents of 0-degree phase shift.

90-degree hybrid (or splitter): a device that pertains to or denotes a current in one of two parallel circuits that have a single-phase current source but unequal impedances and that produces currents of 90-degree phase shift.

degree of polarization: the quantity that characterizes the ratio of the intensity of polarized light to the total intensity of light.

delta (δ)-Eddington approximation: a simple yet accurate method that was proposed for determining monochromatic radiative fluxes in an absorbing-scattering atmosphere; in this method, the governing phase function is approximated by a Dirac-delta function forward-scatter peak and a two-term expansion of the phase function; the fraction of scattering into the truncated forward peak is taken proportional to the square of the phase-function-asymmetry factor, which distinguishes the delta-Eddington approximation from others of a similar nature (http://adsabs.harvard.edu/abs/1976JAtS...33.2452J); one of the approximations of the actual phase function for tissue; in the diffusion approximation of RTT, it is the best function for simulating light transport in tissues characterized by anisotropic scattering.

demodulation: the separation and extraction of modulating low-frequency waves from a modulated carrier wave (high frequency or optical); the device or circuit used for demodulation is called a detector or demodulator.

depth of modulation: for amplitude modulation, this is the ratio of the amplitude of the alternating component of a signal to its mean value.

depolarization: deprivation (destruction) of light polarization.

depolarization length: the length of light beam transport in a scattering-depolarizing medium at which the polarization degree decays to the definite level compared with the totally polarized incident light.

destructive interference: the interference of two waves of equal frequency and opposite phase, resulting in their cancellation where the negative displacement of one always coincides with the positive displacement of the other.

developed speckles: the speckles that are characterized by Gaussian statistics of the complex amplitude, the unity **contrast of intensity fluctuations**, and a negative exponential function of the intensity probability distribution (the most probable intensity value in the corresponding speckle pattern is equal to zero, i.e., destructive interference occurs with the highest probability).

dichroism (diattenuation): a phenomenon related to **pleochroism** of a uniaxial crystal so that it exhibits two different colors when viewed from two different directions under transmitted light; pleochroism is the property possessed by certain crystals that exhibit different colors when viewed from different directions under transmitted light: this is one exhibition of the optical anisotropy caused by the anisotropy of absorption; the varieties of pleochroism are **circular dichroism**, different absorption for light with right and left circular polarization, and **linear dichroism**, different absorption for ordinary and extraordinary rays.

diffraction: a phenomenon associated with a wave motion when a wave train (optical, acoustical, thermal, **photon density**, etc.) passes the edge of an obstacle opaque to the wave motion; the phenomenon is a particular case of interference; the waves are bent at the edge of the obstacle, which acts as a source of secondary waves, all coherent; the interference between a primary wave and a secondary wave produces diffraction bands, which are interference bands.

diffraction of photon density wave (intensity wave): the bending of photon density waves around obstacles in their path; the phenomenon exhibited by wavefronts that, passing the edge of an opaque body, are modulated, thereby causing a redistribution of photon-density-wave amplitude within the front: it is detectable by the presence of minute bands with high and low amplitudes at the edge of a shadow; the phenomenon is a particular case of interference between primary and secondary photon density waves.

diffractometry: measuring techniques based on the phenomenon of wave diffraction.

diffuse photons: the photons that undertake multiple scatter with a broad variety of angles.

diffuse tomography: optical tomography based on reconstruction of the optical macro-inhomogeneity within a scattering medium using diffuse photon pathlength-gating techniques and **back-projection algorithms**.

diffusion: the process by which one gas mixes with another by the movement of the molecules of one gas into another and vice versa; diffusion also occurs when two miscible liquids or solids come in contact with a solvent; the term is also used to describe the passage of molecules through a porous membrane.

diffusion approximation (diffusion theory): the approximated diffusion-type solution of the **RTT**, which is accurate for describing photon migration in infinite, homogeneous, highly scattering media.

diffusion coefficient: the proportionality coefficient between mean-square displacement of a particle within time interval τ: $\langle \Delta r^2 \rangle \sim D\tau$; may be related to molecular or photon diffusion.

diffusion wave spectroscopy (DWS): spectroscopy based on the study of dynamic light scattering in dense media with multiple scattering and related to the investigation of particle dynamics within very short time intervals.

digital electronic autocorrelator: a device that reconstructs with a high accuracy the time-domain autocorrelation function of intensity fluctuations.

digital oscilloscope: a device that analyses with a high accuracy the waveform of **ac** signals.

diode laser: a semiconductor injection laser; **GaAs laser** (830 nm); $GaP_x As_{1-x}$ lasers emit light from 640 nm ($x = 0.4$) to 830 nm ($x = 0$); $Ga_x In_{1-x} As_y P_{1-y}$, lasers, at $y = 2.2x$ and for different values of x, emit in the range from 920 to 1500 nm; $Pb_x S_{1-x}$, $Sn_x Pb_{1-x} Te$, and $Sn_x Pb_{1-x} Se$ lasers, for different values of x, emit in the range from 2.5 to 49 μm.

diode-pumped Nd:YAG: an integrated solid-state laser with an Nd:YAG crystal as a lasing medium and optical pumping provided by a single laser diode or by a laser (light) diode array or matrix.

dipole moment of transition: the mutual displacement and charges of a two-charged particle system (model of molecule); defines the electrical field of the electrically neutral system on distances larger than its size and the action of external fields on the system; when the dipole moment changes, the system emits electromagnetic waves.

dispersion: the state of being dispersed, such as a photon trajectory (general); the variation of the index of refraction of a transparent substance, such as a glass, with the wavelength of light, the index of refraction increases as the wavelength decreases (optics); the separation of white or compound light into its respective colors, as in the formation of a spectrum by a prism (optics); the scattering of values of a variable around the mean or median of a distribution (statistics); a system of dispersed particles suspended in a solid, liquid, or gas (chemistry).

dissector: a transmitting television tube; it can be used as a coordinate-sensitive photodetector.

distribution size function: a function that describes the probability distribution of a particle size value over the size values in the system.

divergence: the "spreading" of a light beam in general, and of a laser beam as it moves away from the laser in particular.

Doppler effect: the apparent change in the frequency of a wave, such as a light wave or sound wave, resulting from a change in the distance between the source of the wave and the receiver.

Doppler interferometry: the dynamic dual-beam interferometry when the reference beam path length is scanned with a constant speed; the Doppler signal induced is the measuring signal for depth profiling of an object placed in the measuring beam; the method is used in partially coherent interferometry or tomography of tissues.

Doppler microscopy: **Doppler spectroscopy** of a medium at a microscopic scale.

Doppler spectroscopy: the spectroscopy based on the study of dynamic light scattering (**Doppler effect**) in media with single scattering and related to investigation of the dynamics (velocity) of particles from the measurements of the Doppler shifts in the frequency of the waves scattered by the moving particles.

double-balanced mixer: an electronic device that mixes two optically detected signals that have the same radio frequency but different amplitudes and phases.

double integrating sphere (DIS) technique: a technique for *in vitro* evaluation of the optical parameters of tissue samples (μ_a, μ_s, and g); it is often combined with collimated transmittance measurements; it implies either sequential or simultaneous measurement of three parameters: total transmittance T_t (using the **integrating sphere**), diffuse reflectance R_d (using the integrating sphere), and collimated transmittance T_c (using a distant detector behind the pinhole at the top of the integrating sphere).

dual-beam coherent interferometry: see **Doppler interferometry**.

dye laser: a laser in which the laser medium is a liquid dye; dye lasers emit in a broad spectral range (e.g., in the visible) and are tunable; wavelengths range from 340 to 960 nm, optical frequency doubling ranges from 217 to 380 nm, and parametric conversion ranges from 1060 to 3100 nm; emitted energy is from 1 mJ to 50 J in periodic pulse mode; mean power is from 0.06 to 20 W; and pulse duration is from 0.007 to 8 μs; pulse frequency from a single pulse to 1 kHz.

dynamic light scattering: light scattering by a moving object that causes a **Doppler shift** in the frequency of the scattered wave relative to the frequency of the incident light.

dynode chain of the PMT: a system of electrodes, each of which serves for the emission of secondary electrons in a vacuum tube.

elastic (static) light scattering: light scattering by static (motionless) objects that occurs elastically, without changes in photon energy or light frequency.

electromagnetic resonance: appears at interaction of the incident radiation with molecules attached to a rough metallic surface; is induced due to collective excitation of conduction electrons in the small metallic structures; also called surface plasmon resonance; **surface-enhanced Raman scattering (SERS)** is based on such electromagnetic effects.

electronic micrograph: micrographs of tissue and/or cell components received with the help of the **electronic microscope**.

electronic microscope: a parallel beam of electrons from an electron gun is passed through a very thin slice of tissue; differential scattering of the electron beam takes place, and an image of tissue microstructure is carried forward in the electron beam; an electron lens is used to focus the electron beam on a fluorescent screen, where a magnified image is formed; the image is registered using an optical camera; the resolving power of the electron microscope is very much greater than that of a light microscope.

electronic transition: if an electron in an atom is activated (given more energy) the electron moves to an energy level farther from the atom nucleus; if an electron moves back to a lower level, energy is given out as electromagnetic radiation.

electronic wave function: the magnitude of the wave function (ψ) represents the varying amplitude of the stationary wave system, in 3D, of an electron situated around a nucleus; associated with the stationary wave is a frequency, ν; ψ^2 is the density of electrons per unit volume; $\psi^2 dV$ is the probability of finding the electron, when it is considered as a particle, in a volume dV; the total volume of the orbital gives a probability of unity; the effective electrical charge associated with a volume dV is $-e\psi^2 dV$, where e is the charge of an electron; the four quantum numbers define possible states of the stationary waves.

electrophoresis: the movement of colloidal particles in an electric field; when two platinum electrodes connected to a dc supply are placed in a lyophobic sol (the disperse phase has no attraction for the continuous phase), the colloidal particles will move to either the cathode or anode depending on the charge on the particle; used for drug delivery in medicine.

emission spectrum: the emission obtained from a luminescent material at different wavelengths when it is excited by a narrow range of shorter wavelengths.

endoscopy: an optical technique and instrumentation for viewing internal organs.

energy: the product of power (watt, W) and time (sec, s); energy is measured in joule (J).

entropy: a measure of the amount of disorder in a system; the more disordered the system, the higher the entropy; an entropy change occurs when a system absorbs or emits heat; the change in entropy dS is measured as the heat change dQ divided by the temperature T at which the change takes place, $dS = dQ/T$.

erbium: yttrium aluminum garnet (Er:YAG) laser: a solid-state laser whose lasing medium is the crystal Er:YAG crystal with an emission in the mid-IR range of 2.79–2.94 μm.

evaporation: the process of changing a liquid into a vapor, usually by applying heat, or by the liquid taking heat from its surroundings; during this process the bulk of the liquid is reduced.

excitation spectrum: the emission spectrum at one wavelength is monitored, and the intensity at this wavelength is measured as a function of the exciting wavelength.

excimer laser: a laser whose lasing medium is an excited molecular complex, an excimer (molecule-dimer); the emission is in the UV; examples are: ArF laser, 193 nm; KrF laser, 248 nm; XeCl laser, 308 nm; and XeF laser, 351 nm.

excited state (energy level): electrons possess energy according to their position in relation to the nucleus of an atom; the closer the electron is to the nucleus the lower the energy; when the energy of an electron changes, it must do so in certain definite steps and not in a continuous way; the position in which electrons may be found according to their energy are called energy levels and sublevels; these levels are counted by their steps outward, and the numbers allotted to them are their quantum numbers.

extinction coefficient: see **attenuation coefficient**.

Fabry-Perot interferometer: the **interferometer** combined of two parallel mirrors (reflecting planes) displace each other by a distance of L (interferometer length); used as a precise optical filter in the super-resolution spectroscopy and as a cavity in lasers.

false color map: a map where each color is distributed through the map and the specific value of the measured parameter is prescribed, for example, the measured velocity of blood flow within the selected skin area; it is used for the fast qualitative estimation of parameter distribution and change.

far-field diffraction zone (far zone): the zone where Fraunhofer diffraction takes place; this is a type of diffraction in which the light source and the receiving screen are effectively at an infinite distance from the diffraction object, i.e., parallel beams of wave trains are used.

Faraday rotator: an optical device that rotates the polarization of light due to the Faraday effect, which in turn is based on a magneto-optic effect; it works because one polarization of the input light is in ferromagnetic resonance with the material that causes its phase velocity to be higher than the other.

fast Fourier transform (FFT) analysis: a fast algorithm for the expression of any periodic function as a sum of sine and cosine functions, as in an electromagnetic wave function.

F/D spectrometer: the spectrometer that uses the frequency-domain (photon-density wave) method for measuring the absorption and scattering spectra of an object (tissue).

femtosecond (fsec) (fs): -10^{-15} sec (s).

fiber: an optical waveguide that uses a phenomenon of total internal reflection for light transportation with low losses and is made from transparent glass, quartz, polymer, or crystal, usually with a circular cross-section; it consists of at least two parts, an inner part or **core** that has a higher refractive index and through which light propagates, and an outer part or **cladding** that has a lower refractive index and provides a totally reflecting interface between core and cladding.

fiber bundle: a flexible bundle of individual optical fibers arranged in an ordered or disordered manner and correspondingly named regular and irregular bundles.

fiber coupler: a fiber optical device that interconnects optical components.

fiber-optic catheter: a flexible single fiber or a fiber bundle used to move light into body cavities and back.

fiber-optic device: any type of device that uses fiber-optical components.

fiber-optic refractometer: a fiber-optic device used to measure the refractive index of a medium (tissue or biological liquid); such a device is usually used to explore the effect of disruption of the total internal reflection and is a robust instrument well suited for biomedical applications.

fiber-optic single-mode x-coupler: a fiber coupler that is made from a single-mode fiber and provides connections between four optical components; it is usually used as a key part of the integrated Michelson interferometer when it connects to a light source, a reference mirror, the reflecting surface under study, and a photodetector.

field of view: the extent of an object that can be imaged or seen through an optical system.

finite-difference method: in numerical analysis, finite differences play an important role they are one of the simplest ways to approximate a differential operator and are extensively used in solving differential equations.

finite-difference time-domain (FDTD): a numerical solution applied to a finite difference in space and time; numerical equivalent of the physical reality under investigation; for example, the solution of Maxwell's equations describing light scattering by a cell.

finite element method: a numerical method for finding an approximate solution to partial differential equations (PDEs) as well as integral equations, such as the **heat** or **radiation transfer equations**; the solution approach is based either on eliminating the differential equation completely (steady state problems), or rendering the PDE into an equivalent ordinary differential equation, which is then solved using standard techniques such as the **finite-difference method**, etc.

flow cytometry: a technique for counting, examining, and sorting microscopic particles (cells) suspended in a stream of fluid; it allows simultaneous multiparametric analysis of the physical and/or chemical characteristics of single cells flowing through an optical and/or electronic detection apparatus.

flowmeter: a device for measuring parameters of a flow, such as flow velocity; for instance blood flow velocity.

fluence rate (total radiant energy fluence rate): the sum of the **radiance** over all angles at a point $\bar{r}$; the quantity that is typically measured in irradiated tissues in units of watts per square centimeter.

fluorescence: the property of emitting light of a longer wavelength on absorption of light energy; essentially occurs simultaneously with the excitation of a sample.

fluorescence anisotropy: transition dipole moments have defined orientations within a molecule; upon excitation with linear polarized light, one preferentially excites those molecules, whose transition dipoles are parallel to the electric field vector of incident light; this selective excitation of an oriented population of molecules results in partially polarized fluorescence, which is described by fluorescence anisotropy.

fluorescence emission spectrum: a fluorescence spectrum measured at a certain excitation wavelength.

fluorescence excitation-emission map: a map presenting the combined data of **fluorescence emission** and **excitation spectra**, where excitation and emission wavelengths are presented on x–y axes with corresponding fluorescence intensity values represented by the isometric lines on the map.

fluorescence excitation spectrum: the intensity of fluorescence measured at a certain emission wavelength as a function of the excitation wavelength.

fluorescence tomography: the **tomography** based on the detection of **fluorescence** signal fluorometer.

fluorophore: a **chromophore** that emits light with a characteristic spectral pattern at its excitation by a proper wavelength.

focal depth: every lens has a range of object positions that give an apparently focused image on a fixed screen; this range is called the depth of focus of the lens.

focal plane: a focusing plane that is perpendicular to the principle axis and also passes through the principle focus; rays parallel to each other, but at an angle to the principle axis, are brought to a focus in the focal plane.

focal spot: the spot obtained at the focus of a lens; the size of the spot depends on the lens and the wavelength, but its diameter is never smaller than the wavelength of light.

form birefringence: birefringence that is caused by the structure of a medium; for example, a system of long dielectric cylinders made from an isotropic substance and arranged in a parallel fashion shows birefringence of form.

forward scattering problem: the modeling of light propagation in a scattering medium by taking into account the experimental geometry, source, and detector characteristics and the known optical properties of a sample, and predicting the measurements and associated accuracies that result.

Fourier optical microscope: a microscope based on the principle that optical density spatial variations in the object plane of the microscope are converted by a **Fourier transform** into spatial frequency variations in the Fourier transform plane in the rear focal plane of the lens; if the optical density changes slowly across the object, the Fourier transform places most of the scattered light near zero angles (low spatial frequency) in the Fourier transform plane (a good model of a cell with clear cytoplasm); if the optical density changes rapidly across the object, the Fourier transform moves more of the energy to larger scattering angles (higher spatial frequency) in the Fourier transform plane (a good model of a cell with highly granular cytoplasm).

Fourier transform: an algorithm for the expression of any periodic function as a sum of sine and cosine functions.

Fourier transform infrared spectroscopy: spectroscopy based on light dispersion by using a Michelson interferometer with a tuned path length difference; in the IR it may provide a 10^2–10^3 higher signal-to-noise ratio, than a grating spectrometer.

fractal dimension: as the complexity of the object structure increases, its fractal dimension increases and is always higher than the topological dimension of the structure; for example, any structure described as a curve (tissue fiber) has a topological dimension of $D = 1$; however, if we make this curve more complex by bending it infinite times, its fractal dimension be equal to two when this curve will densely covers a finite area, or even to three when this curve will "pack" a cube.

fractal object: an object with a self-similar geometry, i.e., each arbitrarily selected part of it is similar to the whole object; **fractal dimension** of the object (structure) is always higher than its topological dimension.

frame grabber: an electronic device that provides video data acquisition and conversion to a digital form.

Franck-Condon principle: an **electronic transition** so fast that the vibrating molecule does not noticeably change its internuclear distance.

Fraunhofer diffraction: a type of diffraction in which the light source and the receiving screen are effectively at an infinite distance from the diffraction object, i.e., parallel beams of wave trains are used.

Fraunhofer diffraction approximation: a description of forward-direction scattering caused by large particles (on the order of 10 μm).

Fraunhofer zone: the zone where Fraunhofer diffraction takes place.

free diffusion: the **diffusion** process that occurs when molecules diffuse in the space free of any membranes and other barriers that hinder diffusion.

frequency-domain technique (method): a spectroscopic or imaging technique (method) that exploits an intensity-modulated light and narrow-band heterodyne detection.

Fresnel diffraction: a type of diffraction in which the light source and the receiving screen are both at a finite distance from the diffraction object, i.e., divergent and convergent beams of wave trains are used.

Fresnel reflection: the reflection of a beam of radiation, such as light, which takes place at the interface between two media of different refractive indexes; not all the radiation is reflected, some may be refracted.

Fresnel zone: the zone where Fresnel diffraction takes place.

GaAs laser: a laser based on the semiconductor material GaAs; the emission is in the NIR, at about 830 nm.

gas-microphone method: relates to opto-acoustic spectroscopy, when an object under study is surrounded by a gas (or combination of gases) that serves as an acoustic coupler between the object and an acoustic receiver such as a microphone; the spectroscopy of the surrounding gas, when an object's optical and acoustical properties are known or fixed, the spectroscopy of the surrounding gas can also be determined.

Gaussian correlation function: the correlation function described by a bell-shaped (Gaussian) curve.

Gaussian light beam: a light beam with a Gaussian shape for the transverse intensity profile; if the intensity at the center of the beam is I_o, then the formula for a Gaussian beam is $I = I_o \exp(-2r^2/w^2)$, where r is the radial distance from the axis and w is the beam "waist"; the intensity profile of such a beam is said to be bell shaped; a laser beam is a Gaussian one; a single-mode fiber also creates a Gaussian beam at its output.

Gaussian size distribution: **distribution size function** of a Gaussian shape.

Gaussian statistics (normal statistics): statistics when a bell-shaped (Gaussian) curve showing a distribution of probability associated with different values of a variate are valid.

Gegenbauer kernel phase function (GK): one of the approximations of the actual phase function for tissue; the **Henyey-Greenstein phase function** is a special case of the **GK**; **GK** is a good function for simulating light transport in a tissue characterized by a high scattering anisotropy, such as blood.

genetic inverse algorithm: genetic algorithms (GAs) are now widely applied in science and engineering as adaptive algorithms for solving practical problems; certain classes of problems are particularly suited for a GA based approach; the general acceptance is that GAs are particularly suited to multidimensional global search problems where the search space potentially contains multiple local minima; unlike other search methods, correlation between the search variables is not generally a problem; the basic GA does not require extensive knowledge of the search space, such as likely solution bounds or functional derivatives (http://gaul.sourceforge.net/intro.html).

Gladstone and Dale law: states that the mean value of the refractive index of a composition represents an average of the refractive indices of its components related to their volume fractions.

Glan-Taylor polarization prism: a type of prism which used as a polarizer or polarizing beamsplitter; the prism is made of two right-angled prisms of calcite (or other birefringent materials), which are separated on their long faces with an air gap; the optical axes of the calcite crystals are aligned parallel to the plane of reflection; total internal reflection of s-polarized light at the air gap ensures that only p-polarized light is transmitted by the device; because the angle of incidence at the gap can be reasonably close to Brewster's angle, unwanted reflection of p-polarized light is reduced.

gold nanoparticles: particles made of gold with dimensions typically of 10–50 nm; they have different chemical and optical properties than those that occur in bulk samples; due to the plasmon-resonant property, high surface reactivity, and their biocompatibility, gold nanoparticles can be used for *in vivo* molecular imaging and therapeutic applications, including optical detection of cancer and phototherapy.

goniophotometry (goniophotometric technique): the technique that measures of the angle-dependent light intensity distribution.

gradient index (GRIN) lens: focuses light through a precisely controlled radial variation of the lens material's index of refraction from the optical axis to the edge of the lens; this allows a GRIN lens with flat or angle polished surfaces to collimate light emitted from an optical fiber or to focus an incident beam into an optical fiber; end faces can be provided with an anti-reflection coating to avoid unwanted back reflection.

grating spectrograph: a spectrograph that uses diffraction grating to produce optical spectra; a diffraction grating is a band of equidistant, parallel lines, usually more than 5000 to the inch, ruled on a glass or polished metal surface for diffracting light to produce optical spectra with a high resolution.

group refractive index: the refractive index associated with the group velocity of a train of waves traveling in a dispersive medium; the group velocity, and correspondingly the group refractive index, depends on the mean wavelength of a train of waves and the rate of change in velocity with wavelength.

Grüneisen parameter: a dimensionless, temperature-dependent factor proportional to the fraction of thermal energy converted into mechanical stress.

halogen lamp: an iodine-cycle tungsten incandescent lamp that is the visible/near infrared (360 nm to >1 μm) light source for spectrophotometry.

hard sphere approximation: the model of mutually impenetrable (hard) spheres; the interparticle forces are zero, except for the fact that two neighboring particles cannot interpenetrate each other.

heat capacity: a measurable physical quantity that characterizes the ability of a body to store heat as it changes in temperature; defined as the rate of change of temperature as heat is added to a body at the given conditions and state of the body (foremost its temperature); expressed in units of joules per Kelvin.

heat (thermal) conduction: the process of heat transfer through a body without visible motion of any part of the body; the process takes place where there is a temperature gradient; heat energy diffuses through the body by the action of particles of high kinetic energy on particles of lower kinetic energy; for solids with covalent bonding, there will be molecules for which motion is restricted to vibrations about fixed positions, and the energy is transferred by high frequency waves.

heat transfer: a variety of processes that provide transfer of heat through a body and its surroundings, such as **heat (thermal) conduction**, heat convection, thermal radiation and absorption, latent heat of fusion, and vaporization.

helix: a connected series of concentric rings of the same radius, joined together to form a cylindrical shape.

hemoglobin spectrum: the main bands are the **Soret band**, the 400–440-nm segment, and the **Q band**, the 540–580-nm segment.

He-Ne (helium neon) laser: a gas laser whose medium is a mixture of He and Ne; lasers with the red emission (632.8 nm) are widely used; lasers with other wavelengths are also available: green (543 nm), yellow (594 nm), orange (604 and/or 612 nm), IR (1152, 1523, and/or 3391 nm).

Henyey-Greenstein phase function (HG): one of the practical semiempirical approximations of the scattering phase function.

hertz (Hz): a unit of frequency that is equal to 1 cycle per second; it is often used to indicate the pulse repetition rate of a laser (e.g., a 10-Hz laser emits 10 pulses per second); 1 kilohertz (kHz) is 10^3 Hz, 1 megahertz (MHz) is 10^6 Hz, 1 gigahertz (GHz) is 10^9 Hz, and 1 terahertz (THz) is 10^{12} Hz.

heterodyne microscopy: a microscopy technique that uses optical heterodyning to enhance the registered signal and **image contrast**.

heterodyne phase system: see **"cross-correlation" measurement device**.

heterodyne spectrum: the spectrum of the intensity fluctuations registered by a photodetector at the intermediate (beat) frequency as a central frequency of the measured spectrum; the intermediate frequency is chosen for technical reasons: it has the best signal-to-noise ratio.

heterodyne system with zero cross-phase detectors: the phase measuring system that uses amplitude modulation at two close radio frequencies, f_1 and f_2.

heterostructure: a semiconductor junction that is composed of layers of dissimilar semiconductor materials with nonequal band gaps; a quantum heterostructure's size restricts the movements of the charge carriers and forces them into a quantum confinement that leads to formation of a set of discrete energy levels with sharper density than for structures of more conventional sizes; important for the fabrication of short-wavelength light-emitting diodes and diode lasers.

histogram: a form that represents the distribution of experimental data as a bar diagram.

hologram: a negative produced by exposing a high resolution photographic plate to two interfering waves: the subject wave, which is formed by illumination of a subject by monochromatic, coherent radiation, as from a laser, and the reference wave, which goes directly from the same light source (laser); when a hologram is placed in a beam of coherent light, a true three-dimensional image of the subject is formed.

holographic microscopy: microscopy that uses holographic principles.

holography: the process or technique of making holograms.

homodyne phase system: a system that does not down convert the radio frequency prior to phase measurements.

homodyne spectrum: the self-beat spectrum of the intensity fluctuations registered by a photodetector; it is like the heterodyne spectrum, but with a central frequency equal to zero, and overlapping negative and positive spectrum wings.

homogeneous medium: a medium that has common physical properties, including optical properties, throughout.

humidity: a measure of the extent to which the atmosphere contains moisture (water vapor).

hydrated: being associated with water molecules.

hydrodynamic radius of a particle: the radius that is determined from the measurements of the translation diffusion coefficient for an ensemble of identical particles in the medium; it is larger than the initial one due to interactions with molecules of the medium.

hydrostatic pressure: the pressure at a point in a liquid is the force per unit area on a very small area round the point; if the point is at depth h in the liquid of density ρ, then pressure $p = \rho g h$; the pressure at a point in a liquid at rest acts equally in all directions; the force exerted on a surface in contact with a liquid at rest is perpendicular to the surface at all points; measured in N/m^2 or Pa (pascal).

hyperosmotic: a term that describes a liquid with a lower concentration of water and higher solute concentration than fluids in a tissue or cell; this term also means that if a cell is hyperosmotic, it absorbs water from the surroundings to dilute the higher solute concentration, thus making the cell isotonic to the environment.

hyperpolarizability: nonlinear **polarizability**, β, characterizes the nonlinear part of the induced dipole moment of the molecule, which is proportional to the squared external electric field with the coefficient of proportionality equal to $(1/2)\beta$.

Jabloski diagram: representation of molecular energy levels and transition rates using the potential curves that are plotted without regard to the variable nuclear distances.

Jones matrix: see **amplitude scattering matrix**.

image-carrying photons: a group of photons that produce an image of a certain macro-inhomogeneity within a scattering medium.

image reconstruction: see **TOAST** and **tomographic reconstruction**.

imaging (image) contrast: pointing differences between two or more objects or points on the object; a parameter that characterizes differentiation (visibility) of the visualized object(s) hidden in the scattering surroundings; contrasting parameters may be used: light intensity, reflectance, polarization degree, fluorescence intensity and life-time, refractive index, reconstructed absorption and scattering coefficients, etc.

imaging resolution: when two objects are close together they might not form two images on the retina of the eye or matrix detector that are distinguishable; the ability to detect two such images of two objects close together is measured by the resolving power of the instrument; for a microscope two objects are resolved if the angular separation of the objects is not less than λ/D, where λ is the wavelength of the light used and D is the diameter of the objective; the smallest separation of two objects, if they are to be resolved, is $0.61\lambda/\text{NA}$, where NA is the **numerical aperture**.

immersion medium (liquid): a liquid that provides optical matching between an objective and a biological object; it enhances the numerical aperture of the objective and the microscope resolution; in addition, optical matching reduces surface reflection and scattering, and consequently allows for the reception of higher **contrast** images.

immersion technique: the technique used to reduce light scattering in an inhomogeneous medium by matching the refractive index of the scatterers and ground substance; immersion liquids with an appropriate refractive index and rate of diffusion are usually used.

impedance: the measure of current flowing in an inductive or capacitive component of a circuit when an alternating potential difference is applied; the magnitude of the impedance varies with the frequency of the **ac**.

index of refraction: a number indicating the speed of light in a given medium as either the ratio of the speed of light in a vacuum to that in the given medium (**absolute index of refraction**) or the ratio of the speed of light in a specified medium to that in the given medium (**relative index of refraction**).

inelastic scattering: from quantum electrodynamics it follows that an individual light-scattering event is considered the absorption of the incident photon, which has the energy $h\nu$, momentum $(h/2\pi)\mathbf{k}$, and polarization p, by a particle of the scattering medium, and then the emission of the photon that has energy $h\nu'$, momentum $(h/2\pi)\mathbf{k}'$, and polarization p'; at $\nu \neq \nu'$ light scattering is accompanied by the redistribution of energy between the radiation and the medium, and is called inelastic, for example, **Raman scattering**; at $\nu = \nu'$, when no redistribution takes place light scattering is called elastic or **Rayleigh scattering**.

infrared spectroscopy: a spectroscopy of middle and far infrared wavelength range the that uses light-excited vibrational-energy states in molecules to get information about the molecular composition, molecular structures, and molecular interactions.

inhomogeneous medium: a medium with a regular or irregular spatial distribution of physical properties, including optical properties.

integrating sphere: a photometric sphere with a highly reflecting white or metallic coating and photodetector inside; used for the precise measurement of diffuse reflectance or total transmittance of scattering materials (tissues); integrating spheres are usually coated with materials that have smooth and high reflectance in the visible and NIR; barium-sulfate, **MgO**, **Spectralon**, and Zenith are most commonly used; for IR applications gold coatings are available.

integration time: the time interval over which measurements are taken; longer integration times allow more averaging in order to filter out background noise and boost the signal-to-noise ratio.

intensity: several measures of light are commonly known as intensity: radiant intensity is a radiometric quantity, measured in watts per steradian (W/sr); luminous intensity is a photometric quantity, measured in lumens per steradian (lm/sr), or candela (cd); **radiance** (**irradiance**) is commonly called "intensity," measured in watts per meter squared (W/m^2).

intensity probability density distribution function: a function that describes the distribution of probability over the values of the light intensity.

interference: the process in which two or more light, sound, or electromagnetic waves of the same frequency combine to reinforce or cancel each other, with the amplitude of the resulting wave being equal to the algebraic sum of the amplitude of the combining waves.

interference fringes: a series of alternating dark and bright bands produced as a result of light interference; with a monochromatic source of light, the bands (fringes) are alternately bright and dark; with white light, the interference bands are colored.

interference of photon density waves (intensity waves): the process in which two or more photon density waves of the same frequency combine to reinforce or cancel each other, with the amplitude of the resulting wave being equal to the algebraic sum of the amplitude of the combining waves.

interference of speckle fields (speckle-modulated fields): the interference of the fields in which amplitudes and phases are randomly modulated due to their interaction (scattering) with inhomogeneous (scattering) media.

interferometer: an instrument that splits a beam of light into a number of coherent beams and then superimposes the beams to obtain interference fringes; the instrument is used to accurately measure wavelengths of light, to examine the hyperfine structure of spectra, to test optical elements for refraction purposes; and to accurately measure distance, displacement, and vibrations.

internal conversion: as a transition between one set of atomic (or molecular) electronic excited levels to another set of the same spin multiplicity (for example, the second singlet state to the first singlet state); it is sometimes called "radiationless deexcitation," because no photons are emitted; it differs from **intersystem crossing** in that, while both are radiationless methods of deexcitation, the molecular spin state for internal conversion remains the same, whereas it changes for intersystem crossing.

intersystem crossing: a photophysical process; an isoenergetic nonradiative transition between two electronic states that have different multiplicities; it often results in a vibrationally excited molecular entity in the lower electronic state, which then usually deactivates to its lowest vibrational level.

invariant embedding method: a method applied to the propagation of various wave types (acoustic, gravity, and electromagnetic) in inhomogeneous media; this method is used to reduce the initial boundary value problems to problems with initial data, permitting the solution of both determinate and statistical problems; it is applicable to both stationary (linear and nonlinear) and nonstationary wave problems.

inverse adding-doubling (IAD) method (technique): a method that provides a tool for the rapid and accurate solution to the inverse scattering problem; it is based on the general method for the transport equation for plane-parallel layers; the term "doubling" means that the reflection and transmission estimates for a layer at certain ingoing and outgoing light angles may be used to calculate both the transmittance and reflectance for a layer twice as thick by means of superimposing one upon the other and summing the contributions of each layer to the total reflectance and transmittance; reflection and transmission in a layer that has an arbitrary thickness are calculated in consecutive order, first for the thin layer with the same optical characteristics (single scattering), then by consecutive doubling of the thickness for any selected layer; the term "adding" indicates that the doubling procedure may be extended to heterogeneous layers for modeling multilayer tissues or taking into account internal reflections related to abrupt changes in refractive index.

inverse MC (IMC) method: the iterative method based on the statistical simulation of photon transport in the scattering media; provides the most accurate solutions to inverse scattering problems; it takes into account the real geometry of the object, the measuring system, and light beams; the main disadvantage is the long computation time.

inverse scattering problem: an attempt to take a set of measurements and error estimates, and only a limited set of parameters describing the sample and experiment, and to deriving the remaining parameters; usually the geometry is known, intensities or their parameters are measured, and the optical properties or sizes of scatterers need to be derived; if these properties are considered to be spatially varying, then the resultant solutions can be presented as a 2D or 3D function of space, i.e., as an image.

ionizing radiation: either particle radiation or electromagnetic radiation in which an individual particle/photon carries enough energy to ionize an atom or molecule by completely removing an electron from its orbit; these ionizations, if enough occur, can be very destructive to living tissue and can cause **DNA** damage and mutations; examples of particle radiation that are ionizing may be energetic electrons, neutrons, atomic ions, or photons; electromagnetic radiation can cause ionization if the energy per photon, or frequency, is high enough, and thus the wavelength is short enough; the amount of energy required varies between molecules being ionized; **x rays** and gamma rays will ionize almost any molecule or atom; far ultraviolet, near ultraviolet, and visible light are ionizing to some molecules; microwaves and radio waves are nonionizing radiation.

IQ circuit: an in-phase quadrature demodulator, a device that allows one to measure the amplitude and phase of an ac signal using the $0°/90°$-phase mixing technique of the receiving and reference signals.

irradiance: a radiometric quantity, measured in watts per meter squared (W/m^2).

irreversible thermodynamics: if the change from initial state to final state of the system is so slow that the process can be assumed to be proceeding through a series of closely spaced quasi-equilibrium states, then such a process is called a reversible process, and the entire time evolution of each of the state variables can be obtained from the conventional theory of thermodynamics; but almost all the processes in which we are most interested are irreversible processes, and the system is not in an equilibrium state during the time the system is evolving; a general theory of nonequilibrium thermodynamics does not exist; the thermodynamics of steady-state processes is relatively well established at least when the system does not deviate from equilibrium substantially.

isobestic point: the point (wavelength) at the spectra having an identical absorption for different forms of molecules.

isotropic scattering: equality of scattering properties along all axes.

KDP: kalium dihydrophosphate; the material widely used in nonlinear optics, for example, for light modulation and frequency doubling.

Kirchhoff approximation: an approximate method for solving wave diffraction problems that is applicable for finding the diffracted field at wave diffraction on inhomogeneities with sizes much larger than the wavelength.

K-space spectral analysis: a near-field wave technique that relies on a series of 2D fast Fourier transforms and that is employed for fast image reconstruction.

Kubelka-Munk model: a two-flux model describing the transportation of radiation in a scattering medium; it employs simple relations for evaluating optical parameters using the diffuse transmittance and reflectance measurements.

laminar flow: occurs when a fluid flows in parallel layers with no disruption between the layers; in fluid dynamics, laminar flow is a flow regime characterized by high momentum diffusion, low momentum convection, and pressure and velocity independence from time; it is the opposite of **turbulent flow**.

Laplace transform: a technique for analyzing linear time-invariant systems such as electrical circuits, harmonic oscillators, optical devices, and mechanical systems; it gives a simple mathematical or functional description to the input or output of a system.

laser: acronym for light amplification by the stimulated emission of radiation; a device that generates a beam of light that is collimated, monochromatic, and coherent.

laser beam: a group of nearly parallel rays generated by a laser; a light beam with a Gaussian shape for the transverse intensity profile (see **Gaussian light beam**).

laser calorimetry: a measuring technique that detects a temperature rise in a sample induced by absorption of a laser beam.

laser Doppler anemometry: the technique of measuring the velocity of flows by the Doppler method using a laser (see **Doppler effect**, **Doppler microscopy**, and **Doppler spectroscopy**).

laser Doppler interferometry: the technique of measuring the velocity of the particles in a flow by the Doppler method using a laser interferometer when a particle's velocity is measured by its traversing of interference fringes.

laser flow cytometry: flow cytometry (see **cytometry** in Glossary 2) with laser excitation of **fluorescence**, **light scattering**, or **polarization** transform of cells under investigation.

laser heating: the heating of an object by laser radiation.

laser interferential retinometer: a device for determining retinal visual acuity in the human eye by projecting the interference fringes produced by a laser interferometer at the retina.

laser power: rate of radiation emission from a laser, normally expressed in watts (W), milliwatts (mW), or microwatts (μW).

laser radiation: the radiation emitted by a laser.

laser speckle contrast analysis (LASCA): the method that uses the spatial statistics of time-integrated speckles; the full-field technique for visualizing capillary blood flow.

latex: a suspension of micron-sized **polystyrene spheres**.

length of thermal diffusivity (thermal length): the length within a medium (tissue) characterizing the distance of heat diffusion at medium heating by a short localized laser or acoustic pulse.

lenslet: a set of spatially distributed lenslike (phase) irregular inhomogeneities.

Light: **ultraviolet (UV)**, **UVC**: 100–280 nm; **UVB**: 280–315 nm; **UVA**: 315–400 nm: **visible**: 400–780 nm (**violet**: 400–450 nm; **blue**: 450–480 nm; **green**: 510–560 nm; **yellow**: 560–590 nm; **orange**: 590–620 nm; **red**: 620–780 nm); **infrared (IR) light**, IRA: 0.78–1.4 μm: **IRB**: 1.4–3.0 μm; **IRC**: 3–1000 μm; **near IR (NIR)**: 0.78–2.5 μm; **middle IR (MIR)**: 2.5–50 μm; and **far IR (FIR)**: 50–2000 μm.

light-emitting diode (LED) (light diode): a semiconductor device that emits light when the forward-directed current passes the *p-n* junction.

lifetime of the excited state: "lifetime" refers to the time the molecule (atom) stays in its excited state before emitting a photon; the lifetime is related to the rate of the excited state of decay, to the facility of the relaxation pathway, radiative and nonradiative; if the rate of spontaneous emission, or any other rate, is fast the lifetime is short; for commonly used fluorescent compounds the typical excited state decay times are within the range of 0.5 to 20 ns.

light guide: an assembly of optical fibers that are bundled but not ordered and that are used for illumination.

light scattering: a change in direction of the propagation of light in a turbid medium caused by reflection and refraction by microscopic internal structures.

light-scattering matrix [LSM (intensity or Mueller matrix)]: the 4×4 matrix that connects the **Stokes vector** of incident light with the **Stokes vector** of scattered light; it describes the polarization state of the scattered light in the far zone that is dependent on the polarization state of the incident light and structural and optical properties of the object.

linear regression: a regression method that allows for the linear relationship between the dependent variable Y and the p independent variables X and a random term ε.

Linnik microscope: see **Linnik-Tolansky interferometer**.

Linnik-Tolansky interferometer: a dual-beam interferometer with a beamsplitter, two reflecting surfaces, and two lenses for focusing beams on the surfaces.

liquid crystal: a substance that exhibits a phase of matter that has properties between those of a conventional liquid, and those of a solid crystal; for instance, a liquid crystal may flow like a liquid, but it has the molecules in the liquid arranged and/or oriented in a crystal-like way.

lithium niobate ($LiNbO_3$): a compound of niobium, lithium, and oxygen; it is a colorless solid material with a trigonal crystal structure; it is transparent for wavelengths between 350 and 5200 nanometers and is used for the manufacture of optical modulators and acoustic wave devices.

local oscillator: the radio- (or optical) frequency oscillator used in heterodyne detecting systems; a local oscillator is stable in frequency and amplitude and has a slightly different frequency than the receiving signal; it is used for converting a high-frequency receiving signal to an intermediate frequency by mixing the local oscillator signal and the receiving signal at an electronic (or photo) detector.

lock-in-amplifier: a low-frequency electronic device that provides synchronous detection of small signals that may have amplitudes a few orders lower than the noise level; the lock-in circuit contains the selective amplifier and a phase detector tuned to the modulation frequency of the detecting signal.

low-pass filter: a filter that rejects the high-frequency components.

low-step scattering: the scattering process in which, on average, each photon undertakes no more than a few scattering events (approximately less than five to ten).

LSM element: one of 16 elements of the light-scattering matrix; each element depends on the scattering angle and wavelength, and the geometrical and optical parameters of the scatterers and their arrangement.

luminescence: light not generated by high temperatures alone; it is different from incandescence, in that it usually occurs at low temperatures and is thus a form of cold body radiation; it can be caused by, for example, chemical reactions, electrical energy, subatomic motions, or stress on a crystal; the following kinds of luminescence are known: **fluorescence**, **phosphorescence**, bioluminescence, photoluminescence, **sonoluminescence**, chemoluminescence, electroluminescence, radioluminescence, mechanoluminescence, triboluminescence, piezoluminescence, thermoluminescence, et al.

Mach-Zehnder interferometer: a dual-beam, four-mirror (two serve as the beamsplitter and beam coupler, and two as reflectors) interferometer typically used as a refractometer, especially for objects occupying a large space.

magnetic resonance imaging (MRI): a noninvasive imaging technique that is based on magnetic resonance methods; it provides a wealth of information about inner structures of the body and, in particular, tumors.

matching substance: a substance used to reduce the boundary effects caused by the complex shape of a scattering object; the scattering properties of such a substance should be similar to the scattering properties of the object under study.

material dispersion: describes the separation of the different wavelengths in a given medium (material) that occurs because the waves are traveling at different velocities in that medium.

Matlab: a high-level language and interactive environment that enables one to perform computationally intensive tasks faster than with traditional programming languages such as C, C++, and Fortran.

mean free path length (MFP): the mean distance between two successive interactions with scattering or absorption experienced by a photon traveling in a scattering-absorption medium.

mechanical stress: the action on a body of any system of balanced forces that results in strain or deformation.

mercury arc lamp: a discharge arc lamp filled with mercury vapor at high pressure; it gives out very bright **UV** and **visible light** at some wavelengths, including 303, 312, 365, 405, 436, 546, and 578 nm.

meridional plane: planes that include the optical axis are meridional planes; it is common to simplify problems in radially symmetric optical systems by choosing object points in the vertical plane only; this plane is then sometimes referred to as the meridional plane.

MgO (magnesium oxide, or magnesia): a white solid mineral that occurs naturally as periclase and is a source of magnesium; it is formed by an ionic bond between one magnesium and one oxygen atom; it is used as a reference white color in photometry and colorimetry; the emissivity value is about 0.9; pressed MgO is used as an optical material; it is transparent from 300 nm to 7 μm; the refractive index is 1.72 at 1 μm.

Michelson interferometer: a dual-beam interferometer with a beamsplitter and two reflecting surfaces; it allows one to realize various types of interference and is widely used in metrology for measurements of lengths, displacements, vibrations, and surface roughness; recently an integrated fiber-optic prototype became very popular (see **fiber-optic single-mode X-coupler**); also widely used in tissue spectroscopy and imaging (see **dual-beam coherent interferometry** and **Doppler interferometry**).

micrometer (i.e., micron or μm): a unit of length that is 10^{-3} millimeter (mm) or 10^{-6} meter (m).

microphone: a device for transforming sound energy into electrical energy; the various types are the carbon microphone, crystal microphone, condenser microphone, and a moving coil or dynamic microphone.

microprofilometer: a device for measuring the roughness of a surface.

microscopy: any technique for producing visible images of structures or details too small to otherwise be seen by the human eye, using a microscope or other magnification tool; more specifically, it is a technique of using a microscope; there are three main branches of microscopy: optical, electron, and scanning probe microscopy; optical and **electronic microscopy** involves the **diffraction, reflection,** or **refraction** of radiation incident upon the subject of study, and the subsequent collection of this scattered radiation in order to build up an image; this process may be carried out by wide-field irradiation of the sample (for example, standard light microscopy and transmission electron microscopy) or by scanning a fine beam over the sample (for example, **confocal microscopy** and scanning electron microscopy); scanning probe microscopy involves the interaction of a scanning probe with the surface or object of interest.

microsecond (μsec) (μs): 10^{-6} sec (s).

micro-spectrophotometric technique: a technique that measures an object's transmittance or reflectance spectra with a high spatial resolution; usually a combination of a microscope and a grating spectrograph with an optical multichannel analyzer (cooled CCD or photodiode array) is used for such measurements.

Mie or **Lorenz-Mie scattering theory**: an exact solution of Maxwell's electromagnetic field equations for a homogeneous sphere.

millisecond (msec) (ms): 10^{-3} sec (s).

minimal erythema dose (MED): the minimal single dose of UV radiation, expressed as energy per unit area J/cm^2, producing a clearly marginated erythema at the irradiated skin site after 24 hours for UVB and 48 hours for UVA.

M-mode OCT image: an image obtained from repeated **A-scans** without moving the incident beam, so it can easily visualize living-object movement and time-dependent changes of tissue structure.

mode-locked laser: a multimode laser with synchronously irradiating modes; the regime is obtained by applying an intracavity high-frequency modulator, with a typical pulse duration of up to a subpicosecond range and a repetition frequency of dozens of megahertz.

modulation: the process of varying the characteristics of an optical wave motion by superimposing on it the characteristics of a second (audio- or radiofrequency) wave motion; there are three main types of modulation: amplitude modulation, frequency modulation, and phase modulation.

modulation frequency: the frequency of the modulating wave.

molecular hyperpolarizability: see **hyperpolarizability**.

monochromatic light: light of one color (wavelength) only or a very limited range of wavelengths; produced by a CW single-frequency (single longitudinal mode) laser.

monodisperse model: a model presenting a disperse medium as monodisperse, such as an ensemble of scatterers with an equal size and refractive index for each scatterer: a healthy eye cornea is a good example of a monodisperse model.

monodisperse system: a disperse system (medium) with a single characteristic parameter, such as an ensemble of scatterers with an equal size and refractive index for each scatterer; a healthy eye cornea is a good example of a monodisperse system, because it consists of dielectric rods with the same refractive index and radius dispersed in a homogeneous ground substance.

Monte Carlo method: a numerical method of statistical modeling; in tissue studies it provides the most accurate simulation of photon transport in samples with a complex geometry, accounting for the specificity of the measuring system and light beam configurations.

Mueller matrix: a 4×4 matrix that transforms an incident **Stokes vector** into the corresponding output Stokes vector of the sample; it fully characterizes the optical polarization properties of the sample; it can be experimentally obtained from measurements with different combinations of source **polarizers** and detection analyzers; at least 16 independent measurements must be acquired to determine a full Mueller matrix.

multichannel optoelectronic near-infrared system for time-resolved image reconstruction (MONSTIR): the noninvasive imaging technique developed at University College London for studying infant brain function that is based on the detection of transmitted pulsed NIR radiation.

multichannel plate: an integrated optical system used for optical amplification (image intensification).

multichannel plate-photomultiplier tube (MCP-PMT): a photomultiplier tube that is integrated with a multichannel plate.

multiflux model: the simplest multiflux model describing transportation of radiation in a scattering medium that employs only two fluxes is the **Kubelka-Munk model**; a more general approach is the discrete ordinates method (or many-flux theory) when the transport equation (**RTT**) can be converted into a matrix differential equation by considering the radiance at many discrete angles; by increasing the number of angles, the matrix solution should approach the exact solution; for laser beam applications, the four-flux model makes use of two diffuse fluxes and forward and backward coherent fluxes; a three-dimensional six-flux model is also available.

multifrequency multiplex (time division multiplex): a process in which measurements on many modulation frequencies are provided concurrently.

multilayered tissue: a tissue that consists of many layers with different structural and optical properties, such as skin, the bladder wall, and wall of bladder.

multimode fiber: a single fiber that allows the excitation (direction) of many modes (rays); e.g., for a fiber with a core diameter of 50 μm, numerical aperture, $NA = 0.2$, and an excitation wavelength of 633 nm, the number of excited modes is equal to 1250.

multiphoton absorption process: a process that needs a very high density of photons ($0.1–10$ MW/cm^2) from a ps-to-fs-pulsed light source; this is because the virtual absorption of a photon of nonresonant energy lasts only for a very short period ($10^{-15}–10^{-18}$ s); during this time a second photon must be absorbed to reach an excited state (http://www.fz-juelich.de/ibi/ibi-1/Two-Photon_Microscopy/).

multiphoton fluorescence: relies on the quasi-simultaneous absorption of two or more photons (of either the same or different energy) by a molecule; during the absorption process, an electron of the molecule is transferred to an excited-state molecular orbit; the molecule (i.e., the fluorophore) in the excited state has a high probability ($>10\%$) to emit a photon during relaxation to the ground state; due to radiationless relaxation in vibrational levels, the energy of the emitted photon is lower compared to the sum of the energy of the absorbed photons (http://www.fz-juelich.de/ibi/ibi-1/Two-Photon_Microscopy/).

multiphoton fluorescence scanning microscopy: the microscopy that employs detection of multiphoton fluorescence at the scanning of a laser beam, inducing the multiphoton signal (see also **two-photon fluorescence microscopy**).

multiple scattering: a scattering process in which, on average, each photon undertakes many scattering events (approximately more than five to ten).

multiwavelength multiplex (wavelength division multiplex): a process in which measurements on many wavelengths are provided concurrently.

nanometer (nm): a unit of length equal to 10^{-9} meter (m).

nanoparticle: a microscopic particle whose size is measured in **nanometres** (nm); it is defined as a particle with at least one dimension <100 nm.

nanosecond (nsec) (ns): 10^{-9} sec (s).

narrow-band filter: an electronic device that selectively damps oscillations of frequencies out of the narrow band while not affecting oscillations of frequencies within this band.

Nd:YAG (neodymium:yttrium aluminium garnet) laser: a solid-state laser whose lasing medium is the crystal Nd:YAG with emission in the NIR at 1064 nm; other less intensive lines at 946, 1319, 1335, 1338, 1356, and 1833 nm are also available.

network analyzer: a two-channel electronic system for measuring amplitude frequency characteristics of a four-terminal network producing modulation swept in the wide-frequency range (for example, 0.3–1000 MHz) and analyzing the detected signal synchronously in the same frequency range.

Nomarski polarizing-interference microscope: an optical microscope with differential interference contrast that incorporates a common path interferometer based on a polarizing prism.

non-Gaussian statistics: a statistically nonuniform process in which the statistical characteristics of the scattered light essentially depend on the observation angle and the degree of nonuniformity of an object.

nonlinear polarization of a material: if the dielectric polarization density (dipole moment per unit volume) P is not linearly proportional to the electric field E, the medium is termed nonlinear and is described by the field of nonlinear optics; to a good approximation (for sufficiently weak fields, assuming no permanent dipole moments are present), P is usually given by a Taylor series in E whose coefficients are the **nonlinear susceptibilities**.

nonlinear regression technique: related to a model $y = f(x, \theta) + \varepsilon$, based on multidimensional x, y data, where f is some nonlinear function with respect to unknown parameters θ; at a minimum, one may like to obtain the parameter values associated with the best fitting curve.

nonlinear susceptibility: the electric susceptibility of a dielectric material is a measure of how easily it polarizes in response to an electric field; this, in turn, determines the electric permittivity of the material and thus influences many phenomena in that medium (for instance, the speed of light); linear susceptibility is defined as the constant of proportionality (which may be a tensor) relating an electric field E, and nonlinear, relating to E^2, E^3, etc., to the induced dielectric polarization density P.

non-Newtonian flow: the flow of a fluid in which the viscosity changes with the applied strain rate; as a result, non-Newtonian fluids may not have a well-defined viscosity.

nonradiative relaxation (nonradiative energy transfer): the relaxation of an excited molecule (losing energy) without emission of light, when the molecule's energy is transformed into the heat, which raises the temperature of the body absorbing the energy by increasing the kinetic energy of the particles composing the body.

nonuniform medium: see **inhomogeneous medium**.

numerical aperture (NA): the light-gathering power of an objective or optical fiber; it is proportional to the sine of the acceptance angle.

objective speckles: the speckles formed in a free space and usually observed on a screen placed at a certain distance from an object.

open-circuit: in electronics, the absence of a load through which electric current would otherwise flow; this can be represented by an infinitely large resistance or **impedance**.

optical activity: the ability of a substance to rotate the plane of polarization of plane- (linear) polarized light (see **chirality**).

optical anisotropy: the difference of optical properties of materials caused by the dependence of light velocity (**refractive index**) on the direction of light propagation and **polarization of light** (see **anisotropic crystal**); it manifests as **birefringence**, **dichroism**, and **optical activity**, as well as **depolarization** at light scattering in a medium, polarized fluorescence, etc.; optical anisotropy may be induced in an optically isotropic medium at external action (mechanical, electrical, magnetic, etc.) that changes its local symmetry; related effects are **photoelasticity**, Kerr effect, Faraday effect, Cotton-Mouton effect, and nonlinear optical activity.

optical attenuator: a device for decreasing the intensity of light; optically neutral or color filters are usually used as attenuators with a fixed or stepwise-variable attenuation; for polarized light an attenuator with a continuously variable attenuation of the rotating polarizer (analyzer) is used.

optical autocorrelator: a device for measuring the autocorrelation function of intensity fluctuations of a scattered optical field.

optical birefringence: see **birefringence**.

optical breakdown: a breakdown in air (and in other transparent media) that is initiated by intense light; the required intensity for optical breakdown depends on the pulse duration; for example, for 1-ps pulses an optical intensity of $\approx 2 \times 10^{13}$ W/cm^2 is required; the high optical intensities can be reached in pulses as generated, e.g., in a **Q-switched laser** (with nanosecond durations) or in a **mode-locked laser** and amplified in a regenerative amplifier (for pulse durations of **picoseconds** or **femtoseconds**).

optical calorimetry: a measuring technique that detects of a temperature rise in a sample induced by light-beam absorption.

optical clearing: controlling optical properties of a scattering medium resulting in the increase of its optical transmittance.

optical coherence interferometry (OCI): see **Doppler interferometry** and **dual-beam coherent interferometry**.

optical coherence microscopy: an **optical microscope** based on a short-focused **OCT**.

optical coherence tomography (OCT): a technique that is based on **Doppler interferometry** in which a partially coherent light source is used and, in addition to the reference beam path length scanning (z-scan) that provides depth profiling of an object, transverse ($x-y$) scanning for 3D images is used; the integrated **single-mode fiber-optic Michelson interferometer** is usually used in OCT; the method is widely used for subsurface tomography of tissue.

optical coherent reflectometry: see **optical coherence tomography (OCT)**.

optical conjugate: two optical points, lines, etc. that are so related as to be interchangeable in certain optical properties; an optical system that provides two points so that a source at one point is brought to focus at the other, and vice versa.

optical darkening effect: controlling of optical properties of a scattering medium resulting in the decrease of its optical transmittance.

optical depth: a measure of transparency, and is defined as the fraction of radiation that is scattered and/or absorbed on a path; the optical depth τ expresses the quantity of light removed from a beam by scattering and/or absorption during its path through a medium.

optical detector: a device that converts optical energy to an electric signal.

optical diffusion tomography: an optical **tomography** that is based on the measurements of CW, pulsed, or modulated light beam transmittance or spatially-resolved reflectance of scattering media with an object (i.e., a tumor) hidden in it; to provide 3D images, synchronous light beam-detector scanning devices or systems with multiple fixed-position light sources and detectors are used; the **back-projection algorithm** is used to provide image reconstruction along the paths of ballistic and/or least scattering photon propagation; the method is used for tomography of thick tissues (breast, brain, arm).

optical fiber cladding: see **fiber**.

optical fiber core: see **fiber**.

optical fiber coupler: see **fiber coupler**.

optical fiber dispersion: in optics, **dispersion** is a phenomenon that causes the separation of a wave into spectral components with different wavelengths, due to the dependence of the wave's speed on its wavelength; dispersion is sometimes called chromatic dispersion to emphasize its wavelength-dependent nature; there are generally two sources of dispersion: material dispersion, which comes from the frequency-dependent response of a material to waves, and waveguide dispersion, which occurs when the speed of a wave in a waveguide (optical **fiber**) depends on its frequency; the transverse modes for waves confined laterally within a finite waveguide generally have different speeds (and field patterns), depending upon the frequency (that is, on the relative size of the wave, the wavelength, compared with the size of the waveguide); dispersion in an optical fiber results in signal degradation, because the varying delay in arrival time between different components of a signal "smears out" the signal in time; a similar phenomenon is modal dispersion, caused by a waveguide that has multiple modes at a given frequency, each with a different speed; a special case of this is polarization mode dispersion, which comes from a superposition of two modes that travel at different speeds due to random imperfections that break the symmetry of the waveguide.

optical Fourier transform: the transform when spatial variations in optical density in the object plane are converted into **spatial frequency** variations in the Fourier transform plane in the rear focal plane of a lens.

optical image: a reconstructed image of an object expressed in terms of local optical parameters, such as absorption and/or scattering coefficients.

optical Kerr effect: the double refraction of light in certain substances that is produced by an external electric field, including high-frequency fields up to the frequencies of IR light.

optical Kerr gate: a transparent cell filled with a substance that shows a Kerr effect and contains two electrodes placed between two polarizers: the cell serves as a high-speed optical shutter.

optical length (optical path length): in a medium with a constant refractive index, the product of the geometric distance and the refractive index; in a medium with a varying refractive index, the integral of the product of an element of length along the path and the local refractive index; optical length is proportional to the phase shift that a light wave undergoes along a path.

optical mean free path (MFP): see **mean free path length**.

optical medical tomography: see **optical diffusion tomography** and **optical coherence tomography (OCT)**.

optical microscopy: see **microscopy**.

optical multichannel analyzer (OMA): a spectrometric instrument that senses incident radiation in several channels at the same time, sorts the radiation from deep ultraviolet to the infrared, and digitizes and stores the information so that it can be processed and analyzed individually by channel.

optical parameters: the physical parameters that characterize the optical properties of an object.

optical parametric oscillator (OPO): a parametric oscillator that oscillates at optical frequencies; it converts an input laser wave (called a "pump") into two output waves of lower frequency (ω_s, ω_i) by means of nonlinear optical interaction; the sum of the output wave frequencies is equal to the input wave frequency: $\omega_s + \omega_i = \omega_p$; the OPO essentially consists of an optical resonator and a nonlinear optical crystal; the optical resonator serves to resonate at least one of the output waves.

optical path: see **optical length (optical path length)**.

optical phantom: a medium that models the transport of visible and infrared light in tissue and is needed to evaluate techniques, to calibrate equipment, to optimize procedures, and for quality assurance.

optical retarder: a device that provides an optical retardation: phase shift or optical path difference; such retarders as the half- or the quarter-wavelength plates provide, respectively, the half-wave or the quarter-wave phase difference.

optical sectioning (slicing): the process of extracting the optical image of a thin layer of tissue; the image is used for **tomographic reconstruction** of a whole body organ.

optical transition: typically an **electronic transition**, where energy is given out as electromagnetic radiation in the optical range.

optical transition lifetime: the radiative lifetime, which is determined by the emission cross section for transition to a lower-lying energy level.

optically thick sample: optical thickness is the depth of a material or medium in which the intensity of light of a given wavelength is reduced by a factor of $1/e$

because of absorption and/or scattering; a sample with high thickness and/or high turbidity that correspond to a few optical thickness depths is optically thick.

optically thin (transparent) sample: a sample with low thickness and/or low turbidity that corresponds to one or less than one optical thickness depth is optically thin.

optoacoustic (OA) interaction: the generation of acoustic waves by the interaction of pulsed or intensity-modulated optical radiation with a sample; actually, several effects can be responsible for such interaction, e.g., the optical inverse piezoelectric effect, optical electrostriction, or optothermal effect.

OA method: the detection of acoustic waves generated via OA interaction with a sample (the term OA primarily refers to the time-resolved technique utilizing pulsed lasers and measuring profiles of pressure in tissue).

OA microscopy: **microscopy** based on detection of an OA signal induced by a sharply focused laser beam.

OA spectroscopy: spectroscopy based on the detection of an OA signal induced by a monochromatic light source (laser) with tuned wavelength.

OA tomography: the **tomography** that is based on the **OA method**.

optode: a transducer that is attached to the distal tip of a fiber-optic sensor; the interaction between the optode and the body is monitored by the fiber-optic sensor.

optogeometric technique: the detection of surface deformation in solids and volume changes in fluids induced by an **optothermal interaction**.

optothermal interaction: the generation of heat waves by the interaction of pulsed or intensity-modulated optical radiation with a sample.

optothermal method: the detection of heat waves generated via interaction of pulsed or intensity-modulated optical radiation with a sample.

optothermal radiometry (OTR): the detection of time-dependent infrared thermal emissions induced by the **optothermal interaction** of light with a sample.

Ornstein-Zernice equation: an equation for the **radial distribution function** $g(r)$ of classical many-particle systems; thermodynamic properties of such systems are determined by the interaction between the particles from which the system is built up; if one knows the radial distribution function, one can calculate all thermodynamic properties of the considered system; light scattering properties of such systems also can be calculated.

osmotic phenomenon: the tendency of a fluid to pass through a semipermeable membrane into a solution where its concentration is lower, thus equalizing the conditions on either side of the membrane.

osmotic pressure: the hydrostatic pressure produced by a solution in a space divided by a differentially permeable membrane due to a differential in the concentrations of a solute.

osmotic stress: the force that a dissolved substance exerts on a semipermeable membrane through which it cannot penetrate, when it is separated from a pure solvent by the membrane.

overtone: a sinusoidal component of a waveform of greater frequency than its fundamental frequency; the term is usually used in acoustics.

oxymetry: the measurement of tissue or blood oxygenation.

packing dimension: one of the most important notions of **fractal dimension**.

packing factor: the fraction of volume in a medium structure that is occupied by particles; it is dimensionless and always less than unity; for practical purposes, a medium structure is often determined by assuming that particles are rigid spheres.

packing function: an analytical expression for molecular (particle) overlap as a function of position; it can be calculated by means of Fourier transforms; overlap functions between pairs of symmetry elements can be combined to give a crystallographic packing function.

paraxial approximation: an approximation used in ray tracing of light through an optical system.

paraxial region: the region where paraxial rays, lying close to the axis of an optical system, propagate.

partial-coherence interferometry: see **Doppler interferometry**, **dual-beam coherent interferometry**, **optical coherence interferometry (OCI)**.

partially-coherence tomography: see **optical coherence tomography (OCT)**.

percolation: concerns the movement and filtering of fluids through porous materials; recent percolation theory, an extensive mathematical model of percolation, has brought new understanding and techniques to a broad range of topics in physics and materials science.

perfusion pump: a fluid propulsion system that provides, for instance, long-term controlled-rate delivery of drugs such as chemotherapeutic agents or analgesics.

permeability coefficient: permeability (P) of molecules across a biological (cell) membrane can be expressed as $P = KD/\Delta x$, where K is the partition coefficient, D is the **diffusion coefficient**, and Δx is the thickness of the membrane; the diffusion coefficient (D) is a measure of the rate of entry into the cell cytoplasm depending on the molecular weight or size of a molecule; K is a measure of the solubility of the substance in lipids; a low value of K describes a molecule like water that is not soluble in lipid.

perturbation method: a method used to find an approximate solution to a problem that cannot be solved exactly, by starting from the exact solution of a related problem; is applicable if the problem at hand can be formulated by adding a "small" term to the mathematical description of the exactly solvable problem; leads to an expression for the desired solution in terms of a power series in some "small" parameter that quantifies the deviation from the exactly solvable problem.

perovskite laser: a neodymium: yttrium aluminum perovskite laser (Nd:YAP); a laser using an yttrium-aluminum-perovskite crystal doped with neodymium as a lasing medium emitting on the wavelength $\lambda = 1341$ nm.

phantom: a standard experimental tissue model (see **optical phantom**).

phase-contrast microscopy (**phase microscopy**): a microscopy that translates the difference in the phase of light transmitted through or reflected by an object into the difference of intensity in the image.

phase-delay measurement device: see **"cross-correlation" measurement device** and **heterodyne phase system**.

phase function: see **scattering phase function**.

phase fluctuations of the scattered field: the fluctuations that are induced by different optical paths for different parts or time periods of a wavefront interacting with an inhomogeneous, generally dynamic medium.

phase lag: a phase shift relative to the incident light modulation phase.

phase object: an object that introduces the difference in phase of the light transmitted through or reflected by an object.

$\lambda/4$-phase plate: see **optical retarder**; a device that provides an optical phase shift of 90° ($\pi/2$ radians) or an optical path difference equal to a quarter of the wavelength; a thin plate of birefringent substance, such as calcite or quartz, is cut parallel to the optical axis of the crystal with a specific thickness that is calculated to give a phase difference of 90° ($\pi/2$ radians) between the emergent ordinary ray and the emergent extraordinary ray for light of a specified wavelength; quarter-wave plates are usually constructed for the wavelengths of sodium light (589 nm); if the angle between the plane of polarization of light incident upon the plate and the optic axis of the plate is 45°, then circularly polarized light is produced and emerges from the plate; if the angle is other than 45°, elliptically polarized light is produced.

phase shift (**phase difference**): the difference in phase between two wave forms; the phase difference is measured by the phase angle between the waves: when two waves have a phase shift (difference) of 90° (or $\pi/2$ radians), one wave is at maximum amplitude when the other wave is at zero amplitude; with a phase difference of 180° (π radians), both waves have zero amplitude at the same time, but one wave is at a crest when the other wave is at a trough.

phase or amplitude cancellation (phased array) method: the basis for this method is the interference of photon-density waves [see **interference of photon density waves (intensity waves)** and **photon-density wave**]; it uses either duplicate sources and a single detector or duplicate detectors and a single source so that the amplitude or phase characteristics can be nulled and the system becomes a differential.

phase plate: see **λ/4-phase plate** and **optical retarder**.

phased-array technique: a spectroscopic or imaging technique that utilizes the **interference of photon density waves (intensity waves)**.

phonon: a quantized mode of vibration occurring in a rigid crystal lattice, such as the atomic lattice of a solid; the study of phonons is an important part of solid state physics, because phonons play a major role in many of the physical properties of solids, including a material's thermal and electrical conductivities; in particular, the properties of long-wavelength phonons give rise to sound in solids—hence the name "phonon," i.e., "voice" in Greek; in insulating solids, phonons are also the primary mechanism by which heat conduction takes place.

phosphorescence: **luminescence** that is delayed with respect to the excitation of a sample.

photoacoustic (PA) method: see **optoacoustic (OA) method**; the term PA primarily describes spectroscopic experiments with CW-modulated light and a photoacoustic cell.

photoacoustic microscopy (PAM): a microscopy utilizing the photoacoustic method and a photoacoustic cell for signal detection.

photobiochemical reaction: a chemical reaction in living matter that is induced by light.

photodetector: see **optical detector**.

photocathode: a cathode that has the property of emitting electrons when activated by light or other radiation.

photoconductive detector: a **photodetector** in which an electric potential is applied across the absorbing region and causes a current to flow in proportion to the irradiance if the photon energy exceeds the energy gap between the valence and the conduction band; for the visible wavelength range—cadmium sulfide, for IR— lead sulfide, silicon doped with arsenide (Si:As), and mercury-cadmium-telluride (HgCdTe) are used as photoconductive materials.

photoelasticity: stress-induced **birefringence** and **dichroism** of a medium.

photomechanical waves: see **laser-generated stress waves**.

photomultiplier [photomultiplying tube (PMT)]: an extremely sensitive detector of light and other radiation consisting of a tube in which the electrons released by radiation striking a photocathode are accelerated to successive dynodes that release several electrons for each incident electron, greatly amplifying the signal obtainable from small quantities of radiation.

photon: a quantum of electromagnetic radiation, usually considered as an elementary particle that has its own antiparticle and that has zero rest mass and charge and a spin of 1.

photon absorption cross section: the ability of a molecule to absorb a photon of a particular wavelength and polarization; although the units are given as an area, it does not refer to an actual size area, at least partially because the density or state of the target molecule will affect the probability of absorption; quantitatively, the number dN of photons absorbed, between the points x and $x + dx$ along the path of a light beam is the product of the number N of photons penetrating to depth x times the number ρ of absorbing molecules per unit volume times the absorption cross section σ_{abs}: $dN/dx = -\rho\sigma_{abs}N$.

photon-correlation spectroscopy: a noninvasive method for studying the dynamics of particles on a comparatively large time scale; the implementation of the single-scattering regime and the use of coherent light sources are of fundamental importance in this case; the spatial scale of testing a colloid structure (an ensemble of biological particles) is determined by the inverse of the wave vector; **quasi-elastic light scattering** spectroscopy, **spectroscopy of intensity fluctuations**, and **Doppler spectroscopy** are synonymous terms related to **dynamic light scattering**.

photon-counting system: a system that makes use of a specific method of photoelectron signal processing and provides sequential detection of single photons; **photomultipliers (PMT)** or **avalanche photodetectors (APD)** are usually used for photon counting; the technique is applicable for detecting very weak signals.

photoelasticity: an experimental method to determine stress distribution in a material; unlike the analytical methods of stress determination, photoelasticity gives a fairly accurate picture of stress distribution even around abrupt discontinuities in a material; the method serves as an important tool for determining the critical stress points in a material and is often used for determining stress concentration factors in irregular geometries.

photon-density wave: a wave of progressively decaying intensity; microscopically, individual photons migrate randomly in a scattering medium, but collectively they form a photon-density wave at a modulation frequency that moves away from a radiation source.

photon diffusion coefficient: see **diffusion coefficient**.

photon (intensity) diffusion wave: see **photon-density wave**.

photon scattering cross section: the ability of a particle to scatter a photon of a particular wavelength and polarization; although the units are given as an area, it does not refer to an actual size area; quantitatively, the number dN of photons scattered, between the points x and $x + dx$ along the path of a light beam, is the product of the number N of photons penetrating to depth x times the number ρ of scattering particles per unit volume times the scattering cross section σ_{sca}: $dN/dx = -\rho\sigma_{sca}N$.

photon shot noise: the noise caused by the irregularity of photoelectron emission; it induces random errors in a photoelectron measuring system; the mean square of photoelectron current fluctuation is defined by the average photocurrent i and the photodetector's bandwidth B_D: $i^2 = 2ei\,B_D$, where e is the charge of the electron; it is difficult to achieve the shot noise limit in practice.

photon transport: a process of photon travel in a homogeneous or inhomogeneous medium with possible macroinhomogeneities; a photon changes its direction due to reflection, refraction, diffraction, or scattering and can be absorbed by an appropriate molecule on its way.

photonic crystal: a periodic optical (nano)structure that affects the propagation of electromagnetic waves (EM) in the same way as the periodic potential in a semiconductor crystal affects the electron motion by defining allowed and forbidden electronic energy bands; the absence of allowed propagating EM modes inside the structures, in a range of wavelengths called a photonic band gap, gives rise to distinct optical phenomena, such as inhibition of spontaneous emission, high-reflecting omni-directional mirrors, and low-loss-waveguiding amongst others; since the basic physical phenomenon is based on **diffraction**, the periodicity of the photonic crystal structure has to be in the same length-scale as half the wavelength of the EM waves, i.e., ~300 nm for photonic crystals operating in the visible part of the spectrum; photonic crystals occur in nature, including biological tissues.

photorefractive technique: the detection of refractive index gradients above and inside a sample using thermal blooming, thermal lensing, probe beam refraction, or interferometry and deflectometry.

photosensitizer: a substance that increases the absorption of another substance at a particular wavelength band.

photothermal flow cytometry: **flow cytometry** that uses photothermal detection abilities.

photothermal microscopy: **microscopy** based on the detection of the photothermal signal induced by a sharply focused laser beams.

photothermal radiometry (PTR): see **optothermal radiometry (OTR)**.

picosecond: (psec) (ps)–10^{-12} sec (s).

piezoceramics: a piezoelectric material that is used to make electromechanical sensors and actuators; lead zirconate titanate (PZT) ceramics are an example; there are several different formulations of the PZT compound, each with different electromechanical properties.

piezodeflector: a device for light beam deflection at certain audio- or radiofrequencies using an acoustooptical effect.

piezo-driver: a device that uses the inverse piezoelectric effect in certain asymmetric crystals, which is obtained by applying a potential difference to a crystal; an alteration in the size of the crystal takes place.

piezoelectric transducer: a device that uses the piezoelectric effect in certain asymmetric crystals; the effect is obtained by applying external pressure to a crystal; positive and negative charges are produced on opposite faces of the crystal, giving rise to a potential difference between the faces; the potential difference operates in the opposite direction if tension is applied instead of pressure; this potential difference is the signal detected in a crystal microphone.

piezooptical coefficient: characterizes the efficiency of stress-induced **birefringence** and **dichroism** of a medium (see **photoelasticity**); indicates whether the material is good or not for stress sensors (**piezoelectric transducer**) and **acousto-optical modulators**.

PIN photodetector: a photodetector based on *p-i-n* semiconductor structure that has a fast response.

pixel: the smallest element of an image that can be individually displayed.

Planck curve (function): gives the intensity radiated by a blackbody as a function of frequency (or wavelength) for a definite body temperature; a blackbody is an object that absorbs all the electromagnetic energy that falls on the object, no matter what the wavelength of the radiation; the area under the curve increases as the temperature is increased (the Stefan-Boltzmann law); the peak in the emitted energy moves to the shorter wavelengths as the temperature is increased (Wien's law).

Planck's constant: (denoted as h) a physical constant that is used to describe the sizes of quanta; it plays a central role in the theory of quantum mechanics and is named after Max Planck, one of the founders of quantum theory; a closely-related quantity is the reduced Planck constant [also known as Dirac's constant $(\hbar = h/2\pi)$]; Planck's constant is also used in measuring energy emitted by light photons, such as in the equation $E = h\nu$, where E is energy, h is Planck's constant, and ν is frequency.

Pockel's cell: a piezoelectric crystal with two plane electrodes for applying an external electric field, placed between two crossed polarizers; the basis of its function is the linear electro-optical effect, which relates to a change in the refractive index of a crystal caused by an external electric field: the phase shift between ordinary and extraordinary rays linearly depends on the electrical field strength; the cell is widely used as an external laser or other light source intensity modulator, as well as an internal laser modulator for giant pulse **Q-switching**.

point spread function (PSF): describes the response of an imaging system to a point source or point object; another commonly used term for the PSF is a system's impulse response; the degree of spreading (blurring) of the point object is a measure for the quality of an imaging system; in functional terms it is the spatial domain version of the modulation transfer function; it is a useful concept in Fourier optics, electron microscopy and other imaging techniques such as 3D microscopy (i.e., **confocal microscopy** and **fluorescence** microscopy).

polarimetry: measurement of the polarization properties of light.

polarizability: the relative tendency of a charge distribution, like the electron cloud of an atom or molecule, to be distorted from its normal shape by an external electric field, which may be caused by the presence of a nearby ion or dipole; the electronic polarizability α is defined as the ratio of the induced dipole moment p of an atom to the electric field E that produces this dipole moment: $p = \alpha E$.

polarization of light (polarized light): a state, or the production of a state, in which rays of light exhibit different properties in different directions; **linear (plane)**: when the electric field vector oscillates in a single, fixed plane all along the beam, the light is said to be linearly (plane) polarized; **elliptical**: when the plane of the electric field rotates, the light is said to be elliptically polarized because the electric field vector traces out an ellipse at a fixed point in space as a function of time; **circular**: when the ellipse happens to be a circle, the light is said to be circularly polarized.

polarization anisotropy: an inequality of polarization properties along different axes.

polarization-gating techniques: techniques for selecting diffuse photon groups with different path lengths, in particular **ballistic** or least-scattering photons, based on their polarization properties; used in polarization-sensitive diffuse or **coherence optical tomography** and spectroscopy.

polarization optical spectroscopy: optical **spectroscopy** using polarizied light as a probe beam and/or detection of transmitted, scattered, or re-emitted polarized light.

polarization optical tomography: optical **tomography** using polarizied light as a probe beam and/or detection of transmitted, scattered, or re-emitted polarized light.

polarizer: a device, often a crystal or prism, that produces polarized light from unpolarized light.

polydisperse system: a **disperse** system (medium) with multiple values of characteristic parameters, such as an ensemble of scatterers with different sizes and refractive indices; a cataract eye lens is a good example of a polydisperse system, because it consists of dielectric balls (aggregated α-crystallins) with various refractive indices and radii dispersed in a homogeneous ground substance.

polydispersion: differently sized (and/or with different refractive indices) dispersed particles suspended in a solid, liquid, or gas.

polymer fiber: a fiber made from transparent polymer materials (see **fiber**).

polystyrene microspheres (beads): used for quality control, calibration, and sizing; widely used for cleanroom certification, filter testing, light-scattering experiments, tissue phantoms design, cell labeling, etc.; nanobeads ranging from 40 to 950 nm, microbeads ranging from 1.00 to 9.00 μm, and megabeads ranging from 10.0 to 175.0 μm are available on the market.

polyvinydene fluoride (PVDF): belongs to piezoelectric materials that are used to make electromechanical sensors and actuators.

porosity: a measure of the void spaces in a material, measured as a fraction, between 0–1.

potassium chromate (K_2CrO_4): the nonscattering, homogeneously absorbing liquid used for constructing phantoms.

power: the rate of energy delivery; it is normally measured in watts, that is, joules per second power-size distribution.

preamplifier: an electronic amplifier that precedes another amplifier to prepare an electronic signal for further amplification or processing.

pressure: the force per unit area applied on a surface in a direction perpendicular to that surface; pressure is scalar and has units of pascals, $1\ Pa = 1\ N/m^2$; pressure is transmitted to solid boundaries or across arbitrary sections of fluid normal to these boundaries or sections at every point.

pressure transient: the analysis of **pressure** changes over time.

probe beam: a light or **laser beam** used for an object or material probing.

probability: the relative frequency with which an event occurs or is likely to occur.

probability density function (probability density distribution): a function that describes the distribution of probability over the values of a variable.

propagation constant: the logarithmic rate of change, with respect to distance in a given direction, of the complex amplitude of any electromagnetic field component.

pulse laser: a laser that generates a single pulse or a set of pulses; a laser with **Q-switching** produces the so-called giant pulses, the **mode-locked laser** produces ultrashort pulses with a high repetition rate.

pump-beam (pulse): laser (light) beam (or pulse) used for the nonlinear material pumping or for interactions of the optical fields with matter in order to provide lasing or spectroscopy.

Q-switching: sometimes known as giant pulse formation, is a technique by which a laser can be made to produce a pulsed output beam; the technique allows the production of light pulses with extremely high (gigawatt) peak power, much higher than would be produced by the same laser if it is operating in a continuous wave mode; compared to **mode-locking**, Q-switching leads to much lower pulse repetition rates, much higher pulse energies, and much longer pulse durations; both techniques are sometimes applied at once.

quadrature mixer: an electronic device that mixes signals with different frequencies by the act of squaring.

quantum detection limit: the limit of detection that is defined by the quantum fluctuations of any light source, including a laser, associated with spontaneous emission and defined by the temperature of the medium that emits the light being detected; such fluctuations, as in the case of **photon shot noise**, cause the irregularity of photoelectron emissions hat induce random errors in a photoelectron measuring system; the mean square of photoelectron current fluctuations also is defined by the average photocurrent i and the photodetector's bandwidth B_{D}: $i^2 = 2ei\,B_{\mathrm{D}}$, where e is the charge of electrons, but the average photocurrent I is proportional to the mean power of quantum fluctuations: it is also difficult to achieve the quantum detection limit in practice.

quantum dot: a semiconductor nanostructure that confines the motion of conduction band electrons, valence band holes, or excitons (bound pairs of conduction band electrons and valence band holes) in all three spatial directions; the confinement can be due to electrostatic potentials (generated by external electrodes, doping, strain and impurities), the presence of an interface between different semiconductor materials (e.g., in core-shell nanocrystal systems), the presence of the semiconductor surface (e.g., semiconductor nanocrystal), or a combination of these; a quantum dot has a discrete quantized energy spectrum; a quantum dot contains a small finite number (of the order of 1–100) of conduction band electrons, valence band holes, or excitons, i.e., a finite number of elementary electric charges.

quantum efficiency of the detector: the ratio of the number of electrons emitted by a photodetector to the number incident at the detector's surface photons.

quantum flux: see **intensity**.

quantum yield: for a radiation-induced process quantum yield is the number of times that a defined event (usually a chemical reaction step) occurs per photon absorbed by the system; a measure of the efficiency with which absorbed light produces some effect; since not all photons are absorbed productively, the typical quantum yield is less than one; quantum yields greater than one are possible for photo-induced or radiation-induced chain reactions, in which a single photon may trigger a long chain of transformations; in optical spectroscopy, the quantum yield is the probability that a given quantum state is formed from the system initially prepared in some other quantum state; for example, a singlet to triplet transition quantum yield is the fraction of molecules that, after being photoexcited into a singlet state, cross over to the triplet state; the fluorescence quantum yield is defined as the ratio of the number of photons emitted to the number of photons absorbed.

quantum-well laser: a diode laser with a quantum-dimension heterostructure as a lasing medium; owing to a high gain, it has a high slope of the watt/ampere characteristic.

quasi-ballistic photons: photons that migrate within a scattering medium along trajectories that are close but not the same as for **ballistic photons**.

quasi-crystalline approximation: first introduced by Lax to break the infinite heirarchy of equations that results in studies of the coherent field in discrete random media; it simply states that the conditional average of a field with the position of one scatterer held fixed is equal to the conditional average with two scatterers held fixed; successful for a range of concentrations from parse to dense and for long and intermediate wavelengths.

quasi-elastic light scattering: see **dynamic light scattering**.

quasi-monochromatic wave: a wave that has a very narrow but nonzero frequency (or wavelength) bandwidth; it can be presented as a group of monochromatic waves with a slightly different wavelength.

quasi-Newton inverse algorithm: the algorithm for finding an extreme point; it builds up an approximation of the inverse Hessian of the function; it is often regarded as the most sophisticated for solving unconstrained problems.

quasi-ordered medium: a medium that has a structure very close to the ordered one but nevertheless is not completely ordered, which is caused by specific interactions between molecules and molecular structures; many of the natural media, including water and some living tissues, are examples of quasi-ordered media.

quasi-periodic (process, signal, function, fluctuations): almost periodic (process, signal, function, fluctuations); almost periodic, it is a property of dynamical systems that appear to retrace their paths through phase space, but not exactly.

radar graph: similar to line graphs, except that they use a radial grid to display data items; a radial grid displays scale value grid lines circling around a central point, which represents zero; higher data values are farther from the center point; the radar graph type gets its name because it resembles a radar screen; the radial grid is not circular but an equilateral polygon.

radial distribution function $g(r)$: the pair distribution function that is a statistical characteristic of the spatial arrangement of the scatterers; used to describe light scattering in a correlated disperse system.

radiance: see **intensity**, **irradiance**.

radiation dosimetry: the measurement or calculation of a radiation dose; the quantity of radiation absorbed by a given mass of material, especially tissue, is dependent upon the strength and distance of the light source and the duration of exposure.

radiation transfer equation (RTE): the integro-differential equation (the Boltzmann or linear transport equation), which is a balance equation describing the flow of particles (e.g., photons) in a given volume element that takes into account their velocity c, location r, and changes due to collisions (i.e., scattering and absorption).

radiation transfer theory (RTT): the theory based on the **radiation transfer equation (RTE)** allowing one to calculate light distributions in the scattering media with absorption.

radio frequency (RF): the part of the electromagnetic spectrum between about 10^6 and 10^9 Hz.

Raman amplifier: based on the **stimulated Raman scattering (SRS)** phenomenon, this process, as with other stimulated emission processes, allows all-optical amplification; **optical fiber** is almost exclusively used as the nonlinear medium for SRS, which is therefore characterized by a resonant frequency downshift of $\sim$13 THz; the SRS amplification process can be readily cascaded, thus accessing essentially any wavelength in the fiber low-loss guiding window.

Raman scattering: the change in wavelength of light scattered while passing through a transparent medium; the collection of new wavelengths is characteristic for the molecular structure of the scattering medium and differs from the fluorescence spectrum in being much less intense and unrelated to an absorption band of the medium; the frequencies of new lines are combinations of the frequency of the incident light and the frequencies of the molecular vibrational and rotational transitions.

Raman shifter: a device based on **stimulated Raman scattering** phenomenon; typically 1st, 2nd, and 3rd Stokes components are induced by a nonlinear medium pumped by a laser whose wavelength should be shifted; for example, the optimum conversion in the $Ba(NO_3)_2$ crystal at pump with a Ti:Sapphire laser (815 to 900 nm) provides a 1047 cm^{-1} shift and extends the laser tuning range to 1300 nm; gaseous and liquid Raman cells are also available; however, among the most efficient Raman crystals suitable for a wide range of pumping pulse durations from picoseconds to nanoseconds; $Ba(NO_3)_2$, $KGd(WO_4)_2$, and $BaWO_4$ are known.

Raman spectroscopy: a spectroscopic technique used in condensed matter (physics, chemistry, and biology) to study **vibrational, rotational**, and other low-frequency modes in a system; it relies on **inelastic scattering**, or **Raman scattering** of monochromatic light, usually from a **laser** in the **visible, near infrared**, or near **ultraviolet** range; **phonons** or other excitations in the system are absorbed or emitted by the laser light, resulting in the energy of the laser **photons** being shifted up or down; the shift in energy gives information about the phonon modes in the system; **infrared spectroscopy** yields similar, but complementary, information.

random medium: a specific state of a nonuniform (inhomogeneous) medium characterized by the irregular spatial distribution of its physical properties, including its optical properties.

random phase screen (RPS): a specific state of a random medium characterized by random spatial variations of the refractive index, which induces corresponding variations in the phase shift of the optical wave transmitted through or reflected by the RPS.

raw experimental data: experimental data before processing.

Rayleigh-Debye theory (approximation): the theory that addresses the problem of calculating the scattering by a special class of arbitrarily shaped particles; it requires that the electric field inside the particle be close to that of the incident field and that the particle can be viewed as a collection of independent dipoles that are all exposed to the same incident field.

Rayleigh distribution: the probability distribution of a random variable x described by the probability density function $p(x) = (x/a^2)\exp(-x^2/2a^2)$, $x \geq 0$; $p(x) = 0$, $x < 0$; the distribution has a positive asymmetry; its mode is at the point $x = a$; the mean value and variance are, respectively, equal to $\langle x \rangle = (\pi/2a)$ and $\sigma^2 = (4 - \pi)a^2/2$.

Rayleigh-Gans theory (approximation): see **Rayleigh-Debye theory (approximation)**.

Rayleigh (resolution) limit: the resolution of an optical device with a circular aperture is limited by the diffraction of light through that aperture; as the aperture increases in diameter, the diffraction spot gets smaller, which increases the resolution of the instrument; in the case of a circular aperture, the diffraction pattern has the shape of a disk surrounded by rings, which is called the Airy disk; if the images of two point sources of light overlap such that the centers of the images are closer than the radius of the Airy disk, the images are considered to be unresolvable; this definition can be written as: $\Delta\theta = 1.22\lambda/D$, where $\Delta\theta$ is the minimum resolvable angular separation of the two objects, λ is the wavelength of the light, and D is the diameter of the aperture.

Rayleigh (scattering) theory: the theory that addresses the problem of calculating scattering by small particles (with respect to the wavelength of the incident light) when individual particle scattering can be described as if it is a single dipole, the scattered irradiance is inversely proportional to λ^4 and increases as a^6, and the angular distribution of the scattered light is isotropic.

reduced scattering coefficient: a lumped property incorporating the **scattering coefficient** μ_s and the **scattering anisotropy factor** g: $\mu_s' = \mu_s(1 - g)$ [cm^{-1}]; μ_s' describes the diffusion of photons in a random walk of step size of $1/\mu_s'$ [cm] where each step involves isotropic scattering; this is equivalent to the description of photon movement using many small steps, $1/\mu_s$, which each involve only a partial (anisotropic) deflection angle if there are many scattering events before an absorption event, i.e., $\mu_a \ll \mu_s'$ (diffusion regime, see **diffusion approximation**); μ_s' is useful in the diffusion regime, which is commonly encountered when treating how visible and near-infrared light propagates through tissues (http://omlc.ogi.edu/classroom/).

reflectance (reflection coefficient): the ratio of the intensity reflected from a surface to the incident intensity; it is a dimensional quantity.

reflecting spectroscopy: the spectroscopy that uses the light back-reflected (scattered) by an object for spectral analysis.

refraction: the change in direction of a ray of light, sound, heat, or the like, in passing obliquely from one medium into another in which its speed is different; the ability of the eye to refract entering light, forming on the retina; the determination of the refractive condition of the eye.

refractive index: see **index of refraction**.

refractive index mismatch: a difference in the index of refraction of two media in contact; a scattering medium that contains scattering particles whose index of refraction is mismatched relative to the index of refraction of the ground substance [see **immersion medium (liquid)** and **immersion technique**].

repetition rate: the number of pulses per second; the repetition rate is measured in hertz.

reproducibility: one of the main principles of the scientific method, and refers to the ability of a test or experiment to be accurately reproduced, or replicated, by someone else working independently.

resistor: a two-terminal electrical or electronic component that resists an electric current by producing a voltage drop between its terminals in accordance with Ohm's law.

retarder: see **optical retarder**.

reverberation: the persistence of sound in a particular space after the original sound is removed; when sound is produced in a space, a large number of echoes build up and then slowly decay as the sound is absorbed by the walls and air, creating reverberation, or reverb.

Riccati-Bessel function: only slightly different from a spherical Bessel function, this function arises in the problem of scattering of electromagnetic waves by a sphere, known as **Mie** scattering.

root mean square (rms): a measure of dispersion in a frequency distribution, it is equal to the square root of the mean of the squares of the deviations from the arithmetic mean of the distribution.

rotational diffusion: the molecular rotational motion is usually only the rotational rocking near the equilibrium orientation; they depend on the interactions with their neighbors, and by jumping in time they are changing orientation; the energy of activation is required for changing the angle of orientation; the Brownian rotational motion can be valid only for comparatively big molecules with the slow changing of orientation angles; in this case the differential character of rotational motion is valid and the rotational diffusion equation can be written; the interaction of molecules between each other can be considered as the friction foresees with the moment P proportional to the angle velocity Ω, $P = \xi\Omega$, where ξ is the rotational coefficient of friction that can be connected with the rotational diffusion coefficient, $D_R = kT/\xi$; in the case of a small macroscopic sphere with radius a, $\xi = 8\pi a^3\eta$, where η is the coefficient of viscosity (http://aph.huji.ac.il/feldman/diel/Diel_Lecture9.ppt).

rotational state (level): the particular pattern of energy levels (and hence of transitions in the rotational spectrum) for a molecule is determined by its symmetry: linear molecules (or linear rotors), symmetric tops (or symmetric rotors), spherical tops (or spherical rotors), and asymmetric tops; rotational spectroscopy (using microwave and/or Raman spectroscopic techniques) studies the absorption and emission electromagnetic radiation by molecules associated with a corresponding change in the rotational quantum number of the molecule.

scatterer: an inhomogeneity or a particle of a medium that refracts or diffracts light or other electromagnetic radiation; light is diffused or deflected as a result of collisions between the wave and particles of the medium; sometimes it is a rough surface or a random-phase screen, also called a scatterer.

scattering: the process in which a wave or beam of particles is diffused or deflected by collisions with particles of the medium it transverses.

scattering angle: related to a photon scattered by a particle so that its trajectory is deflected by a deflection (scattering) angle θ in the **scattering plane** and/or by the azimuthal angle of scattering φ in the plane perpendicular to the scattering plane.

scattering anisotropy factor: the amount of forward direction retained after a single scattering event; if a photon is scattered by a particle so that its trajectory is deflected by an angle θ, then the component of the new trajectory aligned in the forward direction is presented as $\cos\theta$; there is an average deflection angle, and the mean value of $\langle\cos\theta\rangle$ is defined as the anisotropy (http://omlc.ogi.edu/classroom/).

scattering coefficient: a particle with a particular geometrical size redirects incident photons into new directions and so prevents the forward on-axis transmission of photons, this process constitutes **scattering**; the scattering coefficient $\mu_s[\text{cm}^{-1}]$ describes a medium containing many scattering particles at a concentration described as a volume density $\rho[\text{cm}^3]$; the scattering coefficient is essentially the cross-sectional area $\sigma_{sca}[\text{cm}^{-1}]$ per unit volume of medium: $\mu_s = \rho\sigma_{sca}$ (http://omlc.ogi.edu/classroom/).

scattering indicatrix: an angular dependence of the scattered light intensity; for thin samples, the normalized scattering indicatrix is equal to the **scattering phase function**.

scattering medium: a medium in which a wave or beam of its particles is diffused or deflected by collisions with particles.

scattering phase function: the function that describes the scattering properties of the medium and is, in fact, the probability density function for scattering in the direction $\bar{s}'$ of a photon traveling in the direction $\bar{s}$; it characterizes an elementary scattering act: if scattering is symmetric relative to the direction of the incident wave, then the phase function depends only on the scattering the angle θ (angle between directions $\bar{s}$ and $\bar{s}'$).

scattering plane: a plane defined by positions of a light source, a scattering particle, and a detector.

scattering spectrum: the spectrum of scattered light; it can be differential, measured, or calculated for a certain scattering angle, or integrated within an angle (field) of view of the measuring spectrometer.

second-harmonic generation (SHG): (also called frequency doubling) a nonlinear optical process in which photons interacting with a nonlinear material are effectively "combined" to form new photons with twice the energy, and therefore twice the frequency and half the wavelength of the initial photons; in the past several years, SHG has been extended to biological applications: to the imaging of molecules that are intrinsically second-harmonic-active in live cells, such as collagen, and for studying biological molecules by labeling them with second-harmonic-active tags, in particular as a means to detect conformational change at any site and in real time.

self-beating: the signal produced by photomixing the electric components of a scattered field.

semilogarithmic scale: for example, functions of the kind $y = Be^{-\varphi x}$ are used to describe the attenuation of light intensity with distance x and may be plotted on a semilogarithmic scale; taking $\log_{10}$ of both sides gives $\log_{10} y = \log_{10} B - \varphi x$ $\log_{10} e = \log_{10} B - 0.434\varphi x$; plotting $\log y$ vs x will therefore give a straight line of slope $0.434 \times \varphi$.

shear rate: the rate of shear **deformation**; for the ease of it is just a gradient of velocity.

shear stress: a **stress** state where the stress is parallel or tangential to a face of the material, as opposed to normal stress when the stress is perpendicular to the face; for a Newtonian fluid wall shear stress is proportional to shear rate, where the coefficient of proportionality is the viscosity of the fluid.

short-circuit: in electronics, a circuit with a load of an infinitely low resistance or **impedance** through which electric current flows.

shot noise: a type of electronic noise that occurs when the finite number of particles that carry energy, such as electrons in an electronic circuit or photons in an optical device, is small enough to give rise to detectable statistical fluctuations in a measurement; it is important in electronics and photoelectronics; the strength of this noise increases with the average magnitude of the current or intensity of the light; often, however, as the signal increases more rapidly as the average signal becomes stronger, shot noise often is only a problem with small currents and light intensities.

Siegert formula: the formula that, for Gaussian statistics, relates the intensity **autocorrelation function** to the first-order autocorrelation function.

signal oscillator: used in heterodyne detecting systems for notation of the receiving signal, which can be presented as the radio- (or optical) frequency oscillator and has a slightly different frequency than that for the **local oscillator** [used for converting a high-frequency receiving signal to an intermediate frequency by mixing the local oscillator signal and receiving signal at an electronic (or photo-) detector].

signal-to-noise ratio: the ratio of a received (the detector) signal (an electric impulse) to noise (an electric disturbance in a measuring system that interferes with or prevents reception of a signal).

single-frequency laser: a laser that generates a single frequency (one longitudinal mode).

single-integrating sphere "comparison" technique: this technique uses a single integrating sphere containing no baffles but three ports that can be opened for light transmission, or closed or covered by a sample or reference standards for the calibration (comparison) of reflectance or transmittance measurements; an additional two ports are used to illuminate samples by a collimated light beam and collect the scattered light by a fiber bundle placed at the "north pole" of the sphere; this technique has an advantage over the conventional **double integrating sphere technique** in that no corrections are required for sphere properties.

single-mode fiber: a fiber in which only a single mode can be excited; for a fiber with a numerical aperture 0.1 and a wavelength of 633 nm the single mode can be excited if the core diameter is less than 4.8 μm.

single-mode fiber-optic Michelson interferometer: a **Michelson interferometer** integrated with a **fiber-optic single-mode X-coupler**, which optically connects a light source, reference mirror, object, and photodetector.

single-mode laser: a laser that produces a light beam with a Gaussian shape of the transverse intensity profile without any spatial oscillations (see **Gaussian light beam**); in general, such lasers generate many optical frequencies (so-called longitudinal modes), which have the same transverse Gaussian shape.

single-photon counting mode: see **photon-counting system**.

single scattering: the scattering process that occurs when a wave undertakes no more than one collision with particles of the medium in which it propagates.

single scattering approximation: the approximation that assumes tissue is sufficiently thin that single scattering accurately estimates the reflection and transmission for the slab.

singlet state: one of the two ways in which the **spin** of two electrons in an atom or molecule can be combined in atomic physics, the other being a **triplet state**; a single electron has spin 1/2, and a pair of electron spins can be combined to form a state of total spin 1 (triplet state) and a state of spin 0 (singlet state); singlet state is an excited state of a molecule that, upon absorbing light, can release energy as heat or light (**fluorescence**) and thus return to the initial (ground) state; it may alternatively assume a slightly more stable, but still excited state (triplet state), with an electron still dislocated as before but with reversed spin.

singular eigenfunction method: the method for rigorous solving of the transport equation which is solved using the Green's functions in terms of the singular eigenfunctions and their orthogonality relations together with the appropriate boundary conditions; the convergence of the numerical results is fast and the analytical expressions are simple for solving numerically.

small angular (angle) approximation: a useful simplification of the laws of trigonometry, which is only approximately true for finite angles, but correct in the limit as the angle approaches zero; it involves linearization of the trigonometric functions (truncation of their Taylor series); this approximation is useful in many areas of physical science, including optics, where it forms the basis of the **paraxial approximation**.

S-matrix: see **LSM [light-scattering matrix (intensity or Mueller matrix)]**.

snake photons: photons that travel in near-forward paths, having undergone few scattering events, all of which are in the forward or near-forward direction; consequently, they retain the image bearing characteristics to some extent.

soft scattering particles: the refractive index of these particles, n_s, is close to the refractive index of the ground (interstitial) substance, n_0 ($n_s \geq n_0$).

sonoluminescence: the emission of short bursts of light (**luminescence**) from imploding bubbles in a liquid when excited by sound.

sonophoresis: a process that exponentially increases the absorption of topical compounds (transdermal delivery) into the epidermis, dermis, and skin appendages; it occurs because ultrasound waves stimulate microvibrations within the skin epidermis and increase the overall kinetic energy of molecules making up topical agents; it is widely used in hospitals to deliver drugs through the skin; pharmacists compound the drugs by mixing them with a coupling agent (gel, cream, ointment) that transfers ultrasonic energy from the ultrasound transducer to the skin; the ultrasound probably enhances drug transport by cavitation, microstreaming, and heating; it is also used in physical therapy.

Soret band: a very strong absorption band in the blue region of the optical absorption spectrum of a haem protein.

spatial correlation: see **correlation**; valid for the spatial variables.

spatial frequency: a spatial harmonic in the Fourier transform of a periodic or aperiodic (random) spatial distribution.

spatial resolution: a measure of the ability of an optical imaging system to reveal the details of an image, i.e., to resolve adjacent elements.

spatially modulated laser beam: a laser beam with regular interference fringes or irregular speckle modulation.

spatially resolved reflectance technique (SRR): a technique that uses two or more fibers to illuminate an object and collect the back-reflected light; the positions of the illuminating and light-collecting fibers can be fixed or scanned along the object's surface perpendicular or have some angle to the object's surface.

specific heat capacity: also known simply as specific heat; an intensive quantity, meaning it is a property of the material itself, and not the size or shape of the sample; its value is affected by the microscopic structure of the material; commonly, the amount is specified by mass; for example, water has a mass-specific heat capacity of about 4186 joules per Kelvin per kilogram; volume-specific and molar-specific heat capacities are also used; the specific heat of virtually any substance can be measured, including pure elements, compounds, alloys, solutions, and composites.

speckle: a single element of a speckle structure (pattern) that is produced as a result of the interference of a large number of elementary waves with random phases that arise when coherent light is reflected from a rough surface or when coherent light passes through a scattering medium.

speckle contrast: see **contrast of the intensity fluctuations**.

speckle correlometry: a technique based on the measurement of the intensity **autocorrelation function**, characterizing the size and distribution of speckle sizes in a speckle pattern, caused, for example, by the scattering of a coherent light beam from a rough surface: the statistical properties of the scattering object's structure can be deduced from such measurements.

speckle interferometry: the technique that uses the **interference of speckle fields**.

speckle photography: the measuring technique that uses a set of sequential photos of the speckle pattern taken at different moments or with different exposures: this is a full-field technique and can be used to study the dynamic properties of a scattering object (see **LASCA**); the updated instruments make use of computer-controlled CCD cameras for averaging and storing the speckle patterns.

speckle statistics of the first order: the statistics that define the properties of speckle fields at each point.

speckle statistics of the second order: the statistics that show how fast the intensity changes from point to point in a speckle pattern, i.e., they characterize the size and the distribution of speckle sizes in the pattern.

speckle structure: see **speckle**.

Spectrolon: a very white reflective plastic used as the "white reference" in spectral measurements and in **integrating sphere** spectrometers.

spectrophotometry: the spectroscopic method and instrument for making photometric comparisons between parts of spectra.

spectroscopy: the science that deals with the use of the spectroscope and with spectrum analysis.

spectroscopy of intensity fluctuations: see photon-correlation spectroscopy.

spectrum: the range of frequencies or wavelengths.

spectrum analysis: to ascertain the number and character of the constituents combining to produce a signal spectrogram.

spectrum analyzer: an instrument for making the spectrum analysis of a signal.

specular: pertaining to or having the properties of a mirror.

spin: the angular momentum intrinsic to a body; in classical mechanics, the spin angular momentum of a body is associated with the rotation of the body around its own center of mass; in quantum mechanics, spin is particularly important for systems at atomic length scales, such as individual atoms, protons, or electrons; such particles and the spin of quantum mechanical systems ("particle spin") possesses several nonclassical features, and for such systems, spin angular momentum cannot be associated with rotation but instead refers only to the presence of angular momentum.

standard deviation: see **rms (root mean square)**.

statistics: a mathematical science pertaining to the collection, analysis, interpretation or explanation, and presentation of data; it is applicable to a wide variety of academic disciplines.

statistical approach: an approach based on **statistics** as a mathematical science.

statistically significant: a result is called significant if it is unlikely to have occurred by chance; "a statistically significant difference" simply means there is statistical evidence that there is a difference; the significance of a result is also called its p-value; the smaller the p-value, the more significant the result is said to be; popular levels of significance are 5%, 1%, and 0.1%.

stepper motor: a machine that converts electrical energy into mechanical energy by steps; used as the computer-controlled mechanical drivers of optical stages.

stimulated Raman scattering (SRS): a phenomenon that occurs when a lower frequency "signal" photon induces the inelastic scattering of a higher-frequency "pump" photon in a nonlinear optical medium; as a result, another "signal" photon is produced, with the surplus energy resonantly passed to the **vibrational states** of the nonlinear medium; this process is the basis for the **Raman amplifier**.

Stokes parameters: the four numbers I, Q, U, and V representing an arbitrary polarization of light; I refers to the irradiance or intensity of the light; the parameters Q, U, and V represent the extent of horizontal linear, 45° linear, and circular polarization, respectively.

Stokes-Raman scattering: the energy of the Raman scattered photons is lower than the energy of the incident photons.

Stokes shift: the difference (in wavelength or frequency units) between positions of the band maxima of the absorption and **luminescence** spectra (or **fluorescence**) of the same **electronic transition**; when a molecule or atom absorbs light, it enters an excited electronic state; the Stokes shift occurs because the molecule loses a small amount of the absorbed energy before re-releasing the rest of the energy as fluorescence, depending on the time between the absorption and the reemission; this energy is often lost as thermal energy.

Stokes vector: the vector formed by the four **Stokes parameters**.

Stokes wave: the induced (scattered) wave that has a frequency less than the frequency of the incident radiation.

streak camera (synchroscan streak camera): an instrument for recording the temporal profile of light intensity with a high time resolution (of about 10 ps), displaying it as a spatial profile; synchronous scanning controlled by a reference (**trigger beam**) light pulse is provided.

stress: internal distribution of force per unit area that balances and reacts to external loads applied to a body; stress is a second-order tensor with nine components, but can be fully described with six components due to symmetry in the absence of body moments; stress is often broken down into its shear and normal components as these have unique physical significance; stress can be applied to solids, liquids, and gases; static fluids support normal stress (hydrostatic pressure) but will flow under **shear stress**; moving viscous fluids can support shear stress (dynamic pressure); solids can support both shear and normal stress, with ductile materials failing under shear and brittle materials failing under normal stress; all materials have temperature dependent variations in stress related properties, and **non-Newtonian** materials have rate-dependent variations.

stress amplitude: the value of a **stress**.

stress distribution: **stress** is a second-order tensor with nine components.

structure function: the function that describes the second-order statistics of a random process and is proportional to the difference between values of the **autocorre-**

lation function for zero and arbitrary values of the argument; the structure function is more sensitive to small-scale oscillations.

subject arm of an interferometer: the arm on which an object under study is placed.

subjective speckles: the speckles produced in the image space of an optical system (including an eye).

superluminescent diode: a very bright diode light source with a broad linewidth; it is usually manufactured using a laser diode technology (heterostructure, waveguide, etc.), but without reflecting mirrors (there is an antireflection coating at the diode faces or their out-of-parallelism is provided).

surface-enhanced Raman scattering (SERS): a strong increase in **Raman** signals from molecules if those molecules are attached to submicron metallic structures; for a rough surface due to excitation of **electromagnetic resonances** by the incident radiation, such enhancement may be of a few orders; both the excitation and Raman scattered fields contribute to this enhancement; thus, the SERS signal is proportional to the fourth power of the field enhancement factor.

surface plasmon resonance: also known as surface plasmon polaritons, surface plasmon resonances are surface electromagnetic waves that propagate parallel to a metal/dielectric interface; for electronic surface plasmons to exist, the real part of the dielectric constant of the metal must be negative, and its magnitude must be greater than that of the dielectric; this condition is met in the visible-IR wavelength region for air/metal and water/metal interfaces (where the real dielectric constant of a metal is negative and that of air or water is positive); the excitation of surface plasmons by light is denoted for planar surfaces as for nanometer-sized metallic structures which is called localized surface plasmon resonance; typical metals that support surface plasmons are silver and gold, but metals such as copper, titanium, or chromium can also support surface plasmon generation; surface plasmons have been used to enhance the surface sensitivity of several spectroscopic methods, including **fluorescence**, **Raman scattering** (see **surface-enhanced Raman scattering**), and **second harmonic generation**.

symmetric molecule: refers to molecular geometry; molecules have fixed equilibrium geometries—bond lengths and angles—about which they continuously oscillate through vibrational and rotational motions; a symmetric molecule contains identical bonds; for example, trigonal planar, tetrahedral and linear bonding arrangements often lead to symmetrical, nonpolar molecules that contain polar bonds.

symmetric vibrational mode: for example, a moving linear triatomic molecule being in a movement, when each atom oscillates or vibrates along a line connecting them, may be in symmetric or antisymmetric vibrational mode relative to a central atom.

systematic errors: the errors caused by finite tissue volume, curved surfaces, tissue inhomogeneity when scanning, finite source and detection size, uncertainty in their relative positions, etc.; they can be much larger than random errors induced by a **shot noise**.

swept-laser source: a rapidly tunable laser over a broad optical bandwidth.

tensor: a tensor has slightly different meanings in mathematics and physics; in the mathematical fields of multilinear algebra and differential geometry, a tensor is a multilinear function; in physics and engineering, the same term usually means what a mathematician would call a tensor field: an association of a different (mathematical) tensor with each point of a geometric space, varying continuously with position; in the field of diffusion tensor imaging, for instance, a tensor quantity that expresses the differential permeability of organs to water in varying directions is used to produce scans of the brain; perhaps the most important engineering examples are the **stress** tensor and strain tensor, which are both second-rank tensors, and are related in a general linear material by a fourth-rank-elasticity tensor; the rank of a particular tensor is the number of array indices required to describe such a quantity.

therapeutic (or diagnostic) window: the spectral range from 600 to 1600 nm within which the penetration depth of light beams for most living tissues and blood is the highest; certain phototherapeutic and diagnostic modalities take advantage of this range for visible and NIR light.

thermal blooming: a major effect in high-power laser beams transmitting through gaseous mediums as well as the atmosphere; due to this nonlinear heating effect, the beam pattern is deformed through the propagation path.

thermal diffusivity: the ratio of **heat (thermal) conductivity** to volumetric **heat capacity** in **heat transfer** analysis; expressed in units of $m^2 \, s^{-1}$.

thermal expansion coefficient: the energy that is stored in the intermolecular bonds between atoms changes during **heat transfer**; when the stored energy increases, so does the length of the molecular bond; as a result, solids typically expand in response to heating and contract on cooling; this response to temperature change is expressed as its coefficient of thermal expansion; the coefficient of thermal expansion is used in two ways: as a volumetric thermal expansion coefficient (liquids and solid state) and as a linear thermal expansion coefficient (solid state).

thermal image: pictures created by heat, received by a thermal imager, rather than light; it measures radiated IR energy and converts the data to corresponding maps of temperatures; instruments provide temperature data at each image pixel; images may be digitized, stored, manipulated, processed, and printed out.

thermal length: the length of thermal diffusivity that chacterizes the distance in a medium where heat is diffused during the heating laser pulse.

thermal lensing: the virtual lens that is induced in a transparent material by its local heating, particularly by laser beam absorption; the local changes in the refractive index of a sample induce such a lens for some period; such an effect can be used to estimate tissue optical and thermal properties if a probing laser beam is applied.

thermal relaxation time: the time to dissipate the heat absorbed during a laser pulse.

thermoelastic effect: the generation of mechanical stress (acoustic) waves via the time-dependent thermal expansion of a sample.

third harmonic generation: if a narrow-band optical wave pulse at a frequency ω propagates through a nonlinear medium with a nonzero Kerr **nonlinear susceptibility** $\chi^{(3)}$ due to nonlinearity, one will get a signal at a frequency 3ω (see **second harmonic generation**).

three-photon fluorescence microscopy: the microscopy that employs both **ballistic** and scattered photons at the wavelength of the **third harmonic** of incident radiation; it possesses the same advantages as **two-photon fluorescence microscopy** but ensures a somewhat higher spatial resolution and provides an opportunity to excite chromophores with shorter wavelengths.

time-correlated single-photon counting technique: the time-resolved single-photon counting method and instrument (see **photon-counting system**) used for receiving low-intensity light pulses.

time-dependent radiation transfer theory (RTT): the theory that is based on the time-dependent integro-differential equation (the Boltzmann or linear transport equation), which is a balance equation describing the time-dependent flow of particles (e.g., photons) in a given volume element that takes into account their velocity c, location $\bar{r}$, and changes due to collisions (i.e., scattering and absorption).

time-domain technique: a spectroscopic or imaging technique that uses ultrashort laser pulses.

time-gating: a method for selecting photon groups with different arriving times to a detector within a selected and moveable time window; used in diffuse optical tomography and spectroscopy; may be purely electrical or optical, or a combination of both.

time-of-flight: the mean time of photon travel between two points that account for refractive index and scattering properties of the medium.

time-share control: the regime that ensures that, at one time, an optical signal of only one wavelength passes through the whole system.

tissuelike phantom: see **phantom**.

tissue optical parameters (properties) control: any kind of physical or chemical action, such as mechanical stress or changes in osmolarity, which induces reversible or irreversible changes in the optical properties of a tissue [see **immersion medium (liquid)**, **immersion technique**, **matching substance**, and **mechanical stress**].

TOAST (time-resolved optical absorption and scattering tomography): an image reconstruction package developed at University College London that employs a finite-element-method-forward model and an iterative reconstruction algorithm.

tomographic reconstruction: the mathematical procedure of obtaining 3D images by which the size, shape, and position of a hidden object can be determined.

tomography: imaging by sections or sectioning (the Greek word tomos, meaning "a section" or "a cutting"); a device used in tomography is called a tomograph, while the image produced is a tomogram; the method is used in medicine, biology, and other sciences; in most cases it is based on the mathematical procedure called **tomographic reconstruction**; there are many different types of tomography, including functional magnetic resonance imaging (fMRI), **magnetic resonance imaging (MRI)**, **optical coherence tomography (OCT)**, optical projection tomography (OPT), positron emission tomography (PET), single photon emission computed tomography (SPECT), x-ray tomography.

total internal reflection: the reflection of light at the interface between media of different refractive indexes, when the angle of incidence is larger than a critical angle (determined by the media).

transfer matrix method: this method assumes that light consists of various plane waves traveling with oblique angles through the sample; the latent bulk image is obtained by first calculating the vertical amplitude dependence of the field, resulting from the excitation with one plane wave of definite amplitude; it is is applicable for the analysis of a stratified medium; using the vector version of the transfer matrix algorithm, an arbitrarily polarized light can be simulated.

transillumination digital microscopy (TDM): the light transillumination **microscopy** based on the usage of fast and high resolution CCD cameras and corresponding software; it is applicable for *in vivo* **flow cytometry**.

transition matrix (T-matrix) approach: this approach is similar to the Mie theory used for nonspherical objects such as spheroids; the T-matrix for the spherical particles is diagonal.

transmittance: the ratio of the intensity transmitted through a sample to the incident intensity; it is a dimensionless quantity.

trigger beam: the part of a laser beam used to synchronize the measuring system (for example, the streak camera).

triplet state: see **singlet state**.

t-**test (Student's** *t*-**test)**: a test for determining whether an observed sample mean differs significantly from a hypothetical normal population mean.

tunable laser: most lasers emit at a particular wavelength; in tunable lasers, one can vary the wavelength over some limited spectral range.

turbidity: a cloudiness or haziness of material (biological fluid or tissue), caused by individual particles (suspended scatterers) that are generally invisible to the naked eye, thus being much like milk.

turbulent flow: a flow regime characterized by chaotic, stochastic property changes; this includes low-momentum diffusion, high-momentum convection, and rapid variation of pressure and velocity in space and time; flow that is not turbulent is called **laminar flow**; the dimensionless Reynolds number characterizes whether flow conditions lead to laminar or turbulent flow; e.g., for pipe flow, a Reynolds number above about 2300 will be turbulent.

two-frequency Zeeman laser: a laser with the active medium placed in the axial magnetic field; the laser produces two laser lines with a small frequency separation (about 250 kHz) and mutually orthogonal linear polarizations.

two-photon fluorescence microscopy: the microscopy that employs both **ballistic** and scattered photons at the wavelength of the second harmonic of incident radiation coming to a wide-aperture photodetector exactly from the focal area of the excitation beam.

ultrashort laser pulse: the pulses usually produced by mode-locked lasers (picosecond and subpicosecond range) or their modifications, such as synchronously optically pumped or colliding-pulse mode-locked dye (CPM laser) lasers (femtosecond range), or the titanium-sapphire laser with passive mode locking via a Kerr lens (KLM laser) (10–100 fs).

ultrasonic transducer: a device that converts energy into **ultrasound**; refers to a **piezoelectric transducer** that converts electrical energy into sound; alternative methods for creating and detecting ultrasound include magnetostriction and capacitive actuation; it is used in many applications including medical ultrasonography, and nondestructive testing.

ultrasound: mechanical vibrations with frequencies in the range of 2×10^4 to 10^7 Hz.

uniaxial crystal: an **anisotropic crystal** that exhibits two refractive indices: an "ordinary" index (n_o) for light polarized in the x or y directions, and an "extraordinary" index (n_e) for polarization in the z direction; a uniaxial crystal is "positive" if $n_e > n_o$ and "negative" if $n_e < n_o$; light polarized at some angle to the axes will experience a different phase velocity for different polarization components and cannot be described by a single index of refraction; this is often depicted as an index ellipsoid.

variance: the square of the standard deviation.

vector RTT: **radiation transfer theory (RTT)** accounting for the polarization properties of light and its interaction with a scattering medium.

vibrational spectrum: see **vibrational transition**.

vibrational transition: denotes an energetic transition of a molecule with the change of vibrational quantum number (energetic state, or level); at vibrational transitions, only the absorption or emission of infrared light (**vibrational spectrum**) is possible.

vibronic spectrum: see **vibronic transition**.

vibronic transition: denotes the simultaneous change of a vibrational and electronic quantum number (energetic state or level) in a molecule; according to the separability of electronic and nuclear motion in the Born-Oppenheimer approximation, the vibrational transition and electronic transition may be described separately; the selection rule for vibrational transitions is described by the **Franck-Condon principle**; most processes lead to the absorption and emission of relatively broad bands of visible light (**vibronic spectra**), resulting in the colorful world around us.

vibrometer: an instrument that measures amplitudes and frequencies of the mechanical vibrations of an object.

viscosity of the medium: viscosity arises from the friction between one layer of a fluid in motion relative to another layer of the fluid; it is caused by the cohesive forces between molecules; the viscosity of glycerol is high, but the viscosity of water or ethanol is low.

volume fraction: a fraction dealing with mixtures in which there is a large disparity between the sizes and refractive indices of the various kinds of molecules or particles; it provides an appropriate way to express the relative amounts of the various components; in any ideal mixture, the total volume is the sum of the individual volumes prior to mixing; in nonideal cases the additivity of volume is no longer guaranteed; volumes can contract or expand upon mixing and molar volume becomes a function of both concentration and temperature; this is why mole fractions are a safer unit to use.

waist of a laser beam: the narrowest part of a Gaussian beam.

water-binding mode: denotes biological molecule interaction with water molecules and corresponding changes in molecular-water complex spectra.

watt: a unit of power; one watt is equal to one joule per second.

wavelength: distance between two adjacent peaks in a wave.

wavelet transformation: the representation of a signal in terms of scaled and translated copies (known as "daughter wavelets") of a finite length or fast decaying oscillating waveform (known as the "mother wavelet"); in formal terms, this representation is a wavelet series that is a representation of a square-integrable (real or complex valued) function by a certain orthonormal series generated by a wavelet.

weakly scattering RPS: the RPS whose variance in induced-phase fluctuations in the scattered field is much less than unity.

Wigner phase space distribution function: the complex function that defines the coherence property of an optical field for a given position depending on the wave vector.

white noise: a random signal (or process) with a flat power spectral density; the signal's power spectral density has equal power in any band, at any center frequency, having a given bandwidth; white noise is considered analogous to white light, which contains all frequencies.

Wollaston prism: an optical device invented by William Hyde Wollaston that manipulates polarized light; it separates randomly polarized or unpolarized light into two orthogonal, linearly polarized outgoing beams; a prism consists of two orthogonal calcite prisms cemented together on their base (typically with Canada balsam) to form two right triangle prisms with perpendicular optic axes; outgoing light beams diverge from the prism, giving two polarized rays, with the angle of divergence determined by the prisms' wedge angle and the wavelength of the light; commercial prisms are available with divergence angles from 15° to about 45°.

xenon arc lamp: a discharge arc lamp filled with xenon; it gives out very bright UV and visible light in the range from 200 nm to >1.0 μm.

x ray (or Röntgen rays): a form of electromagnetic radiation with a wavelength in the range of 10 to 0.01 nm; primarily used for diagnostic radiography and crystallography; it is a form of ionizing radiation and can be dangerous.

zigzag or snake photons: low-angle scattered photons having zigzag (or snake) trajectories.

ZnSe crystal: a crystal for **ATR** (attenuated total reflectance) spectroscopy; insoluble with a refractive index of 2.4, a long-wavelength cut-off frequency of 525 cm^{-1}, a depth of penetration at 1000 cm^{-1} of 1.66 μm, and a pH range of samples under study of 5–9.

z-scan: see **A-scan**.

Sources

This glossary was compiled using mostly Refs. 1–7, 25, 40, 75, 87, 129, 130, 132, 135, 136, and the following sources:

1. *Webster's New Universal Unabridged Dictionary*, Barnes & Noble Books, New York, 1994.
2. A. Godman and E. M. F. Payne, *Longman Dictionary of Scientific Usage*, reprint edition, Longman Group, Harlow, UK, 1979.

3. A. M. Prokhorov (ed.), *Physical Encyclopedic Dictionary*, Soviet Encyclopedia, Moscow, 1983.

4. A. M. Prokhorov (ed.), *Physical Encyclopedia*, vol. 1, Soviet Encyclopedia, Moscow, 1988.

5. A. M. Prokhorov (ed.), *Physical Encyclopedia*, vol. 2, Soviet Encyclopedia, Moscow, 1990.

6. A. M. Prokhorov (ed.), *Physical Encyclopedia*, vol. 3, Big Russian Encyclopedia, Moscow, 1992.

7. A. M. Prokhorov (ed.), *Physical Encyclopedia*, vol. 4, Big Russian Encyclopedia, Moscow, 1994.

8. http://en.wikipedia.org

Glossary 2. Medicine, Biology, and Chemistry

abdominal fat: the adipose tissue that contains fat cells and that is found around the abdominal organs such as the **intestines, kidneys,** and **liver**.

abdominal organs: the organs contained in the abdominal region of the body; the **diaphragm** separates the abdomen from the **thorax**; the abdomen is posterior to the thorax; viscera other than the **heart** or **lungs** (e.g., **intestines, kidneys, liver**) are abdominal organs.

ablation: the removal of tissue.

abrasive cream: a cream, containing abrasive (hard mineral) particles, that allows one to provide **skin peeling** and make its relief more smooth and penetrative for **liposomes** and **nanospheres**.

acanthocyte: shrunken **erythrocyte**, also known as a spur cell, the term is derived from the Greek word "acanthi" meaning "thorn"; the acanthocyte cell has five to ten irregular, blunt, fingerlike projections that vary in width, length, and surface distribution; acanthocytes form when erythrocyte **membranes** contein excess **cholesterol** compared to **phospholipid** content, which is caused by the increase in blood cholesterol content or the presence of abnormal plasma lipoprotein composition.

acetic acid: a colorless, pungent, water-miscible liquid, CH_3COOH, used in the production of numerous esters that are solvents and flavoring agents.

acetowhitening effect: the effect caused by acetic acid when used during **colposcopy** to enhance differences in the diffuse reflectance (whitening) of normal and diseased regions of the cervical **epithelium**; transient whitening of tissue after the application of acetic acid serves as a simple and inexpensive method for identifying areas that may eventually develop into **cervical cancer**.

actinic keratosis: a scaly or crusty bump that forms on the skin surface; also called solar keratosis, sun spots, or precancerous spots.

acyl group: a functional group derived by the removal of one or more hydroxyl group from an oxoacid; in organic chemistry, the acyl group is usually derived from a carboxylic acid in the form of RC O OH; it therefore has the formula $RC(=O)-$, with a double bond between the carbon and oxygen atoms (i.e., a carbonyl group), and a single bond between R and the carbon.

adenocarcinoma: a **malignant tumor** originating in **glandular epithelium**.

adenoma: a **benign tumor** originating in **glandular epithelium**.

adenomatous: related to **adenoma** and to some types of **glandular hyperplasia**.

adenosine triphosphate (ATP): a **coenzyme** of fundamental importance found in the cells of all organisms; it provides a means of storing energy for many cellular activities.

adipose tissue: a modification of **areolar tissue** in which globules of **oil** are deposited in some of the cells (**fat cells**); the cells tend to be grouped together and, in mammals, occur in the tissues under the skin and around the **abdominal organs** (**kidneys**, **liver**, etc.).

administration: in medicine the route of administration means the path by which a medicinal substance is brought into contact with the body.

adventitia: the external covering of an organ or other structure, derived from **connective tissue**; especially the external covering of a **blood vessel**.

African frog (*Xenopus laevis*): a frog that occurs naturally in southern Africa; there is a substantial population has been introduced in California.

agarose: made from agar, agarose is a gelatinlike product of certain seaweeds; it is used for solidifying certain culture media, as a substitute for **gelatin**, as an emulsifier, etc.

agglomeration: whereby moist sticky particles collide due to turbulence in a medium and adhere to each other.

aggregation: a heterogeneous mass of independent but similar units (molecules, cells, etc.); the term implies the formation of a whole without an intimate mixing of constituents.

albumin: a group of water-soluble proteins coagulated by heat; they occur in eggwhite, **blood serum**, milk, and in other animal and plant tissues.

albumin blue: is a dye used as a quantitative assay to measure albumin levels in biological samples including serum and urine; the intensity of the fluorescent signal is directly proportional to the albumin concentration of the sample; albumin-bound dye has a greatly increased excitation, thus the background caused by the emission of any free dye is minimal; albumin-bound dye absorbs light at 590 nm and emits fluorescence at 620 nm; long wavelength albumin blue dyes—absorption at 633 nm (AB633) and 670 nm (AB670), are also available and used for selective detection of human serum albumin in plasma and blood.

alcohol (spirit): an organic compound that contains one or more hydroxyl groups ($-OH$): the alcohols are hydroxy derivatives of alkanes; they can be classified according to the number of hydroxyl groups: monohydric, C_2H_5OH, **ethanol**; dihydric, $C_2H_4(OH)_2$, **ethylene glycol**; trihydric, $C_3H_5(OH)_3$, **glycerol**.

Alzheimer's disease: a neurodegenerative disease characterized by progressive cognitive deterioration together with declining activities of daily living and neuropsychiatric symptoms or behavioral changes.

amide: the organic functional group characterized by a carbonyl group (C=O) linked to a nitrogen atom (N); in the midinfrared spectral domain, bands due to the amide I, II, III, and A vibrations have been shown to be sensitive to the secondary structure content of **proteins**.

amino acid: any molecule that contains both amine and carboxyl functional groups; in biochemistry, this term refers to alpha amino acids; these are molecules where the amino and carboxylate groups are attached to the same carbon, which is called the α-carbon; the various alpha amino acids differ in which the side chain is attached to their α-carbon; this can vary in size from just a hydrogen atom in glycine, through a methyl group in alanine, to a large heterocyclic group in **tryptophan**; these amino acids are components of **proteins**; there are twenty standard amino acids used by cells in protein biosynthesis and these are specified by the general genetic code; these amino acids can be biosynthesized from simpler molecules; only obtained from food, essential amino acids are: histidine, isoleucine, leucine, lysine, methionine, **phenylalanine**, threonine, **tryptophan**, and valine.

δ-aminolevulenic acid (ALA): a "pro drug" that leads to the endogenous synthesis of **protoporphyrin IX** in the **cells** and **tissues**: it is applying ALA either systematically or topically.

amphiphilic: a chemical compound possessing both **hydrophilic** and **hydrophobic** properties.

anabolism: the synthesis of complex organic compounds from simpler organic compounds, e.g., the synthesis of proteins from amino acids; the process requires energy, mainly supplied in the form of **ATP** (see **metabolism**).

aneurysm: a permanent cardiac or arterial dilation usually caused by a weakened **vessel wall**.

angioplasty: the "reshaping" of blood vessels to improve blood flow.

anhydrous: having no water.

animal model: refers to a nonhuman animal with a disease or **injury** that is similar to a human condition; these test conditions are often termed as animal models of disease; the use of animal models allows researchers to investigate disease states in ways that would be inaccessible in a human patient; performing procedures on the nonhuman animal imply a level of harm that would not be considered ethical to inflict on a human.

anionic: relating to anions, negatively charged ions.

antibiotic: a drug that kills or prevents the growth of **bacteria**; antibiotics are one in a larger class of antimicrobials that include antiviral, antifungal, and antiparasitic drugs; they are relatively harmless to the host and therefore can be used to treat infections; the term "antibiotic" is also applied to synthetic antimicrobials, such as the sulfa drugs; antibiotics are generally small molecules with a molecular weight less than 2000 Da; they are not **enzymes**.

antigen: any foreign protein, or certain other large molecules, that, when present in a host's tissues, stimulates the production of a specific antibody by the host, a response leading to rejection of the antigen by the host; an antigen invades or is injected into an individual.

antritis: an antral (**antrum**) disorder of which examples include acute antritis; it is also known as or related to acute maxillary sinusitis and nodular antritis that is defined as antral gastritis with endoscopic findings characterized by a miliary pattern and prominent lymphoid follicles in biopsy specimens.

antrum: a general term for cavity or chamber, which may have a specific meaning in reference to certain organs or sites in the body; the antrum of the stomach (gastric antrum) is a portion before the outlet that is lined by mucosa and does not produce acid; the paranasal sinuses can be referred to as the frontal antrum, ethmoid antrum, and maxillary antrum.

anxiety: a generalized anxiety disorder is characterized by excessive, exaggerated anxiety and worry about everyday life events.

aorta: the large **artery** that leaves the left ventricle; it conducts the whole of the arterial blood supply to all parts of the body other than the **lungs**; in humans, it carries blood at the rate of 4 dm^3 per minute.

apatite [hydroxyapatite (HAP)]: the natural HAP crystal, $Ca_5OH(PO_4)_3$; dental **enamel** consists of 87–95% HAP crystals; **bone** consists of 50–60% HAP crystals.

aphakis subject: a subject missing **crystalline lens** of the eye.

apoptosis: the natural, programmed death of a cell (type I cell-death, compare **autophagy**) in response to an external signal a chain of biochemical reactions leading are induced to the death of cells no longer needed (as in embryonic development).

aqueous humor: a watery fluid, similar in composition to **cerebrospinal fluid**; it fills the anterior chamber of the **eyeball** behind the **cornea**; the **iris** and **crystalline lens** lie in it; it is continually secreted by the **ciliary body** and absorbed; it helps maintain the shape of the eyeball and assists in the refraction of light.

areolar tissue: a soft, sometimes spongelike **connective tissue** that consists of an amorphous polysaccharide-containing and jellylike ground matrix in which a loose network of **white fibers**, **yellow fibers**, and **reticulin fibers** are embedded; **fibroblasts** form in and maintain the matrix; areolar tissue is found all over the vertebrate body, binding together organs (by **mesenteries**) and **muscles** (by **sheaths**), and occurring as **subcutaneous tissue**; its function is to support or fill in the space between organs or between other tissues; the **fibrous** nature of the matrix is modified by variation in the concentration of white, yellow, or reticulin fibers; this alters the characteristics of toughness, elasticity, and inextensibility to suit the function of the tissue; many modifications of areolar tissue occur.

arm: in anatomy an arm is one of the upper limbs of a two-legged animal; the term arm can also be used for analogous structures, such as one of the paired upper limbs of a four-legged animal; anatomically, the term arm refers specifically to the segment between the shoulder and the elbow; the segment between the elbow and **wrist** is the **forearm**.

arteriole: a branch of an artery with a diameter less than $1/3$ mm; arteriole walls are formed from smooth muscle under the control of the autonomic nervous system; their function is to control blood supply to the **capillaries**.

arteriosclerosis: an arterial disease that occurs especially in the elderly; it is characterized by inelasticity and thickening of the **vessel walls**, with lessened **blood flow**.

artery: a blood vessel conducting blood from the **heart** to tissues and organs; it is lined with endothelium (smooth flat cells) and surrounded by thick, muscular, elastic walls containing white and yellow **fibrous tissue**.

artifact: see Glossary 1.

astrocyte: a starlike cell of the macroglia of nerve tissue.

astrocytoma: a rather well-differentiated **glioma**, which consists of cells that look like **astrocytes**.

atheroma: fatty degeneration of the inner walls (**intima**) of the arteries in **arteriosclerosis**.

atherosclerotic plaque: a fibrous tissue that also contains **fat** and sometimes calcium; it accumulates in **arteries** and leads to the occlusion of the vessel.

atrium: (plural: atria) refers to a chamber or space; the **blood** collection chamber of a **heart**; in humans there are two atria, one on either side of the heart; on the right side is the atrium that holds blood that needs **oxygen**; it sends blood to the right ventricle, which sends it to the **lungs** for oxygen; after it comes back, it is sent to the left atrium; the blood is pumped from the left atrium and sent to the ventricle where it is sent out of the heart to all the rest of the body.

auscultation: hearing sounds of different body structures with diagnostic purposes.

autophagy (autophagocytosis): a process where cytoplasmic materials are degraded through the lysosomal machinery; the process is commonly viewed as **organelles** and long-lived **proteins** sequestered in a double-**membrane vesicle** inside the **cell**, where the contents are subsequently delivered to the **lysosome** for degradation; autophagy is part of everyday normal cell growth and development; for example, a liver-cell **mitochondrion** lasts around ten days before it is degraded and its contents are reused; autophagy also plays a major role in the destruction of bacteria, viruses, and unnecessary proteins that have begun to aggregate within a cell and may potentially cause problems; when autophagy involves the total destruction of the cell, it is called autophagic cell death (also known as cytoplasmic cell death or type II cell death); this is one of the main types of programmed cell death (compare **apoptosis**); it is a regulated process of cell death in a multicellular organism, or in a colony of individual cells such as yeast.

axillary: pertaining to the cavity beneath the junction of the arm and the body, better known as the armpit.

axon (or nerve fiber): a long, slender projection of a nerve cell, or neuron, that conducts electrical impulses away from the neuron's cell body or soma.

bacteria: (singular: bacterium) unicellular microorganisms; they are typically a few micrometers long and have many shapes including spheres, rods, and spirals; bacteria are ubiquitous in every habitat on Earth, growing in soil, acidic hot springs, radioactive waste, seawater, and deep in the earth's crust; some bacteria can even survive in the extreme cold and vacuum of outer space; there are typically 40 million bacterial cells in a gram of soil and a million bacterial cells in a milliliter of fresh water.

baroreflex: in cardiovascular physiology, the baroreflex or baroreceptor reflex is one of the body's homeostatic mechanisms for maintaining blood pressure; it provides a negative feedback loop in which an elevated blood pressure reflexively causes blood pressure to decrease; similarly, decreased blood pressure depresses the baroreflex, causing blood pressure to rise.

Barrett's esophagus: refers to an abnormal change (metaplasia) in the cells of the lower end of the **esophagus** thought to be caused by damage from chronic acid exposure, or reflux esophagitis; it is considered to be a premalignant condition and is associated with an increased risk of esophageal **cancer**.

basal cell carcinoma: the most common **skin cancer**; risk is increased for individuals with a high cumulative exposure to UV light via sunlight; treatment is with surgery, **topical** chemotherapy, x-ray, **cryosurgery**, **photodynamic therapy**; it is rarely life-threatening but if left untreated can be disfiguring, cause bleeding and produce local destruction (e.g., **eye**, **ear**, nose, **lip**).

baseline: information gathered at the beginning of a clinical study from which variations found in the study are measured; a person's health status before he or she begins a clinical trial; baseline measurements are used as a reference point to determine a participant's response to the experimental treatment.

basement membrane: a very thin sheet of **connective tissue** below the **epithelia**; it usually contains polysaccharide and very fine fibers of **reticulin** and **collagen**.

benign tumor: a nonmalignant **tumor**.

beta-carotene: the provitamin for **retinol** (**vitamin A**); it is converted to retinol in the **liver**; an antioxidant.

bile: a secretion of the **liver**; it is a bitter, slightly alkaline liquid, yellowish-green to golden-brown in color, consisting of bile salts, bile pigments, and other substances dissolved in water; its function is to assist in the digestion of fat and to act as a vehicle for the rejection of toxic or poisonous substances.

bilirubin: a yellow **bile** pigment formed in the breakdown of **heme**.

biocompatible: the quality of not having toxic or injurious effects on biological systems.

biofilm: a complex aggregation of microorganisms marked by the excretion of a protective and adhesive matrix; biofilms are also often characterized by surface attachment, structural heterogeneity, genetic diversity, complex community interactions, and an **extracellular** matrix of polymeric substances.

biological cell: an individual unit of protoplasm surrounded by a plasma **membrane** and usually containing a nucleus; a cell may exhibit all the characteristics of a living organism, or it may be highly specialized for a particular function; cells vary considerably in size and shape, but all have the common features of metabolism; every living organism is composed of cells, and every cell is formed from existing cells, usually by division, but also by fusion of sex cells; a cell may contain more than one nucleus; in **prokaryotic** cells, the genetic material is not contained in a **nucleus**.

biopsy: a medical test involving the removal of cells or tissues for examination; when only a sample of tissue is removed, the procedure is called an incisional biopsy or core biopsy; when an entire lump or suspicious area is removed, the procedure is called an excisional biopsy; when a sample of tissue or fluid is removed with a needle, the procedure is called a needle aspiration biopsy; biopsy specimens are often taken from part of a lesion when the cause of a disease is uncertain or its extent or exact character is in doubt; pathologic examination of a biopsy can determine whether a lesion is benign or malignant, and can help differentiate between different types of cancer; the margins of a biopsy specimen are also carefully examined to see if the disease may have spread beyond the area biopsied; "clear margins," or "negative margins," means that no disease was found at the edges of the biopsy specimen; "positive margins" means that disease was found and additional treatment may be needed.

biospeckle: **speckle** (see Glossary 1) formed by coherent light scattering from a cell or tissue.

bladder: a membranous sac that contains or stores fluid.

blister: when the outer (epidermis) layer of the skin separates from the fiber layer (dermis), a pool of lymph and other bodily fluids are collected between these layers while the skin regrows from underneath; this is a defense mechanism of the human body; blisters can be caused by chemical or physical **injury**; an example of chemical injury would be an allergic reaction; physical injury can be caused by heat, frostbite, or friction.

blood: a fluid tissue contained in a network of vessels or sinuses in humans and animals; the vessels or sinuses are lined with **endothelium**; blood is circulated through the network by muscular action of the vessels or the **heart**; it transports oxygen, **metabolites**, and hormones; it contains soluble colloidal proteins (**blood plasma**) and **blood corpuscles**; it assists in temperature control in mammals.

blood cell: see **blood corpuscle**.

blood corpuscle: one of the various types of cells that circulate in **blood plasma**; also called **blood cell**: **red blood cell (RBC) (erythrocyte)**, **white blood cell (WBC) (leukocyte)**, **platelet**, **thrombocyte**.

blood flow: blood movement along a **blood vessel**.

blood microcirculation: the peripheral **blood** circulation, which is provided by the **capillary** network.

blood perfusion: blood pumping (supplying) through an organ or a tissue.

blood plasma: the clear, waterlike, colorless liquid of **blood**; blood plasma is formed by removing all blood corpuscles from blood; plasma can be clotted.

blood vessel: a tube through which **blood** flows either to or from the **heart**; a general term for a conducting vessel for blood: **artery**, **vein**, **arteriole**, **venule**, and **capillary**.

blood volume: the total blood content within the region of a tissue; includes volumes of both oxygenated and deoxygenated blood.

bone: a connective tissue forming the skeleton; it consists of cells embedded in a matrix of bone salts and **collagen fibers**; the bone salts (mostly calcium carbonate and phosphate) form about 60% of the mass of the bone and give it its tensile strength; the bone cells are interconnected by fine protoplasmic processes situated in narrow channels in the bone, and are nourished by the blood stream; this vascular nature of bone differentiates it from **cartilage**.

brain: the coordinating center of the nervous system.

breathing: the transport of oxygen into the body and carbon dioxide out of the body; aerobic organisms require oxygen to create energy, via respiration, in the form of energy-rich molecules such as glucose.

burn: a type of **injury** to the **skin** caused by heat, cold, electricity, chemicals, or radiation (e.g., a sunburn).

burn scars: there are three major types of burn related scars: keloid, hypertrophic, and contractures; keloid scars are an overgrowth of scar tissue, the scar will grow beyond the site of the **injury**, these scars are generally red or pink and will become a dark tan over time; hypertrophic scars are red, thick, and raised, however they differ from keloid scars in that they do not develop beyond the site of injury or **incision**; a contracture scar is a permanent tightening of skin that may affect the underlying muscles and tendons, limiting mobility and possibly damaging or causing degeneration of the nerves (http://www.burnsurvivor.com/scar_types.html).

butanediol: 1,4-butanediol ($C_4H_{10}O_2$) is an **alcohol** derivative of the alkane butane, carrying two hydroxyl groups; it is a colorless viscous liquid; its molecular mass is 90.12 g/mol; its melting point is 20°C and its boiling point is 230°C.

butilene glycol: 1,3 butilene glycol used in **cosmetics**; prevents loss of moisture/gain of moisture; very safe and nonirritating; FDA and Food Chemical Codex III approved; gives rigidity and gloss to lipsticks; retains fragrance on the skin; gives better smoothness, elasticity, and gloss to hair; it provides more inhibition of microorganisms than other glycols; it has lower oral toxicity than other glycols/**glycerin**; its boiling point: 207.5°C, neutral pH.

calcification: the deposition of lime or insoluble salts of calcium and magnesium in a **tissue**.

calf: the fleshy part at the back of the lower part of a human leg.

cancer: a general term applied to a **carcinoma** or a **sarcoma**; the typical symptoms are a **tumor** or swelling, a discharge, pain, an upset in the function of an organ, general weakness and loss of weight.

canine: a dog or any animal of the Canidae, or dog family, including the wolves, jackals, hyenas, coyotes, and foxes.

capillary: a minute hairlike tube (diameter about 5–20 µm) with a wall consisting of a single layer of flattened cells (**endothelium**); the wall is permeable to substances such as water, oxygen, **glucose**, amino acids, carbon dioxide, and to inorganic ions; the capillaries form a network in all tissues; they are supplied with oxygenated **blood** by **arterioles** and pass deoxygenated blood to **venules**; their function is the exchange of dissolved substances between blood and tissue fluid.

capsular: pertaining to a capsule a membranous, again sac or integument.

carbohydrates: simple molecules that are straight-chain aldehydes or ketones with many hydroxyl groups added, usually one on each carbon atom that is not part of the aldehyde or ketone functional group; carbohydrates are the most abundant biological molecules, and fill numerous roles in living things, such as the storage and transport of energy (starch, **glycogen**) and acting as structural components (cellulose in plants, chitin in animals); additionally, carbohydrates and their derivatives play major roles in immune system function, fertilization, pathogenesis, blood clotting, and development; the basic carbohydrate units are called monosaccharides, such as **glucose**, galactose, and fructose; the general chemical formula of an unmodified monosaccharide is $(C \cdot H_2O)n$, where n is any number of three or greater.

carbonyl: a carbon atom double-bonded to an oxygen atom: C=O.

carcinoma [carcinoma *in situ* (CIS)]: a malignant growth of abnormal epithelial cells.

cardiovibrations (heartbeats): the rhythmic vibrations and sound of the heart pumping blood; it has a double beat caused by the sound of ventricles contracting, followed by a shorter, sharper sound of the semilunar valves closing; the atria do not contribute to the sound of the beat.

carious (caries): caries is a multifunctional dental disease; the following factors influence its progression: dental plaque **biofilm** (contains bacteria that are both acid-producing and survive at low pH, *Mutans streptococci* are believed to be the most important bacteria in the initiation and progress of dental caries); the availability of **glucose** that drives bacterial **metabolism** to produce lactic acid; generally caries is initiated in the **enamel** but it may also begin in **dentine** or cementum; when acid challenges occur repeatedly the eventual collapse of enough enamel crystals will result in cavitation.

caries (carious): in human anatomy, the common carotid **artery** supplies blood to the head and neck; it divides in the neck to form the external and internal carotid arteries.

cartilage: a strong, resilient, skeletal tissue; its simplest and most common form consists of a matrix of a polysaccharide-containing protein in which cartilage cells are embedded (chondroblasts); the matrix is hyaline cartilage, which is without structure and **blood vessels**; it is translucent and clear, and occurs in the cartilaginous rings of the trachea and bronchi; elastic cartilage (yellow fibrocartilage) contains **yellow fibers** in the matrix; it occurs in the external ear and in the epiglottis; white fibrocartilage contains **white fibers** in the matrix; it occurs in the disks of cartilage between the vertebrae; all types of cartilage contain chondroblasts, which deposit the matrix and become enclosed in the matrix as chondrocytes.

catabolism: the decomposition of chemical substances within an organism; the substances they are usually complex organic substances, and their products are simpler organic substances; the process is typically accompanied by a release of energy (see **metabolism**).

cataract: an abnormality of the eye characterized by opacity of the **crystalline lens**.

cataractogenesis: the process of **cataract** formation.

cationic: relating to cations, positively charged ions.

cavitation: a general term used to describe the behavior of voids or bubbles in a liquid.

cell: see **biological cell**.

cell fixation: killing, making rigid, and preserving a **cell** for microscopic study.

cell membrane: the thin, limiting covering of a **cell** or cell part; regulates the ingress of substances into a cell or its parts and may have some other functions that depend on the cell's specialization.

cellular organelle: a part of a **cell** that is a structural and functional unit, e.g., a flagellum is a locomotive organelle, a **mitochondrion** is a respiratory organelle; organelles in a cell correspond to organs in an organism.

centriole: a barrel shaped microtubule structure found in most animal **cells**; the walls of each centriole are usually composed of nine triplets of microtubules; an associated pair of centrioles, spatially arranged at right-angles, constitutes the compound structure known to cell biologists as the centrosome; centrioles are very important in the cell division process.

cerebellum: a region of the **brain** that plays an important role in the integration of sensory perception and motor output; many neural pathways link the cerebellum with the motor **cortex**, which sends information to the **muscles** causing them to move, and the spinocerebellar tract, which provides feedback on the position of the body in space; the cerebellum integrates these pathways, using the constant feedback on body position to fine-tune motor movements.

cerebrospinal fluid (CSF): the clear liquid that fills the cavities of the brain and spinal cord and the spaces between the arachnoid and pia matter; the fluid moves in a slow current down the central canal and up the spinal meninges; it is a solution of blood solutes of low molar mass, such as **glucose** and sodium chloride, but not of the same concentration as in the **blood**; it contains little or no protein and very few cells; its function is to nourish the **nervous tissue** and to act as a buffer against shock the total quantity of CSF in humans is about $100\ \text{cm}^3$.

cervical cancer: a malignant tumor of the **cervix uteri**; e.g., a **cervical intraepithelial neoplasia (CIN)**, CIN I and CIN II are precancerous; CIN III stage corresponds to **carcinoma** *in situ* **(CIS)**; the next stage is an invasive cancer.

cervical intraepithelial neoplasia (CIN): CIN I and CIN II are precancerous, and correspond to slight and moderate **displasia**; CIN III stage corresponds to marked displasia or **carcinoma** *in situ* **(CIS)**.

cervical smear: a thin specimen of the cytologic material taken from the female cervical channel; it is usually received as a smear on a glass plate, and is fixed, and stained before being examined.

cervical tissue: the multilayered tissue consisting of the upper epithelial, basal (basal **membrane**), and stromal layers; depending on the area of the **cervix**, the epithelium may be in one of two forms: squamous or columnar.

cervix uteri: the narrow opening to the uterus; a short tube leading from the vagina to the uterus.

chemical potential: in thermodynamics, the amount by which the energy of the system would change if an additional particle was introduced, with the **entropy** (see Glossary 1) and volume held fixed; if a system contains more than one species of particle, there is a separate chemical potential associated with each species, defined as the change in energy when the number of particles of that species is increased by one; the chemical potential is a fundamental parameter in thermodynamics and it is conjugate to the particle number.

chemiluminescence: the emission of light (luminescence) without emission of heat as the result of a chemical reaction.

chest: the part of the trunk between the neck and the abdomen, containing the cavity and enclosed by the **ribs**, sternum, and certain vertebrae, in which the **heart**, **lungs**, etc., are situated.

cholesterol: a sterol (a combination steroid and **alcohol**) and a **lipid** found in the **cell membranes** of all body **tissues**, and transported in the **blood** plasma of all animals.

choroid: the membranous, pigmented middle layer of the **eyeball** between the **sclera** and the **retina**; it contains numerous **blood vessels**; its function is to absorb light to prevent internal reflection in the eyeball and to provide nourishment for the retina; the choroid is continuous with the **iris** in the front of the eye.

chromatin: the complex of **DNA** and **protein** found inside the nuclei of eukaryotic **cells**; the **nucleic acids** are in the form of double-stranded DNA (a double helix); the major proteins involved in chromatin are histone proteins, although many other chromosomal proteins have prominent roles too; the functions of chromatin are to package DNA into a smaller volume to fit in the cell, to strengthen the DNA, to allow **mitosis** and meiosis, and to serve as a mechanism to control expression.

chromatin filaments: chromatin fibers condensed to 30 nm and consisting of nucleosome arrays in their most compact form.

cicatrix: the new tissue that forms over a **wound** and later contracts into a scar.

ciliary body: a thickened circular structure at the edge of the **choroid** and at the border of the **cornea**; the **iris** and the suspensory ligaments are attached to it; it contains the **ciliary muscle** used in accommodation; it secretes **aqueous humor**.

ciliary muscle: a smooth **muscle** that affects zonular fibers in the **eye** (fibers that suspend the **lens** in position during accommodation), enabling changes in lens shape for light focusing.

ciliary pigmented epithelium: the darkly colored **melanin**-pigmented epithelial layer of **ciliary body**.

clinical trials: the application of the scientific method to human health; researchers use clinical trials to test hypotheses about the effect of a particular intervention upon a **pathological** disease condition; well-run clinical trials use defined techniques and rigorous definitions to answer the researchers' questions as accurately as possible; the most commonly performed clinical trials evaluate new drugs, medical devices, biologics, or other interventions on patients in strict scientifically controlled settings, and are required for regulatory authority approval of new therapies; trials may be designed to assess the safety and efficacy of an experimental therapy, to assess whether the new intervention is better than standard therapy, or to compare the efficacy of two standard or marketed interventions; the trial objectives and design are usually documented in a clinical trial protocol; synonyms are clinical studies, research protocols, and medical research.

coagulation: the process of coagulation or of causing something to coagulate, to cause particles (components) to collect together in a compact mass, e.g., the coagulation of egg white is brought about by heat.

coenzyme: the small organic nonprotein molecules that carry chemical groups between **enzymes**; many coenzymes are phosphorylated water-soluble vitamins; however, nonvitamins may also be coenzymes such as **ATP**; coenzymes are consumed in the reactions in which they are substrates, for example: the coenzyme **NADH** is converted to NAD+ by oxidoreductases; coenzymes are, however, regenerated and their concentration maintained at a steady level in the **cell**.

cold cataract: a temperature-induced reversible **cataract**.

collagen: a tough, inelastic, **fibrous** protein; when boiled, it forms a **gelatin**; on adding **acetic acid** it swells up and dissolves; collagen is formed and maintained in tissues by **fibroblasts**; it forms **white fibers** in **connective tissue**; the tropocollagen or "collagen molecule" subunit is a rod about 300-nm long and a 1.5-nm diameter, made up of three polypeptide strands and subunits with regularly staggered ends that spontaneously self-assemble into even larger arrays in the **extracellular** spaces of tissues; there is some covalent cross linking within the triple helices, and a variable amount of covalent cross linking between tropocollagen helices, to form the different types of collagen found in different mature tissues—similar to the situation found with the α-**keratins** in **hair**; a distinctive feature of collagen is the regular arrangement of **amino acids** in each of the three chains of collagen subunits; in **bone**, entire collagen triple helices lie in a parallel, staggered array; 40-nm gaps between the ends of the tropocollagen subunits probably serve as nucleation sites for the deposition of long, hard, fine crystals of the mineral component, which is (approximately) **hydroxyapatite** with some phosphate, which turns certain kinds of **cartilage** into **bone**; collagen gives bone its elasticity and contributes to fracture resistance.

collagen fibers: bundles of **collagen fibrils** (see **white fibers**, **white fibrous tissue**).

collagen fibrils: **collagen** molecules packed into an organized overlapping bundle.

collagen secondary structure: a **collagen** molecule subunit is a rod made up of three polypeptide strands, each of which is a left-handed helix; these three left-handed helices are twisted together into a clockwise coil, a triple helix, a cooperative quaternary structure stabilized by numerous hydrogen bonds.

colloid structure: dispersion of colloidal particles in a continuous phase (the **dispersion** medium) of a different composition or state; true solutions of materials that have dimensions within the colloidal range (1 nm to 100 nm), e.g., molecules of a very large relative molecular mass such as polymers and proteins, or aggregates of small molecules, as in soaps and detergents under certain conditions (association colloids).

colloid isoelectric point: the pH value of the **dispersion** medium of a colloidal suspension at which the colloidal particles do not move in an electric field.

colon: the first or anterior part of the large intestine; it possesses sacculated walls lined with a smooth **mucous membrane**; contains the lining **glands** that secret **mucus** but no digestive **enzymes**; water is absorbed from the unassimilated liquid material, leaving feces; the colon leads directly into the rectum.

colonic: related to **colon**.

colposcope: an endoscopic instrument that provides *in vivo* examination of the vaginal and cervical mucous with a high magnification.

colposcopy: the *in situ* examination of the vaginal and cervical mucous using the colposcope.

columnar epithelium: **cells** that are taller than they are wide; the **nucleus** is closer to the base of the cell; the small **intestine** is a tubular organ lined with this type of **tissue**; unicellular **glands** called goblet cells are scattered throughout the simple columnar epithelial cells and secrete **mucus**; the free surface of the columnar cell has tiny hairlike projections called microvilli; they increase the surface area for absorption.

computed tomography: the imaging of a selected plane (slice) in the body and 3D computer reconstruction of the image of a whole object on the basis of many individual images (slices) using one of the following methods: x ray, magnetic resonance, positron-emission, or optical imaging (slicing).

conjunctiva: a delicate **mucous membrane** that covers the **cornea**, the front part of the **sclera**, and lining of the eyelids: it protects the cornea.

connective tissue: various body tissues that bind together and support organs and other tissues, e.g., connective tissue surrounds **muscles** and **nerves**, connects **bones** and muscles and underlies the **skin**; **cartilage**, and bone are also connective tissues; typical connective tissue consists of cells scattered in an amorphous mucopolysaccharide matrix in which there are varying amounts of connective tissue fibers (mainly **collagen**, but also **elastin** and **reticulin**).

contrast (ing) agents: see Glossary 1.

copolymer (or **heteropolymer**): a polymer derived from two (or more) monomeric species as opposed to a homopolymer, where only one monomer is used.

coproporphyrin: a **porphyrin** that occurs as several isomers; the III isomer, an intermediate in **heme** biosynthesis, is excreted in the feces and **urine** in such diseases as hereditary coproporphyria and variegate porphyria; the I isomer, a side product, is excreted in congenital erythropoietic porphyria disease; is used as a test to measure **red blood cell** porphyrin levels in evaluating of porphyrin disorders.

cornea: the transparent covering at the front of the **eyeball**; it is the modified continuation of the **sclera**; it refracts light and is the most important element in the refractive system of the eye.

corneocyte: the dead **keratin**-filled **squamous cell** of the **stratum corneum**; synonym: horny cell, keratinised cell (**keratinocyte**).

cornification (keratinization): the conversion of epithelium to the stratified **squamous** type; for instance, the conversion of skin cells into **keratin** or other horny material such as nails or scales.

coronary arteries: the right and left coronary arteries that originate from the beginning (root) of the **aorta**, immediately above the aortic **valve**; the left coronary **artery** originates from the left aortic sinus, while the right coronary artery originates from the right aortic sinus.

cortex (cerebral cortex): the outer layer of the cerebral hemisphere, consisting of **gray matter** and rich in synapses; it is extensive in mammals, with fissures and folds.

cosmetics: the substances used to enhance or protect the appearance or odor of the human body; cosmetics include skincare creams, lotions, powders, perfumes, lipsticks, fingernail polishes, **eye** and facial makeup, permanent waves, **hair** colors, deodorants, baby products, bath **oils**, bubble baths, and many other types of products; the FDA defines cosmetics as: "intended to be applied to the human body for cleansing, beautifying, promoting attractiveness, or altering the appearance without affecting the body's structure or functions."

craniocaudal projection: the projection that shows the direction from the **cranium** to the posterior end of the body.

cranium: a domed, bony case composed of several **bone**s joined by sutures; it encloses and protects the **brain**.

cross-linking: to attach by a cross-link: a bond, atom, or group linking the chains of atoms in a polymer, protein, or other complex organic molecule.

cryogenic: related to treatments using very low temperatures (below $-150°C$, $-238°F$ or 123 K) and the behavior of materials at those temperatures.

cryosection: a frozen sectioning procedure that is used to perform rapid microscopic analysis of a tissue specimen; it is used most often in oncological surgery and tissue research.

cryosurgery (cryotherapy): the application of extreme cold to destroy abnormal or diseased tissue; is used to treat a number of diseases and disorders, especially **skin** conditions; warts, moles, skin tags, solar keratoses, and small skin **cancers** are candidates for cryosurgical treatment; some internal disorders are also treated with cryosurgery, including **liver** cancer, **prostate** cancer, and cervical disorders.

crystalline lens: a transparent structure surrounded by a thin capsule and situated immediately behind the **pupil** of the eye; it has the shape of a biconvex lens; it is attached to the **eyeball** by suspensory ligaments; it refracts light onto the **retina**.

crystallins: the structural proteins that are the components of a mammalian **crystalline lens**.

crystalline: a crystalline material has a regular crystal lattice; it does not necessarily form a single regular crystal, e.g., all metals are crystalline because the atoms have a regular arrangement.

cutaneous: relating to the skin.

cyclophotocoagulation: is a transscleral laser procedure for **glaucoma** treatment; in this procedure, the **ciliary body** is treated with a laser to decrease its production of aqueous—this in turn reduces pressure inside the **eye**; about 20 to 40 laser delivery applications are completed.

cyst: a closed, bladderlike sac formed in tissues; it contains fluid or semifluid matter.

cystitis: an infection of the **bladder**, but the term is often used indiscriminately and covers a range of infections and **irritation**s in the lower urinary system.

cytochrome: the **proteins** that contain iron and act as **coenzymes** in cellular respiratory; they are found abundantly in aerobic organisms; they are oxidized by dissolved **oxygen** in a **cell**, and reduced by oxidizable substances in the cell; they are the main **vehicle** for the use of oxygen in **metabolism**.

cytochrome oxidase: a large transmembrane protein complex found in bacteria and the mitochondrion; it is the last protein in the electron transport chain; it receives an electron from each of four **cytochrome** C molecules, and transfers them to one **oxygen** molecule, converting molecular oxygen to two molecules of **water**; in the process, it translocates four protons, helping to establish a chemiosmotic potential that the **ATP** synthase then uses to synthesize ATP.

cytometry: the methods and instruments for the structural and functional study of **cells** and bacteria; e.g., **flow cytometry** is a technique for automatic measurement and analysis of cells and other small particles suspended in a medium.

cytoplasm: the protoplasm of a **cell** exclusive of the **nucleus**; it is not just a simple, slightly viscous, fluid; in it are situated various structures, called **organelles**, each concerned with different functions of the cell; the **plasma membrane** is part of the cytoplasm.

cytoskeleton: made of **fibrous proteins** (e.g., **microfilaments**, **microtubules**, and intermediate filaments); in many organisms maintains the shape of the **cell**, anchors **organelles**, and controls internal movement of structures.

cytosol: (cf. **cytoplasm**, which also includes the **organelles**) is the internal fluid of the **cell**, and a portion of cell **metabolism** occurs here; **proteins** within the cytosol play an important role in signal transduction pathways and glycolysis; in **prokaryotes**, all chemical reactions take place in the cytosol; in **eukaryotes** the portion of cytosol in the nucleus is called nucleohyaloplasm; the cytosol also surrounds the **cytoskeleton**; the cytosol is a "soup" with free-floating particles, but is highly organized on the molecular level.

decylmethylsulfoxide: a tissue penetrating agent similar to **DMSO**; is also known as n-decylmethylsulfoxide (nDMSO).

dehydration: the removal or loss of water by a **tissue** or a **cell**.

denaturation: the alteration of a **protein** shape through some form of external stress (for example, by applying heat, acid, or alkali), in such a way that it will no longer be able to carry out its cellular function; denatured proteins can exhibit a wide range of characteristics, from loss of solubility to communal **aggregation**.

dental plaque: a biofilm (usually a pale yellow to white color) that builds up on the teeth; if not removed regularly, it can lead to dental cavities (**caries**) or periodontal problems (such as gingivitis).

dentin: a hard, calcified, elastic, yellowish material of the same substance as **bone**, but contains no cells; it is the main structural part of a tooth; dentin is composed of base material that is pierced by mineralized dentinal tubules 1–5 μm in diameter; the tubules' density is in the range of $3–7.5 \times 10^6$ cm^{-2}; they contain organic components and natural **HAP [hydroxyapatite (apatite)]** crystals 2–3.5 nm in diameter and up to 100 nm in length, which intensively scatter light.

deoxyhemoglobin: **hemoglobin** disintegrated with **oxygen**.

dermal papilla: extensions of the **dermis** into the **epidermis**; they sometimes can be perceived at the surface of the **skin**.

dermatitis: **inflammation** of the **skin**.

dermatosis: any disease of the **skin**.

dermis: the inner layer of the **skin**; it is composed of **connective tissue**, **blood** and **lymph vessels**, **muscles**, and **nerves**; **collagen fibers** are abundant in the dermis and run parallel to the surface of the skin; they give the skin elasticity; sweat **glands** and hair follicles are scattered throughout the dermis; the dermis is much thicker than the epidermis and is developed from mesoderm.

desorption: a phenomenon and process opposite of sorption (that is, adsorption or absorption), whereby some of a sorbed substance is released; this occurs in a system being in the state of sorption equilibrium between the bulk phase (fluid, i.e., gas or liquid solution) and an adsorbing surface (solid or boundary separating two fluids); when the concentration (or pressure) of substance in the bulk phase is lowered, some of the sorbed substance changes to the bulk state; in chemistry, especially chromatography, desorption is the ability for a chemical to move with the mobile phase—the more a chemical desorbs, the less likely it will adsorb, thus instead of sticking to the stationary phase, the chemical moves up with the solvent front.

desquamation: the shedding of the outer layers of the **skin**; for example, once the rash of measles fades, there is desquamation.

dextran: a complex, branched polysaccharide made of many **glucose** molecules joined into chains of varying lengths.

diabetes (diabetes mellitus): a metabolic disorder characterized by hyperglycemia (high blood sugar); the World Health Organization (WHO) recognizes three main forms of diabetes: type 1, type 2, and gestational diabetes (occurring during pregnancy), which have similar signs, symptoms, and consequences, but different causes and population distributions; type 1 is usually due to autoimmune destruction of the pancreatic beta cells that produce insulin; type 2 is characterized by tissue-wide insulin resistance and varies widely, it sometimes progresses to loss of beta cell function.

diabetic retinopathy: damage to the **retina** caused by complications of **diabetes mellitus**, which could eventually lead to blindness; it is an ocular manifestation of systemic disease, which affects up to 80% of all diabetics who have had diabetes for 15 years or more.

diaphanography: a **noninvasive method** of examining the breast or other human organ by transillumination, using visible or infrared light.

diaphragm: a dome-shaped sheet of tissue, part **muscle**, part **tendon**, separating the thoracic and abdominal cavities.

diastolic: related to diastole, the period of time when the **heart** relaxes after contraction; ventricular diastole is when the ventricles are relaxing, while atrial diastole is when the **atria** are relaxing.

dioley(o)lphosphatidylethanolamine (DOPE): a neutral lipid, used as the carrier system.

dipropylene glycol: $HOC_3H_6OC_3H_6OH$; molecular weight 134.18; refractive index 1.438–1.442; a colorless, viscous, practically nontoxic, and slightly hygroscopic liquid; its melting point is 78°C, boiling point, 231°C; is miscible in water, alcohols, esters, most organic solvents, and various vegetable oils; is used as a solvent, coupling agent, and chemical intermediate in many fields, including **cosmetics**.

disaggregation: the separation of an aggregate body into its component parts.

dissociation: a general process in which ionic compounds (complexes, molecules, or salts) separate or split into smaller molecules, ions, or radicals, usually in a reversible manner; for instance, reversible dissociation of collagen fibers; dissociation is the opposite of association and recombination.

DMSO: dimethyl sulfoxide is the chemical compound $(CH_3)_2SO$; this colorless liquid is an important polar aprotic solvent; it is readily miscible in a wide range of organic solvents as well as water; it has a distinctive property of penetrating the skin very readily, allowing the handler to taste it; its unique capability of to penetrate living tissues without causing significant damage is most probably related to its relatively polar nature, its capacity to accept hydrogen bonds, and its relatively small and compact structure; this combination of properties results in its ability to associate with water, proteins, **carbohydrates**, **nucleic acid**, ionic substances, and other constituents of living systems (www.dmso.org).

DNA (deoxyribonucleic acid): a long-chain compound formed from many **nucleotides** bonded together as units in the chain; a strand of DNA is formed from molecules of deoxyribose (a sugar) and molecules of phosphoric acid attached alternatively in a chain; it is found only in the chromosomes of animals and plants and in the corresponding structures in bacteria and viruses.

dorsal: the term refers to anatomical structures that are either situated toward or grow off the side of an animal or human; in humans, the top of the hand and top of the foot are considered dorsal.

duct: a tube with an outlet, discharging fluids from one system to another; e.g., the **bile** duct discharges bile from the **liver** into the alimentary canal or milk drains through ducts into a cistern in the **mammary gland**.

ductal carcinoma *in situ*: see **duct** and **carcinoma**.

dura mater (pachymeninx): the tough and inflexible outermost of the three layers of the *meninges* surrounding the brain and spinal cord; the *dura mater* itself has two layers: a superficial layer, which is actually the skull's inner *periosteum*, and a deep layer, the *dura mater proper*.

dysfunction: any disturbance in the function of an organ or body part.

dysplasia: an abnormality in the appearance of cells indicative of an early step toward transformation into a **neoplasia**; it is therefore a preneoplastic or precancerous change; this abnormal growth is restricted to the originating system or location, for example, a dysplasia in the epithelial layer will not invade the deeper tissue, or a dysplasia solely in a red blood cell line (refractory anaemia) will stay within the **bone** marrow and cardiovascular systems; the best known form of dysplasia is the precursor lesions to **cervical cancer**, called **cervical intraepithelial neoplasia (CIN)**; this lesion is usually caused by an infection with the **human papilloma virus (HPV)**.

dysplastic: related to **dysplasia**.

ear: the organ that detects sound; the vertebrate ear shows a common biology from fish to humans, with variations in structure according to order and species; it not only acts as a receiver for sound, but plays a major role in the sense of balance and body position; the word "ear" may be used correctly to describe the whole vertebrate ear, or just the visible portion; in most animals, the visible ear is a flap of tissue that is also called the pinna; in humans, the pinna is more often called the auricle; in biomedical optics the lobe of the human ear used as a convenient model for **noninvasive** blood oxygenation and microcirculation studies; in animals—rat, mouse, rabbit, etc., pinna is used as an *in vivo* model for noninvasive blood studies.

ectodermal dysplasia: a hereditary condition characterized by abnormal development of the skin, hair, nails, teeth, and sweat glands.

edema: the effusion of serous fluid into the interstices of cells in tissue spaces or into body cavities.

elastin: an elastic **fibrous** protein resistant to boiling and acetic acid; it forms highly elastic **yellow fibers** in **connective tissue**; elastin is formed and maintained in tissues by **fibroblasts**.

elastosis: the breakdown of elastic **tissue**; for example, the loss of elasticity in the **skin** of elderly people that results from degeneration of **connective tissue**.

electroosmosis: the motion of a polar liquid through a **membrane** or other porous structure under the influence of an applied electric field; (generally, along charged surfaces of any shape and also through nonmacroporous materials, which have ionic sites and allow for water uptake, the latter is sometimes referred to as "chemical **porosity**") also called electroendosmosis.

electroporation: a short pulse of voltage in the range of 5–200 V/cm^2 applied to a biological **membrane** induces its **porosity** that enhances membrane permeation for big molecules.

enamel: a hard, elastic, white material that contains no cells and that is an almost completely inorganic substance; enamel covers the crown of a tooth; dental enamel consists of 87–95% natural **HAP [hydroxyapatite (apatite)]** crystals; they are organized in keyhole-shaped prisms; these prisms are 4–6 μm wide and extend from the dentine-enamel-junction to the outer surface of the tooth; because of their size, number, and refractive index, the prisms are the main light scatterers in enamel.

encapsulated drugs: an encapsulation of some drugs significantly reduce their toxicity (gastrointestinal, **cutaneous**, etc.) especially at the higher dose level and often increase drug efficiency; various encapsulation technologies are used, including **liposomes**.

endocard (endocardium): the serous membrane that lines the cavities of the heart.

endogenous: means "arising from within"; endogenous substances are those that originate from within an organism, **tissue** or **cell**; in biological systems endogeneity refers to the recipient of **DNA** (usually in prokaryotes); however, due to **homeostasis**, discerning between internal and external influences is often difficult.

endoplasmic reticulum (ER): an elaborate series of membranous sacs that communicate with each other in a three-dimensional network and occur in the endoplasm of a cell; the connection between two sacs is an anastomosis; ER is either rough or smooth surfaced; rough ER carries ribosomes on the outside surface of the sacs; smooth ER carries no ribosomes; the functions of ER include the transfer of materials in cells by providing a circulatory system of channels, the formation of **lysosomes**, and lipid **metabolism**.

endothelium: a single layer of squamous cells lining the **heart**, **blood vessels**, and **lymphatic vessels**; the **cells** are tessellated, i.e., they have wavy boundaries that interdigitate or fit together; endothelium is morphologically similar to **epithelium**, but is derived from mesoderm.

enzyme: a protein produced by a living **cell** and that acts as a catalyst in biochemical changes; there are many different types of enzymes, some of which promote a narrow range of chemical reactions on chemically related substances, while most others promote a single chemical reaction; most of the chemical reactions included in **metabolism** are dependent on enzymes to promote them at the rate required for an organism to function properly; a very small quantity of an enzyme is sufficient to convert a large quantity of a substance; each enzyme has optimum conditions for its action, e.g., a temperature of about 35–40°C, a specific pH, the presence of a **coenzyme** for some reactions, and the absence of inhibiting substances.

epicard (epicardium): the inner serous layer of the pericardium, lying directly upon the **heart**.

epidermal stripping sample: a thin slice of **epidermis** obtained with the use of medical glue and a quartz (glass) or metal plate.

epidermis: the outer layer of the skin is a stratified **epithelium** that varies relatively little in thickness over most of the body (between 75 and 150 µm), except on the **palms** and soles, where its thickness may be 0.4–0.6 mm; the epidermis is conventionally subdivided into (1) **stratum basale**, a basal cell layer of keratinocytes, which is the germinative layer of the epidermis, (2) the **stratum spinosum**, which consists of several layers of polyhedral cells lying above the germinal layer, (3) the **stratum granulosum**, which is a layer of flattened cells containing distinctive cytoplasmic inclusions, keratohyalin granules, and (4) the overlying **stratum corneum**, consisting of lamellae of anucleate thin, flat squames that are terminally differentiated **keratinocytes**.

epidurally: means through the *dura mater*.

episclera: the layer of the eye **sclera**.

epithelial tissue: tissue consisting of a sheet of **cells** held together by a minimal amount of cementlike material between the cells; it covers exposed surfaces and lines the cavities and tubes of the body; beneath most epithelial tissue is a thin sheet of **connective tissue**, the **basement membrane**; besides its protective function, epithelial tissue frequently has a secretory function, in which case it is sometimes known as glandular tissue.

epithelium: a sheet of **epithelial tissue**; epithelium is derived from ectoderm and endoderm.

erythema (skin reddening): an abnormal redness of the **skin** due to local congestion, as in **inflammation**; e.g., the skin's response to UV irradiation.

erythematosus lupus: a chronic disease of unknown cause, occasionally affecting internal organs, characterized by red, scaly patches on the **skin**.

erythematous: relating to, or causing, **erythema**.

erythrocyte: a flattened, disk-shaped (circular biconcave disks, about 8 μm in diameter in humans) **cell** that circulates in **blood**; it contains a respiratory pigment, **hemoglobin**; the cell is readily distorted, elastic, and immotile: mammalian erythrocytes have no nuclei, but the erythrocytes of embryos have nuclei; erythrocytes are formed in red **bone** marrow, are destroyed by erythrophages, and have a relatively short life (average 120 days in humans); there are approximately five million per cubic millimeter in normal human blood.

erythrodermia: the general name of the expressed and usually widespread skin redness (**erythema**), often accompanied by scale of the skin.

esophagus: a tube connecting the **pharynx** with the **stomach**, usually about 25 cm for adults; it is divided into three parts: jugular, **chest**, and **abdominal**.

ethanol: see **alcohol**.

ether: the general name for a class of chemical compounds that contain an ether group, which is an **oxygen** atom connected to two (substituted) alkyl groups; a typical example is the solvent and anesthetic diethyl ether, commonly referred to simply as "ether" (ethoxyethane, $CH_3-CH_2-O-CH_2-CH_3$).

ethylene glycol: a colorless, sweet liquid (see **alcohol**) used chiefly as a solvent.

eukaryotes: animals, plants, **fungi**, and protists are eukaryotes, organisms with a complex cell or **cells**, in which the genetic material is organized into a membrane-bound **nucleus** or nuclei; animals, plants, and fungi are mostly multicellular.

evans blue: a biological dye (stain).

evaporation: the process whereby atoms or molecules in a liquid state gain sufficient energy to enter the gaseous state; it is the opposite process of condensation; evaporation is exclusively a surface phenomena and should not be confused with boiling; most notably, for a liquid to boil, its vapor pressure must equal the ambient pressure, whereas for evaporation to occur, this is not the case.

excision: means "to remove as if by cutting"; in surgery, an excision (or resection) is the complete removal of an organ or a tumor, as opposed to a **biopsy**; an "excisional biopsy" (sometimes called a "tumorectomy") is the removal of a tumor with a minimum of healthy tissue; it is therefore an excision rather than a biopsy.

exogenous: an action or object coming from outside a system; the opposite of **endogenous**; for example, an exogenous **contrast agent** in medical imaging refers to a liquid injected in the patient that enhances visibility of a pathology, such as a **tumor**; an exogenous factor is any material present and active in an individual organism or living **cell**, but that originated outside of that organism, as opposed to an endogenous factor, including both pathogens and therapeutics; **DNA** introduced to cells via transfection or viral infection (transduction) is an exogenous factor; carcinogens are exogenous factors.

extracellular: means "outside the **cell**"; outside the plasma **membranes** and occupied by fluid.

ex vivo: taken from the living organism; pertaining to experiments on animal or human organs that are excised from the living body and kept in conditions very close to the natural ones.

eyeball: the spherical structure composed of supporting tissues in which the photoreceptors and refractive media for concentrating light on the **nervous tissues** are situated; the eyeball is divided into anterior and posterior chambers by the **iris**.

facial tissue: refers to a class of soft, absorbant, disposable paper that is suitable for use on the face.

fat: (1) any substance that can be extracted from tissues by ether, hot ethanol, or gasoline (fat solvents); this is a wide definition covering neutral fats, sterols, steroids, carotenes, and terpens; in this sense, lipids, lipins, and lipoids are fats; (2) true fat or neutral fat, as considered in dietetics, is an ester of **glycerol** with one, two, or three different fatty acids replacing the three hydroxyl groups of the trihydric alcohol, glycerol; (3) any substance that is a true fat and solid below 20°C; this is in contrast to an **oil**; (4) see **adipose tissue**.

fat (fatty) acid: a carboxylic acid often with a long unbranched aliphatic tail (chain), which is either saturated or unsaturated; fatty acids derived from natural **fats** and **oils** may be assumed to have at least 8 carbon atoms, e.g., caprylic acid (octanoic acid); most of the natural fatty acids have an even number of carbon atoms, because their biosynthesis involves acetyl-CoA, a **coenzyme** carrying a two-carbon-atom group; fatty acids are produced by the hydrolysis of the ester linkages in a fat or biological oil (both of which are **triglycerides**), with the removal of **glycerol**.

fat cell: a cell in which a food reserve is deposited in the form of droplets of **oil**; the quantity of oil increases until the oil globule formed distends the cell and pushes the nucleus and **cytoplasm** to one side; a collection of fat cells forms **adipose tissue**.

fatty tissue: see **adipose tissue**.

female breast (mamma): the milk-secreting organ of females; it contains a **mammary gland**.

femoral biceps muscle: the muscle pertaining to the thigh or femur.

fibers: the long strands of scleroprotein; they are either **collagen**-forming **white fibers** or **elastin**-forming **yellow fibers**, or **reticulin**-forming **reticular fibers**; fibers form part of a noncellular matrix around and among **cells**; they are formed and maintained in a tissue by **fibroblasts**; a matrix may consist of an amorphous, jellylike polysaccharide together with the three types of fiber; cells and a matrix form a **connective tissue**; different forms of connective tissue possess varying proportions of the constituents of the matrix.

fibril: a fine fiber or filament; e.g., in **muscles** their diameters are in the range of 5–15 nm with a length of about 1–1.5 µm and in the eye cornea, their diameters are in the range of 26–30 nm with a mean of length up to a few millimeters.

fibril D-periodicity: for example, corneal fibrils are D-periodic (axial periodicity of collagen fibrils, where $D \approx 67$ nm), uniformly narrow ($\approx$30–35 nm in diameter), and indeterminate in length, particularly in older animals; the D-periodicity of the fibril arises from side-to-side associations of triple-helical collagen molecules that are $\approx$300 nm in length (i.e., the molecular length $= 4.4 \times D$) and are staggered by D; the D-stagger of collagen molecules produces alternating regions of protein density in the fibril, which explains the characteristic gapping and overlapping appearance of fibrils negatively contrasted for transmission electron microscopy.

fibroadenoma: a **benign tumor** originating in a glandular **epithelium**, having a conspicuous **stroma** consisting of the proliferating **fibroblasts** and other elements of **connective tissue**.

fibroblast: a **cell** that contributes to the formation of **connective tissue**.

fibrocystic: pertaining to the nature of or having a **fibrous cyst** or **cysts**.

fibroglandular tissue: a glandular tissue that has a large number of **fibers**, such as the tissue of the female breast.

fibroid: (1) resembling a **fiber** or **fibrous tissue**; (2) composed of fibers, as a **tumor**; (3) a tumor largely composed of smooth **muscle**.

fibrous: containing, consisting of, or resembling **fibers**.

fibrous cyst: any **cyst** that is surrounded by or situated in a large amount of **fibrous connective tissue**.

fibrous plaque: a small, flat formation or area of **fibrous tissue**.

fibrous tissue: a tissue mainly consisting of conjunctive **collagen** (or **elastin**) **fibers**, often packed in lamellar bundles.

fissure: a groove, natural division, deep furrow, or cleft found in the brain, spinal cord, and liver; a tear in the anus (anal fissure); in dentistry, a break in the tooth enamel.

fixation: in the fields of **histology**, pathology, and **cell** biology, fixation is a chemical process by which biological **tissues** are preserved from decay; fixation terminates any ongoing biochemical reactions, and may also increase the mechanical strength or stability of the treated tissues.

flagelium: a long, fine, threadlike process on a noncellular or unicellular organism, such as bacteria and spermatozoa; usually the organism possesses only one flagellum or possibly two; flagella are used for locomotion; their movements are in 3D and undulate in a wavelike or helical fashion.

flavin: a complex heterocyclic ketone that is common to the nonprotein part of several important yellow **enzymes**, the flavoproteins.

flavin adenine dinucleotide (FAD): formed as the **flavin** moiety is attached with an adenosine diphosphate; a **coenzyme** for many proteins including monoamine **oxidase**, D-amino acid oxidase, glucose oxidase, xanthine oxidase, and Acyl-CoA dehydrogenase.

flavin mononucleotide (FMN): a prosthetic group found in and amongst other **proteins**, **NADH** dehydrogenase and old yellow **enzyme**; a phosphorylated form of riboflavin.

flow cytometry: a technique for automatic measurement and analysis of **cells** and other small particles suspended in a medium; particles flowing at high speed through a narrow opening are measured individually by optical or electrical methods; in this way, methods, where structural and functional characteristics can be determined quickly and with great precision.

fluorescein: a **fluorophore** commonly used in biological microscopy; has an absorption maximum at 494 nm and emission maximum of 521 nm (in water); has an isoabsorptive point (equal absorption for all pH values) at 460 nm.

foot sole: the thickest layers of **skin** on the human body due to the weight that is continually placed on them; contains significantly less pigment than the skin of the rest of the body; one of two areas of the human body that grow no vellus **hair**; houses a denser population of **sweat glands** than most other regions of skin.

forearm: the lower part of the human **arm**, between the elbow and the **wrist**; an arm consists of the upper arm and the forearm.

formalin: trade name of 37% aqueous solution of formaldehyde; in water formaldehyde converts to the hydrate $CH_2(OH)_2$; preserves or fixes **tissue** or **cells** by irreversibly cross-linking primary amine groups in proteins with other nearby nitrogen atoms in protein or DNA through a $-CH_2-$ linkage; can be used as a disinfectant as it kills most **bacteria** and **fungi** (including their **spores**).

freckles: the small tan spots of **melanin** on the **skin** of people with fair complexions.

front chamber (segment) of the human eye: the **cornea**, an anterior chamber of the **eyeball** filled by the **aqueous humor**, and the **iris** and **crystalline lens** in it.

frontal lobe: (see **lobe**).

functional imaging: an imaging technique of the spatial distribution of blood oxygenation, **blood volume**, blood velocity, or any other functional parameter of a living **tissue**.

fundus: the base of an organ, or the part opposite to or remote from an aperture; e.g., fundus (bottom) of the eye.

fungi cells: a division of the subkingdom *Thallophyta*; its members include the yeasts, mushrooms, moulds, and rusts, i.e., fungal organisms; characteristics of this division are that its members have **eucaryotic cells**, they lack chlorophyll, there are unicellular or coenocytic tubular filaments for the main body of the organism, they are saprophytic or parasitic on plants and animals, and they reproduce by forming spores in very large numbers.

fusogenicity: relates to cell membrane fusion by a physical or chemical action.

FVB/N mouse strain: an inbred mouse strain that was established at the National Institute of Health in 1970 from an outbred colony of Swiss mice; is preferable for transgenic analyses.

gall bladder: a small bladder situated between the lobes of the **liver**; it is connected to the liver through the cystic duct and the hepatic duct; its function is to store **bile**, and its capacity in humans is 30–50 cm^3; the liver secretes bile continuously, but the bile only enters the duodenum during periods of digestion, otherwise the liquid is stored in the gall bladder; the walls are contractile and empty the **gall bladder** when food, especially fat, passes through the duodenum; the contractions are probably activated by a hormone secreted by the intestinal walls.

gallstone (biliary calculus): a calculus, or hard stone, formed in the **gall bladder** or a **bile duct**; it contains cholesterol crystals combined with other substances (e.g., calcium salts); the different types of stones are called porcinement, cholesterol, etc.

gastric juice: a secretion from **glands** in the **stomach** wall that contains hydrochloric acid (0.2–0.5%) and digestive **enzymes** (e.g., pepsin), and in young mammals only, rennin.

gastrointestinal (GI): related to the GI tract, also called the digestive tract, alimentary canal, or gut, is the system of organs that takes in food, digests it to extract energy and nutrients, and expels the remaining waste.

gel: an intermediate stage in the **coagulation** of a sol; a mass of intertwining filaments enclose the whole of the dispersion medium to produce a pseudo-solid; a gel is jellylike in appearance and forms a distortable mass.

gelatin: many substances that form lyophilic sols can be obtained in a jellylike condition; the process is called "gelation"; e.g., gelatin mixed with water forms a colloidal solution; when cooled, this becomes a semisolid.

gingival: pertaining to gingiva, or gums, consist of the mucosal tissue that lays over the jawbone; the gingiva are naturally transparent, they are rendered red in color because of the blood flowing through tissue; the gingiva are connected to the teeth and **bone** by way of the periodontal fibers.

gland: an organ manufacturing substances for secretion; it may be large (e.g., the **liver** or **mammary gland**), or it may be small (e.g., a sweat gland); it functions by taking chemical substances and water from the **blood** and synthesizing the compounds for secretion; glands are either exocrine or endocrine, and their methods of secretion are either holocrine, merocrine, or apocrine; they are also described by their shape (e.g., tubular, racemose, flask-shaped).

glandular tissue: a tissue-bearing **gland**.

glaucoma: a disease of the eye characterized by increased pressure within the **eyeball** and a progressive loss of vision.

glioma: a **tumor** of the **brain** arising from and consisting of **neuroglia**.

globulin: one of the two types of **serum proteins**, the other being **albumin**; this generic term encompasses a heterogeneous series of protein families that have larger molecules, are less soluble in pure water, and migrate less during serum electrophoresis than albumin.

α-globulins: a group of globular **proteins** in **blood plasma**, that are highly mobile in alkaline or electrically charged solutions; they inhibit certain blood protease and inhibitor activity.

β-globulins: a group of globular **proteins** in **blood plasma** that are less mobile in alkaline or electricaly charged solutions than α-**globulins**.

glucose: a sugar, $C_6H_{12}O_6$, that have several optically different forms; the common or dextrorotatory form (dextroglucose or D-glucose) occurs in many fruits, animal tissues, and fluids, etc., and has a sweetness about one-half that of ordinary sugar; the levorotatory form (levoglucose or L-glucose) is rare and not naturally occurring; also called "starch syrup," a syrup containing dextrose, maltose, and dextrine, obtained by the incomplete hydrolysis of starch.

glucose clamp experiment: **blood sugar** monitoring at basal (euglycemic) or elevated (hyperglycemic) levels during variable **insulin infusion**; it measures tissue-specific insulin action and **glucose metabolism**.

glucose tolerance test: the **administration** of **glucose** to determine how quickly it is cleared from the **blood**; used to test for **diabetes**, **insulin** resistance, and sometimes reactive hypoglycemia; the glucose is most often given orally so the common test is technically an **oral glucose tolerance test (OGTT)**.

glycation: the result of a **sugar** molecule, such as **glucose**, bonding to a **protein** or **lipid** molecule without the controlling action of an **enzyme**; glycation may occur either inside the body (**endogenous** glycation) or outside the body (**exogenous** glycation); enzyme-controlled addition of sugars to protein or lipid molecules is termed glycosylation; glycation is a haphazard process that impairs the function of biomolecules, while glycosylation occurs at defined sites on the target molecule and is required in order for the molecule to function.

glycerol (glycerin, glycerine): a colorless, odorless, syrupy, sweet liquid (see **alcohol**) usually obtained by the saponification of natural **fats** and **oils**; used in the manufacture of **cosmetics**, perfumes, inks, and certain glues and cements; it also acts as a solvent; and in medicine in suppositories and **skin** emollients.

glycogen: a polysaccharide that is the principal storage form of **glucose** in animal **cells**; it is found in the form of granules in the **cytosol** in many cell types, and plays an important role in the glucose cycle; it forms an energy reserve that can be quickly mobilized to meet a sudden need for glucose, but one that is less compact than the energy reserves of **triglycerides**.

glyco-lipid: any of the class of lipids that comprise the cerebrosides and gangliosides, that upon hydrolysis yield galactose or a similar sugar, a **fatty acid**, and sphingosine or dihydrosphingosine.

Golgi apparatus (complex): a netlike mass of material in the **cytoplasm** of animal **cells** believed to function in cellular secretion.

grandular: pertaining to **tissue** structures that contain granular inclusions; for example, grandular-cystic **hyperplasia**, grandular **tumor**, grandular-**squamous-cell carcinoma**.

gray matter: a **nervous tissue** found in the central nervous system; it contains numerous **cell** bodies (cytons), dendrites, synapses, terminal processes of axons, **blood vessels** and **neuroglia**; it is internal to **white matter** in the spinal cord and some other parts of the **brain**; it is external to white matter in the cerebral hemisphere and in the **cerebellum**; coordination in the central nervous system is effected in gray matter; brain nuclei and nerve centers are composed of gray matter.

green fluorescent protein (GFP): a **protein**, comprised of 238 **amino acids** (27 kDa), from the jellyfish *Aequorea victoria* that fluoresces green when exposed to blue light; GFP has a unique cylindrical shape consisting of an 11-strand β-barrel with a single alpha helical strand containing the **chromophore** that runs through the center; this barrel permits chromophore formation and protects it from quenching by the surrounding microenvironment; in cell and molecular biology, the GFP gene is frequently used as a reporter of expression; in modified forms it has been used to make biosensors.

ground substance: the homogeneous matrix in which the **fibers** and **cells** of **connective tissue** or other particles are embedded.

gyaluronic acid: natural **moisturizing** component in **tissues**; the quantity of gyaluronic acid in an organism decreases with growing older.

hair: a threadlike outgrowth from the **skin**; each hair is a slender rod composed of dead cells strengthened by keratin, but remaining soft and supple; it grows from a hair follicle and its length varies according to species and the part of the body on which it is growing; a follicle surrounds the hair root and **hair shaft**; it penetrates deep into the **dermis**.

hair follicle: a part of the **skin** that grows hair by packing old cells together; attached to the follicle is a **sebaceous gland**.

hair shaft: a mature hair shaft is nonliving biological fiber; it is composed of a central pith (or medulla), surrounded by a more solid cortex, and is enclosed in a thin, hard, cuticle; inside the hair follicle it is surrounded by the inner and outer root sheaths.

hand: is one of the two intricate, prehensile, multifingered body parts normally located at the end of each arm (medically: "terminating each anterior limb/appendage") of a human or other primate.

head: a part of body that comprises the **brain**, eyes, ears, nose, and mouth (all of which aid in various sensory functions, such as sight, hearing, smell, and taste).

heart: a hollow, muscular organ by which rhythmic contractions and relaxations keeps the blood in circulation throughout the body.

heart beats: contractions of the heart; usually the heart rate that describes the frequency of the cardiac cycle, calculated as the number of heart beats in one minute and expressed as "beats per minute" (bpm); the heart beats up to 120 times per minute in childhood; when resting, the adult human heart beats at about 70 bpm (males) and 75 bpm (females).

heart valve leaflet: valves in the **heart** maintain the unidirectional flow of **blood** by opening and closing, depending on the difference in pressure on each side; the mitral valve is the heart valve that prevents the backflow of blood from the left ventricle into the left **atrium**; it is composed of two leaflets (one anterior, one posterior) that close when the left ventricle contracts; each leaflet is composed of three layers of **tissue**: the atrialis, fibrosa, and spongiosa.

hemangioma: a native abnormality caused by proliferation of **endothelial cells**; formed aggregates consisting chiefly of dilated or newly formed **blood vessels** that look like **tumors**; types are capillary hemangioma, **cavernous hemangioma**, senile hemangioma, and verrucous hemangioma.

hematocrit (Hct): the relative volume of the **red blood cells** in a **blood** sample expressed in percentages.

hematoporphyrin: a complex mixture of monomeric and aggregated **porphyrins** used in the **photodynamic therapy** of **tumors**; a purified component of this mixture is known as dihematoporphyrin **ether**.

hematoporphyrin derivative (HPD): a **photosensitizer** with an excitation band around 620 nm; used in **cancer** diagnostics and **photodynamic therapy**.

heme: an iron-containing substance; the basic unit of the **hemoglobin** molecule; mammals have four heme units in their hemoglobin.

hemodynamics: the physiology branch dealing with the forces involved in the circulation of **blood**.

hemoglobin: a red iron-containing respiratory pigment found in the **blood**; it conveys oxygen to the tissues and occurs in reduced form (**deoxyhemoglobin**) in venous blood and in combination with oxygen (**oxyhemoglobin**) in arterial blood; it consists of **heme** combined with globin, a blood protein; it is chemically related to chlorophyll, **cytochrome**, hemocyanin, and **myoglobin** (see **hemoglobin spectrum**, Glossary 1).

hemolysis: the breaking open of **red blood cells** and the release of **hemoglobin** into the surrounding fluid (**plasma**, *in vivo*).

hemolytic disease: hemolytic disease of the newborn is an alloimmune condition that develops in a fetus, when the IgG antibodies that have been produced by the mother and have passed through the placenta, including ones that attack the **red blood cells** in the fetal circulation; the red cells are broken down and the fetus can develop reticulocytosis and anemia; **hemolysis** leads to elevated **bilirubin** levels; after delivery bilirubin is no longer cleared (via the placenta) from the neonate's **blood** and the symptoms of yellowish skin and yellow discoloration of the whites of the eyes increase within 24 hours after birth.

hemorheological status: the status determined on the basis of **blood** rheology parameters, such as whole blood and plasma viscosity, cell transit time, cell deformability, clogging rate, clogging particle changes.

hemorrhage: a discharge of **blood**, as from ruptured **blood vessels**.

histology: the study of **tissue** sectioned as a thin slice, using a microtome; it can be described as microscopic anatomy.

H_2O_2: hydrogen peroxide is a very pale blue liquid that appears colorless in a dilute solution, slightly more viscous than water; it is a weak acid; it has strong oxidizing properties and is therefore a powerful bleaching agent that has found use as a disinfectant.

homologous series: in chemistry, this is a series of organic compounds with a similar general formula, possessing similar chemical properties due to the presence of the same functional group, and shows a gradation in physical properties as a result of increase in molecular size and mass.

horny-skin layer: the same as **stratum corneum**.

human epidermal membrane (HEM): a skin flap containing epidermis and used to perform *in vitro* permeability experiments under varied experimental conditions for different deliverable agents and drugs; two-chamber diffusion cells are typically used.

human papilloma virus (HPV): a diverse group of **DNA**-based viruses that infect the **skin** and **mucous membranes** of humans and a variety of animals; more than 100 different HPV types have been characterized; some HPV types cause benign skin warts, or papillomas, for which the virus family is named; HPVs associated with the development of such "common warts" are transmitted environmentally or by casual skin-to-skin contact.

humidity: see Glossary 1.

hydration: the absorption of water by tissues and cells; the organic hydration reaction, a reaction in which water is added across a double bond; mineral (component of tooth or **bone** tissue) hydration, a reaction in which water is combined into the crystalline structure of a mineral.

hydraulic conductivity: a property of material that describes the ease with which water can move through pore spaces or fractures; it depends on the intrinsic permeability of the material and on the degree of saturation; saturated hydraulic conductivity describes water movement through saturated media.

hydrocephalus: an abnormal increase in the amount of **cerebospinal fluid (CSF)**.

hydrocortisone: a corticosteroid that is similar to a natural hormone produced by adrenal **glands**.

hydrophilic: that which has an affinity with water.

hydrophobic: that which has little or no affinity with water.

α-hydroxy acids (AHAs): such as glycolic, lactic, or fruit acids are the mildest of the peel formulas and produce light peels.

hydroxyapatite (HAP): see **apatite**.

hydroxyethyl cellulose: is a nonionic, water-soluble polymer that can thicken, suspend, bind, emulsify, and form films.

3-hydroxy-L-kynurenine-0-β-glucoside (3-HKG): an important age-related chromophore of the human-eye lens, protecting it from UVA radiation.

hygroscopic: the ability of a substance to attract water molecules from the surrounding environment through either absorption or adsorption; hygroscopic substances include **glycerol**, **ethanol**, methanol, concentrated sulfuric acid, and concentrated sodium hydroxide; calcium chloride is so hygroscopic that it eventually dissolves in the water it absorbs.

hypaque: a commonly used x-ray contrast medium; as diatrizoate meglumine and as diatrizoate sodium, it is used for gastrointestinal studies, angiography, and urography.

hyperchromaticity: the increase in optical density of **DNA** molecules in solution, which increase upon nuclease digestion due to the release of nucleotides that absorb more UV light; such a chromic shift is also seen during the process of denaturation due to temperature of DNA separation.

hyperdermal: refers exclusively to the skin, when, for instance, intradermal injection is provided; see **cutaneous**.

hyperglycemia: a condition in which an excessive amount of **glucose** circulates in the **blood plasma**; it is primarily a symptom of **diabetes** in which there are elevated levels of blood sugar, or glucose, in the bloodstream; in type I diabetes, hyperglycemia results from malfunctioning in the supply of insulin, the chemical that enables cells to receive energy from glucose; type II diabetes is due to a combination of defective insulin secretion and defective responsiveness to insulin, often termed "reduced insulin sensitivity."

hyperinsulinemic-hypoglycemic clamp: a procedure that suppresses endogenous insulin secretion by hyperinsulinemia- and hypoglycemia-mediated feedback inhibition of beta-cells.

hyperosmotic: see Glossary 1.

hyperplasia: the enlargement of a part due to an abnormal increase in the number of its **cells**.

hyperthermia: an acute condition that occurs when the body produces or absorbs more heat than it can dissipate; it is usually due to excessive exposure to heat; it can be created artificially by drugs or medical devices (based on acoustics, microwaves, light, etc.), in these instances it may be used to treat cancer and other conditions.

hypertonic: a solution that has a higher concentration of solutes than that in a cell is said to be hypertonic; this solution has more solute particles and, therefore, relatively less water than the cell contents.

hypodermic: situated or lying under the **skin**, as **a tissue**; performed or introduced under the skin, e.g., injection by a syringe, etc.

hypoosmotic: describes a cell or other membrane-bound object that has a lower concentration of solutes than its surroundings; for example, a cell in a high-salt-concentration medium is hypoosmotic; water is more likely to move out of the cell by osmosis as a result; this is the opposite of **hyperosmotic**.

hypothesis of Roy and Sherrington: the hypothesis widely accepted to account for the phenomenon of increased neuronal metabolic activity giving rise to the accumulation of vasoactive catabolites, which decrease vascular resistance and thereby increase blood flow until normal homeostasis is reestablished.

hypotonic: conditions or bathing media owing to the osmotic flow of water into the **cell cytoplasm**.

hypoxia: lack of **oxygen** in air, **blood**, or **tissue**.

hysterectomy: the excision of the **uterus**.

immobilize: to deprive mobility.

implant: a material grafted (implanted) or introduced into a **tissue**.

incision: a surgical cut of a **tissue**; the separation of soft tissues using a scalpel.

India ink: used in preparation of phantoms as an absorbing medium.

indocyanine green: a tricarbocyanine type of dye (stain) having a high absorption in NIR (800 nm) and little or no absorption in the visible range; it is used in diagnostics for **blood volume** determination, **hemodynamic**, cardiac output, or hepatic function studies.

infiltrate: to perform infiltration, i.e., to penetrate a cell or tissue with a substance; also refers to the substance infiltrated.

infiltrating: the process of percolation and impregnation of material, cell or tissue by gas, liquid, or solution; also related to **cell** migration; examples: adipose infiltration-appearance of **fat** cells in the places where they are normally absent, calcareous infiltration—see **calcification**, fatty infiltration—a pathological storage of fat drops in cell **cytoplasm**.

inflammation: traditionally Western medicine has recognized the four signs of inflammation as *tumor, rubor, calor, and dolor*—swelling, redness, heat, and pain; besides these physical changes, there are also important psychological ones, including lethargy, apathy, loss of appetite and increasing sensitivity to pain; in response to acute damage or entrance of foreign material, monocytes enlarge and synthesis increases the amount of **enzymes** that help to break down the material; in doing so they are transformed to more active **phagocytes** called **macrophages**; http://freespace.virgin.net/ahcare.qua/index4.html.

Infracyanine25 (IC25): an NIR contrasting agent (see **indocyanine green**).

infusion: the administration of a drug parenterally by the intravenous route, **subcutaneous** or intramuscle injection.

injury: tissue damage, **wound**, **trauma**.

in situ: pertaining to experiments on an object in its original place.

insulin: a polypeptide hormone that regulates **carbohydrate metabolism**; it is produced in the islets of Langerhans in the pancreas; it has effects on fat metabolism and it changes the **liver's** activity in storing or releasing **glucose** and in processing **blood lipids**, and in other **tissues** such as **fat** and **muscle**; insulin is used medically to treat some forms of **diabetes mellitus**.

intact: not changed or diminished; not influenced or swayed.

intercellular: between **cells**, as in an intercellular bridge.

interferons (IFNs): the natural **proteins** produced by the **cells** of the immune system of most vertebrates in response to challenges by foreign agents such as viruses, **bacteria**, parasites, and **tumor** cells; they belong to the large class of glycoproteins known as cytokines and assist the immune response by inhibiting viral replication within other cells of the body.

interfibrillar spacing: the spacing between fibrils.

intermolecular spacing: the spacing between molecules.

interstitial fluid: a solution that bathes and surrounds the **cells** of multicellular animals; it is the main component of the **extracellular** fluid, which also includes **plasma** and transcellular fluid; on average, a subject has about 11 liters of interstitial fluid, providing the cells of the body with nutrients and a means of waste removal.

interstitial space: space where **interstitial fluid** is circulating.

intestine: a part of the alimentary canal, in the shape of a long tube, which is concerned with the digestion and absorption of nutrients and the reabsorption of water from feces; most of the digestion and almost all the absorption takes place in the intestine; the internal surface area of the intestine is increased by folds in the lining and projections on the lining; the intestine is coiled in the abdominal cavity; its length is greater than the length of the body; the anterior part of the intestine that contains **glands** for secreting digestive **enzymes** and receives **ducts** from the large digestive glands.

intima: the innermost **membrane** or lining of some organ or part, especially that of an **artery**, **vein**, or **lymphatic vessel**.

intracellular fluid: see **cytoplasm**.

intracellular motility: the motility of **cytoplasm** components.

intralipid, nutralipid, liposyn: intravenously administered nutrients that are fat emulsions containing soybean oil, egg **phospholipids**, and **glycerol**.

invasive: characterized by invasion; denoting: (1) a procedure that requires insertion of an instrument or device into the body through the **skin** or a body orifice for diagnosis or treatment, (2) a diffusion of **malignant tumor** by its growing into or destruction of the adjacent tissue, (3) spread of infection.

in vitro: in medicine, pertaining to experiments on dead tissue.

in vivo: in medicine, pertaining to experiments on living animals and humans.

ionic strength: characterizes a solution, the concentration of all ions present in a solution; generally multivalent ions contribute strongly to the ionic strength.

iontophoresis: a **noninvasive method** of propelling high concentrations of a charged substance, normally medication or bioactive-agents, transdermally by repulsive electromotive force using a small electrical charge applied to an iontophoretic chamber that contains a similarly charged active agent and its **vehicle**; one or two chambers are filled with a solution that contains an active ingredient and its solvent, termed the vehicle; the positively charged chamber, termed the anode will repel a positively charged chemical, while the negatively charged chamber, termed the cathode, will repel a negatively charged chemical into the skin.

iris: the thin, circular, colored sheet of muscular tissue at the front of the **eyeball**, forming the colored part of the eye; the central opening, the **pupil**, allows light to enter the **eyeball**; the iris controls the amount of light that enters the eyeball and assists in accommodating for near objects.

irritation: the enhanced **inflammatory** reaction of **tissue** on its **injury**.

ischemia: a restriction in **blood** supply, generally due to factors in the blood **vessels**, with resultant damage or dysfunction of **tissue**.

isoosmotic: pertaining to solutions that exert the same **osmotic pressure**.

isopropyl laurate: a synthetic compound derived from **fatty acids**; emollient, **moisturizer**.

isopropyl myristate: $C_{17}H_{34}O_2$; refractive index $n_D = 1.435–1.438$ at 20°C; used in **cosmetic** and **topical** medicinal preparations where good absorption through the **skin** is desired; binding agent, emollient, **moisturizer**, and solvent.

isopropyl palmitate: an ester of palmitic acid from coconut oil used to impart silkiness to the **skin** and **hair**; a synthetic antistatic agent, binding agent, emollient, **moisturizer**, and solvent.

isotonic: (1) noting or pertaining to solutions characterized by equal **osmotic pressure**; (2) noting or pertaining to a solution containing just enough salt to prevent the destruction of the **erythrocytes** when added to the **blood**.

keloid: a kind of **fibrous tumor** that forms hard, irregular, clawlike excrescences upon the **skin**, especially postburn.

keratin: a family of **fibrous** structural proteins; tough and insoluble, they form the hard but nonmineralized structures found in animals and other living objects.

keratinocyte: the principal cell type of **epidermis**; so named because of the family of filamentous proteins, the keratins, that comprise its distinctive **cytoskeleton**.

keratectomy: the **incision** of part of the **cornea**.

keratotomy: the **incision** of the **cornea**.

kidney: either of a pair of bean-shaped glandular organs in the back part of the abdominal cavity that excrete urine; a kidney contains numerous nephrons and their associated blood supply; it consists of two zones, a cortex and **medulla**, encased in a fatty protective capsule.

knee: the lower extremity joint that connects the femur and the tibia; since in humans the knee supports nearly the entire weight of the body, it is vulnerable both to acute **injury** and to the development of osteoarthritis.

labeling: the specific marking of **cells** or cell compartments to track probes and measure functional parameters from molecular- and cellular-based studies to *in vivo* systems to understand how marked components impact human physiology and disease; for instance, in cellular transplantation technology, labeling provides information about location, tracking, and quantifying of implanted cells in *in vivo* systems; a wide variety of labeling probes and systems are available; they are mostly based on fluorescing molecules and **nanoparticles** with a possibility of specific binding to cell and **tissue** compartments; CW and time-resolved **fluorescence** techniques are typically used to monitor these markers.

lamella: a platelike structure, appearing in multiples, that occurs in various situations, such as biology (**connective tissue** structures) or materials sciences.

lamina fusca: the layer of the eye **sclera**.

lamina propia: a thin vascular layer of **areolar connective tissue** beneath the **epithelium** and is part of the **mucous membrane**.

Langer's skin tension lines: the local **skin** tension directed lines caused by bundles of fibroconnective **tissues** within the *reticular dermis*.

larynx: a muscular and cartilaginous structure lined with **mucous membrane** at the upper part of the trachea, in which the **vocal cords** are located.

laser coagulation: a **coagulation** of **tissue** caused by laser heating.

laser cyclophotocoagulation: see **cyclophotocoagulation**.

laser interferential retinometer: see Glossary 1.

laser refractive surgery: a special laser (typically UV **excimer laser**, see Glossary 1) reshapes the **cornea** by the precise and controled removal of corneal **tissue** and therefore changes corneal focusing power.

lecithin: technical lecithin contains 60% natural **phospholipids** (major phosphatidylcholine), 30–35% plant oil, glycerol, et al.; it is a basis for many **nourishing (nutritive) creams** due to its ability to penetrate deep into the **skin**.

lens: see **crystalline lens**.

lens syneresis: water is released from the bound state in the hydration layers of lens proteins and becomes bulk water; this increases the difference in refractive index between the lens proteins and the surrounding fluid.

lesion: an **injury** or an alteration of an organ or **tissue**.

leukoplakia: a condition in which thickened, white patches form on a subject's gums, on the inside of his/her cheeks and sometimes on his/her tongue; these patches can't easily be scraped off; the cause of leukoplakia is unknown, but it's considered to result from chronic **irritation**, caused by tobacco or long-term alcohol use; it is the most common of all chronic mouth lesions, more frequently appears in older men.

ligament: a band of **tissue**, usually white and **fibrous**, serving to connect **bones**, hold organs in place, etc.

limbus: the border, edge, or fringe of a part.

lipid: any substance occurring in plants or animals that is soluble in **ether**, hot **ethanol**, and gasoline (i.e., **fat** solvents); the term includes true **fats**, waxes, sterols, steroids, **phospholipids**, etc.

lipid bilayer or **bilayer lipid membrane**: a membrane or zone of a membrane composed of lipid molecules (usually **phospholipids**); the lipid bilayer is a critical component of all biological membranes, including **cell** membranes; the structure of a bilayer explains its function as a barrier; lipids are **amphiphilic** molecules since they consist of polar head groups and nonpolar **acyl** tails; the bilayer is composed of two opposing layers of lipid molecules arranged so that their hydrocarbon tails face one another to form an oily core, while their charged heads face the aqueous solutions on either side of the membrane; thus, the bilayer consists of the **hydrophobic** core region formed by the acyl chains of the lipids, and membrane interfacial regions that are formed by the polar head groups of lipids; the **hydrophilic** interfacial regions are saturated with water, whereas the hydrophobic core region contains almost no water; because of the oily core, a pure lipid bilayer is permeable only to small hydrophobic solutes, but has a very low permeability to polar inorganic compounds and ionic molecules.

lipophilic: that which has affinity with **lipids**.

liposomes: microscopic spherical vesicles prepared by adding a water solution to a **phospholipid** gel; a liposome is a good model of a cell **organelle**; liposome diameters are usually in the range of 20–100 nm; they are used for drug delivery in medicine and **cosmetics**.

lips: a visible organ at the mouth of humans and many animals; both lips are soft, protruding, movable, and serve primarily for food intake, as a tactile sensory organ, and in articulation of speech.

liquid-crystalline phase: a liquid that has certain crystalline characteristics, especially different optical properties in different directions.

liver: a large, reddish-brown, glandular organ located in the upper right side of the abdominal cavity, divided by fissures into five lobes, and functioning in the secretion of **bile** and various **metabolic** processes.

lobe (cerebral lobe): each cerebral hemisphere is divided, more or less arbitrarily, into different regions, each region being a lobe; the deeper fissures are used to distinguish the lobes; each lobe is named from the part of the **skull** near which it is situated; they are terms of convenience, not of anatomical or physiological significance: frontal lobe, temporal lobe, occipital lobe, etc.

lung: either of the two saclike respiratory organs in the **thorax** of humans; the lungs connect to the larynx via trachea, bronchi, and ramifications of bronchial tubes.

lymph: an alkaline colorless liquid obtained from **blood** by filtration through **capillary** walls; it contains a smaller amount of soluble blood proteins and **white blood cells** than blood, but more **lymphocytes**; it contains no **red blood cells**.

lymph nodes (lymphoid tissues): the tissues that produce **lymphocytes** by division of some **cells**; they are found in lymph **glands**, which are formed from a network of **reticular fibers** that enclose **lymphocytes**, lymphoblasts, and **macrophages**; they also occur in the **spleen**, tonsils, and thymus.

lymphatic (lymph) vessels: the thin-walled tubular vessels resembling **veins** in structure but with thinner walls and more valves; the walls are enclosed by smooth **muscle** and **connective tissue**; lymph vessels drain into lymph **ducts**; lymph vessels act as channels along which pathogens are conducted from infected areas of the body, the pathogens being unable to enter the **blood capillaries**; **lymph nodes** are distributed along the lymph vessels; the lymph flow is maintained by peristaltic contractility of the lymph vessels, aided by the squeezing of the vessels by skeletal muscles, with the **valves** maintaining a flow in one direction only.

lymphocyte: a spherical **white blood cell** with one large nucleus and relatively little **cytoplasm**; two types exist, small and large lymphocytes; they are produced continually in **lymphoid tissues**, such as **lymph nodes**, by cell division; the cells are nonphagocytic, exhibit amoeboid movement, and produce antibodies in the **blood**; they constitute about 25% of all leukocytes in the human body.

lymphotropic agent: an agent that influences the functioning of **lymph vessels**.

lyophilized: related to **tissues**, **blood**, **serum**, or other biological substances that are dried by freezing in a high vacuum; the samples preserved to prevent decay, spoilage, and prepared for future use.

lysed blood: the product of **blood** at its **hemolysis**.

lysosomes: the membrane-bound particles that are smaller than **mitochondrion**, occurring in large numbers in the **cytoplasm** of **cells**; they contain hydrolytic **enzymes** that are released when the cell is damaged; these enzymes assist in the digestion and removal of dead cells, the digestion of food and other substances, and the destruction of redundant **organelles**.

macromolecules: pertaining to conventional polymers and biopolymers (such as **DNA**) as well as nonpolymeric molecules with large molecular mass such as **lipids** or macrocycles.

macrophage: a large phagocytic **cell** with one nucleus; movement is by membranelike pseudopodia; these cells are found in contact with **blood** and **lymph** at the sites of corpuscle formation (e.g., in **bone** marrow, **lymph nodes**, and **spleen**); their function is to remove foreign particles from blood and lymph; macrophages are also found in all loose **connective tissue**, but they only become active when the tissue is damaged; their function is to remove the debris from damaged tissues; they form the reticuloendothelial system; in the inactive state (i.e., in undamaged tissue), the resting form of the cell is called a "histiocyte"; macrophages are closely related to **monocytes**.

magnetic resonance imaging (MRI): see Glossary 1, **magnetic resonance imaging**.

malignant: a clinical term that means to be severe and become progressively worse, as in malignant hypertension; in the context of **cancer**, a malignant **tumor** can invade and destroy nearby tissue and may also spread (metastasize) to other parts of the body.

malignant tissue: an abnormally growing **tissue** that has the tendency to spread to other parts of the body, even when the original growth is removed by surgery; eventually it causes death.

mammary gland: a large **gland** on the ventral surface of the mature female; it is thought to be a modified sweat gland; it consists of clusters of gland cells that can extract the necessary substances from **blood** to produce milk; the milk drains through **ducts** into a cistern; a canal leads from the cistern to a mammary papilla; the growth and activity of the gland is under the control of gonadal hormones and the state of the gland is influenced by the estrous cycle; milk production is stimulated by the pituitary lactogenic hormone.

mammography: x-ray **imaging**, **magnetic resonance imaging (MRI)**, **ultrasound (US)**, and positron-emission imaging of a **female breast**, especially for screening or early detection of **cancer**.

mammogram: an image of a **female breast** obtained by **mammography**.

mannitol (or hexan-1,2,3,4,5,6-hexol [$C_6H_8(OH_6)$]): an osmotic diuretic agent and a weak renal vasodilator; it is a sorbitol isomer; it is used clinically to reduce acutely raised intracranial pressure.

mastopathy: any disease of the **female breast**.

meal tolerance test (MTT): the complete nutrient test (**carbohydrate**, **fat**, and **protein** containing meals) that induces both **glucose** and **insulin** responses; the MTT is a more potent insulin stimulator than glucose alone (see **OGTT**).

media: the middle layer of an **artery** or **lymphatic vessel** wall.

mediolateral projection: the medial and lateral planes of the body.

medulla: the inner, paler-colored region of a **kidney**, surrounded by the cortex; it contains the collecting tubules leading from the uriniferous tubules to the pyramid.

medulloblastomas: most **brain tumors** are named after the type of cells from which they develop; medulloblastomas are **malignant** tumors formed from poorly developed cells at a very early stage of their life; they develop in the **cerebellum**, in a part of the brain called the posterior fossa, but may spread to other parts of the brain; very rarely, medulloblastomas may spread to other parts of the body; if they do spread to other parts of the brain, or to the spinal cord, this is usually through the **cerebrospinal fluid (CSF)**; they are more common in children.

melanin: a dark-brown or black pigment; melanin in **melanosomes** of normal **skin** is an extremely dense, virtually insoluble polymer of high molecular weight and is always attached to a structural protein; mammalian melanin pigments have one of two chemical compositions: eumelanin, a brown polymer, and pheomelanin, a yellow-reddish alkali-soluble pigment.

melanin granular (melanosome): the cytoplasmic **organelles** on which melanin pigments are synthesized and deposited; normal human skin color is primarily related to the size, type, color, and distribution of melanosomes; melanosomes are the product of specialized exocrine glands: **melanocytes**.

melanocytes: the components of the **melanin** pigmentary system, which is made up of melanocytes distributed in various sites: the eye (retinal pigment **epithelium**, uveal tract), the ear (in the stria vascularis), the central nervous system (in leptomeninges), the hair (in the hair matrix), the **mucous membranes**, and the **skin** (at the dermal-epidermal interface, where they rest on the basement membrane); in the skin melanocytes project their dendrites into the **epidermis**, where they transfer melanosomes to **keratinocytes**.

melanoma: a darkly pigmented **tumor**, especially of the **skin** or eye, of **cells** containing **melanin**.

melanoma maligna: a special kind of **melanoma** *in situ* that occurs on the sun damaged **skin** of the face or neck may be described as lentigo maligna **melanoma**.

membrane: (1) a very thin layer of **connective tissue** covering an organ: (2) connective tissue that divides **cells**; (3) a thin layer of cells.

meningiomas: the most common **benign tumors** of the **brain** (95% of benign tumors); however, they can also be **malignant**; they arise from the arachnoidal cap cells of the meninges and represent about 15% of all primary brain tumors; they are more common in females than in males (2:1) and has a peak incidence in the sixth and seventh decades.

meniscus: a disk of **cartilage** between the articulating ends of the **bones** in a joint.

mesentery: (1) sheets of thin **connective tissue** by which the **stomach** and **intestines** are suspended from the dorsal wall of the abdominal cavity; (2) the **tissue** supporting the intestines; the mesenteries carry **blood, lymph vessels**, and **nerves** to the organs of the alimentary canal.

metabolism (metabolic processes): the chemical processes that take place in a living organism or within part of a living organism (e.g., **cell**) are collectively known as metabolism; metabolism consists of **catabolism** and **anabolism**.

metabolite: a substance that takes part in a **metabolic process**; those metabolites that the organism cannot manufacture have to be obtained from the environment; some metabolites are supplied partly by the environment and partly by the organism; the majority of the metabolites in an organism are manufactured by the organism.

methylene blue: a biological dye (stain) showing a phototoxic effect; its absorption bands are at 609 and 668 nm; it is used as a stain in bacteriology and as an oxidation-reduction indicator; it can be activated by light to an excited state, which in turn activates oxygen to yield oxidizing radicals, such radicals can cause **cross-linking** of **amino acid** residues on proteins and achieve some degree of cross-linking.

micelles: an aggregate of **surfactant** molecules dispersed in a liquid **colloid**; a typical micelle in aqueous solution forms an **aggregate** with the **hydrophilic** "head" regions in contact with surrounding solvent, sequestering the **hydrophobic** tail regions in the micelle center; this type of micelle is know as a normal phase micelle (oil-in-water micelle); inverse micelles have the headgroups at the center with the tails extending out (water-in-oil micelle); micelles are approximately spherical in shape; other phases, including shapes such as ellipsoids, cylinders, and bilayers are also possible; the shape and size of a micelle is a function of the molecular geometry of its surfactant molecules and solution conditions such as surfactant concentration, temperature, **pH**, and **ionic strength**; the process of forming micelles is known as micellization and forms part of the phase behaviour of many **lipids** according to their **polymorphism**.

microcirculation: the flow of **blood** from **arterioles** to capillaries or sinusoids to **venules**; blood flows freely between an arteriole and a venule through a vessel channel called a thoroughfare channel; capillaries extend from this channel to structures called precapillary sphincters, which control the flow of blood between the arteriole and capillaries; the precapillary sphincters contain **muscle** fibers that allow them to contract; when the sphincters are open, blood flows freely to the capillary beds, where gases and waste can be exchanged with body **tissue**; when the sphincters are closed, blood is not allowed to flow through the capillary beds and must flow directly from the arteriole to the venule through the thoroughfare channel; it is important to note that blood is supplied to all parts of the body at all times but all capillary beds do not contain blood at all times (http://biology.about.com/library/organs/heart/blmicrocirc.htm).

microfibril: a very fine **fibril**, or fiber like strand, consisting of glycoproteins; its most frequently observed structural pattern is $9+2$ in which two central protofibrils are surrounded by nine others; the cellulose inside plants is one of the examples of nonprotein compounds that are using this term with the same purpose.

microfilaments: the fine, threadlike protein fibers, 3–6 nm in diameter; they are composed predominantly of a contractile protein called actin, which is the most abundant cellular protein; microfilaments' association with the protein myosin is responsible for **muscle** contraction; microfilaments can also carry out cellular movements including gliding, contraction, and cytokinesis.

microtubules: cylindrical tubes, 20–25 nm in diameter; they are composed of subunits of the **protein** tubulin; they act as a scaffold to determine **cell** shape, and provide a set of "tracks" for cell **organelles** and vesicles to move on; microtubules also form the spindle fibers for separating chromosomes during **mitosis**; when arranged in geometric patterns inside **flagella** and cilia, they are used for locomotion.

microvessels: see **capillary**.

mineralization: the process where a substance is converted from an organic substance to an inorganic substance, thereby becoming mineralized.

mitochondrion (*pl.* mitochondria): a threadlike, or rodlike, granular **organelle** in the **cytoplasm** of **cells**, about 0.5 μm in width, and up to 10 μm in length for threadlike mitochondria; mitochondria are bounded by a double **membrane**; the inner membrane is folded inward at a number of places to form cristae; mitochondria contain phosphates and numerous **enzymes** that vary in different tissues; their function is cellular respiration and the release of chemical energy in the form of **ATP** for use in most of the cell's biological functions; the cells of all organisms, except bacteria and blue-green algae, contain mitochondria in varying numbers mitochondria are especially numerous in cells involved in significant metabolic activity, such as **liver** cells; mitochondria are self-replicating.

mitosis: the process by which a **cell** nucleus usually divides into two; the process takes place in four phases: prophase, metaphase, anaphase, and telophase; the daughter nuclei are genetically identical to each other and to the parent nucleus.

modified amino resin (MAR): material used in preparation of tissue **phantoms** (see Glossary 1).

monocyte: a spherical **white blood cell** with an oval nucleus; monocytes are the largest of the white blood cells; the cells are voraciously phagocytic and exhibit amoeboid movement; they are produced in **lymphoid tissues** and constitute about 5% of all leukocytes.

moisturizers: complex mixtures of chemical agents specially designed to make the external layers of the **skin** (**epidermis**) softer and more pliable, by increasing its **hydration**; naturally occurring skin lipids and sterols as well as artificial or natural **oils**, humectants, emollients, lubricants, etc., may be part of the composition of commercial skin moisturizers; they usually are available as commercial products for **cosmetic** and therapeutic uses.

molar mass: the mass of one mole of a chemical element or chemical compound.

monomer (**monomeric form**): the original compound from which a polymer is formed, e.g., ethylene is the monomer from which polyethylene is formed.

mononucleotide (**nucleotide**): a unit in a long-chain molecule of **nucleic acid**; it is a chemical compound formed from one molecule of a sugar (ribose or deoxyribose), one molecule of phosphoric acid, and one molecule of a base (containing an amino group); nucleotides are also found free in **cells** (see **DNA**).

monounsaturated fatty acid: a **fatty acid** with one double-bonded carbon in the molecule, with all of the others single-bonded carbons, in contrast to polyunsaturated fatty acids, which have more than one double bond.

mucin: a mucoprotein that forms **mucus** in solution.

mucinous: pertaining to or containing **mucin**.

mucopolysaccharides (or glycosaminoglycans): are long unbranched polysaccharides that consist of a repeating disaccharide unit; they are synthesized in **endoplasmic reticulum** and **Golgi apparatus**; they form an important component of **connective tissues**; their chains may be covalently linked to a **protein** to form **proteoglycans**.

mucous membrane (**mucosa**): a **membrane** consisting of moist **epithelium** and the **connective tissue** immediately beneath it; it usually consists of simple epithelium, but is stratified near openings to the exterior; it is often ciliated and often contains goblet **cells**; mucosa is found in the lining of the gut and in the urinogenital **ducts**.

mucus: a thin, slimy, viscous liquid secreted by epithelial **cells** in **tissues** or **glands**; it protects and lubricates the surface of structures, e.g., the internal surfaces of the greater part of the alimentary canal are lubricated with mucus.

muscle: an organ of movement which is highly contractile, extensible and elastic; it is composed of **muscular tissue**; a muscle contracts and relaxes; it can also be stretched beyond its normal length, and return to its original length and shape when the stretching force is removed.

muscular tissue: a **tissue** characterized by its ability to contract on being stimulated by a motor nerve; there are three main types of muscular tissue forming three types of muscle: skeletal, smooth, and cardiac.

myelin: an electrically insulating phospholipid layer that surrounds the axons of many neurons; it is an outgrowth of glial cells.

myocard (myocardium): the muscular substance of the **heart**.

myocardial infarction: commonly known as a heart attack, is a disease state that occurs when the blood supply to a part of the **heart** is interrupted; the resulting **ischemia** or **oxygen** shortage causes damage and potential death of heart tissue.

myofibrils: cylindrical **organelles**, found within **muscle cells**; they are bundles of filaments that run from one end of the cell to the other and are attached to the cell surface membrane at each end.

myofilaments: the filaments of **myofibrils** constructed from **proteins**; they consist of two types, thick and thin; thin filaments consist primarily of the protein actin; thick filaments consist primarily of the protein myosin; in striated **muscle**, such as skeletal and cardiac muscle, the actin and myosin filaments each have a specific and constant length.

myoglobin: a variety of **hemoglobin** found in voluntary **muscle fibers**; it has a higher affinity for oxygen than hemoglobin, and thus assists in the transfer of oxygen to **muscles**.

NAD, NAD+, NADH: NAD (nicotinamide adenine dinucleotide); an important **coenzyme** found in **cells**; it plays key roles as carriers of electrons in the transfer of reduction potential; cells produce NAD from niacin, and use it to transport electrons in redox reactions; during this process NAD picks up a pair of electrons and a proton and is thus reduced to NADH, releasing one proton (H^+): MH_2 + NAD+ $\rightarrow$ NADH + H^+ + M + energy, where M is a metabolite; two hydrogen atoms (a hydride ion and a proton H^+) are removed from the metabolite and the proton is released into solution; from the hydride electron pair, one electron is transferred to the positively-charged nitrogen, and one hydrogen attaches to the carbon atom opposite to the nitrogen; the reducing potential stored in NADH can be converted to **ATP** through the aerobic electron transport chain or used for anabolic **metabolism**; ATP is the universal energy currency of cells, and the contribution of NADH to the synthesis of ATP under aerobic conditions is substantial; however, under certain conditions (e.g., **hypoxia**) the aerobic regeneration of oxidized NAD+ is unable to meet the cell's immediate demand for ATP; in contrast, glycolysis does not require **oxygen**, but it does require the anaerobic regeneration of NAD+; the oxidation of NADH to NAD+ in the absence of oxygen is called fermentation.

nanospheres: the **fat** particles used for transportation of biologically active substances to the deep layers of **epidermis** and **hair** follicles.

neck: supports the weight of the **head** and protects the **nerves** that travel from the **brain** down to the rest of the body; the cervical portion of the human spine comprises seven bony segments, typically referred to as C-1 to C-7, with cartilaginous disks between each vertebral body; In addition, the neck is highly flexible and allows the head to turn and flex in all directions.

necrosis: the death or decay of **tissue**.

necrotic: pertaining to **necrosis**.

needle-free injection gun: a device creating the required pressure to ensure the medicine penetrates skin tissue directly without needle and correctly being distributed; traditional systems use compressed gas or a spring device to create the pressure that triggers the injection; a novel gas generator system that produces a few milliseconds-gas sparks with a predetermined pressure profile at the moment the injection is made.

neoplasia: (1) **tumor** growth; (2) the formation and growth of new **tissue**.

neoplasm: a new growth of different or abnormal **tissue**; **tumor**.

neoplastic: pertaining to **neoplasia**, **neoplasm**.

nerve: a bundle of parallel funiculi with associated **connective tissue** and **blood vessels**, enclosed in a sheath of connective tissue that forms a tough external coat called the "epineurium."

nervous tissue: **tissue** that consists of nerve cells and their fibers or of nerve fibers alone, together with accessory cells surrounding the **cells** or **fibers**, and **connective tissues** with **blood vessels**.

neurofibroma: a **tumor** that incorporates all sorts of **cells** and structural elements, **infiltrate** the **nerve** and splay apart the individual nerve fibers; although usually benign, they can sometimes degenerate into **cancer**; single neurofibromas often occur in middle and old age and grow at the margins of the peripheral nerves, displacing the nerve's main body; the vestibulocochlear (acoustic) nerve is the most commonly affected; other cranial nerves and spinal nerves are less commonly involved.

neuroglia: the delicate **connective tissue** elements of **nerve tissue** in the central nervous system.

neutral polymer: one that has no electrical charge or ionizable groups such as polyethylene oxide, cellulose, **sugar**, **dextrans**, polyvinyl alcohol, or polystyrene, there are many other examples; some neutral polymers are water soluble, others are not.

nevus: a general term that refers to a number of different, usually benign, pigmented lesions of the **skin**; most birthmarks and moles fall into the category of nevi.

nonionic: not converted into ions.

noninvasive method: a diagnostic method that avoids **trauma** to the **skin** or insertion of an instrument through a body orifice.

nourishing (nutritive) creams: used in **skin cosmetics** for preventing **transepidermal water loss (TEWL)**; they easy penetrate to the deep layers of **epidermis**; skin **hydration** can be provided by two mechanisms—**osmotic** or physiological; as the hydrating substances **sodium lactate**, **pyrrolidonecarboxylic acid**, derivatives of **amino acids** and **sugars**, **proteins**, **mucopolysaccharides** are usually used; as a **hygroscopic** component **glycerol** often use (usually less than 10% in composition), at present glycerol usually replaced by a **propylene glycol**.

nuclear envelope: the main structural elements of the **nucleus**; it is a double **membrane** that encloses the entire **organelle** and keeps its contents separated from the cellular **cytoplasm**.

nuclear pores: because the **nuclear envelope** is impermeable to most molecules, pores are required to allow movement of molecules across the envelope; these pores cross both membranes of the envelope, providing a channel that allows free movement of small molecules and ions; movement through the pores is required for both gene expression and chromosomal maintenance.

nucleic acid: a complex, high-molecular-weight biochemical **macromolecule** composed of nucleotide chains that convey genetic information; the most common nucleic acids are **DNA** and **RNA**; nucleic acids are found in all living **cells** and viruses.

nucleolus: a "sub-organelle" of the **cell nucleus**, which itself is an **organelle**; a main function of the nucleolus is the production and assembly of ribosome components; the nucleolus is roughly spherical, and is surrounded by a layer of condensed **chromatin**; no **membrane** separates the nucleolus from the nucleoplasm.

nucleus: a membrane-enclosed **organelle** found in most eukaryotic cells; it contains most of the cell's genetic material, organized as multiple long linear **DNA** molecules in complex with a large variety of **proteins** such as histones to form chromosomes; the genes within these chromosomes make up the cell's nuclear genome; the function of the nucleus is to maintain the integrity of these genes and to control the activities of the cell by regulating gene expression.

occlusion: a term indicating that the state of something, which is normally open, is now totally closed; in medicine, the term is often used to refer to **blood vessels**, **arteries**, or **veins** that have become totally blocked to any **blood flow**; for issues of artery occlusion, see **stenosis** and **atheroma**; in dentistry, occlusion refers to the manner in which the teeth from upper and lower arches come together when the mouth is closed.

occlusion spectroscopy: the most important **blood** parameters such as **hemoglobin**, **glucose**, **oxygen** saturation, etc., influence the optical transmission growth over systolic **occlusion** and, therefore, may be extracted from the detailed analysis of the time evolution of optical transmission; this forms a basis for a kind of **noninvasive** measurements, i.e., occlusion spectroscopy.

oil: a neutral liquid, soluble in ether, hot **ethanol**, and gasoline, but not in water; it contains carbon and hydrogen, is capable of combustion, and has a marked viscosity; the main types of oils are essential oils, fixed oils, mineral oils; oils are esters of **glycerol** with unsaturated **fatty acids**, of which the most usually occurring are **oleic acid**, linoleic acid, and linolenic acid; oleic acid has one double bond, linoleic has two double bonds, and linolenic has three double bonds; a neutral **fat**, liquid below 20°C, is usually called an oil; it contains a higher proportion of **unsaturated fatty acids** than a solid fat.

ointment: a viscous semisolid preparation used **topically** on a variety of body surfaces; these include the **skin** and the **mucous membrane**.

oleic acid: a **monounsaturated fatty acid** found in various animal and vegetable sources; it has the formula $C_{18}H_{34}O_2$ (or $CH_3(CH_2)_7CH=CH(CH_2)_7COOH$); it comprises 55–80% of olive **oil**.

olfactory tract: a narrow white band, triangular on the coronal section, the apex being directed upward, that lies in the olfactory sulcus on the inferior surface of the **frontal lobe** of the **brain**, and divides posteriorly into a medial and lateral striae.

optic (optical) nerve: the second cranial **nerve**; it is connected to the **retina** and simulated by light; the sensory nerve of sight.

optical biopsy: a measurement of the localized optical properties of **tissues** for diagnostic purpose.

optical clearing: making a **tissue** more translucent by reducing light scattering through matching the refractive index of the scatterers and ground substances; immersion liquids (**osmolytes**) with the appropriate refractive index and the rate of diffusion are usually used (see **immersion technique**, Glossary 1, and **optical immersion technique**).

optical clearing agent (OCA): chemical agents used for controlling the optical properties of **cells** and **tissues** with the result of the increase of their optical transmittance and reduction of the backreflectance.

optical immersion technique: based on impregnation of a **tissue** by a biocompatible chemical agent with a refractive index higher than an interstitial refractive index or **topical** application of a **hyperosmotic** agent inducing tissue **dehydration**; both processes cause an increase of refractive index of interstitial space relating to other tissue compartments and make up tissue more optically transparent (less scattering); for **cell** systems, such as **blood**, an addition to **plasma** a biocompatible chemical agent with a refractive index higher than plasma causes an increase of blood optical transmittance.

oral glucose tolerance test (OGTT): see **glucose tolerance test**.

organelle: a part of a **cell** that is a structural and functional unit, e.g., a **mitochondrion** is a respiratory organelle; organelles in a cell correspond to organs in an organism.

osmolality: a measure of the **osmoles** of solute per kilogram of solvent.

osmolarity: a measure of the **osmoles** of solute per liter of solution; if the concentration is very low, osmolarity and **osmolality** are considered equivalent; in calculations for these two measurements, salts are presumed to dissociate into their component ions; for example, a mole of **glucose** in solution is one osmole, whereas a mole of sodium chloride in solution is two osmoles (one mole of sodium and one mole of chloride), both sodium and chloride ions affect the osmotic pressure of the solution.

osmole (Osm): a unit of measurement that defines the number of moles of a chemical compound that contribute to a solution's **osmotic stress** (pressure).

osmolyte: an osmotically active liquid (molecules) (see **osmotic phenomenon**, **osmotic stress**, Glossary 1).

osmolytic: pertaining to **osmolyte**.

ovalbumin: the main **protein** found in egg white, making up 60–65% of the total protein; is made up of 385 **amino acids**, and its relative molecular mass is 45 kD; it is a glycoprotein with 4 sites of glycosylation.

oxidase: a type of dehydrogenase; the hydrogen removed from the substrate combines with molecular oxygen.

oxidative stress: caused by an imbalance between the production of reactive **oxygen** and a biological system's ability to readily detoxify the reactive intermediates or easily repair the resulting damage; all forms of life maintain a reducing environment within their **cells**; the cellular redox environment is preserved by **enzymes** that maintain the reduced state through a constant input of metabolic energy; disturbances in this normal redox state can cause toxic effects through the production of peroxides and free radicals that damage all components of the cell, including **proteins**, **lipids**, and **DNA**; in humans, oxidative stress is involved in many diseases, such as atherosclerosis, Parkinson's disease and **Alzheimer's disease** and it may also be important in aging; however, reactive oxygen species can be beneficial, as they are used by the immune system as a way to attack and kill pathogens and as a form of cell signaling.

oxygen: chemical element with the chemical symbol O and atomic number 8; it is usually bonded to other elements covalently or ionically; an important example of common oxygen-containing compound is water (H_2O); dioxygen (O_2) is the second most common component of the atmosphere (about 21% by volume) and produced predominantly through photolysis (light-driven splitting of water) during photosynthesis in cyanobacteria, green algae, and plants; oxygen is essential for cellular respiration in all aerobic organisms; triatomic oxygen (ozone, O_3) forms through radiation in the upper layers of the atmosphere and acts as a shield against UV radiation.

oxygenated blood: **blood** saturated by oxygen.

oxyhemoglobin: **hemoglobin** combined with oxygen.

pacemaker: a local rhythm driver; the region of the **heart** or the skeletal **muscles** around a **vessel** where the nervous impulse that starts the contraction of the heart or **blood vessel** muscles is sent out.

pain: a subjective experience; the system that carries information about **inflammation**, damage or near-damage in **tissue**, to the spinal cord and **brain**.

palm: flat of the **hand**.

papillary: related to papilla; papillary **dermis** is the part of the dermis that lies immediately below the **epidermis**, it has vertically oriented **connective tissue** fibers and a rich supply of **blood vessels**; papillary **muscles** of the **heart** serve to limit the movements of the mitral and tricuspid **valves**; papillary **tumors** are the tumors shaped like a small mushroom, with its stem attached to the **epithelial** layer (inner lining) of an organ; papillary tumors are the most common of all **thyroid cancers** ($>70\%$); papillary thyroid cancer forms in cells in the thyroid and grows in small fingerlike shapes, it grows slowly, is more common in women than in men, and often occurs before age 40; papillary **carcinoma** typically exhibits as an irregular, solid or cystic mass that arises from otherwise normal thyroid tissue; papillary serous carcinoma is an aggressive cancer that usually affects the **uterus**/endometrium, peritoneum, or ovary.

parakeratosis: a disorder of the **horny layer** of the **skin epidermis** manifested by the appearance of **cell** nuclei in this layer; it can be seen in chronic **dermatitis**, such as **psoriasis**.

parakeratotic: pertaining to **parakeratosis** (e.g., parakeratotic focus); the **cell** structure near such a focus is substantially disordered, or consists of parakeratotic scales.

pars conv.: pars (partes) convalescent; a part of convalescent tissue.

partially permeable membrane: also termed a semipermeable **membrane**, a selectively permeable membrane or a differentially permeable membrane, is a membrane that allows certain molecules or ions to pass through it by **diffusion** and occasionally specialized "facilitated diffusion"; the rate of passage depends on the pressure, concentration, and temperature of the molecules or solutes on either side, as well as the permeability of the membrane to each solute; depending on the membrane and the solute, permeability may depend on solute size, solubility, properties, or chemistry; an example of a semipermeable membrane is a **lipid bilayer**, on which is based the plasma membrane that surrounds all biological **cells**.

pathological: pertaining to pathology, the study and diagnosis of disease through examination of organs, **tissues**, **cells** and body fluids; the term encompasses both the medical specialty which uses tissues and body fluids to obtain clinically useful information, as well as the related scientific study of disease processes.

peeling: a body treatment technique used to improve and smooth the texture of the facial **skin** using physical (mechanical, acoustical, laser, etc.) or chemical action; for instance chemical solution causes the skin to blister and eventually peel off; the regenerated skin is usually smoother and less wrinkled than the old skin; α-**hydroxy acids (AHAs)** are naturally occurring organic carboxylic acids such as glycolic acid, a natural constituent of sugar cane juice and lactic acid and found in sour milk and tomato juice, is the mildest of the peel formulas and produce light peels for treatment of fine wrinkles, areas of dryness, uneven pigmentation and acne.

percutaneous: pertains to any medical procedure where access to inner organs or other tissue is done through the skin, for instance via needle-puncture of the skin, rather than by using an "open" approach where inner organs or tissue are exposed; phototherapy is another example of percutaneous treatment .

perfusion: oxygen perfusion see **blood perfusion**.

peripapillary: surrounding a papilla; papilla is a projection occurring in various animal tissues and organs.

perivascular: around the blood vessels; for instance, perivascular lymphatics.

peroxisome: a specialized **organelle** containing the oxidizing **enzymes** that degrade peroxides.

petrolatum: a semisolid mixture of hydrocarbons obtained from petroleum; used in medicinal **ointments** and for lubrication.

pH: a measure of the acidity or alkalinity of a solution; solutions with a pH less than 7 are considered acidic, while those with a pH greater than 7 are considered basic (alkaline); pH 7 is defined as neutral because it is the pH of pure water at $25°C$; pH is formally dependent upon the activity of hydrogen ions (H^+), but for very pure dilute solutions.

phagocyte: a **white blood cell** that engulfs foreign bodies, particularly pathogens, by enclosing the body in **cytoplasm** through a process of extending pseudopodia around it (the amoeboid movement for engulfing); in mammals, **polymorphs**, **monocytes**, and **macrophages** are phagocytes; macrophages can be phagocytes of other **WBCs**; phagocytes are an important part of the defense mechanism of most animals against invading pathogens.

phenols: a class of chemical compounds consisting of a hydroxyl group ($-OH$) attached to an aromatic hydrocarbon group; the simplest of the class is phenol (C_6H_5OH).

phenylalanine: an essential alpha-**amino acid**; it exists in two forms, a D and an L form, which are enantiomers (mirror-image molecules) of each other; it has a benzyl side chain; its name comes from its chemical structures consisting of a phenyl group substituted for one of the hydrogens in the side chain of alanine; because of its phenyl group, phenylalanine is an aromatic compound.

Philly mice: a new model for genetic **cataracts**, in which there is an apparent defect in **lens membrane** permeability.

phonophoresis: the use of **ultrasound** to enhance the delivery of topically applied drugs.

phosphate-buffered saline (PBS): a **saline** solution with phosphates added to keep the **pH** approximately constant.

phospholipids: a class of **lipids**, and a major component of all biological **membranes**, along with glycolipids, **cholesterol**, and **proteins**; understanding of the **aggregation** properties of these molecules is known as lipid **polymorphism** and forms part of current academic research.

photo-aging: this condition is most noticeable in women who have spent hours in the sun without the benefit of sunscreen; the most obvious symptoms of photo-aging are: dark age spots on the face and décolleté; deep wrinkles around the eyes; fine lines; leathery skin; a gradual thickening of the skin; uneven complexion.

photobleaching: removal of color from a sample by irradiating it with light of a certain wavelength and intensity; in **photochemotherapy**, the **photosensitizer** can be photobleached, either permanently and/or transiently, by the treatment light; the term "photobleaching" is variously used to denote actual photochemical destruction of the photosensitizer or simply decreased optical absorbance and/or fluorescence, which may not be equal and which does not necessarily involve molecular decomposition.

photochemical therapy (photochemotherapy): the branch of therapy that deals with the biochemical action of light on a tissue photosensitized by the appropriate chemical or a chemical that induces the photosensitive agent in **tissue**, e.g., **photodynamic therapy**, **PUVA therapy**.

photocoagulation: the **coagulation** (clotting) of **tissue** using a laser (or lamp) that produces light in the visible (green) wavelength that is selectively absorbed by **hemoglobin**, which is the pigment in **red blood cells**, in order to seal off bleeding **blood vessels**; photocoagulation has diverse uses such as in **cancer** treatment it is used to treat tumors to destroy blood vessels entering a **tumor** and deprive it of nutrients; in the treatment of a detached **retina** it is used to destroy abnormal blood vessels in the retina and to treat tumors in the eye, etc.; NIR light that is selectively absorbed by not very intensive water and fat bands also is used for tissue coagulation, for instance in the treatment of gastric **ulcers**.

photodestruction: intensive or focused laser beams used in the destruction of a **tissue**, **cell**, or their part (**coagulation**, **ablation**), or photochemically by light with a moderate intensity (**necrosis**).

photodisruption: a localized breakdown of semitransparent biological **tissues** that do not strongly absorb light in the visible range by an intensive tightly focused femtosecond laser pulse; the nonlinearity of the process ensures absorption and, therefore, material alterations are confined to the extremely small focal volume; typically submicrometer-sized photodisrupted regions can be produced inside single **cells**; femtosecond pulses deposit very little energy but still causing breakdown, therefore producing surgical photodisruption, while minimizing collateral damage.

photodynamic therapy (PDT): therapy of **malignant lesions** that involves administration to the patient of a **photosensitizer**, a time delay to allow adequate concentration of the drug in the **tumor**, followed by irradiation of the target **tissue** volume by light of a wavelength appropriate to activate the **photosensitizer** effectively; the consequent photochemical damage results in **tissue necrosis** by directly killing tumor cells and/or by vascular damage leading to ischemic necrosis; for most photosensitizers, it is believed that the PDT effect is mediated by the production of highly active singlet oxygen, $^1O_2$, formed by energy transfer from the excited-state photosensitizer to molecular oxygen in the tissue.

Photofrin II: the effective biological photodynamic dye for red light [see, **hematoporphyrin derivative (HPD)**]; its molecular weight is about 500; it has an extinction coefficient of about 5000 cm^{-1} M^{-1} at 626 nm when dissolved in dextrose.

photorefractive surgery: see **laser refractive surgery**.

photothermal therapy: therapy based on the thermal reaction of a living **tissue** and a **cell** to light that is intensive enough to produce thermal effects; laser-induced thermotherapy (LITT) includes laser-induced hyperthermia (LIHT) using temperatures from 42 to 60°C, high-temperature laser-induced **coagulation** (LIC) for temperatures above 60°C, and laser-induced interstitial thermotherapy (LIITT) for coagulation of deep tissues using special fiber optic probes; LIITT is a safe procedure with minimum physical strain for the patient.

physiological solution: there are a number of physiological solutions that provide safety and normal functioning of biological cells, tissues, and organs; they contain electrolytes and organic acids at concentrations similar to that found in animal or human **serum**; **saline** is a physiological solution of sodium chloride (NaCl) in sterile water, used frequently for intravenous infusion, rinsing contact lenses, and nasal irrigation; saline solutions are available in various concentrations for different purposes; normal saline is the solution of 0.9% w/v of NaCl; it has a slightly higher degree of **osmolality** compared to **blood** (hence, though it is referred to as being **isotonic** with blood in clinical contexts, this is a technical inaccuracy), about 300 mOsm/L.

pigment: any substance whose presence in the **tissues** or **cells** colors them.

pigmentary glaucoma: a form of **glaucoma** that usually presents in young males, 20 to 50 years old; in fact, all patients with pigmentary glaucoma will necessarily have pigmentary dispersion syndrome prior to the onset of glaucoma (i.e., actual **optic nerve** damage and peripheral vision loss); the mechanism of glaucoma development in this syndrome is the deposition of **pigment** from the **iris** into the trabecular meshwork (primary site of fluid egress), essentially "plugging" the microscopic spaces through which fluid escapes.

pigmentation: many **tissues** and organs, such as **skin**, **iris**, **retina**, etc., as well as blood contain **pigments**, such as **melanin** or **hemoglobin**, in specialized cells called **melanocytes** or **erythrocytes**; many conditions affect the levels or nature of pigments in **cells**; for instance, albinism is a disorder affecting the low level of melanin production in animals and humans; pigment color differs from structural color in that it is the same for all viewing angles, whereas structural color is the result of selective reflection or interference, usually because of multilayer structures and light scattering.

plague: an infectious, epidemic disease of high mortality caused by the **bacterium** *Pasteurella pestis*.

plasma: the clear, waterlike, colorless liquid of **blood** and other body liquids.

plasma-membrane: see **cell membrane**.

plasmid: a **DNA** molecule separated from the chromosomal DNA and capable of autonomous replication; it is typically circular and double-stranded, occurs in **bacteria**, sometimes in eukaryotic organisms.

plastic surgery: surgical techniques that change the appearance and function of a person's body; some of these operations are called "**cosmetic**," and others are called "reconstructive."

platelets: the very small, nonnucleated, round or oval disks that are fragments of **cells** from red **bone** marrow; they are found only in mammalian **blood**; there are approximately 200,000–400,000 per mm^3 in human **blood**; they initiate blood clotting by disintegrating and releasing thrombokinase.

polar aprotic solvent: a solvent that does not contain an $O-H$ or $N-H$ bond; acetone ($CH_3-C(=O)-CH_3$) is the polar aprotic solvent.

polyethylene glycol (PEG): any of a series of polymers that have the general formula $HOCH_2(CH_2OCH_2)_nCH_2OH$ or $H(OCH_2CH_2)_nOH$ and a molecular weight of from about 200 to 20,000; they are obtained by condensation of **ethylene glycol** or ethylene oxide and water and used as an emulsifying agent and lubricant in ointments, creams, etc., PGs with a high molecular weight are used as effective **osmolytes**.

polyglycerylmethacrylate: used in drugs and **cosmetic** preparations for personal care/use.

polymorph (polymorphonuclear leukocyte): a polynucleated, irregularly shaped **white blood cell** that exhibits amoeboid movement; the nucleus consists of two or more lobes (in humans up to five) joined by threads; the number of lobes increases with the age of the cell; in a healthy person, the distribution of polymorphs by the number of lodes remains constant; any variation indicates a diseased condition; the cells are all active **phagocytes**; they are produced continually in **bone** marrow and constitute about 70% of all **leukocytes** in humans; the **cytoplasm** of polymorphs in humans is granular; some granulations stain with acid dyes (eosinophils), some with basic dyes (basophils), and some with neutral dyes (neutrophils); all three types increase in number during infection.

polymorphism (pleomorphism): the multiple possible states for a single property, for instance, the property of amphiphiles that gives rise to various **aggregations** of **lipids**; it is also defined as the occurrence of two or more structural forms.

polyorganosiloxane (POS, silicone): the host media for a solid-state **tissue phantom**.

polyp: an abnormal growth of **tissue (tumor)** projecting from a **mucous membrane**; if it is attached to the surface by a narrow elongated stalk it is said to be pedunculated; if no stalk is present it is said to be sessile; polyps are commonly found in the **colon**, **stomach**, nose, **urinary bladder**, and **uterus**; they may also occur elsewhere in the body where mucous membranes exist like the **cervix** and small **intestine**.

polypropylene glycol (PPG): the polymer of **propylene glycol**; chemically it is a polyether; the term polypropylene glycol or PPG is reserved for low to medium range molar mass polymer when the nature of the end-group, which is usually a hydroxyl group, still matters.

pons: a structure located on the **brain** stem; in humans it is above the medulla, below the midbrain, and anterior to the **cerebellum**.

porosity: a measure of the void spaces in a material, and is measured as a fraction, between 0–1, or as a percent between 0–100%; the term porosity is used in multiple fields including biology, for instance, porosity of biological **membranes**.

porphyrin: a heterocyclic macrocycle derived from four pyrrolelike subunits interconnected via their α-carbon atoms via methine bridges ($=CH-$); the macrocycle, therefore, is highly conjugated, and consequently deeply colored; the macrocycle has 26 π-electrons; many porphyrins occur in nature, they are pigments found in both animals and plants.

Porphyromonas gingivalis: is a gram-negative oral anaerobe found in periodontal lesions and associated with adult periodontal disease.

port wine stain (cavernous hemangioma): a **skin** discoloration characterized by a deep red to purple color (see **hemangioma**).

postmenopausal: after menopause; the period of permanent cessation of menstruation, usually occurring between the ages of 45 and 50.

post mortem: occurring after death; colloquial expression for an examination of the body after death (autopsy).

precancerous: a **tissue** lesion that carries the risk of turning into **cancer**; it is a preliminary stage of cancer; these precancerous lesions can have several causes: UV radiation, genetics, exposure to such cancer-causing substances as arsenic, tar or x-ray radiation.

preembryos: a stage of the human life cycle in in-vitro fertilization; an oocyte (egg) is fertilized (but not yet implanted) and forms a preembryo, also called a blastocyte, usually on day five or six.

premenopausal: prior to menopause, the period of permanent cessation of menstruation, usually occurring between the ages of 45 and 50.

presbyopia: the **eye**'s diminished ability to focus that occurs with aging; the most widely held theory is that it arises from the loss of elasticity of the **crystalline lens**, although changes in the lens's curvature from continual growth and loss of power of the **ciliary muscles** have also been postulated as its cause.

Prevotella intermedia: an obligatory anaerobic, black-pigmented, gram-negative rod that is frequently associated with periodontal disease: adult periodontitis, acute necrotizing ulcerative gingivitis, and pregnancy gingivitis; this organism is also involved in extraoral infections such as nasopharyngeal infection and intraabdominal infection; it coaggregates with *Porphyromonas gingivalis*.

Prevotella nigrescens: a genospecie that is very close to *Prevotella intermedia*; *Prevotella intermedia* is likely to be more associated with periodontal sites, whereas *Prevotella nigrescens* seems to be more frequently recovered from healthy gingivae.

prickle cells layer: the layer between the **stratum granulosum** and **stratum basale**, characterized by the presence of prickle **cells**—cells with delicate radiating processes connecting with similar cells, being a dividing **keratinocyte** of the **stratum spinosum** of the **epidermis**.

prokaryotes: are organisms without a **cell nucleus**, or any other membrane-bound **organelles**; most are unicellular, but some prokaryotes are multicellular; the **bacteria** are the prokaryotes.

proliferative disorder: the growth or production of **cells** by multiplication of parts.

Propionibacterium acnes: a relatively slow growing, (typically) aerotolerant anaerobe gram-positive bacterium that is linked to the skin condition acne; this bacteria is largely commensal and thus present on most people's skin; and lives on

fatty acids in the **sebaceous glands** and the **sebum** secreted by them; it is named after its ability to generate propionic acid.

propylene glycol (PG): a colorless, viscous, hygroscopic liquid, $CH_3CHOHCH_2OH$, used chiefly as a lubricant and as a solvent for **fats**, **oils**, and waxes.

prostate (prostate gland): the muscular, **glandular** organ that surrounds the urethra of males at the base of the **bladder**.

protein: the result of **amino acids** joined together in a chain by peptide bonds between their amino and carboxylate groups; an amino acid residue is one amino acid that is joined to another by a peptide bond; each different protein has a unique sequence of amino acid residues, this is its primary structure; just as the letters of the alphabet can be combined to form an almost endless variety of words, amino acids can be linked in varying sequences to form a huge variety of proteins.

proteoglycans: a special class of glycoproteins that are heavily glycosylated; they consist of a core **protein** with one or more covalently attached glycosaminoglycan chain(s); these chains are long, linear **carbohydrate** polymers that are negatively charged under physiological conditions, due to the occurrence of sulphate and uronic acid groups.

protoporphyrin IX (Pp IX): pertaining to carbonic acids: its absorbing bands are the same as for other porphyrins (see **hemoglobin spectra**, Glossary 1), e.g., in diethyl ester solution, Pp IX has the following peaks: 403 nm (Soret band), and 504, 535, 575, and 633 (Q bands); Pp IX is the immediate **heme** precursor; exogenous administration of 5-aminolaevulinic acid (ALA), an early precursor in heme synthesis, induces accumulation of endogenous photoactive porphyrins, particularly Pp IX; induced Pp IX is used in **cancer** diagnostics and **photodynamic therapy**.

psoralene: pertaining to furocumarins; its absorbing peaks lie in the UV at 295 and 335 nm; used in **photochemical therapy** of **psoriasis** and other **dermatosis** (**PUVA**).

psoriasis: a common chronic **skin** disease characterized by scaly patches (psoriasis focus or psoriatic plaque).

psoriatic: pertaining to **psoriasis**.

pulse wave: a wave of pressure sent down the **arteries** by every contraction of the ventricle; the increased pressure can be felt if the **artery** is pressed against a **bone** (usually in the wrist); the pressure wave travels much faster than the flow of **blood** through the artery; the pulse becomes fainter the farther it is from the **heart**; in the **capillaries** it completely disappears.

pupil: the opening of the **iris** of the **eyeball**; radiating muscles dilate the pupil and a ring of **muscle** (a sphincter) a round it constricts the pupil; the regulation of the size of the pupil is a reflex action caused by the stimulus of light on the **optic nerve**.

PUVA therapy: a **photochemical therapy** method based on impregnation of the diseased **skin** by a **psoralen** as a **photosensitizer** and on use of UVA radiation to provide the phototoxic effect (reduction of **cell** abnormal proliferation due to **cross-linking** of **DNA** molecules in the cell nuclei); used for treatment of **psoriasis** and other **skin** disease.

pyloric: pertaining to the region of the **stomach** that connects to the duodenum.

pyrrolidonecarboxylic acid: 2-pyrrolidone-5-carboxylic acid (PCA) is a cyclic derivative of glutamic acid, physiologically present in mammalian **tissues**.

radial artery: the main **artery** of the lateral aspect of the **forearm**.

raffinose: a complex **carbohydrate**, a trisaccharide composed of galactose, fructose, and **glucose**.

raft tissue: the organotypic **tissue** culture systems permitting the growth of differentiated **keratinocytes** *in vitro* or even creating of skin-equivalent tissue model composed of dermis with type I **collagen** and **fibroblast cells** and **epidermis** of differentiated keratinocytes.

red blood cell (RBC): see **erythrocyte**.

rehydration: the replenishment of water and electrolytes lost through **dehydration**.

ren: see **kidney**.

respiratory chain: in aerobic respiration, electrons are transferred from metabolites to molecular **oxygen** through a series of redox reactions mediated by an electron transport chain; the resulting free energy is used for the formation of **ATP** and **NAD**; in anaerobic respiration, analogous reactions take place with an inorganic compound other than oxygen as an ultimate electron acceptor.

reticular fibers: very thin, almost inextensible threads of **reticulin**; they form a network of intercellular **fibers** around and among the **cells** of many **tissues**, e.g., in many large organs such as the **liver** and **kidney**, and also in tissues, such as **nerves** and **muscles**; they especially support and unite **reticular tissue**.

reticular layer of dermis (*reticular dermis*): the lower layer of the **dermis**; it is made primarily of coarse **collagen** and elastic fibers, it is denser than the **papillary dermis**; it strengthens the **skin**, providing structure and elasticity; it also supports other skin components such as **sweat glands** and **hair** follicles.

reticular tissue: a **tissue** consisting of a network of **reticular fibers** around and among **cells**, with **lymph** in the intercellular spaces; it occurs in **muscles**, **nerves**, and the larger **glands**.

reticulin: a tough **fibrous** protein, similar to **collagen**, but more resistant to higher temperatures and chemical reagents; it occurs in vertebrate **connective tissue** as

reticular fibers; reticulin is formed in embryos and also in **wounds**; it often changes to collagen.

retina: the innermost coat of the posterior part of the **eyeball** that receives the image produced by the **crystalline lens**; it is continuous with the **optic nerve** and consists of several layers, one of which contains the rods and cones sensitive to light.

retinal: pertaining to **retina**.

retinal nerve fiber layer (RNFL): formed by the expansion of the fibers of the **optic nerve**.

retinol (vitamin A): a fat-soluble, yellow **oil** stored in the **liver**; it is not excreted and can accumulate in the body to produce toxic effects; retinol is used in the body to produce visual purple, the pigment in rods of the **retina**; a deficiency impairs vision and also causes **epithelial cells** to become flattened and heaped up on one another; this leads to xerophthalmia and also to the formation of hard, rough **skin**.

rhodamine: a family of related chemical compounds; examples are Rhodamine 6G, Rhodamine B, and Rhodamine 123; they are used as dyes; they fluoresce and can thus be measured easily and inexpensively; they are generally toxic, and are soluble in water, methanol, and ethanol; Rhodamine B (excitation 510 nm/fluorescence 580 nm) is used in biology as a staining fluorescent dye; Rhodamine 123 (excitation 480 nm/fluorescence 540 nm) is used in biochemistry to inhibit mitochondrion function.

rheumatic arthritis: a chronic disease marked by **inflammation** of the joints; it is frequently accompanied by marked deformities and is ordinarily associated with manifestations of a general or systemic affliction.

rib: one of a series of curved **bones** that are articulated with the vertebrae and occur in pairs (12 in humans) on each side of the vertebrate body; certain pairs are connected with the sternum and form the thoracic wall.

ribosome: in the **cytoplasm** of a **cell** any of several minute, angular, or spherical particles composed of protein and **RNA**.

Ringer's solution: an aqueous solution of the chlorides of sodium, potassium, and calcium that is **isotonic** to animal **tissue** and is used topically as a **physiological solution** and, in experiments, to bathe animal tissues.

RNA (ribonucleic acid): a **nucleic acid** polymer consisting of nucleotide monomers that acts as a messenger between **DNA** and **ribosomes**, and is also responsible for making proteins out of amino acids; RNA polynucleotides contain ribose sugars and are predominantly uracil unlike DNA; it is transcribed (synthesized) from DNA by **enzymes** called RNA polymerases and further processed by other enzymes; RNA serves as the template for translation of genes into proteins, transferring amino acids to the ribosome to form proteins, and also translating the transcript into proteins.

rouleaux: for a condition wherein the **blood cells** clump together to form what looks like stacks of coins.

saccharose (sucrose): a disaccharide (**glucose** + fructose) with the molecular formula $C_{12}H_{22}O_{11}$; it is best known for its role in human nutrition.

saline: a salt solution that is used for medical treatment; this solution is designed to have the same **osmotic pressure** as **blood**.

saliva: a viscid, colorless, watery fluid secreted into the mouth by the salivary **glands**; it functions in tasting, chewing, and swallowing food; it keeps the mouth moist and starts the digestion of starches.

sarcoma: a malignant growth of abnormal **cells** in **connective tissue**.

scalp: the anatomical area bordered by the face anteriorly and the neck to the sides and posteriorly.

scar: the areas of **fibrous tissue** that replace normal **skin** (or other tissue) after **injury**; a scar results from the biologic process of **wound** repair; thus, scarring is a natural part of the healing process.

Scheimpflug camera: a camera that is based on the Scheimpflug principle; this technique allows the assessment of the anterior segment of the **eye**, from the front of the **cornea** to the back of the **lens**, in a sagittal plane; the Scheimpflug principle allows for quantification of the light scatter.

sciatic nerve: a large **nerve** that runs down the lower limbs; it is the longest single nerve in the body.

sclera (sclerotic): a dense, white, **fibrous membrane**, which, with the **cornea**, forms the external covering of the **eyeball**; scleral regions: limbal, equatorial, and posterior pole region.

scleroderma: a disease in which all the layers of the **skin** become hardened and rigid.

sclerotomy: surgical **incision** of the sclerotic coat of the eye.

sea collagen: used in **cosmetics**; sea **collagen** is a better choice than bovine collagen because of its affinity to the **skin** and its richness in trace elements; deep skin **moisturizer**, prevents and reduces **wrinkles** and lines by redensifying and restructuring the skin.

sebaceous gland: a tiny sebum-producing **gland** found everywhere except on the palms, lips, and soles of the feet; the thicker density of **hair**, the more sebaceous glands are found; they are classified as holocrine glands.

sebum: an oily substance secreted by the **sebaceous glands**; it is made of **fat** (**lipids**) and the debris of dead fat-producing cells; in the **glands**, sebum is produced within specialized **cells** and is released as these cells burst; sebum is odorless, but its bacterial breakdown can produce odors.

sedimentation: the motion of molecules in solutions or particles in suspensions in response to an external force such as gravity, centrifugal force or electric force; sedimentation may pertain to objects of various sizes, ranging from suspensions of dust and pollen particles to cellular suspensions and solutions of single molecules such as **proteins** and peptides.

semen: the viscid, whitish fluid produced in the male reproductive organ; it contains **spermatozoa**.

sensory nerve: **nerves** that receive sensory stimuli, such as how something feels and if it is painful; they are made up of nerve fibers, called sensory fibers (mechanoreceptor fibers sense body movement and pressure placed against the body, and nociceptor fibers sense tissue **injury**).

serum: **blood plasma** with clotting factors removed.

sheath: a protective covering fitting closely to a structure or a part of an organism, especially an elongated structure or part.

silicon oils: polymerized siloxanes are silicon analogues of carbon based organic compounds, and can form (relatively) long and complex molecules based on silicon rather than carbon; chains of alternating silicon are formed: oxygen atoms or siloxane, rather than carbon atoms.

silicon waxes: a semicrystalline with a melting point of 53°C to 75°C to liquid; a clear, light-straw to white and off-white colored flake; they are semiocclusive or occlusive formulations, lubricants, emollients, water-repellents, replacement for petrolatum, thickeners, **moisturizers**, emulsifiers for water-in-oil and water-in-silicone emulsions (up to 80% water content).

skeletal muscle: a type of striated **muscle**, usually attached to the skeleton; skeletal muscles are used to create movement, by applying force to **bone**s and joints via contraction; they generally contract voluntarily (via somatic nerve stimulation), although they can contract involuntarily through reflexes.

skin: the external protective covering on a body, joined by **connective tissue** to the **muscles**; it consists of an inner **dermis** and an outer **epidermis**.

skin appendages: structures associated with the skin such as **hair**, **sweat glands**, **sebaceous glands** and nails; they have their roots in the **dermis** or even in the hypodermis.

skin barrier function: protects internal organs from the environment, resides in the uppermost thin heterogeneous layer called **stratum corneum**, which is composed of dead protein-rich cells and intercellular lipid domains; this two-compartment structure is renewed continuously and when the barrier function is damaged, it is repaired immediately; under low humidity, the stratum corneum becomes thick, the lipid content in it increases and water impermeability is enhanced; the heterogeneous field in the epidermis induced by ions, such as calcium and potassium, regulates the self-referential, self-organizing system to protect the living organism, http://www.scipress.org/journals/forma/pdf/1503/15030227.pdf.

skin flap: a tear of the skin away from the body, which leaves one side of the skin still attached.

skin flap window: a special window surgically made in the skin area void of blood vessels and an implanted glass plate allows for prolonged *in vivo* studies of skin vessels seen through this window.

skin irritation: some physical and chemical exposures to the **skin** may cause **dermatitis** with redness, itching, and discomfort.

skin microdermabrasion: a quick, **noninvasive** procedure used to resurface the **skin**; it gently removes only the very top layers of damaged skin by "sand blasting" them with tiny crystals; the technique exfoliates and gently resurfaces the skin, promoting the formation of new smoother, clearer skin.

skin stripping: a mechanical disruption and reduction of the **stratum corneum** and partially of the living **epidermis**, which are the outermost layers of the **skin**; medical adhesive tapes and medical glues with such substrates as glass, quartz, and metal plates are typically used; the technique is used for study of drug delivery and protective filters distribution in the skin.

skull: the part of the skeleton consisting of the **cranium** and the facial skeleton; the latter includes the sense capsules, the jaws, the hyoid **bone**, and the **cartilage** of the larynx; the skull may also be divided into the neurocranium and the viscerocranium.

slit-lamp: an optical device that consists of a high-intensity light source that can be focused to shine as a slit; it is used in conjunction with a microscope; the lamp facilitates an examination, which looks at the anterior segment, or frontal structures, of the human **eye**, which including the eyelid, **sclera**, **conjunctiva**, **iris**, natural **crystalline lens**, and **cornea**; the binocular slit-lamp examination provides a stereoscopic magnified view of the eye structures in striking detail, enabling exact anatomical diagnoses to be made for a variety of eye conditions.

sodium fluorescein: probably the most commonly used dye in the biological world; it is a **protein** dye, so some caution is required in its use within the living body; sodium **fluorescein** has its peak absorption at 450 nm and produces a yellow/green emission when stimulated by light in the blue region; fluorescent angiography is a technique for examining the **blood** circulation of the **retina** using the dye tracing method that involves the injection of sodium fluorescein into the systemic circulation, and then an angiogram is obtained by photographing the fluorescence emitted after illumination of the retina with blue light.

sodium lactate: natural salt that is derived from a naturally fermented product, lactic acid that is produced naturally in foods such as cheese, yogurt, hard salami, pepperoni, sourdough bread and many others by the action of lactic acid starter cultures (also known as a "good" bacteria); sodium lactate can correct the normal acid-base balance in patients whose **blood** has become too acidic; it can also help treat overdoses of certain medications by increasing removal of the drug from the body.

sodium lauryl sulfate: a detergent and **surfactant** found in many personal care products (soaps, shampoos, toothpaste, etc.).

somatosensory: pertaining to the sense of touch that is mediated by the somatosensory system; touch may simply be considered one of the five human senses; however, when a person touches something or somebody this gives rise to various feelings: the perception of pressure (shape, softness, texture, vibration, etc.), relative temperature and sometimes pain; thus the term "touch" is actually the combined term for several senses; in medicine, the colloquial term "touch" is usually replaced with somatic senses, to better reflect the variety of mechanisms involved; the somatosenses include: **cutaneous** (**skin**), kinesthesia (movement) and visceral (internal) senses; visceral senses have to do with sensory information from within the body, such as **stomach** aches.

sonophoresis: see **phonophoresis**.

spherocytes: the sphere-shaped **erythrocytes**; an auto-hemolytic anemia (a disease of the blood) characterized by the production of spherocytes; it is caused by a molecular defect in one or more of the **proteins** of the erythrocyte **cytoskeleton** (usually ankyrin, sometimes spectrin); because the **cell** skeleton has a defect, the **blood cell** contracts to its most surface-tension efficient and least flexible configuration: a sphere, rather than the more flexible donut-shape.

spleen: a highly vascular, glandular, ductless organ situated in humans at the cardiac end of the **stomach**; it serves chiefly in the formation of **lymphocytes**, in the destruction of worn-out **erythrocytes**, and as a reservoir for red corpuscles and platelets.

spore: a reproductive structure that is adapted for dispersion and surviving for extended periods of time in unfavorable conditions; spores form part of the life cycles of many plants, algae, fungi, and some protozoans.

squames: flat, keratinized, dead **cells** shed from the outermost layer of a stratified **squamous epithelium**.

squamous cell carcinomas: a form of **carcinoma cancer** that may occur in many different organs, including the **skin**, mouth, **esophagus**, prostate, **lungs**, and **cervix**; it is a **malignant tumor** of **epithelium** that shows **squamous cell** differentiation.

squamous epithelium: an **epithelium** characterized by its most superficial layer consisting of flat, scalelike cells called squamous cells; it may possess only one layer of these cells, in which case it is referred to as simple squamous epithelium, or it may possess multiple layers, referred to then as stratified squamous epithelium; both types perform differing functions, ranging from nutrient exchange to protection.

Staphylococcus: any of several spherical bacteria of the genus *Staphylococcus*, occurring in pairs, tetrads, and irregular clusters, certain species of which, such as *S. aureus* can be pathogenic for man.

Staphylococcus toxin: some ***Staphylococci*** produce a toxin, which is responsible for food poisoning; this toxin is heat stable; bacteria can be killed during processing but the toxin may remain behind.

stasis: stopping of **blood flow** or flows of other biological fluids in the organism.

stenosis: a narrowing of a canal (as in the walls of **arteries** or a cardiac **valve**).

steroid: a terpenoid **lipid** characterized by a carbon skeleton with four fused rings; different steroids vary in the functional groups attached to these rings; hundreds of distinct steroids are found in plants, animals, and fungi; all steroids are derived either from the sterol lanosterol (animals and fungi) or the sterol cycloartenol (plants); both sterols are derived from the cyclization of the triterpene squalene.

stomach: a saclike enlargement of the alimentary canal that forms an organ for storing, diluting, and digesting food; it is situated between the **esophagus** and duodenum and divided into a **fundus**, cardiac portion, pyloric portion, and pylorus.

stratum basale: see **epidermis**.

stratum corneum: see **epidermis**.

stratum granulosum: see **epidermis**.

stratum spinosum: see **epidermis**.

stromal layer (stroma): the supporting framework of an organ, as distinguished from the parenchyma, e.g., the main layer of the eye **sclera** and **cornea**.

subcutaneous: see **hypodermic**.

subdermis (subdermal): the **skin** layer that primarily consists of globular **fat cells**.

subepidermal: situated immediately below the **epidermis**.

submucous: the **tissue** layer under the **mucous membrane**.

sucrose: see **saccharose**.

sugar: a white, crystalline **carbohydrate**, soluble in water and sweet to the taste; sugars are classified as reducing or nonreducing, according to their reaction with Fehling's solution, and also as monosaccharides or disaccharides, according to their structure; **glucose**, fructose, galactose, and mannose are monosaccharides, and sucrose is a disaccharide.

sulci: the superficial fissures that increase the surface area of the **cerebral cortex**; the *pia mater* dips down into the fissures.

sulfonated tetraphenyl porphines (TPPSn): are photosensitizing dyes that localize in cell **lysosomes**; extralysosomal location of hydrophylic $TPPS_3$ and $TPPS_4$ in close proximity to the plasma membrane is also found; the Soret band of the dye is 400–440 nm, the emission maxima at 655 nm (dye) and 610 nm (photoproduct).

sunscreen cream: a cream for protecting the **skin** from the sunlight, especially for blocking UVC and UVB rays.

superior sagittal sinus: also known as the superior longitudinal sinus, occupies the attached or convex margin of the falx cerebri.

surfactant: a wetting agent that lowers the surface tension of a liquid that allows easier spreading and lowers the interfacial tension between two liquids.

sweat glands: in humans, there are two kinds of sweat **glands**, which differ greatly in both the composition of the sweat and its purpose; eccrine sweat glands are distributed over the entire body surface but are particularly abundant on the **palms** of **hands**, soles of feet, and on the forehead; these glands produce sweat that is composed chiefly of water with various salts and are used for body temperature regulation; apocrine sweat glands develop during the early to middle puberty ages approximately around the age of 15, releasing more than normal amounts of sweat for approximately a month and subsequently regulate and release normal amounts of sweat after a certain period of time; they are located wherever there is body **hair**.

swelling: the enlargement of organs caused by the accumulation of excess fluid in **tissues**, called **edema**; it can occur throughout the body (generalized), or only in some part or organ that is affected (localized); it is considered one of the five characteristics of **inflammation**.

synergetic (synergistic): refers to the phenomenon in which two or more discrete influences or agents acting together create an effect greater than that predicted by knowing only the separate effects of the individual agents.

T84: the carcinoma cell line.

tendon: a cord of **white fibrous tissue**; it usually attaches **muscle** to **bones**.

Tenon's capsule: adherent to **episcleral tissue**.

thalamus: a pair and symmetric part of the brain; it constitutes the main part of the diencephalons; in the caudal (tail) to oral (mouth) sequence of neuromeres, the diencephalons is located between the mesencephalon (cerebral peduncule, belonging to the brain stem) and the telencephalon.

thermodynamic activity: ions in solution are in constant motion; this movement is temperature dependent, i.e., as water becomes hotter the particles within it move faster and, conversely, as it becomes cooler they slow down.

thigh: in humans the thigh is the area between the pelvis and buttocks and the **knee**; anatomically, it is part of the lower limb; the single **bone** in the thigh is called the femur; this bone is very thick and strong (due to the high proportion of cortical bone), and forms a ball and socket joint at the hip, and a condylar joint at the knee.

thorax: see **chest**.

thrombocyte: a small, spindle-shaped, nucleated **cell**; the cell readily disintegrates, releasing thrombokinase and initiating **blood** clotting.

thyroid: one of the larger endocrine **glands** in the body; this gland is found in the **neck** just below the Adam's apple; the thyroid controls how quickly the body burns energy, makes **proteins** and how sensitive the body should be to other hormones.

tissue: an aggregate of similar **cells** and cell products forming a definite kind of structural material.

tissue phantom: see Glossary 1, **phantom**.

tissue shrinkage: the loss of volume and weight caused, for instance, by **tissue dehydration**.

titanium dioxide (TiO_2) **particles**: an insoluble white powder, is used extensively in many commercial products, including paint, cosmetics, plastics, paper, and food as an anticaking or whitening agent; it is produced and used in the workplace in varying particle-size fractions, including fine and ultrafine sizes.

TMP (**trimethylolpropanol**): ester of methyl phosphoric acid; a lubricator.

tonometer: an instrument for determining pressure or tension, particularly that for measuring tension within the **eyeball**.

tooth: the hard body composed of **dentin** surrounding a sensitive pulp and covered on the crown with **enamel**.

topical: an application of medication to body surfaces such as the **skin** or **mucous membranes**; some **hydrophobic** chemicals such as steroid hormones can be absorbed into the body after being applied to the skin in the form of a cream, gel, or lotion; **transdermal** patches have become a popular means of administering some drugs for birth control, hormone replacement therapy, and prevention of motion sickness; in dentistry, a topical medication may also mean one that is applied to the surface of teeth.

total hemoglobin: the sum concentration of the **oxy-** and **deoxyhemoglobin**.

toxin: any of a group of poisonous, usually unstable compounds generated by microorganisms or plants, or of animal origin; certain toxins are produced by specific pathogenic microorganisms and are the causative agents in various diseases; some are capable of inducing the production of antibodies in certain animals.

trabeculae: the rodlike **cells** or a row of cells forming supporting structures lying across spaces or lumina, e.g., outgrowths of the cell wall across the lumen of tracheids, the supporting meshwork in spongy **bone**.

trachea: a common biological term for an airway through which respiratory air transport takes place in organisms.

transdermal: means through **skin**.

transepidermal water lost (TEWL): describes the total amount of water lost through the **skin**, a loss that occurs constantly by passive diffusion through the **epidermis**; although TEWL is a normal physiological phenomenon, if it rises too high, the skin can become **dehydrated**, which disrupts form and function, and potentially leads to infection or transepidural passage of deleterious agents.

transpupillary: through the **eye pupil**.

transscleral: through the **eye sclera**.

trauma: an often serious and body-altering physical **injury**, such as the removal of a limb.

trazograph: a derivative of 2,4,6-triiodobenzene acid, molecular weight of about 500; a water-soluble colorless liquid usually used at concentrations of 60 or 76% as an intravenous x-ray contrasting agent; very good agent for **optical clearing** of **fibrous tissue** owing to its high **osmolarity** and high index of refraction.

tremor: an unintentional, somewhat rhythmic, to-and-fro **muscle** movement (oscillations) involving one or more parts of the body; it is the most common of all involuntary movements and can affect the **hands**, **arms**, **head**, face, vocal cords, trunk, and legs; most tremors occur in the hands; in some people, tremor is a symptom of another neurological disorder.

triphenylmethane: a biological dye (stain).

trypan blue: a vital stain that is used to color dead **tissues** or **cells** blue; it is a diazo dye; live cells or tissues with intact cell **membranes** will not be colored; since cells are very selective in the compounds that pass through the membrane, in a viable cell trypan blue is not absorbed it traverses the membrane in a dead cell, hence, dead cells are shown as a distinctive blue color under a microscope.

tryptophan: a colorless, crystalline, aromatic essential amino acid that occurs in the seeds of some leguminous plants; it is released from proteins by tryptic digestion and is important in the nutrition of animals.

tubular structure: a structure consisting of tubes.

tumor: an abnormal or diseased swelling in any part of the body, especially a more or less circumscribed overgrowth of new **tissue** that is autonomous, differs more or less in structure from the part in which it grows, and serves no useful purpose; **neoplasm**.

tympanic membrane: a **membrane** separating the tympanium or middle ear from the passage of the external ear; eardrum.

type I collagen: the most abundant **collagen** of the human body; it is present in **scar tissue**, the end product when tissue heals by repair; it is found in **tendons**, the endomysium of **myofibrils** and the organic part of **bone**.

tyrosine: a crystalline amino acid that results from the hydrolysis of proteins.

ulcer: a sore open either to the surface of the body or to a natural cavity, and accompanied by the disintegration of **tissue**, the formation of pus, etc.

ultrasound gel: a viscous gel for medical ultrasound transmission used for diagnostic and therapeutic ultrasound applications; acoustically corrects US energy transmission for frequencies used.

unsaturated fatty acid: a **fatty acid** in which there are one or more double bonds in the fatty acid chain; a fat molecule is **monounsaturated** if it contains one double bond, and polyunsaturated if it contains more than one double bond; where double bonds are formed, hydrogen atoms are eliminated; thus, a saturated fat is "saturated" with hydrogen atoms; the greater the degree of unsaturation in a fatty acid (i.e., the more double bonds in the fatty acid), the more vulnerable it is to lipid peroxidation (rancidity); antioxidants can protect unsaturated fat from lipid peroxidation; unsaturated fats also have a more enlarged shape than saturated fats.

urea: an organic compound of carbon, nitrogen, **oxygen**, and hydrogen, with the formula CON_2H_4 or $(NH_2)_2CO$; urea is also known as carbamide.

urinary bladder: a sac for storing **urine**; it is a diverticulum of the hindgut; urine is conducted to the **bladder** by a ureter; the exit to the bladder is closed by a sphincter **muscle**.

urine: a yellowish, slightly acid, watery fluid; waste matter excreted by the **kidneys**.

urocanic acid: 4-imidazoleacrylic acid, found in the **skin epidermis**; it has high absorption in the UV range with a peak at 260 nm.

uroporphyrin: any of several porphyrins produced by oxidation of uroporphyrinogen; one or more are excreted in excess in the **urine** in several of the porphyries.

uterine: of or to do with the **uterus**, e.g., the uterine walls.

uterus: an organ in which an embryo develops and is nourished; it has walls of unstriated **muscle** that increase greatly in thickness during pregnancy and whose contractions expel the fetus at birth; the uterus is lined with endometrium, which undergoes modification during pregnancy and is also modified under control of sex hormones during the estrus cycle; the uterus is connected through the **cervix** to the vagina.

UV skin filter: a **sunscreen cream** or lotion based on chemical formulations and/or reflecting nanoparticles that filter broadband UV radiation and helps shield the **skin** from the UVA and UVB rays that do skin damage every day.

vacuole: (1) a cavity within a **cell**, often containing a watery liquid or secretion; (2) a minute cavity or vesicle in organic **tissue**.

valve: a structure that allows fluids to flow through it in one direction only; this is done by closing the vessel, or canal, to stop backward flow [see **lymphatic (lymph) vessels**].

vascularization: consisting of or containing **vessels** that conduct **blood** and **lymph**.

vascular: related to **vessels**.

vasculature: arrangement of **blood vessels** in the body or in an organ or body part; the **vascular** network of an organ.

vasoconstriction: constriction of the **blood** or **lymph vessels**, as by the action of a **nerve**.

vasodilation: where **blood vessels** in the body become wider following the relaxation of the smooth **muscle** in the vessel wall; this reduces blood pressure—since there is more room for the blood; vasodilation also occurs in superficial blood vessels of warm-blooded animals when their ambient environment is hot; this process diverts the flow of heated blood to the skin of the animal, where heat can be more easily released into the atmosphere; the opposite physiological process is **vasoconstriction**.

vehicles: the nonliving means of transportation; pertaining to transportation of drugs by various solutes.

vein: a **blood vessel** that conducts **blood** from the **tissues** and organs back to the **heart**; the vein is lined with **endothelium** (smooth flat cells) and surrounded by muscular and **fibrous tissue**; the walls are thin and the diameter large compared with an **artery**; the vein contains **valves** that allow blood to flow only toward the heart.

vein *femoralis* **(femoral)**: the vein pertaining to the thigh or femur.

ventricle: a chamber in **brain** or **heart**; in a heart a chamber that collects **blood** from an **atrium** (another heart chamber that is smaller than a ventricle) and pumps it out of the heart.

venule: a small **vein** that collects **blood** from **capillaries**; it joins other venules to form a vein; a venule has more **connective tissue** than a capillary **muscle**; the permeability of the venule wall to blood is similar to that of a capillary wall.

verografin: a water-soluble colorless liquid usually used at concentrations of 60% or 76% as an intravenous x-ray contrasting agent; very good agent for **optical clearing** of **fibrous tissue**, owing to its high **osmolarity** and high index of refraction; an analog of **trazograph**.

vesicle: a relatively small and enclosed compartment, separated from the **cytosol** by at least one **lipid bilayer**; if there is only one lipid bilayer, they are called unilamellar vesicles; otherwise they are called multilamellar; vesicles store, transport, or digest cellular products and waste.

vessel: a tube or duct, such as an **artery** or **vein**, containing or conveying **blood** or some other body fluid.

videokeratoscope: a keratoscope fitted with a video camera; keratoscope is an instrument marked with lines or circles by means of which the corneal reflex can be observed.

visual acuity: acuteness or clearness of vision, especially form vision, which is dependent on the sharpness of the **retinal** focus within the **eye**, the sensitivity of the nervous elements, and the interpretative faculty of the **brain**.

vital activity (function): any function of the body, **tissue**, **cell**, etc., that is essential for life.

vitality: the peculiarity distinguishing the living from the nonliving; capacity to live and develop.

vitreopathy: a pathology of vitreous body.

vitreous humor: the transparent gelatinous substance filling the **eyeball** behind the **crystalline lens**, called vitreous body.

vocal chord: either of the two pairs of folds of **mucous membrane** projecting into the cavity of the **larynx**.

volar: pertaining to both the **palm** and sole of feet.

volatile solvents: liquids that vaporize at room temperature; these organic solvents can be inhaled for psychoactive effects and are present in many domestic and industrial products such as glue, aerosol, paints, industrial solvents, lacquer thinners, gasoline, and cleaning fluids; some substances are directly toxic to the **liver**, **kidney**, or **heart**, and some produce peripheral neuropathy (nerve damage usually affecting the feet and legs) or progressive **brain** degeneration.

white blood cell (WBC) (leukocyte): a nucleated, motile, colorless cell found in the **blood** and **lymph** of animals; it contains no respiratory pigments; it is either a **lymphocyte**, a **polymorph**, or a **monocyte**; in humans, there are approximately 8000 WBCs per cubic millimeter.

white fibers: see **white fibrous tissue**.

white fibrous tissue: a **connective tissue** that consists of a matrix of very fine, white wavy fibers arranged parallel to each other, in bundles and unbranching, with **fibroblasts** embedded in the bundle; the tissue is tough and inelastic; it is found pure in **tendons**; the **white fibers** are composed of **collagen**.

white matter: the **nervous tissue** found in the central nervous system; it consists of tracts of medullated **nerve** fibers in the **brain** and spinal cord; it also contains **blood vessels** and **neuroglia**; it is mainly external to **gray matter**, but is internal to **gray matter** in the cerebral hemispheres and in the **cerebellum**; the medullated fibers give the tissue its shiny white appearance.

WHO: World Health Organization.

whole blood: **blood** that contains all its natural components: **blood, cells**, and **plasma**.

Wister rat: an animal strain widely used in experimental studies.

wound: a type of physical **trauma** wherein the **skin** is torn, cut, or punctured (an open wound), or where blunt force trauma causes a contusion (a closed wound); in pathology, it specifically refers to a sharp **injury** that damages the **dermis** of the skin.

wrinkle: a ridge or crease of a surface; usually refers to the skin of an organism; in skin a wrinkle or fold may be permanent; skin wrinkles typically appear as a result of the aging processes such as glycation or, temporarily, as the result of prolonged (more than a few minutes) immersion in water; wrinkling in skin is caused by habitual facial expressions, aging, sun damage, smoking, poor **hydration**, and various other factors.

wrist: in human anatomy, the wrist is the flexible and is a narrowing connection between the **forearm** and the **hand**; the wrist is essentially a double row of small short **bone**s, called carpals, intertwined to form a malleable hinge.

yellow fibers: see **yellow elastic tissue**.

yellow elastic tissue: a **connective tissue** that consists of a matrix of coarse **yellow elastic fibers** that branch regularly and anastomosely with **fibroblasts** in the matrix; **elastin** is the principal constituent of this tissue; the tissue rarely occurs in a pure form, usually containing **white fibers**; yellow elastic fibers are numerous in the **lungs** and in the walls of **arteries**, where elastic supporting tissues are required; yellow elastic tissue occurs in ligaments, where an extensible tissue is required.

Yucatan micropigs: strain of hairless small animals widely used in experimental studies.

Sources

This glossary was compiled using mostly Refs. 2, 7, 26, 57, and the following

1. *Webster's New Universal Unabridged Dictionary*, Barnes & Noble Books, New York, 1994.
2. A. Godman and E. M. F. Payne, *Longman Dictionary of Scientific Usage*, reprint edition, Longman Group, Harlow, UK, 1979.

3. *Stedman's Medical Dictionary*, Williams & Wilkins, Baltimore, MD, 1995.

4. K. Jimbow, W. C. Quevedo, T. B. Fitzpatrick, and G. Szabo, "Biology of Melaninocytes," in *Dermatology in General Medicine*, T. B. Fitzpatrick, A. Z. Eisen, K. Wolff, I. M. Freedberg, and K. F. Austen (eds.), McGraw-Hill, New York, 1993, pp. 261–288.

5. http://en.wikipedia.org

6. http://www.medterms.com

7. http://www.disabled-world.com/artman/publish/glossary.shtml

8. http://cancerweb.ncl.ac.uk/cgi-bin/omd?action=Home&query=

9. http://www.online-medical-dictionary.org/link.asp

10. http://www.stedmans.com/

References

1. G. Müller, B. Chance, R. Alfano, et al. (eds.), *Medical Optical Tomography: Functional Imaging and Monitoring*, vol. IS11, SPIE Press, Bellingham, WA, 1993.

2. G. Müller and A. Roggan (eds.), *Laser-Induced Interstitial Thermotherapy*, vol. PM25, SPIE Press, Bellingham, WA, 1995.

3. V. V. Tuchin (ed.), *Selected Papers on Tissue Optics: Applications in Medical Diagnostics and Therapy*, vol. MS102, SPIE Press, Bellingham, WA, 1994.

4. B. Chance, M. Cope, E. Gratton, N. Ramanujam, and B. Tromberg, "Phase Measurement of Light Absorption and Scatter in Human Tissue," *Rev. Sci. Instrum.*, vol. 69, no. 10, 1998, pp. 3457–3481.

5. A. V. Priezzhev, V. V. Tuchin, L. P. Shubochkin, *Laser Diagnostics in Biology and Medicine*, Nauka, Moscow, 1989.

6. V. V. Tuchin, *Lasers and Fiber Optics in Biomedical Science*, Saratov Univ. Press, Saratov, 1998.

7. A. Katzir, *Lasers and Optical Fibers in Medicine*, Academic Press, San Diego, 1993.

8. V. V. Tuchin and J. A. Izatt (eds.), *Coherence Domain Optical Methods in Biomedical Science and Clinical Applications II, III, Proc. SPIE* 3251, 1998; 3598 (1999).

9. V. V. Tuchin, "Lasers and Fiber Optics in Biomedicine," *Laser Physics*, vol. 3, 1993, pp. 767–820; 925–950.

10. V. V. Tuchin, "Lasers Light Scattering in Biomedical Diagnostics and Therapy," *J. Laser Appl.*, vol. 5, nos. 2, 3, 1993, pp. 43–60.

11. D. H. Sliney and S. L. Trokel, *Medical Lasers and Their Safe Use*, Academic Press, New York, 1993.

12. L. E. Preuss and A. E. Profio (eds.), "Special Section on Optical Properties of Mammalian Tissue," *Appl. Opt.*, vol. 28, no. 12, 1989, pp. 2207–2357.

13. J. M. Shmitt, A. Knüttel, and R. F. Bonnar, "Measurement of Optical Properties of Biological Tissues by Low-Coherence Reflectometry," *Appl. Opt.*, vol. 32, 1993, pp. 6032–6042.

14. "Special Section on Lasers in Biology and Medicine," *IEEE J. Quantum Electr.*, vol. 20, no. 12, 1984, pp. 1342–1532; vol. 23, no. 10, 1987, pp. 1701–1855; vol. 26, no. 12, 1990, pp. 2146–2308.

15. O. Minet, G. Mueller, and J. Beuthan (eds.), *Selected Papers on Optical Tomography, Fundamentals and Applications in Medicine*, vol. MS 147, SPIE Press, Bellingham, 1998.

16. A. Katzir (ed.), "Special Section on Biomedical Optics," *Opt. Eng.*, vol. 31, no. 7, 1992, pp. 1399–1486; vol. 32, no. 2, 1993, pp. 216–367.

17. H. Podbielska, C. K. Hitzenberger, and V. V. Tuchin (eds.), "Special Section on Interferometry in Biomedicine," *J. Biomed. Opt.*, vol. 3, no. 1, 1998, pp. 5–79; no. 3, 1998, pp. 225–266.

18. V. V. Tuchin, H. Podbielska, C. K. Hitzenberger (eds.), "Special Section on Coherence Domain Optical Methods in Biomedical Science and Clinics," *J. Biomed. Opt.*, vol. 4, no. 1, 1999, pp. 94–190.

19. T. J. Dougherty (ed.), "Special Issue on Photodynamic Therapy," *J. Clin. Laser Med. Surg.*, vol. 14, 1996, pp. 219–348.

20. V. S. Letokhov, "Laser Biology and Medicine," *Nature*, vol. 316, no. 6026, 1985, pp. 325–328.

21. J. M. Brunetaud, V. Maunoury, and D. Cochelard, "Lasers in Digestive Endoscopy," *J. Biomed. Opt.*, vol. 2, no. 1, 1997, pp. 42–52.

22. A. V. Priezzhev, T. Asakura, and J. D. Briers, *Optical Diagnostics of Biological Fluids III, Proc. SPIE* 3252, 1998.

23. J. G. Fujimoto and M. S. Patterson (eds.), *Advances in Optical Imaging and Photon Migration, OSA Trends in Optics and Photonics*, vol. 21, Optical Society of America, Washington, DC, 1998.

24. V. V. Tuchin, "Light Scattering Study of Tissues," *Physics—Uspekhi*, vol. 40, no. 5, 1997, pp. 495–515.

25. V. P. Zharov and V. S. Letokhov, *Laser Opto-Acoustic Spectroscopy*, Springer-Verlag, New York, 1989.

26. S. Bown, G. Buonaccorsi (eds.), "Special Issue on VI Biennial Meeting of the International Photodynamic Association," *Lasers Med. Sci.*, vol. 12, no. 3, 1997, pp. 180–284.

27. H. J. Geschwind, "Recent Developments in Laser Cardiac Surgery," *J. Biomed. Opt.*, vol. 1, no. 1, 1996, pp. 28–30.

28. W. Rudolph and M. Kempe, "Topical Review: Trends in Optical Biomedical Imaging," *J. Modern Opt.*, vol. 44, no. 9, 1997, pp. 1617–1642.

29. G. J. Mueller and D. H. Sliney (eds.), *Dosimetry of Laser Radiation in Medicine and Biology*, vol. IS5, SPIE Press, Bellingham, WA, 1989.

30. A. Mahadevan-Jansen and R. Richards-Kortum, "Raman Spectroscopy for Detection of Cancers and Precancers," *J. Biomed. Opt.*, vol. 1, no. 1, 1996, pp. 31–70.

31. B. B. Das, F. Liu, and R R. Alfano, "Time-Resolved Fluorescence and Photon Migration Studies in Biomedical and Random Media," *Rep. Prog. Phys.*, vol. 60, 1997, pp. 227–292.

32. M. Motamedi (ed.), "Special Section on Photon Migration in Tissue and Biomedical Applications of Lasers," *Appl. Opt.*, vol. 32, 1993, pp. 367–434.

33. A. Yodh, B. Tromberg, E. Sevick-Muraca, and D. Pine (eds.), "Special Section on Diffusing Photons in Turbid Media," *Appl. Opt.*, vol. 36, 1997, pp. 9–231.

34. T. Durduran, A. G. Yodh, B. Chance, and D. A. Boas, "Does the Photon-Diffusion Coefficient Depend on Absorption?" *J. Opt. Soc. Am. A*, vol. 14, no. 12, 1997, pp. 3358–3365.

35. D. Kessel (ed.), *Selected Papers on Photodynamic Therapy*, vol. MS82, SPIE Press, Bellingham, WA, 1993.

36. S. L. Jacques, "Strengths and Weaknesses of Various Optical Imaging Techniques," Saratov Fall Meeting'01, Internet Plenary Lecture, Saratov, Russia, 2001, http://optics.sgu.ru/SFM.

37. M. J. C. van Gemert, S. L. Jacques, H. J. C. M. Sterenborg, and W. M. Star, "Skin Optics," *IEEE Tranc. Biomed. Eng.*, vol. 36, no. 12, 1989, pp. 1146–1154.

38. M. J. C. van Gemert, J. S. Nelson, T. E. Milner, et al., "Non-Invasive Determination of Port Wine Stain Anatomy and Physiology for Optimal Laser Treatment Strategies," *Phys. Med. Biol.*, vol. 42, 1997, pp. 937–949.

39. H. J. C. M. Sterenborg, M. J. C. van Gemert, W. Kamphorst, et al., "The Spectral Dependence of the Optical Properties of Human Brain," *Lasers Med. Sci.*, vol. 4, 1989, pp. 221–227.

40. W.-F. Cheong, S. A. Prahl, and A. J. Welch, "A Review of the Optical Properties of Biological Tissues," *IEEE J. Quantum Electr.*, vol. 26, no. 12. 1990, pp. 2166–2185. Updated by W.-F. Cheong, further additions by L. Wang and S. L. Jacques, August 6, 1993.

41. S. L. Jacques, "Monte Carlo Modeling of Light Transport in Tissues," in *Tissue Optics*, A. J. Welch and M. C. J. van Gemert (eds.), Academic Press, New York, 1992.

42. H. Niemz, *Laser-Tissue Interactions. Fundamentals and Applications*, Springer-Verlag, Berlin, 1996.

43. R. G. Johnston, S. B. Singham, and G. C. Salzman, "Polarized Light Scattering," *Comments Mol. Cell. Biophys.*, vol. 5, no. 3, 1988, pp. 171–192.

44. J. R. Lakowicz (ed.), *Time-Resolved Laser Spectroscopy in Biochemistry, Proc. SPIE* 1204, Pt. 1-2, 1990.

45. V. V. Tuchin, H. Podbielska, and B. Ovryn (eds.), *Coherence-Domain Methods in Biomedical Science and Clinical Applications, Proc. SPIE* 2981, 1997.

46. A. Kienle, L. Lilge, M. S. Patterson, R. Hibst, R. Steiner, and B. C. Wilson, "Spatially Resolved Absolute Diffuse Reflectance Measurements for Noninvasive Determination of the Optical Scattering and Absorption Coefficients of Biological Tissue," *Appl. Opt.*, vol. 35, no. 13, 1996, pp. 2304–2314.

47. J. R. Mourant, I. J. Bigio, J. Boyer, et al., "Elastic Scattering Spectroscopy as a Diagnostic Tool for Differentiating Pathologies in the Gastrointestinal Tract: Preliminary Testing," *J. Biomed. Opt.*, vol. 1, no. 2, 1996, pp. 192–199.

48. A. Roggan, M. Friebel, K. Dorschel, A. Hahn, and G. Mueller, "Optical Properties of Circulating Human Blood in the Wavelength Range 400–2500 nm," *J. Biomed. Opt.*, vol. 4, no. 1, 1999, pp. 36–46.

49. A. M. K. Nilsson, G. W. Lucassen, W. Verkruysse, S. Andersson-Engels, and M. J. C. van Gemert, "Changes in Optical Properties of Human Whole Blood *In Vitro* Due to Slow Heating," *Photochem. Photobiology*, vol. 65, no. 2, 1997, pp. 366–373.

50. F. A. Marks, "Optical Determination of the Hemoglobin Oxygenation State of Breast Biopsies and Human Breast Cancer Xenografts in Unde Mice," *Proc. SPIE* 1641, 1992, pp. 227–237.

51. M. Bassani, F. Martelli, G. Zaccanti, and D. Contini, "Independence of the Diffusion Coefficient from Absorption: Experimental and Numerical Evidence," *Opt. Lett.*, vol. 22, 1997, pp. 853–855.

52. M. S. Patterson, "Noninvasive Measurement of Tissue Optical Properties: Current Status and Future Prospects," *Comments Mol. Cell. Biophys.*, vol. 8, 1995, pp. 387–417.

53. B. Chance, K. Kang, L. He, H. Liu, and S. Zhou, "Precision Localization of Hidden Absorbers in Body Tissues with Phased-Array Optical Systems," *Rev. Sci, Instrum.*, vol. 67, 1996, pp. 4324–4332.

54. H. J. S. M. Sterenborg and J. C. Van der Leun, "Change in Epidermal Transmission Due to UV-Induced Hyperplasia in Hairless Mice: a First Approximation of the Action Spectrum," *Photodermatology*, vol. 5, 1988, pp. 71–82.

55. M. Ferrari, D. Delpy, and D. A. Benaron (eds.), "Special Section on Clinical Near Infrared Spectroscopy/Imaging," *J. Biomed. Opt.*, vol. 1, no. 4, 1996, pp. 361–434; vol. 2, no. 1, 1997, pp. 7–41; no. 2, pp. 147–175.

56. G. Yoon, A. J. Welch, M. Motamedi, et al., "Development and Application of Three-Dimensional Light Distribution Model for Laser Irradiated Tissue," *IEEE J. Quantum Electr.*, vol. 23, no. 10, 1987, pp. 1721–1733.

57. R. R. Anderson and J. A. Parrish, "Optical Properties of Human Skin," in *The Science of Photomedicine*, J. D. Regan and J. A. Parrish (eds.), Plenum Press, New York, 1982, pp. 147–194.

58. A. Dunn, C. Smithpeter, A. J. Welch, and R. Richards-Kortum, "Finite-Difference Time-Domain Simulation of Light Scattering from Single Cells," *J. Biomed. Opt.*, vol. 2, no. 3, 1997, pp. 262–266.

59. J. M. Schmitt, A. H. Gandjbakhche, and R. F. Bonnar, "Use of Polarized Light to Discriminate Short-Photons in a Multiply Scattering Medium," *Appl. Opt.*, vol. 31, 1992, pp. 6535–6546.

60. B. V. Bronk, W. P. van de Merwe, and M. Stanley, "*In Vivo* Measure of Average Bacterial Cell Size From a Polarized Light Scattering Function," *Cytometry*, vol. 13, 1992, pp. 155–162.

61. V. V. Bakutkin, I. L. Maksimova, P. I. Saprykin, V. V. Tuchin, and L. P. Shubochkin, "Light Scattering by the Human Eye Sclera," *J. Appl. Spectrosc. (USSR)*, vol. 46, no. 1, 1987, pp. 104–107.

62. I. L. Maksimova, V. V. Tuchin, and L. P. Shubochkin, "Light Propagation in Anisotropic Biological Objects," in *Laser Beams*, Khabarovsk Technical Inst. Press, Khabarovsk, USSR, 1985, pp. 91–95.

63. I. L. Maksimova, V. V. Tuchin, L. P. Shubochkin, "Polarization Features of Eye's Cornea," *Opt. Spectrosc. (USSR)*, vol. 60, no. 4, 1986, pp. 801–807.

64. I. L. Maksimova, V. V. Tuchin, and L. P. Shubochkin, "Light Scattering Matrix of Crystalline Lens," *Opt. Spectrosc. (USSR)*, vol. 65, no. 3, 1988, pp. 615–619.

65. G. B. Altshuler and V. N. Grisimov, "Effect of Waveguide Transport of Light in Human Tooth," *USSR Acad. Sci. Reports*, vol. 310, no. 5, 1990, pp. 1245–1248.

66. J. R. Zijp and J. J. ten Bosch, "Angular Dependence of He-Ne-Laser Light Scattering by Bovine Human Dentine," *Archs Oral Biol.*, vol. 36, no. 4, 1991, pp. 283–289.

67. A. V. Priezzhev, V. V. Tuchin, and L. P. Shubochkin, "Laser Microdiagnostics of Eye Optical Tissues and Form Elements of Blood," *Bullet. USSR Acad. Sci., Phys. Ser.*, vol. 53, no. 8, 1989, pp. 1490–1495.

68. I. L. Maksimova, A. P. Mironychev, S. V. Romanov, et al., "Methods and Equipment for Laser Diagnostics in Ophthalmology," *Bullet. USSR Acad. Sci., Phys. Ser.*, vol. 54, no. 10, 1990, pp. 1918–1923.

69. A. N. Korolevich, A. Ya. Khairulina, and L. P. Shubochkin, "Scattering Matrix of a Monolayer of Optically "Soft" Particles at their Dense Package," *Opt. Spectrosc. (USSR)*, vol. 68, 1990, pp. 403–409.

70. E. E. Gorodnichev and D. B. Rogozkin, "Small Angle Multiple Scattering in Random Inhomogeneous Media, *JETP*, vol. 107, 1995, pp. 209–235.

71. H. Rinneberg, "Scattering of Laser Light in Turbid media, Optical Tomography for Medical Diagnostics," in *The Inverse Problem*, H. Lübbig (ed.), Akademie Verlag, Berlin, 1995, pp. 107–141.

72. A. J. Welch and M. C. J. van Gemert (eds.), *Tissue Optics*, Academic Press, New York, 1992.

73. V. L. Kuzmin and V. P. Romanov, "Coherent Effects at Light Scattering in Disordered Systems," *Physics—Uspekhi*, vol. 166, no. 3, 1996, pp. 247–278.

74. K. M. Yoo, F. Liu, and R R. Alfano, "Biological Materials Probed by the Temporal and Angular Profiles of the Backscattered Ultrafast Laser Pulses," *J. Opt. Soc. Am. B.*, vol. 7, 1990, pp. 1685–1693.

75. S. M. Rytov, Yu. A. Kravtsov, and V. I. Tatarskii, *Wave Propagation through Random Media*, vol. 4 of *Principles of Statistical Radiophysics*, Springer-Verlag, Berlin, 1989.

76. V. V. Tuchin (ed.), SPIE CIS Selected Papers: *Coherence-Domain Methods in Biomedical Optics*, vol. 2732, SPIE Press, 1996.

77. V. V. Tuchin, "Coherence-Domain Methods in Tissue and Cell Optics," *Laser Physics*, vol. 8, no. 4, 1998, pp. 807–849.

78. H. Z. Cummins and E. R. Pike (eds.), *Photon Correlation and Light Beating Spectroscopy*, Plenum Press, New York, 1974.

79. H. Z. Cummins and E. R. Pike (eds.), *Photon Correlation Spectroscopy and Velocimetry*, Plenum Press, New York, 1977.

80. M. H. Kao, A. G. Yodh, and D. J. Pine, "Observation of Brownian Motion on the Time Scale of Hydrodynamic Interactions," *Phys. Rev. Lett.*, vol. 70, 1993, pp. 242–245.

81. P. D. Kaplan, A. D. Dinsmore, A. G. Yodh, and D. J. Pine, "Diffuse-Transmission Spectroscopy: a Structural Probe of Opaque Colloidal Mixtures," *Phys. Rev. E.*, vol. 50, 1994, pp. 4827–4835.

82. J. D. Briers, "Laser Doppler and Time-Varying Speckle: a Reconciliation," *J. Opt. Soc. Am. A.*, vol. 13, 1996, pp. 345–350.

83. J. D. Briers and S. Webster, "Laser Speckle Contrast Analysis (LASCA): a Nonscanning, Full-Field Technique for Monitoring Capillary Blood Flow," *J. Biomed. Opt.*, vol. 1, 1996, pp. 174–179.

84. A. F. Fercher, "Optical Coherence Tomography," *J. Biomed. Opt.*, vol. 1, 1996, pp. 157–173.

85. B. Beauvoit, T. Kitai, H. Liu, and B. Chance, "Time-Resolved Spectroscopy of Mitochondria, Cells, and Rat Tissues under Normal and Pathological Conditions," *Proc. SPIE* 2326, 1994, pp. 127–136.

86. A. R. Young, "Chromophores in Human Skin," *Phys. Med. Biol.*, vol. 42, 1997, pp. 789–802.

87. F. A. Duck, *Physical Properties of Tissue: a Comprehensive Reference Book*, Academic Press, London, 1990.

88. B. Chance (ed.), *Photon Migration in Tissue*, Plenum Press, New York, 1989.

89. K. Frank and M. Kessler (eds.), *Quantitative Spectroscopy in Tissue*, PMI Verlag, Frankfurt am Main, 1992.

90. B. W. Henderson and T. J. Dougherty (eds.), *Photodynamic Therapy: Basic Principles and Clinical Applications*, Marcel-Dekker, New York, 1992.

91. H.-P. Berlien and G. J. Mueller (eds.), *Applied Laser Medicine*, Springer-Verlag, Berlin, 2003.

92. N. N. Zhadin and R. R. Alfano, "Correction of the Internal Absorption Effect in Fluorescence Emission and Excitation Spectra from Absorbing and Highly Scattering Media: Theory and Experiment," *J. Biomed. Opt.*, vol. 3, no. 2, 1998, pp. 171–186.

93. A. Kienle, M. S. Patterson, N. Dognitz, R. Bays, G. Wagnieres, and H. van de Bergh, "Noninvasive Determination of the Optical Properties of Two-Layered Turbid Medium," *Appl. Opt.*, vol. 37, 1998, pp. 779–791.

94. J. R. Mourant, J. Boyer, A. H. Hielscher, and I. J. Bigio, "Influence of the Scattering Phase Function on Light Transport Measurements in Turbid Media Performed with Small Source-Detector Separations," *Opt. Lett.*, vol. 21, no. 7, 1996, pp. 546–548.

95. J. R. Mourant, J. P. Freyer, A. H. Hielscher, A. A. Eick, D. Shen, and T. M. Johnson, "Mechanisms of Light Scattering from Biological Cells Relevant to Noninvasive Optical-Tissue Diagnostics," *Appl. Opt.*, vol. 37, 1998, pp. 3586–3593.

96. R. Drezek, A. Dunn, and R. Richards-Kortum, "Light Scattering from Cells: Finite-Difference Time-Domain Simulations and Goniometric Measurements," *Appl. Opt.*, vol. 38, no. 16, 1999, pp. 3651–3661.

97. J. R. Zijp and J. J. ten Bosch, "Anisotropy of Volume-Backscattered Light," *Appl. Opt.*, vol. 36, 1997, pp. 1671–1680.

98. H. Moseley (ed.), "Special Issue on Optical Radiation Technique in Medicine and Biology," *Phys. Med. Biol.*, vol. 24, 1997, pp. 759–996.

99. M. D. Morris (ed.), "Special Section on Biomedical Applications of Vibrational Spectroscopic Imaging," *J. Biomed. Opt.*, vol. 4, 1999, pp. 6–34.

100. K. Okada and T. Hamaoka, "Special Section on Medical Near-Infrared Spectroscopy," *J. Biomed. Opt.*, vol. 4, 1999, pp. 391–428.

101. A. V. Priezzhev and T. Asakura (eds.), "Special Section on Optical Diagnostics of Biological Fluids," *J. Biomed. Opt.*, vol. 4, 1999, pp. 35–93.

102. J. M. Schmitt, "Optical Coherence Tomography (OCT): a Review," *IEEE J. Select. Tops Quant. Electr.*, vol. 5, 1999, pp. 1205–1215.

103. D. Benaron, I. Bigio, E. Sevick-Muraca, and A. G. Yodh (eds.), "Special Issue Honoring Professor Britton Chance," *J. Biomed. Opt.*, vol. 5, 2000, pp. 115–248; pp. 269–282.

104. A. Carden and M. D. Morris, "Application of Vibration Spectroscopy to the Study of Mineralized Tissues (review)," *J. Biomed. Opt.*, vol. 5, 2000, pp. 259–268.

105. R. J. McNichols and G. L. Coté, "Optical Glucose Sensing in Biological Fluids: an Overview," *J. Biomed. Opt.*, vol. 5, 2000, pp. 5–16.

106. L. Beloussov, F.-A. Popp, V. L. Voeikov, and R. van Wijk (eds.), *Biophotonics and Coherent Systems*, Moscow Univ. Press, Moscow, 2000.

107. R. K. Wang, "Modelling Optical Properties of Soft tissue by Fractal Distribution of Scatterers," *J. Modern Opt.*, vol. 47, no. 1, 2000, pp. 103–120.

108. J. G. Fujimoto, W. Drexler, U. Morgner, F. Kartner, and E. Ippen, "Optical Coherence Tomography: High Resolution Imaging Using Echoes of Light," *Optics & Photonics News*, January, 2000, pp. 24–31.

109. J. G. Fujimoto and M. E. Brezinski, "Optical Coherence Tomography Imaging," in *Biomedical Photonics Handbook*, Tuan Vo-Dinh (ed.), CRC Press, Boca Rotan, Florida, 2003, pp. 13-1–29.

110. J. Welzel, "Optical Coherence Tomography in Dermatology: a Review," *Skin Res. Technol.*, vol. 7, 2001, pp. 1–9.

111. A. M. Sergeev, L. S. Dolin, and D. H. Reitze, "Optical Tomography of Biotissues: Past, Present, and Future," *Optics & Photonics News*, July, 2001, pp. 28–35.

112. J. D. Briers, "Laser Doppler, Speckle and Related Techniques for Blood Perfusion Mapping and Imaging," *Physiol. Meas.*, vol. 22, 2001, pp. R35–R66.

113. W. V. Meyer, A. E. Smart, and R. G. W. Brown (eds.), "Special Issue on Photon Correlation and Scattering," *Appl. Opt.*, vol. 40, no. 24, 2001, pp. 3965–4242.

114. P. T. C. So, C. Y. Dong, B. R. Masters, and K. M. Berland, "Two-Photon Excitation Fluorescence Microscopy," in *Annual Review of Biomedical Engineering*, Annual Reviews, Palo Alto, CA. 2000.

115. R. K. Wang, J. C. Hebden, and V. V. Tuchin, "Special Issue on Recent Developments in Biomedical Optics," *Phys. Med. Biol.*, vol. 49, no. 7, 2004, pp. 1085–1368.

116. V. V. Tuchin, J. A. Izatt, and J. G. Fujimoto (eds.), *Coherence Domain Optical Methods in Biomedical Science and Clinical Applications IV-VIII, Proc. SPIE* 3915, 2000; 4251, 2001; 4619, 2002; 4956, 2003; 5316, 2004; *Coherence Domain Optical Methods and Optical Coherence Tomography in Biomedicine IX, X, Proc. SPIE* 5690, 2005; 6079, 2006.

117. V. V. Tuchin, and D. A. Zimnyakov, and A. B. Pravdin (eds.), *Saratov Fall Meeting, Optical Technologies in Biophysics and Medicine, Proc. SPIE* 4001, 2000.

118. V. V. Tuchin (ed.), *Saratov Fall Meeting, Optical Technologies in Biophysics and Medicine II-VII, Proc. SPIE* 4241, 2001; 4707, 2002; 5068, 2003; 5474, 2004; 5771, 2005; 6163, 2006; 6535, 2007.

119. A. Periasamy (ed.), *Methods in Cellular Imaging*, Oxford University Press, New York, 2001.

120. D. B. Murphy, *Fundamentals of Light Microscopy and Electronic Imaging*, Wiley-Liss, New York, 2001.

121. P. Sebbah (ed.), *Waves and Imaging through Complex Media*, Kluwer Academic Publishers, New York, 2001.

122. A. Diaspro (ed.), *Confocal and Two-Photon Microscopy: Foundations, Applications, and Advances*, Wiley-Liss, New York, 2002.

123. J. M. Chalmers and P. R. Grifiths (eds.), *Handbook of Vibrational Spectroscopy*, John Wiley & Sons, Chichester, 2002.

124. Q. Luo, B. Chance, and V. V. Tuchin (eds.), *Photonics and Imaging in Biology and Medicine, Proc. SPIE* 4536, Bellingham, WA, 2002.

125. Q. Luo, V. V. Tuchin, M. Gu, L. V. Wang (eds.), *Photonics and Imaging in Biology and Medicine, Proc. SPIE* 5254, Bellingham, WA, 2003.

126. B. Masters (ed.), *Selected Papers on Optical Low-Coherence Reflectometry and Tomography*, vol. MS165, SPIE Press, Bellingham, WA, 2002.

127. B. E. Bouma and G. J. Tearney (eds.), *Handbook of Optical Coherence Tomography*, Marcel-Dekker, New York, 2002.

128. D. R. Vij and K. Mahesh (eds.) *Lasers in Medicine*, Kluwer Academic Publishers, Boston, Dordrecht, and London, 2002.

129. V. V. Tuchin (ed.), *Handbook of Optical Biomedical Diagnostics*, vol. PM107, SPIE Press, Bellingham, WA, 2002.

130. Tuan Vo-Dinh (ed.), *Biomedical Photonics Handbook*, CRC Press, Boca Raton, 2003.

131. B. R. Masters (ed.), *Selected Papers on Multiphoton Excitation Microscopy*, vol. MS175, SPIE Press, Bellingham, WA. 2003.

132. R. G. Driggers (ed.), *Encyclopedia of Optical Engineering*, Marcel-Dekker, New York, 2003. www.dekker.com/servlet/product/productid/E-EOE/

133. U. Utzinger and R. Richards-Kortum, "Fiber-Optic Probes for Biomedical Optical Spectroscopy," *J. Biomed. Opt.*, vol. 8, 2003, pp. 121–147.

134. R. R. Alfano and B. R. Masters (eds.), *Biomedical Optical Biopsy and Optical Imaging: Classic Reprints on CD-ROM Series*, Optical Society of America, Washington, DC, 2004.

135. V. V. Tuchin, L. V. Wang, and D. A. Zimnyakov, *Optical Polarization in Biomedical Applications*, Springer-Verlag, New York, 2006.

136. V. V. Tuchin (ed.), *Coherent-Domain Optical Methods: Biomedical Diagnostics, Environmental and Material Science*, Kluwer Academic Publishers, Boston, vol. 1 & 2, 2004.

137. B. R. Masters and T. P. C. So, *Handbook of Multiphoton Excitation Microscopy and other Nonlinear Microscopies*, Oxford University Press, New York, 2004.

138. L. V. Wang, G. L. Coté, and S. L. Jacques (eds.), "Special Section on Tissue Polarimetry," *J. Biomed. Opt.*, vol. 7, no. 3, 2002, pp. 278–397.

139. D. A. Zimnyakov and V. V. Tuchin, "Optical Tomography of Tissues (overview)," *Quantum Electron.*, vol. 32, no. 10, 2002, pp. 849–867.

140. W. R. Chen, V. V. Tuchin, Q. Luo, and S. L. Jacques, "Special Issue on Biophotonics," *J. X-Ray Sci. and Technol.*, vol. 10, nos. 3-4, 2002, pp. 139–243.

141. P. French and A. I. Ferguson (eds.), "Special Issue on Biophotonics," *J. Phys. D: Appl. Phys.*, vol. 36, no. 14, 2003, pp. R207–R258; 1655–1757.

142. A. F. Fercher, W. Drexler, C. K. Hitzenberger, and T. Lasser, "Optical Coherence Tomography—Principles and Applications," *Rep. Progr. Phys.*, vol. 66, 2003, pp. 239–303.

143. E. D. Hanlon, R. Manoharan, T.-W. Koo, K. E. Shafer, J. T. Motz, M. Fitzmaurice, J. R. Kramer, I. Itzkan, R. R. Dasari, and M. S. Feld, "Prospects for *In Vivo* Raman Spectroscopy," *Phys. Med. Biol*, vol. 45, 2000, pp. R1–R59.

144. R. R. Ansari and J. Sebag (eds.), "Ophthalmic Diagnostics," *J. Biomed. Opt.*, vol. 9, no. 1, 2004, pp. 8–179.

145. M. I. Mishchenko, J. W. Hovenier, and L. D. Travis (eds.), *Light Scattering by Nonspherical Particles*, Academic Press, San Diego, 2000.

146. M. I. Mishchenko, L. D. Travis, and A. A. Lacis, *Scattering, Absorption, and Emission of Light by Small Particles*, Cambridge Univ. Press, Cambridge, 2002.

147. D. A. Zimnyakov (ed.), *Saratov Fall Meeting, Coherent Optics of Ordered and Random Media*, Proc. SPIE 4242, 2001; 4705, 2002; 5067, 2003; 5475, 2004.

148. C. F. Bohren and D. R. Huffman, *Absorption and Scattering of Light by Small Particles*, Wiley, New York, 1983.

149. G. C. Salzmann, S. B. Singham, R. G. Johnston, and C. F. Bohren, "Light Scattering and Cytometry," in *Flow Cytometry and Sorting*, 2nd ed.,

M. R. Melamed, T. Lindmo, and M. L. Mendelsohn (eds.), Wiley-Liss, New York, 1990, pp. 81–107.

150. V. Backman, R. Gurjar, K. Badizadegan, R. Dasari, I. Itzkan, L. T. Perelman, and M. S. Feld, "Polarized Light Scattering Spectroscopy for Quantitative Measurement of Epithelial Cellular Structures *In Situ*," *IEEE J. Sel. Top. Quant. Elect.*, vol. 5, 1999, pp. 1019–1027.

151. J. R. Mourant, M. Canpolat, C. Brocker, O. Esponda-Ramos, T. M. Johnson, A. Matanock, K. Stetter, and J. P. Freyer, "Light Scattering from Cell: the Contribution of the Nucleus and the Effects of Proliferative Status," *J. Biomed. Opt.*, vol. 5, no. 2, 2000, pp. 131–137.

152. J. R. Mourant, R. R. Gibson, T. M. Johnson, S. Carpenter, K. W. Short, Y. R. Yamada, and J. P. Freyer, "Methods for Measuring the Infrared Spectra of Biological Cells," *Phys. Med. Biol.*, vol. 48, 2003, pp. 243–257.

153. R. Drezek, M. Guillaud, T. Collier, I. Boiko, A. Malpica, C. Macaulay, M. Follen, and R. Richards-Kortum, "Light Scattering from Cervical Cells throughout Neoplastic Progression: Influence of Nuclear Morphology, DNA Content, and Chromatin Texture," *J. Biomed. Opt*, vol. 8, 2003, pp. 7–16.

154. J. M. Schmitt and G. Kumar, "Turbulent Nature of Refractive-Index Variations in Biological Tissue," *Opt. Lett.*, vol. 21, 1996, pp. 1310–1312.

155. D. A. Zimnyakov, V. V. Tuchin, and A. A. Mishin, "Spatial Speckle Correlometry in Applications to Tissue Structure Monitoring," *Appl. Opt.*, vol. 36, 1997, pp. 5594–5607.

156. J. M. Schmitt and G. Kumar, "Optical Scattering Properties of Soft Tissue: a Discrete Particle Model," *Appl. Opt.*, vol. 37, no. 13, 1998, pp. 2788–2797.

157. J. W. Goodman, *Statistical Optics*, Wiley-Interscience Publication, New York, 1985.

158. S. Ya. Sid'ko, V. N. Lopatin, and L. E. Paramonov, *Polarization Characteristics of Solutions of Biological Particles*, Nauka, Novosibirsk, 1990.

159. A. G. Borovoi, E. I. Naats, and U. G. Oppel, "Scattering of Light by a Red Blood Cell," *J. Biomed. Opt.*, vol. 3, no. 3, 1998, pp. 364–372.

160. M. Born and E. Wolf, *Principles of Optics*, 7th ed., Cambridge Univ., Cambridge, 1999.

161. R. D. Dyson, *Cell Biology: a Molecular Approach*, Allyn and Bacon, Boston, 1974.

162. P. Latimer, "Light Scattering and Absorption as Methods of Studying Cell Population Parameters," *Ann. Rev. Biophys. Bioeng.*, vol. 11, no. 1, 1982, pp. 129–150.

163. K. Sokolov, R. Drezek, K. Gossagee, and R. Richards-Kortum, "Reflectance Spectroscopy with Polarized Light: is it Sensitive to Cellular and Nuclear Morphology," *Opt. Express*, vol. 5, 1999, pp. 302–317.

164. A. N. Yaroslavsky, I. V. Yaroslavsky, T. Goldbach, and H.-J. Schwarzmaier, "Influence of the Scattering Phase Function Approximation on the Optical Properties of Blood Determined from the Integrating Sphere Measurements," *J. Biomed. Opt.*, vol. 4, no. 1, 1999, pp. 47–53.

165. G. Kumar and J. M. Schmitt, "Micro-Optical Properties of Tissue," *Proc. SPIE* 2679, 1996, pp. 106–116.

166. J. R. Mourant, T. M. Johnson, S. Carpenter, A. Guerra, T. Aida, and J. P. Freyer, "Polarized Angular Dependent Spectroscopy of Epithelial Cells and Epithelial Cell Nuclei to Determine the Size Scale of Scattering Structures," *J. Biomed. Opt.*, vol. 7, no. 3, 2002, pp. 378–387.

167. M. J. Hogan, J. A. Alvarado, and J. Weddel, *Histology of the Human Eye*, W. B. Sanders Co., Philadelphia, 1971.

168. Q. Zhou and R. W. Knighton, "Light Scattering and Form Birefringence of Parallel Cylindrical Arrays that Represent Cellular Organelles of the Retinal Nerve Fiber Layer," *Appl. Opt.*, vol. 36, no. 10, 1997, pp. 2273–2285.

169. G. Videen and D. Ngo, "Light Scattering Multipole Solution for a Cell," *J. Biomed. Opt.*, vol. 3, 1998, pp. 212–220.

170. J. R. Mourant, T. M. Johnson, V. Doddi, and J. P. Freyer, "Angular Dependent Light Scattering from Multicellular Spheroids," *J. Biomed. Opt.*, vol. 7, no. 1, 2002, pp. 93–99.

171. K. S. Shifrin, *Physical Optics of Ocean Water*, American Institute of Physics, New York, 1988.

172. V. V. Tuchin, I. L. Maksimova, D. A. Zimnyakov, I. L. Kon, A. H. Mavlutov, and A. A. Mishin, "Light Propagation in Tissues with Controlled Optical Properties," *J. Biomed. Opt.*, vol. 2, 1997, pp. 401–417.

173. V. V. Tuchin and D. M. Zhestkov, "Tissue Structure and Eye Lens Transmission and Scattering Spectra," *Proc. SPIE* 3053, 1997, pp. 123–128.

174. A. Brunsting and P. F. Mullaney, "Differential Light Scattering from Spherical Mammalian Cells," *Biophys. J.*, vol. 10, 1974, pp. 439–453.

175. J. Beuthan, O. Minet, J. Helfmann, M. Herring, and G. Mueller, "The Spatial Variation of the Refractive Index in Biological Cells," *Phys. Med. Biol.*, vol. 41, no. 3, 1996, pp. 369–382.

176. F. H. Silver, *Biological Materials: Structure, Mechanical Properties, and Modeling of Soft Tissues*, New York Univ. Press, New York, 1987.

177. R. G. Kessel, *Basic Medical Histology: The Biology of Cells, Tissues, and Organs*, Oxford Univ. Press, New York, 1998.

178. F. P. Bolin, L. E. Preuss, R. C. Taylor, and R. J. Ference, "Refractive Index of Some Mammalian Tissues using a Fiber Optic Cladding Method," *Appl. Opt.*, vol. 28, 1989, pp. 2297–2303.

179. R. Graaff, J. G. Aarnoudse, J. R. Zijp, P. M. A. Sloot, F. F. M. de Mul, J. Greve, and M. H. Koelink, "Reduced Light Scattering Properties for Mixtures of Spherical Particles: a Simple Approximation Derived from Mie Calculations," *Appl. Opt.*, vol. 31, 1992, pp. 1370–1376.

180. L. T. Perelman, V. Backman, M. Wallace, G. Zonios, R. Manoharan, A. Nusrat, S. Shields, M. Seiler, C. Lima, T. Hamano, I. Itzkan, J. Van Dam, J. M. Crawford, and M. S. Feld, "Observation of Periodic Fine Structure in Reflectance from Biological Tissue: a New Technique for Measuring Nuclear Size Distribution," *Phys. Rev. Lett.*, vol. 80, 1998, pp. 627–630.

181. H. C. van de Hulst, *Light Scattering by Small Particles*, Wiley, New York, 1957 [reprint, Dover, New York, 1981].

182. H. C. van de Hulst, *Multiple Light Scattering. Tables, Formulas and Applications*, Academic Press, New York, 1980.

183. A. Ishimaru, *Wave Propagation and Scattering in Random Media*, IEEE Press, New York, 1997.

184. C. Chandrasekhar, *Radiative Transfer*, Dover, Toronto, Ontario, 1960.

185. V. V. Sobolev, *Light Scattering in Planetary Atmospheres*, Pergamon Press, Oxford, 1974.

186. E. P. Zege, A. P. Ivanov, and I. L. Katsev, *Image Transfer through a Scattering Medium*, Springer-Verlag, New York, 1991.

187. A. Z. Dolginov, Yu. N. Gnedin, and N. A. Silant'ev, *Propagation and Polarization of Radiation in Cosmic Media*, Gordon and Breach, Basel, 1995.

188. M. I. Mishchenko, L. D. Travis, and A. A. Lacis, *Multiple Sacattering of Light by Particles*: *Radiative Transfer and Coherent Backscattering*, Cambridge University Press, New York, 2006.

189. E. J. Yanovitskij, *Light Scattering in Inhomogeneous Atmospheres*, Springer-Verlag, Berlin, 1997.

190. G. E. Thomas and K. Stamnes, *Radiative Transfer in the Atmosphere and Ocean*, Cambridge University Press, New York, 1999.

191. D. J. Durian, "The Diffusion Coefficient Depends on Absorption," *Opt. Lett.*, vol. 23, 1998, pp. 1502–1504.

192. A. Ishimaru, "Diffusion of Light in Turbid Material," *Appl. Opt.*, vol. 28, 1989, pp. 2210–2215.

193. T. J. Farrell, M. S. Patterson, and B. C. Wilson, "A diffusion Theory model of Spatially Resolved, Steady-State Diffuse Reflectance for the Noninvasive Determination of Tissue Optical Properties *In Vivo*," *Med. Phys.*, vol. 19, 1992, pp. 881–888.

194. M. Keijzer, W. M. Star, and P. R. M. Storchi, "Optical Diffusion in Layered Media," *Appl. Opt.*, vol. 27, pp. 1988, pp. 1820–1824.

195. G. Yoon, S. A. Prahl, and A. J. Welch, Accuracies of the Diffusion Approximation and its Similarity Relations for Laser Irradiated Biological Media," *Appl. Opt.*, vol. 28, 1989, pp. 2250–2255.

196. K. M. Yoo, F. Liu, and R. R. Alfano, "When Does the Diffusion Approximation Fail to Describe Photon Transport in Random Media?" *Phys. Rev. Lett.*, vol. 64, no. 22, 1990, pp. 2647–2650.

197. I. Dayan, S. Halvin, and G. H. Weiss, "Photon Migration in a 2-Layer Turbid Medium—a Diffusion Analysis," *J. Modern Opt.*, vol. 39, no. 7, 1992, pp. 1567–1582.

198. L. V. Wang and S. L. Jacques, "Source of Error in Calculation of Optical Diffuse Reflectance from Turbid Media Using Diffusion Theory," *Comput. Meth. Progr. Biomed.*, vol. 61, 2000, pp. 163–170.

199. F. Martelli, M. Bassani, L. Alianelli, L. Zangheri, and G. Zaccanti, "Accuracy of the Diffusion Equation to Describe Photon Migration through an

Infinite Medium: Numerical and Experimental Investigation," *Phys. Med. Biol.*, vol. 45, 2000, pp. 1359–1373.

200. S. Del Bianko, F. Martelli, and G. Zaccanti, "Penetration Depth of Light Re-emitted by a Diffusive Medium: Theoretical and Experimental Investigation," *Phys. Med. Biol.*, vol. 47, 2002, pp. 4131–4144.

201. R. Graaff and K. Rinzema, "Practical Improvements on Photon Diffusion Theory: Application to Isotropic Scattering," *Phys. Med. Biol.*, vol. 46, 2001, pp. 3043–3050.

202. D. C. Sahni, E. B. Dahl, and N. G. Sjostrand, "Diffusion Coefficient for Photon Transport in Turbid Media," *Phys. Med. Biol.*, vol. 48, 2003, pp. 3969–3976.

203. T. Khan and H. Jiang, "A New Diffusion Approximation to the Radiative Transfer Equation for Scattering Media with Spatially Varying Refractive Indices," *J. Opt. A: Pure Appl. Opt.*, vol. 5, 2003, pp. 137–141.

204. R. C. Haskell, L. O. Svaasand, T.-T. Tsay, T. C. Feng, M. N. McAdams, and B. J. Tromberg, "Boundary Conditions for the Diffusion Equation in Radiative Transfer," *J. Opt. Soc. Am. A*, vol. 11, no. 10, 1994, pp. 2727–2741.

205. A. Kienle and M. S. Patterson, "Improved Solutions of the Steady-State and Time-Resolved Diffusion Equations for Reflectance from a Semi-Infinite Turbid Media," *J. Opt. Soc. Am. A*, vol. 14, 1997, pp. 246–254.

206. T. J. Farrell and M. S. Patterson, "Experimental Verification of the Effect of Refractive Index Mismatch on the Light Fluence in a Turbid Medium," *J. Biomed. Opt.*, vol. 6, no. 4, 2001, pp. 468–473.

207. M. Motamedi, S. Rastegar, G. LeCarpentier, and A. J. Welch, "Light and Temperature Distribution in Laser Irradiated Tissue: The Influence of Anisotropic Scattering and Refractive Index," *Appl. Opt.*, vol. 28, 1989, pp. 2230–2237.

208. S. R. Arridge, M. Schweiger, M. Hiraoka, and D. T. Delpy, "A Finite Element Approach for Modelling Photon Transport in Tissue," *Med. Phys.*, vol. 20, 1993, pp. 299–309.

209. W. M. Star, "Comparing the P3-approximation with diffusion theory and with Monte Carlo Calculations of Light Propagation in a Slab Geometry," in *Dosimetry of Laser Radiation in Medicine and Biology*, G. J. Mueller and D. H. Sliney (eds.), vol. IS5, SPIE Press, Bellingham, WA, 1989, pp. 146–154.

210. W. M. Star, "Light Dosimetry *In Vivo*," *Phys. Med. Biol.*, vol. 42, 1997, pp. 763–787.

211. D. J. Dickey, R. B. Moore, D. C. Rayner, and J. Tulip, "Light Dosimetry Using the P3 Approximation," *Phys. Med. Biol.*, vol. 46, 2001, pp. 2359–2370.

212. B. Phylips-Invernizzi, D. Dupont, and C. Caze, "Bibliographical Review for Reflectance of Diffusing Media, *Opt. Eng.*, vol. 40, no. 6, 2001, pp. 1082–1092.

213. V. V. Tuchin, S. R. Utz, and I. V. Yaroslavsky, "Tissue Optics, Light Distribution, and Spectroscopy," *Opt. Eng.*, vol. 33, 1994, pp. 3178–3188.

214. S. M. Ermakov and G. A. Mikhailov, *Course on Siatistical Modeling*, Nauka, Moscow, 1982.

215. B. C. Wilson and G. A. Adam, "Monte Carlo Model for the Absorption and Flux Distributions of Light in Tissue," *Med. Phys.*, vol. 10, 1983, pp. 824–830.

216. S. A. Prahl, M. Keijzer, S. L. Jacques, and A. J. Welch, "Monte Carlo Model of Light Propagation in Tissues," in *Dosimetry of Laser Radiation in Medicine and Biology*, G. J. Mueller and D. H. Sliney (eds.), vol. IS5, SPIE Press, Bellingham, WA, 1989, pp. 102–111.

217. M. Keijzer, S. L. Jacques, S. A. Prahl, and A. J. Welch, "Light Distribution in Artery Tissue: Monte Carlo Simulation for Finite-Diameter Laser Beams," *Lasers Surg. Med.*, vol. 9, 1989, pp. 148–154.

218. M. Keijzer, R. R. Richards-Kortum, S. L. Jacques, and M. S. Feld, "Fluorescence Spectroscopy of Turbid Media: Autofluorescence of the Human Aorta," *Appl. Opt.*, vol. 28, no. 20, 1989, pp. 4286–4292.

219. S. T. Flock, B. C. Wilson, D. R. Wyman, and M. S. Patterson, "Monte Carlo Modeling of Light–Propagation in Highly Scattering Tissues I: Model Predictions and Comparison with Diffusion Theory," *IEEE Trans. Biomed. Eng.*, vol. 36, no. 12, 1989, pp. 1162–1168.

220. S. T. Flock, B. C. Wilson, and M. S. Patterson, "Monte Carlo Modeling of Light-Propagation in Highly Scattering Tissues II: Comparison with Measurements in Phantoms," *IEEE Trans. Biomed. Eng.*, vol. 36, no. 12, 1989, pp. 1169–1173.

221. J. M. Schmitt, G. X. Zhou, E. C. Walker, and R. T. Wall, "Multilayer Model of Photon Diffusion in Skin," *J. Opt. Soc. Am. A*, vol. 7, 1990, pp. 2141–2153.

222. S. L. Jacques, "The Role of Skin Optics in Diagnostic and Therapeutic Uses of Lasers," in *Lasers in Dermatology*, Springer-Verlag, Berlin, 1991, pp. 1–21.

223. H. Key, E. R. Davies, P. C. Jackson, and P. N. T. Wells, "Optical Attenuation Characteristics of Breast Tissues at Visible and Near-Infrared Wavelengths," *Phys. Med. Biol.*, vol. 36, no. 5, 1991, pp. 579–590.

224. I. V. Yaroslavsky and V. V. Tuchin, "Light Propagation in Multilayer Scattering Media. Modeling by the Monte Carlo Method," *Opt. Spectrosc.*, vol. 72, 1992, pp. 505–509.

225. L.-H. Wang and S. L. Jacques, "Hybrid Model of the Monte Carlo Simulation and Diffusion Theory for Light Reflectance by Turbid Media," *J. Opt. Soc. Am. A.*, vol. 10, 1993, pp. 1746–1752.

226. R. Graaff, M. H. Koelink, F. F. M. de Mul, et al., "Condensed Monte Carlo Simulations for the Description of Light Transport," *Appl. Opt.*, vol. 32, no. 4, 1993, pp. 426–434.

227. V. V. Tuchin, S. R. Utz, and I. V. Yaroslavsky, "Skin Optics: Modeling of Light Transport and Measuring of Optical Parameters," in *Medical Optical Tomography: Functional Imaging and Monitoring*, G. Müller, B. Chance, R. Alfano, et al. (eds.), vol. IS11, SPIE Press, Bellingham, WA, 1993, pp. 234–258.

228. R. Graaff, A. C. M. Dassel, M. H. Koelink, et al., "Optical Properties of Human Dermis *In Vitro* and *In Vivo*," *Appl. Opt.*, vol. 32, 1993, pp. 435–447.

229. S. L. Jacques and L. Wang, "Monte Carlo Modeling of Light Transport in Tissues," in *Optical-Thermal Response of Laser-Irradiated Tissue*, A. J. Welch and M. J. C. van Gemert (eds.), Plenum Press, New York, 1995, pp. 73–100.

230. L.-H. Wang, S. L. Jacques, L.-Q. Zheng, "MCML–Monte Carlo Modeling of Light Transport in Multi-Layered Tissues," *Comput. Meth. Progr. Biomed.*, vol. 47, 1995, pp. 131–146.

231. S. R. Arridge, M. Hiraoka, and M. Schweiger, "Statistical Basis for the Determination of Optical Pathlength in Tissue," *Phys. Med. Biol.*, vol. 40, 1995, pp. 1539–1558.

232. T. L. Troy, D. L. Page, and E. M. Sevick-Muraca, "Optical Properties of Normal and Diseased Breast Tissues: Prognosis for Optical Mammography," *J. Biomed. Opt.*, vol. 1, no. 3, 1996, pp. 342–355.

233. E. Okada, M. Firbank, M. Schweiger, et al., "Theoretical and Experimental Investigation of Near-Infrared Light Propagation in a Model of the Adult Head," *Appl. Opt.*, vol. 36, no. 1, 1997, pp. 21–31.

234. V. G. Kolinko, F. F. M. de Mul, J. Greve, and A. V. Priezzhev, "On Refraction in Monte-Carlo Simulations of Light Transport through Biological Tissues," *Med. Biol. Eng. Comp.* vol. 35, 1997, pp. 287–288.

235. L.-H. Wang, "Rapid Modeling of Diffuse Reflectance of Light in Turbid Slabs," *J. Opt. Soc. Am. A.*, vol. 15, no. 4, 1998, pp. 936–944.

236. C. R. Simpson, M. Kohl, M. Essenpreis, and M. Cope, "Near-Infrared Optical Properties of *Ex Vivo* Human Skin and Subcutaneos Tissues Measured Using the Monte Carlo Inversion Technique," *Phys. Med. Biol.*, vol. 43, 1998, pp. 2465–2478.

237. J. Laufer, C. R. Simpson, M. Kohl, M. Essenpreis, and M. Cope, "Effect of Temperature on the Optical Properties of *Ex Vivo* Human Dermis and Subdermis," *Phys. Med. Biol.* vol. 43, 1998, pp. 2479–2489.

238. P. M. Ripley, J. G. Laufer, A. D. Gordon, R. J. Connell, and S. G. Bown, "Near-Infrared Optical Properties of *Ex Vivo* Human Uterus Determined by the Monte Carlo Inversion Technique," *Phys. Med. Biol.*, vol. 44, 1999, pp. 2451–2462.

239. M. L. de Jode, "Monte Carlo Simulations of Light Distributions in an Embedded Tumour Model: Studies of Selectivity in Photodynamic Therapy," *Lasers Med. Sci.*, vol. 15, 2000, pp. 49–56.

240. R. Jeraj and P. Keall, "The Effect of Statistical Uncertainty on Inverse Treatment Planning Based on Monte Carlo Dose Calculation," *Phys. Med. Biol.*, vol. 45, 2000, pp. 3601–3613.

241. I. V. Meglinskii, "Monte Carlo Simulation of Reflection Spectra of Random Multilayer Media Strongly Scattering and Absorbing Light," *Quant. Electron.*, vol. 31, no. 12, 2001, pp. 1101–1107.

242. C. K. Hayakawa, J. Spanier, F. Bevilacqua, A. K. Dunn, J. S. You, B. J. Tromberg, and V. Venugopalan, "Perturbation Monte Carlo Methods to Solve Inverse Photon Migration Problems in Heterogeneous Tissues," *Opt. Lett.*, vol. 26, no. 17, 2001, pp. 1335–1337.

243. I. V. Meglinski and S. J. Matcher, "Quantitative Assessment of Skin Layers Absorption and Skin Reflectance Spectra Simulation in Visible and Near-Infrared Spectral Region," *Physiol. Meas.*, vol. 23, 2002, pp. 741–753.

244. S. J. Preece and E. Claridge, "Monte Carlo Modelling of the Spectral Reflectance of the Human Eye," *Phys. Med. Biol.*, vol. 47, 2002, pp. 2863–2877.

245. D. A. Boas, J. P. Culver, J. J. Stott, and A. K. Dunn, "Three Dimensional Monte Carlo Code for Photon Migration through Complex Heterogeneous Media Including the Adult Human Head," *Optics Express*, vol. 10, no. 3, 2002, pp. 159–170.

246. I. V. Meglinski and S. J. Matcher, "Computer Simulation of the Skin Reflectance Spectra, *Comput. Meth. Progr. Biomed.*, vol. 70, 2003, pp. 179–186.

247. F. F. M. de Mul, "Monte-Carlo Simulations of Light Scattering in Turbid Media," Chapter 12 in *Coherent-Domain Optical Methods: Biomedical Diagnostics, Environmental and Material Science*, V. V. Tuchin (ed.), Kluwer Academic Publishers, Boston, vol. 1, 2004, pp. 465–532.

248. A. V. Voronov, E. V. Tret'akov, and V. V. Shuvalov, "Fast Path-Integration Technique Simulation of Light Propagation through Highly Scattering Objects," *Quant. Electr.*, vol. 34, no. 6, 2004, pp. 547–553.

249. M. J. Wilson and R. K. Wang, "A Path-Integral Model of Light Scattered by Turbid Media," *J. Phys. B: At. Mol. Opt. Phys.*, vol. 34, 2001, pp. 1453–1472.

250. L. T. Perelman, J. Wu, I. Itzkan, and M. S. Feld, "Photon Migration in Turbid Media Using Path Integrals," *Phys. Rev. Lett.*, vol. 72, 1994, pp. 1341–1344.

251. A. Y. Polishchuk and R. R. Alfano, "Fermat Photons in Turbid Media: An Exact Analytic Solution for Most Favorable Paths—A Step Toward Optical Tomography," *Opt. Lett.*, vol. 20, 1995, pp. 1937–1939.

252. S. L. Jacques, "Path Integral Description of Light Transport in Tissue," *Ann. NY Acad. Sci.*, vol. 838, 1998, pp. 1–13.

253. V. V. Lyubimov, A. G. Kalintsev, A. B. Konovalov, O. V. Lyamtsev, O. V. Kravtsenyuk, A. G. Murzin, O. V. Golubkina, G. B. Mordvinov, L. N. Soms, and L. M. Yavorskaya, "Application of the Photon Average Trajectories Method to Real-Time Reconstruction of Tissue Inhomogeneities

in Diffuse Optical Tomography of Strongly Scattering Media," *Phys. Med. Biol.*, vol. 47, 2002, pp. 2109–2128.

254. A. H. Gandjbakhche, V. Chernomordik, J. C. Hebden, and R. Nossal, "Time-Dependent Contrast Functions for Quantitative Imaging in Time-Resolved Transillumination Experiments," *Appl. Opt.*, vol. 37, 1998, pp. 1973–1981.

255. A. N. Yaroslavsky, S. R. Utz, S. N. Tatarintsev, and V. V. Tuchin, "Angular Scattering Properties of Human Epidermal Layers," *Proc. SPIE* 2100, 1994, pp. 38–41.

256. M. A. Everett, E. Yeargers, R. M. Sayre, and R. L. Olson, "Penetration of Epidermis by Ultraviolet Rays," *Photochem. Photobiol.*, vol. 5, 1966, pp. 533–542.

257. M. Keijzer, J. M. Pickering, and M. J. C. van Gemert, "Laser Beam Diameter for Port Wine Stain Treatment," *Lasers Surg. Med.*, vol. 11, 1991, pp. 601–605.

258. M. J. C. van Gemert, D. J. Smithies, W. Verkruysse, et al., "Wavelengths for Port Wine Stain Laser Treatment: Influence of Vessel Radius and Skin Anatomy," *Phys. Med. Biol.*, vol. 42, 1997, pp. 41–50.

259. A. Kienle and R. Hibst, "A New Optimal Wavelength for Treatment of Port Wine Stains?" *Phys. Med. Biol.*, vol. 40, 1995, pp. 1559–1576.

260. A. Kienle, L. Lilge, and M. S. Patterson, "Investigation of Multi-Layered Tissue with *In Vivo* Reflectance Measurements," *Proc. SPIE* 2326, 1994, pp. 212–214.

261. V. V. Tuchin, Yu. N. Scherbakov, A. N. Yakunin, and I. V. Yaroslavsky, "Numerical Technique for Modeling of Laser-Induced Hyperthermia," in *Laser-Induced Interstitial Thermotherapy*, G. Müller and A. Roggan (eds.), SPIE Press, Bellingham, WA, 1995, pp. 100–113.

262. Yu. N. Scherbakov, A. N. Yakunin, I. V. Yaroslavsky, and V. V. Tuchin, "Thermal Processes Modeling During Uncoagulating Laser Radiation Interaction with Multi-Layer Biotissue. 1. Theory and Calculating Models. 2. Numerical Results," *Opt. Spectrosc.*, vol. 76, no. 5, 1994, pp. 754–765.

263. S. Willmann, A. Terenji, I. V. Yaroslavsky, T. Kahn, P. Hering, and H.-J. Schwarzmaier, "Determination of the Optical Properties of a Human Brain Tumor Using a New Microspectrophotometric Technique," *Proc. SPIE* 3598, 1999, pp. 233–239.

264. A. N. Yaroslavsky, P. C. Schulze, I. V. Yaroslavsky, R. Schober, F. Ulrich, and H.-J. Schwarzmaier, "Optical Properties of Selected Native and Coagulated Human Brain Tissues *In Vitro* in the Visible and Near Infrared Spectral Range," *Phys. Med. Biol.*, vol. 47, 2002, pp. 2059–2073.

265. W. M. Star, B. C. Wilson, and M. C. Patterson, "Light Delivery and Dosimetry in Photodynamic Therapy of Solid Tumors," in *Photodynamic Therapy, Basic Principles and Clinical Applications*, B. W. Henderson and T. J. Dougherty (eds.), Marcel-Dekker, New York, 1992, pp. 335–368.

266. B. Nemati, H. G. Rylander III, and A. J. Welch, "Optical Properties of Conjuctiva, Sclera, and the Ciliary Body and Their Consequences for Transs-

cleral Cyclophotocoagulation," *Appl. Opt.* , vol. 35, no. 19, 1966, pp. 3321–3327.

267. B. Nemati, A. Dunn, A. J. Welch, and H. G. Rylander III, "Optical Model for Light Distribution during Transscleral Cyclophotocoagulation," *Appl. Opt.*, vol. 37, no. 4, 1998, pp. 764–771.

268. M. J. C. van Gemert, A. J. Welch, J. W. Pickering, et al., "Wavelengths for Laser Treatment of Port Wine Stains and Telangiectasia," *Lasers Surg. Med.*, vol. 16, 1995, pp. 147–155.

269. I. N. Minin, *Theory of Radiative Transfer in Atmosphere of Planets*, Nauka, Moscow, 1988.

270. W. Cai, B. B. Das, F. Liu, et al., "Time-Resolved Optical Diffusion Tomographic Image Reconstruction in Highly Scattering Media," *Proc. Math. Acad. Sci. USA*, vol. 93, 1996, pp. 13561–13564.

271. S. R. Arridge and J. C. Hebden, "Optical Imaging in Medicine II: Modelling and Reconstruction," *Phys. Med. Biol.*, vol. 42, 1997, pp. 841–854.

272. M. S. Patterson, B. Chance, and B. C. Wilson, "Time Resolved Reflectance and Transmittance for the Non-Invasive Measurement of Tissue Optical Properties," *Appl. Opt.*, vol. 28, 1989, pp. 2331–2336.

273. S. L. Jacques, "Time-Resolved Reflectance Spectroscopy in Turbid Tissues," *IEEE Trans. Biomed. Eng.*, vol. 36, 1989, pp. 1155–1161.

274. S. J. Matcher, M. Cope, and D. T. Delpy, "*In Vivo* Measurements of the Wavelength Dependence of Tissue-Scattering Coefficients Between 760 and 900 nm Measured with Time-Resolved Spectroscopy," *Appl. Opt.*, vol. 36, no. 1, 1997, pp. 386–396.

275. W. Cui, N. Wang, and B. Chance, "Study of Photon Migration Depths with Time–Resolved Spectroscopy," *Opt. Lett.*, vol. 16, 1991, pp. 1632–1634.

276. M. Ferrari, Q. Wei, L. Carraresi, et al., "Time-Resolved Spectroscopy of the Human Forearm," *J. Photochem. Photobiol. B: Biol.*, vol. 16, 1992, pp. 141–153.

277. A. H. Hielscher, H. Liu, B. Chance, et al., "Time-Resolved Photon Emission from Layered Turbid Media," *Appl. Opt.*, vol. 35, 1996, pp. 719–728.

278. E. B. de Haller and C. Depeursinge, "Simulation of the Time-Resolved Breast Transillumination," *Med. Biol. Eng. Comp.*, vol. 31, 1993, pp. 165–170.

279. S. Andersson-Engels, R. Berg, S. Svanberg, and O. Jarlman, "Time-Resolved Transillumination for Medical Diagnostics," *Opt. Lett.*, vol. 15, 1990, pp. 1179–1181.

280. L. Wang, P. P. Ho, C. Liu, et al., "Ballistic 2–D Imaging through Scattering Walls using an Ultrafast Optical Kerr gate, *Science.*, vol. 253, 1991, pp. 769–771.

281. B. B. Das, K. M. Yoo, and R. R. Alfano, "Ultrafast Time-Gated Imaging in Thick Tissues: a Step toward Optical Mammography," *Opt. Lett.*, vol. 18, 1993, pp. 1092–1094.

282. V. V. Lubimov, "Image Transfer in a Slab of Scattering Medium and Estimation of the Resolution of Optical Tomography uses the First Arrived Photons of Ultrashort Pulses," *Opt. Spectrosc.*, vol. 76, 1994, pp. 814–815.

283. Y. Q. Yao, Y. Wang, Y. L. Pei, et al., "Frequency-Domain Optical Imaging of Absorption and Scattering Distributions by Born Iterative Method," *J. Opt. Soc. Am. A.*, vol. 14, no. 1, 1997, pp. 325–342.

284. R. Cubeddu, A. Pifferi, P. Taroni, et al., "Time-Resolved Imaging on a Realistic Tissue Phantom: μ_s' and μ_a Images Versus Time-Integrated Images," *Appl. Opt.*, vol. 35, 1996, pp. 4533–4540.

285. A. Yodh and B. Chance, "Spectroscopy and Imaging with Diffusing Light," *Physics Today*, March, 1995, pp. 34–40.

286. S. R. Arridge, M. Cope, and D. T. Delpy, "Theoretical Basis for the Determination of Optical Pathlengths in Tissue: Temporal and Frequency Analysis," *Phys. Med. Biol.*, vol. 37, 1992, pp. 1531–1560.

287. E. B. de Haller, "Time-Resolved Transillumination and Optical Tomography," *J. Biomed. Opt.*, vol. 1, no. 1, 1996, pp. 7–17.

288. H. Heusmann, J. Kolzer, and G. Mitic, "Characterization of Female Breast *In Vivo* by Time Resolved and Spectroscopic Measurements in Near Infrared Spectroscopy," *J. Biomed. Opt.*, vol. 1, no. 4, 1996, pp. 425–434.

289. K. Suzuki, Y. Yamashita, K. Ohta, et al., "Quantitative Measurement of Optical Parameters in Normal Breast using Time-Resolved Spectroscopy: *In Vivo* Results of 30 Japanese Women," *J. Biomed. Opt.*, vol. 1, no. 3, 1996, pp. 330–334.

290. A. Taddeucci, F. Martelli, M. Barilli, et al., "Optical Properties of Brain Tissue," *J. Bimed. Opt.*, vol. 1, no. 1, 1996, pp. 117–130.

291. R. K. Wang and M. J. Wilson, "Vertex/Propagator Model for Least-Scattered Photons Traversing a Turbid Medium," *J. Opt. Soc. Am. A*, vol. 18, no. 1, 2001, pp. 224–231.

292. J.-M. Tualle, E. Tinet, J. Prat, and S. Avrillier, "Light Propagation Near-Turbid–Turbid Planar Interfaces, *Opt. Communs*, vol. 183, 2000, pp. 337–346.

293. Y. Tsuchiya, "Photon Path Distribution and Optical Responses of Turbid Media: Theoretical Analysis Based on the Microscopic Beer-Lambert Law," *Phys. Med. Biol.*, vol. 46, 2001, pp. 2067–2084.

294. G. Zacharakis, A. Zolindaki, V. Sakkalis, G. Filippidis, T. G. Papazoglou, D. D. Tsiftsis, and E. Koumantakis, "*In Vitro* Optical Characterization and Discrimination of Female Breast Tissue During Near Infrared Femtosecond Laser Pulses Propagation," *J. Biomed. Opt.*, vol. 6, no. 4, 2001, pp. 446–449.

295. R. Elaloufi, R. Carminati, and J.-J. Greffet, "Time-Dependent Transport through Scattering Media: from Radiative Transfer to Diffusion," *J. Opt. A: Pure Appl. Opt.*, vol. 4, 2002, pp. S103–S108.

296. D. Arifler, M. Guillaud, A. Carraro, A. Malpica, M. Follen, and R. Richards-Kortum, "Light Scattering from Normal and Dysplastic Cervical Cells at Different Epithelial Depths: Finite-Difference Time-Domain Modeling with

a Perfectly Matched Layer Boundary Condition," *J. Biomed. Opt.*, vol. 8, no. 3, 2003, pp. 484–494.

297. V. Chernomordik, A. H. Gandjbakhche, J. C. Hebden, and G. Zaccanti, "Effect of Lateral Boundaries on Contrast Functions in Time-Resolved Transillumination Measurements," *Med. Phys.*, vol. 26, no. 9, 1999, pp. 1822–1831.

298. V. Chernomordik, A. Gandjbakhche, M. Lepore, R. Esposito, and I. Delfino, "Depth Dependence of the Analytical Expression for the Width of the Point Spread Function (Spatial Resolution) in Time-Resolved Transillumination," *J. Biomed. Opt.*, vol. 6, no. 4, 2001, pp. 441–445.

299. V. Chernomordik, D. W. Hattery, I. Gannot, G. Zaccanti, and A. Gandjbakhche, "Analytical Calculation of the Mean Time Spent by Photons Inside an Absorptive Inclusion Embedded in a Highly Scattering Medium," *J. Biomed. Opt.*, vol. 7, no. 3, 2002, pp. 486–492.

300. V. Chernomordik, D. W. Hattery, D. Grosenick, H. Wabnitz, H. Rinneberg, K. T. Moesta, P. M. Schlag, and A. Gandjbakhche, "Quantification of Optical Properties of a Breast Tumor Using Random Walk Theory, *J. Biomed. Opt.*, vol. 7, no. 1, 2002, pp. 80–87.

301. I. V. Yaroslavsky, A. N. Yaroslavsky, J. Rodriguez, and H. Battarbee, "Propagation of Pulses and Photon-Density Waves in Turbid Media," Chapter 3, in *Handbook of Optical Biomedical Diagnostics*, vol. PM107, V. V. Tuchin (ed.), SPIE Press, Bellingham, WA, 2002, pp. 217–263.

302. J. Rodriguez, I. V. Yaroslavsky, H. Battarbee, and V. V. Tuchin, "Time-Resolved Imaging in Diffusive Media," Chapter 6, in *Handbook of Optical Biomedical Diagnostics*, vol. PM107, V. V. Tuchin (ed.), SPIE Press, Bellingham, WA, 2002, pp. 357–404.

303. S. Fantini and M. A. Franceschini, "Frequency-Domain Techniques for Tissue Spectroscopy and Imaging," Chapter 7, in *Handbook of Optical Biomedical Diagnostics*, vol. PM107, V. V. Tuchin (ed.), SPIE Press, Bellingham, WA, 2002, pp. 405–453.

304. D. J. Papaioannou, G. W. Hooft, S. B. Colak, and J. T. Oostveen, "Detection Limit in Localizing Objects Hidden in a Turbid Medium Using an Optically Scanned Phased Array," *J. Biomed. Opt.*, vol. 1, no. 3, 1996, pp. 305–310.

305. B. W. Pogue and M. S. Patterson, "Error Assessment of a Wavelength Tunable Frequency Domain System for Noninvasive Tissue Spectroscopy," *J. Biomed. Opt.*, vol. 1, no. 3, 1996, pp. 311–323.

306. J. B. Fishkin, O. Coquoz, E. R. Anderson, et al., "Frequency-Domain Photon Migration Measurements of Normal and Malignant Tissue Optical Properties in a Human Subject," *Appl. Opt.*, vol. 36, no. 1, 1997, pp. 10–20.

307. B. J. Tromberg, L. O. Svaasand, T.-T. Tsay, and R. C. Haskell, "Properties of Photon Density Waves in Multiple-Scattering Media," *Appl. Opt.*, vol. 32, 1993, pp. 607–616.

308. B. J. Tromberg, O. Coquoz, J. B. Fishkin, et al., "Non-Invasive Measurements of Breast Tissue Optical Properties using Frequency-Domain Photon Migration," *Phil. Trans. R. Soc. Lond. B.*, vol. 352, 1997, pp. 661–668.

309. D. A. Boas, M. A. O'Leary, B. Chance, and A. G. Yodh, "Scattering and Wavelength Transduction of Diffuse Photon Density Waves," *Phys. Rev. E.*, vol. 47, 1993, pp. R2999–R3002.

310. D. A. Boas, M. A. O'Leary, B. Chance, and A. G. Yodh, "Scattering of Diffuse Photon Density Waves by Spherical Inhomogeneities within Turbid Media: Analytic Solution and Applications," *Proc. Natl. Acad. Sci. USA.*, 91, 1994, pp. 4887–4891.

311. J. R. Lakowicz and K. Berndt, "Frequency-Domain Measurements of Photon Migration in Tissues," *Chem. Phys. Lett.*, vol. 166, 1990, pp. 246–252.

312. M. S. Patterson, J. D. Moulton, B. C. Wilson, et al., "Frequency-Domain Reflectance for the Determination of the Scattering and Absorption Properties of Tissue," *Appl. Opt.*, vol. 30, 1991, pp. 4474–4476.

313. J. M. Schmitt, A. Knüttel, and J. R. Knutson, "Interference of Diffusive Light Waves," *J. Opt. Soc. Am. A.*, vol. 9, 1992, pp. 1832–1843.

314. J. B. Fishkin and E. Gratton, "Propagation of Photon-Density Waves in Strongly Scattering Media Containing an Absorbing Semi-Infinite Plane Bounded by a Strait Edge," *J. Opt. Soc. Am. A.*, vol. 10, 1993, pp. 127–140.

315. L. O. Svaasand, B. J. Tromberg, R. C. Haskell, et al., "Tissue Characterization and Imaging using Photon Density Waves," *Opt. Eng.*, vol. 32, 1993, pp. 258–266.

316. Yu. T. Masurenko, "Spectral-Correlation Method for Imaging of Strongly Scattering Objects," *Opt. Spectrosc.*, vol. 76, 1994, pp. 816–821.

317. H. B. Jiang, K. D. Paulsen, U. L. Osterberg, and M. S. Patterson, "Frequency-Domain Optical-Image Reconstruction in Turbid Media—an Experimental Study of Single-Target Tetectability," *Appl. Opt.*, vol. 36, 1997, pp. 52–63.

318. S. J. Madsen, P. Wyst, L. O. Svaasand, et al., "Determination of the Optical Properties of the Human Uterus using Frequency-Domain Photon Migration and Steady-State Techniques," *Phys. Med. Biol.*, vol. 39, no. 8, 1994, pp. 1191–1202.

319. X. D. Li, T. Durduran, A. G. Yodh, et al., "Diffraction Tomography for Biochemical Imaging with Diffuse Photon-Density Waves," *Opt. Lett.*, vol. 22, 1997, pp. 573–575.

320. C. L. Matson, N. Clark, L. McMackin, and J. S. Fender, "Three-Dimensional Tumor Localization in Thick Tissue with the Use of Diffuse Photon-Density Waves," *Appl. Opt.*, vol. 36, 1997, pp. 214–220.

321. B. Chance, "Optical Method," *Annual Rev. Biophys. Biophys. Chem.*, vol. 20, 1991, pp. 1–28.

322. B. W. Pogue and M. S. Patterson, "Frequency-Domain Optical Absorption Spectroscopy of Finite Tissue Volumes Using Diffusion Theory," *Phys. Med. Biol.*, vol. 39, 1994, pp. 1157–1180.

323. B. W. Pogue, M. S. Patterson, H. Jiang, and K. D. Paulsen, "Initial Assessment of a Simple System for Frequency Domain Diffuse Optical Tomography," *Phys. Med. Biol.*, vol. 40, 1995, pp. 1709–1729.

324. X. Wu, L. Stinger, and G. W. Faris, "Determination of Tissue Properties by Immersion in a Matched Scattering Fluid," *Proc. SPIE* 2979, 1997, pp. 300–306.

325. S. Fantini, M. A. Franceschini, J. B. Fishkin, et al., "Quantitative Determination of the Absorption and Spectra of Chromophores in Strongly Scattering Media: a Light-Emitting-Diode Based Technique," *Appl. Opt.*, vol. 32, 1994, pp. 5204–5212.

326. M. A. Franceschini, K. T. Moesta, and S. Fantini, "Frequency-Domain Techniques Enhance Optical Mammography: Initial Clinical Results," *Proc. Natl. Acad. Sci. USA*, vol. 94, 1997, pp. 6468–6473.

327. I. V. Yaroslavsky, A. N. Yaroslavskaya, V. V. Tuchin, and H.-J. Schwarzmaier, "Effect of the Scattering Delay on Time-Dependent Photon Migration in Turbid Media," *Appl. Opt.*, vol. 36, no. 22, 1997, pp. 6529–6538.

328. W. W. Mantulin, S. Fantini, M. A. Franceschini, S. A. Walker, J. S. Maier, and E. Gratton, "Tissue Optical Parameter Map Generated with Frequency-Domain Spectroscopy," *Proc. SPIE* 2396, 1995, pp. 323–330.

329. H. Wabnitz and H. Rinneberg, "Imaging in Turbid Media by Photon Density Waves: Spatial Resolution and Scaling Relations," *Appl. Opt.*, vol. 36, no. 1, 1997, pp. 67–73.

330. D. A. Boas, M. A. O'Leary, B. Chance, and A. Yodh, "Detection and Characterization of Optical Inhomogeneities with Diffuse Photon Density Waves: a Signal-to-Noise Analysis," *Appl. Opt.*, vol. 36, 1997, pp. 75–92.

331. A. Knüttel, J. M. Schmitt, and J. R. Knutson, "Spatial Localization of Absorbing Bodies by Interfering Diffusive Photon-Density Waves," *Appl. Opt.*, vol. 32, 1933, pp. 381–389.

332. S. Fantini, M. A. Franceschini, and E. Gratton,"Semi-Infinite-Geometry Boundary Problem for Light Migration in Highly Scattering Media: a Frequency-Domain Study in the Diffusion Approximation," *J. Opt. Soc. Am. B.*, vol. 11, 1994, pp. 2128–2138.

333. J. A. Moon and J. Reintjes, "Image Resolution by Use of Multiply Scattered Light," *Opt. Lett.*, vol. 19, 1994, pp. 521–523.

334. A. Weersink, J. E. Hayward, K. R. Diamond, and M. S. Patterson, "Accuracy of Noninvasive *In Vivo* Measurements of Photosensitizer Uptake Based on a Diffusion Model of Reflectance Spectroscopy," *Photochem. Photobiology*, vol. 66, no. 3, 1997, pp. 326–335.

335. V. V. Tuchin, "Fundamentals of Low-Intensity Laser Radiation Interaction with Biotissues: Dosimetry and Diagnostical Aspects," *Bullet. Russian Acad. Sci., Phys. ser.*, vol. 59, no. 6, 1995, pp. 120–143.

336. Y. Chen, C. Mu, X. Intes, and B. Chance, "Signal-to-Noise Analysis for Detection Sensitivity of Small Absorbing Heterogeneity in Turbid Media with Single-Source and Dual-Interfering-Source," *Optics Express*, vol. 9, no. 4, 2001, pp. 212–224.

337. T. Durduran, J. P. Culver, M. J. Holboke, X. D. Li, L. Zubkov, B. Chance, D. N. Pattanayak, and A. G. Yodh, "Algorithms for 3D Localization and

Imaging Using Near-Field Diffraction Tomography with Diffuse Light," *Optics Express*, vol. 4, no. 8, 1999, pp. 247–262.

338. S. J. Matcher, "Signal Quantification and Localization in Tissue Near-Infrared Spectroscopy," Chapter 9, in *Handbook of Optical Biomedical Diagnostics*, vol. PM107, V. V. Tuchin (ed.), SPIE Press, Bellingham, WA, 2002, pp. 487–584.

339. J. S. Maier, S. A. Walker, S. Fantini, M. A. Franceschini, and E. Gratton, "Possible Correlation between Blood Glucose Concentration and the Reduced Scattering Coefficient of Tissues in the Near Infrared," *Opt. Lett.*, vol. 19, 1994, pp. 2062–2064.

340. M. Kohl, M. Cope, M. Essenpreis, and D. Böcker, "Influence of Glucose Concentration on Light Scattering in Tissue-Simulating Phantoms," *Opt. Lett.*, vol. 19, 1994, pp. 2170–2172.

341. J. T. Bruulsema, J. E. Hayward, T. J. Farrell, M. S. Patterson, L. Heinemann, M. Berger, T. Koschinsky, J. Sandahal-Christiansen, H. Orskov, M. Essenpreis, G. Schmelzeisen-Redeker, and D. Böcker, "Correlation between Blood Glucose Concentration in Diabetics and Noninvasively Measured Tissue Optical Scattering Coefficient," *Opt. Lett.*, vol. 22, no. 3, 1997, pp. 190–192.

342. M. G. Erickson, J. S. Reynolds, and K. J. Webb, "Comparison of Sensitivity for Single-Source and Dual-Interfering-Source Configurations in Optical Diffusion Imaging," *J. Opt. Soc. Am. A*, vol. 14, no. 11, 1997, pp. 3083–3092.

343. V. V. Tuchin, "Coherent Optical Techniques for the Analysis of Tissue Structure and Dynamics," *J. Biomed. Opt.*, vol. 4, no. 1, 1999, pp. 106–124.

344. P. Bruscaglioni, G. Zaccanti, and Q. Wei, "Transmission of a Pulsed Polarized Light Beam through Thick Turbid Media: Numerical Results,"*Appl. Opt.*, vol. 32, 1993, pp. 6142–6150.

345. D. Bicout, C. Brosseau, A. S. Martinez, and J. M. Schmitt, "Depolarization of Multiply Scattering Waves by Spherical Diffusers: Influence of the Size Parameter," *Phys. Rev. E.*, vol. 49, 1994, pp. 1767–1770.

346. M. Dogariu and T. Asakura, "Photon Pathlength Distribution from Polarized Backscattering in Random Media," *Opt. Eng.*, vol. 35, 1996, pp. 2234–2239.

347. A. Dogariu, C. Kutsche, P. Likamwa, G. Boreman, and B. Moudgil, "Time-Domain Depolarization of Waves Retroreflected from Dense Colloidal Media," *Opt. Lett.*, vol. 22, 1997, pp. 585–587.

348. A. H. Hielsher, J. R. Mourant, and I. J. Bigio, "Influence of Particle Size and Concentration on the Diffuse Backscattering of Polarized Light from Tissue Phantoms and Biological Cell Suspensions," *Appl. Opt.*, vol. 36, 1997, pp. 125–135.

349. A. Ambirajan and D. C. Look, "A Backward Monte Carlo Study of the Multiple Scattering of a Polarized Laser Beam," *J. Quant. Spectrosc. Radiat. Transfer*, vol. 58, 1997, pp. 171–192.

350. M. J. Rakovic and G. W. Kattawar, "Theoretical Analysis of Polarization Patterns from Incoherent Backscattering of Light," *Appl. Opt.*, vol. 37, no. 15, 1998, pp. 3333–3338.

351. M. J. Racovic, G. W. Kattavar, M. Mehrubeoglu, B. D. Cameron, L. V. Wang, S. Rasteger, and G. L. Cote, "Light Backscattering Polarization Patterns from Turbid Media: Theory and Experiment," *Appl. Opt.*, vol. 38, 1999, pp. 3399–3408.

352. G. Yao and L. V. Wang, "Propagation of Polarized Light in Turbid Media: Simulated Animation Sequences," *Optics Express*, vol. 7, no. 5, 2000, pp. 198–203.

353. D. A. Zimnyakov, Yu. P. Sinichkin, P. V. Zakharov, and D. N. Agafonov, "Residual Polarization of Non-Coherently Backscattered Linearly Polarized Light: the Influence of the Anisotropy Parameter of the Scattering Medium," *Waves in Random Media*, vol. 11, 2001, pp. 395–412.

354. D. A. Zimnyakov and Yu. P. Sinichkin, "Ultimate Degree of Residual Polarization of Incoherently Backscattered Light of Multiple Scattering of Linearly Polarized Light," *Opt. Spectrosc.*, vol. 91, 2001, pp. 103–108.

355. D. A. Zimnyakov, Yu. P. Sinichkin, I. V. Kiseleva and D. N. Agafonov, "Effect of Absorption of Multiply Scattering Media on the Degree of Residual Polarization of Backscattered Light," *Opt. Spectrosc.*, vol. 92, 2002, pp. 765–771.

356. I. A. Vitkin and R. C. N. Studinski, "Polarization Preservation in Diffusive Scattering from *In Vivo* Turbid Biological Media: Effects of Tissue Optical Absorption in the Exact Backscattering Direction," *Optics Communs*, vol. 190, 2001, pp. 37–43.

357. G. Bal and M. Moscoso, "Theoretical and Numerical Analysis of Polarization for Time-Dependent Radiative Transfer Equations," *J. Quant. Spectrosc. & Radiat. Transf.*, vol. 70, 2001, pp. 75–98.

358. A. A. Kokhanovsky, "Photon Transport in Asymmetric Random Media," *J. Opt. A: Pure Appl. Opt.*, vol. 4, 2002, pp. 521–526.

359. A. A. Kokhanovsky, "Reflection and Polarization of Light by Semi-Infinite Turbid Media: Simple Approximations," *J. Colloid & Interface Sci.*, vol. 251, 2002, pp. 429–433.

360. L. Dagdug, G. H. Weiss, and A. H. Gandjbakhche, "Effects of Anisotropic Optical Properties on Photon Migration in Structured Tissues," *Phys. Med. Biol.*, vol. 48, 2003, pp. 1361–1370.

361. H. H. Tynes, G. W. Kattawar, E. P. Zege, I. L. Katsev, A. S. Prikhach, and L. I. Chaikovskaya, "Monte Carlo and Multicomponent Approximation Methods for Vector Radiative Transfer by Use of Effective Mueller Matrix Calculations," *Appl. Opt.*, vol. 40, no. 3, 2001, pp. 400–412.

362. I. M. Stockford, S. P. Morgan, P. C. Y. Chang, and J. G. Walker, "Analysis of the Spatial Distribution of Polarized Light Backscattering," *J. Biomed. Opt.*, vol. 7, no. 3, 2002, pp. 313–320.

363. S. Bartel and A. H. Hielscher, "Monte Carlo Simulations of the Diffuse Backscattering Mueller Matrix for Highly Scattering Media," *Appl. Opt.*, vol. 39, 2000, pp. 1580–1588.

364. X. Wang and L. V. Wang, "Propagation of Polarized Light in Birefringent Turbid Media: Time-Resolved Simulations," *Optics Express*, vol. 9, no. 5, 2001, pp. 254–259.

365. K. Y. Yong, S. P. Morgan, I. M. Stockford, and M. C. Pitter, "Characterization of Layered Scattering Media Using Polarized Light Measurements and Neural Networks," *J. Biomed. Opt.*, vol. 8, no. 3, 2003, pp. 504–511.

366. I. L. Maksimova, S. V. Romanov, and V. F. Izotova, "The Effect of Multiple Scattering in Disperse Media on Polarization Characteristics of Scattered Light," *Opt. Spectrosc.*, vol. 92, no. 6, 2002, pp. 915–923.

367. X. Wang and L. V. Wang, "Propagation of Polarized Light in Birefringent Turbid Media: A Monte Carlo Study," *J. Biomed. Opt.*, vol. 7, no. 3, 2002, pp. 279–290.

368. S. V. Gangnus, S. J. Matcher, and I. V. Meglinski, "Monte Carlo Modeling of Polarized Light Propagation in Biological Tissues," *Laser Phys.*, vol. 14, 2004, pp. 886–891.

369. C. J. Hourdakis and A. Perris, "A Monte Carlo Estimation of Tissue Optical Properties for the Use in Laser Dosimetry," *Phys. Med. Biol.*, vol. 40, 1995, pp. 351–364.

370. A. Yodh, B. Tromberg, E. Sevick-Muraca, and D. Pine (eds.), "Special Section on Diffusing Photons in Turbid Media," *J. Opt. Soc. Am. A.*, vol. 14, 1997, pp. 136–342.

371. L. O. Svaasand and Ch. J. Gomer, "Optics of Tissue," in *Dosimetry of Laser Radiation in Medicine and Biology*, SPIE Press, Bellingham, vol. IS5, 1989, pp. 114–132.

372. H. Horinaka, K. Hashimoto, K. Wada, and Y. Cho, "Extraction of Quasi-Straightforward–Propagating Photons from Diffused Light Transmitting through a Scattering Medium by Polarization Modulation," *Opt. Lett.*, vol. 20, 1995, pp. 1501–1503.

373. S. P. Morgan, M. P. Khong, and M. G. Somekh, "Effects of Polarization State and Scatterer Concentration Optical Imaging through Scattering Media," *Appl. Opt.*, vol. 36, 1997, pp. 1560–1565.

374. A. B. Pravdin, S. P. Chernova, and V. V. Tuchin, "Polarized Collimated Tomography for Biomedical Diagnostics," *Proc. SPIE* 2981, 1997, pp. 230–234.

375. M. R. Ostermeyer, D. V. Stephens, L. Wang, and S. L. Jacques, "Nearfield Polarization Effects on Light Propagation in Random Media," OSA TOPS 3, Optical Society of America, Washington, DC, 1996, pp. 20–25.

376. R. R. Anderson, "Polarized Light Examination and Photography of the Skin," *Arch. Dermatol.*, vol. 127, 1991, pp. 1000–1005.

377. A. W. Dreher and K. Reiter, "Polarization Technique Measures Retinal Nerve Fibers," *Clin. Vis. Sci.*, vol. 7, 1992, pp. 481–485.

378. N. Kollias, "Polarized Light Photography of Human Skin," in *Bioengineering of the Skin: Skin Surface Imaging and Analysis*, K.-P. Wilhelm, P. Elsner, E. Berardesca, and H. I. Maibach (eds.), CRC Press, Boca Raton, 1997, pp. 95–106.

379. S. G. Demos and R. R. Alfano, "Optical Polarization Imaging," *Appl. Opt.*, vol. 36, 1997, pp. 150–155.

380. G. Yao and L. V. Wang, "Two-Dimensional Depth-Resolved Mueller Matrix Characterization of Biological Tissue by Optical Coherence Tomography," *Opt. Lett.*, vol. 24, 1999, pp. 537–539.

381. B. D. Cameron, M. J. Racovic, M. Mehrubeoglu, G. Kattavar, S. Rasteger, L. V. Wang, and G. Cote, "Measurement and Calculation of the Two-Dimensional Backscattering Mueller Matrix of a Turbid Medium," *Opt. Lett.*, vol. 23, 1998, pp. 485–487; Errata, *Opt. Lett.*, vol. 23, 1998, p. 1630.

382. S. L. Jacques, R. J. Roman, and K. Lee, "Imaging Superficial Tissues with Polarized Light," *Lasers Surg. Med.*, vol. 26, 2000, pp. 119–129.

383. S. L. Jacques, J. C. Ramella-Roman, and K. Lee, "Imaging Skin Pathology with Polarized Light," *J. Biomed. Opt.*, vol. 7, no. 3, 2002, pp. 329–340.

384. M. Moscoso, J. B. Keller, and G. Papanicolaou, "Depolarization and Blurring of Optical Images by Biological Tissue," *J. Opt. Soc. Am.*, vol. 18, no. 4, 2001, pp. 948–960.

385. M. H. Smith, "Optimizing a Dual-Rotating-Retarder Mueller Matrix Polarimeter," *Proc. SPIE* 4481, 2001.

386. M. H. Smith, "Interpreting Mueller Matrix Images of Tissues," *Proc. SPIE* 4257, 2001, pp. 82–89.

387. L. L. Deibler and M. H. Smith, "Measurement of the Complex Refractive Index of Isotropic Materials with Mueller Matrix Polarimetry," *Appl. Opt.*, vol. 40, no. 22, 2001, pp. 3659–3667.

388. X.-R. Huang and R. W. Knighton, "Linear Birefringence of the Retinal Nerve Fiber Layer Measured *In Vitro* with a Multispectral Imaging Micropolarimeter, *J. Biomed. Opt.*, vol. 7, no. 2, 2002, pp. 199–204.

389. A. P. Sviridov, D. A. Zimnyakov, Yu. P. Sinichkin, L. N. Butvina, A. I. Omel'chenko, G. Sh. Makhmutova, and V. N. Bagratashvili, "IR Fourier Spectroscopy of *In-Vivo* Human Skin and Polarization of Backscattered Light in the Case of Skin Ablation by AIG: Nd laser radiation," *J. Appl. Spectrosc.*, vol. 69, 2002, pp. 484–488.

390. A. N. Yaroslavsky, V. Neel, and R. R. Anderson, "Demarcation of Non-melanoma Skin Cancer Margins in Thick Excisions Using Multispectral Polarized Light Imaging," *J. Invest. Dermatol.*, vol. 121, 2003, pp. 259–266.

391. E. E. Gorodnichev, A. I. Kuzovlev, and D. B. Rogozkin, "Depolarization of Light in Small-Angle Multiple Scattering in Random Media," *Laser Physics*, vol. 9, 1999, pp. 1210–1227.

392. I. Freund, M. Kaveh, R. Berkovits, and M. Rosenbluh, "Universal Polarization Correlations and Microstatistics of Optical Waves in Random Media," *Phys. Rev. B.*, vol. 42, no. 4, 1990, pp. 2613–2616.

393. D. Eliyahu, M. Rosenbluh, and I. Freund, "Angular Intensity and Polarization Dependence of Diffuse Transmission through Random Media," *J. Opt. Soc. Am. A.*, vol. 10, no. 3, 1993, pp. 477–491.

394. G. Jarry, E. Steiner, V. Damaschini, M. Epifanie, M. Jurczak, and R. Kaizer, "Coherence and Polarization of Light Propagating through Scattering Media and Biological Tissues," *Appl. Opt.*, vol. 37, 1998, pp. 7357–7367.

395. D. A. Zimnyakov and V. V. Tuchin, "About Interrelations of Distinctive Scales of Depolarization and Decorrelation of Optical Fields in Multiple Scattering," *JETP Lett.*, vol. 67, 1998, pp. 455–460.

396. D. A. Zimnyakov, V. V. Tuchin, and A. G. Yodh, "Characteristic Scales of Optical Field Depolarization and Decorrelation for Multiple Scattering Media and Tissues," *J. Biomed. Opt.*, vol. 4, 1999, pp. 157–163.

397. F. Bettelheim, "On the Optical Anisotropy of Lens Fibre Cells," *Exp. Eye Res.*, vol. 21, 1975, pp. 231–234.

398. J. Y. T. Wang and F. A. Bettelheim, "Comparative Birefringence of Cornea," *Comp. Bichem. Physiol., Part A: Mol. Integr. Physiol.*, vol. 51, 1975, pp. 89–94.

399. R. P. Hemenger, "Birefringence of a Medium of Tenuous Parallel Cylinders," *Appl. Opt.*, vol. 28, no. 18, 1989, pp. 4030–4034.

400. D. J. Maitland and J. T. Walsh, "Quantitative Measurements of Linear Birefringence during Heating of Native Collagen," *Laser Surg. Med.*, vol. 20, 1997, pp. 310–318.

401. H. B. Klein Brink, "Birefringence of the Human Crystalline Lens *in vivo*," *J. Opt. Soc. Am. A*, vol. 8, 1991, pp. 1788–1793.

402. R. P. Hemenger, "Refractive Index Changes in the Ocular Lens Result from Increased Light Scatter," *J. Biomed. Opt.*, vol. 1, 1996, pp. 268–272.

403. V. F. Izotova, I. L. Maksimova, I. S. Nefedov, and S. V. Romanov, "Investigation of Mueller matrices of Anisotropic Nonhomogeneous Layers in Application to Optical Model of Cornea," *Appl. Opt.*, vol. 36, no. 1, 1997, pp. 164–169.

404. J. S. Baba, B. D. Cameron, S. Theru, and G. L. Coté, "Effect of Temperature, pH, and Corneal Birefringence on Polarimetric Glucose Monitoring in the Eye," *J. Biomed. Opt.*, vol. 7, no. 3, 2002, pp. 321–328.

405. G. J. van Blokland, "Ellipsometry of the Human Retina *In Vivo*: Preservation of Polarization," *J. Opt. Soc. Am. A*, vol. 2, 1985, pp. 72–75.

406. H. B. Klein Brink and G. J. van Blokland, "Birefringence of the Human Foveal Area Assessed *In Vivo* with Mueller-Matrix Ellipsometry," *J. Opt. Soc. Am. A*, vol. 5, 1988, pp. 49–57.

407. R. C. Haskell, F. D. Carlson, and P. S. Blank, "Form Birefringence of Muscle," *Biophys. J.*, vol. 56, 1989, pp. 401–413.

408. S. Bosman, "Heat-Induced Structural Alterations in Myocardium in Relation to Changing Optical Properties," *Appl. Opt.*, vol. 32, no. 4, 1993, pp. 461–463.

409. G. V. Simonenko, T. P. Denisova, N. A. Lakodina, and V. V. Tuchin, "Measurement of an Optical Anisotropy of Biotissues" *Proc. SPIE* 3915, 2000, pp. 152–157.

410. G. V. Simonenko, V. V. Tuchin, and N. A. Lakodina, "Measurement of the Optical Anisotropy of Biological Tissues with the Use of a Nematic Liquid Crystal Cell," *J. Opt. Technol.*, vol. 67, no. 6, 2000, pp. 559–562.

411. O. V. Angel'skii, A. G. Ushenko, A. D. Arkhelyuk, S. B. Ermolenko, and D. N. Burkovets, "Scattering of Laser Radiation by Multifractal Biological Structures," *Opt. Spectrosc.*, vol. 88, no. 3, 2000, pp. 444–447.

412. M. R. Hee, D. Huang, E. A. Swanson, and J. G. Fujimoto, "Polarization-Sensitive Low-Coherence Reflectometer for Birefringence Characterization and Ranging," *J. Opt. Soc. Am. B*, vol. 9, 1992, pp. 903–908.

413. J. F. de Boer, T. E. Milner, M. J. C. van Gemert, and J. S. Nelson, "Two-Dimensional Birefringence Imaging in Biological Tissue by Polarization-Sensitive Optical Coherence Tomography," *Opt. Lett.*, vol. 22, no. 12, 1997, pp. 934–936.

414. M. J. Everett, K. Schoenerberger, B. W. Colston, Jr., and L. B. Da Silva, "Birefringence Characterization of Biological Tissue by Use of Optical Coherence Tomography," *Opt. Lett.*, vol. 23, no. 3, 1998, pp. 228–230.

415. J. F. de Boer, T. E. Milner, and J. S. Nelson, "Determination of the Depth Resolved Stokes Parameters of Light Backscattered from Turbid Media Using Polarization Sensitive Optical Coherence Tomography," *Opt. Lett.*, vol. 24, 1999, pp. 300–302.

416. J. F. de Boer and T. E. Milner, "Review of Polarization Sensitive Optical Coherence Tomography and Stokes Vector Determination," *J. Biomed. Opt.*, vol. 7, no. 3, 2002, pp. 359–371.

417. C. K. Hitzenberger, E. Gotzinger, M. Sticker, M. Pircher, and A. F. Fercher, "Measurement and Imaging of Birefringence and Optic Axis Orientation by Phase Resolved Polarization Sensitive Optical Coherence Tomography," *Opt. Express*, vol. 9, 2001, pp. 780–790.

418. S. Jiao and L. V. Wang, "Jones-Matrix Imaging of Biological Tissues with Quadruple-Channel Optical Coherence Tomograthy," *J. Biomed. Opt.*, vol. 7, no. 3, 2002, pp. 350–358.

419. M. G. Ducros, J. F. de Boer, H. Huang, L. Chao, Z. Chen, J. S. Nelson, T. E. Milner, and H. G. Rylander, "Polarization Sensitive Optical Coherence Tomography of the Rabbit Eye," *IEEE J. Sel. Top. Quantum Electron.*, vol. 5, 1999, pp. 1159–1167.

420. M. G. Ducros, J. D. Marsack, H. G. Rylander III, S. L. Thomsen, and T. E. Milner, "Primate Retina Imaging with Polarization-Sensitive Optical Coherence Tomography," *J. Opt. Soc. Am. A*, vol. 18, 2001, pp. 2945–2956.

421. C. E. Saxer, J. F. de Boer, B. H. Park, Y. Zhao, C. Chen, and J. S. Nelson, "High Speed Fiber Based Polarization Sensitive Optical Coherence Tomography of *In Vivo* Human Skin," *Opt. Lett.*, vol. 26, 2001, pp. 1069–1071.

422. B. H. Park C. E. Saxer, S. M. Srinivas, J. S. Nelson, and J. F. de Boer, "*In Vivo* Burn Depth Determination by High-Speed Fiber-Based Polarization Sensitive Optical Coherence Tomography," *J. Biomed. Opt.*, vol. 6, 2001, pp. 474–479.

423. X. J. Wang, T. E. Milner, J. F. de Boer, Y. Zhang, D. H. Pashley, and J. S. Nelson, "Characterization of Dentin and Enamel by Use of Optical Coherence Tomography," *Appl. Opt.*, vol. 38, 1999, pp. 2092–2096.

424. A. Baumgartner, S. Dichtl, C. K. Hitzenberger, H. Sattmann, B. Robl, A. Moritz, A. F. Fercher, and W. Sperr, "Polarization-Sensitive Optical Coherence Tomography of Dental Structures," *Caries Res.*, vol. 34, no. 1, 2000, pp. 59–69.

425. A. Kienle, F. K. Forster, R. Diebolder, and R. Hibst, "Light Propagation in Dentin: Influence of Microstructure on Anisotropy," *Phys. Med. Biol.*, vol. 48, 2003, N7–N14.

426. D. Fried, J. D. B. Featherstone, R. E. Glena, and W. Seka, "The Nature of Light Scattering in Dental Enamel and Dentin at Visible and Near-Infrared Wavelengths," *Appl. Opt.*, vol. 34, no. 7, 1995, pp. 1278–1285.

427. G. B. Altshuler, "Optical Model of the Tissues of the Human Tooth," *J. Opt. Technol.*, vol. 62, 1995, pp. 516–520.

428. R. C. N. Studinski and I. A. Vitkin, "Methodology for Examining Polarized Light Interactions with Tissues and Tissuelike Media in the Exact Backscattering Direction," *J. Biomed. Opt.*, vol. 5, no. 3, 2000, pp. 330–337.

429. K. C. Hadley and I. A. Vitkin, "Optical Rotation and Linear and Circular Depolarization Rates in Diffusively Scattered Light from Chiral, Racemic, and Achiral Turbid Media," *J. Biomed. Opt.*, vol. 7, no. 3, 2002, pp. 291–299.

430. J. Applequist, "Optical Activity: Biot's Bequest," *Am. Sci.*, vol. 75, 1987, pp. 59–67.

431. J. D. Bancroft and A. Stevens (eds.), *Theory and Practice of Histological Techniques*, Churchill Livingstone, Edinburgh, New York, 1990.

432. D. M. Maurice, *The Cornea and Sclera. The Eye*, H. Davson (ed.), Academic Press, Orlando, 1984, pp. 1–158.

433. R. W. Hart and R. A. Farrell, "Light Scattering in the Cornea," *J. Opt. Soc. Am.*, vol. 59, no. 6, 1969, pp. 766–774.

434. L. D. Barron, *Molecular Light Scattering and Optical Activity*, Cambridge Univ., London, 1982.

435. R. L. McCally and R. A. Farrell, "Light Scattering from Cornea and Corneal Transparency," in *Noninvasive Diagnostic Techniques in Ophthalmology*, B. R. Master (ed.), Springer-Verlag, New York, 1990, pp. 189–210.

436. I. L. Maksimova and L. P. Shubochkin, "Light-Scattering Matrices for a Close-Packed Binary System of Hard Spheres," *Opt. Spectrosc.*, vol. 70, no. 6, 1991, pp. 745–748.

437. V. Shankaran, M. J. Everett, D. J. Maitland, and J. T. Walsh, Jr., "Polarized Light Propagation through Tissue Phantoms Containing Densely Packed Scatterers," *Opt. Lett.*, vol. 25, no. 4, 2000, pp. 239–241.

438. V. Shankaran, J. T. Walsh, Jr., and D. J. Maitland, "Comparative Study of Polarized Light Propagation in Biological Tissues," *J. Biomed. Opt.*, vol. 7, no. 3, 2002, pp. 300–306.

439. V. V. Tuchin, "Optics of the Human Sclera: Photon Migration, Imaging and Spectroscopy," OSA TOPS 21, Optical Society of America, Washington, DC, 1998, pp. 99–104.

440. I. L. Maksimova, "Scattering of Radiation by Regular and Random Systems Comprised of Parallel Long Cylindrical Rods," *Opt. Spectrosc.*, vol. 93, no. 4, 2002, pp. 610–619.

441. A. G. Ushenko and V. P. Pishak, "Laser Polarimetry of Biological Tissues: Principles and Applications" in *Coherent-Domain Optical Methods: Biomedical Diagnostics, Environmental and Material Science*, vol. 1, V. V. Tuchin (ed.), Kluwer Academic Publishers, Boston, 2004, pp. 94–138.

442. N. G. Khlebtsov, I. L. Maksimova, V. V. Tuchin, and L. Wang, "Introduction to Light Scattering by Biological Objects," Chapter 1 in *Handbook of Optical Biomedical Diagnostics*, vol. PM107, V. V. Tuchin (ed.), SPIE Press, Bellingham, WA, 2002, pp. 31–167.

443. W. A. Shurcliff, *Polarized Light. Production and Use*, Harvard Univ., Cambridge, Mass., 1962.

444. W. A. Shurcliff and S. S. Ballard, *Polarized Light*, Van Nostrand, Princeton, 1964.

445. E. L. O'Neill, *Introduction to Statistical Optics*, Addison-Wesley, Reading, Mass., 1963.

446. D. S. Kliger, J. W. Lewis, and C. E. Randall, *Polarized Light in Optics and Spectroscopy*, Academic, Boston, 1990.

447. E. Collet, *Polarized Light. Fundamentals and Applications*, Dekker, New York, 1993.

448. R. M. A. Azzam and N. M. Bashara, *Ellipsometry and Polarized Light*, Elsevier Science, Amsterdam, 1994.

449. C. Brosseau, *Fundamentals of Polarized Light: A Statistical Optics Approach*, Wiley, New York, 1998.

450. I. L. Maksimova, S. N. Tatarintsev, and L. P. Shubochkin, "Multiple Scattering Effects in Laser Diagnostics of Bioobjects," *Opt. Spectrosc.*, vol. 72, 1992, pp. 1171–1177.

451. V. F. Izotova, I. L. Maksimova, and S. V. Romanov, "Utilization of Relations Between Elements of the Mueller Matrices for Estimating Properties of Objects and the Reliability of Experiments," *Opt. Spectrosc.*, vol. 80, no. 5, 1996, pp. 753–759.

452. V. V. Tuchin, "Biomedical Spectroscopy," in *Encyclopedia of Optical Engineering*, R. G. Driggers (ed.), Marcel-Dekker, New York, 2003, pp. 166–182; www.dekker.com/servlet/product/DOI/101081EEOE120009763

453. V. V. Tuchin, "Light-Tissue Interactions" in *Biomedical Photonics Handbook*, Tuan Vo-Dinh (ed.), CRC Press, Boca Raton, 2003, pp. 3-1–3-26.

454. D. Fried, "Optical Methods for Caries Detection, Diagnosis, and Therapeutic Intervention," in *Biomedical Photonics Handbook*, Tuan Vo-Dinh (ed.), CRC Press, Boca Raton, 2003, pp. 50-1–50-27.

455. S. E. Braslavsky and K. Heihoff, "Photothermal methods" in *Handbook of Organic Photochemistry*, J. C. Scaiano (ed.), CRC Press, Boca Raton, 1989.

456. V. E. Gusev and A. A. Karabutov, *Laser Optoacoustics*, AIP Press, New York, 1993.

457. A. Mandelis and K. H. Michaelian (eds.), "Special Section on Photoacoustic and Photothermal Science and Engineering," *Opt. Eng.*, vol. 36, no. 2, 1997, pp. 301–534.

458. A. A. Karabutov and A. A. Oraevsky, "Time-Resolved Detection of Optoacoustic Profiles for Measurement of Optical Energy Distribution in Tissues," in *Handbook of Optical Biomedical Diagnostics*, Chapter 10, vol. PM107, V. V. Tuchin (ed.), SPIE Press, Bellingham, WA, 2002, pp. 585–674.

459. A. A. Oraevsky and A. A. Karabutov, "Optoacoustic Tomography," in *Biomedical Photonics Handbook*, Chapter 34, Tuan Vo-Dinh (ed.), CRC Press, Boca Raton, 2003, pp. 34-1–34.

460. S. Nagai and M. Izuchi, "Quantitative Photoacoustic Imaging of Biological Tissues," *Jap. J. Appl. Phys.*, vol. 27, no. 3, 1988, pp. L423–L425.

461. A. M. Ashurov, U. Madvaliev, V. V. Proklov, et al., "Photoacoustic Scanning Microscope," *Sci. Res. Instr.*, no. 2, 1988, pp. 154–157.

462. M. G. Sowa and H. H. Mantsch, "FT-IR Step-Scan Photoacoustic Phase Analysis and Depth Profiling of Calcified Tissue," *Appl. Spectr.*, vol. 48, no. 3, 1994, pp. 316–319.

463. R. A. Kruger and P. Liu, "Photoacoustic Ultrasound: Pulse Production and Detection in 0.5% Liposyn," *Med. Phys.*, vol. 21, no. 7, 1994, pp. 1179–1184.

464. R. A. Kruger, L. Pingyu, Y. Fang, and C. R. Appledorn, "Photoacoustic Ultrasoud-Reconstruction Tomography," *Med. Phys.*, vol. 22, no. 10, 1995, pp. 1605–1609.

465. A. A. Oraevsky, "Laser Optoacoustic Imaging for Diagnosis of Cancer," *IEEE/LEOS Newsletter*, vol. 10, no. 12, 1996, pp. 17–20.

466. A. A. Karabutov, N. B. Podymova, and V. S. Letokhov, "Time-Resolved Laser Optoacoustic Tomography of Inhomogeneous Media," *Appl. Phys. B.*, vol. 63, 1996, pp. 545–563.

467. A. A. Oraevsky, S. J. Jacques, and F. K. Tittel, "Measurement of Tissue Optical Properties by Time-Resolved Detection of Laser-Induced Transient Stress," *Appl. Opt.*, vol. 36, no. 1, 1997, pp. 402–415.

468. R. O. Esenaliev, K. V. Larin, I. V. Larina, M. Motamedi, and A. A. Oraevsky, "Optical Properties of Normal and Coagulated Tissues: Measurements Using Combination of Optoacoustic and Diffuse Reflectance Techniques," *Proc. SPIE* 3726, 1999, pp. 560–566.

469. A. A. Karabutov, E. V. Savateeva, N. B. Podymova, and A. A. Oraevsky, "Backward Mode Detection of Laser-Induced Wide-Band Ultrasonic Tran-

sients with Optoacoustic Transducer," *J. Appl. Phys.*, vol. 87, no. 4, 2000, pp. 2003–2014.

470. V. G. Andreev, A. A. Karabutov, and A. A. Oraevsky, "Detection of Ultrawide-Band Ultrasound Pulses in Optoacoustic Tomography," *IEEE Trans. Ultrason. Ferroelectr. Freq. Control*, vol. 50, no. 10, 2003, pp. 1383–1390.

471. G. Paltauf and H. Schmidt-Kloiber, "Pulsed Optoacoustic Characterization of Layered Media," *J. Appl. Phys.*, vol. 88, no. 3, 2000, pp. 1624–1631.

472. K. P. Köstli, M. Frenz, H. P. Weber, G. Paltauf, and H. Schmidt-Kloiber, "Optoacoustic Infrared Spectroscopy of Soft Tissue," *J. Appl. Phys.*, vol. 88, no. 3, 2000, pp. 1632–1637.

473. K. P. Köstli, M. Frenz, H. P. Weber, G. Paltauf, and H. Schmidt-Kloiber, "Optoacoustic Tomography: Time-Gated Measurement of Pressure Distributions and Image Reconstruction," *Appl. Opt.*, vol. 40, no. 22, 2001, pp. 3800–3809.

474. J. A. Viator, G. Au, G. Paltauf, S. L. Jacques, S. A. Prahl, H. Ren, Z. Chen, and J. S. Nelson, "Clinical Testing of a Photoacoustic Probe for Port Wine Stain Depth Determination," *Lasers Surg. Med.*, vol. 30, 2002, pp. 141–148.

475. R. A. Kruger, W. L. Kiser, D. R. Reinecke, and G. A. Kruger, "Thermoacoustic Computed Tomography Using a Conventional Linear Transducer Array," *Med. Phys.*, vol. 30, 2003, pp. 856–860.

476. R. A. Kruger, W. L. Kiser, D. R. Reinecke, G. A. Kruger, and K. D. Miller, "Thermoacoustic Optical Molecular Imaging of Small Animals," *Molecular Imag.*, vol. 2, 2003, pp. 113–123.

477. C. G. A. Hoelen, F. F. M. de Mul, R. Pongers, and A. Dekker, "Three-Dimensional Photoacoustic Imaging of Blood Vessels in Tissue," *Opt. Lett.*, vol. 23, 1998, pp. 648–650.

478. C. G. A. Hoelen and F. F. M. de Mul, "Image Reconstruction for Photoacoustic Scanning of Tissue Structures," *Appl. Opt.*, vol. 39, no. 31, 2000, pp. 5872–5883.

479. C. G. A. Hoelen, A. Dekker, and F. F. M. de Mul, "Detection of Photoacoustic Transients Originating from Microstructures in Optically Diffuse Media such as Biological Tissue," *IEEE Trans. Ultrason. Ferroelectr. Freq. Control*, vol. 48, no. 1, 2001, pp. 37–47.

480. M. C. Pilatou, N. J. Voogd, F. F. M. de Mul, L. N. A. van Adrichem, and W. Steenbergen, "Analysis of Three-Dimensional Photoacoustic Imaging of a Vascular Tree *In Vitro*," *Rev. Sci. Instrum.*, vol. 74, no. 10, 2003, pp. 4495–4499.

481. R. G. M. Kolkman, E. Hondebrink, W. Steenbergen, T. G. van Leeuwen, and F. F. M. de Mul, "Photoacoustic Imaging of Blood Vessels with a Double-Ring Sensor Featuring a Narrow Angular Aperture," *J. Biomed. Opt.*, vol. 9, no. 6, 2004, pp. 1327–1335.

482. G. Ku and L.-H. V. Wang, "Scanning Electromagnetic-Induced Thermoacoustic Tomography: Signal, Resolution, and Contrast," *Med. Phys.*, vol. 28, 2001, pp. 4–10.

483. X. D. Wang, Y. J. Pang, G. Ku, X. Y. Xie, G. Stoica, and L. V. Wang, "Non-invasive Laser-Induced Photoacoustic Tomography for Structural and Functional *In Vivo* Imaging of the Brain," *Nat. Biotechnol.*, vol. 21, 2003, pp. 803–806.

484. X. D. Wang, Y. J. Pang, G. Ku, G. Stoica, and L. V. Wang, "Three-Dimensional Laser-Induced Photoacoustic Tomography of Mouse Brain with the Skin and Skull Intact," *Opt. Lett.*, vol. 28, no. 19, 2003, pp. 1739–1741.

485. J. J. Niederhauser, D. Frauchiger, H. P. Weber, and M. Frenz, "Real-Time Optoacoustic Imaging Using a Schlieren Transducer," *Appl. Phys. Lett.*, vol. 81, 2002, pp. 571–573.

486. B. P. Payne, V. Venugopalan, B. B. Mikić, and N. S. Nishioka, "Optoacoustic Determination of Optical Attenuation Depth Using Intereferometric Detection," *J. Biomed. Opt.*, vol. 8, no. 2, 2003, pp. 264–272.

487. B. P. Payne, V. Venugopalan, B. B. Mikić, and N. S. Nishioka, "Optoacoustic Tomography Using Time-Resolved Intereferometric Detection of Surface Displacement," *J. Biomed. Opt.*, vol. 8, no. 2, 2003, pp. 273–280.

488. U. Oberheide, I. Bruder, H. Welling, W. Ertmer, and H. Lubatschowski, "Optoacoustic Imaging for Optimization of Laser Cyclophotocoagulation," *J. Biomed. Opt.*, vol. 8, no. 2, 2003, pp. 281–287.

489. G. Schüle, G. Hüttman, C Framme, J. Roider, and R. Brinkmann, "Noninvasive Optoacoustic Temperature Determination at the Fundus of the Eye during Laser Irradiation," *J. Biomed. Opt.*, vol. 9, no. 1, 2004, pp. 173–179.

490. R. E. Imhof, C. J. Whitters, and D. J. S. Birch, "Opto-Thermal *In Vivo* Monitoring of Sunscreens on Skin," *Phys. Med. Biol.*, vol. 35, no. 1, 1990, pp. 95–102.

491. S. A. Prahl, I. A. Vitkin, U. Bruggemann, B. C. Wilson, and R. R. Anderson, "Determination of Optical Properties of Turbid Media Using Pulsed Photothermal Radiometry," *Phys. Med. Biol.*, vol. 37, 1992, pp. 1203–1217.

492. S. L. Jacques, J. S. Nelson, W. H. Wright, and T. E. Milner, "Pulsed Photothermal Radiometry of Port–Wine–Stain Lesions," *Appl. Opt.*, vol. 32, 1993, pp. 2439–2446.

493. I. A. Vitkin, B. C. Wilson, and R. R. Anderson, "Analysis of Layered Scattering Materials by Pulsed Photothermal Radiometry: Application to Photon Propagation in Tissue," *Appl. Opt.*, vol. 34, 1995, pp. 2973–2982.

494. T. E. Milner, D. M. Goodman, B. S. Tanenbaum, and J. S. Nelson, "Depth Profiling of Laser-Heated Chromophores in Biological Tissues by Pulsed Photothermal Radiometry," *J. Opt. Soc. Am. A*, vol. 12, 1995, pp. 1479–1488.

495. T. E. Milner, D. M. Goodman, B. S. Tanenbaum, B. Anvari, and J. S. Nelson, "Noncontact Determination of Thermal Diffusivity in Biomaterials Using Infrared Imaging Radiometry," *J. Biomed. Opt.*, vol. 1, 1996, pp. 92–97.

496. D. Fried, S. R. Visuri, J. D. B. Featherstone, J. T. Walsh, W. Seka, R. E. Glena, S. M. McCormack, and H. A. Wigdor, "Infrared Radiome-

try of Dental Enamel During Er: YAG and Er: YSGG Laser Irradiation," *J. Biomed. Opt.*, vol. 1, no. 4, 1996, pp. 455–465.

497. U. S. Sathyam, and S. A. Prahl, "Limitations in Measurement of Subsurface Temperatures Using Pulsed Photothermal Radiometry," *J. Biomed. Opt.*, vol. 2, no. 3, 1997, pp. 251–261.

498. B. Li, B. Majaron, J. A. Viator, T. E. Milner, Z. Chen, Y. Zhao, H. Ren, and J. S. Nelson, "Accurate Measurement of Blood Vessel Depth in Port Wine Stained Human Skin *In Vivo* Using Pulsed Photothermal Radiometry," *J. Biomed. Opt.*, vol. 9, no. 2, 2004, pp. 299–307.

499. B. Choi, B. Majaron, and J. S. Nelson, "Computational Model to Evaluate Port Wine Stain Depth Profiling Using Pulsed Photothermal Radiometry," *J. Biomed. Opt.*, vol. 9, no. 5, 2004, pp. 961–966.

500. L. Nicolaides, A. Mandelis, and S. H. Abrams, "Novel Dental Dynamic Depth Profilometric Imaging Using Simultaneous Frequency-Domain Infrared Photothermal Radiometry and Laser Luminescence," *J. Biomed. Opt.*, vol. 5, 2000, pp. 31–39.

501. R. J. Jeon, A. Mandelis, V. Sanchez, and S. H. Abrams, "Nonintrusive, Noncontacting Frequency-Domain Photothermal Radiometry and Luminescence Depth Profilometry of Carious and Artificial Subsurface Lesions in Human Teeth," *J. Biomed. Opt.*, vol. 9, no. 4, 2004, pp. 804–819.

502. D. H. Douglas-Hamilton and J. Conia, "Thermal Effects in Laser-Assisted Pre-Embryo Zona Drilling," *J. Biomed. Opt.*, vol. 6, no. 2, 2001, pp. 205–213.

503. D. Lapotko, T. Romanovskaya, and V. Zharov, "Photothermal Images of Live Cells in Presence of Drug," *J. Biomed. Opt.*, vol. 7, no. 3, 2002, pp. 425–434.

504. V. Zharov, "Far-Field Photothermal Microscopy beyond the Diffraction Limit," *Opt. Lett.*, vol. 28, 2003, pp. 1314–1316.

505. V. Zharov, V. Galitovsky, and M. Viegas, "Photothermal Detection of Local Thermal Effects during Selective Nanophotothermolysis," *Appl. Phys. Lett.*, vol. 83, no. 24, 2003, pp. 4897–4899.

506. V. Galitovskiy, P. Chowdhury, and V. P. Zharov, "Photothermal Detection of Nicotine-Induced Apoptotic Effects in a Pancreatic Cancer Cells," *Life Sciences*, vol. 75, 2004, pp. 2677–2687.

507. V. P. Zharov, E. I. Galanzha, and V. V. Tuchin, "Integrated Photothermal Flow Cytometry *In Vivo*," *J. Biomed. Opt.*, vol. 10, 2005, pp. 647–655.

508. V. P. Zharov, E. I. Galanzha, and V. V. Tuchin, "Photothermal Image Flow Cytometry *in Vivo*," *Opt. Lett.*, vol. 30, no. 6, 2005, pp. 107–110.

509. A. D. Yablon, N. S. Nishioka, B. B. Mikić, and V. Venugopalan, "Measurement of Tissue Absorption Coefficients by Use of Interferometric Photothermal Spectroscopy," *Appl. Opt.*, vol. 38, 1999, pp. 1259–1272.

510. M. L. Dark, L. T. Perelman, I. Itzkan, J. L. Schaffer, and M. S. Feld, "Physical Properties of Hydrated Tissue Determined by Surface Interferometry of Laser-Induced Thermoelastic Deformation," *Phys. Med. Biol.*, vol. 45, 2000, pp. 529–539.

511. A. A. Oraevsky, S. L. Jacques, R. O. Esenaliev, and F. K. Tittel, "Pulsed Laser Ablation of Soft Tissues, Gels and Aqueous Solutions at Temperatures Below 100°C," *Lasers Surg. Med.*, vol. 18, no. 3, 1995, pp. 231–240.

512. K. V. Larin, I. V. Larina, and R. O. Esenaliev, "Monitoring of Tissue Coagulation During Thermotherapy Using Optoacoustic Technique," *J. Phys. D: Appl. Phys.*, vol. 38, 2005, pp. 2645–2653.

513. C. H. Schmitz, U. Oberheide, S. Lohmann, H. Lubatschowski, and W. Ertmer, "Pulsed Photothermal Radiometry as a Method for Investigating Blood Vessel-Like Structures," *J. Biomed. Opt.*, vol. 6, no. 2, 2001, pp. 214–223.

514. Z. Zhao, S. Nissilä, O. Ahola, and R. Myllylä, "Production and Detection Theory of Pulsed Photoacoustic Wave with Maximum Amplitude and Minimum Distortion in Absorbing Liquid," *IEEE Trans. Instrum. Measur.*, vol. 47, no. 2, 1998, pp. 578–583.

515. I. V. Larina, K. V. Larin, and R. O. Esenaliev, "Real-Time Optoacoustic Monitoring of Temperature in Tissues," *J. Phys. D: Appl. Phys.*, vol. 38, 2005, pp. 2633–2639.

516. R. O. Esenaliev, I. V. Larina, K. V. Larin, D. J. Deyo, M. Motamedi, and D. S. Prough, "Optoacoustic Technique for Noninvasive Monitoring of Blood Oxygenation: A Feasibility Study," *Appl. Opt.*, vol. 41, no. 22, 2002, pp. 4722–4731.

517. L. V. Wang, "Ultrasound-Mediated Biophotonics Imaging: A Review of Acousto-Optical Tomography and Photo-Acoustic Tomography," *Disease Markers*, vol. 19, 2003, 2004, pp. 123–138.

518. K. Maslov, G. Stoica, and L. V. Wang, "*In vivo* Dark-Field Reflection-Mode Photoacoustic Microscopy," *Opt. Lett.*, vol. 30, no. 6, 2005, pp. 625–627.

519. L. Wang and X. Zhao, "Ultrasound-Modulated Optical Tomography of Absorbing Objects Buried in Dense Tissue-Simulating Turbid Media," *Appl. Opt.*, vol. 36, no. 28, 1997, pp. 7277–7282.

520. L. Wang, "Ultrasonic Modulation of Scattered Light in Turbid Media and a Potential Novel Tomography in Biomedicine," *Photochem. Photobiol.*, vol. 67, no. 1, 1998, pp. 41–49.

521. L. V. Wang and G. Ku, "Frequency-Swept Ultrasound-Modulated Optical Tomography of Scattering Media," *Opt. Let.*, vol. 23, no. 12, 1998, pp. 975–977.

522. J. Selb, S. Lévêque-Fort, A. Dubois, B. C. Forget, L. Pottier, F. Ramaz, and C. Boccara, "Ultrasonically Modulated Optical Imaging," in *Biomedical Photonics Handbook*, Chapter 35, Tuan Vo-Dinh (ed.), CRC Press, Boca Raton, 2003, pp. 35-1–12.

523. M. Kempe, M. Larionov, D. Zaslavsky, and A. Z. Genack, "Acousto-Optic Tomography with Multiply Scattered Light," *J. Opt. Soc. Am. A*, vol. 14, no. 5, 1997, pp. 1151–1158.

524. L.-H. V. Wang, "Mechanisms of Ultrasonic Modulation of Multiply Scattered Coherent Light: An Analytical Mode," *Phys. Rev. Lett.*, vol. 8704, 2001, pp. 3903-(1–4).

525. J. P. Gore and L. X. Xu, "Thermal Imaging for Biological and Medical Diagnostics," in *Biomedical Photonics Handbook*, Chapter 17, Tuan Vo-Dinh (ed.), CRC Press, Boca Raton, 2003, pp. 17-1–12.

526. A. L. McKenzie, "Physics of Thermal Processes in Laser-Tissue Interaction," *Phys. Med. Biol.*, vol. 35, 1990, pp. 1175–1209.

527. A. J. Welch and M. J. C. van Gemert (eds.), *Optical-Thermal Response of Laser Irradiated Tissue*, Plenum Press, 1995.

528. C. H. G. Wright, S. F. Barrett, and A. J. Welch, "Laser-Tissue Interaction," in *Lasers in Medicine*, D. R. Vij and K. Mahesh (eds.), Kluwer, Boston, 2002.

529. S. Weinbaum and L. M. Jiji, "A New Simplified Bioheat Equation for the Effect of Blood Flow on Local Average Tissue Temperature," *J. Biomech. Eng.*, vol. 107, 1985, pp. 131–139.

530. Z. F. Cui and J. C. Barbenel, "The Influence of Model Parameter Values on the Prediction of Skin Surface Temperature: I. Resting and Surface Insulation," *Phys. Med. Biol.*, vol. 35, 1990, pp. 1683–1697.

531. M. Nitzan and B. Khanokh, "Infrared Radiometry of Thermally Insulated Skin for the Assessment of Skin Blood Flow," *Opt. Eng.*, vol. 33, 1994, pp. 2953–2957.

532. L. V. Wang and Q. Shen, "Sonoluminescent Tomography of Strongly Scattering Media," *Opt. Lett.*, vol. 23, no. 7, 1998, pp. 561–563.

533. Q. Shen and L. V. Wang, "Two-Dimensional Imaging of Dense Tissue-Simulating Turbid Media by Use of Sonoluminescence," *Appl. Opt.*, vol. 38, no. 1, 1999, pp. 246–252.

534. O. Khalil, "Non-Invasive Glucose Measurement Technologies: An Update from 1999 to the Dawn of the New Millenium," *Diabetes Technol. Ther.*, vol. 6, no. 5, 2004, pp. 660–697.

535. K. M. Quan, G. B. Christison, H. A. Mackenzie, and P. Hodgson, "Glucose Determination by a Pulsed Photoacoustic Technique: An Experimental Study Using a Gelatin–Based Tissue Phantom," *Phys. Med. Biol.*, vol. 38, 1993, pp. 1911–1922.

536. H. A. MacKenzie, H. S. Ashton, S. Spiers, Y. Shen, S. S. Freeborn, J. Hannigan, J. Lindberg, and P. Rae, "Advances in Photoacoustic Noninvasive Glucose Testing," *Clin. Chem.*, vol. 45, 1999, pp. 1587–1595.

537. A. A. Bednov, A. A. Karabutov, E. V. Savateeva, W. F. March, and A. A. Oraevsky, "Monitoring Glucose *In Vivo* by Measuring Laser-Induced Acoustic Profiles," *Proc. SPIE* vol. 3916, 2000, pp. 9–18.

538. A. A. Bednov, E. V. Savateeva, and A. A. Oraevsky, "Glucose Monitoring in Whole Blood by Measuring Laser-Induced Acoustic Profiles," *Proc. SPIE* vol. 4960, 2003, pp. 21–29.

539. Z. Zhao and R. Myllylä, "Photoacoustic Blood Glucose and Skin Measurement Based on Optical Scattering Effect," *Proc. SPIE*, vol. 4707, 2002, pp. 153–157.

540. M. Kinnunen and R. Myllylä, "Effect of Glucose on Photoacoustic Signals at the Wavelemgth of 1064 and 532 nm in Pig Blood and Intralipid," *J. Phys. D: Appl. Phys.*, vol. 38, 2005, pp. 2654–2661.

541. Z. Zhao, *Pulsed Photoacoustic Techniques and Glucose Determination in Human Blood and Tissue*, Ph.D. Dissertation, Oulu, Finland, University of Oulu, 2002. Available online at: http://herkules.oulu.fi/isbn9514266900/index.html.

542. Glucon, Inc.: http://www.glucon.com/

543. Y. Shen, Z. Lu, S. Spiers, H. A. MacKenzie, H. S. Ashton, J. Hannigan, S. S. Freeborn, and J. Lindberg, "Measurement of the Optical Absorption Coefficient of a Liquid by Use of a Time-Resolved Photoacoustic Technique," *Appl. Opt.*, vol. 39, 2000, pp. 4007–4012.

544. D. C. Klonoff, J. R. Braig, B. B. Sterling, C. Kramer, D. S. Goldberger, and Y. Trebino, "Mid-Infrared Spectroscopy for Non-invasive Blood Glucose Monitoring," *IEEE Laser Electro-Opt. Soc. Newslett.*, vol. 12, 1998, pp. 13–14.

545. P. Zheng, C. E. Kramer, C. W. Barnes, J. R. Braig, and B. B. Sterling, "Non-invasive Glucose Determination by Oscillating Thermal Gradient Spectrometry," *Diabetes. Technol. Ther.*, vol. 2, 2000, pp. 17–25.

546. C. D. Malchoff, K. Shoukri, J. I. Landau, and J. M. Buchert, "A Novel Non-invasive Blood Glucose Monitor," *Diabetes Care*, vol. 25, 2002, pp. 2268–2275.

547. R. O. Esenaliev, Y. Y. Petrov, O. Hartrumpf, D. J. Deyo, and D. S. Prough, "Contineous, Noninvasive Monitoring of Total Hemoglobin Concentration by an Optoacoustic Technique," *Appl. Opt.*, vol. 43, 2004, pp. 3401–3407.

548. I. Petrova, R. O. Esenaliev, Y. Y. Petrov, H.-P. F. Brecht, C. H. Svensen, J. Olsson, D. J. Deyo, and D. S. Prough, "Optoacoustic Monitoring of Blood Hemoglobin Concentration: A Pilot Clinical Study," *Opt. Lett.*, vol. 30, 2005, pp. 1677–1679.

549. R. O. Esenaliev, K. V. Larin, I. V. Larina, and M. Motamedi, "Noninvasive Monitoring of Glucose Concentration with Optical Coherent Tomography," *Opt. Lett.*, vol. 26, no. 13, 2001, pp. 992–994.

550. K. V. Larin, M. S. Eledrisi, M. Motamedi, R. O. Esenaliev, "Noninvasive Blood Glucose Monitoring with Optical Coherence Tomography: a Pilot Study in Human Subjects," *Diabetes Care*, vol. 25, no. 12, 2002, pp. 2263–2267.

551. K. V. Larin, M. Motamedi, T. V. Ashitkov, and R. O. Esenaliev, "Specificity of Noninvasive Blood Glucose Sensing Using Optical Coherence Tomography Technique: a Pilot Study," *Phys Med Biol*, vol. 48, 2003, pp. 1371–1390.

552. D. M. Zhestkov, A. N. Bashkatov, E. A. Genina, and V. V. Tuchin, "Influence of Clearing Solutions Osmolarity on the Optical Properties of RBC," *Proc. SPIE* 5474, 2004, pp. 321–330.

553. B. Yin, D. Xing, Y. Wang, Y. Zeng, Y. Tan, and Q. Chen, "Fast Photoacoustic Imaging System Based on 320-element Linear Transducer Array," *Phys. Med. Biol.*, vol. 49, 2004, pp. 1339–1346.

554. Y. Su, F. Zhang, K. Xu, J. Yao, and R. K. Wang, "A Photoacoustic Tomography System for Imaging of Biological Tissues," *J. Phys. D: Appl. Phys.*, vol. 38, 2005, pp. 2640–2644.

555. P. A. Fomitchov, A. K. Kromine, and S. Krishnaswamy, "Photoacoustic Probes for Nondestructive Testing and Biomedical Applications," *Appl. Opt.*, vol. 41, no. 22, 2002, pp. 4451–4459.

556. M. Jaeger, J. J. Niederhauser, M. Hejazi, and M. Frenz, "Diffraction-Free Acoustic Detection for Optoacoustic Depth Profiling of Tissue Using an Optically Transparent Polyvinylidene Fluoride Pressure Transducer Operated in Backward and Forward Mode," *J. Biomed. Opt.*, vol. 10, no. 2, 2005, pp. 024035-1–7.

557. G. Ku, X. Wang, G. Stoica, and L. V. Wang, "Multiple-Bandwidth Photoacoustic Tomography," *Phys. Med. Biol.*, vol. 49, 2004, pp. 1329–1338.

558. B. Beauvoit, T. Kitai, B. Chance, "Contribution of the Mitochondrial Compartment to the Optical Properties of the Rat Liver: a Theoretical and Practical Approach," *Biophys. J.*, vol. 67, 1994, pp. 2501–2510.

559. V. G. Vereshchagin and A. N. Ponyavina, "Statistical Characteristic and Transparency of Thin Closely Packed Disperse Layer," *J. Appl. Spectr. (USSR)*, vol. 22, no. 3, 1975, pp. 518–524.

560. V. Twersky "Interface Effects in Multiple Scattering by Large, Low Refracting, Absorbing Particles," *J. Opt. Soc. Am.*, vol. 60, no. 7, 1970, 908–914.

561. M. Lax, "Multiple Scattering of Waves II. The Effective Field in Dense System," *Phys. Rev.*, vol. 85, no. 4, 1952, pp. 621–629.

562. L. Tsang, J. A. Kong, and R. T. Shin, *Theory of Microwave Remote Sensing*, Wiley, New York, 1985.

563. K. M. Hong, "Multiple Scattering of Electromagnetic Waves by a Crowded Monolayer of Spheres: Application to Migration Imaging Films," *J. Opt. Soc. Am.*, vol. 70, no. 7, 1980, pp. 821–826.

564. A. Ishimaru and Y. Kuga "Attenuation Constant of a Coherent Field in a Dense Distribution of Particles," *J. Opt. Soc. Am.*, vol. 72, no. 10, 1982, pp. 1317–1320.

565. A. N. Ponyavina, "Selection of Optical Radiation in Scattering by Partially Ordered Disperse Media," *J. Appl. Spectrosc.*, vol. 65, no. 5, 1998, pp. 721–733.

566. T. R. Smith, "Multiple Scattering in the Cornea," *J. Mod. Opt.*, vol. 35, no. 1, 1988, pp. 93–101.

567. V. Twersky, "Absorption and Multiple Scattering by Biological Suspensions," *J. Opt. Soc. Am.*, vol. 60, 1970, pp. 1084–1093.

568. J. M. Steinke and A. P. Shephard, "Diffusion Model of the Optical Absorbance of Whole Blood," *J. Opt. Soc. Am. A*, vol. 5, 1988, pp. 813–822.

569. I. F. Cilesiz and A. J. Welch, "Light Dosimetry: Effects of Dehydration and Thermal Damage on the Optical Properties of the Human Aorta," *Appl. Opt.*, vol. 32, 1993, pp. 477–487.

570. W.-C. Lin, M. Motamedi, and A. J. Welch, "Dynamics of Tissue Optics During Laser Heating of Turbid Media," *Appl. Opt.*, vol. 35, no. 19, 1996, pp. 3413–3420.

571. G. Vargas, E. K. Chan, J. K. Barton, H. G. Rylander III, and A. J. Welch, "Use of an Agent to Reduce Scattering in Skin," *Laser. Surg. Med.*, vol. 24, 1999, pp. 133–141.

572. R. M. P. Doornbos, R. Lang, M. C. Aalders, F. W. Cross, and H. J. C. M. Sterenborg, "The Determination of *In Vivo* Human Tissue Optical Properties and Absolute Chromophore Concentrations Using Spatially Resolved Steady-State Diffuse Reflectance Spectroscopy," *Phys. Med. Biol.*, vol. 44, 1999, pp. 967–981.

573. J. R. Lakowicz, *Principles of Fluorescence Spectroscopy*, 2nd ed., Kluwer Academic/Plenum Publ., New York, 1999.

574. H. Schneckenburger, R. Steiner, W. Strauss, K. Stock, and R. Sailer, "Fluorescence Technologies in Biomedical Diagnostics," Chapter 15 in *Optical Biomedical Diagnostics*, V. V. Tuchin (ed.), SPIE Press, Bellingham, WA, 2002, pp. 825–874.

575. Yu. P. Sinichkin, N. Kollias, G. Zonios, S. R. Utz, and V. V. Tuchin, "Reflectance and Fluorescence Spectroscopy of Human Skin *In Vivo*," Chapter 13 in *Optical Biomedical Diagnostics*, V. V. Tuchin (ed.), SPIE Press, Bellingham, WA, 2002, pp. 725–785.

576. S. Svanberg, "New Developments in Laser Medicine," *Phys. Scripta*, vol. T72, 1997, pp. 69–75.

577. R. R. Richards-Kortum, R. P. Rava, R. E. Petras, M. Fitzmaurice, M. Sivak, and M. S. Feld, "Spectroscopic Diagnosis of Colonic Dysplasia," *Photochem. Photobiol.*, vol. 53, 1991, pp. 777–786.

578. H. J. C. M. Sterenborg, M. Motamedi, R. F. Wagner, J. R. M. Duvic, S. Thomsen, and S. L. Jacques, "*In Vivo* Fluorescence Spectroscopy and Imaging of Human Skin Tumors," *Lasers Med. Sci.*, vol. 9, 1994, pp. 344–348.

579. H. Zeng, C. MacAulay, D. I. McLean, and B. Palcic, "Spectroscopic and Microscopic Characteristics of Human Skin Autofluorescence Emission," *Photochem. Photobiol.*, vol. 61, 1995, pp. 639–645.

580. Yu. P. Sinichkin, S. R. Utz, A. H. Mavlutov, and H. A. Pilipenko, "*In Vivo* Fluorescence Spectroscopy of the Human Skin: Experiments and Models," *J. Biomed. Opt.*, vol. 3, 1998, pp. 201–211.

581. R. Drezek, K. Sokolov, U. Utzinger, I. Boiko, A. Malpica, M. Follen, and R. Richards-Kortum, "Understanding the Contributions of NADH and Collagen to Cervical Tissue Fluorescence Spectra: Modeling, Measurements, and Implications," *J. Biomed. Opt.*, vol. 6, no. 4, 2001, pp. 385–396.

582. L. C. Lucchina, N. Kollias, R. Gillies, S. B. Phillips, J. A. Muccini, M. J. Stiller, R. J. Trancik, and L. A. Drake, "Fluorescence Photography in the Evaluation of Acne," *J. Am. Acad. Dermatol.*, vol. 35, 1996, pp. 58–63.

583. N. S. Soukos, S. Som, A. D. Abernethy, K. Ruggiero, J. Dunham, C. Lee, A. G. Doukas, and J. M. Goodson, "Phototargeting Oral Black-Pigmented Bacteria," *Antimicrob. Agents Chemother.*, vol. 49, 2005, pp. 1391–1396.

584. P. Kask, K. Palo, N. Fay, L. Brand, U. Mets, D. Ullmann, J. Jungmann, J. Pschorr, and K. Gall, "Two-Dimensional Fluorescence Intensity Distribution Analysis: Theory and Applications," *Biophys. J.*, vol. 78, 2000, pp. 1703–1713.

585. D. E. Hyde, T. J. Farrell, M. S. Patterson, and B. C. Wilson, "A Diffusion Theory Model of Spatially Resolved Fluorescence from Depth-Dependent Fluorophore Concentrations," *Phys. Med. Biol.*, vol. 46, 2001, pp. 369–383.

586. K. Sokolov, J. Galvan, A. Myakov, A. Lacy, R. Lotan, and R. Richards-Kortum, "Realistic Three-Dimensional Epithelial Tissue Phantoms for Biomedical Optics," *J. Biomed. Opt.*, vol. 7, no. 1, 2002, pp. 148–156.

587. M. J. Eppstein, D. J. Hawrysz, A. Godavarty, and E. M. Sevick-Muraca, "Three-Dimensional, Bayesian Image Reconstruction from Sparse and Noisy Data Sets: Near-Infrared Fluorescence Tomography," *Proc. Natl. Acad. Sci. USA*, vol. 99, no. 15, 2002, pp. 9619–9624.

588. A. Eidsath, V. Chernomordik, A. Gandjbakhche, P. Smith, and A. Russo, "Three-Dimensional Localization of Fluorescent Masses Deeply Embedded in Tissue," *Phys. Med. Biol.*, vol. 47, 2002, pp. 4079–4092.

589. N. C. Biswal, S. Gupta, N. Ghosh, and A. Pradhan, "Recovery of Turbidity Free Fluorescence from Measured Fluorescence: an Experimental Approach," *Optics Express*, vol. 11, no. 24, 2003, pp. 3320–3331.

590. Q. Liu, C. Zhu, and N. Ramanujam, "Experimental Validation of Monte Carlo Modeling of Fluorescence in Tissues in the UV-Visible Spectrum," *J. Biomed. Opt.*, vol. 8, no. 2, 2003, pp. 223–236.

591. C. Zhu, Q. Liu, and N. Ramanujam, "Effect of Fiber Optic Probe Geometry on Depth-Resolved Fluorescence Measurements from Epithelial Tissues: a Monte Carlo Simulation," *J. Biomed. Opt.*, vol. 8, no. 2, 2003, pp. 237–247.

592. D. Y. Churmakov, I. V. Meglinski, S. A. Piletsky, and D. A. Greenhalgh, "Analysis of Skin Tissues Spatial Fluorescence Distribution by the Monte Carlo Simulation," *Appl. Phys. D*, vol. 36, 2003, pp. 1722–1728.

593. H. Schneckenburger, M. H. Gschwend, R. Sailer, H.-P. Mock, and W. S. L. Strauss, "Time-gated fluorescence microscopy in molecular and cellular biology," *Cell. Mol. Biol.*, vol. 44, 1998, pp. 795–805.

594. O. O. Abugo, P. Herman, and J. R. Lakowicz, "Fluorescence Properties of Albumin Blue 633 and 670 in Plasma and Whole Blood, *J. Biomed. Opt.*, vol. 6, no. 3, 2001, pp. 359–365.

595. J. E. Budaj, S. Achilefu, R. B. Dorshow, and R. Rajagopalan, "Novel Fluorescent Contrast Agents for Optical Imaging of *In Vivo* Tumors Based on a Receptor-Targeted Dye-Peptide Conjugate Platform," *J. Biomed. Opt.*, vol. 6, no. 2, 2001, pp. 122–133.

596. K. Suhling, J. Siegel, D. Phillips, P. M. W. French, S. Leveque-Fort, S. E. D. Webb, and D. M. Davis, "Imaging the Environment of Green Fluorescent Protein," *Biophys. J.*, vol. 83, 2002, pp. 3589–3595.

597. I. Gannot, A. Garashi, G. Gannot, V. Chernomordik, and A. Gandjbakhche, "*In Vivo* Quantitative Three-Dimensional Localization of Tumor Labeled with Exogenous Specific Fluorescence Markers," *Appl. Opt.*, vol. 42, no. 16, 2003, pp. 3073–3080.

598. D. Hattery, V. Chernomordik, M. Loew, I. Gannot, and A. Gandjbakhche, "Analytical Solutions for Time-Resolved Fluorescence Lifetime Imaging in a Turbid Medium Such as Tissue," *J. Opt. Soc. Am. A*, vol. 18, no. 7, 2001, pp. 1523–1530.

599. M. Sadoqi, P. Riseborough, and S. Kumar, "Analytical Models for Time Resolved Fluorescence Spectroscopy in Tissues," *Phys. Med. Biol.*, vol. 46, 2001, pp. 2725–2743.

600. E. Kuwana and E. M. Sevick-Muraca, "Fluorescence Lifetime Spectroscopy in Multiply Scattering Media with Dyes Exhibiting Multiexponential Decay Kinetics," *Biophys. J.*, vol. 83, 2002, pp. 1165–1176.

601. K. Vishwanath, B. Pogue, and M.-A. Mycek, "Quantitative Fluorescence Lifetime Spectroscopy in Turbid Media: Comparison of Theoretical, Experimental and Computational Methods," *Phys. Med. Biol.*, vol. 47, 2002, pp. 3387–3405.

602. C. S. Betz, M. Mehlmann, K. Rick, H. Stepp, G. Grevers, R. Baumgartner, and A. Leunig, "Autofluorescence Imaging and Spectroscopy of Normal and Malignant Mucosa in Patients with Head and Neck Cancer," *Lasers Surg. Med.*, vol. 25, 1999, pp. 323–334.

603. N. Anastassopoulou, B. Arapoglou, P. Demakakos, M. I. Makropoulou, A. Paphiti, and A. A. Serafetinides, "Spectroscopic Characterisation of Carotid Atherosclerotic Plaque by Laser Induced Fluorescence," *Lasers Surg. Med.*, vol. 28, 2001, pp. 67–73.

604. S. K. Chang, M. Y. Dawood, G. Staerkel, U. Utzinger, E. N. Atkinson, R. R. Richards-Kortum, and M. Follen, "Fluorescence Spectroscopy for Cervical Precancer Detection: is there Variance Across the Menstrual Cycle?" *J. Biomed. Opt.*, vol. 7, no. 4, 2002, pp. 595–602.

605. R. Hage, P. R. Galhanone, R. A. Zangaro, K. C. Rodrigues, M. T. T. Pacheco, A. A. Martin, M. M. Netto, F. A. Soares, and I. W. da Cunha, "Using the Laser-Induced Fluorescence Spectroscopy in the Differentiation Between Normal and Neoplastic Human Breast Tissue," *Lasers Med. Sci.*, vol. 18, 2003, pp. 171–176.

606. S. Andersson-Engels, G. Canti, R. Cubeddu, C. Eker, C. Klinteberg, A. Pifferi, K. Svanberg, S. Svanberg, P. Taroni, G. Valentini, and I. Wang, "Preliminary Evaluation of Two Fluorescence Imaging Methods for the Detection and the Delineation of Basal Cell Carcinomas of the Skin," *Lasers Surg. Med.*, vol. 26, 2000, pp. 76–82.

607. T. Wu, J. Y. Qu, T.-H. Cheung, K. W.-K. Lo, and M.-Y. Yu, "Preliminary Study of Detecting Neoplastic Growths *In Vivo* with Real Time Calibrated Autofluorescence Imaging," *Optics Express*, vol. 11, no. 4, 2003, pp. 291–298.

608. L. Rovati and F. Docchio, "Autofluorescence Methods in Ophthalmology," *J. Biomed. Opt.*, vol. 9, no. 1, 2004, pp. 9–21.

609. W. Denk, "Two-Photon Excitation in Functional Biological Imaging," *J. Biomed. Opt.*, vol. 1, no. 3, 1996, pp. 296–304.

610. D. W. Piston, B. R. Masters, and W. W. Webb, "Three-Dimensionally Resolved NAD(P)H Cellular Metabolic Redox Imaging of the *In Situ* Cornea with Two-Photon Excitation Laser Scanning Microscopy," *J. Microscopy*, vol. 178, 1995, pp. 20–27.

611. K. M. Berland, P. T. So, and E. Gratton, "Two-Photon Fluorescence Correlation Spectroscopy: Method and Application to the Intracellular Environment," *Biophys. J.*, vol. 68, 1995, pp. 649–701.

612. S. W. Hell, K. Bahlmann, M. Schrader, et al., "Three-Photon Excitation in Fluorescence Microscopy," *J. Biomed. Opt.*, vol. 1, no. 1, 1996, pp. 71–74.

613. B. R. Masters, P. T. C. So, and E. Gratton, "Multi-Photon Excitation Fluorescence Microscopy and Spectroscopy of *In Vivo* Human Skin," *Biophys. J.*, vol. 72, 1997, pp. 2405–2412.

614. B. R. Masters, "Confocal Laser Scanning Microscopy," in *Coherent-Domain Optical Methods: Biomedical Diagnostics, Environmental and Material Science*, Chapter 21, V. V. Tuchin (ed.), Kluwer Academic Publishers, Boston, vol. 2, 2004, pp. 364–415.

615. P. T. C. So, C. Y. Dong, and B. R. Masters, "Two-Photon Excitation Fluorescence Microscopy," in *Biomedical Photonics Handbook*, Tuan Vo-Dinh (ed.), CRC Press, Boca Rotan, Florida, 2003, pp. 11-1-17.

616. Z. X. Zhang, G. J. Sonek, X. B. Wei, C. Sun, M. W. Berns, and B. J. Tromberg, "Cell Viability and DNA Denaturation Measurements by Two-Photon Fluorescence Excitation in CW Al:GaAs Diode Laser Optical Traps," *J. Biomed. Opt.*, vol. 4, no. 2, 1999, pp. 256–259.

617. Ch. J. Bardeen, V. V. Yakovlev, J. A. Squier, K. R. Wilson, S. D. Carpenter, and P. M. Weber, "Effect of Pulse Shape on the Efficiency of Multiphoton Processes: Implications for Biological Microscopy," *J. Biomed. Opt.*, vol. 4, no. 3, 1999, pp. 362–367.

618. A. K. Dunn, V. P. Wallace, M. Coleno, M. W. Berns, and B. J. Tromberg, "Influence of Optical Properties on Two-Photon Fluorescence Imaging in Turbid Samples," *Appl. Opt.*, vol. 39, no. 7, 2000, pp. 1194–1201.

619. Y. Ozaki, "Medical Application of Raman Spectroscopy," *Appl. Spectrosc. Rev.*, vol. 24, no. 3, 1988, pp. 259–312.

620. L. T. Perelman, M. D. Modell, E. Vitkin, and E. B. Hanlon, "Light Scattering Spectroscopy: from Elastic to Inelastic," Chapter 9, in *Coherent-Domain Optical Methods: Biomedical Diagnostics, Environmental and Material Science*, vol. 1, V. V. Tuchin (ed.), Kluwer Academic Publishers, Boston, 2004, pp. 355–395.

621. A. T. Tu, *Raman Spectroscopy in Biology*, John Wiley & Sons Ltd., New York, 1982.

622. G. W. Lucassen, G. N. A. van Veen, and J. A. J. Jansen, "Band Analysis of Hydrated Human Skin Stratum Corneum Attenuated Total Reflectance Fourier Transform Infrared Spectra *In Vivo*", *J. Biomedical Optics*, vol. 3, 1998, pp. 267–280.

623. G. J. Puppels, "Confocal Raman Microspectroscopy," in *Fluorescent and Luminescent Probes for Biological Activity*, W. Mason (ed.), Academic Press, London, 1999, pp. 377–406.

624. G. W. Lucassen, P. J. Caspers, and G. J. Puppels, "Infrared and Raman Spectroscopy of Human Skin *In Vivo*," Chapter 14, in *Optical Biomedical Diagnostics*, V. V. Tuchin (ed.), SPIE Press, Bellingham, 2002, pp. 787–823.

625. R. Petry, M. Schmitt, and J. Popp, "Raman Spectroscopy—a Prospective Tool in the Life Sciences," *Chemphyschem.*, vol. 4, 2003, pp. 14–30.

626. U. Utzinger, D. L. Heintselman, A. Mahadevan-Jansen, A. Malpica, M. Follen, and R. Richards-Kortum, "Near-Infrared Raman Spectroscopy for *In Vivo* Detection of Cervical Precancers," *Appl. Spectrosc.*, vol. 55, 2001, pp. 955–959.

627. C. S. Schatz and R. P. Van Duyne, "Electromagnetic Mechanism of Surface-Enhanced Spectroscopy," in *Handbook of Vibrational Spectroscopy*, J. M. Chalmers and P. R. Grifiths (eds.), John Wiley & Sons Ltd., Chichester, 2002, pp.

628. N. Skrebova Eikje, Y. Ozaki, K. Aizawa, and S. Arase, "Fiber Optic Near-Infrared Raman Spectroscopy for Clinical Noninvasive Determination of Water Content in Diseased Skin and Assessment of Cutaneous Edima," *J. Biomed. Opt.*, vol. 10, 2005, pp. 014013-1-13.

629. J. R. Mourant, R. R. Gibson, T. M. Johnson, S. Carpenter, K. W. Short, Y. R. Yamada, and J. P. Freyer, "Methods for Measuring the Infrared Spectra of Biological Cells," *Phys. Med. Biol.*, vol. 48, 2003, pp. 243–257.

630. M. Kohl, M. Essenpreis, and M. Cope, "The Influence of Glucose Concentration upon the Transport of Light in Tissue-Simulating Phantoms," *Phys. Med. Biol.*, vol. 40, 1995, pp. 1267–1287.

631. J. Qu and B. C. Wilson, "Monte Carlo Modeling Studies of the Effect of Physiological Factors and other Analytes on the Determination of Glucose Concentration *In Vivo* by Near Infrared Optical Absorption and Scattering Measurements," *J. Biomed. Opt.*, vol. 2, no. 3, 1997, pp. 319–325.

632. G. C. Beck, N. Akgun, A. Ruck, and R. Steiner, "Developing Optimized Tissue Phantom Systems for Optical Biopsies," *Proc. SPIE* 3197, 1997, pp. 76–85.

633. G. C. Beck, N. Akgun, A. Ruck, and R. Steiner, "Design and Characterization of a Tissue Phantom System for Optical Diagnostics," *Lasers Med. Sci.*, vol. 13, 1998, pp. 160–171.

634. D. D. Royston, R. S. Poston, and S. A. Prahl, Optical properties of scatering and absorbing materials used in the development of optical phantoms at 1064 nm," *J. Biomed. Opt.*, vol. 1, no. 1, 1996, pp. 110–123.

635. J. J. Burmeister, H. Chung, and M. A. Arnold, "Phantoms for noninvasive blood glucose sensing with near infrared transmission spectroscopy," *Photochem. Photobiol.*, vol. 67, no. 1, 1998, pp. 50–55.

636. A. B. Pravdin, S. P. Chernova, T. G. Papazoglu, and V. V. Tuchin, "Tissue Phantoms," Chapter 5 in *Handbook of Optical Biomedical Diagnostics*, vol. PM107, V. V. Tuchin (ed.), SPIE Press, Bellingham, WA, 2002, pp. 311–352.

637. R. A. J. Groenhuis, H. A. Ferwerda, and J. J. Ten Bosch, "Scattering and Absorption of Turbid Materials Determined from Reflection Measurements. 1. Theory," *Appl. Opt.*, vol. 22, 1983, pp. 2456–2462.

638. R. A. J. Groenhuis, J. J. Ten Bosch, and H. A. Ferwerda, "Scattering and Absorption of Turbid Materials Determined from Reflection Measurements. 2. Measuring Method and Calibration," *Appl. Opt.*, vol. 22, 1983, pp. 2463–2467.

639. D. Chursin, V. Shuvalov, and I. Shutov, "Optical Tomograph with Photon Counting and Projective Reconstruction of the Parameters of Absorbing 'Phantoms' in Extended Scattering Media," *Quantum Electronics*, vol. 29, no. 10, 1999, pp. 921–926.

640. G. Wagnieres, S. Cheng, M. Zellweger, N. Utke, D. Braichotte, J. Ballini, and H. Bergh, "An Optical Phantom with Tissue-Like Properties in the Visible for use in PDT and Fluorescence Spectroscopy," *Phys. Med. Biol.*, vol. 42, 1997, pp. 1415–1426.

641. S. Chernova, A. Pravdin, Y. Sinichkin, V. Kochubey, V. Tuchin, and S. Vari, "Correlation of Fluorescence and Reflectance Spectra of Tissue Phantoms with their Structure and Composition," *Proc. SPIE* 3598, 1999, pp. 294–300.

642. S. Chernova, O. Kasimov, L. Kuznetsova, T. Moskalenko, and A. B. Pravdin, "*Ex Vivo* and Phantom Fluorescence Spectra of Human Cervical tissue," *Proc. SPIE* 4001, 2000, pp. 290–298.

643. S. Chernova, A. Pravdin, Y. Sinichkin, V. Tuchin, and S. Vari, "Layered Gel-Based Phantoms Mimicking Fluorescence of Cervical Tissue," *Proc. OWLS V*, Springer, Berlin, 2000, pp. 301–306.

644. Y. Mendelson and J. Kent, "An *In Vitro* Tissue Model for Evaluating the Effect of Carboxyhemoglobin Concentration on Pulse Oximetry," *IEEE Trans. Biomed. Eng.*, vol. 36, no. 6, 1989, pp. 625–627.

645. V. Sankaran, J. Walsh, and D. Maitland, "Polarized Light Propagation in Biological Tissue and Tissue Phantoms," *Proc. SPIE* 4001, 2000, pp. 54–62.

646. B. Pogue, L. Lilge, M. Patterson, B. Wilson, and T. Hasan, "Absorbed Photodynamic Dose from Pulsed Versus Continuous Wave Light Examined with Tissue-Simulating Dosimeters," *Appl. Opt.*, vol. 36, no. 28, 1997, pp. 7257–7269.

647. M. Wolf, M. Keel, V. Dietz, K. Siebenthal, H. Bucher, and O. Baenziger, "The Influence of a Clear Layer on Near-Infrared Spectrophotometry Mea-

surements Using a Liquid Neonatal Head Phantom," *Phys. Med. Biol.*, vol. 44, 1999, pp. 1743–1753.

648. S. J. Matcher, "Signal Quantification and Localization in Tissue Near-Infrared Spectroscopy", Chapter 9 in *Handbook of Optical Biomedical Diagnostics*, vol. PM107, V. V. Tuchin (ed.), SPIE Press, Bellingham, WA, 2002, pp. 487–586.

649. R. R. Anderson and J. A. Parrish, "The Optics of Human Skin," *J. Invest. Dermatology*, vol. 77, 1981, pp. 13–19.

650. M. Hammer, A. Roggan, D. Schweitzer, and G. Müller, "Optical Properties of Ocular Fundus Tissues—an *In Vitro* Study Using the Double-Integrating-Sphere Technique and Inverse Monte Carlo Simulation," *Phys. Med. Biol.*, vol. 40, 1995, pp. 963–978.

651. W. M. Star, "The Relationship between Integrating Sphere and Diffusion Theory Calculations of Fluence Rate at the Wall of a Spherical Cavity," *Phys. Med. Biol.*, vol. 40, 1995, pp. 1–8.

652. S. A. Prahl, M. J. C. van Gemert, and A. J. Welch, "Determining the Optical Properties of Turbid Media by Using the Adding-Doubling Method," *Appl. Opt.*, vol. 32, 1993, pp. 559–568.

653. P. Marquet, F. Bevilacqua, C. Depeursinge, and E. B. de Haller, "Determination of Reduced Scattering and Absorption Coefficients by a Single Charge-Coupled-Device Array Measurement. 1. Comparison between Experiments and Simulations," *Opt. Eng.*, vol. 34, 1995, pp. 2055–2063.

654. F. Bevilacqua, P. Marquet, C. Depeursinge, and E. B. de Haller, "Determination of Reduced Scattering and Absorption Coefficients by a Single Charge-Coupled-Device Array Measurement. 2. Measurements on Biological Tissue," *Opt. Eng.*, vol. 34, 1995, pp. 2064–2069.

655. F. Bevilacqua, D. Piguet, P. Marquet, J. D. Gross, B. J. Tromberg, and C. Depeursinge, "*In Vivo* Local Determination of Tissue Optical Properties," *Proc. SPIE* 3194, 1997, pp. 262–268.

656. I. V. Yaroslavsky and V. V. Tuchin, "An Inverse Monte Carlo Method for Spectrophotometric Data Processing," *Proc. SPIE*, vol. 2100, 1994, pp. 57–68.

657. R. Marchesini, A. Bertoni, S. Andreola, et al., "Extinction and Absorption Coefficients and Scattering Phase Functions of Human Tissues *In Vitro*," *Appl. Opt.*, vol. 28, 1989, pp. 2318–2324.

658. S. L. Jacques, C. A. Alter, and S. A. Prahl, "Angular Dependence of the He-Ne Laser Light Scattering by Human Dermis," *Lasers Life Sci.*, vol. 1, 1987, pp. 309–333.

659. I. Driver, C. P. Lowdell, and D. V. Ash, "*In Vivo* Measurement of the Optical Interaction Coefficients of Human Tumours at 630 nm," *Phys. Med. Biol.*, vol. 36, 1991, pp. 805–813.

660. V. G. Peters, D. R. Wyman, M. S. Patterson, and G. L. Frank, "Optical Properties of Normal and Diseased Human Tissues in the Visible and Near Infrared," *Phys. Med. Biol.*, vol. 35, 1990, pp. 1317–1334.

661. M. Seyfried, "Optical Radiation Interaction with Living Tissue," in *Radiation Measurement in Photobiology*, Academic, New York, 1989, pp. 191–223.

662. A. Roggan, O. Minet, C. Schröder, and G. Müller, "The Determination of Optical Tissue Properties with Double Integrating Sphere Technique and Monte Carlo Simulations," *Proc. SPIE* 2100, 1994, pp. 42–56.

663. J. W. Pickering, C. J. M. Moes, H. J. C. M. Sterenborg, et al., "Two Integrating Spheres with an Intervening Scattering Sample," *J. Opt. Soc. Am. A.*, vol. 9, 1992, pp. 621–631.

664. J. W. Pickering, S. A. Prahl, N. van Wieringen, et al., "Double–Integrating Sphere System for Measuring the Optical Properties of Tissue," *Appl. Opt.*, vol. 32, 1993, pp. 399–410.

665. A. N. Yaroslavsky, I. V. Yaroslavsky, T. Goldbach, and H.-J. Schwarzmaier, "Inverse Hybrid Technique for Determining the Optical Properties of Turbid Media from Integrating-Sphere Measurements," *Appl. Opt.*, vol. 35, no. 34, 1996, pp. 6797–6809.

666. H.-J. Schwarzmaier, A. N. Yaroslavsky, I. V. Yaroslavsky, et al., "Optical Properties of Native and Coagulated Human Brain Structures," *Proc. SPIE* 2970, 1997, pp. 492–499.

667. E. K. Chan, B. Sorg, D. Protsenko, M. O'Neil, M. Motamedi, and A. J. Welch, "Effects of Compression on Soft Tissue Optical Properties," *IEEE J. Select. Tops Quant. Electr.*, vol. 2, no. 4, 1996, pp. 943–950.

668. E. Chan, T. Menovsky, and A. J. Welch, "Effect of Cryogenic Grinding of Soft-Tissue Optical Properties," *Appl. Opt.*, vol. 35, no. 22, 1996, pp. 4526–4532.

669. I. Fine, E. Loewinger, A. Weinreb, and D. Weinberger, "Optical Properties of the Sclera," *Phys. Med. Biol.*, vol. 30, 1985, pp. 565–571.

670. L.-H. Wang and S. L. Jacques, "Use of Laser Beam with an Oblique Angle of Incidence to Measure the Reduced Scattering Coefficient of a Turbid Medium," *Appl. Opt.*, vol. 34, 1995, pp. 2362–2366.

671. S.-P. Liu, L.-H. Wang, S. L. Jacques, and F. K. Tittel, "Measurement of Tissue Optical Properties by the Use of Oblique-Incidence Optical Fiber Reflectometry," *Appl. Opt.*, vol. 36, 1997, pp. 136–143.

672. A. N. Yaroslavsky, A. Vervoorts, A. V. Priezzhev, I. V. Yaroslavsky, J. G. Moser, and H.-J. Schwarzmaier, "Can Tumor Cell Suspension Serve as an Optical Model of Tumor Tissue in situ?" *Proc. SPIE* 3565, 1999, pp. 165–173.

673. A. N. Yaroslavsky, I. V. Yaroslavsky, and H.-J. Schwarzmaier, "Small-Angle Approximation to Determine Radiance Distribution of a Finite Beam Propagating through Turbid Medium," *Proc. SPIE*, vol. 3195, 1998, pp. 110–120.

674. D. W. Ebert, C. Roberts, S. K. Farrar, W. M. Johnston, A. S. Litsky, and A. L. Bertone, "Articular Cartilage Optical Properties in the Spectral Range 300–850 nm," *J. Biomed. Opt.*, vol. 3, 1998, pp. 326–333.

675. D. K. Sardar, M. L. Mayo, and R. D. Glickman, "Optical Characterization of Melanin," *J. Biomed. Opt.*, vol. 6, 2001, pp. 404–411.

676. M. Hammer and D. Schweitzer, "Quantitative Reflection Spectroscopy at the Human Ocular Fundus," *Phys. Med. Biol.*, vol. 47, 2002, pp. 179–191.

677. T. L. Troy and S. N. Thennadil, "Optical Properties of Human Skin in the Near Infrared Wavelength Range of 1000 to 2200 nm," *J. Biomed. Opt.*, vol. 6, 2001, pp. 167–176.

678. Y. Du, X. H. Hu, M. Cariveau, X. Ma, G. W. Kalmus, and J. Q. Lu, "Optical Properties of Porcine Skin Dermis between 900 nm and 1500 nm," *Phys. Med. Biol.*, vol. 46, 2001, pp. 167–181.

679. S. A. Prahl, "Light Transport in Tissues," PhD Thesis, Univ. of Texas, Austin, 1988.

680. S. A. Prahl, "The Inverse Adding-Doubling Program," htttp://omlc.ogi.edu/software/iad/index.html.

681. O. Khalil, S.-j. Yeh, M. G. Lowery, X. Wu, C. F. Hanna, S. Kantor, T.-W. Jeng, J. S. Kanger, R. A. Bolt, and F. F. de Mul, "Temperature Modulation of the Visible and Near Infrared Absorption and Scattering Coefficients of Human Skin," *J. Biomed. Opt.*, vol. 8(2), 2003, pp. 191–205.

682. T. J. Pfefer, L. S. Matchette, C. L. Bennett, J. A. Gall, J. N. Wilke, A. J. Durkin, and M. N. Ediger, "Reflectance-Based Determination of Optical Properties in Highly Attenuating Tissue," *J. Biomed. Opt.*, vol. 8(2), 2003, pp. 206–215.

683. F. Thueler, I. Charvet, F. Bevilacqua, M. St. Ghislain, G. Ory, P. Marquet, P. Meda, B. Vermeulen, and C. Depeursinge, "*In Vivo* Endoscopic Tissue Diagnostics Based on Spectroscopic Absorption, Scattering, and Phase Function Properties," *J. Biomed. Opt.*, vol. 8, no. 3, 2003, pp. 495–503.

684. S. L. Jacques, "Simple Monte Carlo Code," http://omlc.ogi.edu/software/index.html.

685. G. Kumar and J. M. Schmitt, "Optimal Probe Geometry for Near-Infrared Spectroscopy of Biological Tissue," *Appl. Opt.*, vol. 36, no. 10, 1997, pp. 2286–2293.

686. A. Kienle, F. K. Forster, and R. Hibst, "Influence of the Phase Function on Determination of the Optical Properties of Biological Tissue by Spatially Resolved Reflectance," *Opt. Lett.*, vol. 26, 2001, pp. 1571–1573.

687. C. K. Hayakawa, J. Spanier, F. Bevilacqua, A. K. Dunn, J. S. You, B. J. Tromberg, and V. Venugopalan, "Perturbation Monte Carlo Methods to Solve Inverse Photon Migration Problems in Heterogeneous Tissues," *Opt. Lett.*, vol. 26, 2001, pp. 1335–1337.

688. F. Bevilacqua and C. Depeursinge, "Monte Carlo Study of Diffuse Reflectance at Source-Detector Separations Close to One Transport Mean Free Path," *J. Opt. Soc. Am. A*, vol. 16(2), 1999, pp. 2935–2945.

689. W. Steenbergen, R. Kolkman, and F. de Mul, "Light-Scattering Properties of Undiluted Human Blood Subjected to Simple Shear," *J. Opt. Soc. Am. A*, vol. 16, no. 12, 1999, pp. 2959–2967.

690. S. T. Flock, B. C. Wilson, and M. S. Patterson, "Total Attenuation Coefficient and Scattering Phase Function of Tissues and Phantom Materials at 633 nm," *Med. Phys.*, vol. 14, 1987, pp. 835–841.

691. A. Roggan, K. Dörschel, O. Minet, D. Wolff, and G. Müller, "The Optical Properties of Biological Tissue in the Near Infrared Wavelength Range— Review and Measurements," in *Laser-Induced Interstitial Thermotherapy*, vol. PM25, G. Müller and A. Roggan (eds.), SPIE Press, Bellingham, WA, 1995, pp. 10–44.

692. S. Nickell, M. Hermann, M. Essenpreis, T. J. Farrell, U. Krämer, and M. S. Patterson, "Anisotropy of Light Propagation in Human Skin," *Phys. Med. Biol.*, vol. 45, 2000, pp. 2873–2886.

693. S. Stolik, J. A. Delgado, A. Pérez, and L. Anasagasti, "Measrement of the Penetration Depths of Red and Near Infrared Light in Human "*Ex Vivo*" Tissues," *J. Photochem. Photobiol. B: Biol.*, vol. 57, 2000, pp. 90–93.

694. S. Tauber, R. Baumgartner, K. Schorn, and W. Beyer, "Lightdosimetric Quantitative Analysis of the Human Petrous Bone: Experimental Study for Laser Irradiation of the Cochlea," *Laser Sur. Med.*, vol. 28, 2001, pp. 18–26.

695. F. Bevilacqua, D. Piguet, P. Marquet, J. D. Gross, B. J. Tromberg, and C. Depeursinge, "*In Vivo* Local Determination of Tissue Optical Properties: Applications to Human Brain," *Appl. Opt.*, vol. 38, 1999, pp. 4939–4950.

696. J. Mobley and Tuan Vo-Dinh, "Optical Properties of Tissues," in *Biomedical Photonics Handbook*, Tuan Vo-Dinh (ed.), CRC Press, Boca Raton, 2003, pp. 2-1–2-75.

697. A. Roggan, D. Schäder, U. Netz, J.-P. Ritz, C.-T. Germer, and G. Müller, "The Effect of Preparation Technique on the Optical Parameters of Biological Tissue," *Appl. Phys. B*, vol. 69, 1999, pp. 445–453.

698. W. Gottschalk, Ein Messverfahren zur Bestimmung der Optischen Parameter Biologischer Gevebe *In Vitro*, Dissertation 93 HA8984 Universitaet Fridriciana, Karlsruhe, 1992.

699. N. Ghosh, S. K. Mohanty, S. K. Majumder, and P. K. Gupta, "Measurement of Optical Transport Properties of Normal and Malignant Human Breast Tissue," *Appl. Opt.*, vol. 40, 2001, pp. 176–184.

700. R. Hornung, T. H. Pham, K. A. Keefe, M. W. Berns, Y. Tadir, and B. J. Tromberg, "Quantitative Near-Infrared Spectroscopy of Cervical Dysplasia In Vivo," *Hum. Reprod.*, vol. 14, 1999, pp. 2908–2916.

701. E. Gratton, S. Fantini, M. A. Franceschini, G. Gratton, and M. Fabiani, "Measurements of Scattering and Absorption Changes in Muscle and Brain," *Phil. Trans. R. Soc. Lond. B*, vol. 352, 1997, pp. 727–735.

702. T. J. Farrell, M. S. Patterson, and M. Essenpreis, "Influence of Layered Tissue Architecture on Estimates of Tissue Optical Properties Obtained from Spatially-Resolved Diffuse Reflectometry," *Appl. Opt.*, vol. 37, 1998, pp. 1958–1972.

703. A. N. Bashkatov, "Controlling of Optical Properties of Tissues at Action by Osmotically Active Immersion Liquids," Cand. Science Thesis, Saratov State Univ., Saratov, 2002.

704. E. A. Genina, A. N. Bashkatov, V. I. Kochubey, and V. V. Tuchin, "Optical Clearing of Human *Dura Mater*," *Opt. Spectrosc.*, vol. 98, no. 3, 2005, pp. 470–476.

705. A. N. Bashkatov, E. A. Genina, V. I. Kochubey, and V. V. Tuchin, "Optical Properties of the Subcutaneous Adipose Tissue in the Spectral Range 400–2500 nm," *Opt. Spectrosc.*, vol. 99, no. 5, 2005, pp. 836–842.

706. A. N. Bashkatov, E. A. Genina, V. I. Kochubey, V. V. Tuchin, E. E. Chikina, A. B. Knyazev, and O. V. Mareev, "Optical Properties of Mucous Membrane in the Spectral Range 350 to 2000 nm," *Opt. Spectrosc.*, vol. 97, no. 6, 2004, pp. 978–983.

707. S. Fantini, S. A. Walker, M. A. Franceschini, M. Kaschke, P. M. Schlag, and K. T. Moesta, "Assessment of the Size, Position, and Optical Properties of Breast Tumors *In Vivo* by Noninvasive Optical Methods," *Appl. Opt.*, vol. 37, 1998, pp. 1982–1989.

708. S. Fantini, D. Hueber, M. A. Franceschini, E. Gratton, W. Rosenfeld, P. G. Stubblefield, D. Maulik, and M. R. Stankovic, "Non-Invasive Optical Monitoring of the Newborn Piglet Brain using Continuous-Wave and Frequency-Domain Spectroscopy," *Phys. Med. Biol.*, vol. 44, 1999, 1543–1563.

709. J. F. Black, J. K. Barton, G. Frangineas, and H. Pummer, "Cooperative Phenomena in Two-Pulse Two-Color Laser Photocoagulation of Cutaneous Blood Vessels," *Proc. SPIE* 4244, 2001, pp. 13–24.

710. S. L. Jacques, "Origins of Tissue Optical Properties in the UVA, Visible and NIR Regions," in *Advances in Optical Imaging and Photon Migration*, R. R. Alfano and J. G. Fujimoto (eds.), OSA TOPS 2, Optical Society of America, Washington, DC, 1996, pp. 364–371.

711. D. Levitz, L. Thrane, M. H. Frosz, P. E. Andersen, C. B. Andersen, S. Andersson-Engels, J. Valanciunaite, J. Swartling, and P. R. Hansen, "Determination of Optical Scattering Properties of Highly-Scattering Media in Optical Coherence Tomography Images," *Optics Express* vol. 12, 2004, pp. 249–259, http://www.opticsexpress.org/abstract.cfm?URI=OPEX-12-2-249.

712. A. Knüttel and M. Boehlau-Godau, "Spatially Confined and Temporally Resolved Refractive Index and Scattering Evaluation in Human Skin Performed with Optical Coherence Tomography," *J. Biomed. Opt.*, vol. 5, 2000, pp. 83–92.

713. A. Knüttel, S. Bonev, and W. Knaak, "New Method for Evaluation of *In Vivo* Scattering and Refractive Index Properties Obtained with Optical Coherence Tomography," *J. Biomed. Opt.*, vol. 9, 2004, pp. 265–273.

714. M. J. Holboke, B. J. Tromberg, X. Li, N. Shah, J. Fishkin, D. Kidney, J. Butler, B. Chance, and A. G. Yodh, "Three-Dimensional Diffuse Optical Mammography with Ultrasound Localization in a Human Subject," *J. Biomed. Opt.*, vol. 5, 2000, pp. 237–247.

715. B. J. Tromberg, N. Shah, R. Lanning, A. Cerussi, J. Espinoza, T. Pham, L. Svaasand, and J. Butler, "Non-invasive *In Vivo* Characterization of Breast Tumors using Photon Migration Spectroscopy," *Neoplasia*, vol. 2, 2000, pp. 26–40.

716. I. V. Turchin, E. A. Sergeeva, L. S. Dolin, and V. A. Kamensky, "Estimation of Biotissue Scattering Properties from OCT Images Using a Small-Angle Approximation of Transport Theory," *Laser Physics*, vol. 13, 2003, pp. 1524–1529.

717. L. S. Dolin, F. I. Feldchtein, G. V. Gelikonov, V. M. Gelikonov, N. D. Gladkova, R. R. Iksanov, V. A. Kamensky, R. V. Kuranov, A. M. Sergeev, N. M. Shakhova, and I. V. Turchin, "Fundamentals of OCT and Clinical Applications of Endoscopic OCT," Chapter 17, in *Coherent-Domain Optical Methods: Biomedical Diagnostics, Environmental and Material Science*, vol. 2, V. V. Tuchin (ed.), Kluwer Academic Publishers, Boston, 2004, pp. 211–270.

718. I. V. Turchin, V. A. Kamensky, E. A. Sergeeva, and N. M. Shakhova, "OCT Image Processing Algorithm for Differentiation Biological Tissue Pathologies," *13 International Laser Physics Workshop*, Book of Abstracts, Trieste, Italy, 2004, p. 189.

719. M. Firbank, M. Hiraoka, M. Essenpreis, and D. T. Delpy, "Measurement of the Optical Properties of the Skull in the Wavelength Range 650–950 nm," *Phys. Med. Biol.*, vol. 38, 1993, pp. 503–510.

720. N. Ugryumova, S. J. Matcher, and D. P. Attenburrow, "Measurement of Bone Mineral Density via Light Scattering," *Phys. Med. Biol.*, vol. 49, 2004, pp. 469–283.

721. A. I. Kholodnykh, I. Y. Petrova, K. V. Larin, M. Motamedi, and R. O. Esenaliev, "Precision of Measurement of Tissue Optical Properties with Optical Coherence Tomography," *Appl. Opt.*, vol. 42, 2003, pp. 3027–3037.

722. P. Rol, P. Niederer, U. Dürr, P.-D. Henchoz, and F. Fankhauser, "Experimental Investigation on the Light Scattering Properties of the Human Sclera," *Laser Light Ophthalmol.*, vol. 3, 1990, pp. 201–212.

723. P. O. Rol, Optics for Transscleral Laser Applications: Dissertation No. 9655 for Doctor of Natural Sciences, Swiss Federal Institute of Technology, Zurich, Switzerland, 1992.

724. A. N. Yaroslavsky, I. V. Yaroslavsky, T. Goldbach, and H.-J. Schwarzmaier, "Optical Properties of Blood in the Near-Infrared Spectral Range," *Proc. SPIE* 2678, 1996, pp. 314–324.

725. A. N. Yaroslavsky, A. V. Priezzhev, J. Rodriguez, I. V. Yaroslavsky, and H. Battarbee, "Optics of Blood," in *Handbook of Optical Biomedical Diagnostics*, Chapter 2, vol. PM107, V. V. Tuchin (ed.), SPIE Press, Bellingham, WA, 2002, pp. 169–216.

726. A. N. Bashkatov, E. A. Genina, V. I. Kochubey, and V. V. Tuchin, "Optical Properties of Human Skin, Subcutaneous and Mucous Tissues in the Wavelength Range from 400 to 2000 nm," *J. Phys. D: Appl. Phys.*, vol. 38, 2005, pp. 2543–2555.

727. L. O. Reynolds and N. J. McCormick, "Approximate Two-Parameter Phase Function for Light scattering," *J. Opt. Soc. Am.*, vol. 70, 1980, pp. 1206–1212.

728. P. W. Barber and S. C. Hill, *Light Scattering by Particles: Computational Methods*, World Scientific, Singapore, 1990.

729. A. N. Yaroslavsky, I. V. Yaroslavsky, T. Goldbach, and H.-J. Schwarzmaier, "Different Phase Function Approximations to Determine Optical Properties of Blood: A Comparison," *Proc. SPIE* 2982, 1997, pp. 324–330.

730. M. Hammer, D. Schweitzer, B. Michel, E. Thamm, and A. Kolb, "Single Scattering by Red Blood Cells," *Appl. Opt.*, vol. 37, no. 31, 1998, 7410–7418.

731. I. J. Bigio and J. R. Mourant, "Ultraviolet and Visible Spectroscopies for Tissue Diagnostics: Fluorescence Spectroscopy and Elastic-Scattering Spectroscopy," *Phys. Med. Biol.*, vol. 42, 1997, pp. 803–814.

732. L. T. Perelman and V. Backman, "Light Scattering Spectroscopy of Epithelial Tissues: Principles and Applications," Chapter 12, in *Optical Biomedical Diagnostics*, vol. PM107, V. V. Tuchin (ed.), SPIE Press, Bellingham, WA, 2002, pp. 675–724.

733. V. Backman, M. Wallace, L. T. Perelman, R. Gurjar, G. Zonios, M. G. Müller, Q. Zhang, T. Valdez, J. T. Arendt, H. S. Levin, T. McGillican, K. Badizadegan, M. Seiler, S. Kabani, I. Itzkan, M. Fitzmaurice, R. R. Dasari, J. M. Crawford, J. Van Dam, and M. S. Feld, "Detection of Preinvasive Cancer Cells. Early-Warning Changes in Precancerous Epithelial Cells Can be Spotted *In Situ*," *Nature*, vol. 406, no. 6791, 2000, pp. 35–36.

734. C. Yang, L. T. Perelman, A. Wax, R. R. Dasari, and M. S. Feld, "Feasibility of Field-Based Light Scattering Spectroscopy," *J. Biomed. Opt.*, vol. 5, 2000, pp. 138–143.

735. G. Zonios, L. T. Perelman, V. Backman, R. Manoharan, M. Fitzmaurice, and M. S. Feld. "Diffuse Reflectance Spectroscopy of Human Adenomatous Colon Polyps *In Vivo*," *Appl. Opt.*, vol. 38, 1999, pp. 6628–6637.

736. G. Marguez, L. V. Wang, S.-P. Lin, J. A. Swartz, and S. Thomsen, "Anisotropy in the Absorption and Scattering Spectra of the Chicken Breast Tissue," *Appl. Opt.*, vol. 37, no. 4, 1998, pp. 798–804.

737. V. V. Tuchin, X. Xu, and R. K. Wang, "Dynamic Optical Coherence Tomography in Optical Clearing, Sedimentation and Aggregation Study of Immersed Blood," *Appl. Opt.-OT*, vol. 41, no. 1, 2002, pp. 258–271.

738. A. N. Bashkatov, E. A. Genina, V. I. Kochubey, N. A. Lakodina, and V. V. Tuchin, "Optical Clearing of Human Cranial Bones by Administration of Immersion Agents," NATO Advanced Study Inst. on Biophotonics: From Fundamental Principles to Health, Environment, Security and Defense Applications, Ottawa, Ontario, Canada, September 29–October 9, 2004.

739. A. N. Bashkatov, E. A. Genina, V. I. Kochubey, N. A. Lakodina, and V. V. Tuchin, "Optical Properties of Human Cranial Bones in the Spectral Range from 800 to 2000 nm," *Proc. SPIE* 6163, 2006, pp. 616310-1–11.

740. L. Reynolds, C. Johnson, and A. Ishimaru, "Diffuse Reflectance from a Finite Blood Medium: Applications to the Modeling of Fiber Optic Catheters," *Appl. Opt.*, vol. 15, 1976, pp. 2059–2067.

741. J. M. Steinke and A. P. Shepherd, "Comparison of Mie Theory and the Light Scattering of Red Blood Cells," *Appl. Opt.*, vol. 27, 1988, pp. 4027–4033.

742. D. K. Sardar and L. B. Levy, "Optical Properties of Whole Blood," *Lasers Med. Sci.*, vol. 13, 1998, pp. 106–111.

743. R. N. Pittman, "*In Vivo* Photometric Analysis of Hemoglobin," *Annals Biomed. Eng.*, vol. 14, 1986, pp. 119–137.

744. M. A. Bartlett and H. Jiang, "Effect of Refractive Index on the Measurement of Optical Properties in Turbid Media," *Appl. Opt.*, vol. 40, 2001, pp. 1735–1741.

745. D. Arifler, M. Guillaud, A. Carraro, A. Malpica, M. Follen, and R. Richards-Kortum, "Light Scattering from Normal and Dysplastic Cervical Cells at Different Epithelial Depths: Finite-Difference Time-Domain Modeling with a Perfectly Matched Layer Boundary Condition," *J. Biomed. Opt.*, vol. 8, 2003, pp. 484–494.

746. S. Cheng, H. Y. Shen, G. Zhang, C. H. Huang, and X. J. Huang, "Measurement of the Refractive Index of Biotissue at Four Laser Wavelengths," *Proc. SPIE* 4916, 2002, pp. 172–176.

747. H. Liu and S. Xie, "Measurement Method of the Refractive Index of Biotissue by Total Internal Reflection," *Appl. Opt.*, vol. 35, 1996, pp. 1793–1795.

748. V. V. Tuchin, D. M. Zhestkov, A. N. Bashkatov, and E. A. Genina, "Theoretical Study of Immersion Optical Clearing of Blood in Vessels at Local Hemolysis," *Optics Express*, vol. 12, 2004, pp. 2966–2971.

749. R. Barer, K. F. A. Ross, and S. Tkaczyk, "Refractometry of Living Cells," *Nature*, vol. 171, no. 4356, 1953, pp. 720–724.

750. M. Haruna, K. Yoden, M. Ohmi, and A. Seiyama, "Detection of Phase Transition of a Biological Membrane by Precise Refractive-Index Measurement Based on the Low Coherence Interferometry," *Proc. SPIE* 3915, 2000, pp. 188–193.

751. D. J. Faber, M. C. G. Aalders, E. G. Mik, B. A. Hooper, M. J. C. van Gemert, and T. G. van Leeuwen, "Oxygen Saturation-Dependent Absorption and Scattering of Blood," *Phys. Rev. Lett.*, vol. 93, 2004, pp. 028102-1–4.

752. V. V. Tuchin, R. K. Wang, E. I. Galanzha, N. A. Lakodina, and A. V. Solovieva, "Monitoring of Glycated Hemoglobin in a Whole Blood by Refractive Index Measurement with OCT," Conference Program CLEO/QELS, Baltimore, June 1–6, Optical Society of America, Washington, DC, 2003, p. 120.

753. V. V. Tuchin, R. K. Wang, E. I. Galanzha, J. B. Elder, and D. M. Zhestkov, "Monitoring of Glycated Hemoglobin by OCT Measurement of Refractive Index," *Proc. SPIE* 5316, 2004, pp. 66–77.

754. G. Mazarevica, T. Freivalds, and A. Jurka, "Properties of Erythrocyte Light Refraction in Diabetic Patients," *J. Biomed. Opt.*, vol. 7, 2002, pp. 244–247.

755. S. F. Shumilina, "Dispersion of Real and Imaginary Part of the Complex Refractive Index of Hemoglobin in the Range 450 to 820 nm," *Bullet. Beloruss. SSR Acad. Sci., Phys.-Math. Ser.*, no. 1, 1984, pp. 79–84.

756. J. Hempe, R. Gomez, R. McCarter, and S. Chalew, "High and Low Hemoglobin Glycation Phenotypes in Type 1 Diabetes. A Challenge for Interpretation of Glycemic Control," *J. Diabetes Complications* vol. 16, 2002, pp. 313–320.

757. M. V. Volkenshtein, *Molecualar Optics*, Moscow, Fizmatlit, 1951.

758. G. V. Maksimov, O. G. Luneva, N. V. Maksimova, E. Matettuchi, E. A. Medvedev, V. Z. Pashchenko, and A. B. Rubin, "Role of Viscosity and Permeability of the Erythrocyte Plasma Membrane in Changes in Oxygen-Binding Properties of Hemoglobin During Diabetes Mellitus," *Bull. Exp. Biol. Med.*, vol. 140, no. 5, 2005, pp. 510–513.

759. A. N. Bashkatov, E. A. Genina, V. I. Kochubey, Yu. P. Sinichkin, A. A. Korobov, N. A. Lakodina, and V. V. Tuchin, "*In Vitro* Study of Control of Human Dura Mater Optical Properties by Acting of Osmotical Liquids," *Proc. SPIE* 4162, 2000, pp. 182–188.

760. A. N. Bashkatov, E. A. Genina, V. I. Kochubey, and V. V. Tuchin, "Estimation of Wavelength Dependence of Refractive Index of Collagen Fibers of Scleral Tissue," *Proc. SPIE* 4162, 2000, pp. 265–268.

761. A. N. Bashkatov, E. A. Genina, V. I. Kochubey, M. M. Stolnitz, T. A. Bashkatova, O. V. Novikova, A. Yu. Peshkova, and V. V. Tuchin, "Optical Properties of Melanin in the Skin and Skin-Like Phantoms," *Proc. SPIE* 4162, 2000, pp. 219–226.

762. Y. Kamai and T. Ushiki, "The Three-Dimensional Organization of Collagen Fibrils in the Human Cornea and Sclera," *Invest. Ophthalmol. & Visual Sci.*, vol. 32, 1991, pp. 2244–2258.

763. V. N. Grisimov, "Refractive Index of the Ground Material of Dentin," *Opt. Specrosc.*, vol. 77, 1994, pp. 272–273.

764. X. Wang, T. E. Milner, M. C. Chang, and J. S. Nelson, "Group Refractive Index Measurement of Dry and Hydrated Type I Collagen Films Using Optical Low-Coherence Reflectometry," *J. Biomed. Opt.*, vol. 1, no. 2, 1996, pp. 212–216.

765. W. V. Sorin and D. F. Gray, "Simalteneous Thickness and Group Index Measurements Using Optical Low-Coherence Refractometry," *IEEE Photon. Technol. Lett.*, vol. 4, 1992, pp. 105–107.

766. X. J. Wang, T. E. Milner, R. P. Dhond, W. V. Sorin, S. A. Newton, and J. S. Nelson, "Characterization of Human Scalp Hairs by Optical Low-Coherence Reflectometry," *Opt. Lett.*, vol. 20, 1995, pp. 524–526.

767. G. J. Tearney, M. E. Brezinski, J. F. Southern, B. E. Bouma, M. R. Hee, and J. G. Fujimoto, "Determination of the Refractive Index of Highly Scattering Human Tissue by Optical Coherence Tomography," *Opt. Lett.*, vol. 20, 1995, pp. 2258–2260.

768. M. Ohmi, Y. Ohnishi, K. Yoden, and M. Haruna, "*In Vitro* Simalteneous Measurement of Refractive Index and Thickness of Biological Tissue by the Low Coherence Interferometry," *IEEE Trans. Biomed. Eng.*, vol. 47, 2000, pp. 1266–1270.

769. X. Wang, C. Zhang, L. Zhang, L. Xue, and J. Tian, "Simalteneous Refractive Index and Thickness Measurement of Biotissue by Optical Coherence Tomography," *J. Biomed. Opt.*, vol. 7, 2002, pp. 628–632.

770. S. A. Alexandrov, A. V. Zvyagin, K. K. M. B. D. Silva, and D. D. Sampson, "Bifocal Optical Coherence Refractometry of Turbid Media," *Opt. Lett.*, vol. 28, 2003, pp. 117–119.

771. A. V. Zvyagin, K. K. M. B. D. Silva, S. A. Alexandrov, T. R. Hillman, J. J. Armstrong, T. Tsuzuki, and D. D. Sampson, "Refractive Index Tomography of Turbid Media by Bifocal Optical Coherence Refractometry," *Optics Express*, vol. 11, 2003, pp. 3503–3517.

772. Y. L. Kim, J. T. Walsh Jr., T. K. Goldstick, and M. R. Glucksberg, "Variation of Corneal Refractive Index with Hydration," *Phys. Med. Biol.*, vol. 49, 2004, pp. 859–868.

773. W. Drexler, C. K. Hitzenberger, A. Baumgartner, O. Findl, H. Sattmann, and A. F. Fercher, "Investigation of Dispersion Effects in Ocular Media by Multiple Wavelength Partial Coherence Interferometry," *Exp. Eye Res.*, vol. 66, 1998, pp. 25–33.

774. R. C. Lin, M. A. Shure, A. M. Rollins, J. A. Izatt, and D. Huang, "Group Index of the Human Cornea at 1.3-μm Wavelength Obtained In Vitro by Optical Coherence Domain Reflectometry," *Opt. Lett.*, vol. 29, 2004, pp. 83–85.

775. G. V. Gelikonov, V. M. Gelikonov, S. U. Ksenofontov, A. N. Morosov, A. V. Myakov, Yu. P. Potapov, V. V. Saposhnikova, E. A. Sergeeva, D. V. Shabanov, N. M. Shakhova, and E. V. Zagainova, "Compact Optical Coherence Microscope," Chapter 20, in *Coherent-Domain Optical Methods: Biomedical Diagnostics, Environmental and Material Science*, vol. 2, V. V. Tuchin (ed.), Kluwer Academic Publishers, Boston, 2004, pp. 345–362.

776. J. M. Schmitt, M. Yadlowsky, and R. F. Bonner, "Subsurface Imaging of Living Skin with Optical Coherence Microscopy," *Dermatology*, vol. 191, 1995, pp. 93–98.

777. G. Vargas, K. F. Chan, S. L. Thomsen, and A. J. Welch, "Use of Osmotically Active Agents to Alter Optical Properties of Tissue: Effects on the Detected Fluorescence Signal Measured through Skin," *Lasers Surg. Med.*, vol. 29, 2001, pp. 213–220.

778. D. W. Leonard and K. M. Meek, "Refractive Indices of the Collagen Fibrils and Extrafibrillar Material of the Corneal Stroma," *Biophys. J.*, vol. 72, 1997, pp. 1382–1387.

779. K. M. Meek, S. Dennis, and S. Khan, "Changes in the Refractive Index of the Stroma and its Extrafibrillar Matrix When the Cornea Swells," *Biophys. J.*, vol. 85, 2003, pp. 2205–2212.

780. R. A. Farrell and R. L. McCally, "Corneal Transparency" in *Principles and Practice of Ophthalmology*, D. A. Albert and F. A. Jakobiec (eds.), W. B. Saunders, Philadelphia, PA, 2000, pp. 629–643.

781. D. E. Freund, R. L. McCally, and R. A. Farrell, "Effects of Fibril Orientations on Light Scattering in the Cornea," *J. Opt. Soc. Am. A.*, vol. 3, 1986, pp. 1970–1982.

782. R. A. Farrell, D. E. Freund, and R. L. McCally, "Hierarchical Structure and Light Scattering in the Cornea," *Mat. Res. Soc. Symp. Proc.*, vol. 255, 1992, pp. 233–246.

783. R. A. Farrell, D. E. Freund, and R. L. McCally, "Research on Corneal Structure," *Johns Hopkins APL Techn. Digest.*, vol. 11, 1990, pp. 191–199.

784. M. S. Borcherding, L. J. Blasik, R. A. Sittig, J. W. Bizzel, M. Breen, and H. G. Weinstein, "Proteoglycans and Collagen Fiber Organization in Human Corneoscleral Tissue," *Exp Eye Res.*, vol. 21, 1975, pp. 59–70.

785. M. Spitznas, "The Fine Structure of Human Scleral Collagen," *Am. J. Ophthalmol.*, vol. 71, no. 1, 1971, pp. 68–75.

786. Y. Huang and K. M. Meek, "Swelling Studies on the Cornea and Sclera: the Effect of pH and Ionic Strength," *Biophys. J.*, vol. 77, 1999, pp. 1655–1665.

787. S. Vaezy and J. I. Clark, "Quantitative Analysis of the Microstructure of the Human Cornea and Sclera Using 2-D Fourier Methods," *J. Microsc.*, vol. 175, no. 2, 1994, pp. 93–99.

788. Z. S. Sacks, R. M. Kurtz, T. Juhasz, and G. A. Mourau, "High Precision Subsurface Photodisruption in Human Sclera," *J. Biomed. Opt.*, vol. 7, no. 3, 2002, pp. 442–450.

789. F. A. Bettelheim, "Physical Basis of Lens Transparency," in *The Ocular Lens: Structure, Function and Pathology*, H. Maisel (ed.), Marcel-Dekker, New York, 1985.

790. S. Zigman, G. Sutliff, and M. Rounds, "Relationships between Human Cataracts and Environmental Radiant Energy. Cataract Formation, Light scattering and Fluorescence," *Lens Eye Toxicity Res.*, vol. 8, 1991, pp. 259–280.

791. J. Xu, J. Pokorny, and V. C. Smith, "Optical Density of the Human Lens," *J. Opt. Soc. Am. A.*, vol. 14, no. 5, 1997, pp. 953–960.

792. B. K. Pierscionek and R. A. Weale, "Polarising Light Biomicroscopy and the Relation between Visual Acuity and Cataract," *Eye*, vol. 9, 1995, pp. 304–308.

793. B. K. Pierscionek, "Aging Changes in the Optical Elements of the Eye," *J. Biomed. Opt.*, vol. 1, no. 3, 1996, pp. 147–156.

794. J. A. van Best and E. V. M. J. Kuppens, "Summary of Studies on the Blue–Green Autofluorescence and Light Transmission of the Ocular Lens," *J. Biomed. Opt.*, vol. 1, no. 3, 1996, pp. 243–250.

795. F. A. Bettelheim, A. C. Churchill, W. G. Robinson, Jr., and J. S. Zigler, Jr., "Dimethyl Sulfoxide Cataract: a Model for Optical Anisotropy Fluctuations," *J. Biomed. Opt.*, vol. 1, no. 3, 1996, pp. 273–279.

796. N.-T. Yu, B. S. Krantz, J. A. Eppstein, K. D. Ignotz, M. A. Samuels, J. R. Long, and J. F. Price, "Development of Noninvasive Diabetes Screening Device Using the Ratio of Fluorescence to Rayleigh Scattered Light," *J. Biomed. Opt.*, vol. 1, no. 3, 1996, pp. 280–288.

797. M. J. Costello, T. N. Oliver, and L. M. Cobo, "Cellular Architecture in Aged-Related Human Nuclear Cataracts," *Invest. Ophthal. & Vis. Sci.*, vol. 3, no. 11, 1992, pp. 2244–2258.

798. I. L. Maksimova, D. A. Zimnyakov, and V. V. Tuchin, "Controlling of Tissue Optical Properties I. Spectral Characteristics of Eye Sclera," *Opt. Spectrosc.*, vol. 89, 2000, pp. 78–86.

799. D. A. Zimnyakov, I. L. Maksimova, and V. V. Tuchin, "Controlling of Tissue Optical Properties II. Coherent Methods of Tissue Structure Study," *Opt. Spectrosc.*, vol. 88, 2000, pp. 1026–1034.

800. J. Dillon, "The Photophysics and Photobiology of the Eye," *J. Photochem. Photobiol. B: Biol.*, vol. 10, 1991, pp. 23–40.

801. G. B. Benedek, "Theory of Transparency of the Eye," *Appl. Opt.*, vol. 10, no. 3, 1971, pp. 459–473.

802. A. Tardieu and M. Delaye, "Eye Lens Proteins and Transparency from Light Transmission Theory to Solution X-ray Structural Analysis," *Ann. Rev. Biophys. Chem.*, vol. 17, 1988, pp. 47–70.

803. A. V. Krivandin, "On the Supramolecular Structure of Eye Lens Crystallins. The Study by Small-Angle X-ray Scattering," *Biophysica*, vol. 46, no. 6, 1997, pp. 1274–1278.

804. S. Vaezy and J. I. Clark, "Characterization of the Cellular Microstructures of Ocular Lens Using 2-D Power Law Analysis," *Ann. Biomed. Eng.*, vol. 23, 1995, pp. 482–490.

805. J. M. Ziman, *Models of Disorder: The Theoretical Physics of Homogeneously Disordered Systems*, Cambridge Univer. Press, London, New York, Melbourne, 1979.

806. M. S. Wertheim, "Exact Solution of the Percus-Yevick Integral Equation for Hard Spheres," *Phys. Rev. Lett.*, vol. 10, no. 8, 1963, pp. 321–323.

807. J. L. Lebovitz, "Exact Solution of Generalized Percus-Yevick Equation for a Mixture of Hard Spheres," *Phys. Rev.*, vol. 133, no. 4A, 1964, pp. 895–899.

808. R. J. Baxter, "Ornstein-Zernike Relation and Percus-Yevick Approximation for Fluid Mixtures," *J. Chem. Phys.*, vol. 52, no. 9, 1970, pp. 4559–4562.

809. A. P. Ivanov, V. A. Loiko, and V. P. Dik, *Light Propagation in Densely Packed Disperse Media*, Nauka i Tekhnika, Minsk, 1988.

810. V. G. Vereshchagin and A. N. Ponyavina, "Statistical Characteristic and Transparency of Thin Closely Packed Disperse Layer," *Zh. Prikl. Spektr. (J. Appl. Spectrosc.)*, vol. 22, no. 3, 1975, pp. 518–524.

811. N. L. Larionova, I. L. Maksimova, and V. V. Tuchin, "The Scattering Spectra and Color of Disperse Systems of Weakly Absorbing Particles," *Opt. Spectrosc.*, vol. 93, no. 2, 2002, pp. 273–281.

812. Z. S. Sacks, D. L. Craig, R. M. Kurtz, T. Juhasz, and G. Mourou, "Spatially Resolved Transmission of Highly Focused Beams Through Cornea and Sclera Between 1400 and 1800 nm," *Proc. SPIE* 3726, 1999, pp. 522–527.

813. T. J. T. P. van den Berg and K. E. W. P. Tan, "Light Transmittance of the Human Cornea from 320 to 700 nm for Different Ages," *Vision Res.*, vol. 33, 1994, pp. 1453–1456.

814. A. N. Korolevich, A. Ya. Khairulina, and L. P. Shubochkin, "Influence of Large Biological Cells Aggregation on Elements of the Light Scattering Matrix," *Opt. Spectrosc.*, vol. 77, 1994, pp. 278–282.

815. V. F. Izotova, I. L. Maksimova, and S. V. Romanov, "Analysis of accuracy of laser polarization nephelometer," *Opt. Spectrosc.*, Vol. 80, pp. 1001–1007 (1996).

816. P. S. Hauge, "Recent Developments in Instruments in Ellipsometry," *Surface Science*, vol. 96, 1980, pp. 108–140.

817. W. P. van de Merwe, D. R. Huffman, and B. V. Bronk, "Reproducibility and Sensitivity of Polarized Light Scattering for Identifying Bacterial Suspension," *Appl. Opt.*, vol. 28, 1989, pp. 5052–5057.

818. B. V. Bronk, S. D. Druger, J. Czege, and W. van de Merwe, "Measuring Diameters of Rod-Shaped Bacteria *In Vivo* with Polarized Light Scattering," *Biophys. J.*, vol. 69, 1995, pp. 1170–1177.

819. B. G. de Grooth, L. W. M. M. Terstappen, G. J. Puppels, and J. Greve, "Light-Scattering Polarization Measurements as a New Parameter in Flow Cytometry," *Cytometry*, vol. 8, 1987, pp. 539–544.

820. R. M. P. Doornbos, A. G. Hoekstra, K. E. I. Deurloo, B. G. de Grooth, P. M. A. Sloot, and J. Greve, "Lissajous-Like patterns in Scatter Plots of Calibration Beads," *Cytometry*, vol. 16, 1994, pp. 236–242.

821. O. J. Lokberg, "Speckles and Speckle Techniques for Biomedical Applications," *Proc. SPIE*, vol. 1524, 1991, pp. 35–47.

822. J. C. Dainty (ed.), *Laser Speckle and Related Phenomena*, 2nd ed., Springer-Verlag, New York, 1984.

823. S. A. Akhmanov, Yu. E. D'yakov, and A. S. Chirkin, *Introduction to Statistical Radiophysics and Optics*, Nauka, Moscow, 1981.

824. J. C. Dainty, "The Statistics of Speckle Patterns," in *Progress in Optics XIV*, E. Wolf (ed.), vol. 14, North Holland, 1976, pp. 3–48.

825. D. A. Zimnyakov, "Coherence Phenomena and Statistical Properties of Multiply Scattered Light," Chapter 4, in *Handbook of Optical Biomedical Diagnostics*, vol. PM107, V. V. Tuchin (ed.), SPIE Press, Bellingham, WA, 2002, pp. 265–319.

826. E. I. Galanzha, G. E. Brill, Y. Aisu, S. S. Ulyanov, and V. V. Tuchin, "Speckle and Doppler Methods of Blood and Lymph Flow Monitoring," Chapter 16, in *Handbook of Optical Biomedical Diagnostics*, vol. PM107, V. V. Tuchin (ed.), SPIE Press, Bellingham, WA, 2002, pp. 881–937.

827. D. A. Zimnyakov, J. D. Briers, and V. V. Tuchin, "Speckle Technologies for Monitoring and Imaging of Tissuelike Phantoms," Chapter 18, in *Handbook of Optical Biomedical Diagnostics*, vol. PM107, V. V. Tuchin (ed.), SPIE Press, Bellingham, WA, 2002, pp. 987–1036.

828. S. J. Kirkpatrick and D. D. Duncan, "Optical Assessment of Tissue Mechanics," Chapter 19, in *Handbook of Optical Biomedical Diagnostics*, vol. PM107, V. V. Tuchin (ed.), SPIE Press, Bellingham, WA, 2002, pp. 1037–1084.

829. D. A. Zimnyakov and V. V. Tuchin, "Speckle Correlometry" in *Biomedical Photonics Handbook*, Tuan Vo-Dinh (ed.), CRC Press, Boca Raton, 2003, pp. 14-1–14-23.

830. D. A. Zimnyakov, "Light Correlation and Polarization in Multiply Scattering Media: Industrial and Biomedical Applications," Chapter 1 in *Coherent-Domain Optical Methods: Biomedical Diagnostics, Environmental and Material Science*, V. V. Tuchin (ed.), Kluwer Academic Publishers, Boston, vol. 1, 2004, pp. 3–41.

831. Q. Luo, H. Cheng, Z. Wang, and V. V. Tuchin, "Laser Speckle Imaging of Cerebral Blood Flow," Chapter 5 in *Coherent-Domain Optical Methods: Biomedical Diagnostics, Environmental and Material Science*, V. V. Tuchin (ed.), Kluwer Academic Publishers, Boston, vol. 1, 2004, pp. 165–195.

832. V. P. Ryabukho, "Diffraction of Interference Fields on Random Phase Objects," Chapter 7 in *Coherent-Domain Optical Methods: Biomedical Diagnostics, Environmental and Material Science*, V. V. Tuchin (ed.), Kluwer Academic Publishers, Boston, vol. 1, 2004, pp. 235–318.

833. I. V. Fedosov, S. S. Ulyanov, E. I. Galanzha, V. A. Galanzha, and V. V. Tuchin, Laser Doppler and Speckle Techniques for Bioflow Measuremenys," Chapter 10 in *Coherent-Domain Optical Methods: Biomedical Diagnostics, Environmental and Material Science*, V. V. Tuchin (ed.), Kluwer Academic Publishers, Boston, vol. 1, 2004, pp. 397–435.

834. D. A. Zimnyakov, V. V. Tuchin, S. R. Utz, "Investigation of Statistical Properties of Partly Developed Speckle-Fields in Application to Skin Structure Diagnostics," *Opt. Spectrosc.*, vol. 76, 1994, pp. 838–844.

835. S. S. Ul'yanov, D. A. Zimnyakov, and V. V. Tuchin, "Fundamentals and Applications of Dynamic Speckles Induced by Focused Laser Beam Scattering," *Opt. Eng.*, vol. 33, no. 10, 1994, pp. 3189–3201.

836. S. S. Ul'yanov, V. P. Ryabukho, and V. V. Tuchin, "Speckle Interferometry for Biotissue Vibration measurement," *Opt. Eng.*, vol. 33, no. 3, 1994, pp. 908–914.

837. V. P. Ryabukho, V. L. Khomutov, V. V. Tuchin, D. V. Lyakin, and K. V. Konstantinov, "Laser Interferometer with an Object Sharply Focused Beam as a Tool for Optical Tomography," *Proc. SPIE* 3251, 1998, pp. 247–252.

838. A. P. Shepherd and P. Å. Öberg (eds.), *Laser Doppler Blood Flowmetry*, Kluwer, Boston, 1990.

839. M. E. Fein, A. H. Gluskin, W. W. Y. Goon, B. D. Chew, W. A. Crone, and H. W. Jones, "Evaluation of Optical Methods of Detecting Dental Pulp Vitality," *J. Biomed. Opt.*, vol. 2, no. 1, 1997, pp. 58–73.

840. F. F. M. de Mul, M. H. Koelink, A. L. Weijers, et al., "Self-Mixing Laser-Doppler velocimetry of Liquid Flow and Blood Perfusion of Tissue," *Appl. Opt.*, vol. 31, 1992, pp. 5844–5851.

841. M. H. Koelink, *Direct-Contact and Self-Mixing Laser Doppler Blood Flow Velocimetry*, PhD Thesis, Twente University, Enschede, The Netherlands, 2000.

842. J. Serup and B. E. Jemee (eds.), *Handbook of Non–Invasive Methods and the Skin*, CRC Press, Boca Raton et al., 1995.

843. V. P. Ryabukho, Yu. A. Avetisyan, A. E. Grinevich, D. A. Zimnyakov, and L. I. Golubentseva, "Effects of Speckle-Fields Correlation at Diffraction of Spatially-Modulated Laser Beam on a Random Phase screen," *Pis'ma Zh. Tekh. Fiz.*, vol. 20, no. 11, 1994, pp. 74–78.

844. V. P. Ryabukho, A. A. Chaussky, and V. V. Tuchin, "Interferometric Testing of the Random Phase Objects by Focused Spatially-Modulated Laser Beam," *Photon. Optoelectron.*, vol. 3, 1995, pp. 77–85.

845. V. P. Ryabukho, A. A. Chausskii, and O. A. Perepelitsyna, "Interference-Pattern Image Formation in an Optical System with a Random Phase Screen in the Space–Frequency Plane," *Opt. Spectrosc.*, vol. 92, 2002, pp. 191–198.

846. V. P. Ryabukho, A. A. Chaussky, V. L. Khomutov, and V. V. Tuchin, "Interferometric Testing of the Random Phase Objects (Biological Tissue Models) by a Spatially-Modulated Laser Beam," *Proc. SPIE* 2732, 1996, pp. 100–117.

847. E. Yu. Radchenko, G. G. Akchurin, V. V. Bakutkin, V. V. Tuchin, and A. G. Akchurin, "Measurement of Retinal Visual Acuity in Human Eyes," *Proc. SPIE* 4001, 1999, pp. 228–237.

848. S. Jutamulia and T. Asakura (eds.), Special Section on Optical Engineering in Ophthalmology, *Opt. Eng.*, vol. 34, no. 3, 1995, pp. 640–789.

849. R. R. Ansari, "Quasi-Elastic Light Scattering in Ophthalmology," Chapter 11 in *Coherent-Domain Optical Methods: Biomedical Diagnostics, Environmental and Material Science*, V. V. Tuchin (ed.), Kluwer Academic Publishers, Boston, vol. 1, 2004, pp. 437–464.

850. H. S. Dhadwal, R. R. Ansari, and M. A. DellaVecchia, "Coherent Fiber Optic Sensor for Early Detection of Cataractogenesis in the Human Eye Lens," *Opt. Eng.*, vol. 32, 1993, pp. 233–238.

851. M. Dieckman and K. Dierks, "Diagnostics Methods and Tissue Parameter Investigations Together with Measurement Results (*In Vivo*)," *Proc. SPIE* 2126, 1995, pp. 331–345.

852. S. S. Ul'yanov, "New Type of Manifestation of the Doppler Effect: an Application to Blood and Lymph Flow Measurements," *Opt. Eng.*, vol. 34, 1995, pp. 2850–2855.

853. S. S. Ul'yanov, V. V. Tuchin, A. A. Bednov, G. E. Brill, and E. I. Zakharova "The Application of Speckle-Interferometry Method for the Monitoring of Blood and Lymph Flow in Microvessels," *Lasers Med. Sci.*, vol. 11, 1996, pp. 97–107.

854. A. A. Bednov, S. S. Ulyanov, V. V. Tuchin, G. E. Brill, E. I. Zakharova, "Investigation of Lymph Flow Dynamics by Speckle-Interferometry Method," *Izvestiya VUZ, Appl. Nonlinear Dynamics*, vol. 4, no. 3, 1996, pp. 42–51; English translation: *Proc. SPIE* 3177, 1997, pp. 89–96.

855. S. S. Ulyanov, "Speckled Speckle Statistics with a Small Number of Scatterers: Implication for Blood Flow Measurement," *J. Biomed. Opt.*, vol. 3, 1998, pp. 237–245.

856. P. Starukhin, S. Ulyanov, E. Galanzha, and V. Tuchin, "Blood-Flow Measurements with a Small Number of Scattering Events," *Appl. Opt.*, vol. 39, no. 10, 2000, pp. 2823–2829.

857. S. S. Ulyanov and V. V. Tuchin, "Use of Low-Coherence Speckled Speckles for Bioflow Measurements," *Appl. Opt.*, vol. 39, no. 34, 2000, pp. 6385–6389.

858. I. V. Fedosov, V. V. Tuchin, E. I. Galanzha, A. V. Solov'eva, and T. V. Stepanova, "Recording of Lymph Flow Dynamics in Microvessels Using Correlation Properties of Scattered Coherent Radiation," *Quant. Electron.*, vol. 32, no. 11, 2002, pp. 970–974.

859. N. Konishi and H. Fujii, "Real-Time Visualization of Retinal Microcirculation by Laser Flowgraphy," *Opt. Eng.*, vol. 34, 1995, pp. 753–757.

860. Y. Tamaki, M. Araie, E. Kawamoto, S. Eguchi, and H. Fujii, "Noncontact, Two-Dimensional Measurement of Retinal Microcirculation Using Laser Speckle Phenomenon," *Inv. Ophthalmol. & Visual Sci.*, vol. 35, 1994, pp. 3825–3834.

861. T. J. H. Essex and P. O. Byrne, "A Laser Doppler Scanner for Imaging Blood Flow in Skin," *J. Biomed. Eng.*, vol. 13, 1991, pp. 189–194.

862. K. Wårdell, I. M. Braverman, D. G. Silverman, and G. E. Nilsson, "Spatial Heterogeneity in Normal Skin Perfusion Recorded with Laser Doppler Imaging and Flowmetry," *Microvascular Res.*, vol. 48, 1994, pp. 26–38.

863. J. D. Briers, G. Richards, and X. W. He, "Capillary Blood Flow Monitoring Using Speckle Contrast Analysis (LASCA)," *J. Biomed. Opt.*, vol. 4, no. 1, 1999, pp. 164–175.

864. G. Dacosta, "Optical remote sensing of heartbeats," *Opt. Communs*, Vol. 117, pp. 395–398 (1995).

865. D. A. Zimnyakov and V. V. Tuchin, "Laser Tomography" in *Lasers in Medicine*, D. R. Vij and K. Mahesh (eds.), Chapter 5, Kluwer Academic Publishers, Boston, Dordrecht, and London, 2002, pp. 147–194.

866. H. Cheng, Q. Luo, Q. Liu, Q. Lu, H. Gong, and S. Zeng, "Laser Speckle Imaging of Blood Flow in Microcirculation," *Phys. Med. Biol.*, vol. 49, 2004, pp. 1347–1357.

867. H. Cheng, Q. Luo, Z. Wang, H. Gong, S. Chen, W. Liang, and S. Zeng, "Efficient Characterization of Regional Mesentric Blood Flow by Use of Laser Speckle Imaging," *Appl. Opt.*, vol. 42, no. 28, 2004, pp. 5759–5764.

868. B. Choi, N. M. Kang, and J. S. Nelson, "Laser Speckle Imaging for Monitoring Blood Flow Dynamics in the *In Vivo* Redent Dorsal Skin Fold Model," *Microvasc. Res.*, vol. 68, 2004, pp. 143–146.

869. D. A. Weitz and D. J. Pine, "Diffusing-wave spectroscopy," Chapter 16 in *Dynamic Light Scattering. The Method and Some Applications*, W. Brown (ed.), Oxford University Press, New York, 1993, pp. 652–720.

870. I. V. Meglinskii, A. N. Korolevich, and V. V. Tuchin, "Investigation of Blood Flow Microcirculation by Diffusing Wave Spectroscopy," *Critical Reviews in Biomedical Engineering*, vol. 29, no. 3, 2001, pp. 535–548.

871. I. V. Meglinskii and V. V. Tuchin, "Diffusing Wave Spectroscopy: Application for Skin Blood Monitoring," Chapter 4 in *Coherent-Domain Optical Methods: Biomedical Diagnostics, Environmental and Material Science*, V. V. Tuchin (ed.), Kluwer Academic Publishers, Boston, vol. 1, 2004, pp. 139–164.

872. N. A. Fomin, *Speckle Photography for Fluid Mechanic Measurements*: *Experimental Fluid Mechanics*, Springer-Verlag, Berlin, 1998.

873. G. Maret and E. Wolf, "Multiple Light Scattering from Disordered Media. The Effect of Brownian Motion of Scatterers," *Z. Physik B–Condens. Matter*, vol. 65, 1987, pp. 409–413.

874. A. G. Yodh, P. D. Kaplan, and D. J. Pine, "Pulsed Diffusing-Wave Spectroscopy: High Resolution through Nonlinear Optical Gaiting," *Phys. Rev. B*, vol. 42, 1990, pp. 4744–4747.

875. D. A. Boas, L. E. Campbell, and A. G. Yodh, "Scattering and Imaging with Diffusing Temporal Field Correlations," *Phys. Rev. Lett.*, vol. 75, 1995, pp. 1855–1858.

876. D. J. Pine, D. A. Weitz, J. X. Zhu, and E. Hebolzheimer, "Diffusing-Wave Spectroscopy: Dynamic Light Scattering in the Multiple Scattering Limit," *J. Phys. France*, vol. 51, 1990, pp. 2101–2127.

877. X.-L. Wu, D. J. Pine, P. M. Chaikin, J. S. Huang, and D. A. Weitz, "Diffusing-Wave Spectroscopy in Shear Flow," *J. Opt. Soc. Am. B*, vol. 7, no. 1, 1990, pp. 15–20.

878. J. B. Pawley (ed.), *Handbook of Biological Confocal Microscopy*, Plenum Press, New York, 1990.

879. B. R. Masters (ed.), *Confocal Microscopy*, SPIE Milestone Ser. MS131, Bellingham, WA, 1996.

880. T. Wilson (ed.), *Confocal Microscopy*, Academic Press, London, 1990.

881. T. Wilson, "Confocal Microscopy," in *Biomedical Photonics Handbook*, Tuan Vo-Dinh (ed.), CRC Press, Boca Rotan, Florida, 2003, pp. 10-1–18.

882. T. F. Watson, "Application of High-Speed Confocal Imaging Techniques in Operative Dentistry," *Scanning*, vol. 16, 1994, pp. 168–173.

883. B. R. Masters and A. A. Thaer, "Real Time Scanning Slit Confocal Microscopy of the *In Vivo* Human Cornea," *Appl. Opt.*, vol. 33, 1994, pp. 695–701.

884. B. R. Masters and A. A. Thaer, "*In Vivo* Real-Time Confocal Microscopy of Wing Cells in the Human Cornea: a New Benchmark for *In Vivo* Corneal Microscopy," *Bioimages*, vol. 3, no. 1, 1995, pp. 7–11.

885. M. Rajadhyaksha, M. Grossman, D. Esterowitz, R. H. Webb, and R. R. Anderson, "*In Vivo* Confocal Scanning Laser Microscopy of Human Skin: Melanin Provides Strong Contrast," *J. Invest. Dermatol.*, vol. 104, 1995, pp. 946–952.

886. M. Rajadhyaksha and J. M. Zavislan, "Confocal Reflectance Microscopy of Unstained Tissue *In Vivo*," *Retinoids*, vol. 14, no. 1, 1998, pp. 26–30.

887. M. Rajadhyaksha, R. R. Anderson, and R. H. Webb, "Video-Rate Confocal Scanning Laser Microscope for Imaging Human Tissues *In Vivo*" *Appl. Opt.*, vol. 38, 1999, pp. 2105–2115.

888. B. Masters, "Confocal Microscopy of Biological Tissues," *Proc. SPIE* 2732, 1996, pp. 155–167.

889. M. Bohnke and B. R. Masters, "Confocal Microscopy of the Cornea," *Prog. Retinal Eye Res.*, vol. 18, no. 5, 1999, pp. 553–628.

890. D. C. Beebe and B. Masters, "Cell Lineage and the Differentiation of Corneal Epithelial Cells," *Invest. Ophthalmol. & Vis. Sci.*, vol. 37, no. 9, 1996, pp. 1815–1825.

891. B. R. Masters, "Three-Dimensional Confocal Microscopy of the Living *In Situ* Rabbit Cornea," *Optics Express*, vol. 3, no. 9, 1998, pp. 351–355; www.osa.org.

892. B. R. Masters, G. Gonnord, and P. Corcuff, "Three-Dimensional Microscopic Biopsy of *In Vivo* Human Skin: A New Technique Based on a Flexible Confocal Microscope," *J. Microsc.*, vol. 185, 1997, pp. 329–338.

893. Y. Kimura, P. Wilder-Smith, T. Krasieva, A. M. A. Arrastia-Jitosho, L.-H. L. Liaw, and K. Matsumoto, "Visualization and Quantification of Dentin Structure Using Confocal Laser Scanning Microscopy," *J. Biomed. Opt.*, vol. 2, no. 3, 1997, pp. 267–274.

894. M. Kempe, A. Z. Genak, W. Rudolph, and P. Dorn, "Ballistic and Diffuse Light Detection in Confocal and Heterodyne Imaging Systems," *J. Opt. Soc. Am. A*, vol. 14, no. 1, 1997, pp. 216–223.

895. M. Kempe, W. Rudolph, and E. Welsch, "Comparative Study of Confocal and Heterodyne Microscopy for Imaging through Scattering Media," *J. Opt. Soc. Am. A.*, vol. 13, no. 1, 1996, pp. 46–52.

896. I. V. Meglinsky, A. N. Bashkatov, E. A. Genina, D. Yu. Churmakov, and V. V. Tuchin, "The Enhancement of Confocal Images of Tissues at Bulk Optical Immersion," *Quantum Electronics*, vol. 32, no. 10, 2002, pp. 875–882.

897. I. V. Meglinsky, A. N. Bashkatov, E. A. Genina, D. Yu. Churmakov, and V. V. Tuchin, "Study of the Possibility of Increasing the Probing Depth by

the Method of Reflection Confocal Microscopy upon Immersion Clearing of Near-Surface Human Skin Layers," *Laser Physics*, vol. 13, no. 1, 2003, pp. 65–69.

898. A. N. Yaroslavsky, J. Barbosa, V. Neel, C. DiMarzio, and R. R. Anderson, "Combining Multispectral Polarized Light Imaging and Confocal Microscopy for Localization of Nonmelanoma Skin Cancer," *J. Biomed. Opt.*, vol. 10, no. 10, 2005, pp. 014011-1–6.

899. D. Huang, E. A. Swanson, C. P. Lin, J. S. Schuman, W. G. Stinson, W. Chang, M. R. Hee, T. Flotte, K. Gregory, C. A. Puliafito, and J. G. Fujimoto, "Optical coherence tomography," *Science* vol. 254, 1991, pp. 1178–1181.

900. J. A. Izatt, M. D. Kulkarni, K. Kobayashi, et al., "Optical Coherence Tomography for Biodiagnostics," *Opt. Photon. News*, vol. 8, no. 5, 1997, pp. 41–47, 65.

901. A. F. Fercher, C. K. Hitzenberger, and W. Drexler, "Ocular Partial-Coherence Interferometry," *Proc. SPIE* 2732, 1996, pp. 210–228.

902. A. F. Fercher, W. Drexler, and C. K. Hitzenberger, "Ocular Partial-Coherence Tomography," *Proc. SPIE* 2732, 2996, pp. 229–241.

903. J. M. Schmitt, "Array Detection for Speckle Reduction in Optical Coherence Microscopy," *Phys. Med. Biol.*, vol. 42, 1997, pp. 1427–1439.

904. V. M. Gelikonov, G. V. Gelikonov, N. D. Gladkova, et al., "Coherent Optical Tomograhy of Microscopic Inhomogeneities in Biological Tissues," *JETP's Lett.*, vol. 61, 1995, pp. 149–153.

905. J. M. Schmitt and A. Knüttel, "Model of Optical Coherence Tomography of Heterogeneous Tissue," *J. Opt. Soc. Am. A*, vol. 14, 1997, pp. 1231–1242.

906. G. Häusler, J. M. Herrmann, R. Kummer, and M. W. Linder, "Observation of Light Propagation in Volume Scatterers with 10^{11}-Fold Slow Motion," *Opt. Lett.*, vol. 21, 1996, pp. 1087–1089.

907. G. J. Tearny, M. E. Brezinsky, B. E. Bouma, et al., "Optical Coherence Tomography," *Science*, vol. 276, 1997, pp. 2037–2039.

908. Z. Chen, T. Milner, S. Srinivas, et al., "Noninvasive Imaging of In-Vivo Blood Flow Velocity Using Optical Doppler Tomography," *Opt. Lett.*, vol. 22, 1997, pp. 1119–1121.

909. J. G. Fujimoto, C. Pitris, S. A. Boppart, and M. E. Brezinski, "Optical Coherence Tomography: an Emerging Technology for Biomedical Imaging and Optical Biopsy," *Neoplasia*, vol. 2, 2000, pp. 9–25.

910. J. M. Schmitt, "Restoration of Optical Coherence Images of Living Tissue Using the CLEAN Algorithm," *J. Biomed. Opt.*, vol. 3, no. 1, 1998, pp. 66–75.

911. B. W. Colston, Jr., M. J. Everett, L. B. DaSilva, L. L. Otis, P. Stroeve, and H. Nathel, "Imaging of Hard- and Soft-Tissue Structure in the Oral Cavity by Optical Coherence Tomography," *Appl. Opt.*, vol. 37, no. 16, 1998, pp. 3582–3585.

912. J. M. Schmitt, S. L. Lee, and K. M. Yung, "An Optical Coherence Microscope with Enhanced Resolving Power in Thick Tissue," *Opt. Communs*, vol. 142, 1997, pp. 203–207.

913. J. M. Schmitt and S. H. Xiang, "Cross-Polarized Backscatter in Optical Coherence Tomography of Biological Tissue," *Opt. Lett.*, vol. 23, no. 13, 1998, pp. 1060–1062.

914. J. K. Barton, T. E. Milner, T. J. Pfefer, et al., "Optical Low-Coherence Reflectometry to Enhance Monte Carlo Modeling of Skin," *J. Biomed. Opt.*, vol. 2, no. 2, 1997, pp. 226–234.

915. H. Brunner, R. Lazar, and R. Steiner, "Optical Coherence Tomography (OCT) of Human Skin with a Slow-Scan CCD-Camera," OSA TOPS 6, Optical Society of America, Washington, DC, 1996, pp. 50–55.

916. E. Lankenau, J. Welzel, R. Birngruber, and R. Engelhardt, "*In vivo* Tissue Measurements with Optical Low Coherence Tomography," *Proc. SPIE* 2981, 1995, pp. 78–84.

917. C. K. Hitzenberger, W. Drexler, A. Baumgartner, and A. F. Fercher, "Dispersion Effects in Partial Coherence Interferometry," *Proc. SPIE* 2981, 1997, pp. 29–36.

918. A. G. Podoleanu, M. Seeger, G. M. Dobre, et al., "Transversal and Longitudinal Images from the Retina of the Living Eye Using Low Coherence Reflectometry," *J. Biomed. Opt.*, vol. 3, no. 1, 1998, pp. 12–20.

919. G. Häusler and M. W. Lindner, ""Coherence Radar" and "Spectral Radar"— New Tools for Dermatological Diagnosis," *J. Biomed. Opt.*, vol. 3, no. 1, 1998, pp. 21–31.

920. A. Baumgartner, C. K. Hitzenberger, H. Sattmann, et al., "Signal and Resolution Enhancements in Dual Beam Optical Coherence Tomography of the Human Eye," *J. Biomed. Opt.*, vol. 3, no. 1, 1998, pp. 45–54.

921. W. Drexler, O. Findl, R. Menapace, et al., "Dual Beam Optical Coherence Tomography: Signal Identification for Ophthalmologic Diagnosis," *J. Biomed. Opt.*, vol. 3, no. 1, 1998, pp. 55–65.

922. B. Bouma, L. E. Nelson, G. J. Tearney, et al., "Optical Coherence Tomographic Imaging of Human Tissue at 1.55 μm and 1.81 μm Using Er- and Tm-Dopted Fiber Sources," *J. Biomed. Opt.*, vol. 3, no. 1, 1998, pp. 76–79.

923. R. Walti, M. Bohnke, R. Gianotti, et al., "Rapid and Precise *In Vivo* Measurement of Human Corneal Thickness with Optical Low-Coherence Reflectometry in Normal Human Eyes," *J. Biomed. Opt.*, vol. 3, no. 3, 1998, pp. 253–258.

924. F. I. Feldchtein, G. V. Gelikonov, V. M. Gelikonov, et al., "*In vivo* OCT Imaging of Hard and Soft Tissue of the Oral Cavity," *Optics Express*, vol. 3, no. 6, 1998, pp. 239–250; www.osa.org.

925. J. M. Schmitt, "OCT Elastography: Imaging Microscopic Deformation and Strain in Tissue," *Optics Express*, vol. 3, 1998, pp. 199–211; www.osa.org.

926. X. Wang, T. Milner, Z. Chen, and J. S. Nelson, "Measurement of Fluid-Flow-Velocity Profile in Turbid Media by the Use of Optical Doppler Tomography," *Appl. Opt.*, vol. 36, no. 1, 1997, pp. 144–149.

927. Z. Chen, T. Milner, X. Wang, et al., "Optical Doppler Tomography: Imaging *In Vivo* Blood Flow Dynamics Following Pharmacological Intervention and Photodynamic Therapy," *Photochem. Photobiol.* vol. 67, no. 1, 1998, pp. 56–60.

928. J. A. Izatt, M. D. Kulkarni, and S. Yazdanfar, "*In Vivo* Bidirectional Color Doppler Flow Imaging of Picoliter Blood Volumes Using Optical Coherence Tomography," *Opt. Lett.*, vol. 22, no. 18, 1997, pp. 1439–1441.

929. D. A. Boas, K. K. Bizheva, and A. M. Siegel, "Using Dynamic Low-Coherence Interferometry to Image Brownian Motion within Highly Scattering Media," *Opt. Lett.*, vol. 23, no. 5, 1998, pp. 319–321.

930. V. G. Kolinko, F. F. M. de Mul, J. Greve, and A. V. Priezzhev, "Feasibility of Picosecond Laser-Doppler Flowmetry Provides Basis for Time-Resolved Doppler Tomography of Biological Tissue," *J. Biomed. Opt.*, vol. 3, no. 2, 1998, pp. 187–190.

931. B. Masters, "Early Development of Optical Low-Coherence Reflectometry and Some Recent Biomedical Applications," *J. Biomed. Opt.*, vol. 4, no. 2, 1999, pp. 236–247.

932. R. K. Wang and V. V. Tuchin, "Optical Coherence Tomography: Light Scattering and Imaging Enhancement," Chapter 13 in *Coherent-Domain Optical Methods: Biomedical Diagnostics, Environmental and Material Science*, V. V. Tuchin (ed.), Kluwer Academic Publishers, Boston, vol. 2, 2004, pp. 3–60.

933. P. E. Andersen, L. Thrane, H. T. Yura, A. Tycho, and T. M. Jørgensen, "Optical Coherence Tomography: Advanced Modeling," Chapter 14 in *Coherent-Domain Optical Methods: Biomedical Diagnostics, Environmental and Material Science*, V. V. Tuchin (ed.), Kluwer Academic Publishers, Boston, vol. 2, 2004, pp. 61–118.

934. C. K. Hitzenberger, "Absorption and Dispersion in OCT," Chapter 15 in *Coherent-Domain Optical Methods: Biomedical Diagnostics, Environmental and Material Science*, V. V. Tuchin (ed.), Kluwer Academic Publishers, Boston, vol. 2, 2004, pp. 119–161.

935. A. Podoleanu, "En-Face OCT Imaging," Chapter 16 in *Coherent-Domain Optical Methods: Biomedical Diagnostics, Environmental and Material Science*, V. V. Tuchin (ed.), Kluwer Academic Publishers, Boston, vol. 2, 2004, pp. 163–209.

936. J. F. de Boer, "Polarization Sensitive Optical Coherence Tomography: Phase Sensitive Interferometry for Multi-Functional Imaging," Chapter 18 in *Coherent-Domain Optical Methods: Biomedical Diagnostics, Environmental and Material Science*, V. V. Tuchin (ed.), Kluwer Academic Publishers, Boston, vol. 2, 2004, pp. 271–314.

937. Z. Chen, "Optical Doppler Tomography," Chapter 19 in *Coherent-Domain Optical Methods: Biomedical Diagnostics, Environmental and Material Science*, V. V. Tuchin (ed.), Kluwer Academic Publishers, Boston, vol. 2, 2004, pp. 315–342.

938. S. Neerken, G. W. Lucassen, T. (A. M.) Nuijs, E. Lenderink, and R. F. M. Hendriks, "Comparison of Confocal Laser Scanning Microscopy and Optical Coherence Tomography," Chapter 19 in *Coherent-Domain Optical Methods: Biomedical Diagnostics, Environmental and Material Science,* V. V. Tuchin (ed.), Kluwer Academic Publishers, Boston, vol. 2, 2004, pp. 417–439.

939. F. Reil and J. E. Thomas, "Heterodyne Techniques for Characterizing Light Fields," Chapter 8 in *Coherent-Domain Optical Methods: Biomedical Diagnostics, Environmental and Material Science,* V. V. Tuchin (ed.), Kluwer Academic Publishers, Boston, vol. 1, 2004, pp. 319–351.

940. S. Roth and I. Freund, "Second Harmonic Generation in Collagen," *J. Chem. Phys.,* vol. 70, 1979, pp. 1637–1643.

941. I. Freund, M. Deutsch, and A. Sprecher, "Connective Tissue Polarity," *Biophys. J.,* vol. 50, 1986, pp. 693–712.

942. P. J. Campagnola, H. A. Clark, W. A. Mohler, A. Lewis, and L. M. Loew, "Second-Harmonic Imaging Microscopy of Living Cells," *J. Biomed. Opt.,* vol. 6, no. 3, 2001, pp. 277–286.

943. P. J. Campagnola, A. C. Millard, M. Terasaki, P. E. Hoppe, S. J. Malone, and W. A. Mohler, "Three-Dimensional High-Resolution Second-Harmonic Generation Imaging of Endogenous Structural Proteins in Biological Tissues," *Biophys. J.,* vol. 82, no. 2, 2002, pp. 493–508.

944. P. Stoller, B.-M. Kim, and A. M. Rubenchik, "Polarization-Dependent Optical Second-Harmonic Imaging of a Rat-Tail Tendon," *J. Biomed. Opt.,* vol. 7, no. 2, 2002, pp. 205–214.

945. P. Stoller, K. M. Reiser, P. M. Celliers, and A. M. Rubenchik, "Polarization-Modulated Second-Harmonic Generation in Collagen," *Biophys. J.,* vol. 82, no. 2, 2002, pp. 3330–3342.

946. A. T. Yeh, B. Choi, J. S. Nelson, and B. J. Tromberg, "Reversible Dissosiation of Collagen in Tissues," *J. Invest. Dermatol.,* vol. 121, 2003, pp. 1332–1335.

947. T. Yasui, Y. Tohno, and T. Araki, "Characterization of Collagen Orientation in Human Dermis by Two-Dimensional Second-Harmonic-Generation Polarimetry," *J. Biomed. Opt.,* vol. 9, no. 2, 2004, pp. 259–264.

948. M. Han, L. Zickler, G. Giese, M. Walter, F. H. Loesel, and J. F. Bille, "Second-Harmonic Imaging of Cornea after Intrastromal Femtosecond Laser Ablation," *J. Biomed. Opt.,* vol. 9, no. 4, 2004, pp. 760–766.

949. V. V. Tuchin, *Optical Clearing of Tissues and Blood,* vol. PM 154, SPIE Press, 2005.

950. A. P. Ivanov, S. A. Makarevich, and A. Ya. Khairulina, "Propagation of Radiation in Tissues and Liquids with Densely Packed Scatterers," *J. Appl. Spectrosc. (USSR),* vol. 47, no. 4, 1988, pp. 662–668.

951. G. A. Askar'yan, "The Increasing of Laser and Other Radiation Transport through Soft Turbid Physical and Biological Media," *Sov. J. Quant. Electr.,* vol. 9, no. 7, 1982, pp. 1379–1383.

952. F. Veretout, M. Delaye, and A. Tardieu, "Molecular Basis of Lens Transparency. Osmotic Pressure and X-ray Analysis of α-Crystallin Solutions," *J. Mol. Biol.*, vol. 205, 1989, pp. 713–728.

953. R. Barer and S. Joseph, "Refractometry of Living Cells," *Q. J. Microsc. Sci.*, vol. 95, 1954, pp. 399–406.

954. B. A. Fikhman, *Microbiological Refractometry*, Medicine, Moscow, 1967.

955. E. Eppich, J. Beuthan, C. Dressler, and G. Müller, "Optical Phase Measurements on Biological Cells," *Laser Physics*, vol. 10, 2000, pp. 467–477.

956. B. Chance, H. Liu, T. Kitai, and Y. Zhang, "Effects of Solutes on Optical Properties of Biological Materials: Models, Cells, and Tissues," *Anal. Biochem.*, vol. 227, 1995, pp. 351–362.

957. H. Liu, B. Beauvoit, M. Kimura, and B. Chance, "Dependence of Tissue Optical Properties on Solute-Induced Changes in Refractive Index and Osmolarity," *J. Biomed. Opt.*, vol. 1, 1996, pp. 200–211.

958. V. V. Tuchin, "Optical Immersion as a New Tool to Control Optical Properties of Tissues and Blood," *Laser Phys.*, vol. 15, no. 8, 2005, pp. 1109–1136.

959. V. V. Tuchin, "Optical Clearing of Tissue and Blood Using Immersion Method," *J. Phys. D: Appl. Phys.*, vol. 38, 2005, pp. 2497–2518.

960. A. N. Bashkatov, V. V. Tuchin, E. A. Genina, Yu. P. Sinichkin, N. A. Lakodina, and V. I. Kochubey, "The Human Sclera Dynamic Spectra: *In Vitro* and *In Vivo* Measurements," *Proc. SPIE* 3591, 1999, pp. 311–319.

961. V. V. Tuchin, J. Culver, C. Cheung, S. A. Tatarkova, M. A. DellaVecchia, D. Zimnyakov, A. Chaussky, A. G. Yodh, and B. Chance, "Refractive Index Matching of Tissue Components as a New Technology for Correlation and Diffusing-Photon Spectroscopy and Imaging," *Proc. SPIE* 3598, 1999, pp. 111–120.

962. V. V. Tuchin (ed.), "Controlling of Tissue Optical Properties: Applications in Clinical Study," *Proc. SPIE* 4162, 2000.

963. V. V. Tuchin, "Controlling of Tissue Optical Properties," *Proc. SPIE* 4001, 2000, pp. 30–53.

964. V. V. Tuchin, "Advances in Immersion Control of Optical Properties of Tissues and Blood," *Proc. SPIE* 5254, 2003, pp. 1–13.

965. V. V. Tuchin, A. N. Bashkatov, E. A. Genina, Yu. P. Sinichkin, and N. A. Lakodina, "*In Vivo* Investigation of the Immersion-Liquid-Induced Human Skin Clearing Dynamics," *Technical Physics Lett.*, vol. 27, no. 6, 2001, pp. 489–490.

966. R. K. Wang, X. Xu, V. V. Tuchin, and J. B. Elder, "Concurrent Enhancement of Imaging Depth and Contrast for Optical Coherence Tomography by Hyperosmotic Agents," *J. Opt. Soc. Am. B*, vol. 18, 2001, pp. 948–953.

967. R. K. Wang and V. V. Tuchin, "Enhance Light Penetration in Tissue for High Resolution Optical Imaging Techniques by the Use of Biocompatible Chemical Agents," *J. X-Ray Science and Technology*, vol. 10, 2002, pp. 167–176.

968. R. K. Wang and J. B. Elder, "Propylene Glycol as a Contrast Agent for Optical Coherence Tomography to Image Gastrointestinal Tissue," *Lasers Surg. Med.*, vol. 30, 2002, pp. 201–208.

969. A. N. Bashkatov, E. A. Genina, and V. V. Tuchin, "Optical Immersion as a Tool for Tissue Scattering Properties Control" in *Perspectives in Engineering Optics*, K. Singh and V. K. Rastogi (eds.), Anita Publications, New Delhi, 2003, pp. 313–334.

970. V. V. Tuchin, "Optical Spectroscopy of Tissue," in *Encyclopedia of Optical Engineering*, R. G. Driggers (ed.), Marcel-Dekker, New York, 2003, pp. 1814–1829.

971. R. K. Wang, X. Xu, Y. He, and J. B. Elder, "Investigation of Optical Clearing of Gastric Tissue Immersed with Hyperosmotic Agents," *IEEE J. Select. Tops. Quant. Electr.*, vol. 9, 2003, pp. 234–242.

972. X. Xu and R. K. Wang, "Synergetic Effect of Hyperosmotic Agents of Dimethyl Sulfoxide and Glycerol on Optical Clearing of Gastric Tissue Studied with Near Infrared Spectroscopy," *Phys. Med. Biol.*, vol. 49, 2004, pp. 457–468.

973. M. H. Khan, B. Choi, S. Chess, K. M. Kelly, J. McCullough, and J. S. Nelson, "Optical Clearing of *In Vivo* Human Skin: Implications for Light-Based Diagnostic Imaging and Therapeutics," *Lasers Surg. Med.*, vol. 34, 2004, pp. 83–85.

974. F. Zhou and R. K. Wang, "Theoretical Model on Optical Clearing of Biological Tissue with Semipermeable Chemical Agents," *Proc. SPIE* 5330, 2004, pp. 215–221.

975. V. V. Tuchin and A. B. Pravdin, "Dynamics of Skin Diffuse Reflectance and Autofluorescence at Tissue Optical Immersion," in *Materials on European Workshop "BioPhotonics 2002,"* October 18–20, 2002, Heraklion, Crete, Foundation for Research and Technology–Hellas, Heraklion, CD-edition.

976. D. Y. Churmakov, I. V. Meglinski, and D. A. Greenhalgh, "Amending of Fluorescence Sensor Signal Localization in Human Skin by Matching of the Refractive Index," *J. Biomed. Opt.*, vol. 9, 2004, pp. 339–346.

977. Y. He, R. K. Wang, and D. Xing, "Enhanced Sensitivity and Spatial Resolution for *In Vivo* Imaging with Low-Level Light-Emitting Probes by Use of Biocompatible Chemical Agents," *Opt. Lett.*, vol. 28, no. 21, 2003, pp. 2076–2078.

978. E. I. Galanzha, V. V. Tuchin, Q. Luo, H. Cheng, and A. V. Solov'eva, "The action of Osmotically Active Drugs on Optical Properties of Skin and State of Microcirculation in Experiments," *Asian J. Physics*, vol. 10, no. 4, 2001, pp. 503–511.

979. G. Vargas, A. Readinger, S. S. Dosier, and A. J. Welch, "Morphological Changes in Blood Vessels Produced by Hyperosmotic Agents and Measured by Optical Coherence Tomography," *Photochem. Photobiol.*, vol. 77, no. 5, 2003, pp. 541–549.

980. E. I. Galanzha, V. V. Tuchin, A. V. Solovieva, T. V. Stepanova, Q. Luo, and H. Cheng, "Skin Backreflectance and Microvascular System Functioning at the Action of Osmotic Agents," *J. Phys. D: Appl. Phys.*, vol. 36, 2003, pp. 1739–1746.

981. M. Brezinski, K. Saunders, C. Jesser, X. Li, and J. Fujimoto, "Index Matching to Improve OCT Imaging through Blood," *Circulation*, vol. 103, 2001, pp. 1999–2003.

982. X. Xu, R. K. Wang, J. B. Elder, and V. V. Tuchin, "Effect of Dextran-Induced Changes in Refractive Index and Aggregation on Optical Properties of Whole Blood," *Phys. Med. Biol.*, vol. 48, 2003, pp. 1205–1221.

983. B. Grzegorzewski and E. Kowaliáska, "Optical Properties of Human Blood Sediment," *Acta Physica Polonica A*, vol. 101, no. 1, 2002, pp. 201–209.

984. B. Grzegorzewski, E. Kowaliáska, A. Gãrnicki, and A. Gutsze, "Diffraction Measurement of Erythrocyte Sedimentation Rate," *Optica Applicata*, vol. 32, no. 1, 2002, pp. 15–21.

985. A. K. Amerov, J. Chen, G. W. Small, and M. A. Arnold, "The Influence of Glucose upon the Transport of Light through Whole Blood," *Proc. SPIE* 5330, 2004, pp. 101–111.

986. A. N. Bashkatov, E. A. Genina, Yu. P. Sinichkin, V. I. Kochubey, N. A. Lakodina, and V. V. Tuchin, "Estimation of the Glucose Diffusion Coefficient in Human Eye Sclera," *Biophysics*, vol. 48, no. 2, 2003, pp. 292–296.

987. A. N. Bashkatov, E. A. Genina, Yu. P. Sinichkin, V. I. Kochubey, N. A. Lakodina, and V. V. Tuchin, "Glucose and Mannitol Diffusion in Human *Dura Mater*," *Biophysical J.*, vol. 85, no. 5, 2003, pp. 3310–3318.

988. E. A. Genina, A. N. Bashkatov, Yu. P. Sinichkin, V. I. Kochubey, N. A. Lakodina, G. B. Altshuler, and V. V. Tuchin, "*In Vitro* and *In Vivo* Study of Dye Diffusion into the Human Skin and Hair Follicles," *J. Biomed. Opt.* vol. 7, 2002, pp. 471–477.

989. V. V. Tuchin, E. A. Genina, A. N. Bashkatov, G. V. Simonenko, O. D. Odoevskaya, and G. B. Altshuler, "A Pilot Study of ICG Laser Therapy of *Acne Vulgaris*: Photodynamic and Photothermolysis Treatment," *Lasers Surg. Med.*, vol. 33, no. 5, 2003, pp. 296–310.

990. E. A. Genina, A. N. Bashkatov, G. V. Simonenko, O. D. Odoevskaya, V. V. Tuchin, and G. B. Altshuler, "Low-Intensity ICG-Laser Phototherapy of *Acne Vulgaris*: A Pilot Study," *J. Biomed. Opt.*, vol. 9, no. 4, 2004, pp. 828–834.

991. Yu. P. Sinichkin, S. R. Utz, and H. A. Pilipenko, "*In Vivo* Human Skin Spectroscopy: I Remittance Spectra," *Opt. Spectrosc.*, vol. 80, no. 2, 1996, pp. 228–234.

992. Yu. P. Sinichkin, S. R. Utz, L. E. Dolotov, H. A. Pilipenko, and V. V. Tuchin, "Technique and Device for Evaluation of the Human Skin Erythema and Pigmentation," *Radioengineering*, no. 4, 1997, pp. 77–81.

993. L. E. Dolotov, Yu. P. Sinichkin, V. V. Tuchin, S. R. Utz, G. B. Altshuler, and I. V. Yaroslavsky, "Design and Evaluation of a Novel Portable Erythema-Melanin-Meter," *Lasers Surg. Med.*, vol. 34, no. 2, 2004, pp. 127–135.

994. B. C. Wilson, M. S. Patterson, and L. Lilge, "Implicit and Explicit Dosimetry in Photodynamic Therapy: a New Paradigm," *Lasers Med. Sci.* vol. 12, 1997, pp. 182–199.

995. Y. Ito, R. P. Kennan, E. Watanabe, and H. Koizumi, "Assessment of Heating Effects in Skin During Contineous Wave Near Infrared Spectroscopy," *J. Biomed. Opt.*, vol. 5, 2000, pp. 383–390.

996. S.-j. Yeh, O. Khalil, Ch. F. Hanna, and S. Kantor, "Near-Infrared Thermo-Optical Response of the Localized Reflectance of Intact Diabetic and Non-diabetic Human Skin," *J. Biomed. Opt.*, vol. 8, 2003, pp. 534–544.

997. A. T. Yeh, B. Kao, W. G. Jung, Z. Chen, J. S. Nelson, and B. J. Tromberg, "Imaging Wound Healing Using Optical Coherence Tomography and Multiphoton Microscopy in an *In Vitro* Skin-Equivalent Tissue Model," *J. Biomed. Opt.*, vol. 9, no. 2, 2004, pp. 248–253.

998. T. Sakuma, T. Hasegawa, F. Tsutsui, and S. Kurihara, "Quantitative Analysis of the Whiteness of Atypical Cervical Transformation Zone," *J. Reprod. Med.*, vol. 30, 1985, pp. 773–776.

999. Ya. Holoubek, "Note on Light Attenuation by Scattering: Comparison of Coherent and Incoherent (Diffusion) Approximations," *Opt. Eng.*, 37, 1998, pp. 705–709.

1000. J. S. Balas, G. C. Themelis, E. P. Prokopakis, I. Orfanudaki, E. Koumantakis, and E. S. Helidonis, "*In Vivo* Detection and Staging of Epithelial Dysplasias and Malignancies Based on the Quantitative Assessment of Acetic Acid-Tissue," *J. Photochem. Photobiol.*, vol. 53, 1999, pp. 153–157.

1001. A. Agrawal, U. Utzinger, C. Brookner, C. Pitris, M. F. Mitchell, and R. Richards-Kortum, "Fluorescence Spectroscopy of the Cervix: Influence of Acetic Acid, Cervical Mucus, and Vaginal Medications," *Lasers Surg. Med.*, vol. 25, 1999, pp. 237–249.

1002. R. A. Drezek, T. Collier, C. K. Brookner, A. Malpica, R. Lotan, R. Richards-Kortum, and M. Follen, "Laser Scanning Confocal Microscopy of Servical Tissue before and after Application of Acetic Acid," *Am. J. Obstet. Gynecol.*, vol. 182, 2000, pp. 1135–1139.

1003. B. W. Pogue, H. B. Kaufman, A. Zelenchuk, W. Harper, G. C. Burke, E. E. Burke, and D. M. Harper, "Analysis of Acetic Acid-Induced Whitening of High-Grade Squamous Intraepithelial Lesions," *J. Biomed. Opt.*, vol. 6, 2001, pp. 397–403.

1004. B. Choi, T. E. Milner, J. Kim, J. N. Goodman, G. Vargas, G. Aguilar, and J. S. Nelson, "Use of Optical Coherence Tomography to Monitor Biological Tissue Freezing During Cryosurgery," *J. Biomed. Opt.*, vol. 9, 2004, pp. 282–286.

1005. G. N. Stamatas and N. Kollias, "Blood Stasis Contributions to the Perception of Skin Pigmentation," *J. Biomed. Opt.*, vol. 9, 2004, pp. 315–322.

1006. M. Rajadhyaksha, S. Gonzalez, and J. M. Zavislan, "Detectability of Contrast Agents for Confocal Reflectance Imaging of Skin and Microcirculation," *J. Biomed. Opt.*, vol. 9, 2004, pp. 323–331.

1007. J. K. Barton, N. J. Halas, J. L. West, and R. A. Drezek, "Nanoshells as an Optical Coherence Tomography Contrast Agent," *Proc. SPIE* 5316, 2004, pp. 99–106

1008. R. K. Wang and V. V. Tuchin, "Enhance Light Penetration in Tissue for High Resolution Optical Techniques by the Use of Biocompatible Chemical Agents," *Proc. SPIE* 4956, 2003, pp. 314–319.

1009. R. K. Wang, Y. He, and V. V. Tuchin, "Effect of Dehydration on Optical Clearing and OCT Imaging Contrast after Impregnation of Biological Tissue with Biochemical Agents," *Proc. SPIE* 5316, 2004, pp. 119–127.

1010. M. Lazebnik, D. L. Marks, K. Potgieter, R. Gillette, and S. A. Boppart, "Functional Optical Coherence Tomography of Stimulated and Spontaneous Scattering Changes in Neural Tissue," *Proc. SPIE* 5316, 2004, pp. 107–112.

1011. X. Xu, R. Wang, and J. B. Elder, "Optical Clearing Effect on Gastric Tissues Immersed with Biocompatible Chemical Agents Investigated by Near Infrared Reflectance Spectroscopy," *J. Phys. D: Appl. Phys.*, vol. 36, 2003, pp. 1707–1713.

1012. Y. He and R. K. Wang, "Dynamic Optical Clearing Effect of Tissue Impregnated with Hyperosmotic Agents and Studied with Optical Coherence Tomography," *J. Biomed. Opt.*, vol. 9, 2004, pp. 200–206.

1013. N. Guzelsu, J. F. Federici, H. C. Lim, H. R. Chauhdry, A. B. Ritter, and T. Findley, "Measurement of Skin Strech via Light Reflection," *J. Biomed. Opt.*, vol. 8, 2003, pp. 80–86.

1014. A. F. Zuluaga, R. Drezek, T. Collier, R. Lotan, M. Follen, and R. Richards-Kortum, "Contrast Agents for Confocal Microscopy: How Simple Chemicals Affect Confocal Images of Normal and Cancer Cells in Suspension," *J. Biomed. Opt.*, vol. 7, 2002, pp. 398–403.

1015. H. Schneckenburger, A. Hendinger, R. Sailer, W. S. L. Strauss, and M. Schmitt, "Laser-Assisted Optoporation of Single Cells," *J. Biomed. Opt.*, vol. 7, 2002, pp. 410–416.

1016. B. Grzegorzewski and S. Yermolenko, "Speckle in Far–Field Produced by Fluctuations Associated with Phase Separation," *Proc. SPIE* 2647, 1995, pp. 343–349.

1017. C.-L. Tsai and J. M. Fouke, "Noninvasive Detection of Water and Blood Content in Soft Tissue from the Optical Reflectance Spectrum," *Proc. SPIE* 1888, 1993, pp. 479–486.

1018. L. D. Shvartsman and I. Fine, "Optical Transmission of Blood: Effect of Erythrocyte Aggregation," *IEEE Trans. Biomed. Eng.*, vol. 50, 2003, pp. 1026–1033.

1019. O. Cohen, I. Fine, E. Monashkin, and A. Karasik, "Glucose Correlation with Light Scattering Patterns—a Novel Method for Non-Invasive Glucose Measurements," *Diabetes Technol. Ther.*, vol. 5, 2003, pp. 11–17.

1020. A. N. Yaroslavskaya, I. V. Yaroslavsky, C. Otto, G. J. Puppels, H. Duindam, G. F. J. M. Vrensen, J. Greve, and V. V. Tuchin, "Water Exchange in Human Eye Lens Monitored by Confocal Raman Microspectroscopy," *Biophysics*, vol. 43, no. 1, 1998 pp. 109–114.

1021. V. Tuchin, I. Maksimova, D. Zimnyakov, I. Kon, A. Mavlutov, and A. Mishin, "Light Propagation in Tissues with Controlled Optical Properties," *Proc. SPIE* 2925, 1996, pp. 118–14.

1022. A. N. Bashkatov, E. A. Genina, Yu. P. Sinichkin, N. A. Lakodina, V. I. Kochubey, and V. V. Tuchin "Estimation of Glucose Diffusion Coefficient in Scleral Tissue," *Proc. SPIE* 4001, 2000, pp. 345–355.

1023. E. A. Genina, A. N. Bashkatov, N. A. Lakodina, S. A. Murikhina, Yu. P. Sinichkin, and V. V. Tuchin "Diffusion of Glucose Solution through Fibrous Tissues: *In Vitro* Optical and Weight Measurements," *Proc. SPIE* 4001, 2000, pp. 255–261.

1024. B. O. Hedbys and S. Mishima, "The Thickness-Hydration Relationdhip of the Cornea," *Exp. Eye Res.*, vol. 5, 1966, pp. 221–228.

1025. A. I. Kholodnykh, K. Hosseini, I. Y. Petrova, R. O. Esenaliev, and M. Motamedi, *In vivo* OCT Assessment of Rabbit Corneal Hydration and Dehydration, *Proc. SPIE* 4956, 2003, pp. 295–298.

1026. X. Xu and R. K. Wang, "The Role of Water Desorption on Optical Clearing of Biotissue: Studied with Near Infrared Reflectance Spectroscopy," *Med. Phys.*, vol. 30, 2003, pp. 1246–1253.

1027. J. Jiang and R. K. Wang, "Comparing the Synergetic Effects of Oleic Acid and Dimethyl Sulfoxide as Vehicles for Optical Clearing of Skin Tissue *In Vitro*," *Phys. Med. Biol.*, vol. 49, 2004, pp. 5283–5294.

1028. V. V. Tuchin, T. G. Anishchenko, A. A. Mishin, and O. V. Soboleva, "Control of Bovine Sclera Optical Characteristics with Various Osmolytes," *Proc. SPIE* 2982, 1997, pp. 284–290.

1029. I. L. Kon, V. V. Bakutkin, N. V. Bogomolova, S. V. Tuchin, D. A. Zimnyakov, and V. V. Tuchin, "Trazograph Influence on Osmotic Pressure and Tissue Structures of Human Sclera," *Proc. SPIE* 2971, 1997, pp. 198–206.

1030. D. A. Zimnyakov, V. V. Tuchin, and K. V. Larin, "Speckle Patterns Polarization Analysis as an Approach to Turbid Tissue Structure Monitoring," *Proc. SPIE* 2981, 1997, pp. 172–180.

1031. A. N. Bashkatov, E. A. Genina, Yu. P. Sinichkin, and V. V. Tuchin, "The Influence of Glycerol on the Transport of Light in the Skin," *Proc. SPIE* 4623, 2002, pp. 144–152.

1032. V. V. Tuchin, I. L. Maksimova, A. N. Bashkatov, Yu. P. Sinichkin, G. V. Simonenko, E. A. Genina, and N. A. Lakodina, "Eye Tissues Study—Scattering and Polarization Effects," *OSA TOPS*, Optical Society of America, Washington, DC, 1999, pp. 255–258.

1033. V. V. Tuchin, A. N. Bashkatov, E. A. Genina, and Yu. P. Sinichkin, "Scleral Tissue Clearing Effects," *Proc. SPIE* 4611, 2002, pp. 54–58.

1034. A. V. Papaev, G. V. Simonenko, and V. V. Tuchin, "A Simple Model for Calculation of Polarized Light Transmission Spectrum of Biological Tissue Sample," *J. Opt. Technol.*, vol. 71, no. 5, 2004, pp. 3–6.

1035. S. Yu. Shchyogolev, "Inverse Problems of Spectroturbidimetry of Biological Disperse Systems: an Overview," *J. Biomed. Opt.*, vol. 4, 1999, pp. 490–503.

1036. V. V. Tuchin, X. Xu, and R. K. Wang, "Sedimentation of Immersed Blood Studied by OCT," *Proc. SPIE* 4241, 2001, pp. 357–369.

1037. V. V. Tuchin, X. Xu, R. K. Wang, and J. B. Elder, "Whole Blood and RBC Sedimentation and Aggregation Study using OCT," *Proc. SPIE* 4263, 2001, pp. 143–149.

1038. A. N. Bashkatov, E. A. Genina, I. V. Korovina, Yu. P. Sinichkin, O. V. Novikova, and V. V. Tuchin, "*In Vivo* and *In Vitro* Study of Control of Rat Skin Optical Properties by Action of 40%-Glucose Solution," *Proc. SPIE* 4241, 2001, pp. 223–230.

1039. A. N. Bashkatov, E. A. Genina, I. V. Korovina, V. I. Kochubey, Yu. P. Sinichkin, and V. V. Tuchin, "*In Vivo* and *In Vitro* Study of Control of Rat Skin Optical Properties by Acting of Osmotical Liquid," *Proc. SPIE* 4224, 2000, pp. 300–311.

1040. A. N. Bashkatov, A. N. Korolevich, V. V. Tuchin, Yu. P. Sinichkin, E. A. Genina, M. M. Stolnitz, N. S. Dubina, S. I. Vecherinski, and M. S. Belsley, "*In Vivo* Investigation of Human Skin Optical Clearing and Blood Microcirculation under the Action of Glucose Solution," *Asian J. of Physics*, vol. 15, no. 1, 2006, pp. 1–14.

1041. E. V. Cruz, K. Kota, J. Huque, M. Iwaku, and E. Hoshino, "Penetration of Propylene Glycol into Dentine," *Int. Endodontic J.*, vol. 35, 2002, pp. 330–336.

1042. A. N. Bashkatov, D. M. Zhestkov, E. A. Genina, and V. V. Tuchin, "Immersion Optical Clearing of Human Blood in the Visible and Near Infrared Spectral Range," *Opt. Spectrosc.*, vol. 98, no. 4, 2005, pp. 638–646.

1043. D. M. Zhestkov, A. N. Bashkatov, E. A. Genina, and V. V. Tuchin, "Influence of Clearing Solutions Osmolarity on the Optical Properties of RBC," *Proc. SPIE* 5474, 2004, pp. 321–330.

1044. S. P. Chernova, N. V. Kuznetsova, A. B. Pravdin, and V. V. Tuchin, "Dynamics of Optical Clearing of Human Skin *In Vivo*," *Proc. SPIE* 4162, 2000, pp. 227–235.

1045. P. L. Walling and J. M. Dabney, "Moisture in Skin by Near-Infrared Reflectance Spectroscopy," *J. Soc. Cosmet. Chem.*, vol. 40, 1989, pp. 151–171.

1046. K. A. Martin, "Direct Measurement of Moisture in Skin by NIR Spectroscopy," *J. Soc. Cosmet. Chem.*, vol. 44, 1993, pp. 249–261.

1047. K. Wichrowski, G. Sore, and A. Khaiat, "Use of Infrared Spectroscopy for *In Vivo* Measurement of the Stratum Corneum Moisturization after Application of Cosmetic Preparations," *Int. J. Cosmet. Sci.*, vol. 17, 1995, pp. 1–11.

1048. J. M. Schmitt, J. Hua, and J. Qu, "Imaging Water Absorption with OCT," *Proc. SPIE* 3598, 1999, pp. 36–46.

1049. K. F. Kolmel, B. Sennhenn, and K. Giese, "Investigation of Skin by Ultraviolet Remittance Spectroscopy," *British J. Dermatol.*, vol. 122, no. 2, 1990, pp. 209–216.

1050. H.-J. Schwarzmaier, M. P. Heintzen, W. Müller, et al., "Optical Density of Vascular Tissue before and after 308-nm Excimer Laser Irradiation," *Opt. Eng.*, vol. 31, 1992, pp. 1436–1440.

1051. R. Splinter, R. H. Svenson, L. Littman, et al., "Computer Simulated Light Distributions in Myocardial Tissues at the Nd-YAG Wavelength of 1064 nm," *Lasers Med. Sci.*, vol. 8, 1993, pp. 15–21.

1052. V. V. Tuchin, "Control of Tissue and Blood Optical Properties," in *Biophotonics—Principles and Applications*, NATO Advanced Study Institute, September 29–October 9, 2004, Ottawa, Canada, *Advances in Biophotonics*, B. W. Wilson, V. V. Tuchin, and S. Tanev (eds.), IOS Press, Amsterdam, 2005, pp. 79–122.

1053. S. Tanev, V. V. Tuchin and P. Paddon, "Light Scattering Effects of Gold Nanoparticles in Cells: FDTD Modeling," *Laser Physics Letters*, vol. 3, no. 12, 2006, pp. 594–598.

1054. S. Tanev, W. Sun, N. Loeb, P. Paddon, and V. Tuchin, "The Finite-Difference Time-Domain Method in the Biosciences: Modelling of Light Scattering by Biological Cells in Absorptive and Controlled Extra-cellular Media," in *Biophotonics—Principles and Applications*, NATO Advanced Study Institute, September 29–October 9, 2004, Ottawa, Canada, *Advances in Biophotonics*, B. W. Wilson, V. V. Tuchin, and S. Tanev (eds.), IOS Press, Amsterdam, 2005, pp. 45–78.

1055. B. Choi, L. Tsu, E. Chen, T. S. Ishak, S. M. Iskandar, S. Chess, and J. S. Nelson, "Determination of Chemical Agent Optical Clearing Potential Using *In Vitro* Human Skin," *Lasers Surg. Med.*, vol. 36, 2005, pp. 72–75.

1056. V. V. Tuchin, G. B. Altshuler, A. A. Gavrilova, A. B. Pravdin, D. Tabatadze, J. Childs, and I. V. Yaroslavsky, "Optical Clearing of Skin Using Flashlamp-Induced Enhancement of Epidermal Permeability," *Lasers Surg. Med.*, vol. 38, 2006, pp. 824–836.

1057. A. A. Gavrilova, D. Tabatadze, J. Childs, I. Yaroslavsky, G. Altshuler, A. B. Pravdin, and V. V. Tuchin, "*In vitro* optical clearing of rat skin using lattice of photoinduced islands for enhancement of transdermal permeability," *Proc. SPIE* 5771, 2005, pp. 344–348.

1058. O. F. Stumpp and A. J. Welch, "Injection of Glycerol into Porcine Skin for Optical Skin Clearing with Needle-Free Injection Gun and Determination of Agent Distribution Using OCT and Fluorescence Microscopy," *Proc. SPIE* 4949, 2003, pp. 44–50.

1059. O. F. Stumpp, A. J. Welch, T. E. Milner, and J. Neev, "Enhancement of Transdermal Skin Clearing Agent Delivery Using a 980 nm Diode Laser," *Lasers Surg. Med.*, vol. 37, 2005, pp. 278–285.

1060. M. H. Khan, S. Chess, B. Choi, K. M. Kelly, and J. S. Nelson, "Can Topically Applied Optical Clearing Agents Increase the Epidermal Damage Threshold and Enhance Therapeutic Efficacy," *Lasers Surg. Med.*, vol. 35, 2004, pp. 93–95.

1061. M. H. Khan, C. Przeklasa, B. Choi, K. M. Kelly, and J. S. Nelson, "Laser Assisted Tattoo Removal in Combination with Topically Applied Optical Clearing Agents," *25th Annual Meeting of the American Society for Laser Medicine and Surgery*, March 30–April 3, 2005, Lake Buena Vista, Florida, Abstracts, *Lasers Surg. Med.*, Suppl. 17, March 2005, p. 85.

1062. R. J. McNichols, M. A. Fox, A. Gowda, S. Tuya, B. Bell, and M. Motamedi, "Temporary Dermal Scatter Reduction: Quantitative Assessment and Imlications for Improved Laser Tattoo Removal," *Lasers Surg. Med.*, vol. 36, 2005, pp. 289–296.

1063. R. Cicchi, F. S. Pavone, D. Massi, and D. D. Sampson, "Contrast and Depth Enhacement in Two-Photon Microscopy of Human Skin *Ex Vivo* by Use of Optical Clearing Agents," *Opt. Express*, vol. 13, 2005, pp. 2337–2344.

1064. D. A. Zimnyakov, V. V. Tuchin, A. A. Mishin, et al., "*In Vitro* Human Sclera Structure Analysis Using Tissue Optical Immersion Effect," *Proc. SPIE* 2673, 1996, pp. 233–243.

1065. V. V. Tuchin, D. A. Zimnykov, I. L. Maksimova, G. G. Akchurin, A. A. Mishin, S. R. Utz, and I. S. Peretochkin, "The Coherent, Low-Śoherent and Polarized Light Interaction with Tissues undergo the Refractive Indices Matching Control," *Proc. SPIE* 3251, 1998, pp. 12–21.

1066. A. Kotyk and K. Janaček, *Membrane Transport: an Interdisciplinary Approach*, Plenum Press, New York, 1977.

1067. A. Pirie and van R. Heyningen, *Biochemistry of the Eye*, Blackwell Scientific Publications, Oxford, 1966.

1068. I. S. Grigor'eva and E. Z. Meilikhova (eds.), *Handbook of Physical Constants*, Energoatomizdat, Moscow, 1991.

1069. I. K. Kikoin (ed.), *Handbook of Physical Constants*, Atomizdat, Moscow, 1976.

1070. H. Schaefer and T. E. Redelmeier, *Skin Barier: Principles of Percutaneous Absorption*, Karger, Basel, 1996.

1071. F. Pirot, Y. N. Kalia, A. L. Stinchcomb, G. Keating, A. Bunge, and R. H. Guy, "Characterization of the Permeable Barrier of Human Skin *In Vivo*," *Proc. Natl. Acad. Sci. USA*, vol. 94, 1997, pp. 1562–1567.

1072. I. H. Blank, J. Moloney, A. G. Emslie, et al., "The Diffusion of Water Across the Stratum Corneum as a Function of its Water Content," *J. Invest. Dermatol.*, vol. 82, 1984, pp. 188–194.

1073. T. von Zglinicki, M. Lindberg, G. H. Roomans, and B. Forslind, "Water and Ion Distribution Profiles in Human Skin," *Acta Derm. Venerol. (Stockh)*, vol. 73, 1993, pp. 340–343.

1074. G. Altshuler, M. Smirnov, and I. Yaroslavsky, "Lattice of Optical Islets: a Novel Treatment Modality in Photomedicine," *J. Phys. D: Appl. Phys.*, vol. 38, 2005, pp. 2732–2747.

1075. P. Michailova, *Medical Cosmetics*, Moscow, Medicine, 1984.

1076. M. Kirjavainen, A. Urtti, I. Jaaskelainen, et al., "Interaction of Liposomes with Human Skin *In Vitro*—the Influence of Lipid Composition and Structure," *Biochem. Biophys. Acta*, vol. 1304, 1996, pp. 179–189.

1077. K. D. Peck, A.-H. Ghanem, and W. I. Higuchi, "Hindered Diffusion of Polar Molecules Through and Effective Pore Radii Estimates of Intact and Ethanol Treated Human Epidermal Membrane," *Pharmaceutical Res.*, vol. 11, 1994, pp. 1306–1314.

1078. T. Inamori, A.-H. Ghanem, W. I. Higuchi, and V. Srinivasan, "Macromolecule Transport in and Effective Pore Size of Ethanol Pretreated Human Epidermal Membrane," *Intern. J. Pharmaceutics*,vol. 105, 1994, pp. 113–123.

1079. M. Sznitowska, "The influence of Ethanol on Permeation Behavior of the Porous Pathway in the Stratum Corneum," *Int. J. Pharmacol.*, vol. 137, 1996, pp. 137–140.

1080. A. K. Levang, K. Zhao, and J. Singh, "Effect of Ethanol/Propylene Glycol on the *In Vitro* Percutaneous Absorption of Aspirin, Biophysical Changes and Macroscopic Barrier Properties of the Skin," *Int. J. Pharm.*, vol. 181, 1999, pp. 255–263.

1081. D. Bommannan, R. O. Potts, and R. H. Guy, "Examination of the Effect of Ethanol on Human Stratum Corneum *In Vivo* Using Infrared Spectroscopy," *J. Control Release*, vol. 16, 1991, pp. 299–304.

1082. C. A. Squier, M. J. Kremer, and P. W. Wertz, "Effect of Ethanol on Lipid Metabolism and Epidermal Permeability Barrier of Skin and Oral Mucosa in The Rat," *J. Oral Pathol. Med.*, vol. 32, 2003, pp. 595–599.

1083. U. Jacobi, J. Bartoll, W. Sterry, and J. Lademann, "Orally Administered Ethanol: Transepidermal Pathways and Effects on the Human Skin Barrier," *Arch. Dermatol. Res.*, vol. 296, 2005, pp. 332–338.

1084. http://www.dmso.org.

1085. J. Lademann, N. Otberg, H. Richter, H.-J. Weigmann, U. Lindemann, H. Schaefer, and W. Sterry, "Investigation of Follicular Penetration of Topically Applied Substances," *Skin Pharmacol. Appl. Skin Physiol.*, vol. 14, 2001, pp. 17–22.

1086. J. Lademann, U. Jacobi, H. Richter, N. Otberg, H.-J. Weigmann, H. Meffert, H. Schaefer, U. Blume-Peytavi, and W. Sterry, "*In Vivo* Determination of UV-Photons Entering into Human Skin," *Laser Phys.*, vol. 14, 2004, pp. 234 - 237.

1087. J. Lademann, A. Rudolph, U. Jacobi, H.-J. Weigmann, H. Schaefer, W. Sterry, and M. Meinke "Influence of Nonhomogeneous Distribution of Topically Applied UV Filters on Sun Protection Factors," *J. Biomed. Opt.*, vol. 9, 2004, pp. 1358–1362.

1088. S. Lee, D. J. McAuliffe, N. Kollias, T. J. Flotte, and A. G. Doukas "Photomechanical Delivery of 100-nm Microspheres Through the Stratum Corneum: Implications for Transdermal Drug Delivery," *Laser Surg. Med.*, vol. 31, 2002, pp. 207–210.

1089. S. Lee, T. Anderson, H. Zhang, T. J. Flotte, and A. G. Doukas, "Alteration of Cell Membrane by Stress Waves *In Vitro*," *Ultrasound Med. & Biol.*, vol. 22, 1996, pp. 1285–1293.

1090. S. Lee, D. J. McAuliffe, H. Zhang, Z. Xu, J. Taitelbaum, T. J. Flotte, and A. G. Doukas, "Stress-Waves-Induced Membrane Permiation of Red Blood Cells is Faciliated by Aquaporins," *Ultrasound Med. & Biol.*, vol. 23, 1997, pp. 1089–1094.

1091. D. J. McAuliffe, S. Lee, H. Zhang, T. J. Flotte, and A. G. Doukas, "Stress-Waves-Assisted Transport through the Plasma Membrane *In Vitro*," *Laser Surg. Med.*, vol. 20, 1997, pp. 216–222.

1092. C. L. Gay, R. H. Guy, G. M. Golden, V. H. W. Mak, and M. L. Francoeur, "Characterization of Low-Temperature (i.e., <65°C) Lipid Transitions in Human Stratum Corneum," *J. Invest. Dermatol.*, vol. 103, 1994, pp. 233–239.

1093. J. S. Nelson, J. L. McCullough, T. C. Glenn, W. H. Wright, L.-H. L. Liaw, and S. L. Jacques, "Mid-Infrared Laser Ablation of Stratum Corneum Enhances *In Vitro* Percutaneous Transport of Drugs," *J. Invest. Dermatol.*, vol. 97, 1991, pp. 874–879.

1094. J.-Y. Fang, W.-R. Lee, S.-C. Shen, Y.-P. Fang, and C.-H. Hu "Enhancement of Topical 5-Aminolaevulinic Acid Delivery by Erbium:YAG Laser and Microdermabrasion: A Comparison with Iontophoresis and Electroporation," *British J. Dermatol.*, vol. 151, 2004, pp. 132–140.

1095. U. Jacobi, E. Waibler, W. Sterry, and J. Lademann, "*In Vivo* Determination of the Long-Term Reservoir of the Horny Layer Using Laser Scanning Microscopy," *Laser Phys.*, 15, no. 4, 2005, pp. 565 – 569.

1096. E. Waibler, "Investigation of the long-term reservoir of the stratum corneum—Quantification, localization and residence time," Summary of the doctoral thesis, January 22, 2005, Charité-Universitätsmedizin, Berlin.

1097. S. Mordon, C. Sumian, and J. M. Devoisselle, "Site-Specific Methylene Blue Delivery to Pilosebaceous Structures Using Highly Porous Nylon Microspheres: An Experimental Evaluation," *Lasers Surg. Med.*, vol. 33, 2003, pp. 119–125.

1098. D. A. Zimnyakov and Yu. P. Sinichkin, "A study of Polarization Decay as Applied to Improved Imaging in Scattering Media," *J. Opt. A: Pure Appl. Opt.*, vol. 2, 2000, pp. 200–208.

1099. M. Gu, X. Gan, A. Kisteman, and M. G. Xu, "Comparison of Penetration Depth Between Two-Photon Excitation and Single-Photon Excitation in Imaging Through Turbid Tissue Media," *Appl. Phys. Lett.*, vol. 77, 2000, pp. 1551–1553.

1100. E. Beaurepaire, M. Oheim, and J. Mertz, "Ultra-Deep Two-Photon Fluorescence Excitation in Turbid Media," *Opt. Commun.*, vol. 188, 2001, pp. 25–29.

1101. B. R. Masters and P. T. C. So, "Confocal Microscopy and Multi-Photon Excitation Microscopy of Human Skin *In Vivo*," *Opt. Express*, vol. 8, 2001, pp. 2–10.

1102. K. König and I. Riemann, "High-Resolution Multiphoton Tomography of Human Skin with Subcellular Spatial Resolution and Picosecond Time Resolution," *J. Biomed. Opt.*, vol. 8, 2003, pp. 432–439.

1103. A. V. Priezzhev, O. M. Ryaboshapka, N. N. Firsov, and I. V. Sirko, "Aggregation and Disaggregation of Erythrocytes in Whole Blood: Study by Backscattering Technique," *J. Biomed. Opt.*, vol. 4, no. 1, 1999, pp. 76–84.

1104. A. H. Gandjbakhche, P. Mills, and P. Snabre, "Light-Scattering Technique for the Study of Orientation and Deformation of Red Blood Cells in a Concentrated Suspension," *Appl. Opt.*, vol. 33, 1994, pp. 1070–1078.

1105. A. V. Priezzhev, N. N. Firsov, and J. Lademann, "Light Backscattering Diagnostics of Red Blood Cells Aggregation in Whole Blood Samples," Chapter 11 in *Handbook of Optical Biomedical Diagnostics*, vol. PM107, V. V. Tuchin (ed.), SPIE Press, Bellingham, WA, 2002, pp. 651–674.

1106. S. M. Bertoluzzo, A. Bollini, M. Rsia, and A. Raynal, "Kinetic Model for Erythrocyte Aggregation," *Blood Cells, Molecules, and Diseases*, vol. 25, no. 22, 1999, pp. 339–349.

1107. S. Chien, "Physiological and Pathophysiological Significance of Hemorheology," in *Clinical Hemorheology*, S. Chien, J. Dormandy, E. Ernst, and A. Matarai (eds.), Martinus Nijhoff, Dordrecht, 1987, pp. 125–134.

1108. D. H. Tycko, M. H. Metz, E. A. Epstein, and A. Grinbaum, "Flow-Cytometric Light Scattering Measurement of Red Blood Cell Volume and Hemoglobin Concentration," *Appl. Opt.*, vol. 24, 1985, pp. 1355–1365.

1109. M. Yu. Kirillin and A. V. Priezzhev, "Monte Carlo Simulation of Laser Beam Propagation in a Plane Layer of the Erythrocytes Suspension: Comparison of Contributions from Different Scattering Orders to the Angular Distribution of Light Intensity," *Quant. Electr.*, vol. 32, no. 10, 2002, pp. 883–887.

1110. N. G. Khlebtsov and S. Yu. Shchyogolev, "Account for Particle Nonsphericity at Determination of Parameters of Disperse Systems by a Turbidity Spectrum Method. 1. Characteristic Functions of Light Scattering by Nonspherical Particle Systems in Rayleigh-Gans Approximation," *Opt. Spectrosc.*, vol. 42, 1977, pp. 956–962.

1111. A. Ya. Khairullina and S. F. Shumilina, "Determination of Size Distribution Function of the Erythrocytes According to Size by the Spectral Transparency Method," *J. Appl. Spectrosc.*, vol. 19, 1973, pp. 1078–1083.

1112. J. Beuthan, O. Minet, M. Herring, G. Mueller, and C. Dressler, "Biological Cells as Optical Phase-Filters—A Contribution to Medical Functional Imaging," *Minimal Invasive Medizin*, vol. 5, no. 2, 1994, pp. 75–78.

1113. K. V. Larin, T. Akkin, M. Motamedi, R. O. Esenaliev, and T. E. Millner, "Phase-Sensitive Optical Low-Coherence Reflectometry for Detection of Analyte Concentration," *Appl. Opt.*, vol. 43, 2004, pp. 3408–3414.

1114. L. Heinemann, U. Kramer, H. M. Klotzer, M. Hein, D. Volz, M. Hermann, T. Heise, and K. Rave, "Non-Invasive Task Force: Noninvasive Glucose Measurement by Monitoring of Scattering Coefficient During Oral Glucose Tolerance Tests," *Diabetes Technol. Ther.*, vol. 2, 2000, pp. 211–220.

1115. M. Essenpreis, A. Knüttel, D. Boecker, inventors; Boehringer Mannheim GmbH, assignee: "Method and Apparatus for Determining Glucose Concentration in a Biological Sample," US patent 5,710,630, January 20, 1998.

1116. F. O. Nuttall, M. C. Gannon, W. R. Swaim, and M. J. Adams, "Stability Over Time of Glycohemoglobin, Glucose, and Red Blood Cells Survival in Hemologically Stable People without Diabetes," *Metabolism*, vol. 53, no. 11, 2004, pp. 1399–1404.

1117. K. V. Larin, I. V. Larina, M. Motamedi, V. Gelikonov, R. Kuranov, and R. O. Esenaliev, "Potential Application of Optical Coherent Tomography for Non-invasive Monitoring of Glucose Concentration," *Proc. SPIE* 4263, 2001, pp. 83–90.

1118. D. W. Schmidtke, A. C. Freeland, A. Heller, and R. T. Bonnecaze, "Measurements and Modeling of the Transient Difference Between Blood and Subcutaneous Glucose Concentrations in the Rat After Injection of Insulin," *Proc. Natl. Acad. Sci. USA*, vol. 95, 1998, pp. 294–299.

1119. M. Han, L. Zickler, G. Giese, M. Walter, F. H. Loesel, and J. F. Bille, "Second-Harmonic Imaging of Cornea after Intrastromal Femtosecond Laser Ablation," *J. Biomed. Opt.*, vol. 9, no. 4, 2004, pp. 760–766.

1120. B. Chance, Q. Luo, S. Nioka, D. C. Alsop, and J. A. Detre, "Optical Investigations of Physiology: a Study of Intrinsic and Extrinsic Biomedical Contrast," *Phil. Trans. R. Soc. Lond. B*, vol. 352, 1997, pp. 707–716.

1121. Q. Luo, S. Nioka, and B. Chance, "Functional Near-Infrared Imager," *Proc. SPIE* 2979, 1997, pp. 84–93.

1122. S. J. Matcher and C. E. Cooper, "Absolute Quantification of Deoxy-haemoglobin Concentration in Tissue Near Infrared Spectroscopy," *Phys. Med. Biol.*, vol. 39, 1994, pp. 1295–1312.

1123. H. R. Heekeren, R. Wenzel, H. Obrig, et al., "Functional Human Brain Mapping During Visual stimulation using near-infrared light," *Proc. SPIE* 2979, 1997, pp. 847–858.

1124. M. B. Lilledahl, O. A. Haugen, M. Barkost, and L. O. Svaasand, "Reflection Spectroscopy of Atherosclerotic Plaque," *J. Biomed. Opt*, vol. 11, no. 2, 2006, pp. 021005-1–7.

1125. V. Ntziachristos, X. H. Ma, M. Schnall, A. Yodh, and B. Chance, "Concurrent Multi-Channel Time-Resolved NIR with MR Mammography: Instrumentation and Initial Clinical Results," in *Advances in Optical Imaging and Photon Migration*, J. G. Fujimoto and M. S. Patterson (eds.), OSA TOPS 21, Optical Society of America, Washington, DC, 1998, pp. 284–288.

1126. F. E. W. Schmidt, M. E. Fry, J. C. Hebden, and D. T. Delpy, "The Development of a 32-Channel Time-Resolved Optical Tomography System," in *Advances in Optical Imaging and Photon Migration*, J. G. Fujimoto and M. S. Patterson (eds.), OSA TOPS 21, Optical Society of America, Washington, DC, 1998, pp. 120–122.

1127. S. Ijichi, T. Kusaka, K. Isobe, F. Islam, K. Okubo, H. Okada, M. Namba, K. Kawada, T. Imai, and S. Itoh, "Quantification of Cerebral Hemoglobin as a Function of Oxygenation Using Near-infrared Time-resolved Spectroscopy in a Piglet Model of Hypoxia," *J. Biomed. Opt.*, vol. 10, no. 2, 2005, pp. 024026-1–9.

1128. NIM Inc., 3508 Market St., Philadelphia, PA 19104.

1129. G. G. Akchurin, D. A. Zimnyakov, and V. V. Tuchin, "Optoelectronic Module for Laser Microwave Modulation Spectroscopy and Tomography of Biological Tissues," *Critical Rev. in Biomed. Eng.*, vol. 1, no. 1, 2000, pp. 46–53.

1130. H. Y. Ma, C. W. Du, and B. Chance, "A Homodyne Frequency-Domain Instrument—I&Q Phase Detection System," *Proc. SPIE* 2979, 1997, pp. 826–837.

1131. B. Chance, E. Anday, S. Nioka, et al., "A Novel Method for Fast Imaging of Brain Function, Non-invasively, with Light," *Optics Express*, vol. 2, 1998, pp. 411–423.

1132. S. Nioka, S. Zhou, E. Anday, W. Thayer, D. Kurth, M. Papadopoulos, Y. Chen, and B. Chance, "Phazed Array Functional Imaging of Neonate's Meurological Disorders," in *Advances in Optical Imaging and Photon Migration*, J. G. Fujimoto and M. S. Patterson (eds.), OSA TOPS 21, Optical Society of America, Washington, DC, 1998, pp. 262–265.

1133. B. Chance, E. Anday, E. Conant, S. Nioka, S. Zhou, and H. Long, "Rapid and Sensitive Optical Imaging of Tissue Functional Activity, and Breast," in *Advances in Optical Imaging and Photon Migration*, J. G. Fujimoto and M. S. Patterson (eds.), OSA TOPS 21, Optical Society of America, Washington, DC, 1998, pp. 218–225.

1134. R. M. Daneu, Y. Wang, X. D. Li, et al.,"Regional Imager for Low-resolution Functional Imaging of the Brain with Diffusing Near-infrared Light," *Photochem. Photobiol.*, vol. 67, 1998, pp. 33–40.

1135. J. H. Choi, M. Wolf, V. Toronov, U. Wolf, C. Polzonetti, D. Hueber, L. P. Safonova, R. Gupta, A. Michalos, W. Mantulin, and E. Gratton, "Noninvasive Determination of the Optical Properties of Adult brain: Near-infrared Spectroscopy Approach," *J. Biomed. Opt.*, vol. 9 , no. 1, 2004, pp. 221–229.

1136. J. Zhao, H. S. Ding, X. L. Hou, C. L. Zhou, and B. Chance, "In Vivo Determination of the Optical Properties of Infant Brain using Frequency-domain Near-infrared Spectroscopy," *J. Biomed. Opt.*, vol. 10, no. 2, 2005, pp. 024028-1–7.

1137. H. Fang, M. Ollero, E. Vitkin, L. M. Kimerer, P. B. Cipolloni, M. M. Zaman, S. D. Freedman, I. J. Bigio, I. Itzkan, E. B. Hanlon, and L. T. Perelman, "Noninvasive Sizing of Subcellular Organelles with Light Scattering Spectroscopy," *IEEE J. Sel. Top. Quant. Elect.*, vol. 9, no. 2, 2003, pp. 267–276.

1138. H.-J. Schnorrenberg, R. Haßner, M. Hengstebeck, K. Schlinkmeier, and W. Zinth, "Polarization Modulation Can Improve Resolutionin Diaphanography," *Proc. SPIE* 2326, 1995, pp. 459–464.

1139. D. A. Zimnyakov and Yu. P. Sinichkin, "A Study of Polarization Decay as Applied to Improved Imaging in Scattering Media," *J. Opt. A: Pure Appl. Opt.* vol. 2, 2000, pp. 200–208.

1140. S. G. Demos, W. B. Wang, and R. R. Alfano, "Imaging Objects Hidden in Scattering Media with Fluorescence Polarization Preservation of Contrast Agents," *Appl. Opt.*, vol. 37, 1998, pp. 792–797.

1141. S. G. Demos, W. B. Wang, J. Ali, and R. R. Alfano, "New Optical Difference Approaches for Subsurface Imaging of Tissues," in *Advances in Optical Imaging and Photon Migration*, J. G. Fujimoto and M. S. Patterson (eds.), OSA TOPS 21, Optical Society of America, Washington, DC, 1998, pp. 405–410.

1142. A. Muccini, N. Kollias, S. B. Phillips, R. R. Anderson, A. J. Sober, M. J. Stiller, and L. A. Drake, "Polarized Light Photography in the Evaluation of Photoaging," *J. Am. Acad. Dermatol.*, vol. 33, 1995, pp. 765–769.

1143. Yu. P. Sinichkin, D. A. Zimnyakov, D. N. Agafonov, and L. V. Kuznetsova, "Visualization of Scattering Media upon Backscattering of a Linearly Polarized Nonmonochromatic Light," *Opt. Spectrosc.*, vol. 93, 2002, pp. 110–116.

1144. S. L. Jacques, K. Lee, and J. Roman, "Scattering of Polarized Light by Biological Tissues," *Proc. SPIE* 4001, 2000, pp. 14–28.

1145. J. S. Tyo, "Enhancement of the Point-spread Function for Imaging in Scattering Media by Use of Polarization-Difference Imaging," *J. Opt. Soc. Amer. A*, vol. 17, 2000, pp. 1–10.

1146. D. A. Zimnyakov, Yu. P. Sinichkin, and V. V. Tuchin, "Polarization Reflectance Spectroscopy of Biological Tissues: Diagnostical Applications," *Izv. VUZ Radiphysics*, vol. 47, 2005, pp. 957–975.

1147. A. P. Sviridov, V. Chernomordik, M. Hassan, A. C. Boccara, A. Russo, P. Smith, and A. Gandjbakhche, "Enhancement of Hidden Structures of Early Skin Fibrosis Using Polarization Degree Pattern and Pearson Correlation Analysis," *J. Biomed. Opt.*, vol. 10, no. 5, 2005, pp. 051706-1–6.

1148. A. Myakov, L. Nieman, L. Wicky, U. Utzinger, R. Richards-Kortum, and K. Sokolov, "Fiber Optic Probe for Polarized Reflectance Spectroscopy In Vivo: Design and Performance," *J. Biomed. Opt.*, vol. 7, no. 3, 2002, pp. 388–397.

1149. R. H. Newton, J. Y. Brown, and K. M. Meek, "Polarised Light Microscopy Technique for Quantitative Mapping Collagen Fibril Orientation in Cornea," *Proc. SPIE* 2926, 1996, pp. 278–284.

1150. S. Inoué, "Video Imaging Processing Greatly Enhance Contrast, Quality, and Speed in Polarization-based Microscopy," *J. Cell Biol.*, vol. 89, 1981, pp. 346–356.

1151. R. Oldenbourg and G. Mei, "New Polarized Light Microscope with Precision Universal Compensator," *J. Microscopy*, vol. 180, no. 2, 1995, pp. 140–147.

1152. T. T. Tower and R. T. Tranquillo, "Alignment Maps of Tissues: I. Microscopic Elliptical Polarimetry," *Biophys. J.*, vol. 81, 2001, pp. 2954–2963.

1153. T. T. Tower and R. T. Tranquillo, "Alignment Maps of Tissues: II. Fast Harmonic Analysis for Imaging," *Biophys. J.*, vol. 81, 2001, pp. 2964–2971.

1154. D. A. Yakovlev, S. P. Kurchatkin, A. B. Pravdin, E. V. Gurianov, M. Yu. Kasatkin, and D. A. Zimnyakov, "Polarization Monitoring of Structure and Optical Properties of the Heterogenous Birefringent Media: Application in the Study of Liquid Crystals and Biological Tissues," *Proc. SPIE* 5067, 2003, pp. 64–72.

1155. X. Gan, S. P. Schilders, and M. Gu, "Image Enhancement through Turbid Media under a Microscope by Use of Polarization Gating Methods," *J. Opt. Soc. Am. A*, vol. 16, 1999, pp. 2177–2184.

1156. X. Gan and M. Gu, "Image Reconstruction through Turbid Media under a Transmission-mode Microscope," *J. Biomed. Opt.*, vol. 7, no. 3, 2002, pp. 372–377.

1157. N. Huse, A. Schönle, and S. W. Hell, "Z-polarized Confocal Microscopy," *J. Biomed. Opt.*, vol. 6, no. 3, 2001, pp. 273–276.

1158. A. Asundi and A. Kishen, "Digital Photoelastic Investigations on the Tooth-bone Interface," *J. Biomed. Opt.*, vol. 6, 2001, pp. 224–230.

1159. A. Kishen and A. Asundi, "Photomechanical Investigations on Post Endodontically Rehabilitated Teeth," *J. Biomed. Opt.*, vol. 7, no. 2, 2002, 262–270.

1160. D. B. Tata, M. Foresti, J. Cordero, P. Tomashefsky, M. A. Alfano, and R. R. Alfano, "Fluorescence Polarization Spectroscopy and Time-resolved Fluorescence Kinetics of Native Cancerous and Normal Rat Kidney Tissues," *Biophys. J.*, vol. 50, 1986, pp. 463–469.

1161. A. Pradhan, S. S. Jena, B. V. Laxmi, and A. Agarwal, "Fluorescence Depolarization of Normal and Diseased Skin Tissues," *Proc. SPIE* 3250, 1998, pp. 78–82.

1162. S. K. Mohanty, N. Ghosh, S. K. Majumder, and P. K. Gupta, "Depolarization of Autofluorescence from Malignant and Normal Human Breast Tissues," *Appl. Opt.*, vol. 40, no. 7, 2001, pp. 1147–1154.

1163. N. Ghosh, S. K. Majumder, and P. K. Gupta, "Polarized Fluorescence Spectroscopy of Human Tissue," *Opt. Lett.*, vol. 27, 2002, pp. 2007–2009.

1164. Y. Aizu and T. Asakura, "Bio-speckle Phenomena and their Application to the Evaluation of Blood Flow," *Opt. Laser Technol.*, vol. 23, 1991, pp. 205–219.

1165. B. Ruth, "Measuring the Steady-state Value and the Dynamics of the Skin Blood Flow Using the Non-contact Laser Method," *Med. Eng. Phys.*, vol. 16, 1994, pp. 105–111.

1166. E. N. D. Stenov and P. Å. Öberg, "Design and Evaluation of a Fibre-optic Sensor for Limb Blood Flow Measurements," *Physiol. Meas.*, vol. 15, no. 3, 1994, pp. 261–270.

1167. S. C. Tjin, S. L. Ng, and K. T. Soo, "New Side-projected Fiber Optic Probe for *In Vivo* Flow Measurements," *Opt. Eng.*, vol. 35, no. 11, 1996, pp. 3123–3129.

1168. S. C. Tjin, D. Kilpatrick, and P. R. Johnston, "Evaluation of the Two-fiber Laser Doppler Anemometer for *In Vivo* Blood Flow Measurements: Experimental and Flow Simulation Results," *Opt. Eng.*, vol. 34, no. 2, 1995, pp. 460–469.

1169. R. R. Ansari, "Ocular Static and Dynamic Light Scattering: A Non-invasive Diagnostic Tool for Eye Research and Clinical Practice," *J. Biomed. Opt.*, vol. 9, no. 1, 2004, pp. 22–37.

1170. B. Chu, *Laser Light Scattering: Basic Principles and Practice*, Academic Press, New York, 1991.

1171. T. Tanaka and G. B. Benedek, "Observation of Protein Diffusivity in Intact Human and Bovine Lenses with Application to Cataract," *Invest. Ophthal. Vis. Sci.*, vol. 14, no. 6, 1975, pp. 449–456.

1172. S. E. Bursell, P. C. Magnante, and L. T. Chylack, "*In Vivo* Uses of Quasi-elastic Light Scattering Spectroscopy as a Molecular Probe in the Anterior Segment of the Eye," *Noninvasive Diagnostic Techniques in Ophthalmology*, B. R. Masters (ed.), Springer-Verlag, New York, 1990, pp. 342–365.

1173. L. Rovati, F. Fankhauser II, and J. Rick, "Design and Performance of a New Ophthalmic Instrument for Dynamic Light Scattering in the Human eye," *Rev. Sci. Instrum.*, vol. 67, no. 7, 1996, p. 2620.

1174. D. A. Boas and A. G. Yodh, "Spatially Varying Dynamical Properties of Turbid Media Probed with Diffusing Temporal Light Correlation," *J. Opt. Soc. Am. A.*, vol. 14, no. 1, 1997, pp. 192–215.

1175. D. A. Boas, I. V. Meglinsky, L. Zemany, et al., "Diffusion of Temporal Field Correlation with Selected Applications," SPIE CIS Selected Paper 2732, 1996, pp. 34–46.

1176. A. G. Yodh and N. Georgiades, "Diffusing-wave Interferometry," *Opt. Communs*, vol. 83, 1991, pp. 56–59.

1177. I. V. Meglinsky, D. A. Boas, A. G. Yodh, B. Chance, and V. V. Tuchin, "The Development of Intensity Fluctuations Correlation Method for Noninvasive Monitoring and Quantifying of Blood Flow Parameters," *Izvestija VUZ Applied Nonlinear Dynamics*, vol. 4, no. 6, 1996, pp. 72–81.

1178. A. Ya. Khairulina, "The Informativity of the Autocorrelation Function of the Time Domain Fluctuations of the Backscattered by Erythrocytes Suspension Radiation," *Opt. Spectrosc.*, vol. 80, no. 2, 1996, pp. 268–273.

1179. G. Yu, G. Lech, C. Zhou, B. Chance, E. R. Mohler III, and A. G. Yodh, "Time-Dependent Blood Flow and Oxygenation in Human Sceletal Muscles Measured with Noninvasive Near-Infrared Diffuse Optical Spectroscopies," *J. Biomed. Opt.*, vol. 10, no. 2, 2005, pp. 024027-1–7.

1180. K. U. Frerichs and G. Z. Feuerstein, "Laser Doppler Flowmetry: A Review of its Application for Measuring Cerebral and Spinal Cord Blood Flow," *Mol. Chem. Neuropathol.*, vol. 12, 1990, pp. 55–61.

1181. G. V. Belcaro, U. Hoffman, A. Bollinger, and A. N. Nicolaides, *Laser Doppler*, Med-Orion Publishing Company, London, 1994.

1182. E. Berardesca, P. Elsner, and H. I. Maibach (eds.), *Bioengineering of the Skin: Cutaneous Blood Flow and Erythema*, CRC Press, Roca Raton, 1995.

1183. C. E. Riva, B. L. Petring, R. D. Shonat, and C. J. Pournaras, "Scattering Process in LDV from Retinal Vessels," *Appl. Opt.*, vol. 28, 1989, pp. 1078–1083.

1184. E. R. Ingofsson, L. Tronstad, E. V. Hersh, and C. E. Riva, "Efficacy of Laser Doppler Flowmetry in Determining Pulp Vitality of Human Teeth," *Endod. Dent. Traumatol.*, vol. 10, 1994, pp. 83–87.

1185. A. V. Priezzhev, B. A. Levenko, and N. B. Savchenko, "Investigation of Blood Flow Dynamics in the Embryogenesis of *Macropodus Opercularis*," *Biophysics*, vol. 40, no. 6, 1995, pp. 1373–1378.

1186. J. K. Barton and S. Stromski, "Flow Measurements without Phase Information in Optical Coherence Tomography Images," *Optics Express*, vol. 13, no. 14, 2005, pp. 5234–5239.

1187. F. F. M. de Mul, M. H. Koelink, M. L. Kok, et al., "Laser Doppler Velocimetry and Monte Carlo Simulations on Models for Blood Perfusion in Tissue," *Appl. Opt.*, vol. 34, no. 28, 1995, pp. 6595–6611.

1188. D. Y. Zang, P. Wilder-Smith, J. E. Millerd, and A. M. A. Arrastia, "Novel Approach to Laser Doppler Measurement of Pulpal Blood Flow," *J. Biomed. Opt.*, vol. 2, 1997, pp. 304–309.

1189. E. Logean, L. F. Schmetterer, and C. E. Riva, "Optical Doppler Velocimetry at Various Retinal Vessel Depths by Variation of the Source Coherence Length," *Appl. Opt.*, vol. 39, no. 16, 2000, pp. 2858–2862.

1190. D. V. Kudinov and A. V. Priezzhev, "Numerical Simiulation of Light Scattering in a Turbid Medium with Moving Particles as Applied to Medical Optical Tomography," *Moscow Univ. Phys. Bull.*, vol. 53, no. 3, 1998, pp. 39–45.

1191. A. Serov, B. Steinacher, and T. Lasser, "Full-field Laser Doppler Perfusion Imaging and Monitoring with an Intelligent CMOS camera," *Optics Express*, vol. 13, 2005, pp. 3681–3689.

1192. A. Serov and T. Lasser, "High-speed Laser Doppler Perfusion Imaging Using an Integrating CMOS Image Sensor," *Optics Express*, vol. 13, no. 17, 2005, pp. 6416–6428.

1193. A. Serov and T. Lasser, "High-speed Laser Doppler Imaging of Blood Flow in Biological Tissue," *Proc. SPIE* 6163, 2006, pp. 00–00.

1194. Y. Aizu, K. Ogino, T. Sugita, et al., "Evaluation of Blood Flow at Ocular Fundus by Using Laser Speckle," *Appl. Opt.*, vol. 31, 1992, pp. 3020–3029.

1195. B. Zang, C. M. Pleass, and C. S. Ih, "Feature Information Extraction from Dynamic Biospeckle," *Appl. Opt.*, vol. 33, 1994, pp. 231–237.

1196. P. Zakharov, S. Bhat, P. Schurtenberger, and F. Scheffold, "Multiple Scattering Suppression in Dynamic Light Scattering Based on a Digital Camera Detection Scheme," *Appl. Opt.* vol. 45, 2006, pp. 1756–1764.

1197. A. K. Dunn, H. Bolay, M. A. Moskowitz, and D. A. Boas, "Dynamic Imaging of Cerebral Blood Flow using Laser Speckle," *J. Cereb. Blood Flow Metab.*, vol. 21, 2001, pp. 195–201.

1198. S. Yuan, A. Devor, D. A. Boas, and A. K. Dunn, "Determination of Optimal Exposure Time for Imaging of Blood Flow Changes with Laser Speckle Contrast Imaging," *Appl. Opt.*, vol. 44, 2005, pp. 1823–1830.

1199. K. R. Forrester, C. Stewart, J. Tulip, C. Leonard, and R. C. Bray, "Comparison of Laser Speckle and Laser Doppler Perfusion Imaging: Measurement in Himan Skin and Rabbit Articulat Tissue," *Med. Biol. Eng. Comput.*, vol. 40, 2002, pp. 687–697.

1200. K. R. Forrester, J. Tulip, C. Leonard, C. Stewart, and R. C. Bray, "A Laser Speckle Imaging Technique for Measuring Tissue Perfusion," *IEEE Trans. Biomed. Eng.*, vol. 51, 2004, pp. 2074–2084.

1201. Q. Liu, Z. Wang, and Q. Luo, "Temporal Clustering Analysis of Cerebral Blood Flow Activation Maps Measured by Laser Speckle Contrast Imaging," *J. Biomed. Opt.*, vol. 10, no. 2, 2005, pp. 024019-1–7.

1202. A. C. Völker, P. Zakharov, B. Weber, F. Buck, and F. Scheffold, "Laser Speckle Imaging with an Active Noise Reduction Scheme," *Optics Express*, vol. 13, no. 24, 2005, pp. 9782–9787.

1203. B. Weber,C. Burger, M. T. Wyss, G. K. von Schulthess, F. Scheffold, and A. Buck, "Optical Imaging of the Spatiotemporal Dynamics of Cerebral Blood Flow and Oxidative Metabolism in the Rat Barrel Cortex," *Europ. J. Neurosci.*, vol. 20, 2004, pp. 2664–2671.

1204. A. Serov, W. Steenbergen, and F. de Mul, "Prediction of the Photodetector Signal Generated by Doppler-induced Speckle Fluctuations: Theory and Some Validations," *J. Opt. Soc. Am. A*, vol. 18, 2001, pp. 622–639.

1205. R. Bonner and R. Nossal, "Model for Laser Doppler Measurements of Blood Flow in Tissue," *Appl. Opt.*, vol. 20, 1981, pp. 2097–2107.

1206. H. Bolay, U. Reuter, A. K. Dunn, Z. Huang, D. A. Boas, and A. M. Moskowitz, "Intrinsic Brain Activity Triggers Trigeminal Meningeal Afferernts in a Migraine Model," *Nat. Med.*, vol. 8, 2002, pp. 136–142.

1207. Z. Wang, Q. M. Luo, H. Y. Cheng, W. H. Luo, H. Gong, and Q. Lu, "Blood flow activation in rat somatosensory cortex under sciatic nerve stimulation revealed by laser speckle imaging," *Prog. Nat. Sci.*, vol. 13, 2003, pp. 522–527.

1208. A. C. Ngai, J. R. Meno, and H. R. Winn, "Simultaneous Measurements of Pial Arteriolar Diameter and Laser-Doppler Flow during Somatosensory Stimulation," *J. Cereb. Blood Flow Metab.*, vol. 15, 1995, pp. 124–127.

1209. T. Matsuura and I. Kanno, "Quantitative and Temporal Relationship between Local Cerebral Blood Flow and Neuronal Activation induced by Somatosensory Stimulation in Rats," *Neurosci. Res.*, vol. 40, 2001, pp. 281–290.

1210. H. Y. Cheng, Q. M. Luo, S. Q. Zeng, S. B. Chen, J. Cen, and H. Gong, "Modified Laser Speckle Imaging Method with Improved Spatial Resolution," *J. Biomed. Opt.*, vol. 8, no. 3, 2003, pp. 559–564.

1211. M. Henning, D. Gerdt, and T. Spraggins, "Using a Fiber-Optic Pulse Sensor in Magnetic Resonance Imaging," *Proc. SPIE* 1420, 1991, pp. 34–40.

1212. S. M. Khanna, R. Danliker, J.-F. Willemin, et al., "Cellular Vibration and Motility in the Organ of Corti," *Acta Oto-laryngologica*, Suppl. 467, 1989.

1213. S. M. Khanna, C. J. Koester, J. F. Willemin, et al., "A Noninvasive Optical System for the Study of the Function of Inner Ear in Living Animals," *Proc. SPIE* 2732, 1996, pp. 64–81.

1214. N. Stasche, H.-J. Foth, K. Hoermann et al, "Middle Ear Transmission Disorders—Tympanic Membrane Vibration Analysis by Laser-Doppler-Vibrometry," *Acta Oto-laryngologica*, vol. 114, 1994, pp. 59–63.

1215. M. Maeta, S. Kawakami, T. Ogawara, and Y. Masuda, "Vibration Analysis of the Tympanic Membrane with a Ventilation Tube and a Perforation by Holography," *Proc. SPIE* 1429, 1991, pp. 152–161.

1216. H. D. Hong and M. Fox, "Noninvasive Detection of Cardiovascular Pulsations by Optical Doppler Techniques," *J. Biomed. Opt.*, vol. 2, no. 4. 1997, pp. 382–390.

1217. J. Hast, R. Myllylä, H. Sorvoja, and J. Miettinen, "Arterial Pulse Shape Measurement Using Self-Mixing Effect in a Diode Laser," Quantum Electron., vol. 32, no. 11, 2002, pp. 975–980.

1218. J. Hast, Self-Mixing Interferometry and its Applications in Noninvasive Pulse Detection, PhD Dissertation, Oulu University Press, Oulu, Finland, 2003.

1219. V. Tuchin, A. Ampilogov, A. Bogoroditsky, et al., "Laser Speckle and Optical Fiber Sensors for Micromovements Monitoring in Biotissues," *Proc. SPIE* 1420, 1991, pp. 81–92.

1220. S. Yu. Kuzmin, S. S. Ul'yanov, V. V. Tuchin, and V. P. Ryabukho, "Speckle and Speckle-Interferometric Methods in Cardiodiagnostics," *Proc. SPIE* 2732, 1996, pp. 82–99.

1221. M. Conerty, J. Castracane, E. Saravia, et al., "Development of Otolaryngological Interferometric Fiber Optic Diagnostic Probe," *Proc. SPIE* 1649, 1992, pp. 98–105.

1222. S. S. Ul'yanov and V. V. Tuchin, "The Analysis of Space-Time Projection of Differential and Michelson-type Output Signal for Measurement," *Proc. SPIE* 1981, 1992, pp. 165–174.

1223. R. Berkovits and S. Feng, "Theory of Speckle-Pattern Tomography in Multiple-Scattering Media," *Phys. Rev. Lett.*, vol. 65, 1990, pp. 3120–3123.

1224. D. A. Zimnyakov and V. V. Tuchin, "Fractality of Speckle Intensity Fluctuations," *Appl. Opt.*, vol. 35, 1996, pp. 4325–4333.

1225. D. A. Zimnyakov, V. V. Tuchin, and A. A. Mishin, "Visualization of Biotissue Fractal Structures Using Spatial Speckle-Correlometry Method," *Izvestiya VUZ, Appl. Nonlinear Dynamics*, vol. 4, 1996, pp. 49–58.

1226. D. A. Zimnyakov, V. V. Tuchin, S. R. Utz, and A. A. Mishin, "Speckle Imaging Methods Using Focused Laser Beams in Applications to Tissue Mapping," *Proc. SPIE* 2433, 1995, pp. 411–420.

1227. D. A. Zimnyakov and V. V. Tuchin, "About "Two-Modality" of Speckle Intensity Distributions for Large-Scale Phase Scatterers," *Lett. J. Technical Phys.*, vol. 21, 1995, pp. 10–14.

1228. D. A. Zimnyakov and V. V. Tuchin, ""Lens-like" Local Scatterers Approach to the Biotissue Structure Analysis," *Proc. SPIE* 2647, 1995, pp. 334–342.

1229. D. A. Zimnyakov, V. P. Ryabukho, and K. V. Larin, ""Micro-Lens" Effect Manifestation in Focused Beam Diffraction on Large Scale Phase Screens," *Lett. J. Technical Phys.*, vol. 20, 1994, pp. 14–19.

1230. D. A. Zimnyakov, "Scale Effects in Partially Developed Speckle Structure. The Case of Gaussian Phase Screens," *Opt. Spectrosc.*, vol. 79, 1995, pp. 155–162.

1231. D. A. Zimnyakov, V. V. Tuchin, and S. R. Utz, "Human Skin Epidermis Structure Investigation Using Coherent Light Scattering," *Proc. SPIE* 2100, 1994, pp. 218–224.

1232. D. A. Zimnyakov, V. V. Tuchin, S. R. Utz, and A. A. Mishin, "Human Skin Image Analysis Using Coherent Focused Beam Scattering," *Proc. SPIE* 2329, 1995, pp. 115–125.

1233. D. A. Zimnyakov, V. V. Tuchin, A. A. Mishin, and K. V. Larin, "Correlation Dimension of Speckle Fields for Scattering Structures with Fractal Properties," *Izvestija VUZ. Applied Nonlinear Dynamics*, vol. 3, no. 6, 1995, pp. 126–134; English translation: *Proc. SPIE* 3177, 1997, pp. 158–164.

1234. S. J. Jacques and S. Kirkpatrick, "Acoustically Modulated Speckle Imaging of Biological Tissues," *Opt. Let.*, vol. 23, no. 11, 1998, pp. 879–881.

1235. S. Kirkpatrick and M. J. Cipolla, "High Resolution Imaged Laser Speckle Strain Gauge for Vascular Applications," *J. Biomed. Opt.*, vol. 5, no. 1, 2000, pp. 62–71.

1236. D. D. Duncan and S. Kirkpatrick, Processing Algorythms for tracking Speckle Shifts in Optical Elastography of Biological Tissues," *J. Biomed. Opt.*, vol. 6, no. 4, 2001, pp. 418–426.

1237. A. Kishen, V. M. Murukeshan, V. Krishnakumar, and A. Asundi, "Analysis on the Nature of Thermally Induced deformation in Human dentine by Electronic Speckle Pattern Interferometry (ESPI)," *J. of Dentistry*, vol. 29, 2001, pp. 531–537.

1238. J. Lademann, H.-J. Weigmann, W. Sterry, V. Tuchin, D. Zimnyakov, G. Müller, and H. Schaefer, "Analysis of the penetration Process of Drigs and Cosmetic Products into the Skin by Tape Strippings in Combination with Spectroscopic Measurements," *Proc. SPIE* 3915, 2000, pp. 194–201.

1239. P. Zaslansky, J. D. Currey, A. A. Friesem, and S. Weiner, "Phase Shifting Speckle Interferometry for Determination of Strain and Young's Modulus of Mineralized Biological Materials: A Study of Tooth Dentin Compression in Water," *J. Biomed. Opt.*, vol. 10, no. 2, 2005, pp. 024020-1–13.

1240. V. P. Tychinsky, "Coherent Phase Microscopy of Intracellular Processes," *Physics—Uspekhi*, vol. 44, 2001, pp. 617–629.

1241. V. P. Tychinsky, "Microscopy of Subwave Structures," *Physics—Uspekhi*, vol. 166, 1996, pp. 1219–1229.

1242. C. Dressler, E. V. Perevedentseva, J. Beuthan, O. Minet, E. Balanos, G. Graschew, and G. Mueller, "Research on Human Carcinoma Cells in Different Physiological States Using the Laser Phase Microscopy," *Proc. SPIE* 3726, 1999, pp. 397–402.

1243. P. Corcuff, C. Bertrand, and J. L. Leveque, "Morphometry of Human Epidermis *In Vivo* by Real-Time Confocal Microscopy," *Arch. Dermatol. Res.*, vol. 285, 1993, pp. 475–481.

1244. V. B. Karpov, "Study of Biological Samples with a Laser Fourier Holographic Microscopy," *Laser Physics*, vol. 4, 1994, pp. 618–623.

1245. S. C. W. Hyde, N. P. Barry, R. Jones, J. C. Dainty, and P. M. W. French, "Sub-100 pm Depth-Resolution Holographic Imaging through Scattering Media in the Near-Infrared," *Opt. Lett.*, vol. 20, 1996, pp. 2320–2322.

1246. C. Dunsby and P. French, "Techniques for Depth-Resolved Imaging through Turbid Media Including Coherence-Gated Imaging," *J. Phys. D: Appl. Phys.*, vol. 36, no. 14, 2003, pp. R207–R227.

1247. P. French, "Low-Coherence Holography," in *Coherent-Domain Optical Methods: Biomedical Diagnostics, Environmental and Material Science*, V. V. Tuchin (ed.), Kluwer Academic Publishers, Boston, vol. 1, 2004, pp. 199–234.

1248. V. V. Tuchin, V. V. Ryabukho, D. A. Zimnyakov, et al., "Tissue Structure and Blood Microcirculation Monitoring by Speckle Intereferometry and Full-Field Correlometry," *Proc. SPIE* 4251, 2001, pp. 148–155.

1249. V. V. Tuchin, L. I. Malinova, V. P. Ryabukho, et al., "Optical Coherence Techniques for Study of Blood Sedimentation and Aggregation," *Proc. SPIE* 4619, 2002, pp. 149–156.

1250. S. N. Roper, M. D. Moores, G. V. Gelikonov, F. I. Feldchtein, N. M. Beach, M. A. King, V. M. Gelikonov, A. M. Sergeev, and D. H. Reitze, "*In vivo* Detection of Experimentally Induced Cortical Dysgenesis in the Adult Rat Neocortex Using Optical Coherence Tomography," *J. Neurosci. Meth.*, vol. 80, 1998, pp. 91- 98.

1251. W. Drexler, U. Morgner, F. X. Kartner, C. Pitris, S. A. Boppart, X. D. Li, E. P. Ippen, and J. G. Fujimoto, "*In Vivo* Ultrahigh Resolution Optical Coherence Tomography," *Opt. Lett.*, vol. 24, 1999, pp. 1221–1223.

1252. M. Wojtkowski, R. Leitgeb, A. Kowalczyk, T. Bajraszewski, and A. F. Fercher, "*In Vivo* Human Retinal Imaging by Fourier Domain Optical Coherence Tomography," *J. Biomed. Opt.*, vol. 7, 2002, pp. 457–463.

1253. R. Leitgeb, C. K. Hitzenberger, and A. F. Fercher, "Performance of Fourier Domain vs. Time Domain Optical Coherence Tomography," *Opt. Express*, vol. 8, 2003, pp. 889–894.

1254. M. A. Coma, M. V. Sarunic, C. Yang, and J. A. Izatt, "Sensitivity Advantage of Swept Source and Fourier Domain Optical Coherence Tomography," *Optics Express*, vol. 11, no. 18, 2003, pp. 2183–2189.

1255. A. Maheshwari, M. A. Choma, and J. A. Izatt, "Heterodyne Swept-Source Optical Coherence Tomography for Complete Complex Conjugate Ambiguity Removal," *Proc. SPIE* 5690, 2005, pp. 91–95.

1256. R. V. Kuranov, V. V. Sapozhnikova, I. V. Turchin, E. V. Zagainova, V. M. Gelikonov, V. A. Kamensky, L. B. Snopova, and N. N. Prodanetz, "Complementary Use of Cross-Polarization and Standard OCT for Differential Diagnosis of Pathological Tissues," *Opt. Express*, vol. 10, 2002, pp. 707–713.

1257. S. J. Matcher, C. P. Winlove, and S. V. Gangnus, "Collagen Structure of Bovine Intervertebral Disc Studied Using PolarizationSensitive Optical Coherence Tomography," *Phys. Med. Biol.*, vol. 49, 2004, pp. 1295–1306.

1258. N. Ugrumova, D. P. Attenburrow, C. P. Winlove, and S. J. Matcher, "The collagen Structure of Equine Articular Cartilage, Characterized Using Polarization-Sensitive Optical Coherence Tomography," *J. Phys. D: Appl. Phys.*, vol. 38, 2005, pp. 2612–2619.

1259. L. Vabre, A. Dubois, and A. C. Boccara, "Thermal-Lifgt-Full-Field Optical Coherence Tomography," *Opt. Lett.*, vol. 27, 2002, pp. 530–533.

1260. A. Dubois, K. Grieve, G. Moneron, R. Lecaque, L. Vabre, and A. C. Boccara, "Ultra-High Resolution Full-FieldOptical Coherence Tomography," *Appl. Opt.*, vol. 43, 2004, pp. 2874–2883.

1261. H.-W. Wang, A. M. Rollins, and J. A. Izatt, "High Speed, Full Field Optical Coherence Tomography," *Proc. SPIE* 3598, 1999, pp. 204–212.

1262. A. M. Sergeev, V. M. Gelikonov, G. V. Gelikonov, F. I. Feldchtein, R. V. Kuranov, N. D. Gladkova, N. M. Shakhova, L. B. Snopova, A. V. Shakhov, I. A. Kuznetzova, A. N. Denisenko, V. V. Pochinko, Yu. P. Chumakov, and O. S. Streltzova, "*In Vivo* Endoscopic OCT Imaging of Precancer and Cancer States of Human Mucosa," *Opt. Express*, vol. 1, 1997, pp. 432–440.

1263. A. Eigensee, G. Häusler, J. M. Herrmann, and M. W. Lindner, "A New Method of Short-Coherence Interferometry in Human Skin (*In Vivo*) and in Solid Volume Scatterers," *Proc. SPIE* 2925, 1996, pp. 169–178.

1264. L. Poupinet and G. Jarry, "Heterodyne Detection for Measuring Extinction Coefficient in Mammalian Tissue," *J. Optics (Paris)*, vol. 24, 1993, pp. 279–285.

1265. G. Jarry, L. Poupinet, J. Watson, and T. Lepine, "Extinction Measurements in Diffusing Mammalian Tissue with Heterodyne Detection and a Titanium: Sapphire Laser," *Appl. Opt.*, vol. 34, 1995, pp. 2045–2050.

1266. H. Inaba, "Photonic Sensing Technology is Opening New Fronties in Biophotonics," *Opt. Rev.*, vol. 4, 1997, pp. 1–10.

1267. B. Devaraj, M. Usa, K. P. Chan, T. Akatsuka, and H. Inaba, "Recent Advances in Coherent Detection Imaging (CDI) in Biomedicine. Laser Tomography of Human Tissue *In Vivo* and *In Vitro*," *IEEE J. Selected Topics Quant. Electron.*, vol. 2, 1996, pp. 1008–1016.

1268. B. Devaraj, M. Takeda, M. Kobayashi, et al., "*In Vivo* Laser Computed Tomographic Imaging of Human Fingers by Coherent Detection Imaging Method Using Different Wavelengths in Nar Ifrared Rgion," *Appl. Phys. Lett.*, vol. 69, 1996, pp. 3671–3673.

1269. V. Prapavat, J. Mans, R. Schutz, et al., "*In Vivo*-Investigations on the Detection of Chronical Polyarthritis Using a CW-Transillumination Method in Interphalangeal Joints," *Proc. SPIE* 2626, 1995, pp. 360–366.

1270. A. Wax and J. E. Thomas, "Optical Heterodyne Imaging and Wigner Phase Space Distributions," *Opt. Lett.*, vol. 21, 1996, pp. 1427–1429.

1271. M. Friebel, A. Roggan, G. Müller, and M. Meinke, "Determination of Optical Properties of Human Blood in the Spectral Range 250 to 1100 nm Using Monte Carlo Simulation with Hematocrit-Dependent Effective Scattering Phase Functions," *J. Biomed. Opt.*, vol. 11, no. 3, 2006, pp. 034021-1–10.

1272. S. C. Gebhart, W. C. Lin, and A. Mahadevan-Jansen, "*In Vitro* Determination of Normal and Neoplastic Human Brain Tissue Optical Properties Using Inverse Adding-Doubling," *Phys. Med. Biol.*, vol. 51, 2006, pp. 2011–2027.

1273. E. Salomatina, B. Jiang, J. Novak, and A. N. Yaroslavsky, "Optical Proper-
      ties of Normal and Cancerous Human Skin in the Visible and Near Infrared
      Spectral Range," *J. Biomed. Opt.* (accepted for publication).
1274. A. L. Clark, A. Gillenwater, R. Alizadeh-Naderi, A. K. El-Naggar, and
      R. Richards-Kortum, "Detection and Diagnosis of Oral Neoplasia with an
      Optical Coherence Microscope," *J. Biomed. Opt.*, vol. 9, no. 6, 2004, pp.
      1271–1280.
1275. A. M. Zysk, E. J. Chaney, and S. A. Boppart, "Refractive Index of
      Carcinogen-Induced Rat Mammary Tumours," *Phys. Med. Biol.*, vol. 51,
      2006, pp. 2165–2177.
1276. L. Oliveira, A. Lage, M. Pais Clemente, and V. V. Tuchin, "Concentration
      Dependence of the Optical Clearing Effect Created in Muscle Immersed in
      Glycerol and Ethylene Glycol," *Proc. SPIE* 6535, 2007.
1277. X. Ma, J. Q. Lu, H. Ding, and X. H. Hu, "Bulk Optical Parameters of Porcine
      Skin Dermis Tissues at Eight Wavelengths from 325 to 1557 nm," *Opt. Lett.*,
      vol. 30, 2005, pp. 412–414.
1278. H. Ding, J. Q. Lu, K. M. Jacobs, and X. H. Hu, "Determination of Refractive
      Indices of Porcine Skin Tissues and Intralipid at Eight Wavelengths between
      325 and 1557 nm," *J. Opt. Soc. Am. A*, vol. 22, 2005, pp. 1151–1157.
1279. H. Ding, J. Q. Lu, W. A. Wooden, P. J. Kragel, and X. H. Hu, "Refractive
      Indices of Human Skin Tissues at Eight Wavelengths and Estimated Disper-
      sion Relations between 300 and 1600 nm," *Phys. Med. Biol.*, vol. 51, 2006,
      pp. 1479–1489.
1280. D. Chan, B. Sculz, M. Rübhausen, S. Wessel, and R. Wepf, "Structural In-
      vestigations of Human Hairs by Spectrally Resolved Ellipsometry," *J. Bio-
      med. Opt.*, vol. 11, no. 1, 2006, pp. 014029-1–6.
1281. M. Friebel and M. Meinke, "Determination of the Complex Refractive In-
      dex of Highly Concentrated Hemoglobin Solutions Using Transmittance
      and Reflectance Measurements," *Biomed. Opt.*, vol. 10, 2005, pp. 064019.
1282. M. Friebel and M. Meinke, "Model Function to Calculate the Refractive
      Index of Native Hemoglobin in the Wavelength Range of 250–1100 nm De-
      pendent on Concentration," *Appl. Opt.*, vol. 45, no. 12, 2006, pp. 2838–
      2842.
1283. J. J. J. Dirckx, L. C. Kuypers, and W. F. Decraemer, "Refractive Index of
      Tissue Measured with Confocal Microscopy," *J. Biomed. Opt.*, vol. 10, no.
      4, 2005, pp. 044014-1–8.

Index

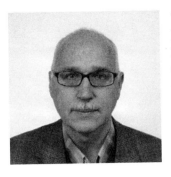

Valery V. Tuchin was born February 4, 1944. He received his degrees MS in Radiophysics and Electronics (1966), Candidate of Sciences in Optics (PhD, 1973), and Doctor of Science in Quantum Radiophysics (1982) from Saratov State University, Saratov, Russia. He is a Professor and holds the Optics and Biomedical Physics Chair, and he is a director of Research-Educational Institute of Optics and Biophotonics at Saratov State University. Prof. Tuchin also heads the Laboratory of Laser Diagnostics of Technical and Living Systems of Precision Mechanics and Control Institute, Russian Academy of Sciences. He was dean of the Faculty of Physics of Saratov University from 1982 to 1989.

His research interests include biomedical optics, biophotonics and laser medicine, nonlinear dynamics of laser and biophysical systems, physics of optical and laser measurements. He has authored more than 300 peer-reviewed papers and books, including his latest, *Handbook of Optical Biomedical Diagnostics* (SPIE Press, Vol. PM107, 2002; Translation to Russian, Fizmatlit, Moscow, 2007), *Coherent-Domain Optical Methods for Biomedical Diagnostics, Environmental and Material Science* (Kluwer Academic Publishers, Boston, USA, vol. 1 & 2, 2004), *Optical Clearing of Tissues and Blood* (SPIE Press, Vol. PM 154, 2005), and *Optical Polarization in Biomedical Applications*, Springer, 2006 (Lihong Wang, and Dmitry Zimnyakov – co-authors). He is a holder of more than 25 patents.

Prof. Tuchin currently teaches courses on optics, tissue optics, laser and fiber optics in biomedicine, optical measurements in biomedicine, laser dynamics, biophysics and medical physics for undergraduate and postgraduate students. Since 1992, Prof. Tuchin has been the instructor of SPIE and OSA short courses on biomedical optics for an international audience of engineers, students and medical doctors; and he is an editorial board member of *J. of Biomedical Optics* (SPIE), *Lasers in the Life Sciences*, *J. of X-Ray Science and Technology, J. of Biophotonics, J. on Biomedical Photonics* (China), and the Russian journals *Izvestiya VUZ, Applied Nonlinear Dynamics, Quantum Electronics* and *Laser Medicine*. He is a member of the Russian Academy of Natural Sciences and the International Academy of Informatization, a member of the board of SPIE/RUS and a fellow of SPIE. He has been awarded the title and scholarship "Soros Professor" (1997–1999), and the Russian Federation Scholarship for the outstanding scientists (1994–2003); and Honored Science Worker of the Russian Federation (since 2000). Since 2005 Prof. Tuchin is a vice-president of Russian Photobiology Society. In 2007 he has been awarded by SPIE Educator Award.

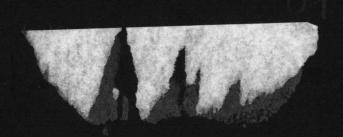